KIRK L. PETERSON, M.D.

Professor of Medicine
Edith and William Perlman
   Professor of Clinical Cardiology
University of California, San Diego,
   School of Medicine
San Diego, California

PASCAL NICOD, M.D.

Professor of Medicine
University of Lausanne
   School of Medicine
Chairman, Department of Internal
   Medicine
Centre Hospitalier Universitaire Vaudois
Lausanne, Switzerland

CARDIAC CATHETERIZATION

Methods, Diagnosis, and Therapy

W.B. SAUNDERS COMPANY
A Division of Harcourt Brace & Company
Philadelphia
London   Toronto   Montreal   Sydney   Tokyo

W.B. SAUNDERS COMPANY
A Division of Harcourt Brace & Company

The Curtis Center
Independence Square West
Philadelphia, Pennsylvania 19106

Library of Congress Cataloging-in-Publication Data

Cardiac catheterization: methods, diagnosis, and therapy / [edited by] Kirk L.
Peterson, Pascal Nicod—1st ed.

p. cm.

ISBN 0–7216–3064–2

1. Cardiac catheterization.   I. Peterson, Kirk L.   [DNLM: 1. Heart
  Diseases—diagnosis.   2. Heart Diseases—therapy.   3. Heart
  Catheterization—methods.   WG 210 1997]

RC683.5.C25C36 1997   616.1'20754—dc20

DNLM/DLC   95–3944

CARDIAC CATHETERIZATION: Methods, Diagnosis, and Therapy   ISBN 0–7216–3064–2

Printed in the United States of America.

Last digit is the print number: 9   8   7   6   5   4   3   2   1

Hans Peter Krayenbühl, M.D. (October 19, 1933–July 29, 1993)
Professor of Medicine
Formerly, Chief, Cardiology, Medical Policlinic
University of Zurich
Zurich, Switzerland

Over the last four decades cardiac catheterization and angiography have defined with precision the underlying pathophysiology and pathoanatomy of patients with both acquired and congenital cardiovascular diseases. With the development of interventional techniques, the cardiac catheterization laboratory has now evolved into an important environment for treatment of many forms of heart disease. To this discipline that evolved in parallel in North America, Europe, and Asia after World War II, Professor Hans Peter Krayenbühl was a highly esteemed and internationally recognized contributor. Beginning with his precise studies in the 1970s of myocardial contractility, using catheter micromanometry and quantitative cine angiography, followed by his detailed analyses during the 1900s of the mechanics of left ventricular systolic and diastolic function in valvular heart disease, both before and after corrective surgery, and extending over the last decade of his career to innovative studies of coronary dynamics and flow, Professor Krayenbühl brought to his medical scholarship an insatiable curiosity, imaginative intellect, and supremely critical analysis. He wrote and coauthored more than 380 contributions to the cardiovascular disease literature during his lifetime.

While systematically contributing major research papers, Hans Peter, as many of us knew him, found time and energy to foster the development and creativity of professional cardiovascular societies on both sides of the Atlantic. He was an Honorary Fellow of the Council on Clinical Cardiology, American Heart Association; an International Fellow of the American Heart Association; and a Fellow of the European Society of Cardiology. During his tenure as President of the European Society of Cardiology, 1988 to 1990, this organization experienced a renaissance as an educational and professional resource for the world of cardiology. In November 1992 he was invited to give the Paul Dudley White International Lecture of the American Heart Association in New Orleans, Louisiana.

Hans Peter was an engaging and warm personality, always interested in sharing ideas and generous to his collaborators. Directly behind his obvious physical energy and intellectual zeal was an appealing sense of humor and genuine modesty. To be remembered especially was his enthusiasm for taking his dear Colette and visiting guests to a favorite Dixieland jazz bar in the old town of Zurich, where he tapped his toes with zest.

Considering Professor Krayenbühl's collegial personality, special talents, and contributions, it is no surprise that cardiologists from many countries, including many who did not speak his native tongue, came to Zurich to benefit from his professional tutelage. He trained personally a number of outstanding physicians, from within and outside Switzerland, who, themselves, continue to make important contributions to the art and science of cardiology.

In recognition of Professor Krayenbühl's esteemed and notable achievements in the areas of cardiac hemodynamics, imaging, pathophysiology, and treatment, this textbook is dedicated to this warmly remembered, highly respected, and deeply missed colleague.

CONTRIBUTORS

James K. Alexander, M.D.
Professor of Medicine (Cardiology); Baylor College of Medicine, Houston, Texas.
Catheterization and Angiography in Chronic Obstructive Pulmonary Disease

William Auger, M.D.
Associate Professor of Medicine, University of California, San Diego, School of Medicine; Associate Director, Pulmonary Vascular Program, University of California, San Diego, Medical Center, San Diego, California.
Pulmonary Angioscopy; Catheterization and Angiography in Pulmonary Hypertension

Christophe Bauters, M.D.
Associate Professor of Medicine, University of Lille, Lille, France.
Coronary Balloon Angioplasty: Methods and Results

Michel E. Bertrand, M.D.
Professor of Medicine, University of Lille, Lille, France.
Coronary Balloon Angioplasty: Methods and Results

Valmik Bhargava, Ph.D.
Associate Project Bio-Engineer, University of California, San Diego; Research Engineer, Cardiology Section, San Diego Veterans Affairs Medical Center, San Diego, California.
Measurement of Blood Flow; Left and Right Contrast Ventriculography: Methods for Quantitation of Volume and Mass; Catheterization and Angiography in Coronary Heart Disease; Catheterization and Angiography in Dilated Cardiomyopathy and Heart Failure

Colin M. Bloor, M.D.
Professor of Pathology and Director, Molecular Pathology Graduate Program, Department of Pathology, University of California, San Diego, School of Medicine, La Jolla; Attending Pathologist, University of California, San Diego, and Medical Center, Veterans Affairs Medical Center, San Diego, California.
Myocardial Biopsy Preparation and Interpretation

Kelly R. Branch, B.S.
Research Assistant, San Diego Cardiac Center, San Diego, California.
Supported Circulation in the Cardiac Catheterization Laboratory

Maurice Buchbinder, M.D.C.M.
Director, Interventional Cardiology, Sharp Hospital, San Diego, and Scripps Hospital, La Jolla, California.
Coronary Plaque Ablation and Atherectomy: Methods and Results

Peng-Sheng Chen, M.D.
Associate Professor, University of California, Los Angeles; Staff Cardiologist, Cedars-Sinai Medical Center, Los Angeles, California.
Catheterization in Disorders of Cardiac Rhythm

Jonathan Clague, M.D., M.R.C.P.
Senior Registrar, St. George's Hospital Medical School, London, United Kingdom.
Coronary Stents: Types and Results

Bruno Cotter, M.D.
Clinical and Research Fellow, Division of Cardiology, University of California, San Diego, Medical Center, San Diego, California.
Catheter Retrieval of Foreign Objects

Howard C. Dittrich, M.D.
Associate Professor of Medicine, Division of

Cardiology, Department of Medicine,
University of California, San Diego, San Diego,
California.
*Myocardial Biopsy: Techniques, Indications, and
Complications*

Gregory K. Feld, M.D.
Associate Professor, University of California,
San Diego, School of Medicine; Director,
Cardiac Electrophysiology Program, University
of Califoria, San Diego, Medical Center, San
Diego, California.
Catheterization in Disorders of Cardiac Rhythm

Martin Fromer, M.D.
Assistant Professor, University of Lausanne
School of Medicine; Director,
Electrophysiology Laboratory, Division of
Cardiology, Centre Hospitalier Universitaire
Vaudois, Lausanne, Switzerland.
Implantable Cardioverter-Defibrillators

Gabriel Gregoratos, M.D.
Professor of Medicine (Cardiology) and
Associate Head, Division of Cardiovascular
Medicine, University of California, Davis, Davis;
Director, Clinical Cardiology, University of
California, Davis, Medical Center, Sacramento,
California.
*Cardiac Catheterization: Basic Techniques and
Complications; Catheterization and Angiography in
Congenital Heart Disease of the Adult*

Parviz Haghighi, M.D.
Clinical Professor of Pathology, University of
California, San Diego, School of Medicine;
Staff Pathologist, Veterans Affairs Medical
Center, San Diego, California.
Myocardial Biopsy: Preparation and Interpretation

Otto M. Hess, M.D.
Professor, Department of Cardiology,
University Hospital, Zurich, Switzerland.
*Assessment of Systolic Left Ventricular Function;
Assessment of Diastolic Left Ventricular Function*

Brian E. Jaski, M.D.
Clinical Associate Professor, University of
California, San Diego; Medical Director,
Advanced Heart Failure and Cardiac
Transplant, and Co-Director, Cardiac
Catheterization Laboratory, Sharp Memorial
Hospital, San Diego, California.
*Supported Circulation in the Cardiac Catheterization
Laboratory*

Lukas Kappenberger, M.D.
Professor of Cardiology, University of Lausanne
Medical School; Professor and Chief, Division
of Cardiology, Centre Hospitalier Universitaire
Vaudois, Lausanne, Switzerland.
*Cardiac Pacing: Modes, Indications, and
Implantation Techniques; Implantable Cardioverter-
Defibrillators*

Morton J. Kern, M.D.
Professor of Medicine, St. Louis University;
Director, J. G. Mudd Cardiac Catheterization
Laboratory, St. Louis University Health Science
Center, St. Louis, Missouri.
Measurement of Coronary Blood Flow

Marvin A. Konstam, M.D.
Professor of Medicine and Radiology, Tufts
University School of Medicine; Director, Adult
Cardiac Catheterization Laboratory, New
England Medical Center, Boston,
Massachusetts.
Assessment of Right Ventricular Function

Hans P. Krayenbühl, M.D. *(deceased)*
Formerly Professor of Medicine and Chief of
Cardiology, Medical Policlinic, University of
Zurich, Zurich, Switzerland
Assessment of Systolic Left Ventricular Function

Jean-Marc LaBlanche, M.D.
Professor of Medicine, University of Lille, Lille,
France.
Coronary Balloon Angioplasty: Methods and Results

Philip A. Ludbrook, M.B., B.S.
Professor of Medicine (Cardiology) and
Radiology, Cardiovascular Division, Barnes
Hospital at Washington University School of
Medicine, St. Louis, Missouri.
Measurement of Coronary Blood Flow

G. B. John Mancini, M.D.
Eric W. Hamber Professor and Head,
Department of Medicine, University of British
Columbia; Staff, Faculty of Medicine,
Vancouver Hospital and Health Sciences
Centre, Vancouver, British Columbia, Canada.
Digital Cardiac Angiography

Kenneth Moser, M.D.
Professor of Medicine, and Director,
Pulmonary and Critical Care Division,
University of California, San Diego, School of
Medicine, San Diego, California.
*Pulmonary Angioscopy; Catheterization and
Angiography in Pulmonary Hypertension*

Pascal Nicod, M.D.
Professor of Medicine, University of Lausanne
School of Medicine; Chairman, Department of
Internal Medicine, Centre Hospitalier
Universitaire Vaudois, Lausanne, Switzerland.
*Catheterization and Angiography in Dilated
Cardiomyopathy and Heart Failure; Catheterization
and Angiography in Hypertrophic Cardiomyopathies;
Catheterization and Angiography in Restrictive and
Constrictive Disorders of the Heart; Catheter
Retrieval of Foreign Objects*

Kirk L. Peterson, M.D.
Professor of Medicine, Edith and William
Perlman Professor of Clinical Cardiology,
University of California, San Diego, School of
Medicine, San Diego, California.
*Cardiac Catheterization and Angiography: Evolution
of Use and Practice; Measurement and
Interpretation of Intracardiac, Venous, and Arterial
Physiologic Waveforms; Radiographic
Angiocardiography: Equipment and Contrast Agents;
Pulmonary Angioscopy; Catheterization and
Angiography in Valvular Heart Disease;
Catheterization and Angiography in Coronary Heart
Disease; Catheterization and Angiography in
Pulmonary Hypertension; Catheterization and
Angiography in Congenital Heart Disease of the
Adult; Thrombolysis, Coronary Angiography, and
Coronary Angioplasty in Acute Coronary Syndromes;
Coronary Plaque Ablation and Atherectomy:
Methods and Results; Catheter Balloon Valvuloplasty*

Ralf Polikar, M.D.
Privat-Docent, University of Lausanne School
of Medicine, Centre Hospitalier Universitaire
Vaudois, Lausanne; Chief, Department of
Internal Medicine, Hôpital de Nyon, Nyon,
Switzerland.
*Catheterization and Angiography in Hypertrophic
Cardiomyopathies; Catheterization and Angiography
in Restrictive and Constrictive Disorders*

Mark Reisman, M.D.
University of Washington; Director of
Cardiovascular Research, Swedish Medical
Center, Seattle, Washington.
*Coronary Plaque Ablation and Atherectomy:
Methods and Results*

Urs Scherrer, M.D.
Associate Professor, Department of Internal
Medicine, Centre Hospitalier Universitaire
Vaudois, Lausanne, Switzerland.
*Catheterization and Angiography in Hypertrophic
Cardiomyopathies*

Jürg Schlaepfer, M.D.
Centre Hospitalier Universitaire Vaudois,
Lausanne, Switzerland.
*Cardiac Pacing: Modes, Indications, and
Implantation Techniques*

Ralph Shabetai, M.D.
Professor of Medicine, University of California
School of Medicine, University of California,
San Diego; Chief, Cardiology Section, San
Diego, Veterans Affairs Medical Center, San
Diego, California.
*Measurement of Blood Flow; Myocardial Biopsy:
Techniques, Indications and Complications;
Catheterization and Angiography in Dilated
Cardiomyopathy and Heart Failure; Catheterization
and Angiography in Restrictive and Constrictive
Disorders of the Heart*

C. Todd Sherman, M.D.
Assistant Professor of Clinical Medicine,
University of Calfornia, Los Angeles, Center
for Health Sciences, Los Angeles, California.
Coronary Angioscopy

Deborah Shure, M.D.
Associate Professor of Medicine, Washington
University, St. Louis, Missouri.
Pulmonary Angioscopy

Ulrich Sigwart, M.D. F.R.C.P., F.A.C.C., F.E.S.C.
Professor of Medicine, University of
Dusseldorf, and Recognized Teacher,
University of London; Director, Department of
Invasive Cardiology; Royal Brompton Hospital,
London, United Kingdom.
Coronary Stents: Types and Results

Richard W. Smalling, M.D., Ph.D.
Professor of Medicine and Co-director, Division
of Cardiology, University of Texas Medical
School at Houston; Director, Clinical
Cardiology, and President, Medical Staff,
Hermann Hospital, Houston, Texas.
*Coronary Angiography: Methods, Quantitations and
Comparison with Other Imaging Modalities*

James E. Udelson, M.D.
Associate Professor of Medicine and Radiology,
Tufts University School of Medicine; Director,
Nuclear Cardiology Laboratory, and Associate,
Cardiac Catheterization Laboratory, New
England Medical Center, Boston,
Massachusetts.
Assessment of Right Ventricular Function

Peter Vollenweider, M.D.
Department of Internal Medicine, Centre
Hospitalier Universitaire Vaudois, Lausanne,
Switzerland.
*Catheterization and Angiography in Hypertrophic
Cardiomyopathies*

Frank C. P. Yin, M.D., Ph.D.
Professor of Medicine and Biomedical
Engineering, The Johns Hopkins University
School of Medicine, Baltimore, Maryland.
Assessment of Cardiac Pressure and Wall Forces

PREFACE

Anyone who has ever worked in any science knows how much aesthetic joy he has obtained. That is, in the actual activity of science, in the process of making a discovery, however humble it is, one can't help feeling an awareness of beauty. The subjective experience, the aesthetic satisfaction, seems exactly the same as the satisfaction one gets from writing a poem or a novel, or composing a piece of music. I don't think anyone has succeeded in distinguishing between them. The literature of scientific discovery is full of this aesthetic joy.

C.P. SNOW
"THE MORAL UN-NEUTRALITY
OF SCIENCE"
1960

More than 5 years ago, I set out to organize this text on cardiac catheterization and angiography. By then I had spent close to 25 years of my adult professional life learning, applying, and teaching this remarkable discipline of medical science and technology. While working in the cardiac catheterization laboratory I observed repeatedly the wondrous marriage of physics, physiology, and biochemistry to the fundamental needs of patients seeking help for symptoms and signs of heart disease.

With each individual studied, I could never separate the sophisticated science and technology from the humanistic and altruistic impulses that perforce underlie the work of a physician. To measure an abnormal physiologic parameter with precision, to visualize with high spatial resolution an impediment to circulatory function, to witness a suspected but not yet proven abnormal electrophysiologic pathway, all performed for the benefit of a member of my species, engendered intense feelings of gratification. As the discipline evolved, I reveled further in

the opportunity to apply catheter techniques to the relief of heart disease. I often mused privately, "How can the 'literary intellectual' question the redeeming value of science and technology?"

In this spirit of wonder, and desiring to share my experiences with this craft, I invited a number of outstanding contributors from both sides of the Atlantic Ocean (many of whom I either learned from, collaborated with, or taught as a faculty member at the University of California, San Diego, School of Medicine) to cooperate in writing a relatively comprehensive text on cardiac catheterization and angiography. Most accepted my entreaties, and for their cooperation and scholarly efforts I am most grateful. I am indebted especially to my coeditor, Professor Pascal Nicod, who, following his 5 years at UCSD, took on the task of writing and editing a number of chapters despite his new responsibilities at the University of Lausanne School of Medicine, Switzerland.

A number of physicians influenced my own intellectual growth in cardiology and thus served as the crucible out of which this work was forged. James K. Alexander was a delightfully charismatic and stimulating teacher of the crafts of cardiac diagnosis and hemodynamic research while I served as a postgraduate fellow at Baylor College of Medicine in Houston, Texas, in the late 1960s. While at the University of California, San Diego, from 1970 onward, I benefited enormously from the flourishing research and teaching environment for the cardiovascular sciences, created and nurtured by Eugene Braunwald until his departure to the Harvard Medical School in 1972. Over the following two decades, this climate prevailed under the ever-stimulating and creative leadership of John Ross, Jr., and served to augment further my interest in cardiac diagnosis and myocardial mechanics. During

ix

this latter period, I cannot overlook the productive and pleasurable sabbatical leave that I spent in Switzerland in 1979–1980. While I was there, Wilhelm Rutishauser of the University of Geneva graciously helped me set up an experimental animal model of mitral regurgitation and engendered much of my subsequent interest in videodensitometry and digital cardiac imaging. At the University of Zurich, the late Hans Peter Krayenbühl allowed me the opportunity to pursue studies on left atrial function and ultimately provided access to the catheterization laboratories at the Kantonspital in Zurich, where Andreas Gruntzig generously demonstrated to me his new technique of coronary angioplasty. All of these people and venues contributed, both directly and indirectly, to the ultimate production of this book.

It is my hope that both the novice as well as the already mature cardiologist will find this text a useful resource for augmenting their knowledge of the science and art of cardiac catheterization and angiography. Hopefully, through the collective efforts of all of the authors, this text more fully catalogues our knowledge of a branch of medicine that impacted enormously the diagnosis and therapy of cardiovascular disease during the twentieth century.

KIRK L. PETERSON, M.D.

and limitations. *In* Kaltenbach M, Rentrop P, Grüntzig AR (eds): Transluminal Coronary Angioplasty and Intracoronary Thrombolysis. Berlin, Springer-Verlag, 1982, pp 110–124.

62. Penny WF, Schmidt DA, Safian RD, et al: Insights into the mechanism of luminal improvement after directional coronary atherectomy. Am J Cardiol 1991: 67:435.

63. Peterson KL, Rivera I, McDaniel M, et al: Percutaneous transluminal coronary rotational ablation: Serial follow-up by quantitative angiography. *In* Serruys PW, Strauss BH, King SB III (eds): Restenosis After Intervention with New Mechanical Devices. Dordrecht, The Netherlands, Kluwer Academic, 1992, pp 313–330.

64. Lategola M, Rahn H: A self-guiding catheter for cardiac and pulmonary arterial catheterization and occlusion. Proc Soc Exp Biol Med 1953; 84:667–669.

65. Dotter CT, Straube KR: Flow-guided cardiac catheterization. Am J Roentgenol 1962; 88:27–31.

66. Fogerty TJ, Cranley JJ, Krause RJ, et al: A method for extraction of arterial emboli and thrombus. Surg Gynecol Obstet 1963; 116:241–244.

67. Rashkind W, Miller W: Creation of an atrial septal defect without thoracotomy: A palliative approach to complete transposition of the great arteries. JAMA 1966; 196:991–992.

68. Swan HJC, Ganz W, Forrester JS, et al: Catheterization in the heart in man with use of flow-directed balloon tipped catheters. N Engl J Med 1970; 283:447–451.

69. Dotter CT, Judkins MJ: Transluminal treatment of arteriosclerotic obstruction: Description of a new technique and a preliminary report of its application. Circulation 1964; 30:654–670.

70. Zeitler E, Schoop W, Zahnow W: The treatment of occlusive arterial disease by transluminal catheter angioplasty. Radiology 1971; 99:19.

71. Zeitler E, Grüntzig AR, Schoop W (eds): Percutaneous Vascular Recanalization. New York, Springer-Verlag, 1978.

72. Zeitler E: Percutaneous dilatation and recanalization of iliac and femoral arteries. Cardiovasc Intervent Radiol 1980; 3:207.

73. Portmann W: Ein neuer Korsett-Ballonkatheter zur transluminalen Rekanalisation nach Dotter unter besonderer Berücksichtigung von Obliterationen an den Beckenarterien. Radiol Diagn 1973; 14:239.

74. Grüntzig AR: Perkutane Dilatation von Coronarstenosen-Beschreibung eines neuen Kathetersystems. Klin Wochenschr 1976; 54:543.

75. Grüntzig AR, Myler RK, Hanna EH, Turina MI: Coronary transluminal angioplasty [abstract]. Circulation 1977; 55/56:III-84.

76. Grüntzig AR: Transluminal dilatation of coronary artery stenosis [letter]. Lancet 1978; 1:263.

77. Grüntzig AR, Myler RK, Stertzer SH, et al: Coronary percutaneous transluminal angioplasty: Preliminary results [abstract]. Circulation 1978; 58:II-56.

78. Grüntzig AR, Senning A, Siegenthaler WE: Nonoperative dilatation of coronary artery stenosis: Percutaneous transluminal coronary angioplasty. N Engl J Med 1979; 301:61.

79. Simpson JB, Baim DS, Robert EW, Harrison DC: A new catheter system for coronary angioplasty. Am J Cardiol 1982; 49:1216.

80. Simpson JB, Johnson DE, Thapliyal HV, et al: Transluminal atherectomy: A new approach to the treatment of atherosclerotic vascular disease. Circulation 1985; 72:III-146.

81. Simpson JB, Selmon MR, Robertson GC, et al: Transluminal atherectomy for occlusive peripheral vascular disease. Am J Cardiol 1988; 61:96G–101G.

82. Spears JR, Reyes VP, Wynne J, et al: Percutaneous coronary laser balloon angioplasty: Initial results of a multicenter experience. J Am Coll Cardiol 1990; 16:293.

83. Litback F, Eigler NL, Margolis JR, et al: Percutaneous excimer laser coronary angioplasty. Am J Cardiol 1990; 66:1027.

84. Siegel RJ, DonMichael TA, Fishbein MC, et al: In vivo ultrasound arterial recanalization of atherosclerotic total occlusions. J Am Coll Cardiol 1990; 15:345–351.

85. Fourier JL, Bertrand ME, Auth DC, et al: Percutaneous coronary rotational angioplasty in humans: Preliminary report. J Am Coll Cardiol 1989; 14:1278–1282.

86. Kan J, White RI, Mitchell SE, Gardner TJ: Percutaneous balloon valvuloplasty: A new method for treating congenital pulmonary valve stenosis. N Engl J Med 1982; 307:540.

87. Pepine CJ, Gessner JH, Feldman RL: Percutaneous balloon valvuloplasty for pulmonic valve stenosis in the adult. Am J Cardiol 1982; 50:1442.

88. Lababidi Z, Wu JR: Percutaneous balloon valvuloplasty. Am J Cardiol 1983; 52:560.

89. Lababidi Z, Wu JR, Walls JT: Percutaneous balloon aortic valvuloplasty: Results in 23 patients. Am J Cardiol 1984; 53:194.

90. Cribier A, Saoudi N, Berland J, et al: Percutaneous transluminal valvuloplasty of acquired aortic stenosis in elderly patients: An alternative to valve replacement? Lancet 1986; 1:63–67.

91. Inoue K, Ouraki T, Nakamura T, et al: Clinical application of transvenous mitral commissurotomy by a new balloon catheter. J Thorac Cardiovasc Surg 1984; 87:394.

92. Lock JE, Khalilullah M, Shrivastava S, et al: Percutaneous catheter commissurotomy in rheumatic mitral stenosis. N Engl J Med 1985; 313:1515.

93. Al Zaibag MA, Ribeiro PA, Al Kasab S: Percutaneous balloon valvotomy in tricuspid stenosis. Br Heart J 1987; 57:51.

94. Ribeiro PA, Al Zaibag MA, Al Kasab SA, et al: Percutaneous double balloon valvotomy in tricuspid stenosis. Am J Cardiol 1988; 61:660.

95. de Lezo JS, Pan M, Sancho M, et al: Percutaneous transluminal balloon dilatation of discrete subaortic stenosis. Am J Cardiol 1986; 58:619.

96. Lock JE, Bass JL, Amplatz K, et al: Balloon dilatation angioplasty of aortic coarctations in infants and children. Circulation 1983; 68:109.

97. Lock JE, Castaneda-Zuniga WR, Fuhrman BP, et al: Balloon dilatation angioplasty of hypoplastic and stenotic pulmonary arteries. Circulation 1983; 67:962.

98. Waldman JD, Schoen FJ, Kirkpatrick SE, et al: Balloon dilatation of porcine bioprosthetic valve in the pulmonary position. Circulation 1987; 76:109.

99. McKay CR, Waller BF, Hong R, et al: Problems encountered with catheter balloon valvuloplasty of bioprosthetic aortic valves. Am Heart J 1988; 115:463.

100. Calvo OL, Sobrino N, Gamallo C, et al: Balloon percutaneous valvuloplasty for stenotic bioprosthetic valves in mitral position. Am J Cardiol 1987; 60:736.

101. Feit F, Stecy PJ, Nachamie MS: Percutaneous balloon valvuloplasty for stenosis of a porcine bioprosthesis in the tricuspid valve position. Am J Cardiol 1986; 58:363.

102. Scherlag BJ, Lau SH, Helfant RH, et al: Catheter technique for recording His bundle activity in man. Circulation 1969; 39:13.

103. Castellanos A Jr, Chapunoff E, Castillo C, et al: His bundle electrograms in two cases of Wolff-Parkinson-White (pre-excitation) syndrome. Circulation 1970; 41:399.

104. Scheinman MM, Morady F, Hess DS, et al: Catheter-induced ablation of the atrioventricular junction to control refractory supraventricular arrhythmias. JAMA 1982; 248:851.
105. Gallagher JJ, Svenson RH, Kasell JH, et al: Catheter technique for closed-chest ablation of the atrioventricular conduction system. N Engl J Med 1982; 306:194.
106. Belhassen B, Miller HI, Geller E, Laniado S: Transcatheter electrical shock ablation of ventricular tachycardia. J Am Coll Cardiol 1986; 7:1347–1455.

Chapter 2

Cardiac Catheterization
Basic Techniques and Complications

GABRIEL GREGORATOS

The first step toward the successful performance of a cardiac catheterization is the complete and thorough precatheterization evaluation of the patient. The physician performing the procedure must do a complete history and physical examination and become thoroughly familiar with all previously collected information, including noninvasive (electrocardiographic, echocardiographic, and nuclear studies) and invasive data—this point cannot be overemphasized. Particularly in patients with coronary artery disease, information regarding coronary anatomy obtained during previous catheterization and angiocardiography is an invaluable asset that helps the operator perform the catheterization efficiently and in a timely fashion.

On the basis of the available information obtained during precatheterization evaluation, the operator must develop a plan for the procedure. This step is necessary in all catheterizations, but it is especially important for patients with valvular or congenital heart disease. The plan—written or simply developed in the mind of the operator—includes all aspects of the procedure: vascular access, types of catheters to be used, whether to perform a combined right and left heart catheterization or a left heart catheterization alone, whether to use a retrograde or transseptal approach to the left heart, the sequence of data acquisition and angiocardiographic examinations, the performance of special procedures (e.g., coronary sinus catheterization and indicator-dilution studies), and any special requirements that a particular patient may have (e.g., chronic anticoagulant therapy).

It is necessary for the operator to communicate the cardiac catheterization plan to the nurses and technologists assisting with the procedure. Special patient requirements (such as oxygen administration and special medications to be given during the procedure) must be discussed with the nurses in detail. Similarly, the specific technical details of the procedure must be discussed with the technologist ahead of time. It is necessary to establish which of the many different procedures available in most laboratories (Table 2–1) will be undertaken and in what sequence. For example, whether cardiac output determination will be performed by the Fick method, the thermodilution method, or the indocyanine green dye dilution method must be determined. The proposed method of recording transvalvular gradients, other specialized data acquisitions, and the sequence of an-

Table 2–1. **Commonly Performed Procedures During Cardiac Catheterization**

Intracardiac and intravascular pressure recording
Oxygen consumption and carbon dioxide production
   measurements
Arterial and mixed venous oxygen content measurement
Hemoglobin oxygen saturation measurements (shunt
   detection)
Indicator-dilution studies
   Qualitative (shunt detection)
   Quantitative (cardiac output determination and shunt
     quantification)
Thermodilution studies (cardiac output determination)
Intracardiac electrical signal recording
Exercise studies
Pacing (atrial or ventricular) studies
Angiocardiographic studies (cine- or cut-film technique)
   Selective ventriculography (right or left)
   Selective atrial angiography (right or left)
   Aortography
   Pulmonary angiography
   Coronary arteriography
   Iliofemoral arteriography
   Renal arteriography
Angioscopic studies
Intravascular ultrasound studies
Therapeutic interventions

giocardiographic studies also must be discussed with the technologist.

It is only with meticulous attention to detail and proper planning that a cardiac catheterization can be performed quickly and efficiently and that the data acquired will be valid and useful in further patient management.

PATIENT PREPARATION

As with any invasive procedure, all patients experience a variable degree of anxiety before cardiac catheterization. It is necessary for the operator to discuss frankly and in some detail with the patient the indications, risks, and pro-

cedural details of the catheterization. Informed consent must be obtained verbally and in writing (Fig. 2–1). Although the explanation of the procedure must be thorough, complete, and honest, the operator must endeavor to allay the patient's anxiety. In general, the discomfort of the procedure (which is usually slight) and the risks should be stated fairly and not minimized. It is good practice to advise patients that major and minor complications may be encountered and to specifically mention the three major complications of death, stroke, and heart attack. The operator will then emphasize that major complications are rare and that in large series[1] the incidence of these major complications was approximately 1 in 500 cases. He or she will

---

Your doctor has requested you receive a specialized heart test that will include the following part(s) as marked:

☐ right heart catheterization (placement of a hollow tube to the right side of the heart through a vein)
☐ left heart catheterization (placement of a hollow tube to the left side of the heart through an artery)
☐ left ventricular cineangiogram (taking X-ray moving pictures of the heart beating)
☐ selective coronary cineangiography (taking X-ray moving pictures of the arteries nourishing the heart)
☐ selective coronary bypass graft cineanigiography (taking X-ray moving pictures of coronary bypass grafts)
☐ other _____

You may be given a sedative to help you relax during the procedure, but you will remain conscious. The procedure will be done in a room with special X-ray and electronic equipment to perform the procedure and monitor your safety. The skin over a large artery or vein or both in your groin or arm will be anesthetized (numbed). A thin hollow tube called a catheter will be placed into the artery or vein or both and guided to your heart using X-ray. Using the catheter, measurements of your heart's function will be made and X-ray movies may be taken of your heart and its arteries, as specifically listed above. The X-ray movies involve use of contrast medium (x-ray dye) which may produce a brief heat sensation or other chest discomfort for a few seconds. To further test your heart function or treat abnormalities, medicine may be given during the procedure. At the end of the procedure the catheter(s) will be removed and bleeding controlled by pressure or sutures. You will then be asked to rest in bed.

Though complications of this procedure are unusual, they may occasionally occur. When they do occur they are usually mild, but it is possible for a severe complication to happen, such as heart attack, stroke, heart damage, blood vessel blockage or tear, limb loss, bleeding, reaction to the X-ray dye, irregular heart rhythm, infection, or death. All due care will be taken to attempt to prevent complications and emergency treatment will be available if needed.

———

I have read or had read to me the above information and understand it. My doctor has discussed this procedure and its indications and possible complications with me and answered all my questions regarding it. Other approaches to my care have been discussed with me and I understand why this procedure is recommended now.

[ ]   patient speaks English
[ ]   patient does not speak English; translation by _____

DATE _____   PATIENT or patient's legal representative and relationship to patient

TIME _____   INFORMANT and printed name of informant (must be physician)

                   TRANSLATOR or Witness (if patient can't sign)*

*If the patient can make a mark, the patient should do so witnessed by a University employee. If the patient is physically incapable of signing, a University employee, and if possible, the patient's spouse or relative should sign in witness of the patient's having given verbal consent.

Figure 2–1. Informed consent form used at the Medical Center of the University of California, Davis. This is a multipurpose form, and the physician obtaining the consent must specify which procedures are to be performed. (Courtesy of University of California, Davis Medical Center, Sacramento, CA.)

then mention lesser complications such as arrhythmia, vascular injury or thrombosis, and contrast media reactions and report their incidence as usually less than 1 in 100 cases.

We have found it most useful to have a follow-up by a registered nurse who further discusses the procedure with the patient after informed consent has been obtained. Others have found that showing the patient a brief film or video describing the procedure can further reduce preoperative anxiety and provide significant benefit.[2]

Mild preoperative sedation is generally practiced in all cardiac catheterization laboratories. Although some invasive cardiologists elect to administer a sedative such as diazepam or midazolam intravenously on patient arrival in the catheterization laboratory, it is often preferable to premedicate patients orally at least an hour before the procedure so that on arrival in the laboratory, the patient has obtained maximum benefit from the premedication. It is important to recognize that sedatives may affect hemodynamics. This is particularly relevant in patients with congenital and valvular heart disease. The combination of meperidine, promethazine, and chlorpromazine used for many years for premedication of children undergoing cardiac catheterization has been found to produce significant pulmonary vasoconstriction and systemic vasodilation in animal models[3]; therefore, I prefer to premedicate adult patients simply with 5 mg of diazepam and 25 to 50 mg of diphenhydramine an hour or so before the procedure. If, despite this premedication, the patient arrives in the catheterization laboratory manifestly anxious, the oral premedication may be supplemented with 0.5 to 1 mg of midazolam intravenously. It is important to prevent patient oversedation and especially hypoventilation and hypoxemia. As more and more critically ill patients are brought to the catheterization laboratory for diagnostic studies and interventional procedures, the risk of excessive sedation must always be kept in mind. Other important areas to be addressed before the procedure include the management of chronic anticoagulant therapy, the continuation or discontinuation of certain medications, and the management of urinary output.

Generally, it is unnecessary to discontinue heparin infusion before diagnostic transfemoral cardiac catheterization if the need for anticoagulation appears to be major (such as in unstable angina). If the activated partial thromboplastin time (APTT) is at about two times the control, the technique should not induce hemorrhagic complications. If necessary, heparin anticoagu-

lation can be promptly reversed with the administration of protamine sulfate. On the other hand, chronic anticoagulation with oral warfarin presents a greater risk and must be managed differently. To perform a cardiac catheterization by the transfemoral approach, it is preferable to have the International Normalized Ratio (INR) at 2 or less. Usually, warfarin can be discontinued 48 hours before the date of the procedure and, if necessary, may be supplemented with an intravenous infusion of heparin before the catheterization if a transfemoral approach is planned. However, cardiac catheterization can be performed safely by the brachial cutdown technique in patients on chronic warfarin therapy with the INR in the therapeutic range of 2 to 3.5. If it becomes necessary to reverse an excessively high prothrombin time, fresh frozen plasma may be used, and vitamin K_1, which would make subsequent anticoagulation with warfarin difficult, should be avoided.

With reference to chronic medications, diuretics and digitalis may be withheld the morning of the procedure, although clearly this will vary from patient to patient. The withholding of digitalis to minimize the risk of digitoxic arrhythmias has been handed down from the days when most catheterizations involved patients with valvular heart disease and atrial fibrillation. The withholding of diuretics the morning of the procedure is based on frequent experiences with patients in heart failure who have received excessive diuretic therapy and arrive in the catheterization laboratory in a hypovolemic state. As a result, the hemodynamic data obtained can be spurious, and the reduced urinary output may increase the risk of iodinated contrast media nephropathy. Hypovolemia also increases the difficulty in accessing the central venous system and may require special maneuvers (see later).

Most patients undergo diuresis during catheterization as a result of fluid administration and the osmotic diuretic effect of contrast media. Some male patients (especially those with prostatic hypertrophy) find it difficult to void in the supine position. An indwelling urinary bladder catheter may be inserted before the cardiac catheterization in all patients who may be expected to develop voiding problems. Other preparations include fasting. It is customary to keep a patient fasting from midnight on for a morning catheterization. If the procedure is scheduled for late afternoon, a clear liquid breakfast is allowed at 7 A.M. and the patient is kept fasting thereafter. Except for patients in profound heart failure, maintenance fluids may be initiated intravenously in the form of 5%

dextrose in half-normal saline at a rate of 50 to 75 mL/hr during the hours they are kept fasting before cardiac catheterization. In addition to providing fluids, a good intravenous access is most helpful should drug administration become necessary before catheter insertion.

The routine precatheterization orders employed at the Medical Center of the University of California, Davis can be found in Figure 2–2.

VASCULAR ACCESS

Most cardiac catheterization procedures are performed via the percutaneous transfemoral (arterial and venous) approach. A smaller but still significant number of procedures are performed via the right brachial artery and basilic vein approach, primarily by direct surgical exposure of the vessels but, occasionally, percutaneously as well. Transseptal catheterization of the left heart and direct left ventricular apical puncture are reserved for specific indications, although the former technique is experiencing a modest revival.[4, 5] The transbronchial and posterior paraspinal approaches to left heart catheterization are of historical interest only as they were associated with a high rate of morbidity and mortality and therefore have been abandoned. Access to the right heart via the percutaneous right internal jugular vein approach, although common in the critical care unit, is used relatively infrequently in the catheterization laboratory and is reserved primarily for the performance of endomyocardial biopsy or for the insertion of a balloon-tipped flotation monitoring catheter during the performance of mitral or aortic valvuloplasty. In this section, the various methods of vascular access are described in some detail.

Percutaneous Transfemoral Approach

On arrival in the catheterization laboratory, the appropriately premedicated patient is placed on the radiographic table top, which should be padded with a 1- or 2-inch-thick foam rubber pad. Electrocardiographic monitoring leads are attached to the patient, and a preliminary rhythm strip is obtained as part of the catheterization record. Critically ill patients are provided with oxygen by either nasal cannula or mask, and a pulse oximeter is attached to one of the patient's fingers to monitor oxygenation continuously. Blood pressure is obtained by sphygmomanometry and also entered in the catheterization record before any other procedure is undertaken. At this point an assessment is made as to the adequacy of the patient's premedication, and, if necessary, additional sedation is administered intravenously as noted previously. The right groin area is surgically prepped and scrubbed with a solution of 1% povidone-iodine (Betadine) for 3 minutes. The area is then dried with sterile gauze pads, and the patient is draped with a sterile, specially manufactured fenestrated drape (Femoral drape, transparent area right side, Argon Company, Athens, TX). Meanwhile, the operator will have surgically washed and scrubbed his or her hands and will be sterilely gloved and gowned. When performing a catheterization by percutaneous vascular access, the operator may or may not wear a cap and mask. On the other hand, a cap and mask are required when a surgical cutdown in the antecubital fossa is performed. The left femoral artery and vein may be used equally well; however because most operators are right handed, most laboratories are set up routinely for the right groin approach.

The next step for the operator is to identify the femoral artery and vein in the inguinal region. The femoral artery usually can be palpated in the middle of the inguinal ligament, which courses from the anterosuperior iliac spine to the pubic tubercle (Fig. 2–3). Once the inguinal ligament and the femoral artery are identified, the course of the artery is determined by palpating the vessel for 2 to 3 cm below the inguinal ligament with the second and third fingers of the left hand. While maintaining these two fingers on the femoral artery at all times, the operator establishes local analgesia by first inducing a small intradermal wheal directly over the artery with 1% lidocaine using a short 26-gauge needle. This needle is then exchanged for a 1 1/2-inch 22-gauge needle, and additional lidocaine infiltration is carried out. The skin and subcutaneous tissues overlying the femoral artery and its adjacent vein are thoroughly anesthetized. Infiltration should be made cephalad to the level of the inguinal ligament on either side of the femoral artery and vein. It is important to aspirate at every new needle position before injecting lidocaine to ascertain that the artery or vein has not been entered. Should this happen, the needle is immediately withdrawn, and firm pressure is applied over the vessel for 2 minutes. This is usually adequate to induce hemostasis even in anticoagulated patients. The discomfort to the patient associated with lidocaine injection can be minimized by slow injection and by the use of a buffered lidocaine solution.[6] Once adequate lidocaine analgesia has been obtained, again the course of the artery is identified and

I. Cardiac Catheterization scheduled for _____ (date) at _____ (time).

II. Check all items that apply

_____ 1. NPO after midnight except for medications.

_____ 2. Clear liquid breakfast; NPO thereafter except for medications.

_____ 3. Patient to take all regular medications, except:

Hold _____   Hold _____

_____ 4. Hold all regular medications.

_____ 5. Other

III. Premedications at _____ (time) or to be called.

_____   _____

_____   _____

_____   _____

IV. Precath labs required (within 72 hours): ECG, CBC, PT, CHEM-7

V. Cardiology fellow to obtain consent for:

_____ 1. Right Heart Catheterization   _____ 2. Left Heart Catheterization

_____ 3. Left Ventriculography   _____ 4. Graft Angiography

_____ 5. Selective Coronary Angiography

_____ 6. Other Procedures: (_____)

VI. Prep and shave both groins.

VII. Start IV at _____ (time), in left arm with 20-gauge Intracath. Start 1000 mL bag D5/0.5 N.S.

at _____ (time) and run at _____ mL/h.

VIII. Have patient void before sending to Catheterization Lab.

IX. Send dentures, glasses, and all charts with patient to Catheterization Lab.

X. Send patient (on stretcher) to Catheterization Lab at _____ (time).

XI. LIST ALL ALLERGIES:

_____   _____   _____

XII. Additional and/or special orders:

Figure 2–2. Standard pre-cardiac catheterization orders.

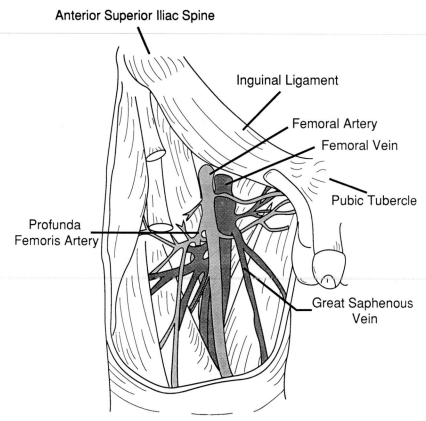

Figure 2–3. Relations of arteries and veins in the right femoral triangle. Note the femoral vein position deep to the femoral artery as the vessels course caudally from the inguinal ligament. (From Romanes GJ [ed]: Cunningham's Textbook of Anatomy, 12th ed. London, Oxford University Press, 1981; by permission of Oxford University Press.)

a small transverse skin incision is made with a no. 11 surgical blade to a depth of 2 to 3 mm. This incision is placed approximately 2 to 3 cm distal to the inguinal ligament and directly over the femoral artery pulse. A second similar skin nick is then placed at the same level approximately 1 cm medial to the artery; this second nick generally will overlie the femoral vein (see Fig. 2–3).

Although the location of the skin incisions as described usually coincides with the femoral skin crease, this is not a constant landmark. It is therefore always necessary to identify the inguinal ligament whose anatomic location is constant and prepare the skin for vascular puncture at a level of 2 to 3 cm caudad to this structure. The location of the puncture site is critical. High location at or above the inguinal ligament can result in major complications, including local and retroperitoneal hematomas, because of the inability to compress the vessels adequately once the catheters have been removed. Puncturing the vessels low, more than 3 cm caudad to the inguinal ligament, may result

in entering the femoral artery at the point of its bifurcation into the profunda and superficial vessels. Similarly, distal puncture of the femoral vein increases the risk of placing the puncture at the entry point of the saphenous vein. Generally, puncture at bifurcation sites increases the risk of vessel injury and vessel thrombosis. Furthermore, the femoral artery overlies in part the femoral vein distal to the inguinal ligament, and a low puncture site increases the possibility that the venipuncture may pass through the femoral artery, thereby setting the stage for development of an arteriovenous communication when the catheters are removed.

Once the skin incisions have been appropriately placed, a small mosquito clamp is introduced, and the skin and subcutaneous tissues are gently separated with blunt dissection. The intent of this is to form a tunnel through which the catheter will pass easily. This blunt dissection is carried out until the hemostat passes through the superficial fascia, which is usually 0.5 to 1 cm deep to the skin in the average-sized adult. It is important to avoid injury to either vessel by excessively deep and vigorous blunt dissection. This is a particular risk in patients who are thin.

Femoral Vein Access

Vascular access is then accomplished by a standard Seldinger approach.[7] The femoral artery is again palpated over a 2- to 3-cm course below the inguinal ligament, applying a slight lateral traction on the vessel with the left hand. The Seldinger needle (Fig. 2–4) is then inserted into the skin incision overlying the femoral vein and advanced cephalad and very slightly medially with the needle at a 45-degree angle relative to the skin (Fig. 2–5). The intent is to puncture the femoral vein 0.5 to 1 cm medial to the femoral artery pulse. The puncture is carried out with a firm, quick motion that transfixes the femoral vein with the needle passing through both the anterior and posterior walls of the vessel. It is not uncommon at this point for the needle to reach the periosteum of the femoral head, which can be quite sensitive if not previously adequately anesthetized. If the patient experiences discomfort at this point, the Seldinger obturator is removed and an additional 1 to 2 mL of lidocaine is injected via the can-

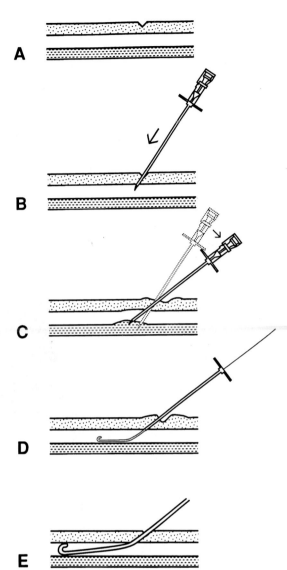

Figure 2–5. Schematic representation of Seldinger technique for vascular access. *A,* A small skin incision has been placed directly over the vessel. *B,* The Seldinger needle is introduced at a 45-degree angle, with a quick motion designed to transfix both anterior and posterior vessel walls. *C,* The hub of the needle is depressed closer to the plane of the skin, and the obturator is removed. *D,* The cannula is then slowly withdrawn until its tip is lying in the vessel lumen and free flow of blood is obtained. A J-tip flexible guide wire is introduced through the cannula and is seen to lie in the vessel lumen. *E,* The Seldinger cannula has been removed, with the guide wire remaining in the lumen to allow insertion of either a catheter or a sheath-dilator assembly.

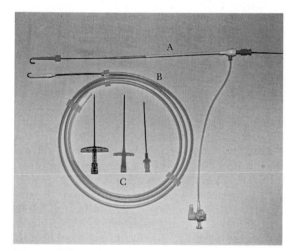

Figure 2–4. Vascular access equipment. **A,** 7-French 0.038-inch catheter sheath introducer system with backbleed valve, side-arm, and three-way stopcock attached (Cordis Corporation, Miami, FL). There is a vessel dilator and 45-cm J-guide wire within the sheath. **B,** Guide wire (Argon Company, Athens, TX) (in its tubular container), J-tipped, fixed-core, Teflon-coated 0.035-inch × 150 cm. **C,** Vascular entry needles. The Seldinger needle consists of two components: an outer blunt cannula and an inner sharp obturator with rounded edges. *Left,* Standard Seldinger, 18-gauge, 2-7/8 inch (Manan Med Products, Northbrook, IL). *Center,* Modified Seldinger, 18-gauge, 2 3/4-inch (UMI Corporation, Ballston Spa, NY). *Right,* Guide wire introducer needle (thin-walled) 18-gauge, 2 3/4-inch (UMI).

nula in the vicinity of the periosteum. A 10-mL syringe is then attached to the cannula (from which the obturator has already been removed), and the whole syringe-needle assembly is tilted downward so that the needle forms only a 20- to 30-degree angle with the skin surface. Gentle suction is applied to the syringe, and the syringe-needle assembly is very slowly withdrawn. It is important to control the assembly with both hands. The right hand is holding the syringe and applying gentle suction, whereas the left hand is controlling the cannula by holding it by its flange. When the tip of the Seldinger cannula is free within the femoral vein lumen, free flow of blood will enter the syringe. At this point all withdrawing motion is stopped, the needle held steady with the left hand, and the syringe is disconnected. A 0.035- or 0.038-inch J-guide wire is then introduced into the needle and advanced 15 to 20 cm (see Fig. 2–5). The introduction of the J-guide wire into the needle can be accomplished either by using the plastic introducer supplied with it or by straightening the J-tip by hyperextending the wire between the thumb and index finger of the right hand. This procedure requires practice but is easy to master. If difficulty is encountered in locating the femoral vein and the patient is believed to be hypovolemic with venous collapse, he or she should be asked to perform a moderate Valsalva maneuver, which will distend the vein and make it easier to locate. The initial passage of the J-guide wire through the needle into the femoral and iliac vein should be smooth with no resistance encountered. If the operator feels any resistance, further wire advancement should be stopped, and fluoroscopy should be used immediately to locate the tip of the wire. Occasionally, the wire advancement is arrested by entry in a small side branch. Simply pulling back the guide wire for 1 to 2 cm, rotating it, and then readvancing solves this problem. If, however, resistance to wire advancement is encountered just as the wire is exiting the needle, this implies arrest of the forward progress because of wire tip impingement on the back or one of the sidewalls of the femoral vein. In extreme circumstances the wire may occasionally double up on itself right after it exits the Seldinger cannula. If this happens, the wire should be gently pulled back and removed. Great care must be taken not to amputate the distal soft part of the guide wire against the cannula. In general, if difficulties are encountered advancing the wire beyond the tip of the cannula, the wire should be removed, a syringe reattached, and free flow of blood re-established. Occasionally, slightly angling the cannula medially or laterally or further depressing it against the skin of the patient's thigh will provide the necessary orientation to allow the guide wire to exit the cannula and enter the venous channel freely. Once the J-tip is seen to traverse the iliac vein and enter the inferior vena cava (IVC) just above its bifurcation, fluoroscopy will show the guide wire to be just lateral to the right border of the spine. At this point while holding the guide wire steady, the Seldinger cannula is removed, and moderate pressure is exerted over the entry point to prevent backbleeding. The cannula is removed over the length of the guide wire, which is then wiped with a saline-moistened gauze pad. Although an end-hole catheter can then be introduced directly over the wire into the femoral vein, the current practice is to insert a sheath-dilator assembly with a back-bleed valve and side-arm connector (see Fig. 2–4). This is preferable because backbleeding is avoided and the side-arm allows for the injection of fluids or drugs, and the use of a sheath allows for multiple catheter exchanges without having to resort to further use of guide wires, and it eliminates the need of maintaining pressure over the puncture site at the time of each exchange. Insertion of the sheath-dilator assembly is generally simple and easy unless one is dealing with a patient who is very obese or who has had several prior catheterizations that produced a great deal of scar tissue overlying the femoral vessels. As the sheath-dilator assembly is introduced over the wire, it is helpful for an assistant to hold the guide wire straight and taut, because otherwise it may be carried forward by the dilator and "buckle" in the subcutaneous tissues. The operator holds the sheath-dilator assembly with the right hand while continuing to exert moderate pressure over the puncture site to prevent backbleeding. The sheath-dilator assembly is advanced gently and with a rotating motion through the skin and subcutaneous tissues and into the femoral vein. If resistance is encountered, it may be occasionally helpful to remove the dilator from the sheath and make a pass first with the dilator alone and then with the sheath-dilator assembly. If the sheath is shown to wrinkle after an unsuccessful attempted insertion, it should be discarded and a new sheath should be used. On completion of the insertion process, the dilator and guide wire are removed and a syringe is attached to the side-arm to establish free backflow of blood through the sheath and side-arm. Next, the sheath is flushed and filled through its side-arm with heparinized saline, and the stopcock is shut off.

In many laboratories, a standard 18-gauge thin-walled (see Fig. 2–4) needle is used instead of the Seldinger needle for venous and arterial puncture. The technique is similar to the Seldinger approach described earlier except that the needle is inserted connected to a 10-mL syringe, and gentle continuous suction is ex-

CONTENTS

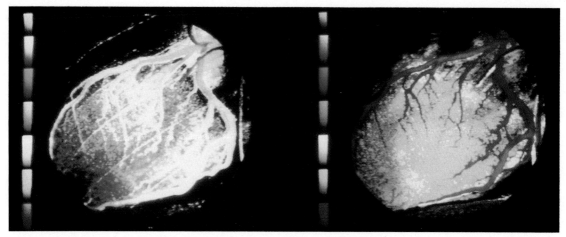

Figure 10–8. Color-coded and intensity-modulated parametric image from a patient with normal coronary flow reserve. Colors encode temporal characteristics of the contrast medium bolus (contrast medium appearance in first cycle = red, second cycle = yellow, etc.). Intensity reflects the amount of contrast medium (and flow) in the myocardium. The left panel depicts flow at rest. The right panel was obtained after intracoronary injection of papaverine to induce maximal hyperemia.

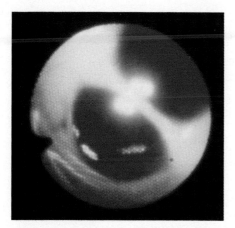

Figure 15–4. A normal pulmonary artery bifurcation as viewed through an angioscope; note the smooth, pale, glistening appearance of the intima; bright red blood fills the lumen.

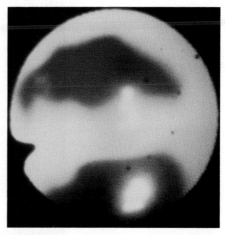

Figure 15–5. Roughening and irregularity of the contour of the pulmonary artery, believed to be secondary to partial recanalization, as visualized by the angioscope positioned just proximal to a bifurcation.

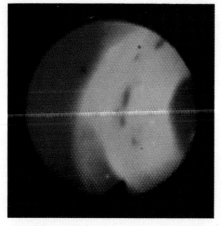

Figure 15–6. Pitting of the internal vessel surface, believed to be due to intimal fibrosis and organization of laminated clot. Blood in the lumen has been displaced by the inflated balloon at the tip of the angioscope.

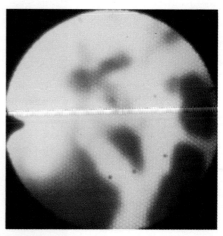

Figure 15–7. Bands and webs, remnants of an organized thromboembolic clot, as visualized through the angioscope.

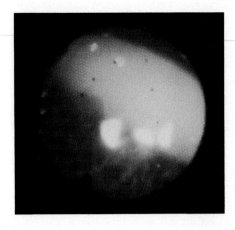

Figure 15–8. Pitted thromboembolic material incorporated into the vessel wall. White spots in the image represent reflected light off the inflated balloon at the tip of the angioscope. The small red dots are due to broken optical fibers that do not transmit light.

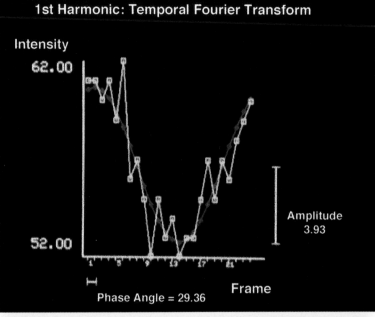

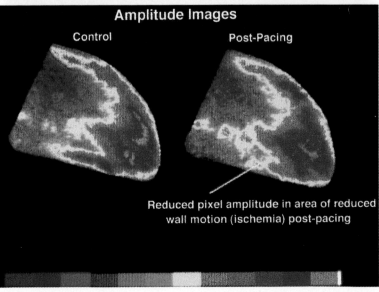

Figure 19–13. A, Plot of gray scale (intensity) versus time (cineframe) throughout the cardiac cycle for a single pixel. The first harmonic of a temporal Fourier transform is shown, in red, superimposed. Amplitude and phase angle for the first harmonic are displayed. *B,* Parametric image display of the amplitudes calculated, pixel by pixel over the left ventricular region of interest. Pseudocolor coding below shows low amplitudes as purple, whereas high amplitudes are shown as shades of red. The ventricle was filmed in the right anterior oblique projection. Note the reduced pixel amplitudes on the control injection along the high inferior wall in the area of an old inferoposterior myocardial infarction. During the immediate postpacing ischemia, the area of reduced amplitudes along the inferior wall enlarges, indicating reduced wall motion in this region.

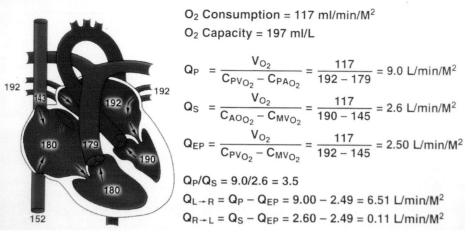

$$O_2 \text{ Consumption} = 117 \text{ ml/min/M}^2$$
$$O_2 \text{ Capacity} = 197 \text{ ml/L}$$

$$Q_P = \frac{V_{O_2}}{C_{PVO_2} - C_{PAO_2}} = \frac{117}{192 - 179} = 9.0 \text{ L/min/M}^2$$

$$Q_S = \frac{V_{O_2}}{C_{AOO_2} - C_{MVO_2}} = \frac{117}{190 - 145} = 2.6 \text{ L/min/M}^2$$

$$Q_{EP} = \frac{V_{O_2}}{C_{PVO_2} - C_{MVO_2}} = \frac{117}{192 - 145} = 2.50 \text{ L/min/M}^2$$

$$Q_P/Q_S = 9.0/2.6 = 3.5$$
$$Q_{L \to R} = Q_P - Q_{EP} = 9.00 - 2.49 = 6.51 \text{ L/min/M}^2$$
$$Q_{R \to L} = Q_S - Q_{EP} = 2.60 - 2.49 = 0.11 \text{ L/min/M}^2$$

Figure 25–6. Schematic diagram of blood oxygenation in the heart in the presence of a relatively large interatrial septal defect with left-to-right shunting of oxygenated blood and normal pulmonary vascular resistance. A step-up in oxygen content is noted in the right atrium. Note the equations used for calculation of pulmonary blood flow (QP), systemic blood flow (QS), and effective pulmonary blood flow (QEP).

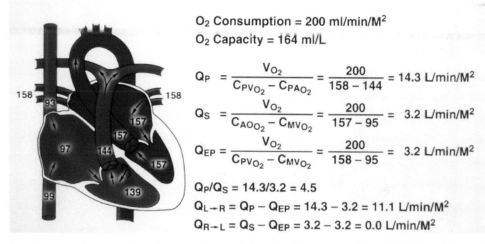

$$O_2 \text{ Consumption} = 200 \text{ ml/min/M}^2$$
$$O_2 \text{ Capacity} = 164 \text{ ml/L}$$

$$Q_P = \frac{V_{O_2}}{C_{PVO_2} - C_{PAO_2}} = \frac{200}{158 - 144} = 14.3 \text{ L/min/M}^2$$

$$Q_S = \frac{V_{O_2}}{C_{AOO_2} - C_{MVO_2}} = \frac{200}{157 - 95} = 3.2 \text{ L/min/M}^2$$

$$Q_{EP} = \frac{V_{O_2}}{C_{PVO_2} - C_{MVO_2}} = \frac{200}{158 - 95} = 3.2 \text{ L/min/M}^2$$

$$Q_P/Q_S = 14.3/3.2 = 4.5$$
$$Q_{L \to R} = Q_P - Q_{EP} = 14.3 - 3.2 = 11.1 \text{ L/min/M}^2$$
$$Q_{R \to L} = Q_S - Q_{EP} = 3.2 - 3.2 = 0.0 \text{ L/min/M}^2$$

Figure 25–7. Schematic diagram of blood oxygenation in the heart in the presence of a relatively large left-to-right shunt at the ventricular level and normal pulmonary vascular resistance. Sometimes, in the presence of tricuspid regurgitation, the step-up is detectable at the low right atrial level. Alternatively, with a high membranous ventricular septal defect, the step-up may be detectable in the pulmonary artery.

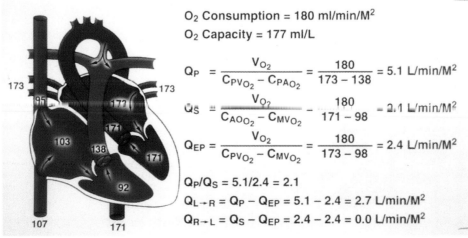

$$O_2 \text{ Consumption} = 180 \text{ ml/min/M}^2$$
$$O_2 \text{ Capacity} = 177 \text{ ml/L}$$

$$Q_P = \frac{V_{O_2}}{C_{PVO_2} - C_{PAO_2}} = \frac{180}{173 - 138} = 5.1 \text{ L/min/M}^2$$

$$Q_S = \frac{V_{O_2}}{C_{AOO_2} - C_{MVO_2}} = \frac{180}{171 - 98} = 2.1 \text{ L/min/M}^2$$

$$Q_{EP} = \frac{V_{O_2}}{C_{PVO_2} - C_{MVO_2}} = \frac{180}{173 - 98} = 2.4 \text{ L/min/M}^2$$

$$Q_P/Q_S = 5.1/2.4 = 2.1$$
$$Q_{L \to R} = Q_P - Q_{EP} = 5.1 - 2.4 = 2.7 \text{ L/min/M}^2$$
$$Q_{R \to L} = Q_S - Q_{EP} = 2.4 - 2.4 = 0.0 \text{ L/min/M}^2$$

Figure 25–8. Schematic diagram of blood oxygenation in the heart in the presence of a patent ductus arteriosus and normal pulmonary vascular resistance. The arterial admixture of venous blood is best detected near the site of the shunt but may also be notable above the pulmonic valve and into the right pulmonary artery.

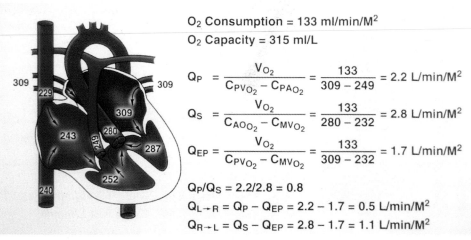

$$O_2 \text{ Consumption} = 133 \text{ ml/min/M}^2$$

$$O_2 \text{ Capacity} = 315 \text{ ml/L}$$

$$Q_P = \frac{V_{O_2}}{C_{PVO_2} - C_{PAO_2}} = \frac{133}{309 - 249} = 2.2 \text{ L/min/M}^2$$

$$Q_S = \frac{V_{O_2}}{C_{AOO_2} - C_{MVO_2}} = \frac{133}{280 - 232} = 2.8 \text{ L/min/M}^2$$

$$Q_{EP} = \frac{V_{O_2}}{C_{PVO_2} - C_{MVO_2}} = \frac{133}{309 - 232} = 1.7 \text{ L/min/M}^2$$

$$Q_P/Q_S = 2.2/2.8 = 0.8$$

$$Q_{L \to R} = Q_P - Q_{EP} = 2.2 - 1.7 = 0.5 \text{ L/min/M}^2$$

$$Q_{R \to L} = Q_S - Q_{EP} = 2.8 - 1.7 = 1.1 \text{ L/min/M}^2$$

Figure 25–9. Schematic diagram of blood oxygenation in a heart with tetralogy of Fallot and bidirectional shunting at the high ventricular septal level. Left-to-right shunting is relatively small owing to obstruction to the pulmonary vascular bed by pulmonary stenosis. Right-to-left shunting is facilitated by aortic override of the ventricular septum.

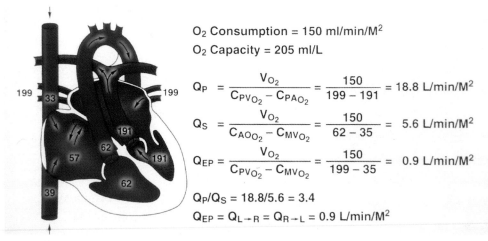

$$O_2 \text{ Consumption} = 150 \text{ ml/min/M}^2$$

$$O_2 \text{ Capacity} = 205 \text{ ml/L}$$

$$Q_P = \frac{V_{O_2}}{C_{PVO_2} - C_{PAO_2}} = \frac{150}{199 - 191} = 18.8 \text{ L/min/M}^2$$

$$Q_S = \frac{V_{O_2}}{C_{AOO_2} - C_{MVO_2}} = \frac{150}{62 - 35} = 5.6 \text{ L/min/M}^2$$

$$Q_{EP} = \frac{V_{O_2}}{C_{PVO_2} - C_{MVO_2}} = \frac{150}{199 - 35} = 0.9 \text{ L/min/M}^2$$

$$Q_P/Q_S = 18.8/5.6 = 3.4$$

$$Q_{EP} = Q_{L \to R} = Q_{R \to L} = 0.9 \text{ L/min/M}^2$$

Figure 25–10. Schematic diagram of blood oxygenation in a heart with D-transposition of the great vessels and an atrial septal defect. Note that the pulmonary and systemic circuits function in parallel; effective pulmonary blood flow (Q_{EP}) is dependent on the intracardiac shunt. In the absence of left ventricular outflow obstruction, pulmonary blood flow is increased.

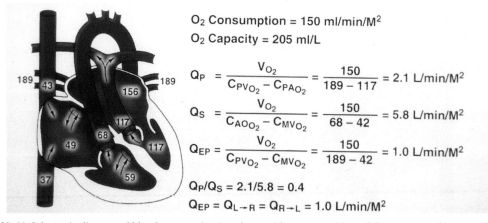

$$O_2 \text{ Consumption} = 150 \text{ ml/min/M}^2$$

$$O_2 \text{ Capacity} = 205 \text{ ml/L}$$

$$Q_P = \frac{V_{O_2}}{C_{PVO_2} - C_{PAO_2}} = \frac{150}{189 - 117} = 2.1 \text{ L/min/M}^2$$

$$Q_S = \frac{V_{O_2}}{C_{AOO_2} - C_{MVO_2}} = \frac{150}{68 - 42} = 5.8 \text{ L/min/M}^2$$

$$Q_{EP} = \frac{V_{O_2}}{C_{PVO_2} - C_{MVO_2}} = \frac{150}{189 - 42} = 1.0 \text{ L/min/M}^2$$

$$Q_P/Q_S = 2.1/5.8 = 0.4$$

$$Q_{EP} = Q_{L \to R} = Q_{R \to L} = 1.0 \text{ L/min/M}^2$$

Figure 25–11. Schematic diagram of blood oxygenation in a heart with D-transposition of the great vessels, an atrial septal defect, a ventricular septal defect, and subpulmonic stenosis. In this case, Q_{EP} contributes approximately the same proportion of Q_S. Because of the subpulmonic stenosis, pulmonary blood flow is reduced and Q_P/Q_S is diminished.

METHODS

Chapter 1

Cardiac Catheterization and Angiography
Evolution of Use and Practice

KIRK L. PETERSON

Through most of the the twentieth century, the diagnosis and therapy of cardiovascular diseases have been dependent on the pathophysiologic and pathoanatomic information uncovered by cardiac catheterization and angiography. These methods have evolved from the simplest measurement of the height of a fluid column in a venous structure to the insertion of sophisticated, miniaturized diagnostic and therapeutic devices into essentially all anatomic loci of the human heart. The story of this evolution, particularly as witnessed over the last 50 years, epitomizes the advances made in our understanding of normal and abnormal physiologic processes; moreover, it confirms the success of human ingenuity and applied technology in improving the clinical outcomes of patients with life-threatening cardiovascular illnesses.

EARLY HISTORY

Beginning in 1844, Claude Bernard, a French physiologist, catheterized the arterial and venous systems in a series of animal experiments. It was not until 1876 that Bernard reported these experiments in *Leçons sur la Chaleur Animal,* published in Paris.[1] Adolph Fick, presumably aware of Bernard's experiments, proposed cardiac catheterization as a method of estimating the total cardiac output.[2, 3] Subsequently, Otto Frank in 1895[4] and E. H. Starling[5] and Dalen Richards[6] in 1918 used the concepts of Bernard and Fick in their surprisingly sophisticated publications on cardiac physiology and drug action.

The application of cardiac catheterization to human studies awaited the foresight and fortitude of Werner Forssmann, a German urologic surgeon. Forssmann first experimented with cadavers and proved that a catheter could easily be passed into the right atrium for central administration of pharmacologic agents. In 1929, at a small German hospital in Eberswald, and while defying his superiors and deceiving his nurse assistant, Forssmann documented the first passage of a catheter into the human heart by recording a radiograph of his own chest in the hospital radiology department.[7, 8] Forssmann later wrote amusingly about the event in his autobiography[8, 9]:

I decided to override Schneider's prohibition and go ahead with the experiment on my own heart, secretly and quickly. But I needed an assistant, the surgical nurse. I had to win her over or I would have no access to the necessary sterile instruments.

I let a few days go by and then started to prowl around Nurse Gerda Ditzen like a sweet-toothed cat around the cream jug. I knew I'd be able to carry out my black deed only during afternoon siesta while everyone in the hospital was dozing, so I made a point of dawdling in the canteen after lunch, hoping to meet Nurse Gerda as she left the nurses' dining room. We often lent each other books, so it was easy to find something to gossip about; and she'd invite me back to her little office next to the operating room for a cup of coffee. When, about a fortnight after my conversation with Schneider, she said with a sigh, "What a pity we can't do the experiment together!" I decided the time had come.

The following afternoon the good lady was sitting in her cubicle when I breezed in, whistling cheerfully. "Nurse Gerda, I want you to give me a set of instruments for a venesection under local anesthesia, and a ureteral catheter."

She started up suspiciously. "But no one in the

ward's scheduled for a venesection. You're not planning to do that experiment of yours against boss's orders are you?"

"Nurse Gerda, you need know nothing about what I'm going to do. But supposing I were to do the experiment—it'd be quite safe."

She eyed me closely. "Are you absolutely sure there's no danger?"

"Absolutely."

"All right then, do it to me, I put myself in your hands."

"Well, why not? you'll be the first person in history to undergo such an experiment."

Of course, I had no intention of going through with this, but it was the only way to get the instruments. She got everything ready in the little operating room, then sat down and held out her left arm. When I suggested she lie down on the operating table she flatly refused at first. But I reminded her how, as she knew from her own experience, patients sometimes collapse from even the smallest dose of novacaine, and so I preferred her to be lying down for the anesthetic. She gave in, and with the speed of light I strapped her legs down so tightly that she couldn't reach the buckle; I then tied down her hand. Amazingly enough she accepted my explanation that I had to take all these precautions against her falling off the table since I had no one to assist me. I'd pushed the instrument tray behind her head so she couldn't see what I was doing. In the twinkling of an eye I had anesthetized my left elbow. Now I went back to her and began to iodize her elbow ceremoniously, and then to lay a sterile cloth over it, all very slowly and deliberately in order to kill time. When my anesthetic began to take effect I quickly made an incision in my skin, inserted a Deschamps aneurysm needle under the vein, opened it and pushed the catheter about a foot inside. I packed it with gauze and laid a sterile split over it. Then I released Nurse Gerda's right hand and loosened the straps around her knees.

"There we are, it's ready now. Please call the X-ray nurse."

Only then did she realize what had happened. She started to yell at me for having deceived her. It wasn't far to the X-ray room, but we had to go down into the basement, and by the time we arrived Nurse Eva was waiting for us. Upon my instruction she placed me behind the fluoroscope screen.

News spread like wildfire in a hospital. Suddenly Romeis burst in, half asleep and his hair all tousled: "You idiot, what the hell are you doing?" He was so desperate he almost tried to pull the catheter out of my arm. I had to give him a few kicks in the shin to calm him down.

In the immediate years that followed, Forssmann's historic self-experiment was met,

for the most part, with ridicule[3] and avoidance[8] by his professional colleagues. Klein in Prague, however, was an exception; he recognized the technique's potential and reported on the use of a catheter to obtain mixed venous samples for calculation of the cardiac output by the Fick principle.[8, 10]

MILESTONES

Right Heart Catheterization

Once the feasibility of right heart catheterization was established, the most prolific investigators in the early application of that procedure to humans were André F. Cournand and Dickinson Richards, Jr., working together at New York City's Bellevue Hospital. In 1956, because of their innovative contributions, Forssmann, Cournand, and Richards received jointly the Nobel Prize for Medicine. Cournand, in 1941, reported on the catheterization of the right auricle of humans[11] and, later, as part of a wartime program to study shock, published preliminary reports on pressures in the right side of the heart and the pulmonary artery.[12, 13] Near contemporaneously on the other side of the Atlantic Ocean, McMichael and Sharpey-Schafer of Great Britain studied the effects of posture, venous pressure change, atropine, and adrenaline on cardiac output, using the Fick method.[14] James V. Warren, while working as part of a group at Grady Hospital in Atlanta, soon applied the technique to sampling of hepatic and renal venous blood for analysis of regional blood flow to those organs.[15, 16] This same group also first described the use of right heart catheterization to study the hemodynamics of atrial septal defects.[17] Later in the 1940s, Bing and colleagues,[18] Dexter and coworkers,[19] and Cournand and associates[20] all reported on the use of cardiac catheterization of the right heart to study the physiologic abnormalities in congenital heart disease. Dexter's laboratory in Boston made a particularly notable contribution by describing the oxygen content[21] and the phasic and mean pressure characteristics[22] of the pulmonary "capillary" wedge position (obtained by wedging a catheter into the periphery of the pulmonary vasculature).

Left Heart Catheterization

In the early 1950s, Zimmerman and colleagues[23] in Cleveland, Ohio, and Limon-Lason and Bouchard in Mexico[24] first reported the passage of a catheter retrograde across the aortic valve into the left ventricle following insertion into a peripheral artery. Shortly thereafter, in 1953, Seldinger published a study of the use of percutaneous insertion of catheters into peripheral arteries,[25] a technique that could also be applied to peripheral veins; it significantly simplified the surgical skills necessary for performance of cardiac catheterization. A further major development in the 1950s, attributed primarily to John Ross, Jr., was atrial transseptal catheterization, a technique for entering the left atrium and left ventricle via the right femoral vein.[26–29] This technique used a long needle, curved at its tip and introduced into the right atrium through a slightly shorter catheter, to puncture the area of the foramen ovale, whereupon the outer coaxial catheter was advanced over the needle and into the left atrium. The near identity of the pulmonary capillary wedge and the left atrial pressure pulses in most patients and the ease, safety, and success of entering the left ventricle retrograde made for relatively infrequent use of atrial transseptal catheterization of the left heart. However, a resurgence of need for the atrial transseptal technique has emerged in recent years as a consequence of the development of balloon mitral valvuloplasty.

CARDIAC ANGIOGRAPHY

The early approaches to contrast angiography of the heart evolved in parallel with the development of techniques for cardiac catheterization. Forssmann himself had injected contrast medium into the central circulation, but the resultant images were said to be suboptimal. Augustin Castellano in 1937 at a professional meeting in Havana, Cuba, presented a series of cardiac angiograms recorded after injection of iodinated contrast medium into the venous system.[3] George Robb and Israel Steinberg[30] in New York later gained recognition in the United States for their technique of injecting relatively large amounts of iodinated contrast medium through large-bore needles placed into peripheral veins, followed by radiographs taken with a single-plane or biplane film changer. Film-changer (Schonander) images were perfected by radiologists at the Karolinska Institute in Sweden and provided superior spatial resolution with minimal blurring; however, the temporal resolution of the beating heart was suboptimal. Subsequently, selective injection of contrast medium through low-resistance, relatively large-bore catheters allowed superior definition of abnormal anatomic structures and often avoided superimposition of upstream

structures. Catheters were positioned by the operator while they were viewing the cardiac image directly on the input phosphor of an image intensifier. Radiation exposure to the patient (and operator) was relatively high owing to the nonpulsed, constant-potential x-ray source.

The most important innovation in cardiac angiography, emerging in the late 1950s and early 1960s, was selective coronary arteriography. Previous attempts at imaging the coronary arteries had used nonselectve injection of a large bolus of contrast medium into the ascending aortic root, at times attempted during periods of bradycardia or asystole induced by acetylcholine,[31] occlusion aortography,[32] diastolic-phase dye injections,[33] increased intrabronchial pressure,[34] or hypotension induced by pacing.[35] These efforts to visualize radiographically the coronary arteries were never applied broadly until Mason Sones, in 1959, discovered by accident that contrast medium could be safely injected through a catheter engaged selectively into a coronary artery.[36, 37] Also, the development of pulsed x-ray sources, high-speed cineangiography, and high-resolution image intensifiers allowed recording of the dynamic characteristics of contrast medium passage through the coronary arterial tree on 35mm cinefilm with levels of radiation acceptable to both patient and operator. Within a brief period after Sones's initial development of the technique, selective cine-coronary angiography was being performed throughout the world and indisputably set the stage for new approaches to coronary artery revascularization surgery.[38–44] In the 1960s, Ricketts and Abrams[45] and others[46, 47] described percutaneous techniques for performing cinearteriography of the coronary arterial tree. Preshaped catheters, particularly those designed by Dr. Melvin Judkins, found wide applicability, and they remain even today the most commonly used catheters in a diagnostic heart catheterization laboratory.

Quantitative methods to assess cardiac angiographic images first appeared in the late 1950s.[48, 49] An oft-cited seminal contribution was that of Harold Dodge and colleagues, who reported a validation study on the use of biplane angiocardiograms for measurement of diastolic and systolic left ventricular volumes.[50] Similar approaches were developed thereafter for quantification of left atrial and right ventricular volumes.[51, 52] Digital processing by high-speed computers of coronary arteriograms was then employed for improved quantification of atherosclerotic lesion severity[53]; measurements of minimal and mean lesion diameter, lesion length, and percentage of luminal stenosis all have since become important end-points in trials that assess the effects of various types of lifestyle, dietary, pharmacologic, and mechanical interventions in coronary atherosclerosis.[54–63]

BALLOON CATHETER APPLICATIONS

The 1960s and 1970s also witnessed the development of a number of diagnostic and therapeutic techniques based on inflatable balloons mounted on the end of a catheter. Lategola and Rahn[64] in 1953, followed by Dotter and Straube in 1962,[65] reported on self-guided or flow-guided catheters for cardiac and pulmonary arterial catheterization and occlusion. In addition, when arterial catheters began to be inserted via a brachial arteriotomy, balloon-tipped catheters were used to extract arterial thrombi and emboli after catheter removal.[66] Then, in 1966, Rashkind and Miller[67] used a balloon, inflated at the end of a catheter, to rupture the tissue around the foramen ovale to provide palliative shunting for infants with transposition of the great arteries. This technique has subsequently been applied to a number of congenital lesions where malformations impede adequate access of desaturated systemic venous blood to the pulmonary circuit.

The most ubiquitous use of balloon catheter technology in cardiac catheterization awaited an application by H. J. C. Swan and colleagues[68] to bedside hemodynamic monitoring. These investigators at the Cedars of Lebanon Hospital in Los Angeles used simple balloon-guided pulmonary artery catheterization, without fluoroscopy, to study and monitor the right and left heart filling pressures and cardiac output. Not only did measurements by the balloon flotation catheter allow definition of the trends in circulatory hemodynamics in response to pharmacologic, electrical, and mechanical interventions, but they served to prognosticate clinical outcome in patients with acute myocardial infarction, to detect early circulatory compromise in patients undergoing both noncardiac and cardiac surgery, and to define sources of pulmonary hypertension in patients with cardiopulmonary disorders. The technique also has been used to investigate the hemodynamic effects of essentially all new cardiovascular drugs (antiarrhythmic agents, systemic arterial and venous vasodilators, inotropic stimulants) of the last 2 decades. Finally, the development of balloon flotation catheters significantly reduced the time, necessary operator dexterity, and complications associated with the acquisition of right heart hemodynamic measurements in the catheterization laboratory.

INTERVENTIONAL CARDIOLOGY

The 1960s and 1970s also witnessed the explosive development of catheter techniques for treatment of vascular and valvular obstruction, now commonly known as the discipline of interventional cardiology. Dotter and Judkins,[69] in 1962, first reported the use of coaxial catheters for dilating lesions in peripheral arteries. This approach never gained recognition because of associated complications, although it was pursued more vigorously in Europe by Zeitler and colleagues.[70–72] Nevertheless, it was Zeitler's trainee, Andreas Grüntzig, who in the early 1970s recognized the potential of a caged latex balloon catheter, first described by Portmann,[73] to dilate atherosclerotic obstructions in peripheral vessels. Grüntzig[74] developed for peripheral arterial dilation a double-lumen catheter with a polyvinylchloride distensible balloon near its tip; subsequently, he miniaturized the catheter for the coronary circulation. After extensive animal experimentation, the technique was first applied by Grüntzig[75, 76] to the coronary circulation of humans in 1977 at the University Hospital (Kantonspital) in Zurich, Switzerland. Catheter balloon angioplasty soon thereafter emerged as a major therapeutic technique for treatment of both peripheral and coronary arterial atherosclerosis.[77–79] Its success and limitations have inspired in the last decade the design and construction of other angioplastic devices, including guillotine-like shavers for plaque removal,[80, 81] laser balloon catheters,[82] excimer laser ablation catheters,[83] ultrasound ablation catheters,[84] and diamond-studded burrs for high-speed rotational ablation of atherosclerotic plaque.[85]

The additional promise of catheter balloon dilation for valvular heart disease and obstructive lesions of the great vessels was first realized for pulmonary valve stenosis in the early 1980s by Kan,[86] Pepine,[87] and Lababidi[88] and their colleagues. Dramatic reductions in transvalvular pressure gradients were noted and within a short period led to use of the technique for all four native cardiac valves, as well as in congenital coarctation of the aorta and discrete subaortic stenosis. Lababidi and associates[89] first applied catheter balloon valvuloplasty to the treatment of congenital aortic stenosis, and Cribier and colleagues[90] in Paris initially described the use of the technique in calcific aortic stenosis. In the same period catheter balloon valvuloplasty for mitral stenosis was first described by

Inoue and coworkers[91]; Lock and colleagues[92] also reported early on a series in which the technique was used to treat rheumatic mitral stenosis. Tricuspid stenosis soon thereafter was successfully treated by catheter balloon dilation, using a double-balloon technique.[93, 94] Membranous, discrete subaortic stenosis was reported to be successfully treated by balloon dilation in 1986 by de Lezo and colleagues[95] and treatment of coarctation by Lock and associates in 1983.[96] The latter investigator published the initial report on the use of catheter balloon dilation angioplasty of hypoplastic and stenotic pulmonary arteries.[97] Catheter balloon dilation of porcine heterograft bioprostheses was also reported in the late 1980s in all four native valve positions.[98–101]

INTRACARDIAC ELECTROPHYSIOLOGY

The last 25 years have also seen the rapid evolution of techniques for studying the normal and abnormal physiology of the electrical conduction system in the heart. Beginning with the first report of an electrode catheter recording of a His bundle electrogram in humans by Scherlag and associates[102] in 1969, electrophysiologists proceeded to demonstrate abnormal conduction through both native and anomalous tissue[103] and have now used such measurements for assessing the antiarrhythmic effect of numerous pharmacologic agents. Moreover, these techniques have spawned the development of surgical as well as catheter techniques for ablation of electrical pathways believed to be the underlying source of cardiac arrhythmias.[104–106] Miniaturized implantable pacemakers, with highly sophisticated electrical circuits that can be elaborately programmed for electrocardiographic monitoring and stimulation and connected to well-insulated leads placed transvenously into the right heart, have now been developed. Finally, these same technologies are being applied to the development and application of implantable defibrillators that provide prompt detection and conversion of life-threatening ventricular arrhythmias.

The development of the cardiac catheter, despite its already enormous influence on the characterization and treatment of human heart disease, has not yet reached full maturity. Even in the face of significant advances in noninvasive diagnostic techniques, the continuing dependence of adult and pediatric cardiologists on cardiac catheterization and angiography for precise and accurate diagnoses and the increasing use of catheter-based therapies ensure the future of the cardiac catheterization and angiography laboratory in specialty health care facilities. If he were with us now, the audacious Werner Forssmann would only marvel at the evolution of a discipline he founded some 67 years ago.

REFERENCES

1. Bernard Claude: Lecons sur la Chaleur Animal. Paris, Baillere et Fils, 1876.
2. Rashkind WJ, Wagner HR, Tait N: Historical aspects of interventional cardiology: Past, present, and future. Tex Heart Inst J 1986; 13:363–367.
3. Leachman RD, Dear WE, Garcia E: The changing role of the cardiac catheterization laboratory. Tex Heart Inst J 1988; 15:77–79.
4. Frank O: Zur Dynamik Dei Hertzmuskels. Z Biol 1895; 32:370–396.
5. Starling EH: The Linacre Lecture on the Law of the Heart. London, Longmans Green, 1918.
6. Dale HH, Richards AN: The vasodilator action of histamine and of some other substances. J Physiol 1918; 52:110–141.
7. Forssmann W: Die sondierung des rechten herzens. Klin Wochenschr 1929; 8:2085–2087.
8. Warren JV: Fifty years of invasive cardiology. Am J Med 1980; 69:10–12.
9. Forssmann W: Experiments on Myself: Memoirs of a Surgeon in Germany. New York, St. Martin's Press, 1974, pp 84–85.
10. Klein O: Determining human cardiac output (minute volume) using Fick's principle (extraction of mixed venous blood by cardiac catheterization). Med Wochenschr 1930; 77:1311–1312.
11. Cournand A, Ranges HA: Catheterization of the right auricle in man. Proc Soc Exp Biol Med 1941; 46:462–466.
12. Cournand A, Lauson HD, Bloodfield RA, et al: Recording of right heart pressures in man. Proc Soc Exp Biol Med 1944; 55:34–36.
13. Cournand A, Riley RL, Bradley SE, et al: Studies of the circulation in clinical shock. Surgery 1943; 13:964–966.
14. McMichael J, Sharpey-Schafer EP: Cardiac output in man by direct Fick method: Effects of posture, venous pressure change, atropine and adrenaline. Br Heart J 1944; 6:33–40.
15. Warren JV, Brannon ES: A method of obtaining blood samples directly from the hepatic vein in man. Proc Soc Exp Biol Med 1944; 55:144–146.
16. Warren JV, Brannon ES, Merrill AJ: A method of obtaining renal venous blood in unanesthetized persons with observations on the extraction of oxygen and sodium para amino hippurate. Science 1944; 100: 108–110.
17. Brannon ES, Weens HS, Warren JV: Atrial septal defect: Study of hemodynamics by the technique of right heart catheterization. Am J Med Sci 1945; 210: 480–491.
18. Bing RJ, VanDam LD, Gray FD: Physiological studies in congenital heart disease. Part I. Bull Johns Hopkins Hosp 1947; 80:107–120.
19. Dexter L, Haynes FW, Burwell CS, et al: Studies of congenital heart disease. Part I: Technique of venous catheterization as a diagnostic procedure. J Clin Invest 1947; 26:547–551.

20. Cournand A, Baldwin JS, Himmelstein A: Cardiac Catheterization in Congenital Heart Disease: A Clinical and Physiological Study in Infants and Children. New York, Commonwealth Fund, 1949.

21. Dexter L, Burwell CS, Haynes FW, Seibel RE: Oxygen content of pulmonary "capillary" blood in unanesthetized human beings. J Clin Invest 1946; 25:913.

22. Hellems HK, Haynes FW, Dexter L: Pulmonary "capillary" pressure in man. J Appl Physiol 1949; 2:24.

23. Zimmerman HA, Scott RW, Becker ND: Catheterization of the left side of the heart in man. Circulation 1950; 1:357.

24. Limon-Lason R, Bouchard A: El cateterismo intracardico—cateterizacion de las cavidades izquierdas en el hombre: Registro simultaneo de presion y electrocardiograma intracavetarios. Arch Inst Cardiol Mexico 1950; 21:271.

25. Seldinger SI: Catheter replacement of the needle in percutaneous arteriography: A new technique. Acta Radiol 1953; 39:368.

26. Ross J Jr: Catheterization of the left heart through the interatrial septum: A new technique in its experimental evaluation. Surg Forum 1958; 9:297.

27. Ross J Jr: Transseptal left heart catheterization: A new method of left atrial puncture. Ann Surg 1959; 149:395.

28. Ross J Jr, Braunwald E, Morrow AG: Transseptal left atrial puncture: A new method for the measurement of left atrial pressure in man. Am J Cardiol 1959; 3:653.

29. Cope C: Technique for transseptal catheterization of the left atrium: Preliminary report. J Thoracic Surg 1959; 37:482.

30. Robb GP, Steinberg I: Visualization of chambers of heart, pulmonary circulation, and great blood vessels in man: A practical method. Am J Roentgenol 1939; 41:1–17.

31. Arnulf G, Chacornac R: Communication to La Societe de Chirurgie de Lyon, November 14, 1957. In Arnulf G: L'arteriographie methodique des arteres coronaires grace a l'utilisation de l'acetyl-choline: Donnees experimentales et cliniques. Bull Acad Natl Med (Paris) 1958; 661:25–26.

32. Dotter Ct, Frische LH: Visualization of the coronary circulation by occlusion aortography: A practical method. Radiology 1958; 71:502–523.

33. Richards LS, Thal AP: Phasic dye injection control system for coronary arteriography in the human. Surg Gynecol Obstet 1958; 107:739.

34. Nordenstrom B: Contrast examination of the cardiovascular system during increased intrabronchial pressure. Acta Radiol Suppl 1960: 200:110.

35. Bilgutay AM, Gannon P, Sterns LP, et al: Coronary arteriography: New method under induced hypotension by pacing—experimental and clinical application. Arch Surg 1964; 89:899.

36. Sones FM Jr, Shirey EK, Proudfit WL, Westcott RN: Cine-coronary arteriography. Circulation 1959; 20:773.

37. Sones FM Jr, Shirey EK: Cine-coronary arteriography. Mod Concepts Cardiovasc Dis 1962; 31:735–738.

38. Bailey CP, May A, Lemmon WM: Survival after coronary endarterectomy in man. JAMA 1957; 164:641.

39. Longmire WP Jr, Cannon JA, Kattus AA: Direct-vision coronary endarterectomy for angina pectoris. N Engl J Med 1958; 259:993.

40. Johnson WD, Flemma RJ, Lepley D Jr, et al: Extended treatment of severe coronary artery disease: A total surgical approach. Ann Surg 1969; 170:460.

41. Favaloro RG, Effler DB, Groves LK: Severe segmental obstruction of the left main coronary artery and its divisions: Surgical treatment by the saphenous vein graft technic. J Thorac Cardiovasc Surg 1970; 60:469.

42. Green GE, Stertzer SH, Gordon RB, et al: Anastomosis of the internal mammary artery to the distal left anterior descending coronary artery. Circulation 1970: 41:79.

43. Garrett HE, Dennis EW, DeBakey ME: Aortocoronary bypass with saphenous vein grafts: Seven-year follow-up. JAMA 1973; 223:729.

44. Sabiston DC Jr: The coronary circulation. Johns Hopkins Med J 1974; 134:314.

45. Ricketts JH, Abrams HL: Percutaneous selective coronary cine arteriography. JAMA 1962; 181:620.

46. Judkins MP: Selective coronary arteriography: A percutaneous transfemoral technique. Radiology 1967: 89:815.

47. Amplatz K, Formanek G, Stranger P, Wilson W: Mechanics of selective coronary artery catheterization via the femoral approach. Radiology 1967; 89:1040.

48. Dodge HT, Tannenbaum HL: Left ventricular volume in normal man and alterations with disease [abstract]. Circulation 1956; 14:927.

49. Chapman CB, Baker O, Reynolds J, Bonte FJ: Use of biplane cinefluorography for measurement of ventricular volume. Circulation 1958; 18:1105.

50. Dodge HT, Sandler H, Ballew DW, Lord JD Jr: The use of biplane angiocardiography for the measurement of left ventricular volume in man. Am Heart J 1960; 60:762.

51. Arvidsson H: Angiocardiographic observations in mitral disease with special reference to volume variations in the left atrium. Acta Radiol Stockholm 1958; Suppl 158:111.

52. Arcilla RA, Tsai P, Thilenius O, et al: Angiographic method for volume estimation of right and left ventricles. Chest 1971; 60:446.

53. Brown BG, Bolson E, Frimer M, Dodge HT: Quantitative coronary arteriography: Estimation of dimensions, hemodynamic resistance, and atheroma mass of coronary artery lesions using the arteriogram and digital computation. Circulation 1977; 55:329.

54. Brensike JF, Levy RI, Kelsey SF, et al: Effects of therapy with cholestyramine on progression of coronary arteriosclerosis: Results of the NHLBI Type II Coronary Intervention Study. Circulation 1984; 69:313.

55. Blankenhorn DH, Nessim, SA, Johnson RL, et al: Beneficial effects of combined colestipol-niacin therapy on coronary atherosclerosis and coronary venous bypass grafts. JAMA 1987; 257:3233.

56. Buchwald H, Varco RL, Matts JP, et al: Effect of partial ileal bypass surgery on mortality and morbidity from coronary heart disease in patients with hypercholesterolemia. N Engl J Med 1990; 323:946.

57. Brown G, Albers JJ, Fisher LD, et al: Regression of coronary artery disease as a result of intensive lipid-lowering therapy in men with high levels of apolipoprotein B. N Engl J Med 1990; 323:1298.

58. Ornish D, Brown SE, Scherwitz LW, et al: Can lifestyle changes reverse coronary heart disease? Lancet 1990; 336:129.

59. Blankenhorn DH, Azen SP, Kramschb DM, et al: The Monitored Atherosclerosis Regression Study (MARS): Coronary angiographic changes with lovastatin therapy. Ann Intern Med 1993; 119:969.

60. Waters D, Higginson L, Gladstone P, et al: Effect of monotherapy with an HMG-CoA reductase inhibitor on the progression of coronary atherosclerosis as assessed by serial quantitative arteriography: The Canadian Coronary Atherosclerosis Intervention Trial. Circulation 1994; 89:959.

61. Serruys PW, Booman F, Troost GJ, et al: Computerized quantitative coronary angiography applied to percutaneous transluminal coronary angioplasty: Advantages

erted until the femoral vein is entered. The purported advantages of this technique are that only the anterior wall of the vessel is punctured, in contrast with the Seldinger technique, which results in a puncture of both the anterior and posterior vessel walls. On the other hand, the thin-walled needle has a cutting edge and probably inflicts more damage to the vessel wall. This is probably of no clinical relevance in puncturing the femoral vein but may be significant if this type of needle is used to puncture the femoral artery multiple times. My preference remains the standard Seldinger technique.

Although access to the right femoral vein was described earlier, the left femoral vein may be used equally well. One need only be aware of the normal landmarks and the fact that the femoral vein lies medial to the femoral artery and follow the same technique as described earlier. When accessing the left femoral vessels, the operator will find it more convenient to stand on the left side of the patient, palpate the femoral artery with the right hand, and use the left hand to insert the needle. Once the sheath is in place, all further manipulation is carried out from the right side of the patient and table.

Femoral Artery Access

Puncture of the right femoral artery is carried out via the more laterally placed skin nick described previously. The technique is essentially the same as that described for the femoral vein and in fact may be easier because the operator is palpating the femoral arterial pulse and delineating the course and direction of the artery. The Seldinger needle again is inserted at a 45-degree angle to the skin and directed cephalad in a direction in line with the two fingertips outlining the course of the femoral artery. Again, needle insertion is performed in a gentle but steady manner attempting to transfix the femoral artery in one quick motion. Once the artery is transfixed, it is common for transmitted pulsations to be felt (and seen) by the operator via the needle. At this point the obturator is removed and the needle is depressed to a 20- to 30-degree angle relative to the frontal plane and slowly withdrawn. No syringe is attached when an arterial puncture is performed; therefore, the needle flange can be held with both hands for better control. Once the tip of the cannula enters the arterial lumen, vigorous pulsatile arterial blood flow will be seen. The operator has a long (150-cm) 0.035- or 0.038-inch J-guide wire ready and immediately inserts it into the Seldinger cannula hub and advances it into the vessel. Again, if the arterial puncture has

been properly performed and there is no peripheral vascular obstructive disease present, the guide wire will pass easily and with no resistance for 15 to 20 cm. Fluoroscopy should then be employed and the J-guide wire advanced further up the iliac artery beyond the aortic bifurcation, where it will be seen to lie slightly to the left of the center of the patient's spine. Once this is achieved, the Seldinger cannula is removed, and firm pressure is exerted over the entry point of the wire to prevent backbleeding. The guide wire is wiped with a moistened gauze pad and a sheath-dilator assembly with a back-bleed valve and a side-arm is introduced into the femoral artery in the same manner as described earlier. The guide wire and dilator are then removed, and blood is aspirated via the side-arm and the sheath flushed well with heparinized saline. Systemic anticoagulation is usually carried out at this point; in most laboratories 3000 to 5000 U of heparin sodium is administered intravenously before the procedure is continued. The patient is then ready to have catheters introduced into both femoral vessels for the performance of right and left heart catheterization.

Considerable difficulty may be encountered in advancing the guide wire initially in elderly patients with significant peripheral vascular disease and arterial tortuosity. If any resistance is encountered in advancing the wire, all forward motion should cease. If the patient complains of discomfort, the possibility of subintimal dissection must be entertained. It is critical for the operator to understand that guide wires should not be forced, and any resistance encountered must be investigated. Often, when a standard J-guide wire will not progress up the iliac artery, use of specialized guide wires will allow access into the arterial system. The Terumo (Terumo Radifocus Guide Wire M, Terumo Corporation, Tokyo, Japan) wire with its reduced frictional characteristics has been a most helpful addition in traversing tortuous and diseased iliofemoral vessels, as have the Wholey (Wholey Hi Torque Floppy Guide Wire System, Advanced Cardiovascular Systems, Mountain View, CA) and the Bentson (Teflon covered) (Bentson Spring Guide Wire, Argon) wires. If, despite these attempts, the guide wire cannot be advanced beyond a certain point several centimeters from the cannula tip, or if the patient experiences any discomfort, the Seldinger cannula should be removed, the wire wiped with a moistened gauze pad and a 5-French dilator introduced very carefully over the wire to a point just proximal to the obstruction. The guide wire is then removed and the dilator is aspirated to ensure its location within the artery and carefully flushed. A small amount of contrast medium is then injected gently under fluoroscopic visualization; this will generally outline the artery and the reason for the difficulty in advancing the guide wire into the abdominal aorta. Once the anatomic problem is identified, additional measures can be taken to bypass the obstructed area. If a subintimal dissection is identified, it is best not to continue the procedure from this artery but move on to the left femoral or the right brachial artery. The patient should be observed carefully for extension of the dissection or arterial compromise, both potential but extremely uncommon sequelae of a wire-induced subintimal dissection.

Brachial Vessel Cutdown Approach

When it is decided that cardiac catheterization must be carried out by vascular access from an upper extremity, the right brachial artery and one of the right brachial veins are the preferred access sites. Right heart catheterization can be performed well from the left upper extremity (in fact, the first passage of a catheter into the right atrium by Werner Forssmann in 1929 was through a left antecubital vein), but left heart catheterization may be difficult in some patients because entry into the ascending aorta from the left subclavian artery can be particularly tortuous.

Patient preparation is as described for the transfemoral technique. However, in this instance the right antecubital fossa is widely shaved and the entire upper extremity from wrist to the axilla is surgically prepped with 1% povidone-iodine solution. The patient is asked to hold his or her arm in the air without touching the armboard, and once the prep has been completed, a knitted sterile stockinette is sterilely introduced over the patient's hand and rolled up the extremity. The sterile, sheathed arm is then laid on a sterile towel on the armboard in a supinated position, and additional sterile draping is carried out to cover the patient's entire body, including the right shoulder and right axilla. Particular care must be taken to sterilely drape the area between the armboard and the table adjacent to the patient's right axilla.

The operator then identifies by palpation the brachial artery and cuts a hole 3 inches in diameter in the stockinette overlying the antecubital fossa. Local analgesia is then induced. For brachial cases I prefer to use 2% lidocaine because of the longer duration of the analgesia. With a short 26-gauge needle, an intradermal

wheal is raised directly over the brachial artery pulse approximately 0.5 to 1 cm above the flexor crease. In sequence, using a 1 1/2-inch 22-gauge needle, the skin, subcutaneous tissues, deep fascia, and muscles are anesthetized approximately 3 cm on either side of the brachial artery pulse. Ideally, a median cubital vein or the median basilic vein will have been previously identified, and the skin and subcutaneous tissues overlying the veins will have been included in the area anesthetized. If the patient has no obvious median basilic vein, it is best to avoid the lateral cubital vein, which drains into the cephalic, because the latter enters the axillary vein at a sharp angle, making catheter manipulation difficult (Fig. 2–6). If no median cubital veins are noted, one of the two deep brachial venae comitantes that usually run on either side of the brachial artery (Fig. 2–7) can be used.

The next step is to perform a skin incision using a no. 15 surgical blade. The incision should be wide, at least 3 to 4 cm in length, transverse to the long axis of the extremity, and include the brachial pulse and the median cubital vein identified previously. Care must be taken to carry the incision only through the dermis so as not to inadvertently injure the

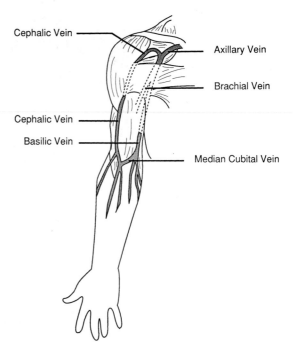

Figure 2–6. Schematic representation of superficial upper extremity veins. Note the acute angle the cephalic vein makes as it enters the axillary vein. The median cubital and median basilic veins provide a much more direct route to the axillary vein. (From Romanes GJ [ed]: Cunningham's Textbook of Anatomy, 12th ed. London, Oxford University Press, 1981; by permission of Oxford University Press.)

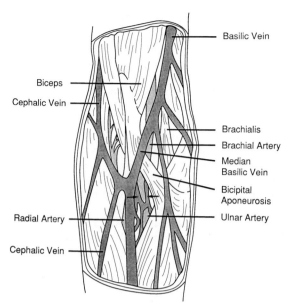

Basilic Vein

Biceps

Cephalic Vein

Brachialis

Brachial Artery

Median
Basilic Vein

Bicipital
Aponeurosis

Radial Artery

Ulnar Artery

Cephalic Vein

Figure 2–7. Schematic representation of the vascular anatomy of the antecubital fossa. Note that the brachial artery courses under the bicipital aponeurosis, which must be retracted to provide better access to the artery. Also note the two venae comitantes *(opposed arrows)* coursing on either side of the brachial artery. These small veins may be used for right heart access if the superficial veins are unsuitable. (From Romanes GJ [ed]: Cunningham's Textbook of Anatomy, 12th ed. London, Oxford University Press, 1981; by permission of Oxford University Press.)

superficial veins that lie in the areolar tissue directly below the dermis. Once the incision has been made, further dissection is carried out bluntly using a small curved mosquito hemostat. The plane of the dissection is always parallel to the long axis of the upper extremity to avoid injury to the nerves and vessels within the incision. Usually, one of the superficial median cubital veins is easily identifiable. Dissection is carried out on either side of the vein that is freed also from the underlying areolar tissue. Tags of 3-0 black silk are carried around the vein with the help of a curved hemostat and are anchored to the sterile drapes proximally and distally. Eventually, the distal tag is used to ligate the vein, but it is preferable to delay this until after the catheter has been inserted because ligation of the vein occasionally provokes venospasm. The tags may also be used to good advantage to retract the vein medially or laterally because it often overlies the brachial artery at this level (see Fig. 2–7). Blunt dissection is then carried into deeper layers; it is important to dissect one layer at a time, avoiding the development of a ''hole'' directly over the brachial artery. Dissection is continuously monitored by palpating the brachial artery pulse. Often at the level of the incision the brachial artery will be lying partially

beneath the bicipital aponeurosis (see Fig. 2–7), which needs to be retracted laterally to free up the vessel. Great care must be taken to avoid shearing off one of the small branches of the artery at this level (e.g., the inferior ulnar collateral). Also, care must be taken not to injure the median nerve, which usually lies just medial to the brachial artery at this level. Optimal position for the operator performing the cutdown is to stand between the patient's arm and chest because this position provides the best line of sight of the antecubital fossa structures. Once the layers overlying the brachial artery have been dissected away, the vessel is further freed on either side and inferiorly with the use of the curved mosquito clamp or a small right-angle vascular clamp. Before the brachial artery is brought to the surface of the incision, it should be cleared of surrounding fat and fascia for a distance of at least 2 cm. It is then brought to the surface with a curved hemostat or the earlier-mentioned right-angle vascular clamp and tagged proximally and distally with two lengths of silicone elastomer surgical tape, which are also anchored to the surrounding drapes with small hemostats.

If a superficial basilic or median cubital vein was not isolated initially, the operator searches for a vena comitans either medial or lateral to the brachial artery. These are very delicate venous structures, and great care must be taken not to injure them. A small plexus of veins that frequently joins the two venae comitantes and overlies the brachial artery must frequently be either retracted or ligated and divided before the artery can be totally freed.

It is then time to insert the catheters. The previously isolated vein is raised by the two black silk tags, and a small straight forceps is placed underneath it to form a ''bridge.'' The vein is then grasped with a small forceps *without teeth* and compressed in the vertical direction so as to increase its anteroposterior profile. While the vein is held gently with the forceps, a small venotomy is performed transversely using a no. 11 surgical blade with the cutting edge pointing up. The size of the venotomy should not exceed 25% to 33% of the overall anteroposterior diameter of the vessel. The previously selected catheter, which has been washed and flushed, can then be introduced into the vein with the help of a small plastic catheter introducer (Catheter Introducer, Becton Dickinson Co., Rutherford, NJ). The catheter is advanced quickly but gently 20 to 30 cm to allow its tip to reach the axillary or proximal subclavian vein as quickly as possible. Leaving the tip of the catheter in the more distal smaller vessel is another potential cause of venospasm. Similarly, it is important to keep all catheter surfaces moist, and it is my practice to place a moistened 4 × 4 gauze pad over the vein at all times. If resistance is encountered in advancing the catheter, forward motion stops, the catheter is withdrawn 3 to 4 cm and rotated, and another pass is attempted. Most commonly, resistance in advancing the catheter at this point is the result of the catheter tip entering a small side branch. Occasionally, especially in patients with multiple prior catheterizations or who have received multiple intravenous infusions, part of the superficial basilic system may be thrombosed, and this will account for inability to advance the catheter. In this instance this approach should be abandoned, and the catheter should be introduced via one of the deep brachial veins. The basilic vein is then ligated distally, and the proximal tag remains anchored to the sterile drapes with sufficient tension to prevent backbleeding.

Before the arterial catheter is introduced, the patient is systemically heparinized with 5000 U of heparin sodium intravenously; 3000 to 5000 U of heparin can be infused into the distal brachial artery through the arteriotomy. However, the systemic route is preferable, because it appears that the likelihood of vascular complications increases with the number of catheter introductions through the arteriotomy.

After the patient has been heparinized, the artery is double-wrapped with the elastomer surgical tape. The patient must be warned in advance that when arterial blood flow to the forearm is interrupted, a certain amount of numbness and discomfort of the forearm and hand must be expected. This is usually mild, and if the patient has been warned, it does not pose a major problem. The brachial artery is again grasped in a similar manner with a small forceps without teeth and compressed in a vertical direction to increase its anteroposterior profile. A very small transverse (perpendicular to the long axis of the vessel) arteriotomy is carried out again with a no. 11 surgical blade, the tip of which is introduced into the anterior wall with an upward cutting motion. A longitudinal arteriotomy is *not* advisable because it will often result in stenosis of the vessel when repaired. The correct arteriotomy is small and should never exceed 25% of the arterial diameter. It is important that the arteriotomy be performed in a "clean" manner, and one must avoid multiple stabbing attempts that may result in separation of the arterial wall layers and make repair at the end of the procedure more difficult. The previously selected left heart catheter, which has been wiped and flushed, is then inserted into

the artery via the arteriotomy. It is important at this point for an assistant to concomitantly relax the proximal elastomer tape, otherwise injury to the intima can be produced by the catheter tip pressing against the occluded lumen. Because intimal injury appears to be a major cause of vascular complications, the use of a closed-end catheter with a rounded smooth tip (e.g., NIH catheter) is preferable. Once the catheter tip has been advanced 10 to 15 cm, the proximal elastomer tape is again tightened and anchored with a hemostat to the sterile drape. The catheter is aspirated and copiously flushed with a heparinized flush solution and connected to the pressure measuring system with intermittent flushing capabilities. When properly performed with adequate local analgesia, brachial arterial and venous cutdown and catheterization of the right and left heart by this approach are virtually painless.

Percutaneous entry into the brachial artery is practiced by many operators and has been reported to be safe and efficacious.[8] However, catheter manipulation through a sheath with a hemostatic valve in the brachial artery can present difficulties. Furthermore, anatomic variability of the brachial artery bifurcation may increase the risk of complications.[9] For these reasons the brachial artery approach is most frequently by the cutdown technique described earlier.

Percutaneous Internal Jugular Vein Approach

As stated earlier, the internal jugular vein is used only occasionally in the catheterization laboratory, usually when the right heart chambers are markedly dilated or when it is anticipated that a monitoring pulmonary artery flotation catheter will be necessary during and after an interventional procedure. Access to the internal jugular vein is described briefly in this section. The right internal jugular vein should be used exclusively, because percutaneous access into the left internal jugular vein may be accompanied by injury to the thoracic duct that drains into it.

The patient is placed on the radiographic table and is asked to rotate his or her head to the left. The neck is extended with no pillow under the patient's head. If the patient is believed to be even mildly hypovolemic, access to the right internal jugular vein will be facilitated by elevating the legs on several pillows to increase venous return to the right side of the heart and distend the vein. The right side of the neck is prepped and sterilely draped. The operator must then identify the sternocleidomastoid triangle because the right internal jugular vein usually courses under the medial border of the clavicular head of the sternocleidomastoid muscle (Fig. 2–8). Once the apex of the sternocleidomastoid triangle is identified, lidocaine infiltration is carried out by the usual procedure. With the use of a 1 1/2-inch 22-gauge needle connected to the lidocaine-containing syringe, further infiltration and simultaneous exploration are carried out for the right internal jugular vein. The needle is inserted at the apex of the sternocleidomastoid triangle and directed posteriorly and caudally toward the patient's right nipple at an angle approximately 30 degrees relative to the plane of the skin. Care must be exercised to avoid injecting the carotid sheath because this may cause tamponade of the vein and create difficulty in its cannulation. The needle is advanced slowly while gentle suction is exerted with the syringe. If the vein cannot be located easily and venous collapse due to hypovolemia is suspected, having the patient perform a moderate Valsalva maneuver can be helpful by causing further distention of the internal jugular vein. Once the vein has been located, the needle is disconnected from the syringe and left in situ as a guide. The risk of air embolism is minimal, particularly if the patient's lower extremities are elevated to increase central venous pressure.

Using the exploring needle as a guide, a thin-walled 3-inch 18-gauge needle is then inserted parallel to the exploring needle and advanced until it enters the vein and free blood return is obtained on gentle suction. A 45-cm 0.035-inch J-guide wire is then introduced into the needle and should advance freely down the internal jugular vein into the superior vena cava (SVC). The exploring needle is removed, and a small skin incision is made at the point the thin-walled needle enters the skin using a no. 11 surgical blade that is held parallel and close to the needle and advanced 4 to 5 mm. In sequence, a small straight mosquito clamp is introduced parallel to the needle, and dissection is carried out for approximately 1 cm to separate the fibers of the platysma muscle. Once this is accomplished, while holding the wire in place, the thin-walled needle is removed, the guide wire is wiped with a moistened saline pad, and an 8-French sheath-dilator assembly is introduced into the vein over the guide wire in a standard fashion. As always, care must be taken to avoid wire buckling as the sheath-dilator assembly is advanced. Once the assembly is in the vein, the dilator and guide wire are removed, and aspiration is carried out via the side-arm to ascertain the proper positioning of the sheath, which is then flushed copiously and filled with heparinized saline and is then available for catheter introduction.

CATHETER SELECTION

Right Heart Catheters

A variety of catheters are available for right heart catheterization (Fig. 2–9). In my laboratory, the most commonly used catheter for entry into the right heart chambers is a balloon flotation (Swan-Ganz) catheter. This catheter can be used equally well for right heart catheterization when using the femoral, brachial, internal jugular, or subclavian vein approach. A variety of features have been added to the basic balloon flotation catheter since its introduction,[10] including a thermistor to measure cardiac output by the thermodilution method, additional infusion ports, and pacing electrodes. The advantages of a balloon-tipped catheter include ease of passage through right heart chambers of normal dimensions and its relatively atraumatic nature. This is particularly important when undertaking cardiac catheterization in a patient with complete left bundle branch block (LBBB). In this instance, if one uses a stiff catheter and it impinges on the septum, it is possible to induce complete right bundle branch block (RBBB).

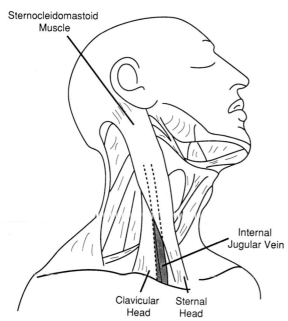

Figure 2–8. Anatomic relations of the right sternocleidomastoid triangle. Note the internal jugular vein coursing under the medial margin of the clavicular head of the sternocleidomastoid muscle.

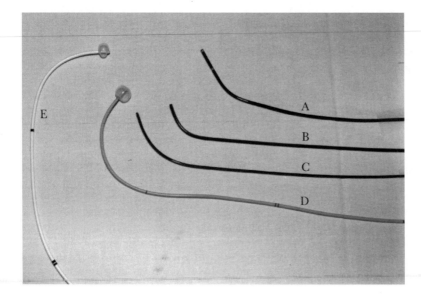

Figure 2–9. Right heart catheters. **A,** 7-French Zucker pacing catheter with end-hole and two distal side-holes. **B,** 7-French Cournand catheter, end-hole. **C,** 6-French NIH, closed-end, six-side-hole angiographic catheter. (**A** through **C** are manufactured by the United States Catheter and Instrument Corporation, Billerica, MA.) **D,** 7.5-French Swan-Ganz balloon-tipped, flow-directed catheter (Edwards Laboratories, Santa Ana, CA). **E,** 8-French Berman angiographic balloon catheter (Arrow International, Reading, PA). Note the eccentric balloon inflation.

The combination of RBBB and LBBB, of course, results in complete heart block and may require emergent pacing. This risk is minimized (but not eliminated) with the use of balloon-tipped catheters. The disadvantages of the Swan-Ganz catheter include its relative softness and lack of "body" that make rotation and manipulation through dilated cardiac chambers more difficult. This is particularly true when using this catheter from the femoral vein approach. If this problem is encountered, the catheter may be stiffened until it reaches the pulmonary artery by the introduction in its distal lumen of a 0.025-inch flexible, Teflon-covered guide wire. Although the frequency response of the pressure measuring lumen of balloon flotation catheters ranges from 10 to 20 Hz and is generally considered adequate for clinical pressure measurements, it may not provide a pulmonary artery wedge pressure waveform of sufficient fidelity to measure transmitral valve gradients in mitral stenosis. In this instance a stiff woven Dacron end-hole catheter may provide better fidelity pressure waveforms. Conversely, in patients with severe pulmonary vascular disease, better wedge pressure recordings are usually obtained with balloon flotation catheters than with straight end-hole catheters.

The second most commonly used right heart catheter in my laboratory is the woven Dacron end-hole Cournand catheter (United States Catheter and Instrument Corporation [USCI], Billerica, MA). This catheter is stiffer than the balloon flotation catheters and has good torque control and body. It must be actively manipulated through the right cardiac chambers under fluoroscopic visualization and usually provides good fidelity pulmonary artery wedge pressure recordings. It is used commonly from both femoral and brachial venous approaches and may also prove difficult to manipulate through markedly dilated right-sided cardiac chambers, in which case passage may be facilitated through the introduction of a 0.035-inch Teflon-coated J-guide wire with a large curve. Another woven Dacron catheter frequently used for right heart catheterization is the Goodale-Lubin catheter, which has an end-hole and two opposed side-holes near its tip. It provides good fidelity pressure recordings but may not give adequate wedge pressure waveforms in patients with pulmonary vascular disease. The Zucker catheter (USCI) is a modified Goodale-Lubin catheter with two electrodes, one at the tip and the second 1 cm proximal to the tip. It is used when the need for atrial or ventricular pacing can be anticipated. Platinum electrode catheters are used for the performance of hydrogen or ascorbate indicator-dilution studies.

Pulmonary and right ventricular angiography is usually performed via a standard closed-end, multiple side-hole NIH catheter (USCI). Other catheters that can be used to good advantage include a specially modified standard pigtail catheter with a large curve (USCI), the Berman angiographic balloon catheter (Arrow Incorporated, Reading, PA) or the Grollman pulmonary angiography catheter, which is a pigtail catheter with a reverse curve at its end to allow rapid insertion in the pulmonary artery.[11]

Left Heart Catheters

The most common catheter used for retrograde left heart catheterization via the femoral artery is the pigtail catheter in either the standard or angled configuration (USCI, Cordis, and others) (Fig. 2–10). This is an excellent catheter that usually traverses normal and mildly stenotic aortic valves easily, gives good fidelity pressure recordings, and can be used for left ventriculography and aortography as well. The angled pigtail catheter is preferred when catheterizing horizontally positioned hearts, in which cases a straight pigtail catheter, after traversing the aortic valve, will probably impinge on the inferior wall of the left ventricle and induce considerable ectopic activity. Other catheters used via the transfemoral approach include the Gensini end-hole and side-hole catheter and the multipurpose coronary arteriography catheter (Cordis and others). In my laboratory the first choice for retrograde left heart catheterization is always the pigtail catheter, and I resort to other catheters only when dealing with severe aortic stenosis that requires special catheter configurations to cross the aortic valve.

Retrograde left heart catheterization via the brachial approach is most commonly conducted with a standard NIH closed-end/multiple side-hole catheter (USCI). The NIH catheter with a standard mild curve is easy to manipulate across a normal aortic valve, and even ventricles with moderate aortic stenosis can most often be suc-

cessfully catheterized with this catheter. I have recently used to good advantage a closed-end pigtail catheter for left heart catheterization via the brachial approach. The stiff end of the 0.035-inch J-guide wire is introduced into this catheter until its tip is straightened and then the catheter is inserted into the brachial arteriotomy and advanced under fluoroscopic control into the proximal subclavian artery. The wire is then removed; the catheter is aspirated and flushed carefully, connected to the pressure measuring system, and then advanced via the innominate artery into the ascending aorta. In patients with severe tortuosity of the subclavian and innominate arteries, a standard open-end pigtail catheter is used via the brachial approach, allowing introduction of a J-guide wire to help manipulate the catheter across the tortuous brachiocephalic vessels. All catheters mentioned earlier provide good fidelity pressure recordings and can be used for left ventriculography and aortography.

In general 6-French and 7-French catheters are currently used for left heart catheterization. With the advent of "high-flow" catheters, these sizes provide more than adequate flow rates to perform high-quality left ventriculography and aortography. Catheters sized 5-French are available for use in smaller-sized patients and pro-

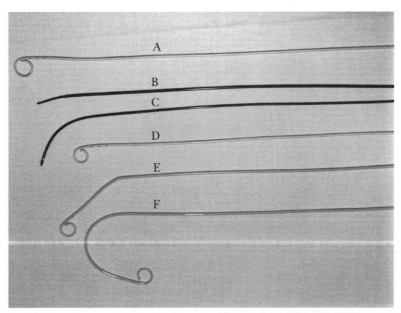

Figure 2–10. Left heart catheters. **A,** 7-French closed-end, six-side-hole pigtail catheter. **B,** 7-French Lehman left ventriculographic closed-end, four-side-hole catheter. **C,** 7-French NIH, closed-end, six-side-hole angiographic catheter. (Catheters **A** through **C** are introduced via open arteriotomy and are manufactured by the United States Catheter and Instrument Corporation [USCI], Billerica, MA.) **D,** 7-French standard open-end, side-hole pigtail catheter. **E,** 7-French 145-degree angulated pigtail catheter. (**D** and **E** are manufactured by Cordis Corporation, Miami, FL.) **F,** 7-French curved tight-radius, open-ended, eight-side-hole pigtail catheter (USCI). This catheter is useful for left ventriculography through a transseptal Mullins Sheath (see text) and for right ventriculography.

vide adequate pressure recording fidelity and adequate, but not ideal, opacification during left ventriculography and coronary arteriography. Additionally, 5-French catheters lack sufficient stiffness and torque control, making their manipulation in all but the most routine cases difficult. For these reasons, 5-French catheters are used infrequently in my laboratory.

TECHNIQUE OF RIGHT HEART CATHETERIZATION

Femoral Vein Approach

Once the sheath has been placed in a femoral vein as described earlier, the appropriately selected catheter is introduced. Right heart catheterization using a balloon flotation catheter is described first.

The appropriately selected and size-matched catheter to the previously inserted sheath is wiped with a wet sponge, the integrity of the balloon is pretested by inflation before insertion, and then the catheter is inserted in the sheath and advanced approximately 10 to 15 cm. At this point blood is aspirated and the catheter is flushed and connected to the pressure monitoring system. Under fluoroscopic visualization and continuous pressure monitoring, the catheter is advanced up the iliac vein into the IVC. Frequently, the catheter tip will enter small venous side branches, and

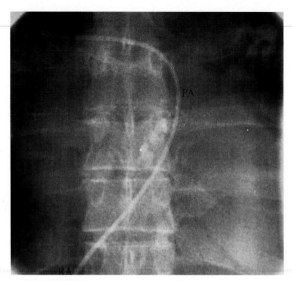

Figure 2–12. Flotation catheter wedged in a right upper lobe pulmonary artery branch. Note the almost-straight line that the catheter assumes (in the anteroposterior projection) from the low right atrium (RA) to the pulmonary artery (PA).

its progress is thereby arrested. This can be avoided by inflating the balloon to half its full capacity. Normally, the catheter passes easily up the IVC and into the right atrium. After pressure recordings are made, the balloon is inflated to its full volume and the catheter is rotated clockwise and advanced to cross the tricuspid valve (Fig. 2–11). After right ventricular pressure recordings are made, the catheter is rotated further clockwise and advanced into the right ventricular outflow tract. In general, if the catheter after crossing the tricuspid valve has been advanced deep into the right ventricular apex, it must be first pulled back until its tip is only 0.5 to 1 cm beyond the valve. At this point further clockwise rotation will move the tip anteriorly, and on fluoroscopic visualization the catheter appears to straighten in the anteroposterior projection. Simultaneously with the clockwise rotation, the catheter is advanced and in most instances passes easily through the right ventricular outflow tract into the main pulmonary artery (Fig. 2–12). Further advancement brings the tip of the catheter and balloon into either the left or right main pulmonary artery branches and then the "wedge" position. If the tricuspid valve annulus approximates the horizontal plane of the body, difficulty may be encountered crossing the tricuspid valve with the earlier described maneuver. In this situation, an alternate maneuver is to impinge the tip of the balloon flotation catheter along the lateral wall of the right atrium and create a

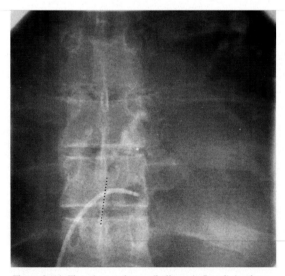

Figure 2–11. Flotation catheter (balloon inflated) in the right ventricular inflow tract. From this point the catheter is rotated clockwise and advanced to cross the right ventricular outflow tract and enter the pulmonary artery. The approximate plane of the tricuspid valve is indicated by the dotted line.

180-degree loop. The balloon-tipped catheter is then rotated clockwise and advanced and usually passes across the tricuspid valve fairly easily. In the presence of a severely enlarged right atrium, this maneuver may not suffice. In this instance, after the catheter tip has impinged on the lateral right atrial wall, it is further advanced until a complete 360-degree loop is formed with the catheter tip pointing medially toward the tricuspid valve, which can then be crossed. With this latter maneuver, as the catheter enters the right ventricle, its tip is pointing superiorly toward the right ventricular outflow tract, and one has only to continue advancing the catheter for the tip to enter the pulmonary artery. In markedly dilated hearts even this maneuver may be unsuccessful and the flotation catheter must be stiffened by inserting a 0.025-inch flexible guide wire in its distal lumen. Care must be exercised not to advance the wire beyond the tip of the catheter to prevent the induction of ectopy.

Occasionally, a catheter appears to be entering the right ventricle but may in fact be in an entirely different location. If an atrial septal defect (or patent foramen ovale) is present, the catheter may pass across the defect and into the left atrium and still superficially appear to be crossing the tricuspid valve (see Chapter 25). Catheter entry into the coronary sinus also mimics the catheter course across the tricuspid valve (Fig. 2–13, *right panel*). In both instances, the catheter tip is oriented posteriorly and as a result enters the coronary sinus or crosses the atrial septal defect. Occasionally, the catheter enters the coronary sinus and courses up into a left SVC draining into the coronary sinus (Fig. 2–13, *left panel*). Careful pressure monitoring may not be of help in localizing the catheter tip in these two situations, but aspiration of a small blood sample and determination of its hemoglobin oxygen saturation clearly indicate if the catheter tip is in the left atrium (saturation >95%), in the coronary sinus (saturation <45%), or in the right atrium (saturation 70% to 75%). Once the balloon catheter is in the wedge position, it is flushed gently with 0.5 to 1 mL of saline, and the pressure waveform is evaluated. Pulmonary artery wedge pressures are obtained both with the balloon inflated and with the balloon deflated, with the catheter in a more distal pulmonary artery radicle, where it functions as an ordinary end-hole catheter. With the balloon deflated and the catheter wedged into a distal pulmonary artery branch, the wedge position can be confirmed by the

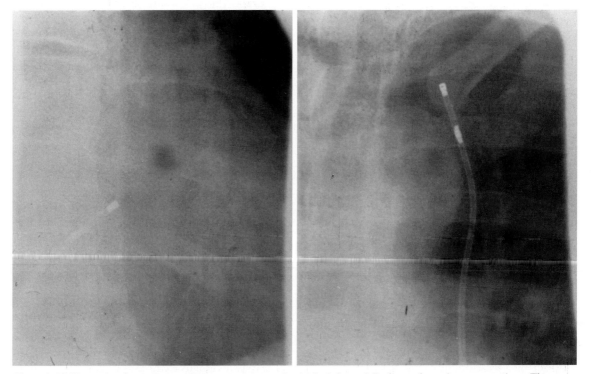

Figure 2–13. Unusual catheter passage (anteroposterior projection). *Left panel,* Zucker catheter in coronary sinus. The appearance is similar to the catheter passage across the tricuspid valve (in anteroposterior projection). *Right panel,* Catheter has been further advanced into a left superior vena cava draining into the coronary sinus. Confirmation of catheter tip location in the coronary sinus is easily made by withdrawal of a markedly desaturated blood sample (saturation <45%).

gentle aspiration of fully oxygenated blood from the pulmonary capillaries. This is not possible when the balloon is inflated and the catheter is wedged into a more proximal pulmonary arterial branch.

When a Cournand catheter is used for right heart catheterization via the femoral approach, catheter manipulation must be gentle because it is much stiffer than the balloon flotation catheter described earlier. Once the Cournand catheter tip is in the right atrium, clockwise rotation and slight advancement usually bring it across the tricuspid valve. Again, if the tricuspid annulus plane is fairly horizontal, the slight curve of the Cournand catheter will not allow the tip to advance across the valve but rather slide up and down the interatrial septum and get caught in the right atrial appendage. In this instance, the first maneuver is to increase the curvature of the Cournand catheter. This is easily accomplished by withdrawing the catheter in the upper part of the IVC and engaging its tip into a hepatic vein. The body of the catheter is then prolapsed into the right atrium, and the tip simultaneously disengages from the hepatic vein. The catheter is then in the right atrium with its end forming a 180-degree loop. The catheter is then rotated clockwise and withdrawn slightly. This maneuver should bring the tip across the tricuspid valve and into the body of the right ventricle. Before further advancement to the pulmonary artery is attempted, it is crucial to have the catheter tip free and not trapped in right ventricular trabeculae near the apex of the chamber. Therefore, the catheter is gently pulled back until the tip is seen to form an almost 90-degree angle with the body of the catheter on fluoroscopic visualization in the anteroposterior projection. Then, and only then, is the catheter further rotated clockwise and advanced into the right ventricular outflow tract and main pulmonary artery. Frequently, having the patient simultaneously take a deep breath aligns the right ventricular outflow tract optimally and facilitates passage of the catheter across it and into the main pulmonary artery.

Obtaining a pulmonary artery wedge pressure with the straight Cournand catheter involves simultaneously advancing the catheter into a distal pulmonary artery radicle while the patient takes a deep breath. In general, better wedge pressure tracings are obtained with the catheter tip in a distal pulmonary artery radicle of an upper or lower lobe away from the cardiac silhouette. Occasionally, having the patient cough at the end of the deep inspiration fixes the catheter in the wedged position. Gentle flushing with 0.5 to 1 mL of heparinized flush at this point often improves the quality of the wedge pressure tracing. It is important for the operator to recognize that vigorous or excessive flushing can cause vascular tone changes just distal to the catheter tip and produce spurious and unreliable wedge pressure waveforms.

Brachial Vein Approach

Catheterization of the right-sided cardiac chambers via the brachial vein is actually simpler and easier than via the femoral vein approach. The only potential difficulty encountered after insertion of a catheter in the median cubital vein is the possibility of venospasm. This happens more commonly in women and other patients with small veins. It is important to have the catheter meticulously cleaned and wiped free of any residue or foreign material that may increase the risk of venospasm. Additionally, it is important to pass the catheter as quickly as possible beyond the small veins and into the axillary or subclavian vein because the tip of a flow-directed catheter with its irregular balloon-tipped surface may contribute to the development of venospasm. It is useful to always maintain a moistened saline sponge over the brachial vein cutdown because introducing a dry catheter into the vein may also provoke local venospasm.

Once the balloon-tipped catheter is in the mid-right atrium, the balloon is inflated and the catheter is advanced and gently rotated counterclockwise. In most instances it then passes promptly across the tricuspid valve, and the curve of the catheter makes its tip point superiorly toward the right ventricular outflow tract and pulmonary artery. Once the catheter tip is in the pulmonary artery, the mechanics of obtaining a pulmonary artery wedge pressure are as described previously.

The procedure is somewhat different when using a Cournand or NIH catheter from the brachial vein approach. Once the catheter has entered the right atrium, it is rotated gently so that the tip points toward the lateral wall and is advanced further until the tip engages the lateral wall and a gentle loop forms resembling the letter J on fluoroscopic visualization. The catheter is then rotated counterclockwise. This disengages the tip from the lateral wall of the right atrium and points it anteriorly, thus avoiding the coronary sinus orifice. Further advancement causes the tip to jump across the tricuspid valve and enter the right ventricle. A few ventricular extrasystoles are a common occurrence at this point. Most often, as the catheter J-loop passes across the tricuspid valve, the tip continues pointing superiorly and therefore slight further advancement will cause the tip to enter the right ventricular outflow tract, cross the pulmonic valve, and enter the pulmonary artery (Fig. 2–14A). Having the patient take a deep breath while advancing the catheter across the right ventricle often facilitates catheter passage in this situation as well.

Right heart catheterization via a left antecubital vein is extremely easy. The natural curve of balloon flotation and Cournand catheters is such that the tip points toward the tricuspid valve when the catheter is in the mid-right atrium. Simple advancement usually brings the tip across the tricuspid valve and through the right ventricular outflow tract (Fig. 2–14B). In most instances it is unnecessary to form the aforementioned J-loop against the lateral right atrial wall when catheter access is via a left antecubital vein.

The operator must always keep in mind that woven Dacron catheters are stiff and may produce myocardial injury. Continuous pressure monitoring should be observed throughout the transit of the catheter across the right ventricle, and should at any time the pressure become damped, all further advance should stop because the catheter is most likely impinging against the right ventricular outflow tract and the potential for perforation exists.

Internal Jugular Vein Approach

Performing right heart catheterization via the right internal jugular vein is almost always ac-complished by the use of a balloon flotation catheter. When the sheath is properly positioned in the right internal jugular vein, the balloon flotation catheter that is introduced has almost a straight-line approach through the right atrium to the tricuspid valve. The balloon is inflated when the catheter is in the mid-right atrium and slight counterclockwise rotation orients the curved tip and balloon anteriorly, at which point it will almost always cross the tricuspid valve easily. Continued advancement then allows the flotation catheter to traverse the right ventricular outflow tract and enter the pulmonary artery. This procedure is usually so easy that it is commonly practiced without the help of fluoroscopic visualization at the bedside in critical care units. However, difficulty may be encountered even using this approach when massive right atrial dilation and severe tricuspid regurgitation are present. In this setting, stiffening the catheter with 0.025-inch guide wire as previously mentioned can be helpful, and fluoroscopic visualization may be essential.

TECHNIQUE OF RETROGRADE LEFT HEART CATHETERIZATION

Femoral Artery Approach

In my laboratory, the standard pigtail catheter is the most common catheter used for left heart catheterization via the femoral artery. The cath-

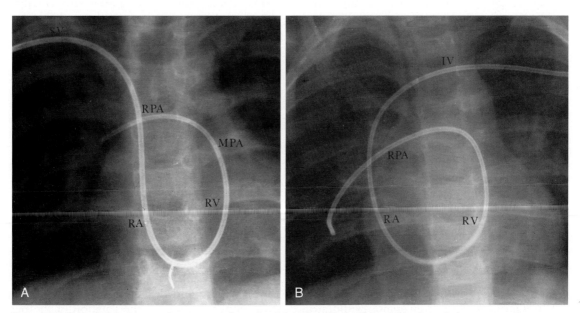

Figure 2–14. Typical right heart catheter course from the right *(A)* and left *(B)* brachial approach (anteroposterior projection). In *A* the catheter tip is in the right pulmonary artery. In *B* the catheter tip is wedged in a small branch of the right lower lobe pulmonary artery. SV, subclavian vein; RA, right atrium; RV, right ventricle; MPA, main pulmonary artery; RPA, right pulmonary artery; IV, innominate vein.

eter is flushed and wiped clean of any residue with a wet 4 × 4 gauze sponge. A 0.035 or 0.038-inch Teflon-coated J-guide wire is introduced into the pigtail catheter and advanced until the guide wire is just inside the catheter tip. The catheter is then grasped with the thumb and forefinger of the right hand, the pigtail is straightened, and the catheter tip is introduced into the prepositioned arterial sheath and advanced within the sheath until all the side-holes are beyond the hemostatic valve. The J-guide wire is then advanced beyond the catheter tip and under fluoroscopic visualization maneuvered beyond the aortic bifurcation to the descending thoracic aorta just above the level of the diaphragm. The wire is then held in this position and the pigtail catheter advanced gently over the wire until its tip also reaches the level of the diaphragm. The guide wire is removed, and the catheter is aspirated twice and flushed vigorously before it is connected to the pressure measuring system. Under continuous pressure monitoring and fluoroscopic visualization the pigtail catheter is then advanced gently up the descending thoracic aorta around the arch and into the ascending aorta. Occasionally, in patients with hypertension or severe aortic regurgitation, the brachiocephalic vessels are dilated and the pigtail catheter will enter the left carotid or the innominate artery. If this occurs, the catheter is withdrawn, slightly rotated so that the pigtail is pointing anteriorly and inferiorly, and readvanced. Occasionally, it may be necessary to reintroduce the guide wire for the pigtail catheter to be advanced around the arch. If the arch proves particularly difficult to traverse, visualizing the guide wire–catheter passage at a 60-degree left anterior oblique projection can be helpful. Once the catheter is in the ascending aorta, a baseline pressure recording is made of central aortic pressure. It is then time to cross the aortic valve retrogradely. Usually, I prefer to conduct this maneuver with fluoroscopic visualization at a 30-degree right anterior oblique projection. The catheter is rotated so that its pigtail is pointing at 2 o'clock and the catheter is gently advanced against the aortic cusps. Often, the catheter passes directly across the aortic valve and into the left ventricle. If this does not happen, several attempts are made with different pigtail orientation. If the valve still cannot be crossed, the pigtail is advanced against the left coronary sinus sufficiently to form a secondary loop (Fig. 2–15). The catheter is then gently withdrawn, and as the secondary loop traverses the aortic cusps the pigtail will fall across the valve into the left ventricle. Changing orientation of the

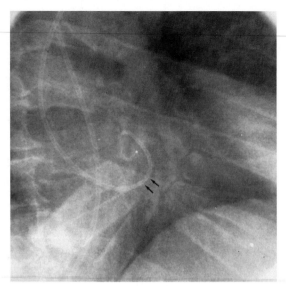

Figure 2–15. Pigtail catheter with secondary loop *(arrows)* in the aortic root. This is a helpful maneuver to cross the aortic valve (see text) (30-degree right anterior oblique projection).

heart and aortic cusps by having the patient take a deep breath and hold it in often proves to be of assistance.

If the patient has severe aortic stenosis, it is almost impossible to cross the aortic valve with a standard pigtail catheter. In this situation, I employ a modification of the technique described by Laskey and coworkers[12]: A straight 0.035-inch Teflon-coated guide wire is introduced into the pigtail; after the catheter has been withdrawn 4 to 5 cm above the aortic cusps, the soft tip of the guide wire is extended beyond the pigtail (which is uncoiled) and advanced to the level of the aortic valve. The orientation of the wire can be controlled by the length it is allowed to protrude from the tip of the catheter. If the pigtail catheter is high up in the ascending aorta, the advancing wire will have a more perpendicular course and be oriented toward the right coronary sinus. Conversely, if the pigtail is only 2 to 3 cm above the aortic cusps, the protruding guide wire will have a more horizontal course and point more toward the left coronary sinus. It is preferable to hold the pigtail catheter fixed and advance the guide wire independently. Care must be exercised not to advance the guide wire into a coronary artery orifice, because the potential for intimal injury and dissection exists. With each pass, minor changes in the rotation of the pigtail catheter and length of wire protruding are introduced so that the entire aortic cusp plane can be explored. With this technique, even severely stenotic aortic valves can be crossed successfully most of the time. In calcified aortic valves, the orifice can often be seen on fluoroscopy and the guide wire aimed accordingly. The operator should remember that despite systemic heparinization, guide wires are thrombogenic. Therefore, the maximum period allowed for catheter-wire manipulation is 9 minutes. Every 3 minutes the wire is removed from the catheter; it is then wiped and cleaned with a heparinized saline sponge and the catheter is vigorously doubly aspirated and flushed before reintroduction of the guide wire. If after two 3-minute sessions the aortic valve has not been crossed, it is my practice to resort to a different catheter. Although specially configured catheters have been devised for crossing severely stenotic valves,[13, 14] they are usually unnecessary. In patients with a very small aortic root, a right coronary Judkins catheter provides the needed guide wire orientation to cross the aortic valve. Conversely, in a markedly dilated root with the initial portion of the ascending aorta being almost horizontal and the plane of the aortic annulus therefore being more vertical than normally, I have found a no. 1 or 2 Amplatz left coronary catheter helpful. With this catheter positioned close to the plane of the aortic cusps, the guide wire assumes a horizontal course and allows exploration of the aortic valve plane to better advantage.

Once the guide wire has crossed the aortic valve, care must be taken to avoid impaling it on ventricular trabeculae. The operator must hold the wire steady and gently advance the guiding catheter (pigtail or other) over it until it crosses the stenotic aortic valve (Fig. 2–16). One must make certain that the wire is free in the left ventricular cavity before advancing the pigtail or other guiding catheter over it because instances of intramyocardial insertion of the catheter have been recorded with this technique. Once the pigtail catheter is in the left ventricle, the wire is removed and the catheter is doubly aspirated, flushed vigorously, and again connected to the pressure measuring system for the recording of pressures and subsequent performance of ventriculography. As previously stated, in horizontally positioned hearts an angled pigtail may be preferable to a standard straight catheter. If the valve is crossed with a Judkins or Amplatz catheter, once pressure recordings have been made, it is my practice to replace this catheter with a pigtail to perform angiographic studies. This is accomplished with a 260-cm, 0.035-inch, J-tip exchange guide wire that is positioned in the left ventricle through the original catheter. The exchange process entails the slow withdrawal of the original catheter from the ventricle while simultaneously advancing the exchange wire to maintain its position. This process is carried out under continuous fluoroscopic visualization of the J-tip to preclude it being pulled inadvertently back across the aortic valve (which would necessitate repetition of the entire process). Once the original guiding catheter is out of the body, the wire is again wiped clean with a moistened gauze pad, and a pigtail catheter is threaded over it and advanced up the aorta. It is necessary to hold the wire position fixed so it will not advance along with the catheter and coil in the left ventricle, causing ventricular ectopy or perforation. Care must be exercised when the pigtail begins to cross the stenotic aortic valve because it is possible for the exchange wire to be prolapsed backward into the aortic root. This can be avoided by continuous fluoroscopic visualization and continuous adjustment of the guide wire position. A 0.038-inch wire that has more body may be used to better advantage in patients with severe calcific aortic stenosis with markedly distorted valve architecture.

Brachial Artery Approach

Retrograde left heart catheterization via the right brachial artery approach is usually accomplished with an NIH closed-end catheter. The catheter is introduced into the brachial artery, as previously described, doubly aspirated and flushed vigorously, and then connected to the pressure measuring system. It is advanced carefully through the brachial and axillary arteries until it enters the subclavian artery, at which point it is in the fluoroscopic field and can be visualized. Any resistance met on catheter advancement should cause the operator to stop, withdraw the catheter 3 or 4 cm, rotate it, and readvance it gently. Once the subclavian artery has been reached, the catheter tip is rotated caudad and gently advanced. Unless there is a great deal of brachiocephalic vessel tortuosity, the catheter will pass easily into the innominate artery and then into the ascending aorta. However, especially in older patients with atherosclerotic and tortuous vessels, a good deal of difficulty may be encountered in entering the ascending aorta. Maneuvers that help traverse the subclavian and innominate arteries include having the patient take a deep breath, shrug his or her right shoulder, turn the head to the extreme left and extend the neck by removing the pillow, as well as extending the right arm by manual traction on the wrist while at the

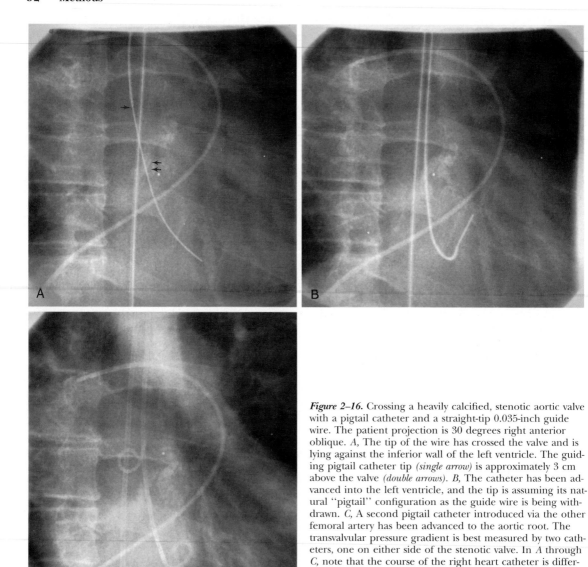

Figure 2–16. Crossing a heavily calcified, stenotic aortic valve with a pigtail catheter and a straight-tip 0.035-inch guide wire. The patient projection is 30 degrees right anterior oblique. *A,* The tip of the wire has crossed the valve and is lying against the inferior wall of the left ventricle. The guiding pigtail catheter tip *(single arrow)* is approximately 3 cm above the valve *(double arrows). B,* The catheter has been advanced into the left ventricle, and the tip is assuming its natural "pigtail" configuration as the guide wire is being withdrawn. *C,* A second pigtail catheter introduced via the other femoral artery has been advanced to the aortic root. The transvalvular pressure gradient is best measured by two catheters, one on either side of the stenotic valve. In *A* through *C,* note that the course of the right heart catheter is different than in Figure 2–14 because of the different projection (right anterior oblique versus anteroposterior).

same time exerting cephalad pressure in the right axilla. If the catheter still cannot pass down the innominate into the ascending aorta at this point, I prefer to exchange the closed-end catheter for an open-end pigtail, which is then advanced over a standard J-guide wire. This maneuver is almost always successful and obviates the risk of plaque disruption and vascular injury by more vigorously manipulating and prolapsing the closed-end catheter, as other operators have suggested.

Once the catheter is in the ascending aorta and the central aortic pressure has been recorded, it is time to cross the aortic valve retrogradely. It can be first attempted to advance the NIH catheter directly into the left ventricle by moving the catheter back and forth while at the

same time rotating it through a 360-degree arc to explore the entire plane of the aortic cusps. If this is unsuccessful, the catheter is looped in one of the aortic sinuses and prolapsed across the aortic valve into the left ventricle. Usually a stable position can be found in the left ventricle when the NIH catheter tip is parallel to the long axis of the ventricle. In some instances, however, this position generates significant ventricular ectopy. An alternative catheter position is to curve the NIH catheter posteriorly just in front of the mitral valve. In this position ventricular ectopy is usually minimized and pressure measurements can be accomplished. However, this position is not ideal for optimal opacification of the left ventricle during angiographic studies. If a closed-end pigtail catheter is used via the brachial artery approach, traversing the aortic valve is accomplished in a similar manner as described in the previous section. In patients with critical aortic stenosis, studied via the brachial artery, my first catheter choice continues to be the 7-French NIH catheter. If I am unsuccessful crossing the aortic valve with this catheter, I will use instead a Lehman ventriculography catheter or, preferably, a standard open-end pigtail catheter with the straight guide wire technique described earlier. Some operators, in this setting, prefer to use a Sones coronary arteriography catheter, which, once across the aortic valve, can be used for ventriculography as well as for pressure measurement. Because angiography with a Sones catheter tends not to be entirely satisfactory because of induction of ventricular extrasystoles, I use it rarely for this purpose.

The left atrium is the least accessible chamber by the retrograde technique. Shirey and Sones[15] reported a retrograde method of left atrial catheterization in 1966 using a specially designed, long-taper side-hole catheter resembling the Sones coronary arteriography catheter. This catheter is prolapsed across the aortic valve so that its tip faces posteriorly on entry into the left ventricle. On pulling back on the redundant catheter loop, the tip frequently crosses the mitral valve and enters the left atrium. Other investigators have described retrograde left atrial catheterization by the transfemoral approach using either specially preformed catheters[16, 17] or a standard pigtail catheter.[18] All of these techniques are cumbersome, so that when direct left atrial catheterization is required, the transseptal technique is commonly used as described in the following section.

TRANSSEPTAL LEFT HEART CATHETERIZATION

Transseptal left heart catheterization was introduced almost simultaneously by Ross[19] and Cope[20] in 1959. Brockenbrough[21] modified the original Ross transseptal needle in 1960 by engrafting a 21-gauge needle tip on the 18-gauge needle body. As a result, this procedure became the preferred method of left heart catheterization in the early to mid-1960s. The frequency of transseptal catheterization declined subsequently because of complications associated with the procedure and general acceptance of evidence indicating that the mean pulmonary artery wedge pressure and mean left atrial pressure are similar.[22, 23] Recently, renewed interest

in this technique[4, 5] has been stimulated by several factors: the increasing number of patients with a mechanical aortic prosthesis who require cardiac catheterization, the development of techniques for balloon mitral valvuloplasty (see Chapter 32), recognition that in the presence of severe pulmonary vascular disease the pulmonary artery wedge pressure may be inaccurate, and improvements in the transseptal equipment and laboratory imaging systems that have increased the safety of transseptal catheterization. An example of major differences between pulmonary artery wedge pressure and direct left atrial pressure obtained transseptally can be seen in Figure 2–17. In this section I describe briefly the essentials of the transseptal technique but must caution the reader that this procedure should be undertaken only after thorough and extensive training has been accomplished. Because of the risk of hemorrhagic complications, transseptal catheterization is never performed on anticoagulated patients.

Before the procedure is begun, the transseptal equipment is assembled and tested. Two different catheter systems are available: the conventional Brockenbrough needle and catheter and the newer Mullins sheath-dilator assembly.[24] With both catheter systems, interatrial septal puncture is carried with the Brockenbrough modification of the Ross needle. This is a 70-cm 18-gauge curved needle that tapers to 21-gauge at its tip (Fig. 2–18). The procedure using the conventional Brockenbrough system is described in the following paragraphs.

Before any vascular access procedure is undertaken, the relative length of the needle and catheter system to be used is ascertained. The Brockenbrough catheter is flushed and the needle is inserted all the way to the catheter tip. Passage of the needle in the catheter ex vivo is facilitated by uncoiling the tight distal catheter curve. Once it is determined that the needle tip is 1 to 2 mm inside the catheter tip, the distance between the proximal end of the catheter and the needle flange is *accurately* determined. Some operators use a small ruler to determine the precise distance between these two points, but it is easier to place the right hand middle and index fingers on the proximal portion of the needle against the needle flange and assess at which point the proximal end of the catheter is touching the index finger. This is carefully committed to memory before proceeding with vascular access.

Initially, a pigtail catheter is introduced percutaneously into the right femoral artery as previously described. The catheter is positioned just above the aortic bifurcation and flushed vigor-

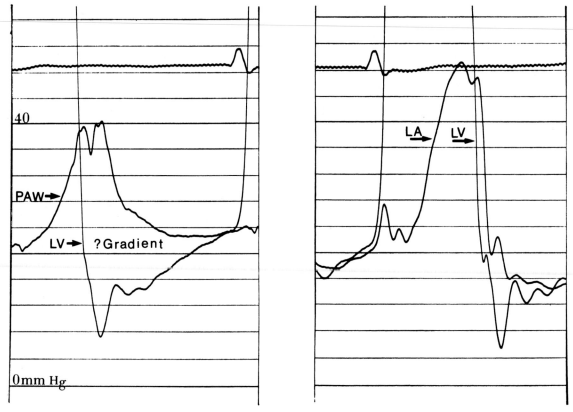

Figure 2–17. Example of the usefulness of transseptal measurement of left atrial pressure. In this patient with an 8-year-old mitral bioprosthesis, the simultaneous pulmonary artery wedge (PAW) and left ventricular (LV) pressures *(left panel)* suggested a moderate transprosthetic pressure gradient of potential importance in association with low cardiac output. The transseptally measured left atrial (LA) pressure *(right panel)* recorded simultaneously with LV pressure shows clearly the absence of prosthetic valve stenosis. Spurious wedge pressure was probably the result of severe pulmonary vascular disease.

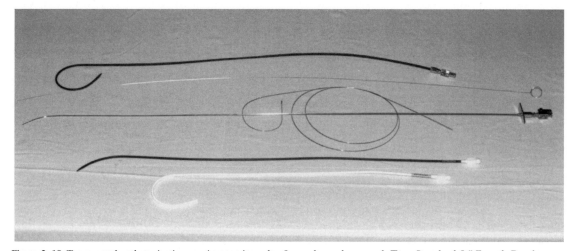

Figure 2–18. Transseptal catheterization equipment in order from above downward. **Top,** Standard 8.5-French Brockenbrough catheter. **Second from top,** Bing stylet, usually inserted in the transseptal needle as it is advanced up the Brockenbrough catheter. **Third from top,** Brockenbrough transseptal needle, 18-gauge with 21-gauge tip. **Fourth from top,** Catheter tip occluder (coiled) used to increase curvature of a Brockenbrough catheter and facilitate passage through the mitral valve. **Bottom,** Mullins dilator and curved sheath assembly, which may be used instead of the Brockenbrough catheter (see text).

ously and left there to provide arterial pressure monitoring. The patient is *not* anticoagulated at this point; therefore, the pigtail catheter must be either manually flushed every 2 to 3 minutes or be connected to an automatic pressure flush system.

The right femoral vein is entered percutaneously and a 0.035-inch J-guide wire introduced and advanced under fluoroscopic visualization through the IVC and right atrium into the lower SVC. The left femoral vein is never used for transseptal catheterization because of the angulated course of the left iliac vein as it joins the IVC. The skin entry point is dilated with an 8-French dilator, and the Brockenbrough catheter is introduced over the wire and advanced gently up the venous system until its tip lies in the SVC. This catheter is fairly stiff and should be advanced gently, particularly as it courses over the pelvic brim. Once the catheter tip has reached the SVC, the guide wire is removed and the catheter aspirated and flushed vigorously. The Brockenbrough needle is then introduced into the open end of the catheter with the Bing stylet within it. It is gently advanced and must be allowed to rotate freely as it courses through the skin and subcutaneous tissues and especially over the pelvic brim, at which point the patient may complain of slight discomfort. As the needle tip approaches the end of the catheter (gauged by means of the previously made measurements), the Bing stylet is removed and the tip of the needle brought to within 2 mm of the catheter tip. The needle hub is then connected to the pressure manifold with a short length of pressure tubing and flushed vigorously. SVC pressure is obtained through the needle and recorded. At this point the needle tip as indicated by the direction of the needle flange is usually oriented straight up (anteriorly) if the patient is lying perfectly flat.

Under continuous fluoroscopic visualization and pressure monitoring, both needle and catheter are withdrawn slowly, being held with both hands in a constant relationship. The right hand is firmly controlling the direction indicator of the needle flange, and during withdrawal from the SVC the direction indicator is slowly rotated clockwise so that it points posteromedially approximately 60 degrees from the horizontal plane. Always maintaining a constant relationship between the needle and catheter and making absolutely certain that the needle tip does not protrude beyond the catheter tip, the operator makes a continuous, slow withdrawal caudally, causing the catheter tip to go over two small "humps." The first is the junction of the SVC and right atrium, and the second is the

bulge of the non-coronary sinus of the aortic root. As the catheter tip moves over this second bulge, it moves slightly toward the patient's left and overlies the vertebral column. Further withdrawal caudally produces an additional movement medially as the catheter tip falls into the fossa ovalis. If the foramen is patent, the catheter may cross directly into the left atrium at this point—this is ascertained by a sudden change in the atrial pressure waveform. In my experience, this happens infrequently.

At this point puncture of the interatrial septum is first considered. However, before proceeding, some operators recommend moving the image intensifier into the right anterior oblique position to confirm that the transseptal needle tip is pointing posterior to the aortic root (identified by a pigtail catheter positioned just above the aortic valve). After flushing the needle carefully, the catheter is advanced slightly to engage the limbic upper margin of the fossa. With the posteromedial orientation of the needle-catheter assembly maintained as described earlier, the catheter is anchored firmly in position with the left hand and the needle is advanced beyond the tip of the catheter to puncture the interatrial septum. Some operators advise an abrupt forward motion of the needle tip to effect this puncture.[25] This is unnecessary, and it is preferable to advance the needle in a more measured manner to engage the septum. The right atrial pressure waveform at this point dampens into usually a straight line but should remain above zero. Further advancement of the needle produces puncture of the paper-thin interatrial septum in the fossa. A distinct "pop" is felt by the operator and immediately the typical left atrial pressure waveform is seen on the monitoring oscilloscopic screen. Entry into the left atrium can be confirmed either by withdrawal of oxygenated blood (hemoglobin oxygen saturation of 95% or higher) or by injection of a small amount of contrast medium through the needle.[26] Although some operators recommend the use of biplane fluoroscopy[4] to more accurately control the interatrial septal puncture, it is usually neither helpful nor necessary. Satisfied that the needle tip is then in the left atrium, one continues to advance the needle and Brockenbrough catheter together, at the same time rotating the tip slightly anteriorly to approximately 30 degrees from the horizontal plane. It is important that as the needle-catheter assembly is manipulated across the interatrial septum, the operator control its motion so that the advancing needle does not injure the opposite wall of the left atrium. Once the operator is satisfied that the catheter tip has crossed the interatrial septum, the needle is held stationary and the catheter advanced a short distance over the tip of the needle and then the needle is gently pulled back and removed. The catheter is connected directly to the pressure manifold (blood is aspirated to remove any clots that may have formed) and flushed vigorously twice. The patient should then be anticoagulated with 5000 U of heparin given intravenously. If the anatomy is not distorted, slight further advancement of the Brockenbrough catheter in the left atrium while imparting it a slight *counterclockwise* rotation will bring it to the level of the mitral valve annulus and across the valve into the left ventricular inflow tract (Fig. 2–19). Often, the catheter will have passed posteriorly into one of the pulmo-

nary veins. It must then be withdrawn 1 to 2 cm into the left atrium and readvanced. If the catheter curve is insufficient to point the tip inferiorly toward the mitral valve orifice, a curved-tip occluder can be inserted in the catheter so as to make the curve tighter and facilitate crossing the mitral valve.

Major problems encountered during transseptal catheterization include inadvertent puncture of the aortic root or the posterior free wall of the right atrium. If the catheter-needle assembly is firmly oriented posteromedially as described earlier, puncture of the aortic root is highly unlikely. Puncture of the posterior right atrial wall and even the aortic root with a 21-gauge needle tip is quite benign in nonanticoagulated patients. However, if this complication

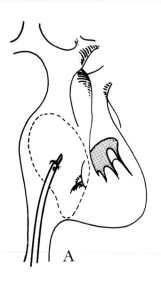

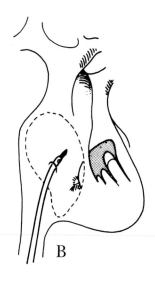

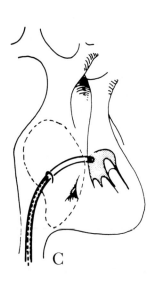

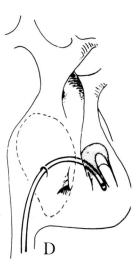

Figure 2–19. Schematic representation of transseptal left heart catheterization. *A,* Needle puncture of interatrial septum at the fossa ovalis. *B,* Catheter and needle are both advanced into the left atrium. *C,* The needle is withdrawn to the level of the interatrial septum, and the catheter is advanced further over the needle into the left atrium. *D,* The transseptal needle is removed, and the catheter is advanced across the mitral valve into the left ventricle.

is unrecognized and the 8.5-French Brocken-brough catheter is advanced either into the pericardium or the aortic root, major and even fatal complications may arise. One should understand that the most important element of this procedure is the proper identification and location of the fossa ovalis. If the fossa is not located on the first pass, the entire procedure must be repeated by removing the needle, reinserting the J-guide wire into the SVC, repositioning the Brockenbrough catheter there, and then repeating the entire process. Under no circumstances should the operator attempt to reposition the catheter-needle assembly in the SVC or advance it in any way. Perforations of the free right atrial wall, right atrial appendage, and coronary sinus may occur during such improper manipulations. Although it is possible to perform a transseptal puncture across the muscular interatrial septum in areas other than the fossa ovalis, this is much harder and catheter manipulation in the left atrium becomes difficult. Additionally, puncture of the interatrial septum in a nonstandard location increases the risk of complications such as coronary sinus perforation and should be avoided in all circumstances.

Additional complications have been reported in the left atrium with laceration of the left atrial appendage or the posterior left atrial wall if the catheter-needle assembly is vigorously advanced across the interatrial septum in an uncontrolled fashion. In general, locating the fossa ovalis becomes more difficult as atrial enlargement progresses. Massive right atrial dilation is one of the major contraindications to performing transseptal left heart catheterization. Marked skeletal deformities and scoliosis of the thoracic spine are other major contraindications.

Left ventriculography can be performed through the standard Brockenbrough catheter. It was originally advocated that angiography be performed only after a catheter-tip occluder was inserted to eliminate its end-hole and minimize the risk of left ventricular intramyocardial contrast media injection. However, this is usually unnecessary because left ventriculography can be performed safely via the Brockenbrough catheter injecting 36 to 42 mL of contrast medium at a rate of 10 to 12 mL/sec, with no complications. Care must be exercised, of course, to ascertain that the catheter tip is not impinging on the inferior left ventricular wall. Conversely, it is known that the catheter tip occluder may be ejected forcefully forward at the time of the pressure injection, causing myocardial damage in the process.

The Mullins transseptal sheath is another commonly used method of transseptal catheterization. It consists of a long curved femoral sheath and a long dilator that can be advanced into the left atrium over a Brockenbrough needle in a manner similar to the one described earlier. After removal of the needle and dilator, the long sheath allows insertion into the left atrium and left ventricle of any conventional catheter. The sharply curved pigtail catheter (USCI) may be helpful in performing high-quality left ventriculography when the Mullins sheath transseptal technique is used.

The advantages and disadvantages of the three major techniques for left heart catheterization are listed in Table 2–2.

TRANSTHORACIC LEFT VENTRICULAR APPROACH

Rarely, retrograde and transseptal left heart catheterization may not be possible when both mitral and aortic valve orifices are protected by mechanical prostheses. Other situations making the retrograde approach to left ventricular catheterization hazardous include the presence of critical aortic stenosis of a homograft, xenograft, or even native aortic valve. Transseptal left heart catheterization may be hazardous in the presence of massive right atrial dilation or thoracic skeletal deformities. In these situations, direct percutaneous transthoracic left ventricular puncture offers a reasonable alternative. This technique has been well established for the purpose of obtaining left ventricular pressure recordings[27] and performing left ventricular angiocardiography.[28] Fortunately, the need for this procedure arises infrequently. In a series of 20,000 cardiac catheterizations reported from the Brompton Hospital in London, left ventricular puncture was performed in only 112 procedures.[29]

The patient is studied in the usual premedicated postabsorptive state. Because bradycardia and hypotension (presumably vasovagal in origin) are reported with some degree of regularity,[30] premedication may include in this instance 1 mg of atropine sulfate intravenously just before the start of the procedure. As a precaution, 2 U of blood typed and crossmatched are available. If the patient is anticoagulated and must remain on anticoagulants, warfarin dosage must be adjusted before the procedure to an INR of not greater than 1.5. For patients anticoagulated with warfarin, 2 U of fresh frozen plasma are available.

The actual procedure is relatively simple.

Table 2–2. **The Three Common Techniques of Left Heart Catheterization**

Techniques	Advantages	Disadvantages
Percutaneous Transfemoral Retrograde Technique	No cutdown or vascular repair required Large femoral artery not susceptible to spasm Arterial access is usually quick and easy	Atherosclerotic obstructions encountered frequently Difficult access in morbidly obese patients Difficult hemostasis in patients with morbid obesity, wide pulse pressure, full anticoagulation Prolonged ($\geq$6–8 hr) bedrest required Late hematomas may develop
Retrograde Technique by Surgical Exposure of Brachial Artery	Atherosclerotic obstructions encountered rarely Better catheter control in difficult manipulations Better hemostasis in anticoagulated patients and in face of wide pulse pressure	Requires surgical cutdown and vascular repair Arteriospasm a common occurrence (especially in women) Vascular complications more common Tortuous brachiocephalic vessels impede catheter passage
Transseptal Technique	Left ventricular catheterization can be accomplished in the face of severe aortic stenosis or mechanical aortic valve prosthesis Direct left atrial pressure may be obtained in instances where "wedge" pressure is unobtainable or suspect Eliminates risk of catheter entrapment and false gradient recording in patients with hypertrophic obstructive cardiomyopathy	Specialized technique requires maintenance of higher skill level Increased morbidity Suspected left atrial thrombus and anticoagulation are absolute contraindications Scoliosis and other skeletal deformities are relative contraindications

With the patient in the supine position, the apical impulse on the chest wall is clearly identified. After surgical preparation of the area, the skin and subcutaneous tissues are infiltrated with 1% lidocaine and the needle is advanced to anesthetize the intercostal tissues, taking care to avoid the inferior margin of the rib. The infiltrating needle is advanced until the cardiac impulse is felt to anesthetize the pericardium.

If pressure recording alone is required, a 2-inch 19-gauge needle connected to the pressure transducer by a length of flexible tubing is used to puncture the chest wall. The needle is advanced toward the right shoulder oriented 20 to 30 degrees posteriorly so that it will enter the left ventricle at the apex in line with its long axis. Passage of the needle through the myocardium is heralded by two or three ectopic beats, and then a clear ventricular pressure tracing appears on the oscilloscope. The needle is held stationary at this point, and simultaneous left ventricular and aortic pressures are recorded through the ventricular needle and a previously introduced retrograde arterial catheter (Fig. 2–20).

If left ventricular angiography is required, a small skin incision is made overlying the apex beat and a 3-inch thin-walled 18-gauge needle is used. Once the needle has entered the left ventricular cavity as described earlier, the pressure tubing is disconnected and a J-tip 0.035-inch guide wire is inserted and advanced into the left ventricle. When the guide wire is seen to be in the left ventricular cavity, the needle is removed and a short 6-French Gensini catheter is inserted over the guide wire under fluoroscopic visualization into the left ventricular cavity. The catheter can be used both for pressure recording and the performance of left ventriculography.

On completion of the diagnostic studies, the catheter is removed and the patient monitored closely for several hours in the post anesthesia care unit. An echocardiogram is performed immediately on completion of the study and again several hours later to detect development of hemopericardium. A chest radiograph is also obtained to make certain that a pneumothorax was not induced. Complications reported with this procedure include cardiac tamponade (2%), pneumothorax (1%), pericardial effusion (4%), vasovagal reactions (6%), and pleuritic or pericardial pain (or both) (9%).

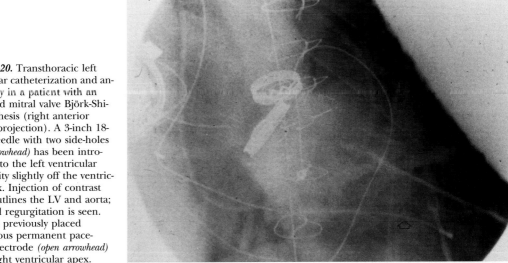

Figure 2–20. Transthoracic left ventricular catheterization and angiography in a patient with an aortic and mitral valve Björk-Shiley prosthesis (right anterior oblique projection). A 3-inch 18-gauge needle with two side-holes (*solid arrowhead*) has been introduced into the left ventricular (LV) cavity slightly off the ventricular apex. Injection of contrast media outlines the LV and aorta; no mitral regurgitation is seen. Note the previously placed transvenous permanent pacemaker electrode (*open arrowhead*) in the right ventricular apex.

TERMINATION OF PROCEDURE AND PATIENT AFTERCARE

At the conclusion of a transfemoral cardiac catheterization, it is generally advisable to reverse heparin anticoagulation with protamine sulfate. This is particularly true if the patient has received 5000 U of heparin at the onset of the procedure. Studies[30] suggest that after a 5000-U bolus of heparin, therapeutic anticoagulation (defined as activated partial thromboplastin time greater than 60 seconds) may last as long as 177 minutes. Lack of protamine reversal of the anticoagulant effect under these circumstances requires prolonged arterial compression time to induce hemostasis and increase the risk of hemorrhagic complications. Conversely, a 3000-U bolus of heparin at the onset of the catheterization procedure has been shown to provide therapeutic anticoagulation for only a maximum of 47 minutes. Therefore, patients undergoing brief-duration, uncomplicated left heart catheterization who receive 3000 U of heparin at the beginning of the procedure need not be given protamine sulfate.

At the conclusion of the study, the arterial catheter is removed and the pressure manifold is connected to the side-arm of the indwelling arterial sheath for continuous pressure monitoring during protamine administration. Protamine is administered slowly in doses of 1 to 2 mg per 200 U of heparin given (25 to 50 mg protamine sulfate for a 5000-U bolus of heparin). The rate of administration is no faster than 10 mg/min. Severe protamine reactions consisting of profound hypotension, dyspnea, and wheezing have been reported following rapid administration of this drug intravenously, especially in diabetic patients who have previously received NPH insulin.[31] Although other investigators have minimized this risk,[32] I prefer to use 3000 U of heparin in insulin-dependent diabetic patients and not reverse the anticoagulant with protamine.

After protamine has been administered and the patient has been monitored for an additional 2 to 3 minutes, three fingers of the left hand are placed on the course of the femoral artery beginning at the skin entry point and cephalad to the level of the inguinal ligament and moderate pressure is applied while the sheath is removed with the right hand. It is useful to allow a single spurt of arterial blood following removal of the sheath (hoping that thrombus material stripped from the surface of the sheath will be expelled) before increasing pressure with the three fingers of the left hand to initially obliterate the pulse and effect hemostasis. An assistant should check for the presence or absence of pedal pulses and pressure on the femoral artery should be adjusted accordingly. During the next 10 to 15 minutes, the pressure is reduced gradually and at 15 to 20 minutes pressure is released completely. The patient is observed an additional 2 to 5 minutes, and then the venous sheath is removed and pressure applied over the femoral vein to effect venous hemostasis as well. In the presence of marked obesity, effecting hemostasis by manual compression may be difficult and the application of a mechanical clamp (Compressar, Instromedix, Beaverton, OR) may be helpful. A trained nurse or technologist must always be in attendance after the clamp has been applied to ascertain that adequate hemostasis is provided and distal limb perfusion is not compromised.

Once hemostasis is accomplished either by manual or clamp pressure, the inguinal area is assessed for the development of a hematoma due to slow subcutaneous blood oozing. If no such evidence is found and the distal pulses are of good quality, a small bandage is applied to the puncture site and the patient is transferred to a stretcher while maintaining the extremity straight. The patient is kept at bedrest overnight and a 5-pound sandbag is placed over the puncture area for the first 6 hours, mainly as a reminder to avoid flexion of the lower extremity at the hip. After 6 hours, if there have been no complications, the patient is allowed to turn from side to side, again maintaining a straight right lower extremity. The patient's head and shoulders may be elevated 30 to 45 degrees as long as this is accomplished by the usual hospital bed control and without the patient exerting any effort.

With the advent of "come and go" procedures, many patients are discharged without the benefit of overnight observation in the hospital. In this situation, we use 6-French arterial catheters and observe the patient a minimum of 8 hours in a holding area. Before discharge, the inguinal area is inspected carefully for evidence of recurrent bleeding, formation of hematoma, or the presence of a bruit suggesting the development of an arteriovenous fistula. Distal limb perfusion is assessed and then the patient is asked to ambulate for 10 to 20 minutes slowly on the floor before being given clearance to go home. Ambulatory catheterization patients are advised to minimize activities for the next 24 hours and are given explicit instructions about what to do should late bleeding occur.

If the cardiac catheterization has been performed via the surgically exposed brachial artery and vein, repair of the arteriotomy and the brachial cutdown is required. In this setting, heparinization is not reversed; in fact, if the procedure has been a lengthy one, additional heparin is given, as mentioned next.

After the arterial catheter has been removed from the brachial artery, the proximal arterial tape is loosened sufficiently to allow one or two arterial blood spurts. The proximal arterial tape is retightened, and the distal tape is in sequence loosened. Retrograde flow from the distal brachial artery should be present via collaterals but is usually not pulsatile. If antegrade and retrograde flow are sluggish, a 3-French Fogarty embolectomy catheter (Shiley Laboratories, Irvine, CA) is used both proximally and distally to remove any thrombus that may have formed during the procedure. Three thousand units of heparin in 10 mL of normal saline are then introduced into the proximal brachial artery through a small, flexible polyethylene tube (2 1/2-inch, 18-gauge external PE cannula, Sureflow intravenous catheter, Terumo Corporation and others) and sequestered there either by tightening the elastomer tape or, preferably, applying a vascular bulldog clamp. Similarly, additional heparin is infused into the distal artery segment and a second bulldog clamp placed on the brachial artery distal to the arteriotomy. The use of vascular clamps to occlude the artery during repair is preferred to simply using traction on the elastomer tape because the latter procedure places considerable tension on the artery and makes repair more difficult. Arterial repair is carried out with the use of 6-0 Tevdek (Tevdek II, Deknatel Division, Queens Village, NY) or Prolene suture material. Various suture techniques are used by different operators. Two stay sutures are placed on either end of the arteriotomy, which is then closed by placing two or three small horizontal mattress sutures. Other operators have recommended a continuous running suture.[33] Another technique that may be advantageous in patients with very small brachial arteries is the subadventitial pursestring suture originally proposed for arterial catheterization of children.[34] The pursestring suture must be placed at the beginning of the procedure before the arteriotomy is performed.

After completion of the arterial repair, the vascular clamps are removed, and the closed arteriotomy is observed for leakage. The radial pulse is palpated. If no radial pulse is detectable, one should wait 2 or 3 minutes because often the brachial artery may be in spasm after repair. If after several minutes there is still no palpable radial pulse, the arteriotomy repair is taken down and the entire procedure repeated, including thorough exploration of the artery both proximally and distally with a Fogarty catheter. If repair again results in an unobtainable or markedly diminished radial pulse, prompt consultation from a vascular surgeon should be obtained while the patient is still on the catheterization table and the incision is open. If the brachial artery has been traumatized during the catheterization, it may require surgical débridement and vein patch angioplasty.[35]

Once the arteriotomy has been closed and the integrity of arterial circulation established, the venous catheter is removed and the vein ligated proximally by means of the proximal silk tag. The wound is then flushed with large quantities of sterile saline, and the edges are trimmed of any devitalized subcutaneous fatty tissue. The wound may be closed with the use of interrupted 3-0 silk vertical mattress sutures or by the use of a subcuticular stitch using an absorbable suture (e.g., 4-0 Dexon "S" with cutting needle, Davis Geck, Inc., Manati, PR), which avoids the subsequent need for suture removal. A dry sterile dressing is applied to the wound after it has been closed and the arm is immobilized on an armboard for the next 24 hours to prevent excessive motion and wound disruption.

Important elements in patient aftercare include the careful monitoring of vital signs for 6 to 12 hours after the procedure as well as of the pulse distal to the point of arterial entry (pedal and radial pulses for transfemoral and brachial catheterizations, respectively). The dressing covering the wound should be observed frequently for any evidence of bleeding, and the patient is usually restarted on all previous medications. In patients who require anticoagulation, heparin infusion may be restarted immediately after brachial artery repair or 4 hours after removal of the catheter from the femoral artery if no delayed bleeding has occurred. Patients receiving contrast medium usually undergo an osmotic diuresis, and fluid replacement is important to prevent hypovolemic hypotension. Patients are instructed to drink at least 1 quart of water or juice by dinnertime. The oral fluid intake is supplemented by a continuous intravenous infusion of 5% dextrose in half-normal saline given at a rate of 100 mL/hr. Obviously, in patients with elevated left ventricular filling pressures and impaired left ventricular function, the administration of fluids should be carefully monitored to prevent development of pulmonary edema.

In general, patients do not experience significant pain following transfemoral catheterization. Most of the discomfort after catheterization is related to low back pain if the patient is made to lie absolutely flat (which is unnecessary, as mentioned earlier). After brachial cutdown, however, a modest amount of discomfort can be expected, and an analgesic such as acetaminophen with codeine may be necessary. Patients are allowed to eat their usual diet and may get out of bed following a brachial cutdown within a couple of hours after the completion of the procedure.

All patients undergoing catheterization should be seen by the primary operator late that afternoon or early evening and be evaluated regarding their general condition as well as the status of the wound. This is also the appropriate time to discuss the findings of catheterization with the patient and his or her family and make initial recommendations about further therapy.

COMPLICATIONS OF CARDIAC CATHETERIZATION

As with any invasive procedure, complications can be expected to occur with cardiac catheterization and angiocardiography. Although uncommon, some complications can be serious and have devastating consequences. The invasive cardiologist must be always keenly aware of the possible development of complications and take every step available to avoid such events.

The first major multicenter report of complications was the result of the cooperative study on cardiac catheterization[36] that was published in 1968. The rate of serious complications reported in this study was 3.4%. The first report of the Registry of the Society for Cardiac Angiography and Interventions (SCA&I)[37] reviewed the incidence of complications in 53,581 patients studied in 66 laboratories over a 14-month period. Major complications were reported to occur in 1.82% of patients studied. A subsequent report of the SCA&I Registry reviewed complications occurring among an additional 222,553 patients undergoing selective coronary arteriography.[1] The rate of major complications in this report was similar at 1.74% of all patients. Major complications were death, myocardial infarction, cerebrovascular accident, major arrhythmias, vascular injury, hemorrhage, contrast medium reactions, and other miscellaneous complications. Patients with valvular heart disease undergoing cardiac catheterization and angiocardiography may be at higher risk for complications. The multicenter Veterans Administration Cooperative Study on valvular heart disease reported an incidence of complications in 6.9% of 1483 patients studied in 13 centers.[38] In addition to valvular disease, the following factors were associated with higher than average risk of death in the SCA&I Registry report: age greater than 60 years, New York Heart Association (NYHA) functional class IV, left main coronary disease, and ejection fraction less than 30%.[39] Gender and catheterization technique (brachial or femoral) did not affect mortality. Patients with severe disease of other organ systems (renal insufficiency, pulmonary insufficiency, insulin-dependent diabetes mellitus, and severe peripheral vascular disease) also appear to be at higher risk of death and other major complications. This section is a brief review of the various complications and the measures that minimize their occurrence.

Vascular Injury

In the recent report of the SCA&I Registry,[1] vascular complications were more common with the brachial approach than with the transfemoral approach (0.96% versus 0.22%). Conversely, hemorrhage was more common with the femoral approach by a factor of 10 (0.10% versus 0.01% for the brachial approach). In another study of 7333 patients undergoing percutaneous transfemoral left heart catheterization procedures, 73 (1%) patients required surgical repair of catheterization-related vascular complications. The overall incidence of vascular complications varied according to the type of procedure performed and was higher for interventional procedures than for simple diagnostic catheterization.[40] In this study 0.6% of patients undergoing diagnostic catheterization required surgical repair of the invaded artery as compared with 0.9% of patients undergoing percutaneous transluminal coronary angioplasty, 5.2% of patients undergoing transfemoral balloon valvuloplasty, and 11.5% of patients who had an intra-aortic balloon pump placement. The types of complications associated with transfemoral left heart catheterization included groin hematoma, false aneurysm, arteriovenous fistula, arterial dissection, and arterial perforation.[41] In a prospective study of 502 patients who underwent cardiac catheterization by the brachial approach, 5.8% were found to have postcatheterization complaints of pain, distal pallor, hypesthesia, or paresthesia; 19% were found to have a reduced wrist blood pressure index of less than 0.85; and 4.5% were found to have occlusion of the brachial artery by angiography.[42] Risk factors associated with a high incidence of brachial artery complications included previous catheterization and valvular disease.

The best way to avoid vascular complications is to pay meticulous attention to technique. As mentioned earlier, proper location of the femoral artery puncture is crucial for the prevention of femoral artery complications. Rapaport and associates[43] have postulated that when femoral artery puncture is carried out below the level of the femoral head, there is subsequent lack of bony support for adequate arterial compression after catheter removal, and this contributes to the development of pseudoaneurysms or arteriovenous fistulas or both. Altin and coworkers[44] confirmed Rapaport and associates' contention when they found that 10 of 11 femoral arterial pseudoaneurysms were located below the level of the femoral head. Dissections and perforations of the iliac artery are avoided by meticulous manipulation of guide wires and catheters as they advance to the abdominal aorta and by not advancing against resistance. Femoral hematomas can be prevented by maintenance of adequate pressure on the femoral artery until all bleeding has stopped. As mentioned previously, hemostasis is difficult in morbidly obese patients, and the brachial artery approach is preferable in these cases.

Brachial artery complications can be minimized again by meticulous attention to technique. A number of factors are important, including performance of a small *clean* arteriotomy, use of a Fogarty embolectomy catheter when antegrade or retrograde blood flow is impaired, and performance of a transverse arteriotomy so that when it is closed, the lumen of the artery will not be compromised.

Cardiac Complications

Cardiac complications can be grouped into three categories: (1) perforation of the heart, (2) myocardial infarction, and (3) induction of arrhythmias or conduction disturbances.

Cardiac perforation is an uncommon complication, although in the first cooperative study[36] 0.8% of patients sustained a perforation of the heart or great vessels. However, most of the patients reported in this study were those with valvular heart disease, and one third of the reported perforations were located in the right atrium and were incident to a transseptal left heart catheterization. Currently, the most common site of cardiac perforation is the right ventricular outflow tract of elderly patients who undergo right heart catheterization by means of a relatively stiff woven Dacron catheter (NIH or Cournand). The use of balloon flotation catheters has reduced (but not eliminated) the risk of cardiac chamber perforation both because of the innate softness of these catheters and because the inflated balloon presents a large surface area and distributes the pressure against the myocardium widely. Perforation of the left ventricle via the retrograde approach is rare and almost always is related to the improper manipulation of a stiff straight-tip guide wire. Cardiac tamponade is the major risk following perforation of a cardiac chamber in an anticoagulated patient. Interventional cardiologists must have the skills and be prepared to perform immediate pericardiocentesis should such a catastrophe be encountered. Right ventricular perforation is also the main complication of endomyocardial biopsy, which is discussed in Chapter 16.

Major arrhythmias requiring therapy occurred in 0.47% of patients reported in the SCA&I Registry.[1] Ventricular tachycardia and ventricular fibrillation were reported in the Coronary Artery Surgery Study (CASS) Registry to occur in 0.54% of all patients undergoing cardiac catheterization.[45]

Generally, supraventricular arrhythmias (atrial fibrillation or supraventricular tachycardia) are the result of injudicious catheter manipulation in the right or left atrium. When atrial fibrillation develops during right heart catheterization, the offending catheter must be pulled back to the vena cava immediately. Often, this is all that is required, and normal sinus rhythm returns within 2 or 3 minutes. If atrial fibrillation persists and ventricular response is rapid, pharmacologic therapy is indicated. Digoxin, 0.5 mg administered intravenously, is my initial drug of choice, but verapamil, adenosine, or β-blockers may be preferable in specific patient circumstances.

Ventricular arrhythmias are more likely to occur with catheter manipulation in the right or left ventricle or during coronary arteriography. The use of balloon flotation catheters for right heart catheterization does minimize the risk of inducing ventricular ectopy as the catheter passes through the right ventricle but does not eliminate it. This is particularly true in critically ill patients with ischemic heart disease. Patel and colleagues[46] reported a 52.3% incidence of cardiac arrhythmias during insertion of balloon flotation catheters in critically ill patients. During coronary arteriography, ventricular tachycardia and ventricular fibrillation may occur suddenly even in patients with no coronary artery disease. This occurrence can be reduced by injecting the minimal amount of contrast medium that produces adequate opacification of the coronary artery. Ventricular arrhythmias can also be minimized by the use of the newer nonionic contrast media that appear to have less direct myocardial depressant effect than the older ionic agents.[47] It is therefore my practice to use preferentially nonionic contrast media, especially in patients who are critically ill and demonstrate hemodynamic instability and propensity to ventricular arrhythmias.[48]

Marked sinus bradycardia, frequently accompanied by hypotension, is usually the result of so-called vasovagal reactions or sinus node hypoperfusion during coronary arteriography. Vasovagal reactions are common and are usually induced by pain or severe anxiety in poorly prepared and nonsedated patients. They are frequently heralded by a feeling of nausea that is followed by bradycardia and hypotension.

The presumed mechanism of these reactions is sudden peripheral vasodilation without the usual compensatory increase in cardiac output.[49] Vasovagal reactions can be treated promptly by cessation of whatever manipulation induced them to begin with, intravenous administration of 0.6 to 1.2 mg of atropine and, if necessary, elevation of the legs or administration of parenteral fluids. In general, prompt recognition and treatment result in rapid reversal of the bradycardia and hypotension. Occasionally, severe sinus bradycardia results from selective coronary arteriography, particularly of the right coronary artery. The expanding use of nonionic contrast media, however, has dramatically reduced the incidence of sinus slowing during coronary arteriographic procedures.

Conduction disturbances occur infrequently during diagnostic cardiac catheterization. Complete heart block was reported to occur in only 7 of the 12,367 procedures reported in the original cooperative study on cardiac catheterization.[36] When complete heart block occurs, it usually develops during right heart catheterization in patients with preexisting LBBB.[50, 51] The mechanism of complete heart block in this situation is transient trauma to the right bundle branch by the catheter as it traverses the right ventricle on its way to the pulmonary artery. The development of RBBB in a patient with preexisting LBBB leads to complete heart block and a variable period of asystole with resultant profound hypotension. The risk of RBBB development in the catheterization laboratory has been reported to be between 3% and 4%.[52] In at least one study the incidence of RBBB has been reported to be much higher (23%) in patients with preexisting conduction disturbances, suggesting that a diseased conduction system may be more vulnerable to catheter-induced trauma.[52] Because of the risk of complete heart block, when one undertakes right heart catheterization in a patient with preexisting LBBB, it is prudent to have standby pacing capabilities available. If the plan is to use a woven Dacron catheter for right heart catheterization, I commonly employ a 7-French Zucker catheter. This catheter can be used both for recording of pressures and right ventricular pacing should it become necessary. The use of a balloon flotation catheter for right heart catheterization has markedly reduced the incidence of transient RBBB during right heart catheterization. The reported 3% incidence of RBBB during right heart catheterization by balloon flotation catheters[53] is high and probably reflects the fact that most recent studies of right heart catheterization complications have been derived from bedside catheterization of critically ill patients in intensive care units without the benefit of fluoroscopic guidance. For these reasons, prophylactic transvenous pacing is not routinely used even in patients with LBBB undergoing right heart catheterization with a balloon flotation catheter. Great care must be taken not to induce right bundle branch trauma with passage of the catheter through the right ventricle. If it appears that reaching the pulmonary artery will be difficult (as in massive right atrial dilation), then a temporary transvenous electrode is inserted into the venous system and left in the IVC or SVC in the event it is required. Alternatively, a flotation catheter with pacing electrodes may be used, although pacing cannot always be established reliably by this method.

Complete heart block has also been reported to occur rarely after left heart catheterization in patients with or without preexisting RBBB.[54–56] Various mechanisms have been postulated for this occurrence, but it appears likely that direct trauma to the interventricular septum as the pigtail catheter crosses the aortic valve and enters the left ventricle is largely responsible. This situation may arise more frequently when the pigtail catheter is prolapsed across the aortic valve, thereby increasing the risk of trauma to the septum.

Significant bradyarrhythmias and high-grade conduction disturbances have been reported in patients with preexisting conduction abnormalities undergoing coronary arteriography.[57] The incidence of these complications has been reduced with the advent of nonionic contrast agents. Although theoretically patients with underlying conduction abnormalities may benefit from prophylactic temporary pacing, the need for this has not been unequivocally demonstrated.[57] Of relevance is a report indicating that the frequency of ventricular arrhythmias was higher in patients who had a prophylactic pacemaker inserted in the right ventricle than among those who did not.[58] Because of these reasons, temporary pacemakers are rarely used during coronary arteriography even in patients with preexisting BBB. When it is decided that a temporary pacemaker is necessary, it is my practice to leave the pacemaker electrode in the IVC, thereby avoiding mechanical ventricular stimulation and, potentially, the induction of ventricular arrhythmias. An experienced operator should be able to advance the pacemaker electrode from the IVC into the right ventricle and effect ventricular capture in less than 10 seconds, should the need arise.

Myocardial infarction as a complication of cardiac catheterization and angiocardiography is uncommon. Its incidence was 0.06% and 0.07% overall in the two reports of the SCA&I Registry.[1, 37] Earlier studies have reported higher rates of 1.2%[59] and 2.6%.[60] The risk for myocardial infarction appears to be the same for the transfemoral and the brachial artery techniques.[1] Predisposing factors include unstable angina, recent infarction, and significant left main coronary artery stenosis.[61] Because soft tissue trauma associated with cardiac catheterization (by both brachial and femoral techniques) causes modest elevations of total serum creatine kinase (CK) activity,[62] the diagnosis of pericatheterization myocardial infarction must be made only in the presence of unequivocal electrocardiographic Q wave development or elevation of serum CK-MB activity.

The mechanisms of pericatheterization myocardial infarction include coronary artery thromboembolism; myocardial hypoperfusion during periods of hypotension or arrhythmias; and ongoing, unrecognized, and untreated myocardial ischemia. Appropriate anticoagulation, double- or triple-drug anti-ischemic therapy (including intravenous nitroglycerin infusion in patients with unstable angina), and blood pressure support are essential elements in preventing myocardial infarction and death during cardiac catheterization. Intra-aortic balloon counterpulsation in unstable patients or patients with suspected left main coronary artery stenosis frequently provides the necessary margin of safety and prevents this complication.

Central Nervous System Complications

A number of central nervous system (CNS) complications have been reported to occur during cardiac catheterization. CNS complications include cerebrovascular accidents, presumably embolic, spinal cord infarction, seizures, and cortical blindness. Most patients who develop a CNS complication and are subsequently studied have clearcut evidence of embolic involvement on computed tomographic or magnetic resonance imaging of the brain.[63]

The risk of cerebrovascular accidents was identical at 0.07% in both reports of the SCA&I Registry.[1, 37] As was the case for myocardial infarction, the incidence of this complication was independent of the technique used. Prevention of CNS embolic complications is largely dependent on full systemic anticoagulation and meticulous attention to technique of catheter aspiration and flushing and guide wire wiping, as previously mentioned. Occasionally, cholesterol emboli may be responsible for CNS complications. It appears that the incidence of cholesterol embolization is increasing largely because of the performance of more invasive procedures on older patients with more severe atherosclerotic disease.[64] Prevention of cholesterol emboli depends on meticulous attention to catheter manipulation technique. Especially in older patients with severely diseased vessels, catheter advancement must be slow and gentle. All catheters (other than pigtail) should be advanced around the aortic arch to the ascending aorta only with the flexible tip of a J-guide wire leading the way. Great care must be exercised in these patients to avoid the inadvertent entry of a catheter (with or without a guide wire in place) into one of the major brachiocephalic vessels. Patients with brachiocephalic bruits are probably at an increased risk of CNS complications and deserve an extra-careful catheterization approach. Spinal cord infarction as a result of cardiac catheterization has been reported, with at least one case documented to be due to cholesterol embolization.[65]

Transient cortical blindness has been reported to occur after vertebral and cerebral angiography. After cardiac catheterization it is an exceedingly uncommon complication that has been reported in only four cases. Of interest is the fact that one these cases involved selective arteriography of an internal mammary artery graft.[66] The mechanism of transient cortical blindness induced by angiography is not well understood. Hypotension, the presence of hypertensive vascular disease, and the amount of contrast material injected all have been implicated. Another mechanism recently suggested is that contrast media may produce a partial and temporary disruption of the blood-brain barrier, accumulating selectively in the striate cortex in sufficient concentration to cause blindness.[66] Because vertebral arteriography has been associated with this complication, it is important to avoid entry and contrast medium injection into a vertebral artery while searching for the internal mammary artery takeoff, usually located directly opposite the origin of the vertebral artery (see Chapter 19).

Pulmonary Complications

Disruption of a pulmonary arterial branch with associated pulmonary hemorrhage is an uncommon, dreaded, and almost uniformly fatal complication seen almost exclusively with the use of balloon flotation catheters. Autopsies of patients dying from this complication have documented evidence of perforation or tear of a small pulmonary artery branch,[67] frequently at a bifurcation point.[68] Factors that predispose to the development of this complication include age greater than 60 years, pulmonary hypertension, systemic anticoagulation, and valvular heart disease.[67]

Several mechanisms have been postulated to explain this complication. Lapin and Murray[69] proposed that perforation occurs in areas of aneurysmal dilation and weakening of the pulmonary artery as a result of chronic pulmonary hypertension. Lateral pressure by the inflated balloon wedged in a bifurcation has also been proposed as a mechanism for pulmonary artery injury.[68] Other proposed mechanisms include balloon overinflation with resulting arterial wall disruption or some mechanism whereby the tip of the catheter injures the artery because of eccentric balloon inflation.[70] The incidence of this complication is low, reported as 0.2%[71] to 0.3%.[72]

The first symptom heralding pulmonary arterial disruption is cough, followed rapidly by brisk hemoptysis. Should this occur during a cardiac catheterization procedure, the first step to be taken is to reverse systemic anticoagulation by means of protamine sulfate. The patient should be placed on his or her side with the affected lung down[67] and should be intubated promptly to establish adequate airway and provide easy access to bronchoscopy. Unless the hemoptysis subsides rapidly, operative intervention with resection of the affected lobe is indicated. It goes without saying that in the face of this catastrophic complication, the cardiac catheterization procedure is interrupted.

Another pulmonary complication is pulmonary edema, which is being seen with increasing frequency as the acuity of patients taken to the catheterization laboratory increases. Commonly, pulmonary edema is the result of acute ischemic injury or volume overload of a patient with impaired left ventricular function. Pulmonary artery wedge pressure should be monitored throughout the performance of left heart angiographic studies in these patients. If the pulmonary artery wedge pressure rises above 25 mm Hg after left ventriculography or coronary arteriography or both, furosemide is administered intravenously along with an intravenous infusion of a vasodilator such as sodium nitroprusside or nitroglycerin (the latter is preferred in patients suspected of an acute ischemic event). Administration of oxygen by mask and raising the patient's torso to at least 45 degrees are also of help in this situation. A decision about whether to continue the study or not depends on the specific needs of the patient, the severity of the pulmonary edema, and the rapidity of its resolution.

Renal Complications

Most renal complications following cardiac catheterization are the result of contrast media nephrotoxicity (see Chapter 7). However, embolic (both thromboembolism and cholesterol embolism) complications have been reported.[73] In the report of the SCA&I Registry, the overall incidence of the radiocontrast-induced complications was 0.23%.[1] However, in the analysis of major complications by technique, contrast medium–related complications were 0.25% in the transfemoral technique group as compared with 0.19% in the brachial approach group. This was a statistically significant difference, which suggests that at least in some of these patients, what was thought to be a contrast medium–induced complication may have been related to embolic injury of the kidneys. The mechanism producing contrast medium–induced nephrotoxicity is unclear despite considerable study. A number of factors have been suggested as contributory or causal: hypotension, proteinuria, preexisting renovascular disease, dosage of the radiocontrast agent, hyperuricemia, and the use of high-osmolar contrast media. In a prospective study of 199 cardiac catheterizations in patients older than 70 years of age, the following independent risk factors for postcatheterization renal dysfunction were identified: total volume of contrast medium more than 200 mL, serum albumin level less than 3.5 gm/dL, diabetes mellitus, serum sodium level lower than 135 mEq/L and baseline creatinine level higher than 1.5 mg/dL.[74] In this study, renal insufficiency (defined as a rise of serum creatinine greater than 0.5 mg/dL above baseline) occurred in 1.2% of patients with no risk factors, in 11.2% of those with one risk factor, and in more than 30% among those with two or more risk factors. In another prospective trial using nonionic contrast media, the risk for nephropathy was found to be relatively constant up to a serum creatinine level of 1.2 mg/dL, with a sharp rise in the probability of nephropathy when the serum creatinine level reached 1.2 mg/dL.[75]

The overall incidence of contrast medium–induced nephropathy (as defined earlier) is approximately 10%. However, in most reported series, this type of renal insufficiency follows a benign course, with very few patients progressing to oliguria or requiring dialysis.[74–76] In the prospective study of Rich and Crecelius,[74] complete or partial resolution of the renal insufficiency occurred in 75% of the cases, whereas moderate renal dysfunction persisted in 24%. Severe deterioration of renal function to a creatinine level of more than 2 mg/dL occurred in only 1.6% of their group of elderly patients. Although pericatheterization mortality tends to be higher in patients with radiocontrast-induced renal insufficiency, most likely this reflects the fact that patients who develop this complication are sicker to begin with.

Although the role of dehydration as a predisposing factor to contrast medium–induced nephropathy remains uncertain, common practice includes adequate hydration of patients before they undergo angiographic studies whenever possible. Additionally, I attempt to minimize the contrast medium volume given to all patients with serum creatinine levels higher than 1.5 mg/dL. The performance of biplane coronary arteriography can effectively reduce by half the amount of contrast medium given. Additionally, left ventriculography is frequently omitted if another technique would allow equally good assessment of left ventricular function without the use of contrast medium. If I anticipate that a patient with a serum creatinine level higher than 1.5 mg/dL will receive a near maximal contrast medium load (3 mL/kg body weight), in addition to good hydration I prepare the patient with an intravenous infusion of 25 gm of mannitol starting approximately 30 minutes before the angiographic studies. Although its value has not been unequivocally proved with randomized trials, the use of mannitol or furosemide or both may be helpful in preventing or minimizing contrast medium–induced renal complications in high-risk patients.[77, 78]

Infection and Febrile Reactions

Febrile reactions have been reported to occur in 3% to 50% of cardiac catheterizations,[79] but more recent studies suggest that this is a rare complication. Thus, only one febrile reaction was reported in 2029 catheterizations reported in the Veterans Administration Cooperative Study on complications in patients with valvular heart disease.[38] The incidence of true bacteremia is probably even lower.[80, 81] As a result, the practice of prescribing prophylactic antibiotic therapy to patients undergoing cardiac catheterization has been largely abandoned. Cardiac catheterization is generally not considered a procedure for which antibiotics should be administered for endocarditis prophylaxis, according to the latest recommendations of the American Heart Association.[82] Meticulous attention to surgical technique and asepsis when performing a brachial artery cutdown probably provides the best protection against endocarditis.

However, it is not considered inappropriate to prescribe antibiotic prophylaxis for cardiac catheterizations performed via brachial artery and vein cutdown in patients with prosthetic cardiac valves or prior history of endocarditis or both.[82]

When fever occurs, it is usually transient and most commonly represents a pyrogenic reaction. It has been long recognized that this type of a febrile reaction is more common when multiple-use intravascular catheters are employed.[83, 84] Residual endotoxin has been detected on catheters even after meticulous sterilization; it is for this reason that most laboratories have converted to single-use disposable catheters.[85]

Miscellaneous Complications

Thrombophlebitis is a rare complication in adults undergoing cardiac catheterization. When it occurs it is almost always localized to an upper extremity superficial vein following its isolation, catheterization, and subsequent ligation. Symptoms are almost always minor and respond to local measures, including elevation of the extremity and hot soaks.

Thrombosis of a femoral vein after percutaneous entry is also rare in adults. I have seen only one instance of femoral vein thrombosis due to development of a large groin hematoma with secondary venous compression. Femoral vein thrombosis following catheterization in infants, however, is considerably more common. In one study the incidence was reported as 15.6% in infants younger than 1 year of age.[86] The rate of deep venous thrombosis appeared to increase with decreasing patient weight and was also higher when an indwelling femoral vein catheter was left in place longer than 24 hours. Of interest is the fact that in some patients the thrombosis spared the catheterized femoral vein and involved only the IVC.

Hypotension during cardiac catheterization may be the result of a vasovagal reaction, hypovolemia, or severe myocardial depression. These entities were discussed earlier. It is essential that when hypotension develops, all catheter manipulation be stopped, and the operator should attempt to ascertain the precise cause for this event and take measures to remedy the hypotension before continuing with the procedure. After conclusion of the catheterization, hypotension may develop as a result of excessive diuresis secondary to the osmotic load of the contrast medium. It should then be treated with generous fluid replacement, as mentioned previously.

Cholesterol embolization has been mentioned earlier as one cause of postcatheterization renal insufficiency. Rarely, multiple cholesterol emboli involve the eye, skin, distal extremities, and brain. It is postulated that this multiple cholesterol embolization syndrome (MCES) results from a shower of cholesterol crystals from ulcerated atherosclerotic plaques provoked by intravascular catheter manipulation or anticoagulant therapy in predisposed patients with severe atherosclerotic vascular disease.[87] Characteristically, patients with MCES demonstrate confusion, impaired visual acuity, livedo reticularis, and ulcerating gangrenous lesions of the distal lower extremities. Treatment of this catastrophic complication is unsatisfactory except for discontinuation of anticoagulants (in an effort to allow a thrombus to form over the ulcerated atherosclerotic plaque) and surgical correction of a major embolic lesion if it is accessible. MCES may occur in patients with soft, friable atherosclerotic plaques even in the absence of intravascular manipulations.

Death

Death during the procedure is a dreaded and uncommon complication of cardiac catheterization and angiography. In the most recent SCA&I Registry report[1] the death rate among 222,553 patients undergoing selective coronary arteriography was 0.1%. This rate was significantly lower than the 0.14% death rate described in the original SCA&I Registry report.[37] Deaths were more common in patients older than 60 years of age, those in NYHA functional class IV, patients with left main coronary artery obstruction, and those with left ventricular ejection fraction under 30%.[1] Technique (brachial versus femoral approach) and gender were not found to be independent risk factors.

Even though the current overall death rate of 0.1% is considerably better than the 1% rate reported in early studies,[59, 60] further reduction probably cannot be anticipated as more severely ill and unstable patients are taken to the catheterization laboratory for diagnostic studies and therapeutic interventions. Particularly relevant to patients with coronary artery disease (who form the bulk of catheterization studies in most laboratories) is the presence of left main coronary artery obstruction. I cannot overemphasize to the beginning angiographer the need for caution in patients suspected of having significant left main coronary obstruction. Gordon and associates[61] found that unstable angina (angina within 24 hours of cardiac catheterization) and distance from catheter tip to left main lesion of 6 mm or less were the only significant independent factors that increased the risk of pericatheterization complications in this subgroup of patients. No relationship was found between the incidence of complications and NYHA functional class, technique used, performance of ventriculography, number of coronary injections, amount of contrast medium injected, severity of left main stenosis, number of major coronary arteries diseased, mean arterial pressure, left ventricular end-diastolic pressure, and left ventricular ejection fraction. This study then suggested two obvious measures to be taken in patients suspected of left main coronary disease to prevent death and major complications. The first is that every attempt should be made to "cool off" the patient by means of medical therapy before taking him or her to the catheterization laboratory. It is self-evident that performing a stressful invasive procedure in patients with active ischemic symptoms may well increase the risk for complications. The second measure relates to the technique of intubating the left main coronary artery. Every effort should be made to keep the catheter tip as far away from the atherosclerotic lesion as possible, and great care should be exercised not to occlude the left main coronary artery even transiently with the catheter tip. A preliminary "cusp" or "flush" injection before the catheter is selectively positioned in the left main artery is strongly advised.

Major complications, including death, have been reported as a result of retrograde catheterization across a mechanical aortic valve prosthesis.[88] This is particularly true of tilting disk valves such as the Björk-Shiley and Medtronic-Hall prostheses. Because the risk of complications is high and transprosthetic left ventricular catheterization induces significant aortic regurgitation that makes hemodynamic assessment of left ventricular function difficult, this technique is not recommended despite reports in the literature of successful studies by this route.[89]

When undertaking cardiac catheterization and angiocardiography on a patient with suspected left main coronary artery obstruction or other factors predisposing to death and major complications, it is well for the invasive cardiologist to coordinate the diagnostic procedure with the cardiac surgery schedule so that, if necessary, the patient may be taken directly to the operating room for revascularization. Other precautions to be observed in patients with major risk factors include minimizing the amount of fluids and contrast medium administered. It is advisable that the right heart catheterization be performed first in all patients be-

lieved to have significant systolic or diastolic left ventricular dysfunction so that the patient's hemodynamics (left ventricular filling pressures and cardiac output) may be optimized by the administration of diuretics or vasodilators or both before the administration of contrast media.

Meticulous attention to technique and rapidity of the catheterization procedure minimize the risk of death and other major complications. Similarly, constant monitoring of patient oxygenation and of arterial and left ventricular filling pressures allows the operator to intervene before the situation has become critical.

GENERAL PRINCIPLES

The specific procedures to be followed for a successful cardiac catheterization are dealt with in detail in other chapters. In this section, I only set the stage and bring to the attention of the reader certain important general principles that must be observed at all times.

The importance of adequate patient preparation cannot be overemphasized. Time spent with the patient before the procedure is time well spent in that it makes a patient more cooperative and the procedure easier. The patient's history and medical status must be carefully examined, and the presence of contraindications (Table 2–3) must be investigated. Although there are few absolute contraindications to car-

Table 2–3. **Contraindications to Cardiac Catheterization**

Absolute
Patient refusal or inability to give informed consent
Lack of patient cooperation
Anticipated patient refusal to undergo subsequent therapeutic intervention(s)

Relative
Any condition that temporarily increases risk of procedure
Recent cerebrovascular accident
Progressive renal insufficiency
Active gastrointestinal hemorrhage
Febrile illness and active infectious process
Severe anemia (hematocrit <25%)
Uncontrolled ventricular arrhythmias
Uncontrolled severe hypertension
End-stage pulmonary or hepatic disease
Coagulopathy and bleeding diathesis
Pulmonary edema
Severe electrolyte imbalance
Digitalis toxic arrhythmias
Lack of cardiosurgical backup
Severe cachexia
Other systemic disease(s) that severely limits life expectancy

diac catheterization, many of the listed relative contraindications are important, and the operator is best advised to consider delaying the procedure until some of these contraindications have been treated and minimized.

To a great extent cardiac catheterization technique is an art. The single major characteristic that distinguishes the expert catheterizer from a mediocre one is the expert's ability to recognize what can and cannot be done safely and when to proceed with a technique or approach and when to desist. In fact, this defines the quality of "gentleness" about which Dr. G. A. H. Miller has so eloquently written.[90] Students of cardiac catheterization are strongly urged to read this reference carefully and incorporate the suggestions therein into their armamentarium.

Dr. Frank Hildner has recently proposed and written about 10 basic axioms for new students of cardiac catheterization, as summarized in Table 2–4.[91] Readers are referred to the article itself and are urged strongly to make these axioms part of their daily practice.

To obtain meaningful hemodynamic data, it is important for the patient to be in a steady-state and as near to euvolemia as possible. The prevailing atmosphere in the laboratory should be one of quiet competence and decorum. Un-

Table 2–4. **Basic Principles of Cardiac Catheterization**

1. Catheterization technique is mostly mental, not physical.
2. Control the catheter—do not let it control you.
3. Never advance the catheter or guide wire without fluoroscopy.
4. Never advance against resistance.
5. Always obtain backbleeding from the catheter before aspiration or flushing.
6. Evaluate data as they are collected and before proceeding to another phase.
7. Never take anything for granted. Double- and triple-check everything.
8. Catheterization is best performed with finesse, not with force.
9. Pain indicates a problem; correct it immediately.
10. Never leave the laboratory without obtaining answers to all questions (but see no. 13).
11. Always go around the aortic arch with the guide wire leading the catheter.
12. Adapt your technique or approach to the individual patient.
13. Know your (and the patient's) limits; learn when to quit.
14. Remember that Murphy's law[93] is always operational in the catheterization laboratory.

Items 1 through 10 adapted from Hildner FJ: Ten basic instructions and axioms for new students of cardiac catheterization. Cathet Cardiovasc Diagn 1991; 22:307–309. Copyright © 1991 John Wiley & Sons, Inc. Reprinted by permission of John Wiley & Sons, Inc.

necessary conversation must be kept to a minimum. Jokes within hearing distance of an awake patient are inappropriate. Inflammatory or anxiety-provoking statements must be avoided. Teaching must be done in a quiet, professional manner. Both the instructor and the trainee share responsibility in making the patient comfortable. It is only with strict adherence to these rules that a patient has a remote chance of being in a steady-state when hemodynamic measurements are made. Another important consideration is the sequence of procedures to be followed. In general, it is best to acquire hemodynamic data (resting and exercise) before angiographic studies because contrast agents exert a variety of influences on the patient's cardiovascular system (see Chapter 7).

Reproducibility of cardiac output measurements is only fair. This is the result in part to normal variations in cardiac output under circumstances that prevail in most laboratories and in part to the inherent errors of available techniques. Changes in cardiac output of $\pm 20\%$ within a 30-minute period are not at all uncommon. Cardiac output and mixed venous oxygen content are almost always higher if measured within 5 minutes of initial catheter positioning in the pulmonary artery than at a later time. Hence, it is crucial to allow time for the patient to "settle down" and achieve as close to a steady-state as possible after instrumentation and before hemodynamic measurements are made.

Pressure measurement techniques are also fraught with error and artifact. Although this subject is addressed in detail in Chapters 3 and 4, the following points adapted from Butler and Oldershaw[92] should always be kept in mind:

1. The pressure or pressure gradient should be stable and reproducible.
2. The contour of the pressure tracing, both height and nadir, should resemble pressure tracings normally obtained in the particular chamber.
3. Pressure tracings should make sense, that is, they should fit the clinical diagnosis and other observations made up to that point.
4. Although modern pressure transducers are electrically stable, it is best that they be calibrated against mercury regularly.

It is the practice in my laboratory to calibrate the transducers with a mercury sphygmomanometer before the beginning of every case, and air zero is rechecked before each pressure recording.

Adequate preparation and meticulous attention to the invasive technique and data acquisition procedures are essential requirements for the efficient and successful completion of cardiac catheterization procedures.

REFERENCES

1. Johnson LW, Lozner EC, Johnson S, et al: Coronary arteriography 1984–1987: A report of the Registry of the Society for Cardiac Angiography and Interventions. Part I: Results and complications. Cathet Cardiovasc Diagn 1989; 17:5–10.

2. Herrmann KS, Kreuzer H: A randomized prospective study on anxiety reduction by preparatory disclosure with and without video film show about a planned heart catheterization. Eur Heart J 1989; 10:753–757.

3. Goldberg SJ, Linde LM, Wolfe RR, et al: The effects of meperidine, promethazine, and chlorpromazine on pulmonary and systemic circulation. Am Heart J 1969; 77:214–221.

4. O'Keefe JH, Vliestra RE, Hauley PC, et al: Revival of the transseptal approach for catheterization of the left atrium and ventricle. Mayo Clin Proc 1985; 60:790–795.

5. Ali Khan MA, Mullins CE, Bash SE, et al: Transseptal left heart catheterization in infants, children, and young adults. Cathet Cardiovasc Diagn 1989; 17:198–201.

6. Sapin P, Petrozzi R, Dehmer GJ: Reduction in injection pain using buffered lidocaine as a local anesthetic before cardiac catheterization. Cathet Cardiovasc Diagn 1991; 23:100–102.

7. Seldinger SI: Catheter replacement of needle in percutaneous arteriography: A new technique. Acta Radiol 1953; 39:368–376.

8. Cohen M, Rentrop KP, Cohen BM, et al: Safety and efficacy of percutaneous entry of the brachial artery versus cutdown and arteriotomy for left-sided cardiac catheterization. Am J Cardiol 1986; 57:682–684.

9. Deligonul V, Gabliani G, Kern MJ, et al: Percutaneous brachial artery catheterization: The hidden hazard of high brachial artery bifurcation. Cathet Cardiovasc Diagn 1988; 14:44–45.

10. Swan HJC, Ganz W, Forrester J, et al: Catheterization of the heart in man with use of a flow-directed balloon-tipped catheter. N Engl J Med 1970; 283:447–451.

11. Grollman JH, Price JE Jr, Gray RK: Percutaneous trans-femoral right heart catheterization. Am J Cardiol 1972; 30:646–647.

12. Laskey WK, Untereker WJ, Kusiak V, et al: A safe and rapid technique for retrograde catheterization of the left ventricle in aortic stenosis. Cathet Cardiovasc Diagn 1982; 8:429–435.

13. Houick GL, Cayler GC, Richardson WR, et al: New type of catheter tip for retrograde catheterization of the left ventricle in congenital aortic stenosis. N Engl J Med 1962; 266:1101–1103.

14. Feldman T, Carroll JD, Chiu YC: An improved catheter design for crossing stenosed aortic valves. Cathet Cardiovasc Diagn 1989; 16:279–283.

15. Shirey EK, Sones FM: Retrograde transaortic and mitral valve catheterization: Physiologic and morphologic evaluation of aortic and mitral valve lesions. Am J Cardiol 1966; 18:745–753.

16. Freeman DJ: New preformed catheter and method for retrograde left atrial or complete left heart catheterization. Cathet Cardiovasc Diagn 1978; 4:305–310.

17. Repa I, Yedlicka JW, Hunter DW, et al: Retrograde left atrial catheterization. Radiology 1989; 173:565–567.

18. Iskandrian AS, Bemis CE, Kimbris D, et al: Retrograde catheterization of the left atrium. Br Heart J 1979; 42:715–718.

19. Ross J: Transseptal left heart catheterization: A new method of left atrial puncture. Ann Surg 1959; 149:395–401.

20. Cope C: Technique for transseptal catheterization of the left atrium: Preliminary report. J Thorac Cardiovasc Surg 1959; 37:482–486.

21. Brockenbrough EC, Braunwald E: A new technique for left ventricular angiography and transseptal left heart catheterization. Am J Cardiol 1960; 6:1062–1064.

22. Luchsinger PC, Seip HW, Patel DJ: Relationship of pulmonary artery wedge pressure to left atrial pressure in man. Circ Res 1962; 11:315–318.

23. Walston A, Kendall ME: Comparison of pulmonary wedge and left atrial pressure in man. Am Heart J 1973; 86:159–164.

24. Mullins CE: Transseptal left heart catheterization: Experience with a new technique in 520 pediatric and adult patients. Pediatr Cardiol 1983; 4:239–246.

25. Bain DS, Grossman W: Percutaneous approach and transseptal catheterization. In Grossman W (ed): Cardiac Catheterization and Angiography, 3d ed. Philadelphia, Lea & Febiger, 1986, p 74.

26. Schoonmaker FW, Vijay NK, Jantz RD: Left atrial and ventricular transseptal catheterization review: Losing skills? Cathet Cardiovasc Diagn 1987; 13:233–238.

27. Brock R, Milstein BB, Ross DN: Percutaneous left ventricular puncture in the assessment of aortic stenosis. Thorax 1956; 11:163–171.

28. Wong CM, Wong PHC, Miller GAH: Percutaneous left ventricular angiography. Cathet Cardiovasc Diagn 1981; 7:425–432.

29. Morgan JM, Gray HH, Gelder C, et al: Left heart catheterization by direct ventricular puncture: Withstanding the test of time. Cathet Cardiovasc Diagn 1989; 16:87–90.

30. Vacek JL, Bellinger RL, Phelix J: Heparin bolus therapy during cardiac catheterization. Am J Cardiol 1988; 62:1314–1317.

31. Stewart WJ, McSweeney SM, Kellet MA, et al: Increased risk of severe protamine reactions in NPH insulin-dependent diabetics undergoing cardiac catheterization. Circulation 1984; 70:788–792.

32. Reed DC, Gascho JA: The safety of protamine sulfate in diabetics undergoing cardiac catheterization. Cathet Cardiovasc Diagn 1988; 14:19–23.

33. Mendel D, Oldershaw P: A Practice of Cardiac Catheterization, 3rd ed. London, Blackwell Scientific Publications, 1980.

34. Husson GS, Blackman MS: Arteriotomy for catheterization of the left side of the heart in children. N Engl J Med 1963; 268:545–546.

35. Mann JW, Davidson JT III: Vein patch angioplasty for brachial artery occlusion after cardiac catheterization. Am Surg 1990; 56:520–522.

36. Braunwald E, Gorlin R: Cooperative study on cardiac catheterization: Total population studied, procedures employed, and incidence of complications. Circulation 1968; 37:Suppl 3:8–16.

37. Kennedy JW: Complications associated with cardiac catheterization and angiography. Cathet Cardiovasc Diagn 1982; 8:5–11.

38. Folland ED, Oprian C, Giacomini J, et al: Complications of cardiac catheterization and angiography in patients with valvular heart disease. Cathet Cardiovasc Diagn 1989; 17:15–21.

39. Lozner EC, Johnson LW, Johnson S, et al: Coronary arteriography 1984–1987: A report of the Registry of the Society for Cardiac Angiography and Interventions. Part II: An analysis of 218 deaths related to coronary arteriography. Cathet Cardiovasc Diagn 1989; 17:11–14.

40. Skillman JJ, Kim D, Bain DS: Vascular complications of percutaneous femoral cardiac interventions: Incidence and operative repair. Arch Surg 1988; 123:1207–1212.

41. Kaufman J, Moglia R, Lacy C, et al: Peripheral vascular complications from percutaneous transluminal coronary angioplasty: A comparison with transfemoral cardiac catheterization. Am J Med Sci 1989; 297:22–25.

42. Hammacher ER, Eikelboom BC, van Lier HJJ, et al: Brachial artery lesions after cardiac catheterization. Eur J Vasc Surg 1988; 2:145–149.

43. Rapaport S, Sniderman DW, Morse SS, et al: Pseudoaneurysm: A complication of faulty technique in femoral arterial punctures. Radiology 1985; 154:529–530.

44. Altin RS, Flicher S, Naidech HJ: Pseudoaneurysm and arteriovenous fistula after femoral artery catheterization: Association with low femoral punctures. AJR 1989; 152:629–631.

45. Epstein AE, Davis KB, Kay GN, et al: Significance of ventricular tachyarryhthmias complicating cardiac catheterization: A CASS Registry Study. Am Heart J 1990; 119:494–501.

46. Patel C, Laboy V, Venus B, et al: Acute complications of pulmonary artery catheter insertion in critically ill patients. Crit Care Med 1986; 14:195–197.

47. Gertz EW, Wisneski JA, Chiu D, et al: Clinical superiority of a new contrast agent (Iopamidol) for cardiac angiography. J Am Coll Cardiol 1985; 5:250–258.

48. Hirshfeld JW, Kussmaul WG, DiBattiste PM, et al: Safety of cardiac angiography with conventional ionic contrast agents. Am J Cardiol 1990; 63:355–361.

49. Wright KE Jr, McIntosh HD: Syncope: A review of pathophysiologic mechanisms. Prog Cardiovasc Dis 1971; 13:580–594.

50. Stein PD, Mathur VS, Herman MV, et al: Complete heart block induced during cardiac catheterization of patients with preexisting bundle branch block. Circulation 1966; 34:783–791.

51. Gupta PK, Haft JI: Complete heart block complicating cardiac catheterization. Chest 1972; 61:185–187.

52. Akhtar M, Damato RN, Gilbert-Leeds CJ, et al: Induction of iatrogenic electrocardiographic patterns during electrophysiologic studies. Circulation 1977; 56:60–65.

53. Sprung CL, Eiser B, Schein RMH, et al: Risk of right bundle branch block and complete heart block during pulmonary artery catheterization. Crit Care Med 1989; 17:1–3.

54. Twidale N, Tonkin A: Ventricular standstill complicating cardiac catheterization. PACE 1987; 10:139–141.

55. Goethals MA, Kersschot IE, Snoeck J: Ventricular standstill during left heart catheterization [letter]. PACE Pacing Clin Electrophysiol 1988; 11:123–124.

56. McBride W, Hillis LD, Lange RA: Complete heart block during retrograde left-sided cardiac catheterization. Am J Cardiol 1989; 63:375–376.

57. Langou RA, Sheps DS, Wolfson S, et al: Intraventricular conduction during coronary arteriography in patients with preexisting conduction abnormalities. Invest Radiol 1977; 12:505–500.

58. Gilchrist IC, Cameron A: Temporary pacemaker use during coronary arteriography. Am J Cardiol 1987; 60:1051–1054.

59. Chahine RA, Herman MV, Gorlin R: Complications of coronary arteriography: Comparison of the brachial to the femoral approach. Ann Intern Med 1972; 76:862.

60. Wilson WJ, Lee GB, Amplatz K: Biplane selective coronary arteriography via percutaneous transfemoral approach. Am J Roentgenol 1967; 100:332–340.

61. Gordon PR, Abrams C, Gash AK, et al: Pericatheterization risk factors in left main coronary artery stenosis. Am J Cardiol 1987; 59:1080–1083.

62. Roberts R, Ludbrook PA, Weiss ES: Serum CPK isoenzymes after cardiac catheterization. Br Heart J 1975; 37:1144–1149.

63. Weissman BM, Aram DM, Levinsohn MW, et al: Neurologic sequelae of cardiac catheterization. Cathet Cardiovasc Diagn 1985; 11:577–583.

64. Colt HG, Begg RJ, Saporito JJ, et al: Cholesterol emboli after cardiac catheterization: Eight cases and a review of the literature. Medicine (Baltimore) 1988; 67:389–400.

65. Blankeship JC, Mirkel S. Spinal cord infarction resulting from cardiac catheterization. Am J Med 1989; 87:239–240.

66. Kinn RM, Breisblatt WM: Cortical blindness after coronary angiography: A rare but reversible complication. Cathet Cardiovasc Diagn 1991; 22:177–179.

67. Paulson DM, Scott SM, Sethi GK: Pulmonary hemorrhage associated with balloon flotation catheters. J Thorac Cardiovasc Surg 1980; 80:453–458.

68. Golden MS, Pinder T, Anderson WT, et al: Fatal pulmonary hemorrhage complicating the use of a flow-directed balloon-tipped catheter in a patient receiving anticoagulant therapy. Am J Cardiol 1973; 32:865–867.

69. Lapin ES, Murray JA: Hemoptysis with flow-directed cardiac catheterization. JAMA 1972; 220:1246.

70. Shin B, Ayella RJ, McAslan TC: Pitfalls of Swan-Ganz catheterization. Crit Care Med 1977; 5:125–127.

71. Boyd KD, Thomas SJ, Gold J, et al: A prospective study of complications of pulmonary artery catheterizations in 500 consecutive patients. Chest 1983; 84:245–249.

72. Haapaniemi J, Gadowski R, Naini M, et al: Massive hemoptysis secondary to flow-directed thermodilution catheters. Cathet Cardiovasc Diagn 1979; 5:151–157.

73. Gaines PA, Kennedy A, Moorehead P, et al: Cholesterol embolization: A lethal complication of vascular catheterization. Lancet 1988; 1:168–170.

74. Rich MW, Crecelius CA: Incidence, risk factors, and clinical course of acute renal insufficiency after cardiac catheterization in patients 70 years of age or older. Arch Intern Med 1990; 15:1237–1242.

75. Davidson CJ, Hlatky M, Morris KG, et al: Cardiovascular and renal toxicity of a nonionic radiographic contrast agent after cardiac catheterization. Ann Intern Med 1989; 110:119–124.

76. Gomes AS, Baker JD, Martin-Paradero V, et al: Acute renal dysfunction after major arteriography. Am J Roentgenol 1985; 145:1249–1253.

77. Berkseth RO, Kjellstrand CM: Radiologic contrast-induced nephropathy. Med Clin North Am 1984; 68:351–370.

78. Snyder HE, Killer DA, Foster JH: The influence of mannitol on toxic reactions to contrast angiography. Surgery 1968; 64:640–642.

79. Frank V, Herz L, Daschner FD: Infection risk of cardiac catheterization and arterial angiography with single- and multiple-use disposable catheters. Clin Cardiol 1988; 11:785–787.

80. Sande MA, Levinson ME, Lukas DS, et al: Bacteremia associated with cardiac catheterization. N Engl J Med 1969; 281:1104–1106.

81. Shawker TH, Kluge RM, Ayella RJ: Bacteremia associated with angiography. JAMA 1974; 229:1090–1092.

82. Dajani AS, Bisno AL, Chung KJ, et al: Prevention of bacterial endocarditis: Recommendations by the American Heart Association. JAMA 1990; 264:2919–2922.

83. Bauer E, Denson P, Faxon D, et al: Endotoxic reactions associated with the reuse of cardiac catheters—Massachusetts. MMWR CDC Surveill Summ 1979; 28:25–27.

84. Brown WJ, Fowler M, Friedman C, et al: Endotoxic reactions associated with the reuse of cardiac catheters—Michigan. MMWR CDC Surveill Summ 1974; 28:189.

85. Kundsin RB, Walter CW: Detection of endotoxin on sterile catheters used for cardiac catheterization. J Clin Microbiol 1980; 11:209–212.

86. Laurin S, Lundström NR: Venous thrombosis after cardiac catheterization in infants. Acta Radiol 1987; 28:241–246.

87. Kawakami Y, Hirose K, Watanabe Y, et al: Management of multiple cholesterol embolization syndrome—a case report. Angiology 1990; 41:248–252.

88. Horstkotte D, Jehle J, Loogen F: Death due to transprosthetic catheterization of a Björk-Shiley prosthesis in the aortic position. Am J Cardiol 1986; 58:566–567.

89. Rigaud M, Dubourg O, Luwaert R, et al: Retrograde catheterization of left ventricle through mechanical aortic prosthesis. Eur Heart J 1987; 8:689–696.

90. Miller GAH: On "gentleness." Cathet Cardiovasc Diagn 1989; 17:246–247.

91. Hildner FJ: Ten basic instructions and axioms for new students of cardiac catheterization. Cathet Cardiovasc Diagn 1991; 22:307–309.

92. Butler PRE, Oldershaw PJ: Measurement of pressure. *In* Mendel D, Oldershaw PJ (eds): A Practice of Cardiac Catheterization, 3rd ed. Oxford, Blackwell Scientific Publications, 1986, pp 186–188.

93. Block A: Murphy's Law and Other Reasons Why Things Go Wrong. London, Methuen, 1977.

Chapter 3

Measurement and Interpretation of Intracardiac, Venous, and Arterial Physiologic Waveforms

KIRK L. PETERSON

The cardiologist performing cardiac catheterization not only must access safely the relevant intracardiac chambers, associated veins, and great vessels but also must analyze carefully the form and fidelity of the physiologic waveforms obtained from these same sites. Interpretation of these waveforms is dependent inherently on an understanding of their mode of acquisition and their normal characteristics. In this chapter, the pressure and flow signals acquired during basal, normal physiologic function are presented. Specific abnormalities in catheter-derived pressure and flow signals, as markers of altered function, are discussed fully in the chapters devoted to individual diseases. Also, the more complex issues surrounding assessment of intracardiac pressure and wall forces are discussed in detail in Chapter 4.

PHYSIOLOGIC SIGNAL RECORDING SYSTEM

All cardiac catheterization suites are equipped with a physiologic recording system(s) that provides, with variable configuration and design, real-time display and hard-copy of intracardiac and intravascular pressure, electrocardio0-graphic, indicator-dilution, and, in some instances, flow velocity, ultrasonic, and impedance waveforms. To minimize radiation exposure, the recording system should be either within the room and shielded from the x-ray source or, alternatively, positioned outside (and hardwired into) the procedure room; the apparatus is attended by a technician or nurse trained in all facets of its operation. A voice communication link between the operating physician and the recording personnel allows ready processing of the signals taken during the procedure. Ide-

ally, oscilloscopic display of all physiologic signals is provided not only at the recorder itself but also on a slave television monitor situated for comfortable line-of-sight viewing by the physician performing the procedure.

Components of a Physiologic Recording System

The three major parts of a modern recording system (Fig. 3–1) include (1) the sensor or transducer (an instrument that picks up the relatively small energies of change in pressure, velocity, sound, motion, electrical polarization, or temperature and converts them into an electrical signal); (2) the amplifier (an electrical device that magnifies the electrical output of the sensor or transducer, according to a preestablished calibration factor); and (3) the display and archival component that serves to make the physiologic signal immediately visible and records the measurements in graphic form for permanent storage either on paper or on a magnetic archival medium (i.e., a floppy disk, hard disk, or digital or analog magnetic tape).

Determinants of Accurate Physiologic Signal Recording

Critical to the accuracy of a recording system is its linearity, sensitivity, and stability over the range of values recorded during the catheterization procedure. *Linearity* refers to a first-order polynomial relation between the magnitude of the input signal and the output of the amplifier. This essential characteristic allows a standard calibration signal to be used to quantitate the magnitude of any given physiologic parameter, such as pressure, velocity, and electrical depolarization. Linearity also implies that if the gain of the display is changed so as to magnify signals

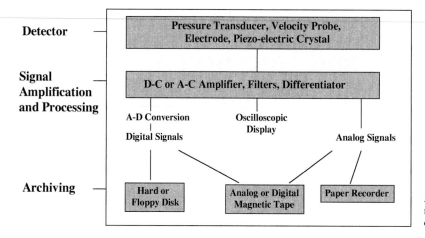

Figure 3–1. Scheme of the components of a physiologic signal recording system.

of relatively small magnitude, then a first-order relation over the full range of values remains intact. *Sensitivity* refers to the ability of the recording system to respond to relatively small changes in the magnitude of the physiologic parameter being measured. For example, in the absence of heart disease, the variations in pressure in the right atrium throughout the cardiac cycle are relatively small (0 to 5 mm Hg). *Stability* refers to a constant electrical output when the magnitude of the physiologic signal is zero; in the case of intracardiac pressure, the reference level for zero pressure, measured by fluid-filled catheter, is taken as the atmospheric pressure outside the body. Thus, the recording system is calibrated so that the baseline (or zero level) is equivalent to the output of the transducer when open to room air. This level must then remain stable during the course of recording for the calibrated voltage change to maintain its validity as a measure of pressure change. Frequent rezeroing of the pressure amplifier and checking on its pressure calibration ensure the accuracy of acquired pressure signals.

The accuracy of physiologic signal recording is also highly dependent on the degree to which the signal is filtered, the presence or absence of extraneous artifacts, and the responsiveness of the system to high-frequency changes in signal magnitude. Pressure acquisition during cardiac catheterization is particularly influenced by the frequency response of the recording system (see Chapter 4 for detailed discussion). An excessively filtered signal often underestimates the peak magnitude of a parameter (e.g., peak rate of tension development [dP/dt]). On the other hand, high-frequency noise may camouflage or obscure a peak value; in this circumstance, careful filtering often serves to "clean up" an unreliable or noisy

recording. Because most extraneous mechanical and electrical noise is random in occurrence, beat averaging of transducer waveforms also reduces noise and shows more clearly the underlying physiologic signal (Fig. 3–2).[1]

The physiologic recording system also must provide a graphic output of measured variables with a high degree of temporal fidelity. For example, the hard-copy output of paper recorders displays time-lines that are then used for calculation and measurement of temporal variables such as the systolic ejection or diastolic filling periods. The accuracy of these time intervals is ensured by using a timing mechanism, a quartz clock, that synchronizes precise time intervals with the time-lines displayed on the graphic recording. Synchronization of waveforms with a time reference, such as the R wave of the electrocardiogram, is important in those recording systems that use digital processing and beat averaging for on-line quantitation of physiologic signals.

Phasic Pressure Measurement

Even though catheter-tip pressure micromanometers, with their superior fidelity, are available, expense and fragility preclude their routine use. Thus, fluid-filled catheters connected to an external strain gauge transducer likely will continue to be used in most catheterization laboratories for an indeterminate time.

STRAIN GAUGE TRANSDUCERS. A strain gauge transducer consists of a chamber that has a stiff diaphragm as one of its walls (Fig. 3–3A). The diaphragm is displaced within the chamber in direct proportion to the force or pressure that is exerted on the side that is exposed to the fluid-filled column through the catheter. The movement of the diaphragm is used to change the resistance of sensing elements or wires that

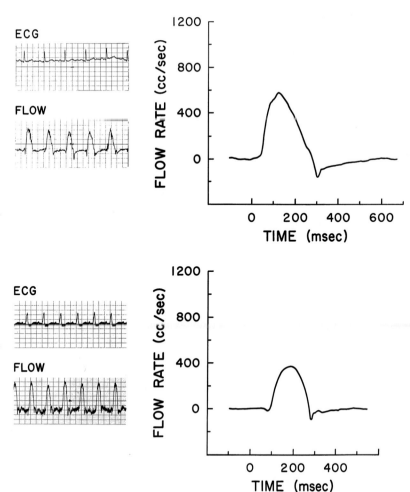

ECG

FLOW

ECG

FLOW

Figure 3–2. *Upper,* Original records of electrocardiogram (ECG) and catheter-tip velocity probe output *(left)* with average flow profile *(right)* obtained by averaging 64 beats and calibrated for flow units by means of a simultaneous indocyanine dye dilution curve. Signals were recorded in a patient with coronary atherosclerosis and mild left ventricular dysfunction. *Lower,* Original records of ECG and catheter-tip velocity output *(left)* and average flow profile *(right),* obtained by averaging 75 beats and calibrated by a simultaneous indocyanine dye dilution curve. Signals were recorded in a patient with primary myocardial disease and severe left ventricular failure with reduced stroke volume. (From Uther JB, Peterson KL, Shabetai R, Braunwald E: Measurement of ascending aortic flow patterns in man. J Appl Physiol, 1972; 34:513–518.)

are attached to it. In a strain gauge transducer, the resistance decreases with stretching. The resistance wires are ordinarily placed in a so-called Wheatstone bridge circuit (Fig. 3–3*B*), where four wires are arranged so that when the diaphragm moves, two of the wires contract while two others stretch.[2] When the diaphragm of the transducer is in the unstretched state (vented on both sides to atmospheric pressure), the four wires are balanced electrically so that no potential difference is present across the circuit. When movement of the diaphragm either stretches or contracts the wires, the circuit then becomes unbalanced, and a potential difference develops that is proportional to the force of the pressure on the diaphragm. The voltage of this potential difference is then fed to an amplifier and subsequently is recorded and archived.

Optimally, to minimize signal distortion and maximize fidelity, the transducer attached to a fluid-filled catheter should contain a minimum of air bubbles. Degassing the solution

used to fill the catheter and transducer improves the measured frequency response of the system. However, this can seldom be accomplished in a busy catheterization laboratory. Also, to minimize the distortion of a fluid-filled system, the catheter should be attached directly to the transducer; alternatively, an interposed connecting tubing should be made as short as possible. Stopcocks positioned between the end of the catheter and the pressure manometer should be minimized or eliminated. Finally, a low band-pass filter (e.g., high-frequency cut-off of 20 to 25 Hz) can be used effectively to remove any artifacts caused by catheter whip or contact with a heart structure.

TRANSDUCER LEVELING AND CALIBRATION. Intracardiac pressures, by convention, are referenced to the atmospheric pressure outside of the body. In addition, calibration and measurement of pressure in the lung and in each cardiac chamber make the assumption that all chambers are positioned at the same level with

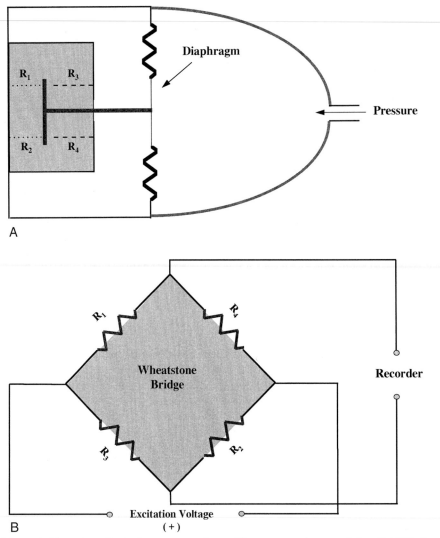

A

B

Figure 3–3. *A,* Schematic illustration of a strain gauge transducer. When pressure is exerted via a fluid-filled catheter onto a relatively stiff diaphragm, its movement, by stretching, reduces resistances R_3 and R_4 and augments resistances R_1 and R_2. (See text for discussion.) *B,* Schematic illustration of a classic Wheatstone bridge circuit. Resistances R_1 through R_4 correspond to those in *A.* When movement of the diaphragm either stretches or contracts the wires and changes their resistance, the circuit then becomes unbalanced, and a potential difference develops that is proportional to the force of the pressure on the diaphragm.

respect to the transducer outside of the body. Any differences in hydrostatic pressure that are dependent on the catheter's anteroposterior position within the heart are ignored. To minimize these differences, the outside transducer should be positioned as close as possible to the *average* height of the heart above the surface on which the patient is lying during the procedure. Several conventions have been used for estimating this level of the heart, including (1) 10 cm above the height of the table; (2) 5 cm below the sternal angle; (3) the mid-chest level; (4) the height of the palpable apex of the heart; and (5) the level of the table itself. Any absolute

reference relative to the height of the table suffers from the variability between individuals of chest anteroposterior dimensions. Thus, in our laboratory, we prefer to set the transducer height at a visual estimate of the mid-chest position when viewed from the side.

To ensure pressure measurement accuracy, it is desirable to calibrate the transducer against an independent pressure source. A standard reference is a column of mercury transmitted into the transducer chamber via a three-way stopcock or multiport manifold. Not only transducer gain but also linearity can be tested in this fashion; this is accomplished by subjecting the transducer to equal increments of pressure (e.g., 25, 50, 75, and 100 mm Hg). Ideally, this mercury manometer calibration should be performed before each case. Moreover, if there is any question about the accuracy of a given pressure measurement, the external calibration can be repeated quickly during the procedure.

Amplifiers for Signal Processing

DIRECT-COUPLED AMPLIFIER. With this type of amplifier the excitation signal is fed directly to the amplifier, and there is no loss of pure or slowly varying direct current (DC) signals. The major disadvantages of the direct-coupled amplifier are its zero level instability and limited gain. However, it does not cause distortion, and it exhibits a uniform response over a broad frequency range.[2]

CARRIER AMPLIFIER. In a traditional design of a carrier amplifier, an oscillator and a capacitance-coupled amplifier are combined; the oscillator energizes the transducer with an alternating-current voltage, and the amplitude of the carrier voltage is modulated in response to the strength of the physiologic signal. The modulated signal then undergoes three stages of processing in the capacitance-coupled amplifier: (1) amplification of the strength of the signal; (2) all other signals, other than those occurring at 2400 Hz, are discarded (excluding 60-cycle and spurious signals) by a tuned circuit; and (3) further amplification. Thereafter, a diode rectifier circuit (which cannot pass alternating-current [AC] voltages) is used to extract the carrier oscillations, followed by a smoothing filter, resulting in a pulsating DC voltage that corresponds to the amplitude variations produced by the transducer. The ultimate DC voltage is then transmitted to a recording device.[2]

For pressure measurements, where stability of both the zero level and gain of the amplifier are essential, the use of AC, as opposed to DC, amplifiers is recommended. Usually, the excitation current is at 2400 cycles per second (Hz) and is supplied by the oscillator section of a carrier amplifier. To balance the transducer, a variable resistance (R balance) and capacitor (C balance) are added to the circuit; they allow setting the zero level on the recording paper to atmospheric pressure.

Pressure Pulses on the Right Side of the Heart

RIGHT ATRIUM. The normal right atrial pressure pulse is characterized by an a wave, gener-

ated during the period of atrial systole, a small c wave generated during the time of closure of the tricuspid valve and isovolumetric systole of the right ventricle, and a v wave generated during the period of right ventricular systole and filling of the right atrium from the systemic veins and coronary sinus. The x descent follows the a wave and coincides with right atrial relaxation. Following the c wave, there is a second pressure decline sometimes referred to as the x' descent; this corresponds to the fall in pressure in the right atrium as the ventricle ejects blood, intrapericardial pressure falls, and right ventricular volume diminishes, and before much filling has yet taken place in the right atrium. The y descent follows the peak of the v wave and begins immediately after the opening of the tricuspid valve (Fig. 3–4). A reciprocal relationship exists between right atrial pressure and flow. Thus, there is essentially no flow present in the right atrium at the peaks of both the a and v waves (see discussion on right atrial flow).

In the right atrium, the a wave is usually dominant to the v wave. The pressure pulse in the right atrium normally exhibits an a wave lower than 8 mm Hg, a v wave of 7 mm Hg or lower, and a mean pressure of 6 mm Hg or lower. Increased resistance to filling of the right ventricle, as in the hypertrophy associated with valvular pulmonic stenosis, leads to atrial hypertrophy and a more forceful atrial contraction. In this circumstance, the dominance of the magnitude of the a wave over the v wave is exaggerated. By contrast, certain conditions lead to a dominance of the v wave over the a wave. In severe right atrial dilation, the force of atrial contraction may be lost related to loss of contractility in atrial musculature. A large communication between the right and left atria, as in an atrial septal defect, leads to these two chambers functioning as a common chamber; in this circumstance the pressure pulse characteristics of the left atrium predominate, and the v wave often exceeds the a wave. Alternatively, in the setting of tricuspid regurgitation, there is exaggerated and early filling of the right atrium during right ventricular systole, and the right atrial pressure pulse becomes dominated by the v wave and "ventricularization" of the right atrial pressure pulse. The slope of the y descent depends on the resistance to filling of the right ventricle itself (right ventricular compliance), obstruction at the level of the tricuspid valve, or restraint of right ventricular filling imposed by pericardial tamponade.

RIGHT VENTRICLE. The right ventricular pressure pulse normally exhibits a peak systolic pres-

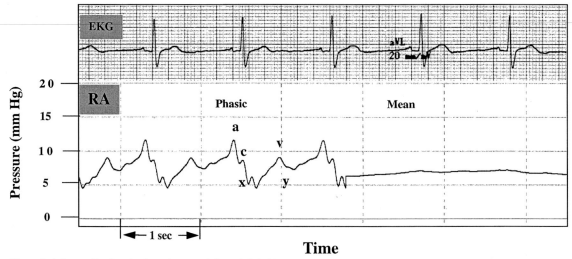

Figure 3–4. Example of a phasic and mean right atrial (RA) pressure pulse in a normal person. The a wave occurs simultaneously with atrial contraction; the v wave occurs during atrial filling; the c wave is coincident with the onset of ventricular contraction; the x descent corresponds to the fall in pressure after atrial contraction and the continued fall during early systole (x'); and the y descent occurs after the opening of the tricuspid valve and with early diastolic filling.

sure equivalent to that in the main pulmonary artery and is 30 mm Hg or lower. The early diastolic pressure is either near atmospheric or, in some instances, subatmospheric, and it then rises with ventricular filling up to a maximum of 7 mm Hg. Generally, the right atrial and right ventricular diastolic pressures are near equivalent. However, during early diastole, there may be a short period of inequality, immediately after the opening of the tricuspid valve, when right ventricular pressure continues to fall despite blood filling the ventricle. This period of so-called suction appears related to continued active relaxation of ventricular muscle and elastic recoil after the completion of ventricular systole (Fig. 3–5). Pressure during the first third of diastole rises rapidly during the period of early diastolic filling. At the beginning of diastasis the resistance to filling significantly increases, and the pressure then rises much more slowly until the onset of atrial systole. Particularly in fluid-filled pressure manometer systems, there may be a pressure "overshoot" at the end of the rapid-filling period, as shown in Figure 3–5. This same kind of artifact, attributable to an underdamped system (see Chapter 4), can also be seen at or near the peak of right ventricular systolic pressure. The period of diastasis is abbreviated as heart rate increases; thus, with rapid heart rates (>100 beats/min), the rapid-filling phase is followed immediately by atrial contraction.

PULMONARY ARTERY. The peak systolic pressure in the pulmonary artery is equivalent to

the peak systolic pressure in the right ventricle. Immediately after the end of ejection, the pulmonic valve closes, and the dicrotic notch is registered on the pressure pulse (Fig. 3–6). Thereafter the pressure falls during diastole, usually to a level that is nearly equivalent to the left atrial mean or pulmonary capillary mean pressures.[3, 4] An exception to this equivalency of the pulmonary artery diastolic pressure with the mean left atrial pressure is (1) an elevated pulmonary vascular resistance associated with vasoconstriction or anatomic compromise of the vascular cross-sectional area at the pulmonary arteriolar level or (2) a relatively rapid heart rate such that during diastole the pulmonary artery pressure does not have time to fall to the level of that in the left atrium. The mean and diastolic pulmonary artery pressures can be elevated in response to any condition that (1) increases, universally or selectively, pulmonary vascular resistance at the arteriolar level; (2) obliterates selectively a significant portion of the pulmonary vascular bed upstream to the arteriolar level, such as multiple large or small thromboemboli; or (3) increases left atrial or pulmonary venous mean pressure, such as left ventricular diastolic dysfunction, mitral stenosis or regurgitation, and fibrosing mediastinitis.

PULMONARY ARTERY (CAPILLARY) WEDGE AND LEFT ATRIAL PRESSURES. Provided it is properly positioned and there is no intervening anatomic obstruction (e.g., pulmonary venous obstruction or cor triatriatum) a fluid-filled, end-hole

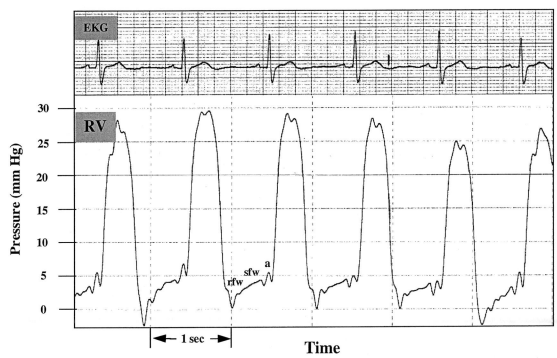

Figure 3–5. Example of a right ventricular (RV) pressure pulse in a normal person. During early diastole, after the opening of the tricuspid valve and despite ventricular filling, the ventricular pressure may fall (often referred to as the period of *ventricular suction*). Thereafter, the period of the rapid filling wave (rfw) occurs, followed by the period of slow filling (sfw) and the a wave of atrial contraction.

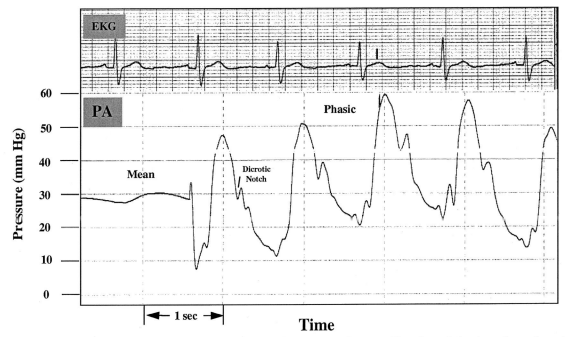

Figure 3–6. Example of a pulmonary artery (PA) pressure pulse in a normal person. Note the variation in peak systolic and end-diastolic pressures with respiration. The dicrotic notch appears shortly after the end of ejection and the closure of the pulmonic valve.

catheter that is wedged into the distal ramifications of the pulmonary artery tree records a pressure pulse that is close, if not identical, to that recorded simultaneously in the left atrium immediately above the mitral valve.[3] A time delay between the left atrial and pulmonary arterial wedge recordings of approximately 140 to 200 msec is generally noted. A balloon occlusion pressure, using a standard flotation catheter with an end-hole, also provides a similar pressure pulse, although the peaks of the a and v waves are often damped compared with the direct left atrial pressure recording. Because it is recorded within the lung itself, the pulmonary artery wedge pressure is much more sensitive to unusual changes in intrathoracic pressure brought about by the respiratory cycle (e.g., obstructive airway disease and assisted mechanical ventilation with positive end-expiratory pressure).

The pulmonary arterial wedge and left atrial pressure pulses are again characterized by a, c, and v waves (Fig. 3–7). In contradistinction to the right atrium, the left atrial pressure pulse exhibits normally a dominant v wave (≤15 mm Hg) and a subordinate a wave (≤12 mm Hg). In the normal pressure pulse, or in the presence of mitral regurgitation without stenosis, there is a rapid fall in pressure during early diastole (y descent) and a slow rise in pressure during late diastole (diastasis), reflecting equilibration between the atrial and ventricular pressures during the slow phase of ventricular filling.

LEFT VENTRICLE. The left ventricular pressure pulse is characterized by a peak systolic pressure that is nearly equivalent to that in the ascending aorta. However, there may be a small early-systolic and mid-systolic impulse gradient that is best appreciated on micromanometer pressure pulses (Fig. 3–8).[5] In the absence of any impediment to left ventricular outflow, this peak pressure occurs at the end of the first third of systole, but it can be influenced by aortic input impedance, as discussed later. The peak positive rate of rise of the left ventricular pressure (peak dp/dt) occurs before the opening of the aortic valve (see Fig. 3–8); peak negative dP/dt occurs near simultaneously with the closure of the aortic valve and marks the beginning of isovolumetric relaxation in the left ventricle.

Following aortic valve closure, the left ventricular pressure declines at a near-monoexponential rate (see Chapters 12 and 19) until the time of opening of the mitral valve. As in the right ventricle, the early diastolic pressure in the left ventricle may continue to fall after mitral valve opening to near-atmospheric levels before exhibiting a relatively rapid increase in response to rapid ventricular filling. Thus, there may exist transiently in early diastole a pressure gradient between the left atrium and the left ventricle. Later in diastole, and particularly seen on fluid-filled catheter tracings, there may be a transient overshoot of pressure at the end of the rapid-filling phase and before it begins to level off during the period of diastasis (slow-filling wave; Fig. 3–9). At end-diastole, the pressure again quickly augments in response to

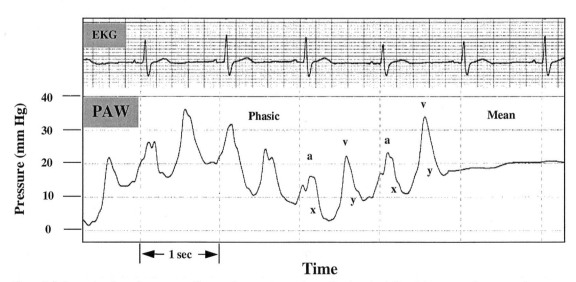

Figure 3–7. Example of a pulmonary capillary wedge pressure pulse, reflecting the left atrial pressure, in a normal person. Note that the v wave is dominant to the a wave; and the c wave is generally damped out by the intervening lung tissue. The *x* descent corresponds to the fall in pressure after atrial contraction and the continued fall during early systole; the *y* descent occurs after the opening of the mitral valve and with early diastolic filling. PAW, pulmonary artery wedge.

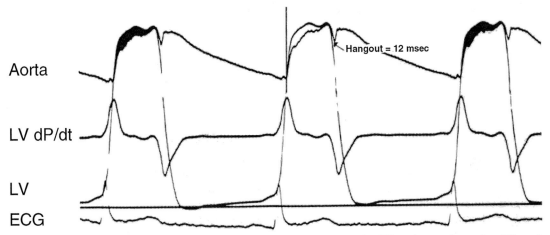

Figure 3–8. Micromanometer tracings recorded simultaneously in the left ventricle (LV) and aorta. An analog differentiation of the LV pressure pulse, LV dP/dt, is also shown along with the electrocardiogram (ECG). The systolic shaded area represents the small impulse gradient between the left ventricle and aorta. Note that peak dP/dt occurs before the opening of the aortic valve. (Modified from Shaver JA, O'Toole JD, Curtiss EJ, et al: Second heart sound: The role of altered greater and lesser circulation. Circulation 1975; American Heart Association Monograph No. 46, 58–67.)

atrial systole. Left ventricular end-diastolic pressure immediately precedes the beginning of isometric contraction in the left ventricular pressure pulse. This point, also known as the *z point,* is situated on the downslope of the left ventricular a wave and marks the crossing over of the left atrial and left ventricular pressures.

In general, the mean pulmonary arterial wedge, mean left atrial, and left ventricular end-diastolic pressures all are near equivalent in magnitude.[3, 4] However, in the presence of severe mitral regurgitation and a left atrium with normal or increased compliance, the v wave may be quite exaggerated and the mean left atrial and pulmonary arterial wedge pressures may exceed the left ventricular end-diastolic pressure. By contrast, in the presence of a relatively noncompliant left ventricle, the a wave in the left atrium and ventricle may be exaggerated. In this circumstance the mean pulmonary capillary and left atrial pressures may be lower than the end-diastolic pressure in the left ventricle.

The left ventricular end-diastolic pressure is found to be elevated (>12 mm Hg) in the following situations: (1) when the ventricle bears an excessive diastolic volume, as in mitral or aortic regurgitation, or a large left-to-right shunt at or distal to the ventricular septum; (2) in the presence of loss of myocardial contractility where the ventricle dilates and moves up its intrinsic diastolic pressure-volume relationship; (3) in the presence of concentric hypertrophy with increased wall thickness where the left ventricular chamber and muscle become less compliant, as in valvular aortic stenosis or long-

standing systemic hypertension; (4) in the presence of a restrictive or infiltrative cardiomyopathy where the ventricular chamber and muscle are likewise much stiffer than normal; and (5) in the presence of constrictive pericardial disease or high-pressure pericardial effusion.

ASCENDING AORTIC PRESSURE. During ejection, the normal pressure in the ascending aorta generally parallels that in the left ventricle, although the left ventricular pressure, at any instant, is slightly higher, reflecting the impulse gradient that propels blood out of the ventricle (see Fig. 3–8). Once the aortic valve closes, the aortic pressure declines somewhat more slowly than the left ventricular pressure, reflecting the accumulated pressure waves from the thoracic aorta and its tributaries and the capacitance of the ascending aorta. This gives rise to a slight ''hanging out'' of the dicrotic notch from its equivalent position on the left ventricular pressure pulse (see Fig. 3–8).[5]

Following the dicrotic notch on the ascending aortic pressure pulse, there is an increase in pressure related to some retrograde flow from the periphery into the ascending aorta and the elastic recoil of the ascending aorta (see Fig. 3–8). However, as blood then runs off into the periphery, there is a gradual decline in systemic arterial pressure until, at the beginning of the next cardiac cycle, the pressure again quickly rises as the left ventricle opens the aortic valve (Fig. 3–10). The rate and magnitude of decline of the ascending aortic pressure during diastole are dependent on the integrity of the aortic valve, the presence or

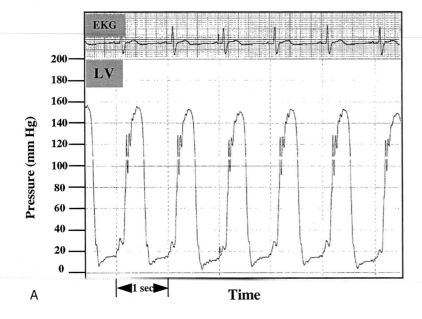

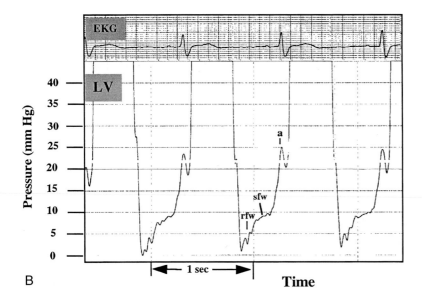

Figure 3–9. A, Fluid-filled catheter tracing in the left ventricle (LV) in a patient with a prominent atrial kick (a wave). Note the mechanical artifact on the upstroke of the tracing at about the time of opening of the aortic valve. *B,* Same patient as in *A.* The left ventricular tracing is now recorded at a higher gain to show more clearly the morphology of the diastolic pressure, including the rapid-filling wave (rfw), the slow-filling wave (sfw), and the atrial kick (a).

absence of an abnormal connection of the aorta into the pulmonary vasculature or the right side of the heart, the presence or absence of a large arteriovenous fistula, and the capacitance and resistance of the peripheral circuit. In all these latter circumstances, a so-called run-off condition can be present that leads to an excessive rate of decline of systemic diastolic arterial pressure to an inordinately low level. Also, in these conditions, there is a wide pulse pressure, reflecting an augmentation of the difference between the peak systolic and end-diastolic pressures in the ascending aortic pressure pulse.

SYSTEMIC ARTERIAL PRESSURE. The systemic arterial pressure generally parallels the configuration of that recorded in the ascending aorta. However, the shape and absolute magnitude of the pressure are influenced significantly by the impedance characteristics of the peripheral arterial vasculature. For example, in a young person with relatively elastic arteries the femoral artery peak systolic pressure, in addition to being delayed compared with that in the ascending aorta, is often augmented by 10 to 15 mm Hg. These differences can become of vital diagnostic importance when a peripheral arte-

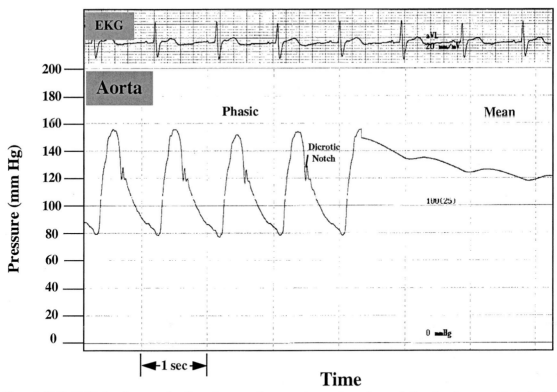

Figure 3–10. Fluid-filled catheter tracing from the ascending aorta in a patient who was believed to be normal but who had a mild elevation of the systolic pressure during the procedure. Note the dicrotic notch, followed successively by a slight rise in aortic pressure and then a continuous fall through the remainder of diastole. (See text for discussion.)

rial pressure is used to estimate that in the ascending aorta (e.g., as in valvular aortic stenosis; see Chapter 20).

Phasic Flow Measurement and Interpretation

Measurement of phasic flow in the heart, the major veins, and the great vessels has been accomplished predominantly by use of electromagnetic flow-velocity probe catheters. These devices also have been used in humans to describe the qualitative (directional) and quantitative flow changes produced by various physiologic, pathologic, and pharmacologic effects.[1, 6–9] They have also been used to measure vascular impedances to pulsatile flow, particularly in the ascending aorta and systemic arterial circuit.[10–12] Analysis of the impedance spectra of these latter signals has allowed a rational understanding of the role of retrograde arterial reflections in the pressure waveforms recorded from the ascending aorta down to the level of the iliac arteries.

RIGHT HEART FLOW. Phasic velocity of flow tracings from both the superior and inferior

venae cavae, recorded simultaneously during normal physiologic conditions in humans with a right atrial pressure pulse, demonstrate that there is a bimodal pattern of flow with the peaks coincident with the x and y descents on the pressure tracing (Fig. 3–11). It has also been conclusively shown, using velocity catheters, that normal inspiration is associated with an augmentation of blood flow velocity in the venae cavae; a consequential increase in right ventricular stroke volume can also be appreciated by velocity tracings recorded in the main pulmonary artery.

LEFT HEART FLOW. Phasic velocity tracings in the pulmonary veins have not been recorded in humans, although it is clear that left atrial volume expands during ventricular systole (during the period of generation of the v wave), and then with the opening of the mitral valve and the y descent, there is a rapid influx of flow out of the pulmonary veins and left atrium into the left ventricle. Then, with atrial systole, there is again an augmentation of flow into the left ventricle, but there may also be simultaneously some regurgitant flow into the pulmonary veins, particularly if the left ventricle is operating on

Flow Velocity (SVC) and Right Atrial Pressure

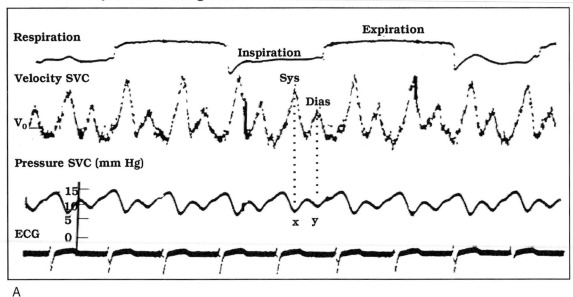

A

Flow Velocity (IVC) and Right Atrial Pressure

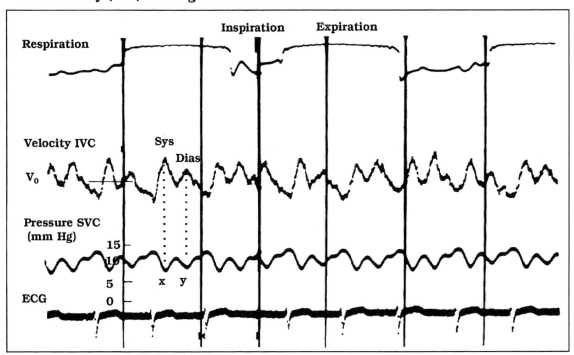

B

Figure 3–11. Tracings of blood flow velocity (by electromagnetic catheter-tip velocity catheter) and simultaneous pressure in the superior vena cava (SVC) *(A)* and inferior vena cava (IVC) *(B)*. The patient exhibited mild congestive cardiac failure. V_0 designates zero flow. Peak systolic flow in both the superior and inferior venae cavae corresponds to the *x* descent of right atrial pressure; the smaller peak during diastole corresponds to the *y* descent of pressure. (Adapted from Shabetai R: The Pericardium. New York, Grune & Stratton, 1981, p 69.)

a relatively stiff portion of its pressure-volume curve.

AORTIC FLOW. The recording of ascending aortic flow in humans, with and without aortic and ventricular pressure, has been used to assess the input impedance into the systemic arterial circuit[10–12]; beat-by-beat indices of left ventricular function, including stroke volume; stroke work, stroke power, and flow velocity; and the force-velocity-length relations of the left ventricle.[13] None of these applications has ever reached a level of routine use, primarily because of complexity and cost. Nevertheless, study of ascending aortic flow has provided significant insight into the normal and abnormal physiology of the left heart and systemic circuit in humans.

LEFT VENTRICULAR VELOCITY OF EJECTION AND FORCE-VELOCITY-LENGTH RELATIONS. An important application of the ascending aortic velocity waveform is its use in calculation of the rate of volume change in the left ventricle. If one knows the end-diastolic volume (as measured by biplane left ventriculography) and assumes that the cross-sectional area of the aorta is constant, then one can use the integral of the aortic velocity waveform to calculate instantaneous left ventricular volume throughout ejection.[13] The peak and mean rate of ejection can also be derived from these data. In humans, we have used aortic velocity tracings, in concert with high-fidelity left ventricular pressure measurements, to construct a comprehensive, three-dimensional force-velocity-length analysis of left ventricular function (Fig. 3–12).

VASCULAR RESISTANCE, IMPEDANCE, AND REFLECTED WAVES. Study of pulsatile flow in the ascending aorta and downstream has been of particular interest because of its interaction with the configuration of the arterial pressure pulse. The ratio of the pressure difference across the arterial circuit and the total flow provides a measure of mean vascular resistance. However, this simple measure is, at best, an approximation of the forces resisting flow and applies only to a constant-flow, nonpulsatile system. Moreover, if the arterial system was a pure resistance,

SHORTENING VELOCITY vs. WALL TENSION & CIRCUMFERENCE

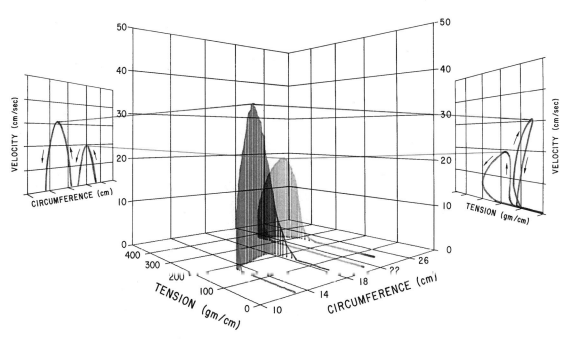

Figure 3–12. Three-dimensional perspective plot of left ventricular velocity, tension, and circumference. The loop of a patient with normal ventricular function is in the foreground; the loop of a patient with impaired ventricular function is in the background, toward the far corner. Each adjacent vertical line in the loop indicates a 5-msec interval. Projections of two-dimensional tension-velocity and velocity-length relations, to the right and left respectively, are also shown. (From Peterson KL, Uther JB, Shabetai R, Braunwald E: Assessment of left ventricular performance in man: Instantaneous tension-velocity-length relations obtained with the aid of an electromagnetic velocity catheter in the ascending aorta. Circulation 1973; 47:924–935.)

then the shape of pressure and flow waves in the root of the aorta would be identical throughout the cardiac cycle. In fact, as the left ventricle contracts, it not only propels blood forward but also distends a variably compliant aorta. In addition, blood moving forward during systole confronts retrograde waves reflected from sites downstream in the vascular tree. These phenomena cause a significant alteration in the configuration of the arterial pressure pulse that is out of phase with the flow waveform.

To characterize this complex interaction, the Fourier analysis is applied to the phasic changes in pressure and flow. Using relevant mathematic techniques, the pressure and flow waves can be broken down to identify a set of sinusoidal waves, or "harmonics," that are equivalent to the observed pulsation. Each harmonic is then described by its modulus (amplitude), phase angle (timing in relation to other harmonics), and frequency. The ratio of the amplitudes of a given pressure harmonic to its corresponding flow harmonic provides the impedance modulus, a measure of vessel resistance that can then be plotted versus the frequency of the individual sinusoidal functions (Fig. 3–13). From this spectrum, a characteristic impedance, Z_c, can be calculated by averaging all impedance moduli

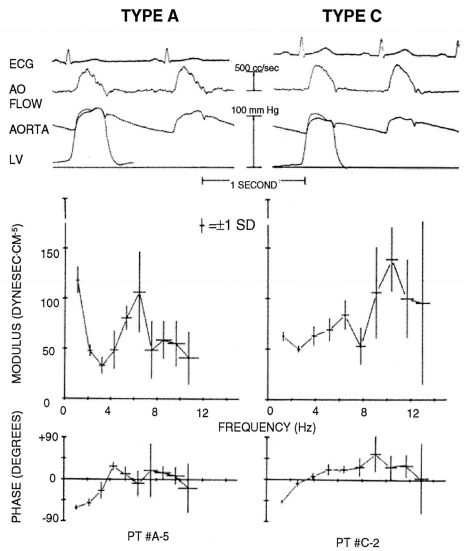

Figure 3–13. Pressure and flow waves and corresponding impedance plots from type A *(left panel)* and type C *(right panel)* beats. Note the later and larger rise in left ventricular (LV) and aortic (AO) pressure in the type A, as opposed to type C, patient. Increased oscillatory behavior of the impedance spectrum of type A suggests that late rise is due to reflected waves. (See text for full discussion.) (From Murgo JP, Westerhof N, Giolma JP, Altobelli SA: Aortic input impedance in normal man: Relationship to pressure waveforms. Circulation 1980; 62:105–116.)

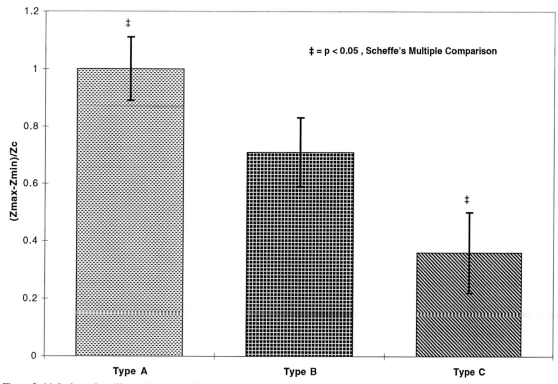

Figure 3–14. Index of oscillatory behavior ($[Z_{max} - Z_{min}]/Z_c$), computed from impedance spectrum, for various types of ascending aortic pressure pulses. (See text for definitions of types A, B, and C.)

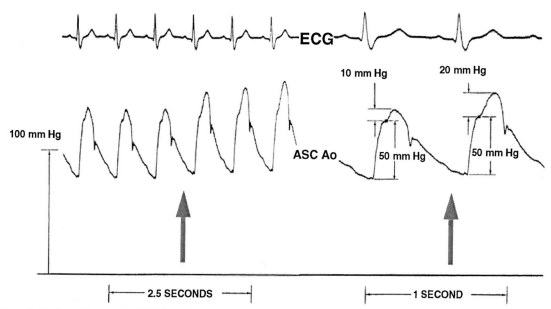

Figure 3–15. Ascending aortic (ASC Ao) micromanometer pressure waveforms taken before and after manual occlusion of the femoral arteries bilaterally. Note the immediate increase in the systolic pressure after compression *(arrows)*. The initial portion of the aortic pulse pressure from upstroke to the inflection point remains unchanged at 50 mm Hg. However, the secondary rise in late systolic pressure (ΔP) increases from 10 to 20 mm Hg, believed to be secondary to an augmentation of the reflected wave from the periphery. (From Murgo JP, Westerhof N, Giolma JP, Altobelli SA: Aortic input impedance in normal man: Relationship to pressure waveforms. Circulation 1980; 62:105–116.)

above 2 Hz. Then, to make interpatient comparisons, a given subject's amplitude spectra are normalized to the characteristic impedance.

Murgo and associates have applied multisensor catheters (two solid-state pressure sensors and one velocity probe) to the analysis of ascending aorta input impedance.[12] They found that ascending aortic pressure pulses can be classified into the following types:

A, where peak systolic pressure (P_{pk}) occurred in late systole and following a well-defined inflection point (P_i) and $\Delta P/PP > 0.12$, where $\Delta P = P_{pk} - P_i$ and PP = total pressure

B, where peak systolic pressure also occurred in late systole, following an inflection point, but $0 < \Delta P/PP \leq 0.12$

C, where peak systolic pressure preceded a well-defined inflection point and $\Delta P/PP \leq 0.00$

Type A and C beats are shown schematically in Figure 3–13. Type A and B patients demonstrated oscillations of the impedance moduli about the characteristic impedance, whereas type C patients manifested flatter impedance spectra. Thus, a later and larger rise in pressure (type A) was associated with a more oscillatory impedance spectrum, attributed to the effect of reflected waves returning from the periphery into the ascending aorta. The degree of arterial reflection was quantitated by an index of the amplitude of oscillation of the impedance moduli around the characteristic impedance, where

$$(Z_{max} - Z_{min})/Z_c$$

and where Z_{max} and Z_{min} are the maximum and minimum impedance moduli in the spectrum and Z_c is the characteristic impedance (Fig. 3–14).

Also, by applying a simplified analog model for the aorta (an elastic tube connected to a pump and terminating in a resistance), Murgo and associates derived the *effective length* (i.e., the distance from the measurement site to the reflection site) from both the impedance spectra and the pressure waveforms; by two different methods this distance was calculated to be between 44 ± 2 (SEM) and 48 ± 2 (SEM) cm. This length approximates the distance between the ascending and the terminal part of the abdominal aorta and the bifurcation into the iliac arteries. They also showed that external compression of the femoral arteries by external manual compression caused an immediate change in the configuration of the ascending aortic pressure pulse compatible with an augmentation of the reflected wave component (Fig. 3–15).

REFERENCES

1. Uther JB, Peterson KL, Shabetai R, Braunwald E: Measurement of ascending aortic flow patterns in man. J Appl Physiol 1972; 34(4):513–518.
2. Camishion RC: Basic Medical Electronics. Boston, Little, Brown, 1964, p 138.
3. Walston A, Kendall ME: Comparison of pulmonary wedge and left atrial pressure in man. Am Heart J 1973; 86:159–164.
4. Lappas D, Lell WA, Gabel JC, et al: Indirect measurement of left atrial pressure in surgical patients: Pulmonary capillary wedge and pulmonary artery diastolic pressures compared with left atrial pressures. Anesthesiology 1973; 38:394–397.
5. Shaver JA, O'Toole JD, Curtiss EJ, et al: Second heart sound: The role of altered greater and lesser circulation. Circulation 1975; American Heart Association Monograph No. 46, 58–67.
6. Gabe IT, Mason DT, Gault JH, et al: Measurement of instantaneous blood flow velocity and pressure in conscious man with a catheter-tip velocity probe. Circulation 1969; 40:603–614.
7. Gabe IT, Mason DT, Gault JH, et al: Effects of respiration on venous return and stroke volume in cardiac tamponade. Br Heart J 1970; 32:592–596.
8. Mason DT, Gabe IT, Mills CJ, et al: Application of the catheter-tip electromagnetic velocity probe in the study of the central circulation in man. Am J Med 1970; 49:465–471.
9. Shabetai R: The Pericardium. New York, Grune & Stratton, 1981.
10. Mills CJ, Gabe IT, Gault JH, et al: Pressure-flow relationships and vascular impedance in man. Cardiovasc Res 1970; 4:405–417.
11. Nichols WW, Conti CR, Walker WE, Milnor WR: Input impedance of the systemic circulation in man. Circ Res 1977; 40:451.
12. Murgo JP, Westerhof N, Giolma JP, Altobelli SA: Aortic input impedance in normal man: Relationship to pressure waveforms. Circulation 1980; 62:105–116.
13. Peterson KL, Uther JB, Shabetai R, Braunwald E: Assessment of left ventricular performance in man: Instantaneous tension-velocity-length relations obtained with the aid of an electromagnetic velocity catheter in the ascending aorta. Circulation 1973; 47:924–935.

Chapter 4

Assessment of Cardiac Pressure and Wall Forces

FRANK C. P. YIN

At the time of cardiac catheterization an accurate assessment of the pressure gradient across a stenotic valve or atherosclerotic lesion is often the critical factor in guiding therapeutic decisions. Likewise, precise measurement of chamber pressures is essential for the evaluation of chamber function, whether one uses isovolumetric indices such as the maximum rate of tension development,[1] the chamber function indices derived from a pump function approach,[2] or the end-systolic pressure-volume approach.[3-5] Evaluation of vascular function in terms of compliance, impedance, or pressure waveform analysis[6-10] also requires accurate measurement of vascular pressures.

Over and above these applications that use pressure directly, there is great interest in assessing accurately the stresses in the wall, because these are necessary to determine regional function and are believed to play a role in the regulation of regional coronary flows.[11] Unlike pressure, which is a scalar quantity, there are many components of wall stresses relating to the directions in which the forces act. Ideally, one would like to be able to measure directly the individual components of these stresses. However, this is not possible with current techniques, because the mechanical coupling with the tissue required by these methods renders the force measurements highly dependent on the degree of coupling.[12-14] Hence, almost all data on wall stresses are predictions based on mathematic models of the heart that incorporate simplified geometries with the cavity pressure serving as the load.[12, 15-22] An alternative to measuring the individual stress components is to obtain some averaged measure of the stresses. Intramyocardial pressure has been proposed as one such index. There is, however, much controversy not only about how best to make this

measurement but also about its interpretation.[23-27]

Recently, another method of indexing wall stresses using an indentation technique has been proposed.[28, 29] This method is based on the observations in isolated tissue that there is a direct relationship between wall stiffness and stress.[30-32] Thus, rather than directly measuring the in-plane stiffness, which would be subject to the same limitations as trying to measure the in-plane forces, small indentations are imposed perpendicular to the wall from which a so-called transverse stiffness (ratio of the indentation stress to strain) is obtained. Transverse stiffness has shown some promise as an index of the summated effect of the in-plane wall stresses in passive and active states.[28, 29] However, as in intramyocardial pressure, neither method provides information about shear stresses or the individual normal stress components.

Even though noninvasive methods such as Doppler ultrasonography are touted for their ability to accurately estimate some pressure gradients, especially across stenotic valves,[33-37] it should be pointed out that this method, similar to the Gorlin formulas for estimating the areas of stenotic valves, is based on a simplified version of the Bernoulli principle of fluid dynamics. This version of the principle is strictly applicable only to steady-state flow of perfect fluids under so-called streamline conditions. A perfect fluid is one that has no viscosity and is incompressible. Streamline flow means that each fluid particle travels along a distinct path that can be traced throughout the entire flow field. Another way to state this is that the flow field must not be turbulent. When the Doppler method is used to estimate the pressure gradients or the pressure half-time from the velocity data just described, it is further assumed that flow acceleration and viscous losses are negligible compared with the connective acceleration. Blood is far from being a perfect fluid—the flows in the heart and large vessels are not steady. Moreover, the flows across stenotic valves and atherosclerotic lesions are the most likely of any flows in the body to be turbulent or to contain eddies. Thus, none of the assumptions on which the Bernoulli principle is based is likely to be operative under conditions in which Doppler estimates of pressure gradients are made. These considerations seem to have been overlooked because being able to make noninvasive estimates of pressure gradients across stenotic valves is currently one of the most widely touted advantages of the Doppler method. Hence, the purportedly good correlations between directly measured and noninvasively estimated pressure gradients across stenotic valves may be more fortuitous than real and should be viewed with considerable circumspection.

Other noninvasive means of estimating central aortic pressure such as calibrated carotid pressure tracings[38, 39] and applanation tonometry[40] also are based on simplifying assumptions that severely limit their applicability. The calibrated carotid tracing assumes a strict one-to-one relationship of the linear interpolation between the diastolic and systolic pressures measured by sphygmomanometry in the brachial artery and the peak and nadir of the carotid tracing. Whether this key assumption is valid under all the conditions one is likely to see in the clinical situation (such as in the presence of aging, hypertension, and atherosclerosis) has yet to be proved conclusively. The principle underlying applanation tonometry is that the portion of the vessel under the probe is flat. If the vessel wall under the probe is either concave outward or inward, the pressure will be overestimated or underestimated, respectively. Because many factors in the tissue between the skin and the vessel can affect how the vessel is deformed by the pressure of the probe on the skin, and because one cannot view the vessel to adjust the contact pressure of the probe to ensure that the region of the vessel under the probe is flat, it is extremely unlikely that this method enables one to obtain accurate estimates of absolute pressures in the large vessels.

Thus, for the most accurate and reliable assessment of pressure—whether in the lumen of a vessel, the cavity of a heart chamber, or the interstitial space in the ventricular wall—there is no substitute for direct measurement with a suitable sensor. Accepting this, it behooves us to understand how to obtain as accurate a measurement as is necessary for each application. To do this requires some understanding of basic

principles of transducer design and how to assess transducer performance and thereby some possible sources of artifact. The remainder of this chapter discusses these issues.

DEFINITIONS

Units of Pressure

Imagine an infinitesimal cube of fluid volume that is acted on by forces. *Pressure* is defined as the force per unit area acting anywhere on the cube. Hence, the units of pressure in the centimeter-gram-second system are dynes/cm^2. In the biologic sciences, however, it is more common to express pressure in units of a millimeter of mercury, which is also called a *Torr*. For smaller values it is convenient to express pressure as centimeters of water. The interconversion among these units is easily remembered if one visualizes the pressure acting at the bottom of a column of fluid with a cross-sectional area of 1 cm^2. If the fluid is mercury with a depth of 1 mm, the pressure at the bottom of the column is 1 mm Hg. Because mercury has a density 13.6 times that of water, this column exerts a pressure equivalent to a column of water 13.6 mm (or 1.36 cm) in depth. The force exerted at the bottom of this column of water is its mass multiplied by the constant of gravitational acceleration, or

$$1.36 \text{ gm} \times 980 \text{ cm/sec}^2 = 1330 \text{ dynes}$$

Thus,

$$1 \text{ Torr} = 1 \text{ mm Hg} = 1330 \text{ dynes/cm}^2$$

Another unit in which pressure is expressed is the kilopascal, abbreviated kPa. Because a pascal is 1 N/m^2, simple algebra reveals that

$$1 \text{ kPa} = 7.5 \text{ mm Hg}$$

Harmonic Content

In discussing the adequacy of a pressure measurement system, one term that is used is the *harmonic* or *harmonic content*. The term *harmonic* means a wave whose frequency is a whole-number multiple of the frequency of another wave. The harmonics of any wave can be obtained by use of the mathematic technique called *Fourier series analysis*. This method is a means of representing any *periodically repeating, time-varying signal* as a sum of an infinite number of sine or cosine waves, or both, each of increasing frequency. Each of these waves is a harmonic of the fundamental wave, which is a sine or cosine wave with a period equal to that of the original signal. In mathematic notation, one can represent a signal x(t) with a period T as

$$x(t) = A_0/2 + \sum_{n=1}^{\infty} A_n\cos(n\omega t) + B_n\sin(n\omega t)$$

where the integer n designates the harmonic number, ω is the fundamental angular frequency ($\omega = 2\pi/T$), and the A_n/B_n represent the magnitudes of the coefficients of the nth harmonic. This equation can be rewritten as

$$x(t) = A_0/2 + \sum_{n=1}^{\infty} M_n\cos(n\omega t - \phi_n)$$

The modulus of the nth harmonic M_n is $(A_n^2 + B_n^2)^{1/2}$ and the phase angle ϕ_n is arctan (B_n/A_n). Stated another way, this equation states that this signal x(t) is composed of a mean term plus a sum of harmonics of sine and cosine waves, each with a period of T/n.

The number of harmonics required to adequately describe the signal of interest is called that signal's harmonic content. Of course, the harmonic content of any wave is, in theory, infinite. Depending on the application, however, a finite number of harmonics is usually sufficient to represent those features of the signal of interest. An example of a measured aortic pressure wave and the synthesized wave resulting from using either the first 2 or 10 harmonics is illustrated in Figure 4–1. Even with only the first 2 harmonics included, the general features of the waveform are evident. When 10 harmonics are included, almost all of the features except the very-high-frequency information near the dicrotic notch are evident. Thus, to reasonably and adequately represent the pressure wave visually, 10 harmonics are sufficient. To more quantitatively express how much

information is included at a given harmonic, one calculates the proportion of power contained at that harmonic relative to the power of the complete wave obtained by integration of the signal. One could, for example, define the harmonic content as the lowest harmonic (or frequency) for which resynthesis of the signal using that and all lower harmonics results in an acceptable proportion, for example, 95% of the total power or variance. Using this definition, the harmonic content of pressure and flow waves was found to be approximately 10,[41] with harmonics up to about 20 required in some instances.

Frequency Response

The *frequency response* of any transducer system describes the amplitude and phase response to an input signal of constant amplitude but increasing frequency. Suppose that a sine wave of given amplitude but increasing frequency is imposed on a pressure recording system. A system with a perfect frequency response would yield a signal with the same amplitude and no time (phase) shift compared with the input signal, regardless of the frequency. In reality, at some frequency the amplitude of the output signal begins to deviate from that of the input signal, and the phase of the output also differs. In general terms, if the amplitude response of the output is greater than the input, the system is underdamped. Conversely, if the output is less than the input, the system is overdamped (see detailed discussion later). Often, rather than specifying all the details of the response, the frequency response is described as the maximum frequency at which the amplitude response is considered to be flat, that is, within 5% of the perfect response.

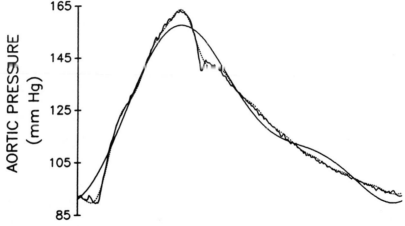

Figure 4–1. Aortic pressure wave measured with a micromanometer system *(jagged solid line)* compared with the synthesized wave resulting from using 2 *(smooth solid line)* and 10 harmonics *(dotted line)*.

AORTIC PRESSURE (mm Hg)

165

145

125

105

85

TYPES OF PRESSURE TRANSDUCERS

Four basic types of pressure transducers are likely to be encountered in either the clinical or research catheterization laboratory: (1) unbonded strain gauge (traditionally used in most catheterization facilities), (2) piezoelectric, (3) fiberoptic, and (4) servo-null micropressure. The basic principle behind all these transducers is the same. The pressure imposed on a primary sensor causes a deformation. A second sensor produces a signal proportional to the deformation that is then sensed by an external device, amplified, and recorded. In the case of the unbonded strain-gauge type of transducer, the primary sensor surface is a stiff metal diaphragm and the secondary sensors are strain gauges connected in a Wheatstone bridge arrangement. As the diaphragm is slightly deformed by the pressure, the gauges are deformed, resulting in changes in resistance. This change in resistance is then amplified and converted to a voltage that can be recorded by an external device. The major advantage of this type of transducer is its high sensitivity and stability and its relatively low cost. The major disadvantage is that the sensing elements cannot be made very small so that some type of coupling (usually via a fluid-filled catheter) is required between the site of pressure measurement and the transducer. As discussed later, this coupling can introduce significant artifacts, and it also limits the frequency response of this type of transducer system.

For piezoelectric-type transducers, piezoelectric crystals rather than wire strain gauges are used to sense displacement of a diaphragm. Otherwise, the principles of operation are the same as for the strain-gauge type. The major advantage of this type of system is that the piezoelectric crystals can be so small that the entire sensor head can be placed at the tip of a catheter. By eliminating the long fluid column, this type of transducer not only significantly increases the frequency response but also decreases the artifacts compared with the strain-gauge type transducers. This type of transducer is more fragile than the strain-gauge types and must be handled with extreme care. Additionally, the hydrophilic nature of the diaphragm-crystal bonding material can cause some transient artifacts as the junction swells when the sensor is first placed in contact with fluid. Thus, a period of stabilization in fluid is recommended before use.[42]

Fiberoptic pressure-measuring transducers employ the concept of measuring the displacement of the diaphragm by optical means. The advent of fiberoptic bundles has enabled the production of catheters containing such bundles to be used for pressure measurement. Basically, the deformation of a diaphragm is determined by two bundles of coated fibers: One bundle serves to transmit the light to the diaphragm, and the second detects the light reflected from the tip. By proper design, it is possible to make the amount of received light proportional to the displacement and hence the pressure. The major advantages of such a system are its small size, enabling placement at the tip of a catheter, and the absence of any electrical currents. The major disadvantage is the rather complex design requirements that result in higher costs than other systems.

The micropipette pressure-measuring systems employ the principle that a small change in conductivity of the fluid at the tip of a micropipette produces a large change in the resistance measured in the micropipette. The micropipette is filled with fluid (usually hypertonic sodium chloride) that has a different conductivity than the medium (e.g., plasma) whose pressure is to be measured. When the tip of the micropipette is placed into the tissue space and plasma enters the tip, a large resistance change occurs in the micropipette. A servo-null system is used to generate a counterbalancing pressure in the micropipette to push the plasma–sodium chloride interface back to its original position. This pressure is that in the plasma. The obvious advantage of this system is the ability to measure pressures in spaces on the order of a few microns in size. There is, however, a limitation of about 25 Hz in frequency response. Moreover, because the micropipettes are usually made of glass, they tend to break if there is much motion in the tissue so that contracting specimens are not easily studied. This problem has been reportedly overcome with the use of plastic micropipettes,[23] but the difficulty is that the plastic pipettes cannot be made as small as the glass ones and are more difficult to penetrate into vessels or tissue space.

ARTIFACTS IN PRESSURE MEASUREMENT

Mechanical Artifacts

Nonlinearity

To obtain absolute units of pressure, it is necessary to perform a calibration against a known source of pressure before or after use of the selected system. This is usually done using a mercury manometer because this is still the standard reference. Usually one imposes a finite set of known pressures on the system and records the deflections of the signal corresponding to this set of references. By assuming that the system is linear in the range of the imposed reference pressures, the intermediate pressures are inferred from linear interpolation. Most modern pressure transducers and amplifier systems are reasonably linear over a wide range of pressures so that the interpolations are likely to be valid. Nevertheless, to be absolutely certain, it is always a good idea to make sure that the calibrations encompass more than the entire expected pressure range because some transducers may have nonlinear responses at the extremes of their working ranges.

Hysteresis

Another potential source of artifact is *hysteresis*. This term refers to a different response depending on whether pressure on the sensor is increasing or decreasing. The presence of hysteresis markedly complicates accurate pressure measurement to such an extent that one should not use sensors with this characteristic. Hysteresis is absent in most sensors unless they get pressurized beyond their safe limits.

Harmonic Distortion

By far the most common type of artifact one is likely to face is that of harmonic distortion. This type of distortion can affect either the amplitude or phase angle, or both, of any harmonic. The amplitudes can either be exaggerated or underestimated, and the phase angles can be either advanced or retarded from their true values. This type of distortion occurs because of the finite masses of the sensing element and the medium between the sensor and the site of pressure measurement. Thus, harmonic distortion can never be completely avoided. For most modern transducers, the mass of the sensing element is so small that the distortion resulting from it is almost negligible. In the case of the external strain-gauge transducers coupled via a fluid column in a catheter to the site of pressure measurement, however, the mass of the fluid is not negligible. Rather, the pressure acting on the mass of fluid and sensor acts like a damped spring-mass system set into oscillation and leads to inevitable distortion.

Figure 4–2 illustrates simultaneous left ventricular pressures recorded with a micromanometer and a fluid-filled system in a human during routine cardiac catheterization. The overestimation of the pressures is clearly seen

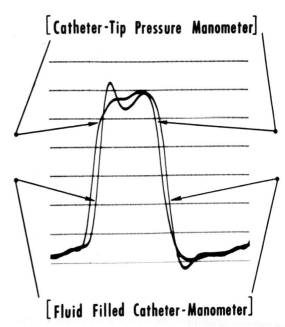

Figure 4–2. Simultaneous left ventricular pressure recorded with a micromanometer and a fluid-filled catheter system. (From Nichols WW, O'Rourke MF: McDonald's Blood Flow in Arteries. London, Edward Arnold, 1990.)

in the wide fluctuations above and below the pressure recorded by the micromanometer late in systole and early in diastole. It is clear that these distortions could result in quite inaccurate estimations of the true pressure.

Orientation Effects

In the definition of pressure presented earlier, it was stated that the pressure is the same in all directions. This is true only in the absence of flow, in which case the pressure measured is a static pressure. If there is flow, the measured pressure depends on the direction of the sensing element relative to the flow, because of the kinetic energy carried by the flowing fluid. The total pressure is the sum of the static and kinetic contributions. Thus, a sensor that is facing the flow records the sum of both the static and kinetic components because the catheter tip essentially stops the flow, converting all of the energy into pressure. Conversely, one that is facing downstream from the flow records a pressure that is the static minus the kinetic term. One that is parallel to the flow records only the static term. The magnitude of the kinetic term is approximately equal to $0.5\rho v^2$ where ρ is the density and v is velocity. In the ascending aorta, where v is about 150 cm/sec, the kinetic term is about 1.17×10^4 dynes/cm^2, or about 9 mm Hg of pressure. Thus, the kinetic contribution may not always be negligible, particularly under conditions when the flow velocity is greatly increased above normal such as with exercise, or in jets created by aortic valve obstruction or with some types of prosthetic valves.

Impact Artifacts

Because all pressure sensors are in reality strain- or deformation-sensitive elements, there is the possibility of artifacts arising if the sensor is touched by anything other than fluid or blood. This type of artifact is more common with the catheter-tipped sensors if they are impacted by tissue. In the ventricle or large vessels this impact artifact is usually easy to recognize because its very high frequency compared with the pressure signal produces a transient "spike" superimposed on the underlying pressure tracing. When one uses these sensors for measuring intramyocardial pressure, however, the artifact becomes less distinct because the intramyocardial pressure is also caused by muscle contraction. One way to ascertain that the pressure is truly a fluid pressure is to rotate the sensor to another orientation. Because there is virtually no flow in the tissue, one should record a true static pressure that is independent of orientation. If one sees an orientation effect, one must surmise that either there is a direct impact effect from the contracting muscle or that one is measuring the pressure where there is considerable flow, such as in a vascular structure. In either instance, a pressure that is affected by orientation is not a reliable estimate of intramyocardial tissue pressure.

When using fluid-filled catheters, one can also see an impact artifact resulting from valves or the ventricular walls hitting the catheter. The resultant pressure transient is transmitted through the column of fluid and produces an artifact if its frequency content is compatible with the frequency response of the system. Another type of artifact results from the "whip" of the catheter itself independent of physical contact with surrounding structures. The rapid motion of the catheter sets up acceleration of the contained fluid, whose effect is then seen in the pressure tracing. Again, these artifacts are usually of higher frequency than the underlying true signal but may be difficult to differentiate from true transients at times in the cardiac cycle such as the dicrotic notch, where high-frequency components normally reside.

Curvature Effects

One type of artifact that has not gotten the attention it deserves relates to curvature of the deformable structure within which the sensor resides. Consider a curved, membranous, fluid-containing structure with a pressure sensor in it. As the membrane is deformed by the action of surrounding structures—or by the process of introducing the sensor—the pressure in the fluid will be affected according to Laplace's law. Compared with the state with flat surfaces, if the surface is deformed so that it is concave inward, the pressure will be higher and vice versa when it is convex inward. Although the pressure measured in the fluid is the reflection of all the forces acting on the cavity, the interpretations of these pressures may be difficult. A good example is the estimation of pleural pressures from a catheter placed within neighboring structures such as the vena cava and esophagus.[43] The estimated pleural pressure is dependent on the curvature of the structure within which the catheter tip is situated. Another area in which the pressure measurements are open to question is that of intramyocardial pressure. One could question the meaning of a single intramyocardial pressure at any localized region in the heart wall. It is not clear what constitutes the "intramyocardial pressure" because the fluid pressure on one side of the curved membrane differs from that on the other side. With any number of adjoining structures, each acted on by potentially different forces and each having potentially different wall properties and curvatures, one can easily imagine a whole array of different fluid pressures. Viewed in this way, it is not at all clear that intramyocardial pressure is a well-defined entity that can be estimated with a single probe, regardless of its size. The need for techniques to calculate average pressures from large numbers of such species underlies the use of wicks and capsules for interstitial pressure measurement.[44] However, these large sensors undoubtedly cause considerable physical distortion of the very small tissue spaces in which the pressure is to be measured, with the result that the meaning of the resulting pressures is seriously open to question. The measurement of intramyocardial or tissue pressure remains clouded by these issues, and no satisfactory solution has been achieved.[25, 27]

Potential Artifacts in Physiologic Measurements

In any particular physiologic application, one or more of the mechanical artifacts may be present. Let us examine some common situations and list the circumstances wherein artifacts may be present. With most high-quality, modern transducer and pressure recording systems, the concerns of nonlinearity and hysteresis should not be issues. If one is careless about handling a transducer, however, such as inadvertently overpressurizing the chamber of a strain-gauge type of system, one can easily damage the diaphragm or the strain gauges. Assuming one has not completely damaged the sensor, a highly nonlinear response will result. Thus, one should periodically confirm that the system in use is behaving as expected.

The issue of harmonic distortion can be avoided with the use of micromanometers. Generally, however, these sensors are too expensive to warrant routine use. Thus, most catheterization laboratories and intensive care settings continue to rely on the unbonded strain-gauge type transducer. As discussed earlier, only with extreme care, including the use of degassed solutions, very stiff catheters and connections, and large-enough bore catheters, can one obtain measurements reasonably free of harmonic distortion. Usually, however, in a busy cardiac catheterization laboratory, meticulous attention to such details is, of necessity, often overlooked. In this setting, numerous potential artifacts can occur. For example, if a small amount of blood or contrast agent is left in the catheter, the decrease in diameter with the former and the increased viscosity of the latter can lead to severe overdamping. In addition, small air bubbles either introduced at the time of flushing or residing in the solutions also degrade the performance. Finally, the use of very small diameter or very soft plastic catheters, such as the flow-directed ones often used for right-sided heart catheterization, leads to artifacts. One only has to recall the often uninterpretable wild fluctuations in signals from right-sided heart catheters to see that such artifacts are indeed manifested.

Although the use of too small a catheter may produce an overdamped signal, the use of too large a catheter may disturb the flow field sufficiently to affect the measurement. For example, if one is recording pressure in a vessel with a catheter that occupies more than about 50% of the cross-sectional area of the vessel, the acceleration of the flow produced by the catheter produces a reading different from that had no catheter been present. A good rule of thumb is to use catheters that occupy less than 20% of the cross sectional area of the vessel. Similarly, if the sensor is positioned in the middle of a jet, depending on whether the sensor is pointed upstream, downstream, or perpendicular to the flow, the reading one obtains will not be representative of the average pressure in that chamber or vessel.

EVALUATING TRANSDUCER PERFORMANCE

Although harmonic distortion can be avoided by using micromanometer or fiberoptic catheter-tip transducers, practical considerations (primarily higher cost and greater fragility) usually preclude their use for routine diagnostic cardiac catheterization. Thus, because fluid-filled systems are still the most common ones used in most cardiac catheterization laboratories, it is useful to discuss in some detail how to assess and then correct for the distortion. To achieve optimal responses from a fluid-filled system, the solutions used to fill the catheter and transducer dome should contain a minimum amount of microbubbles of air. This can be achieved by degassing or boiling the solutions and filling the catheter and transducer extremely slowly (i.e., 1 to 2 mL/hr). Because this is usually precluded in a busy catheterization laboratory, one usually has less than optimal systems. Figure 4–3 compares the normalized amplitude responses of a micromanometer with those of a Statham P23 ID transducer connected to a commonly used 120-cm long, 7-French angiographic catheter and a 7-French flow-directed thermodilution catheter. The phase differences between the latter two systems compared with the micromanometer system, calculated by standard Fourier analysis of the signals, are also shown. All three systems were tested simultaneously in a chamber subjected to a sinusoidal pressure of constant amplitude and increasing frequency. The two fluid-filled systems were prepared in the manner found in most catheterization laboratory settings; that is, all visible air bubbles were carefully removed, but degassed saline was not used. The amplitude response of all three systems are identical only for very low frequencies. As the frequency is successively increased, the micromanometer response remains constant, whereas beginning at frequencies of about 5 and 10 Hz for the flow-directed and angiographic catheter systems, respectively, the responses begin to deviate considerably from that of the micromanometer. At low frequencies both fluid filled systems yield overestimations of the true amplitude, and the phase responses are nearly 180 degrees out of phase. This exaggeration can be considerable at certain frequencies. Thereafter, as frequency is further increased, there is progressive underestimation of the amplitude and a flattening of the phase lag. This type of overestimation followed by underestimation is typical of systems that are underdamped, as discussed in more detail later.

If one does not have the capability to di-

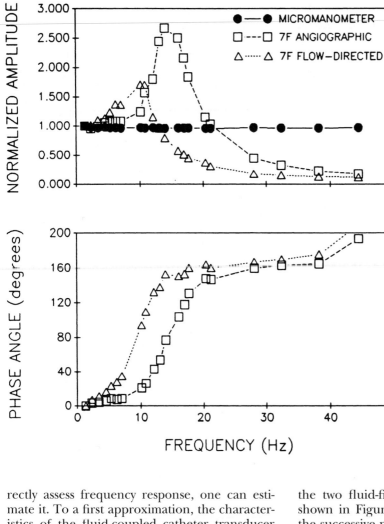

Figure 4–3. Amplitude and phase responses of micromanometer, 7-French angiographic, and 7-French flow-directed catheter systems to a sine wave pressure input of constant amplitude and increasing frequency. The phase of micromanometer (not shown) is zero at all frequencies.

rectly assess frequency response, one can estimate it. To a first approximation, the characteristics of the fluid-coupled catheter transducer system behaves like a damped spring-mass system. Thus, its response is governed by a linear second-order equation whose solution is well known. Before applying the theory, however, one must experimentally determine two important parameters of the pressure system in question—namely the amount of damping and the natural frequency, which is the frequency at which the undamped system would oscillate when set into motion. These parameters can easily be obtained by performing a so-called "pop test." The tip of the catheter is placed in a chamber with a thin rubber membrane cover. The pressure in the chamber is raised to a steady level and is suddenly lowered by "popping" the rubber membrane. We have found that applying a lighted match to the membrane produces a cleaner signal than does mechanically rupturing the membrane. Regardless, the response of the pressure measuring system following the sudden decrease in pressure is recorded at fast speed. The responses of

the two fluid-filled systems to such a test are shown in Figure 4–4. T is the period between the successive peaks, and the ratio between successive peaks or troughs is denoted by

$$\delta = h_{i+1}/h_i$$

Several δs are averaged from which one obtains the logarithmic decrement,

$$\Delta = \ln(\delta)$$

Other parameters necessary to describe this second order system are the damping constant,

$$\beta_o = \Delta/T$$

the undamped natural frequency,

$$\omega_o = (4\pi^2 + \Delta^2)^{1/2}/T$$

and the damping ratio

$$\beta = \beta_o/\omega_o$$

For the two systems we tested, the flow-directed and angiographic catheter systems had undamped natural frequency of 120 and 240 Hz and damping ratios of 0.12 and 0.08, respec-

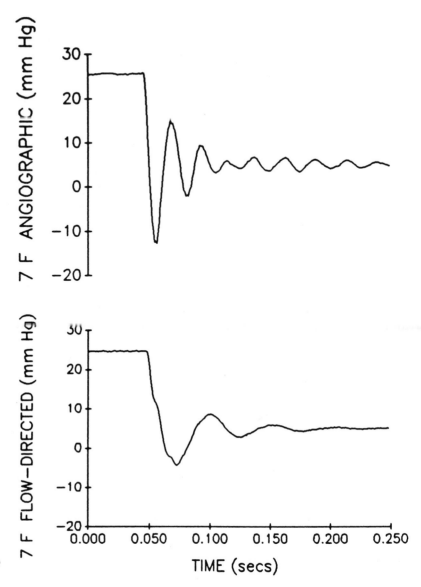

Figure 4–4. The results of the flow-directed and angiographic catheter systems of Figure 4–3 to a transient "pop" test.

tively. The situation with smaller-sized or differing material catheters must be examined but is not likely to be substantially different. Thus, to accurately estimate a signal with a harmonic content much higher than 10 to 20 Hz using any of the fluid-filled catheter systems, one must either use a micromanometer or apply some corrections to the fluid-filled system.

The theoretic solution for a second-order damped spring-mass system set into oscillation by sinusoidal waves of unit amplitude at various damping ratios is illustrated in Figure 4–5. In both panels the abscissa is the driving frequency divided by the undamped natural frequency. The ordinate in the upper panel is the relative (with respect to the input signal) amplitude, and in the lower panel is the phase lag ex-

pressed as degrees. Several features of these graphs are of interest. For a damping ratio of 1.0, which is called *critical,* the relative amplitude decreases almost linearly with frequency. The phase lag is, however, a nonlinear function of frequency. In contrast, for a relative damping ratio of 0.7, which is called *optimal,* the maximum frequency is achieved when the relative amplitude remains at 1. Above this frequency the response falls off. Because of the presence of this largest "flat" range of frequencies, an optimally damped system is quite desirable. The frequency at which the amplitude ratio begins to deviate from 1 is a measure of the upper range of useful frequencies for the system. Note also that the phase lag for optimal damping is nearly linear with frequency. This feature makes

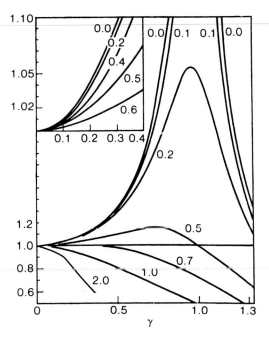

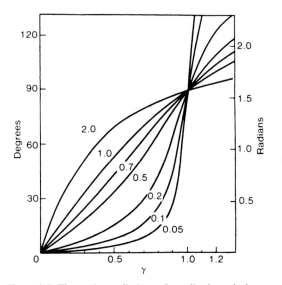

Figure 4–5. Theoretic predictions of amplitude and phase responses of a second-order damped spring-mass system to a sine wave input of constant amplitude and increasing frequency (see text). (From Milnor WR: Hemodynamics, 2nd ed. Baltimore, Williams & Wilkins, 1989.)

that the theoretic predictions are quite close to the experimental observations.

Thus, although it is not difficult to estimate the undamped natural frequency and the relative damping, it is quite difficult, in practice, to appropriately correct for the characteristics of a particular system to obtain a relatively artifact-free estimate of the various pressure harmonics. Because typical fluid-filled systems are highly underdamped rather than being optimally damped, these corrections are highly dependent on the value of the damping ratio and hence are subject to considerable uncertainty. Alternatively, one could, in theory, alter some of the properties of the system to make the damping closer to optimal (such as by using catheters with different wall material and using more viscous fluid in the catheter). Although these alterations may make the damping more optimal, they are also likely to lower the undamped natural frequency and thus decrease the range in which the amplitude response is flat. In actuality, as discussed earlier, uncontrollable factors, such as the presence of minute air bubbles or a small layer of thrombi on the wall of the catheter, will alter the system response so much that it would be difficult to estimate exactly what the system properties were at the instant the recording was made and thus make corrections extremely difficult.

One can increase the range of useful frequencies and minimize the need for phase corrections by greatly increasing the natural frequency and decreasing the damping ratio. Even with extreme care, however, the natural frequencies for fluid-filled systems cannot be increased much higher than 200 Hz. In contrast, micromanometers have very high natural frequencies. For example, the system I use has a natural frequency close to 20,000 Hz. Thus, even though the damping is small, the upper limit for a flat amplitude response could be considerably greater than 100 to 200 Hz. Likewise, with such a high natural frequency and low damping ratio, it is unnecessary to apply any corrections for phase lag. These considerations are the motivation for using such high-frequency-response micromanometer systems when precise pressure recordings are desired.

SELECTING A PRESSURE MEASUREMENT SYSTEM

Based on the considerations discussed thus far, it should be reasonably easy to select the optimal pressure measurement system for a particular application. Aside from the obvious con-

it easy to apply phase corrections to a system that is optimally damped. The other responses shown are for an overdamped and underdamped system. For the former, the amplitude response is less than 1 for almost all frequencies. For the latter, the amplitude response is greater than 1 for a certain range of frequencies. Comparing Figures 4–3 with 4–5, we see siderations of cost, matching the available amplifier and recording system, reliability, and ruggedness, the first technical consideration is the harmonic content of the desired signal. For mean pressures or very-low-frequency content signals, such as in the venous system, any of the systems described should be suitable, and it would not make much sense to use the more complex and expensive systems. For measurement of vascular and ventricular pressures during routine diagnostic catheterization, the strain-gauge systems should suffice as long as one keeps in mind their limitations and, more important, their potential artifacts. For hemodynamic research purposes, there is probably no substitute for a catheter-tipped micromanometer system, because of its superior accuracy combined with good frequency response. Balanced against the advantages, however, are the relatively higher cost and greater fragility of such a system compared with the standard strain-gauge transducers.

For measuring intramyocardial or interstitial pressure, my own bias is that the micropressure systems are probably the most reliable because they produce the least amount of physical distortion to the tissue spaces. Nevertheless, one should still be cognizant of the fact that, despite their relatively small tips, the micropipette inevitably produces some tissue stretching that may result in a disturbed measurement compared with the situation had no sensor been present. Recessed-tipped micromanometer systems have been designed to be free of impact artifacts, although their much larger size compared with the micropressure systems introduces the unknown aspect of greater tissue damage and distortion. Unprotected micromanometers potentially experience impact artifacts and must be used with great care. In addition, their large size with the attendant unavoidable tissue damage and distortion resulting in a difficult to quantify an amount of artifact is also a disadvantage.

REFERENCES

1. Peterson KL, Skloven D, Ludbrook P, et al: Comparison of isovolumic and ejection phase indices of myocardial performance in man. Circulation 1974; 49:1088–1101.
2. Elzinga G, Westerhof N: How to quantify pump function of the heart. Circ Res 1979; 44:303–308.
3. Kass DA, Maughan WL: From "emax" to pressure-volume relations: A broader view. Circulation 1988; 77: 1203–1212.
4. Sagawa K, Maughan L, Suga H, Sunagawa K: Cardiac Contraction and the Pressure-Volume Relationship. New York, Oxford University Press, 1988.
5. Suga H, Kitabatake A, Sagawa K: End-systolic pressure determines stroke volume from fixed end-diastolic volume in the isolated canine left ventricle under a constant contractile state. Circ Res 1979; 44:238–249.
6. Liu ZR, Brin KP, Yin FCP: Estimation of arterial compliance: An improved method and evaluation of current methods. Am J Physiol 1986; 251:H588–H600.
7. Murgo JP, Westerhof N, Giolma JP, Altobelli SA: Effects of exercise on aortic input impedance and pressure wave forms in normal humans. Circ Res 1981; 48:334–343.
8. Murgo JP, Westerhof N, Giolma JP, Altobelli SA: Manipulation of ascending aortic pressure and flow wave reflections with the Valsalva maneuver: Relationship to input impedance. Circulation 1981; 63:122–132.
9. Nichols WW, Conti CR, Walker WE, Milnor WR: Input impedance of the systemic circulation in man. Circ Res 1977; 40:451–458.
10. Ting CT, Brin KP, Lin SJ, et al: Arterial hemodynamics in human hypertension. J Clin Invest 1986; 78:1462–1471.
11. Hoffman JIE, Spaan JAE: Pressure-flow relations in coronary circulation. Physiol Rev 1990; 70:331–390.
12. Burns JW, Covell JW, Myers R, Ross J Jr: Comparison of directly measured left ventricular wall stress calculated from geometric reference figures. Circ Res 1971; 28:611–621.
13. Feigl EO, Simon GA, Fry DL: Auxotonic and isometric cardiac force transducers. J Appl Physiol 1967; 23: 597–600.
14. Huisman RM, Elzinga G, Westerhof N, Sipkema P: Measurement of left ventricular wall stress. Cardiovasc Res 1980; 14:142–153.
15. Falsetti HL, Mates RE, Grant C, et al: Left ventricular wall stress calculated from one-plane cineangiography. Circ Res 1970; 26:71–83.
16. Ghista DN, Sandler H: An analytic elastic-viscoelastic model for the shape and forces in the left ventricle. J Biomech 1969; 2:35–47.
17. Huisman RM, Sipkema P, Westerhof N, Elzinga G: Comparison of models used to calculate left ventricular wall force. Med Biol Eng Comput 1980; 18:133–144.
18. Janz RF, Grimm AF: Finite-element model for the mechanical behavior of the left ventricle. Circ Res 1972; 30:244–252.
19. McHale PA, Greenfield JC Jr: Evaluation of several geometric models for estimation of left ventricular circumferential wall stress. Circ Res 1973; 33:303–312.
20. Mirsky I: Left ventricular stresses in the intact human heart. Biophys J 1969; 9:189–208.
21. Wong AYK, Rautaharju PM: Stress distribution within the left ventricular wall approximated as a thick ellipsoidal shell. Am Heart J 1968; 75:649–662.
22. Yin FCP: Ventricular wall stress. Circ Res 1981; 49: 829–842.
23. Heineman FW, Grayson J: Transmural distribution of intramyocardial pressure measured by micropipette technique. Am J Physiol 1985; 249:H1216–H1223.
24. Nematzadeh D, Rose JC, Schryver T, et al: Analysis of methodology for measurement of intramyocardial pressure. Basic Res Cardiol 1984; 79:86–97.
25. Rabbany SY, Kresh JY, Noordergraaf A: Intramyocardial pressure: Interaction of myocardial fluid pressure and fiber stress. Am J Physiol 1989; 257:H357–H364.
26. Stein PD, Sabbah HN, Marzilli M, Blick EF: Comparison of the distribution of intramyocardial pressure across the canine left ventricular wall in the beating heart during diastole and in the arrested heart. Circ Res 1980; 47:258–267.
27. Halperin HR, Chew PC, Weisfeldt ML, et al: Transverse stiffness: A method for estimation of myocardial wall stress. Circ Res 1987; 61:695–703.

28. Halperin HR, Chew PC, Humphrey JD, Yin FCP: Transverse stiffness can distinguish active from passive wall stress in the isolated ventricular septum. Circulation 1986; 76:II-289.

29. Loeffler L, Sagawa K: A one-dimensional viscoelastic model of cat heart muscle studied by small-length perturbations during isometric contraction. Circ Res 1975; 36:498–512.

30. Spurgeon HA, Thorne PR, Yin FCP, et al: Increased dynamic stiffness of trabeculae carneae from senescent rats. Am J Physiol 1977; 232:H373–H380.

31. Templeton GH, Donald TC, Mitchell JH, Hefner LL: Dynamic stiffness of papillary muscle during contraction and relaxation. Am J Physiol 1973; 224:693–698.

32. Hatle L, Brubakk A, Tromsdal A, Angelsen B: Noninvasive assessment of pressure drop in mitral stenosis by Doppler ultrasound. Br Heart J 1978; 40:131–140.

33. Hatle L, Angelsen B, Tromsdal A: Noninvasive assessment of atrioventricular pressure half-time by Doppler ultrasound. Circulation 1979; 60:1096–1104.

34. Hatle L, Angelsen B, Tromsdal A: Noninvasive assessment of aortic stenosis by Doppler ultrasound. Br Heart J 1980; 43:284–292.

35. Holen J, Aaslid R, Landmark K, Simonsen S: Determination of pressure gradient in mitral stenosis with a noninvasive ultrasound Doppler technique. Acta Med Scand 1976; 199:455–460.

36. Holen J, Simonsen S: Determination of pressure gradient in mitral stenosis with Doppler echocardiography. Br Heart J 1979; 41:529–535.

37. Borow KM, Green LH, Grossman W, Braunwald E: Left ventricular end-systolic stress-shortening and stress-length relations in humans: Normal values and sensitivity to inotropic state. Am J Cardiol 1982; 50:1301–1308.

38. Borow KM, Colan SD, Neumann A: Altered left ventricular mechanics in patients with valvular aortic stenosis and coarctation of the aorta: Effects on systolic performance and late outcome. Circulation 1985; 72:515–522.

39. Kelly R, Karamanoglu M, Gibbs H, et al: Noninvasive carotid pressure wave registration as an indicator of ascending aortic pressure. J Vasc Med Biol 1989; 1: 241–247.

40. Milnor WR: Hemodynamics, 2nd ed. Baltimore, Williams & Wilkins, 1989.

41. Yin FCP, Guzman PA, Brin KP, et al: Effect of nitroprusside on hydraulic vascular loads on the right and left ventricle of patients with heart failure. Circulation 1983; 67:1330–1339.

42. Tsitlik JE, Halperin HR, Guerci AD, et al: Augmentation of pressure in a vessel indenting the surface of the lung. Ann Biomed Eng 1987; 15:259–284.

43. Wiig H, Reed RK, Aukland K: Measurement of interstitial fluid pressure: Comparison of methods. Ann Biomed Eng 1986; 14:139–151.

44. Westerhof N: Physiological hypotheses—intramyocardial pressure: A new concept, suggestions for measurement. Basic Res Cardiol 1990; 85:105–119.

Chapter 5

Measurement of Blood Flow

RALPH SHABETAI
VALMIK BHARGAVA

CARDIAC OUTPUT

Normal Physiology

Before details are presented regarding measurement of cardiac output in the cardiac catheterization laboratory, it is appropriate to review briefly the relevant physiology.[1] The normal cardiac output is often stated to be between 5 and 6 L/min for an average-sized young adult male. However, as we shall see, cardiac output is changed by a number of physiologic factors. Cardiac output is often expressed as cardiac index, that is, cardiac output divided by body surface area. An average body surface area for Western males is 1.73 m²; thus, the normal cardiac index is 3.5 L/min/m². Although cardiac index is in common use, the underlying rationale can be disputed in that it may have been more appropriate to normalize cardiac output by body weight. When normal subjects are studied, more variation is found in cardiac index than in the oxygen saturation of mixed venous blood, which remains at 75% when basal tissue needs for oxygen are adequately met by a normal cardiac output. The variation in cardiac index results in part from errors in estimating body surface area, but in greater part from individual variations in basal metabolic rate. In this regard, it should be noted that cardiac output is directly proportional to metabolic rate.

In cardiac catheterization laboratories in the 1990s, a significant proportion of cardiac catheterization procedures is carried out in older patients. It is therefore important to recognize that cardiac output decreases with age, perhaps by as much as 25 mL/m²/yr.[1, 2] The cardiac index of newborns is lower than that of young children, but this finding is an artifact based on the low body surface area for weight in neonates. By the age of 45 years, cardiac index typically decreases to 3 L/min/m², representing a cardiac output of 5.2 L/min, assuming an average body build. Both heart rate and stroke volume decline with increasing age, but the decline in stroke volume exceeds that in heart rate.

Pathophysiologic Variations

A number of complicating factors may be present in patients coming to the cardiac catheterization laboratory for procedures that include measurement of cardiac output. Important among these factors are anxiety, hypoxia, pulmonary disease, liver disease, hyperthyroidism, and anemia, all of which elevate cardiac output, often by a considerable amount, and sedation or hypovolemia, which may lower cardiac output.

The effects of exercise on cardiac output are discussed in detail in Chapter 20. Here it suffices to mention that normal, young, well-trained people can increase cardiac output sixfold and extraction of oxygen by the tissues threefold, thus increasing oxygen availability to the tissue by a factor of 18.[3] When normal subjects exercise, their increased demand for oxygen is provided in part by increasing cardiac output and in part by increasing oxygen extraction (arteriovenous oxygen difference).

MEASUREMENT TECHNIQUES

Measurement of the cardiac output is a fundamental task in the cardiac catheterization laboratory. The two methods most commonly applied are (1) the direct method of Fick and (2) the use of an extraneous indicator like indocyanine green or cold saline, in place of the naturally occurring indicator, oxygen. The Fick principle states that the uptake of a substance by an organ is the product of blood flow to the organ and the difference in concentration of that substance between the artery supplying it and the vein draining it. In the absence of a pathologic shunt, and for the moment ignoring physiologic shunts, systemic blood flow, integrated over several heart beats, is identical to pulmonary blood flow. Thus, to measure cardiac output by the method of Fick, it suffices to measure pulmonary blood flow.

Fick Principle

According to the Fick principle, which is based on the conservation of mass under steady-state conditions, the rate at which a substance leaves a system is equal to the rate at which it enters. This principle is commonly applied to oxygen transport to derive cardiac output. Consider that blood containing 160 mL/L of oxygen enters the lung from the pulmonary artery and that, while in the lung, 250 mL/min of oxygen are added to the blood such that the concentration of oxygen in blood leaving the lung is 200 mL/L. Under steady-state conditions, the rate at which oxygen leaves the lung via the pulmonary veins is equal to the rate at which it entered the lung from the pulmonary artery plus the rate at which oxygen is added to it by ventilation during its passage through the lung (Fig. 5–1). The derivation of cardiac output, or pulmonary blood flow, based on this principle appears in Equation 1.

$$\text{CO (L} \cdot \text{min}^{-1}) = \frac{\text{O}_2 \text{ consumption (mL} \cdot \text{min}^{-1})}{(\text{C}_{\text{PVO}_2 \text{ or SAO}_2} - \text{C}_{\text{PAO}_2})} \quad (1)$$

where CO = cardiac output, $\text{C}_{\text{PVO}_2 \text{ or SAO}_2}$ = pulmonary vein or systemic artery oxygen con-

centration, and C_{PAO_2} = pulmonary artery oxygen concentration.

In some laboratories, arteriovenous oxygen difference is expressed in milliliters per 100 milliliters (mL%) instead of milliliters per liter, in which case it is necessary to divide the numerator (oxygen consumption) by 10 to obtain cardiac output in liters per minute.

It is not easy to measure oxygen consumption, and significant errors may also creep into the measurement of the oxygen content of arterial and mixed venous blood. It is therefore critically important that persons whose responsibility it is to interpret hemodynamic data thoroughly understand the Fick principle, appreciate the limitations of its application in the cardiac catheterization laboratory, and become familiar with what values to expect on the technician's worksheet. It is unwise simply to look at the bottom line, a practice that may eventually lead to acceptance of an erroneous cardiac output.

The Fick equation asks for the amount of oxygen delivered per unit of time from the lung to the blood. This value cannot be directly determined in the laboratory; instead, one must substitute the rate of oxygen flow into the lungs and assume that, during the period of determination of cardiac output, the amount of oxygen leaving the lungs, and thus entering the blood, is precisely the amount entering the lungs. This balance is true only when lung volume remains constant during the measurement. Regrettably, this often is not the case, but rather changes in lung volume due to factors such as changing

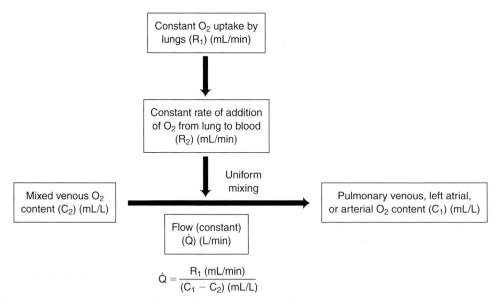

Figure 5–1. Schematic representation of the principles underlying the direct method of Fick for measurement of cardiac output ($\dot{Q}$). R_1 and R_2 are assumed to be equal and are *estimated by* VO_2. $C_1 - C_2$ is the arteriovenous O_2 difference.

patterns of respiration and a shift in patient posture are taking place. This is a major reason why a steady-state is critical to the Fick principle. The Fick principle simply does not hold if the rate of oxygen consumption differs from the rate of its delivery to the blood stream, or if either cardiac output or oxygen consumption changes during the measurement.

When cardiac catheterization was first introduced into clinical practice, enormous efforts were made to ensure the basal steady-state during determination of cardiac output. The day before the procedure was to be carried out, the patient was familiarized with the laboratory, equipment, and personnel and was asked to practice breathing through a respiratory valve with its large, uncomfortable mouthpiece and with the nose clipped to prevent nasal respiration. The procedure proper was carried out early the next morning after a night's fast, so that the output obtained would be the basal output. The pace in today's cardiac catheterization laboratories does not permit any of these approaches. Few patients brought to the laboratory are in a basal state, and many are not even in steady-state when cardiac output is measured.

Measurement of oxygen consumption is time-consuming and demands the best efforts of patient, physician, and technician. Not surprisingly, cardiologists have sought means to obtain cardiac output without measuring oxygen consumption. (The use of indicators other than oxygen are discussed later.) Another way to avoid measuring oxygen consumption is to substitute a predicted value for oxygen consumption for the measured value. The predicted value is obtained from tables in which the influence of age, gender, and heart rate is taken into consideration.[4] The data were derived from careful measurements of normal subjects spanning a wide age range. In reality, it makes no more sense to assume a person's oxygen consumption than to assume the height or weight. When one consults the original sources from which normal values for oxygen consumption are derived, one finds considerable variation, for example, from 110 to 160 ml/min/m². This degree of variability, together with the problems concerning basal and steady-states, significantly undermines the worth of the predicted value of oxygen consumption.

The method of Fick has great advantages over other methods of determining cardiac output in that it yields not only the cardiac output but also oxygen consumption and the oxygen content of mixed venous blood and systemic arterial blood, all of which are of great physiologic and clinical significance. Correctly measured, oxygen consumption identifies the metabolic state and arterial oxygen saturation is a measure of ventilation, whereas cardiac performance is directly related to the content of oxygen in mixed venous blood.

Under basal conditions in normal human subjects, the body tissues extract 25% of the oxygen delivered by the cardiac output, so that the normal value for mixed venous oxygen saturation is 75% of capacity and its partial pressure is 40 mm Hg. When cardiac output is less than normal, the tissues meet their demands for oxygen by increasing extraction; thus, the percentage of saturation and tension of oxygen in mixed venous blood decrease. Conversely, in high output states, the mixed venous oxygen saturation is higher than normal.

Measurement of Oxygen Consumption

To determine the rate of oxygen consumption, it is necessary to measure ventilation and to analyze the oxygen content of expired air. Ventilation can be measured by collecting all the exhaled air over a timed period (usually 3 minutes). The Douglas bag or the Tissot spirometer is most commonly used for this purpose. To collect all the expired air, the patient breathes through a low-resistance respiratory valve attached to a mouthpiece similar to that used by scuba divers. The patient inhales room air through the valve and exhales through it into the collecting system. The mouthpiece is furnished with a large rubber flange around which the patient seals the lips firmly to prevent leakage of air. The mouthpiece also contains two prongs on which the patient can bite to help maintain a comfortable position of the valve. A padded clip is placed on the nose to completely eliminate nasal respiration. The standard Douglas bag has a capacity of 60 L and offers minimal resistance to exhalation. It is provided with a valve and has a small side-arm for removing gas samples for analysis. When the valve is shut, the patient exhales through the connecting tubing and valve into the room air. When the valve is open, all expired air is delivered to the Douglas bag. The initial 2 or 3 minutes are used with the valve turned to room air to familiarize the patient with the apparatus and allow the establishment of a respiratory pattern that will not change during the actual collection. During this preliminary period, ambient air is washed out of the connecting tubing and is replaced by the patient's exhaled air. The valve of the Douglas bag is then turned on and the Douglas bag is allowed to partially fill. The valve is then turned off again and the Douglas bag is disconnected

Table 5–1. **Pressure Correction Factor (mm Hg) for Humidity From Saturated to Dry Gases***

Temperature (°C)	Pressure (mm Hg)	Temperature (°C)	Pressure (mm Hg)	Temperature (°C)	Pressure (mm Hg)	Temperature (°C)	Pressure (mm Hg)
20.0	17.5	24.5	23.0	29.0	30.0	33.5	38.8
20.5	18.0	25.0	23.8	29.5	30.9	34.0	39.9
21.0	18.6	25.5	24.4	30.0	31.8	34.5	41.0
21.5	19.2	26.0	25.2	30.5	32.7	35.0	42.2
22.0	19.8	26.5	25.9	31.0	33.7	35.5	43.4
22.5	20.4	27.0	26.7	31.5	34.7	36.0	44.6
23.0	21.1	27.5	27.5	32.0	35.7	36.5	45.8
23.5	21.7	28.0	28.3	32.5	36.7	37.0	47.0
24.0	22.4	28.5	29.2	33.0	37.7	37.5	48.4

*To find the correction factor (1) read the pressure value corresponding to the room temperature and (2) subtract from the atmospheric pressure.

and completed evacuated. Thereafter, the bag is reconnected after which the valve is turned to the bag, and a stopwatch is started simultaneously. To determine cardiac output at rest, expired air is usually collected for about 3 minutes, after which the valve is returned so the patient is exhaling into the room and, simultaneously, the stopwatch is stopped and the precise time of collection is recorded. A sample of exhaled air is removed from the side-arm of the Douglas bag and its volume is noted, after which the contents of the bag are expressed either into a wet test meter or into a Tissot spirometer to determine the volume of expired air.

When a Tissot spirometer is used on line instead of a Douglas bag, the procedure is similar. The spirometer and its connecting tubing must again be completely rinsed by the patient's expired air to remove all traces of ambient air. Thereafter, the volume of expired air is determined from the initial and final readings on the instrument.

Perhaps the most common cause of an invalid measure of cardiac output by the method of Fick is failure to collect all the expired air. When the nose clip is applied, it must be ascertained that the patient cannot breathe through the nose. As the procedure progresses, care should be taken to ensure that the nose clip has not slipped. The patient is required to maintain a leak-proof seal with the lips while biting on the prongs of the mouthpiece. Leaking around the mouthpiece is a common source of error, and vigilant attention to this detail on the part of the cardiac catheterization team and the patient is mandatory. Less commonly, the leak is in the valve, tubing, or bag, all of which should

be checked before every procedure and monitored by means of a good preventive maintenance program. Ruptured tympanic membrane is a surprising major source of leak, and the physician should ascertain that this condition does not exist before attempting to measure oxygen consumption. In a rigorous laboratory, measurement of oxygen consumption, like other scientific measurements, should be performed in duplicate. When a Douglas bag or Tissot spirometer is used to collect expired air, the physician should insist that air gas analysis be carried out promptly after the collection is complete; otherwise, there is a tendency for gas to diffuse through the theoretically impervious material of the Douglas bag or via leaks in the Tissot spirometer. When the patient has been oversedated, the volume of expired air and the oxygen consumption are lower than normal, even when the measurement has been carried out correctly. If the patient is excited, nervous, febrile, or thyrotoxic, the volume of expired air and the oxygen consumption are often increased above normal levels.

It is unnecessary for the cardiologist to be able to perform the procedures necessary for measuring oxygen consumption, still less to become proficient in performing the chemical analysis. However, all physicians should be familiar with the anticipated values for gas volumes and concentrations so they can check the veracity of the final result (Fig. 5–2).

Strictly speaking, to measure the rate of oxygen consumption, one should know the oxygen content and the volumes of both inspired (room) air and expired air. Oxygen consumption is then given by Equation 2 (see below).

$$\text{Oxygen consumption} = \frac{\text{Volume of inspired air} \cdot \% \, O_2 \, - \, \text{Volume of expired air} \cdot \% \, O_2}{\text{Duration of collection of expired air}} \quad (2)$$

Name: _John Doe_   Date: _September 13, 1993_

Height: _175_ cm   Weight: _69_ kg   BSA: _1.83_ m^2

a.	Barometric pressure:	_756_ mm Hg
b.	Room temperature:	_22°C_ (273 + 22°K)
c.	O_2 fractional concentration in expired air	0.1732
	O_2 fractional concentration in inspired air at STPD	0.2093
d.	CO_2 fractional concentration in expired air	0.0265
	CO_2 fractional concentration in inspired air at STPD	0.0004
e.	Sample volume	0.03 L
f.	Tissot: Final	588 mm
g.	Tissot: Initial	418 mm
h.	Tissot: Difference (**f** − **g**) = 588 − 418	170 mm
j.	Volume collected (**h** × 0.1332*) = 170 × 0.1332	22.6 L
k.	Collection time	3.0 min
m.	Ventilation at ATPS [(**j** + **e**)/**k**] = (total volume)/time = 22.67/3.0	7.56 L/min
n.	Barometric pressure correction for humidity (Table 5–1)	19.8 mm Hg
p.	Ventilation at STPD:	
	m × (**a** − **n**)/760 × 273/(**b** + 273) = 7.56 × (756 − 19.8)/760 × 273/(22 + 273)	6.78 L/min
q.	Fractional concentration of N_2 in expired air:	
	1 − **c** − **d** − **n/a** = 1 − 0.1732 − 0.0265 − 19.8/756 =	0.7741
r.	Haldane correction factor for O_2 (**q** × 0.2647 − **c**) = 0.7741 × 0.2647 − 0.1732	0.0317
s.	Oxygen consumption (**p** × **r** × 1000) = 6.78 × 0.0317 × 1000	215 mL/min
t.	Haldane correction factor for CO_2:	
	(**d** − **q** × 0.0004) = 0.0265 − 0.7741 × 0.0004	0.0262
u.	CO_2 production (**p** × **t** × 1000) = 6.78 × 0.0262 × 1000	177 mL/min
v.	O_2 consumption index (**s/BSA**) = 215/1.83	117 mL/min/m^2
w.	Respiratory gas exchange ratio (**u/s**) = 177/215	0.82

* The calibration factor for each Tissot spirometer is different. In this example it is 0.1332 L/mm.
BSA, body surface area.

Figure 5–2. Example showing the calculation of O_2 consumption and CO_2 production using the Douglas bag and Tissot spirometer method.

However, the volumes of inspired air and expired air are not identical because, during normal basal respiration, the volume of oxygen consumed slightly exceeds the volume of carbon dioxide produced, resulting in a gas exchange ratio (respiratory quotient) less than unity and usually in the vicinity of 0.86. A good method for determining the true volume of inspired air is to measure the concentration of nitrogen in inspired air and expired air. Nitrogen is an inert gas and thus is neither consumed nor produced during respiration. It therefore can be used as a volume indicator according to Equation 3 (see below).

In many laboratories, the difference in the volumes of inspired air and expired air is assumed to be negligible. In this instance nitrogen contents are not measured, but ventilation is simply taken as the volume of air exhaled during the collection period.

The concentrations of oxygen, nitrogen, and carbon dioxide in the inspired room air can be determined from standard tables after ascertaining the barometric pressure and atmospheric temperature. A good-quality barometer is standard equipment in the cardiac catheterization laboratory. The classic earlier studies of oxygen consumption and carbon dioxide production in humans and animals were performed with the micro-Scholander apparatus. With this ingenious device, it was possible to measure oxygen content to an accuracy of 0.002 volume percent (vol%). The technique is time consuming and laborious and requires the services of a highly trained technician. Not surprisingly, it is little used in today's busy cardiac catheterization laboratories. The content of these gases in expired air can be obtained by a variety of devices that are simpler and much faster to use than the micro-Scholander. These include devices

$$\frac{\text{Volume of inspired air at STP (unknown)}}{\text{Volume of expired air at STP (measured)}} = \frac{\% \ N_2 \ \text{in expired air (measured)}}{\% \ N_2 \ \text{in inspired air (known)}} \tag{3}$$

such as the Beckman or Radiometer instruments, which measure the partial pressure of the gases from which their volumetric content can be calculated. Alternatively, instruments such as the Lex-O_2 Con, which contain a fuel cell capable of accurately determining the oxygen content of air samples, may be used. In some laboratories this determination is made on a mass spectrometer. Figure 5–2 gives a step-by-step procedure to calculate oxygen consumption using the Tissot spirometer for exhaled gas volume.

On-line Methods for Measurement of Oxygen Consumption

Although many laboratories still use the Douglas bag or the Tissot spirometer to measure the volume of expired air, in many other laboratories this method has been abandoned in favor of measurement of oxygen consumption on-line, using a system comprising a flowmeter to measure ventilation and gas analyzers to measure the carbon dioxide and oxygen content of the air passing over them. Two methods are available: the open-flow system and the closed-flow system.

In the open-flow system, the patient's head and neck are placed in a large, loose-fitting mask through which air is sucked over the face at a known rate fast enough to prevent any of the expired air from leaking out. The expired air passes through a mixing chamber at the output port, where it is continuously monitored for the concentration of oxygen and carbon dioxide. The purpose of the mixing chamber is to ensure a true mixed-air sample from the alveoli and the anatomic dead space. Knowing the flow rate of the gas and the difference in concentration of oxygen and carbon dioxide in the inspired air and expired air, one can calculate the oxygen consumption and carbon dioxide production from the Fick equation.

In the closed-flow system, the subject breathes through a valve identical to that used for the Douglas bag or Tissot technique, or a pneumotachometer may be used. The expired air is passed into a mixing chamber and, as it leaves, is continuously sampled for oxygen and carbon dioxide concentrations. The oxygen consumption is calculated from the flow rate and the difference in concentration of oxygen between room air and expired air. If the difference in oxygen concentration between room air and expired air is 0.04 mL/mL and the flow rate is 5500 mL/min, oxygen consumption is their product, that is, 220 mL/min. Carbon di-

oxide production is calculated in the same manner.

In the open-flow system, if the oxygen concentration difference of room air combined with the air stream being sucked passed the patient's face at a rate of 50,000 mL/min is 0.44%, oxygen consumption is 0.0044 mL/mL times 50,000 mL/min, which again is 220 mL/min. The open-flow system does not measure ventilation, but in both systems, air flow is measured over a known interval of time at a given pressure, temperature, and humidity, to which appropriate correction factors are applied to express the volume at STP and zero humidity. In closed-flow systems, it is reasonable to assume that the air is fully saturated with water, but in the open-flow system, the humidity must be measured, because expired air represents only a small portion of the total flow. As with the Douglas bag and Tissot methods, the volume of inspired air can be calculated from Equation 3 (see also Fig. 5–2). Oxygen consumption is calculated from the volumes of inspired and expired air and their concentrations of oxygen (Equation 2) after correcting for temperature and pressure.

When the micro-Scholander apparatus was used to analyze samples of expired air, the concentrations of oxygen, carbon dioxide, and nitrogen were directly determined. Most modern systems include analyzers for oxygen and carbon dioxide, but not for nitrogen. Instead, it is assumed that for both inspired air and expired air, any volume not accounted for by oxygen and carbon dioxide must be nitrogen (the Haldane transformation).

The flowmeter is the least accurate link in the system, having a measurement error of 5%. The error in the measurement of gas concentrations is usually within 1%. Thus, the error in measuring oxygen consumption is within 7%.

Blood Gas Analysis

The denominator of the Fick equation requires knowledge of the oxygen content of arterial blood (as a surrogate for pulmonary venous blood) and the oxygen content of samples obtained as a measure of mixed venous oxygen content obtained from the pulmonary artery. Catheterization of the pulmonary artery is necessary for obtaining mixed venous blood because of streamlining in the right heart chambers. Blood returning to the right atrium via the inferior vena cava is relatively highly oxygenated because it includes the highly oxygenated renal venous return. (The kidneys receive about one fourth of the cardiac output but extract oxygen minimally.) The highly oxygenated renal venous blood enters the right atrium via the inferior vena cava, which may contain as much as 2 vol% more oxygen than blood returning via the superior vena cava. On the other hand, because of near-maximal myocardial oxygen extraction, blood returning to the right atrium via the coronary sinus has a very low oxygen content. The oxygen content of blood returning to the heart via the superior vena cava is intermediate in comparison with the inferior vena caval and coronary sinus venous return. These streams of blood containing differing oxygen concentration do not become adequately mixed until the blood enters the pulmonary artery.

When cardiac catheterization was introduced into clinical practice, the standard method for blood gas analysis employed the manometric apparatus of Van Slyke. However, this method is time consuming and requires the services of well-trained, dedicated technicians, who become exposed to the hazards of mercury vapor toxicity. Although the numerous attempts made to develop methods comparable in accuracy to that of Van Slyke have not been totally successful, they are simpler and quicker to perform and are now standard in cardiac catheterization laboratories. Percentage concentration of oxygen in a blood sample can be read by a variety of available oximeters. The percentage saturation of blood with oxygen may also be determined from the oxyhemoglobin dissociation curve at the appropriate pH and temperature. To calculate the arteriovenous oxygen difference for the calculation of cardiac output, it is necessary to convert the percentage of blood oxygen saturation (e.g., 96% for arterial and 75% for mixed venous) into oxygen content. The oxygen capacity of blood (100% saturation) is the concentration of oxygen in blood that is in equilibrium with room air. Oxygen capacity is usually estimated from the relationship that 1 gm of hemoglobin combines with 1.36 mL of oxygen. Therefore, the value of hemoglobin in grams per 100 mL is multiplied by 1.36 to yield oxygen capacity, that is, 100% saturation. Others have stated that the conversion factor should be 1.34 or 1.39. In some laboratories the hematocrit level multiplied by 3 is multiplied by 1.36 to yield oxygen capacity. One advantage of the Van Slyke method, which yielded the result in vol%, not in percentage of saturation, was that oxygen capacity could be determined directly by analyzing a sample that had been equilibrated with room air. The Lex-O_2 Con instrument measures blood oxygen content in units of volume, although with less accuracy than the Van Slyke apparatus. Blood gas samples can also be analyzed by gas chromatography or mass spectroscopy, but these methods are not available in most cardiac catheterization laboratories. The method of Van Slyke used to provide an accuracy of blood gas content up to 0.2 vol%. Thus, the arteriovenous oxygen difference could be determined with an accuracy of 0.4 vol%. This limitation of even the most accurate method for determining blood oxygen content makes the method of Fick grossly inaccurate for measuring very high cardiac output. Consider two patients, both having an oxygen consumption of 250 mL/min. The first patient has an arteriovenous oxygen difference of 0.8 vol%, which because of this limitation could in the extremes be anywhere between 1.2 and 0.4 vol%. Cardiac output could therefore be calculated anywhere between 250/4 and 250/12, that is, any value between 62 and 21 L/min! Consider, on the other hand, another patient who has an arteriovenous oxygen difference of 5 vol%, that is, 5.4 to 4.6 vol%, which would yield a cardiac output between 4.6 and 5.4 L/min.

If one assumes a normal ventilation-to-perfusion ratio in a patient breathing room air at sea level, the theoretic saturation of oxygen in the pulmonary venous blood is 97.4%. In normal subjects, arterial blood is slightly contaminated by venous admixture from sources such as the Thebesian veins and some of the bronchial veins and has a concentration of oxygen slightly less than that in the pulmonary veins. The percentage saturation of a sample of arterial blood can be readily calculated from the oxygen tension using the oxyhemoglobin dissociation curve (Fig. 5–3). Unfortunately, in the range of 75% saturation of oxygen, normal for mixed venous blood, the curve is extremely steep, and therefore small errors in determining the partial pressure of oxygen result in large errors in the estimation of oxygen saturation (see Fig. 5–3). A sample calculation is given in Table 5–2.

Every effort should be made to ensure that the blood samples are collected anaerobically and are free from contaminating saline or excess heparin. (Small syringes of good quality and having a tight plunger are needed.) Heparin is placed in the syringe. Immediately before sampling, the plunger is pulled back to wet the barrel. All excess heparin is expelled, after which the syringe is held nozzle-up. Saline is aspirated from the catheter with another syringe until whole blood appears in the syringe. The aspirating syringe is disconnected from the catheter hub, which is held below heart level so that blood can displace air. A liquid-to-liquid connection of the catheter to the sample sy-

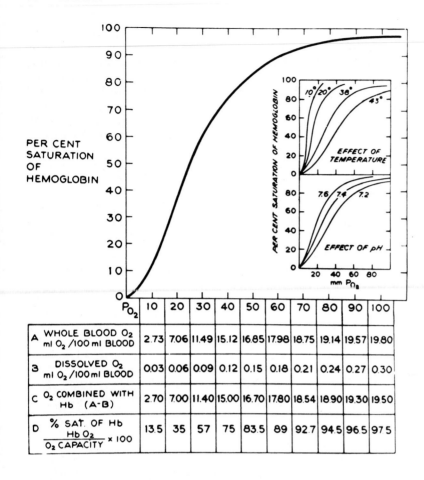

Figure 5–3. Oxygen dissociation curve for hemoglobin. Note that at values of P_{O_2} found in arterial blood, the curve is almost flat; therefore, small errors in P_{O_2} do not cause large errors in the calculated percentage of saturation of oxygen. However, when P_{O_2} is in the range usually found in mixed venous blood samples, the curve is steep and therefore unreliable for determining percent saturation with oxygen. (From Ranney HM, Sharma V: Structure and function of hemoglobin. *In* Williams WJ, Beutler E, Erslev AJ, Lichtman MA (eds): Hematology, 4th ed. New York, McGraw-Hill, 1990, pp 377–397.)

ringe is then made, after which blood is slowly and gently sucked from the catheter. Failure to take these precautions results in air bubbles or froth, which adversely affects accuracy. When 1 to 2 mL has been withdrawn, the sample syringe is disconnected and held nozzle-up. Any air bubble is expelled, and the syringe is capped. The sample should be analyzed promptly. If this is not possible, the sample must be kept on ice and analyzed as soon as possible.

The inherent errors in measurement of oxygen consumption and blood gas analysis mean

Table 5–2. **Example Showing the Calculation of Fick of Cardiac Output from Arteriovenous Oxygen Difference and Oxygen Consumption**

Variable	Calculation
Oxygen consumption	$= 240 \text{ mL} \cdot \text{min}^{-1}$
Hemoglobin content of arterial blood	$= 15.2 \text{ gm} \cdot \text{dL}^{-1}$
Oxygen capacity of arterial blood	$= 15.2 \text{ gm} \cdot 1.36 \text{ mL} \cdot \text{dL}^{-1}/\text{gm}^{-1}$
	$= 20.67 \text{ mL} \cdot \text{dL}^{-1}$
Oxygen percentage of saturation, arterial blood	$= 95\%$
Arterial oxygen content	$= 0.95 \times 20.67 \text{ mL} \cdot \text{dL}^{-1}$
	$= 19.6 \text{ mL} \cdot \text{dL}^{-1}$
Oxygen percentage of saturation, pulmonary arterial	$= 74\%$
Oxygen content, pulmonary arterial	$= 0.74 \cdot 20.67 \text{ mL} \cdot \text{dL}^{-1}$
	$= 15.3 \text{ mL} \cdot \text{dL}^{-1}$
Arteriovenous oxygen difference	$= 19.6 - 15.3 \text{ mL} \cdot \text{dL}^{-1}$
	$= 4.3 \text{ mL} \cdot \text{dL}^{-1}$
Cardiac output	$= 240 \text{ mL} \cdot \text{min}^{-1}/43 \text{ mL} \cdot \text{L}^{-1}$
	$= 5.53 \text{ L} \cdot \text{min}^{-1}$
Body surface area (m²)	$= 1.82 \text{ m}^2$
Cardiac index	$= 3.04 \text{ L} \cdot \text{min}^{-1} \cdot \text{m}^{-2}$

that cardiac output can be measured at best with an accuracy of 10%, more commonly 15%. This error is even larger when the patient is not in true steady-state. It is important to recall that reproducibility does not necessarily imply accuracy. An example of the calculation of cardiac output by the method of Fick is shown in Table 5–2.

Indicator-Dilution Techniques

Strictly speaking, the direct method of Fick is an indicator-dilution method, the indicator being oxygen. More commonly in cardiology, *indicator-dilution* refers to the mean concentration and mean transit time of an artificial substance added to the blood stream. The most commonly employed method is cold saline injected into the superior vena cava and sampled in the pulmonary artery. The resulting change of temperature in the pulmonary artery is detected by a fast thermistor. Another indicator, now less commonly used, is indocyanine green, frequently referred to as *green dye*. The dye is injected into the central circulation, preferably the pulmonary artery, and is detected in a systemic artery. Stewart[5] in 1897 first reported the application of indicator-dilution to the measurement of cardiac output, and Hamilton and Remington[6] later established the accuracy and reproducibility of the method. The principle is that the volume of fluid in a container can be determined accurately if a known mass of indicator is added to the container and is thoroughly dispersed and its final concentration is measured. The volume is given by the ratio of the mass of indicator injected to the final concentration of the added indicator. The principle is also valid when the fluid is in motion, as in the circulatory system.

Green Dye Cardiac Method

Theory

Suppose that at a given instant of time ($t = 0$) when no dye has been previously injected, a mass (m) of dye is injected into a flowing stream that has no recirculation. If the instantaneous flow is $Q(t)$ and the concentration of dye after thorough mixing at the sampling point is $c(t)$, then the area under the curve, that is, the integral of the product of the instantaneous flow $Q(t)$ and concentration $c(t)$ from time 0 to infinity, represents the total contrast medium injected (i.e., m):

$$m = \int_0^\infty Q(t) \cdot c(t) \cdot dt \qquad (4)$$

Assuming that the flow is constant, that is, $Q(t)$ is not a function of time but is Q, then Equation 4 can be written as:

$$m = Q\int_0^\infty c(t) \cdot dt \qquad (5)$$

where the integral term represents the area under the curve. Solving for constant flow Q yields:

$$Q = \frac{m}{\int_0^\infty c(t) \cdot dt} \qquad (6)$$

To apply this principle to the calculation of the cardiac output, recirculation must be excluded, so that the curve represents a single passage of dye from the injection site to the sampling site. The methods by which recirculation is excluded from the curve are described in the following section.

Method

A precise quantity of green dye is mixed in a measured volume of normal saline using the volumetric techniques of quantitative chemistry. A small quantity of this solution is added to volumetric flasks of blood in precisely known concentration, for example, 1 mg/L, 5 mg/L, or 10 mg/L. These samples are inserted into a densitometer or cuvette. The corresponding deflections are recorded on paper to determine a calibration factor (Fig. 5–4).

A measured quantity of the green dye solution (typically 5 mg) is injected into the blood stream in which it becomes uniformly mixed. The blood containing the dye is continuously withdrawn from the sampling site using a Harvard or similar type of pump through a cuvette. The usual injection site is a central vein or the pulmonary artery, and the sampling site is customarily the aorta or any systemic artery. The output of the densitometer, which reads the concentration of dye as it builds up and then decays, is continuously recorded at slow paper speed and is directly input to a green dye cardiac output computer. Approximately 20 to 30 seconds of data are recorded (Fig. 5–5A). The area under the curve is estimated (mg/sec/L). The amount of contrast medium injected (in

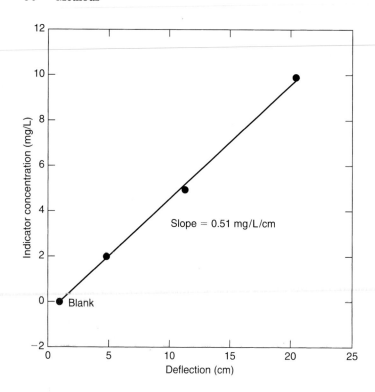

Slope = 0.51 mg/L/cm

Blank

Figure 5–4. Data to calibrate an indicator-dilution curve. Note that at least two concentrations should be used. This technique avoids errors due to faulty dilution and ensures that the curve is linear. The point marked as "blank" is the calibration point with no green dye. Concentrations of 0, 2, 5, and 10 mg/L were used. The slope of the linear regression line is the correction factor.

milligrams) is known; therefore, the cardiac output is calculated as:

$$\text{Cardiac output} = \frac{\text{Amount of dye (mg)} \cdot 60 \ (\text{sec} \cdot \text{min}^{-1})}{\text{Area under curve (mg} \cdot \text{sec} \cdot \text{L}^{-1})} \tag{7}$$

Let us assume, that with an injection of 6 mg of dye, the area under the curve is 72 mg/sec/L. The cardiac output is then estimated as:

$$\text{Cardiac output} = \frac{6 \ (\text{mg}) \cdot 60 \ (\text{sec} \cdot \text{min}^{-1})}{72 \ (\text{mg} \cdot \text{sec} \cdot \text{L}^{-1})} \tag{8}$$

$$= 5.0 \ (\text{L} \cdot \text{min}^{-1})$$

METHODS FOR EXCLUSION OF RECIRCULATION. To calculate the area under the curve for a single passage of the green dye, that is, excluding all recirculation, it is important to identify the exact point at which recirculation began, usually somewhere near the lower third of the downslope of the dye concentration versus time plot, but this point cannot be identified with precision on the linear plot (see Fig. 5–5A). However, because the concentration of green dye at the sampling site decays exponentially, when the data are replotted on a semilogarithmic scale, the instant of recirculation is demarcated by a sharp interruption of the downslope initiating a second rise in the concentration of dye (see Fig. 5–5B). On a semilogarithmic plot, the downslope of the curve is linear until the point of recirculation. The downslope of the semilogarithmic plot can then be linearly extrapolated from the point where circulation begins to the

baseline. The points along the extrapolated downslope are plotted back onto the original curve that had linear coordinates. The area under the curve in square centimeters can then be calculated by integration. Dividing by the paper speed (centimeters per second) and multiplying by the calibration factor (milligram per liter per centimeter) yields the area under the curve in units of milligram per second per liter.

Indocyanine green is nontoxic and stable and has no effect on the cardiovascular system. Its concentration is easily and precisely measured by densitometry. The dye remains in the plasma compartment between the site of injection and the sampling site during its initial passage. It is important to deliver the dye as a bolus. The withdrawal syringe should withdraw arterial blood at a constant rate of at least 30 to 40 mL/min. The length and internal diameter of the connecting tubes must allow an adequate dynamic response to the densitometer but must critically damp excessive pulsations. Cardiac output can be derived on-line from the green dye curve by a computer, but it is important for the operator to see the original analog output of the photo cell and be satisfied that an adequate curve has been obtained before accepting the reading from a cardiac output computer.

In the presence of severe mitral or aortic regurgitation, the downslope of the cardiac output curve becomes extremely prolonged. Cardiac output can then be better estimated by

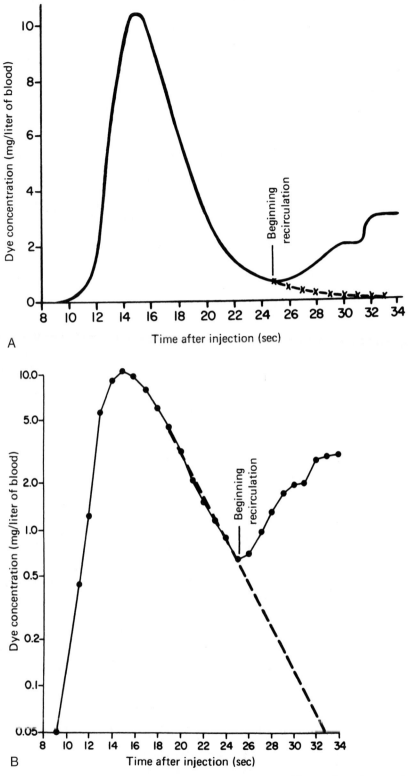

Figure 5–5. *A,* Indicator-dilution curve (indocyanine green). The curve has a rapid upstroke and a smooth downslope as far as the point of recirculation. Cardiac output is inversely proportional to the area under the curve, but it is difficult to pinpoint the exact onset of recirculation. *B,* Indicator-dilution curve depicted in *A* replotted on a semilogarithmic ordinate. The point at which recirculation begins is much more distinct, and the curve may be extrapolated toward zero. The extrapolated curve represents a single circulation of the indocyanine green. The points along the dotted portion of the curve, which assume an exponential disappearance of the indicator, are used in most methods of calculating cardiac output from indicator-dilution curves. (*A* and *B* from Guyton AG, Jones CE, Coleman GG: Circulatory Physiology: Cardiac Output and Its Regulation. Philadelphia, WB Saunders, 1973, pp 40–80.)

injecting the dye into the superior vena cava and sampling from the pulmonary artery. Although this technique invites some error secondary to incomplete mixing, the error is likely to be considerably smaller than errors inherent when one attempts to extrapolate an excessively slow downslope, as would be obtained from a systemic artery in the presence of severe valvular regurgitation. The downslope of the indicator-dilution curve is similarly greatly prolonged in any low cardiac output state. In consequence, the onset of recirculation cannot be identified accurately even after semilogarithmic transformation. Thus, in high cardiac output states, the direct method of Fick is unacceptably inaccurate, whereas in low cardiac output states indicator-dilution curves are unacceptable. Green dye curves can also be obtained by injecting the dye into the left ventricle and sampling from a peripheral artery. Although mixing is probably less complete than when the dye is injected into the pulmonary circulation and sampled from a systemic artery, the resulting cardiac output correlates quite well with cardiac output measured by the direct method of Fick.

Indocyanine green deteriorates with exposure to light; it is therefore important that the dye be used within an hour of preparation. Withdrawal rate through the densitometer should be maintained constant. The length and elasticity of tubing between sampling site and the cuvette should be kept to a minimum to avoid distorting the concentration curve. There should be enough distance from a chamber to allow for the mixing of the dye before it reaches the sampling site. The amount of dye injected must be the quantity introduced in the blood stream, not that delivered by the syringe, that is, minus the quantity left in the stopcock, tubing, and catheter.

Green dye method yields considerable variation in flow measurements ($\pm 20\%$) when compared with the Fick method[7, 8] and with electromagnetic flow estimation.[9] The technique has reproducibility in dogs up to $\pm 12\%$ when measured in two different arteries.[10] These variations occur when the requirements for validity of "complete mixing" and "representative sampling," the classic assumptions of the theory, cannot be met in practice. Mixing errors occur when the total flow across the cross-section of a vascular segment is not proportional to the blood flow through each element of the cross-section. Variations detailed earlier in this section are inherent in the practical estimation of cardiac output using dye dilution techniques, because complete mixing is rarely achieved and sampling errors exist. Differences between the method of Fick and dye dilution techniques are large in patients with low cardiac output.[11] In patients with left-to-right shunt, early recirculation of dye distorts the concentration curve[11] and leads to erroneous results.

To minimize the errors of mixing when using the bolus technique, a cumulative infusion method has been used and shown to be more accurate.[12, 13] In spite of these observations, the difficulties of recovering first-pass information from recirculation of constant infusion makes the bolus injection less popular.

A significant practical disadvantage of measuring cardiac output by green curves is that a considerable volume of blood is withdrawn from the systemic circulation. In studies requiring several determinations of cardiac output and in which the withdrawn blood is discarded, blood loss may become significant. On the other hand, if the blood is to be reinfused, extreme care must be taken to maintain sterility and to avoid the possible infusion of air bubbles or blood clot into the systemic artery. Another disadvantage of the green dye method is that green dye comes in the form of a powder, and the liquid dye must be made up using strict volumetric techniques at the time of cardiac catheterization. Most cardiac catheterization technicians are untrained in volumetric chemistry and therefore the results of cardiac output determined by the green dye method are likely to be inaccurate in most laboratories. All cardiac output determinations during the study as well as the calibration curve must be performed using the original mixture of powder and diluent.

Standard syringes are not sufficiently accurate in calibration for delivering the precise intended dose of green dye. Special calibrated volumetric syringes are therefore required.

Thermodilution Methods

For all the reasons described earlier, quantitative green dye curves for estimating cardiac output are seldom used now in laboratories, their place having been taken by thermodilution. A small thermistor can be incorporated into the tip of a catheter to measure cardiac output by thermodilution. The thermistor is a solid-state material that has a negative coefficient of resistivity; that is, it decreases its electrical resistance when ambient temperature increases. The thermistor is connected to one arm of a standard Wheatstone bridge; the bridge is unbalanced by slight changes in blood temperature. Cardiac output is measured by the thermodilution technique, which is based on the same principle as the green dye dilution method discussed earlier.

In this instance, fluid at low temperature, not a dye, is the indicator.

The system most commonly used was originally described by Forrester and associates.[14] Saline, either iced or at room temperature, is injected through the proximal port of a triple-lumen Swan-Ganz catheter into the superior vena cava or right atrium. The thermistor is positioned in the pulmonary artery. An indicator-dilution curve, exactly equivalent to the green dye curve, is registered as the cool saline passes the thermistor tip. Cardiac output is usually read from an on-line computer. Under carefully controlled conditions, this method can be made to correlate well with the direct method of Fick (Fig. 5–6).[15, 16] As with green dye dilution curves, it is critical that the operator be able to inspect the original thermodilution analog curve and not rely on the digital readout from a computer without seeing the original data. Several curves must be made to check for consistency. As with green dye curves, low cardiac output results in a slow downslope of the indicator-dilution curve with resulting difficulty in detecting the exact onset of recirculation.[17] When cardiac output is low, it is overestimated by the thermodilution technique.[18] Unlike the situation with green dye curves in which the indicator is injected into the pulmonary circulation with sampling from the systemic circulation, cardiac output determined by thermodilution is obtained by injecting and sampling in the pulmonary circulation. Mitral and aortic regurgitation do not directly influence the downslope of the indicator-dilution curve. However, severe tricuspid valve regurgitation results in poor mixing in the right atrium with subsequent loss of indicator to the body tissue before the indicator reaches the pulmonary artery. Therefore, tricuspid regurgitation results not only in a prolonged downslope of the indicator-dilution curve but also in a falsely low cardiac output measure.[19]

In early applications of the thermodilution technique for the measurement of cardiac output, iced saline was rapidly injected into the pulmonary artery with the assumption that saline emerging from the proximal port would also be close to 0°C. It was then necessary to keep the cold saline in ice for an hour before use and to avoid warming of the injecting syringe and its contents by the operator's hand, which would lower the dose of cold and result in underestimation of cardiac output. Currently used systems employ a second transistor placed between the syringe used for injection and the hub of the catheter, allowing measurement of temperature at the injection site as well as in the pulmonary artery. This development allows the much more convenient injection of room-temperature saline rather than iced saline.[20]

Thermodilution has rapidly become the preferred method of measuring cardiac output in the cardiac catheterization laboratory. However, in the rigorous laboratory, the results of cardiac output by thermodilution should be checked from time to time against the direct method of Fick.

In many laboratories, cardiac output is estimated by measuring arteriovenous oxygen dif-

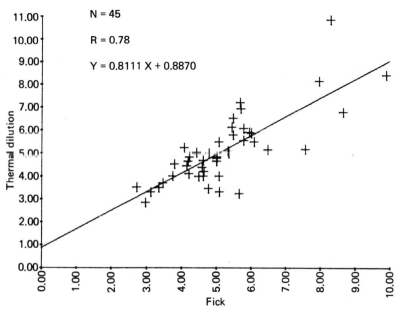

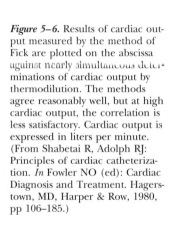

Figure 5–6. Results of cardiac output measured by the method of Fick are plotted on the abscissa against nearly simultaneous determinations of cardiac output by thermodilution. The methods agree reasonably well, but at high cardiac output, the correlation is less satisfactory. Cardiac output is expressed in liters per minute. (From Shabetai R, Adolph RJ: Principles of cardiac catheterization. *In* Fowler NO (ed): Cardiac Diagnosis and Treatment. Hagerstown, MD, Harper & Row, 1980, pp 106–185.)

ference and using a predicted value such as 130 mL/min/m^2 for oxygen consumption. The use of this assumed value for oxygen consumption, however, is fraught with inaccuracies, because considerable variation in basal metabolic rate exists among patients and because many patients in the cardiac catheterization laboratory are not in the basal state. Cardiac output based on the measured arteriovenous oxygen difference but an assumed oxygen consumption can be taken only as a rough estimate of cardiac output. If a thermodilution curve for cardiac output is obtained together with blood samples for measurement of arteriovenous oxygen difference, oxygen consumption can be calculated. Quality control of the adequacy of cardiac output determination in the cardiac catheterization laboratory is best achieved by periodically measuring oxygen consumption, arteriovenous oxygen difference, and the thermodilution curve in the same patient, preferably at rest and after an intervention.

When several thermodilution curves are obtained in rapid sequence from a patient, cardiac output should not vary more than 5%. Frequently, this ideal is not achieved. At least three curves should be obtained, but if variation is more than 5%, additional curves should be done and the most deviant values rejected.

Cardiac Output by Left Ventricular Contrast Angiography

Stroke volume can be obtained by measuring left ventricular end-diastolic and end-systolic volumes from a left ventriculogram. These methods are not discussed further in this chapter because they are discussed in detail in Chapter 8. The method is of particular value in patients with mitral or aortic regurgitation. Total stroke volume is given by the difference between end-diastolic and end-systolic volume, whereas forward stroke volume is given by the indicator-dilution or direct method of Fick. The difference between the two is the regurgitant fraction, which yields a reasonable estimate with a severity of valvular incompetence. Estimation of stroke volume by ventriculography should never be relied on for calculation of regurgitant fraction unless the correlation between the ventriculographic and other methods of measurement with stroke volume have been established for an individual laboratory.

Measurement of Cardiac Output by Flowmeter

In experimental animals, cardiac output is often obtained using an ultrasonic or electromagnetic flowmeter with the transducer placed around the aorta. In the case of the electromagnetic flowmeter, the coil is energized by an intermittent current that creates a magnetic field through which the blood flows. The charged particles in the blood stream flowing through the magnetic field generate a voltage proportional to blood flow velocity.

If the cross-sectional area of the aorta is known, velocity can be converted to volume flow. Flowmeters are practically never used in standard cardiac catheterization, but velocity curves generated via a velocity transducer placed in the aorta or pulmonary artery[21] can be obtained for research purposes. Most reported studies employ an electromagnetic flowmeter, but Doppler devices have also been used. The advantage of the technique is its ability to document beat-to-beat variations in stroke volume.[22, 23] These devices have an inherently low signal-to-noise ratio. Also, the magnetic field is not uniform and catheter motion results in artifacts. Furthermore, aortic cross-sectional area changes during the cardiac cycle. Nevertheless, acceptable waveforms of aortic blood flow velocity can be obtained, and the signal-to-noise ratio can be improved by signal averaging. Stroke volume is proportional to the area under the curve. Currently, the use of flowmeters in the cardiac catheterization laboratory is strictly limited to clinical investigation.

BLOOD FLOW CALCULATIONS IN THE PRESENCE OF SHUNTS

The method of Fick can still be employed when a left-to-right or a right-to-left, or bidirectional, shunt exists between the systemic and pulmonary circulations. The more common shunts include atrial and ventricular septal defects, persistent arterial duct, aortopulmonary window, sinus of Valsalva aneurysm with rupture into the right atrium or right ventricle, coronary artery connection to the right atrium or right ventricle, and aortic to right heart chamber fistula secondary to infective endocarditis and stab wounds that penetrate the pulmonary artery and aorta. When right-sided heart pressures and pulmonary vascular resistance (PVR) are substantially lower than systemic pressures, the shunt is from the systemic to the pulmonary circulation, that is, left to right. When the PVR and right-sided heart pressures are equal to systemic, or nearly so, the flows are balanced and little, if any flow occurs in either direction across the connection. When right-sided heart pressure or PVR exceeds sys-

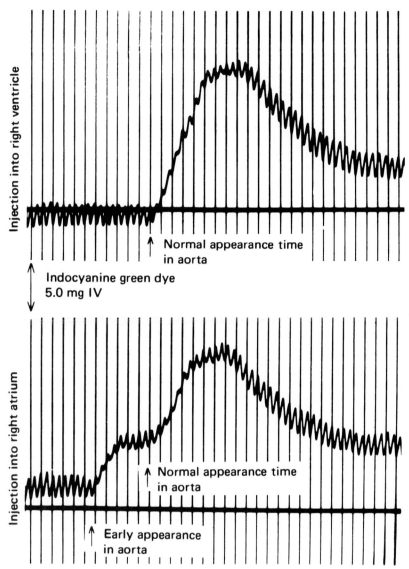

Figure 5–7. Right-to-left shunt detected by indocyanine green dye. The dye is injected as a bolus into a right-sided heart chamber, and its appearance time in a systemic artery is detected with a suitable densitometer. When the dye was injected into the pulmonary artery (distal to the right to left shunt), the curve appeared normal *(top)*. When dye was injected into the right atrium *(bottom)*, a portion of the dye traversed the shunt, bypassed the lung, and caused a premature appearance of dye in the aorta. The first appearance was followed by a second appearance representing that portion of the dye that had traversed the lungs in the usual way. Thus, the upstroke has a double hump. Time lines show 1-second intervals. (From Shabetai R, Adolph RJ: Principles of cardiac catheterization. *In* Fowler NO (ed): Cardiac Diagnosis and Treatment. Hagerstown, MD, Harper & Row, 1980, pp 106–185.)

temic pressure, flow is from right to left through the abnormal connection.

Systemic and Pulmonary Blood Flow in the Presence of an Isolated Left-to-Right Shunt

When a defect allows shunting from left to right, the assumption that integrated pulmonary and systemic blood flow are equal no longer holds, because the pulmonary flow ex-

ceeds the systemic flow by the amount of left-to-right shunt. Nevertheless, the general Fick principle still holds. Thus, pulmonary flow is given by the oxygen consumption in milliliters per minute divided by the arteriovenous oxygen difference in milliliters per liter. Arterial oxygen content can be obtained in the same manner as is used in patients with no shunt. Alternatively, oxygenated blood can be obtained directly from a pulmonary vein or the left atrium, in instances in which the catheter can cross a defect. However, a problem exists with the mixed venous oxygen content because the venous return is mixed with arterial blood at the site of the shunt and all sites distal to it. It has already been emphasized that in subjects without a shunt, the venous blood is not completely mixed until after it has passed through the right heart chambers and has entered the pulmonary artery. Clearly, if a left-to-right shunt exists, there is no source for thoroughly mixed but uncontaminated venous blood. The more proximal the left-to-right shunt, the more severe does this problem become. Thus, if there is a persistent arterial duct, blood drawn from the pulmonary artery will be contaminated with blood coming from the aorta via the duct to the pulmonary artery. However, in the absence of pulmonary valve regurgitation, a close approximation of mixed venous blood can be obtained by averaging several samples withdrawn from the outflow region of the right ventricle. If the shunt is through a ventricular septal defect, the right ventricle becomes an invalid source for mixed venous blood. The next proximal site would then be the right atrium but, as we have seen, blood flow into the right atrium is streamlined and therefore adequate mixing has not taken place. Finally, if the shunt is through an atrial septal defect, there is no source that even approximates mixed venous blood.

A satisfactory solution to the problem is based on the observation that in subjects without a shunt, the oxygen content of pulmonary arterial blood is the same as the oxygen content calculated from the superior vena caval oxygen content multiplied by 3 plus the oxygen content in the inferior cava, the whole divided by 4[24]:

$$MV_{O_2} = \frac{(SV_{CO_2} \cdot 3) + IV_{CO_2}}{4} \quad (9)$$

where MV_{O_2} is mixed venous oxygen content, SV_{CO_2} and IV_{CO_2} and are the oxygen content of the superior and inferior vena cava, respectively.

The total pulmonary blood flow (TPF) is the oxygen consumption divided by the arteriovenous oxygen difference of all blood flowing to the lung, regardless of its source. That is, TPF is the sum of the normal venous return to the lung plus the left-to-right shunt as shown in Equation 10:

$$TPF = \frac{V_{O_2}}{(PV_{O_2} - PA_{O_2})} \quad (10)$$

where V_{O_2} is oxygen consumption and PV_{O_2} and PA_{O_2} are the oxygen content of pulmonary

venous (or systemic arterial) and pulmonary arterial oxygen content.

The effective pulmonary flow (EPF) is the quotient of oxygen consumption and the difference between the oxygen content of pulmonary venous blood and that of mixed venous blood. The mixed venous blood oxygen content is usually calculated as in Equation 9, but in the case of a persistent arterial duct without pulmonary valve regurgitation, right ventricular oxygen content is a close approximation:

$$EPF = \frac{V_{O_2}}{(PV_{O_2} - MV_{O_2})} \quad (11)$$

Left-to-right (L $\rightarrow$ R) shunt (liters per minute) is calculated as TPF minus EPF:

$$L \rightarrow R = TPF - EPF \quad (12)$$

PVR in Equation 13 is given by the ratio of the pressure drop across the pulmonary bed to the TPF as in Equation 10:

$$PVR = \frac{\overline{PAP} - \overline{LAP}}{TPF} \quad (13)$$

where $\overline{PAP}$ is pulmonary arterial mean pressure and $\overline{LAP}$ is left atrial or pulmonary wedge mean pressure. Vascular resistance is commonly expressed in units of dynes per second per cm^5, but the calculation is done from pressure difference in millimeters of mercury and cardiac output in liters per minute. Vascular resistance from these data are more conveniently expressed as clinical (or Wood) units. To convert to dynes per second per cm^5, the value in clinical units is multiplied by 80, although we see no advantage in using this theoretically based unit.

An example of calculation of a simple left-to-right shunt follows:

Source	Pressure (mm Hg)	O₂ Saturation (%)	O₂ Content (vol%)
Pulmonary vein or aorta	5	98	19.7
Pulmonary artery	35/14	88	17.8
Right ventricle	35/4	80	16.1
Right atrium	4	76	15.3
Superior vena cava	4	75	15.1
Inferior vena cava	4	86	17.3

V_{O_2} = mL/min; hemoglobin = 14.8 gm/dL; conversion factor = 1.36.

$$TPF = \frac{250 \text{ mL/min}}{(197 - 178) \text{ mL/L}} = 13.2 \text{ L/min} \quad (14)$$

$$EPF = \frac{250 \text{ mL/min}}{(197 - 157) \text{ mL/L}} = 6.3 \text{ L/min} \quad (15)$$

$$L \rightarrow R = 13.2 - 6.3 = 6.9 \text{ L/min} \quad (16)$$

$$\frac{TPF}{EPF} = \frac{13.2}{6.3} = \frac{2.1}{1} \quad (17)$$

$$PVR = \frac{35 - 5}{13.2} = 2.3 \text{ units} \quad (18)$$
$$= 184 \text{ dynes/sec/cm}^5$$

$$SVR = \frac{100 - 4}{6.3} = 15.2 \text{ units} \quad (19)$$
$$= 1219 \text{ dynes/sec/cm}^5$$

$$\frac{PVR}{SVR} = 0.15 \quad (20)$$

In this case of an isolated left-to-right shunt, it is reasonable to assume that systemic flow is the same as EPF. Systemic vascular resistance (SVR) is calculated using this estimate of systemic blood flow. EPF is then frequently termed *systemic flow* and designated as $\dot{Q}s$. TPF is designated as $\dot{Q}P$.

The magnitude of a left-to-right shunt is frequently expressed as the ratio of TPF to EPF. In the example earlier, the patient had a left-to-right shunt with a pulmonary to systemic flow ratio ($\dot{Q}P/\dot{Q}s$) of 2 to 1 and a PVR to SVR ratio of 0.15.

Right-to-Left Shunt

When blood shunts from the lesser to the greater circulation, the assumption that, in the absence of a concurrent left-to-right shunt, systemic flow and pulmonary flow are equal, no longer holds. Likewise, when shunting is bidirectional, it can no longer be assumed that systemic flow and effective pulmonary flow are the same.

In the case of a simple right-to-left shunt, venous admixture lowers the oxygen content of arterial blood, thereby lessening the arteriovenous oxygen difference across the systemic vascular bed (oxygen content in the aorta minus that in the pulmonary artery) compared with the arteriovenous oxygen content across the pulmonary vascular bed (oxygen content of the pulmonary vein minus that of the pulmonary artery), which is the source of mixed venous blood. Therefore, as shown in the following example, systemic flow exceeds pulmonary flow:

Source	O₂ Saturation (%)	O₂ Content (vol%)
Pulmonary artery	75	17.3
Pulmonary vein	97	22.4
Aorta	82	19.0

$Vo_2 = 250$ mL/min; hemoglobin = 17 gm/dL; conversion factor = 1.36.

$$TPF = EPF = \dot{Q}P$$
$$= \frac{250 \text{ mL/min}}{(22.6 - 17.3) \text{ mL/L}} = 4.9 \text{ L/min} \quad (21)$$

$$SF = \dot{Q}s = \frac{250 \text{ mL/min}}{(224 - 190) \text{ mL/L}} = 7.4 \text{ L/min} \quad (22)$$

$$R \rightarrow L = 7.4 - 4.9 = 2.5 \text{ L/min} \quad (23)$$

$$\frac{\dot{Q}s}{\dot{Q}P} = 1.5 = \frac{1.5}{1} \quad (24)$$

In the case of a bidirectional shunt, TPF, EPF, and systemic flow all differ from each other as in the following example:

Source	O₂ Saturation (%)	O₂ Content (vol%)
Pulmonary vein	97	21.0
Pulmonary artery	80	17.4
Aorta	88	19.2
Superior vena cava	60	13.8
Inferior vena cava	70	15.3

$Vo_2 = 250$ mL/min; hemoglobin = 16 gm/dL; conversion factor = 13.6.

$$TPF = \frac{250 \text{ mL/min}}{(210 - 174) \text{ mL/L}} = 6.9 \text{ L/min} \quad (25)$$

$$EPF = \frac{250 \text{ mL/min}}{(210 - 142) \text{ mL/L}} = 3.7 \text{ L/min} \quad (26)$$

$$SF(\dot{Q}s) = \frac{250 \text{ mL/min}}{(192 - 142) \text{ mL/L}} = 5.0 \text{ L/min} \quad (27)$$

$$L \rightarrow R = 3.2 \text{ L/min} \quad (28)$$

$$R \rightarrow L = 1.3 \text{ L/min} \quad (29)$$

Other methods for detecting shunts are described in Chapter 25). These include angiography and a technique using inhaled hydrogen. Angiography provides only a semiquantitative estimate of the magnitude of a shunt. The hydrogen curve is exquisitely sensitive for the detection and localization of a left-to-right shunt but is of no value in quantification. Green dye curves can also be used to detect and localize a shunt (see Fig. 5–6) but are no longer used for quantification.

REFERENCES

1. Guyton AC, Jones CE, Coleman GC: Cardiac output and its regulation. *In* Circulatory Physiology, 2nd ed. Philadelphia, WB Saunders, 1973, pp 3–20.
2. Brandfondbrenn M, Landowne M, Shock NW: Changes in cardiac output with age. Circulation 1955; 12: 557–566.
3. Epstein SE, Beiser GD, Stampfer M, et al: Characterization of the circulatory response to maximal upright exercise in normal subjects and patients with heart disease. Circulation 1967; 35:1049–1062.
4. Altman PL, Dittmer DS (eds): Biological Handbooks: Respiration and Circulation. Bethesda, MD, FASEB, 1971, pp 43–44.
5. Stewart GN: Researches on the circulation time and on the influences which affect it: The output of the heart. J Physiol 1897; 22:159–183.
6. Hamilton WF, Remington JW: Comparison of the time concentration curves in arterial blood of diffusible and non-diffusible substances when injected at a constant rate and when injected instantaneously. Am J Physiol 1947; 148:35–39.
7. Dow P: Dimensional relationships in dye dilution curves from humans and dogs with an empirical formula for certain troublesome curves. J Appl Physiol 1955; 7: 399–408.
8. Hetzel PS, Swan HJ, Ramirez de Arellano AA, Wood EH: Estimation of cardiac output from first part of arterial dye-dilution curve. J Appl Physiol 1958; 13: 92–97.
9. Smulyan H: Reliability of the indicator-dilution technique. Am Heart J 1961; 62:140–141.
10. Smulyan H, Cuddy RP, Eich R: An evaluation of indicator-dilution technique in the dog. J Appl Physiol 1962; 17:729–734.
11. Hamilton FN, Minzel JC, Schlobohm RM: Measurement of cardiac output by two methods in dogs. J Appl Physiol 1967; 22:362–364.
12. Sleeper JC, Thompson HK Jr, McIntosh HD, Elston RC: Reproducibility of results obtained with indicator-dilution technique for estimating cardiac output in man. Circ Res 1962; 11:712–720.
13. Maramba LC, Javier RP, Hildner FJ, Samet P: A reappraisal of the abnormal indicator dye dilution curves in valvular incompetence and low output states: Recognition of a diagnostic pitfall and a possible preventive measure with specific reference to left-to-right shunt. Am J Med 1971; 50:20–23.
14. Forrester JS, Ganz W, Diamond G, et al: Thermodilution cardiac output determination with a single flow-directed catheter. Am Heart J 1972; 83:306–311.
15. Fegler G: The reliability of the thermal dilution method for determination of the cardiac output and blood flow in central veins. Q J Exp Physiol 1957; 42:254–266.
16. Reddy PS, Curtiss EI, Bell B, et al: Determinants of variation between Fick and indicator-dilution estimates of cardiac output during diagnostic cardiac catheterization: Fick versus dye cardiac outputs. J Lab Clin Med 1976; 87:568–576.
17. Hillis LD, Firth BG, Winniford MD: Comparison of thermodilution and indocyanine green in low cardiac output or left-sided regurgitation. Am J Cardiol 1986; 57:1201–1202.
18. Uan Ghondelle A, Ditchey RV, Groves BM, et al: Thermodilution method overestimates low cardiac output in humans. Am J Physiol 1983; 245(Heart Circ Physiol 14):H690–H692.
19. Lipkin DP, Poole-Wilson PA: Measurement of cardiac output during exercise by the thermodilution and direct Fick techniques in patients with chronic congestive heart failure. Am J Cardiol 1985; 56:321–324.
20. Elkayam U, Berkley R, Azen S, et al: Cardiac output by thermodilution technique: Effect of injectate's volume and temperature on accuracy and reproducibility in the critically ill patient. Chest 1983; 84:418–422.
21. Gabe IT, Gault JH, Ross J Jr, et al: Measurement of instantaneous blood flow velocity and pressure in conscious man with a catheter tip velocity probe. Circulation 1969; 40:603–614.
22. Uther JB, Peterson KL, Shabetai R, Braunwald E: Measurement of force-velocity-length relationships in man with an electromagnetic flowmeter catheter. Adv Cardiol 1974; 12:198–209.
23. Shabetai R, Fowler NO, Guntheroth WG: The hemodynamics of cardiac tamponade and constrictive pericarditis. Am J Cardiol 1970; 26:480–489.
24. Miller HC, Brown DJ, Miller GAH: Comparison of formulae used to estimate oxygen saturation in mixed venous blood from caval samples. Br Heart J 1974; 36:446–451.

Chapter 6

Measurement of Coronary Blood Flow

MORTON J. KERN
PHILIP A. LUDBROOK

FUNCTIONAL ANATOMY OF THE CORONARY CIRCULATION

Human coronary circulation may be considered as three units: (1) epicardial arteries, (2) muscular and nonmuscular capillary arterioles, and (3) venous conduits (Fig. 6–1). Each unit responds differently, at times in opposite directions, to a variety of physiologic stimuli. The large epicardial vessels serve as conduits for blood flow, providing nutritive perfusion to the metabolic units of myocardium. The muscular arteriolar system modulates capillary blood flow, proportioning the overall coronary blood flow to different regions of the myocardium according to immediate demands. Capillary flow is thus regulated by various stimuli, both intrinsic and extrinsic, which act on the muscular precapillary arteriolar resistance vessels. The regulatory units (muscular arterioles) respond profoundly to moment-to-moment changes in metabolic demand and other pharmacologic and physiologic stimuli (Fig. 6–2). Oxygen supply is balanced with myocardial oxygen demand

CORONARY BLOOD FLOW AND MYOCARDIAL ISCHEMIA

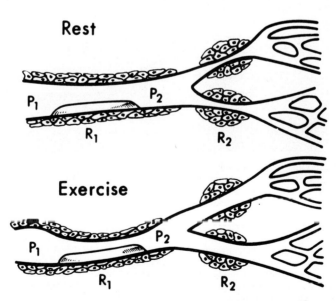

Figure 6–1. Diagrammatic schema of coronary arterial vascular bed showing the epicardial artery (R_1), muscular precapillary arteriole (R_2), and capillary bed *(right)*. P_1 and P_2 represent pressure measured in the epicardial vessel before and after an atherosclerotic plaque. Physiologic changes may influence luminal dimensions at one or more of the resistance circuits; for example, the lower figure shows one effect of exercise causing dynamic narrowing of the R_1 (epicardial) vessel with dilation of the R_2 vessels. (From Epstein SE, Talbot TL: Dynamic coronary tone in precipitation, exacerbation, and relief of angina pectoris. Am J Cardiol 1981; 48:797–803. *Reprinted with permission from American Journal of Cardiology.*)

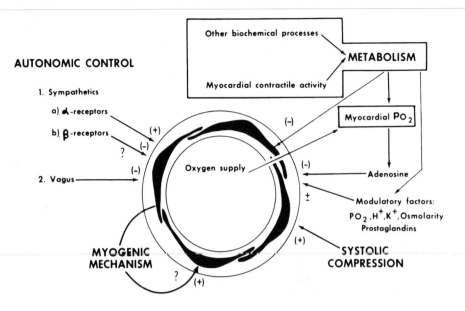

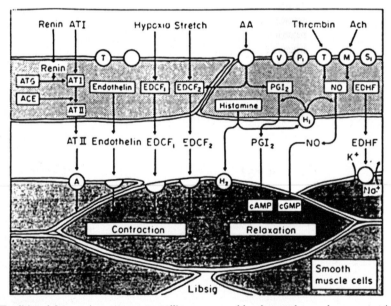

Figure 6–2. Upper, Traditional four major systems controlling coronary blood smooth muscle vasoconstriction: (1) metabolism and myocardial oxygen tension and other modulators, including concentration of hydrogen, potassium, osmolarity, and prostaglandins; (2) systolic compression, controlling coronary blood flow for a limited part of the cardiac cycle; (3) the myogenic mechanism, playing a role through indicators that are not well defined; and (4) autonomic control. (*Upper* from Berne RM, Rubio R: Coronary circulation. *In* Berne RM [ed]: Handbook of Physiology, vol 1: Cardiovascular System. Bethesda, MD, American Physiologic Society, 1979, p 873.) *Lower,* The contribution of endothelial cells to smooth muscle vasoconstriction and vasorelaxation is mediated by various factors. AT I is converted in endothelial cells to AT II, which, in turn, acts on AT receptors to promote contraction. Many of the endothelial-derived vasoactive substances are displayed on this diagram: AA, arachidonic acid; ACE, angiotensin-converting enzyme inhibitor; ATG, angiotensinogen; Ach, acethylcholine; AT, angiotensin; cAMP and cGMP, cyclic adenosine and guanosine monophosphate; EDCF, endothelial-derived constricting factor; EDHF, endothelial-derived hyperpolarizing factor; NO, nitric oxide; PGI, prostacycline). (*Lower* from Lücher TF: Endothelial Vasoactive Substances in Cardiovascular Disease. Basel, Switzerland, S. Karger AG, 1988, pp 1–21.)

via the process of autoregulation.[1] As blood traverses the capillary bed and oxygen and nutrients are extracted, metabolic byproducts are removed via capillary venules into the large coronary veins and, finally, for most of the blood draining from the left ventricle, into the coronary sinus. The great cardiac vein has been regarded, with some limitations (see later), as a conduit that drains the flow traversing the anterior left ventricular region, and approximates, therefore, left anterior descending coronary artery flow.[2]

Epicardial Arteries

The ostia of the epicardial arteries originate from the sinuses of Valsalva at the root of the aorta. The size of the left main coronary artery ranges from 2 to 5.5 mm in diameter and from 2 to 40 mm in length.[3, 4] The left main coronary artery divides into two major branches, the left anterior descending and circumflex coronary arteries, supplying most of the left ventricular myocardium. "Normal" anatomic variations are common, including a short, medium-sized, or long left anterior descending artery supplying the proximal anterior portion of the left ventricle, the entire left ventricle to the apex, or the entire left ventricle, apex, and part of the inferior wall, respectively.

The distribution of the circumflex artery also varies considerably. If dominant, it may supply most of the lateral and inferior portions of the left ventricle and continue in the inferior interventricular groove as the posterior descending branch, supplying the inferior aspect of the interventricular septum. Conversely, if small, it may supply only the basal portion of the lateral wall, with most of the inferior wall being supplied by the right coronary artery. Septal perforating branches, which perfuse the interventricular septum and the conduction system of the heart, arise principally from the left anterior descending and posterior descending arteries. The atrioventricular nodal branch may arise from either the circumflex or right coronary arteries (in keeping with left or right coronary dominance).

Numerous anatomic variations of the coronary circulation have been observed.[3, 4] Although specific congenital anomalies have been described,[5] associated alterations in the physiologic behavior of the coronary arteries have not been reported, apart from instances of sudden death in patients with anomalous left main arteries interposed between the aorta and the pulmonary artery. For further details of coronary anatomy and anomalies, see Chapter 9.

Functional Attributes of Epicardial Arteries

Epicardial coronary arteries are the largest conduits for blood flow to the myocardium. These conduits are ringed by smooth muscle, the vasoconstrictor activity of which is modulated by factors acting directly on smooth muscle (such as nitroglycerin) and by stimuli originating from the endothelial cells (such as acetylcholine and endothelium-derived relaxing factor).[6–8] The contribution of normal epicardial vessels to total coronary resistance is small; they are sensitive to metabolic and neurogenic stimuli, but their vasoactive responses are of limited physiologic significance. However, segmental or generalized spasm of epicardial vessels may occur, producing abrupt myocardial ischemia in the subtended area of myocardium.

Left ventricular epicardial vessels conduct blood predominantly during diastole and in early systole. During late diastole, the epicardial coronary arteries expand to comprise a capacitance bed, which may be further augmented by vasodilation.[9, 10] Small branches from the epicardial vessels penetrate perpendicularly into the intramural myocardium. Septal branches originating from the left anterior descending coronary artery generally perfuse the anterior two thirds of the interventricular septum, whereas the perforating branches of the posterior descending extend upward to supply the posterior one third of the septum. These septal branches supply the conduction system in a dual fashion. Communications between anterior and posterior descending arteries beyond the atrioventricular nodal branch are often the source of strategically important collateral vessels. The intramural coronary network penetrates in a circumferential fashion around the subendocardial myocardium, with intercommunicating anastomoses supplying the subendocardial musculature[10] and providing the anatomic basis for collateral development.

Capillaries and Arterioles

The capillary bed permits transit of oxygen, electrolytes, and nutrients from blood to interstitium, with simultaneous return of carbon dioxide and products of aerobic and anaerobic metabolism from the tissue bed to the blood stream.

In human and most mammalian hearts, the capillary wall consists of media only, as compared with epicardial vessels, which are distinguished by three layers: the intima, the media, and the adventitia.[11] The precapillary sphincter constitutes a dynamic flow-regulating gate, modulating blood flow to the capillary bed. Precapillary sphincters and small arterioles respond to vasoconstrictor and vasodilator stimuli and limit or redirect flow to different myocardial regions of the myocardium. Hypoxia, acidosis, hyperosmolarity, adenosine, and other metabolic factors are known to influence capillary flow profoundly.[12] Capillary density and distribution may be altered in various disease states, such as left ventricular hypertrophy, myocardial infarction, and cardiomyopathy, and by exercise conditioning.[13, 14]

Myocardial Venous Drainage

The capillary venous bed converges on venules that in turn drain the left ventricle through three principal venous channels.[15] The epicardial veins converge and drain through the coronary sinus, located in the atrioventricular groove, into the right atrium. The ostium of the coronary sinus is located immediately posterior and cranial to the lower part of the tricuspid valve annulus. Anterior superficial cardiac veins drain the right ventricular myocardium directly into the right atrium. Small thebesian veins drain venous blood from the atria, interatrial septum, and portions of the left and right ventricles and interventricular septum directly into all four cardiac chambers.

The pattern of venous drainage from the anterior wall of the left ventricle varies considerably. Flow in the anterior great cardiac vein has been regarded as a clinically useful indicator of myocardial blood flow.[16, 17] In the dog, however, the proportion of myocardial flow draining via the anterior cardiac vein may be altered during ischemia.[17] Under these circumstances, anterior cardiac vein flow may not reflect myocardial flow accurately. This may also be the case in humans. Further, venous flow may not necessarily reflect arterial flow in the face of interventions known to modify coronary flow dynamics in humans. Autonomic regulation of resistance vessels and coronary flow has been reviewed by Young and associates[18]; coronary microcirculatory physiology has been reviewed also by Chilian and colleagues[19] (see also Fig. 6–2).

The anatomic features of the coronary circulation contribute to the observed variance between coronary flow measurements obtained with use of the several techniques to be discussed. The relationship between flow velocity and absolute flow in an epicardial artery is proportional to the diameter of the artery. The location and size of major side branches may interfere with epicardial intracoronary velocity measurements. Flow from venous side branches draining into the coronary sinus is responsible for most of the error associated with measurement of coronary blood flow by means of the coronary sinus thermodilution technique. Even small movements of the thermistors across the entrances of venous branches into the coronary sinus may also lead to substantial error in measured flow.

PHYSIOLOGY OF CORONARY BLOOD FLOW

Coronary blood flow is regulated physiologically by several principal factors: myocardial metabolism (including myocardial tissue oxygen tension [Po_2] and other biochemical modulators), systolic compression, direct myogenic influences, and autonomic mechanisms[12] (see Fig. 6–2). "Autoregulation" is the physiologic process by which myocardial blood flow is modulated in proportion to myocardial oxygen demand, which in turn is determined principally by heart rate, contractility, and left ventricular wall stress. Such changes in coronary blood flow in response to metabolic demands are controlled by various factors, including adenosine, acidosis, tissue Pco_2, osmolality, and circulating prostaglandins. Autonomic control of coronary flow is mediated by α-adrenergic vasoconstriction and β-adrenergic vasodilation. Myogenic mechanisms are poorly understood but probably involve endothelium-derived factors. Local control of coronary blood flow has been reviewed extensively.[20]

Metabolic Control Factors

The link between coronary blood flow and the metabolic requirements of the heart has not been well defined. Under basal conditions, myocardial oxygen utilization ($M\dot{V}o_2$) is 8 to 10 mL/100 gm of myocardium per minute, and coronary blood flow is approximately 75 to 80 mL/100 gm per minute; both increase many times when cardiac work (defined as cardiac output × mean aortic pressure) is increased. The type of work performed is a major factor determining $M\dot{V}o_2$. Because the heart is primarily a volume pump, oxygen needs are reduced at equivalent external workloads when cardiac output is increased without changing afterload. In the basal state, the heart consumes 1 or 2 ml/100 gm of myocardium per minute more oxygen than does resting skeletal muscle.

Coronary vasodilation may also be induced by low myocardial tissue, increasing myocardial

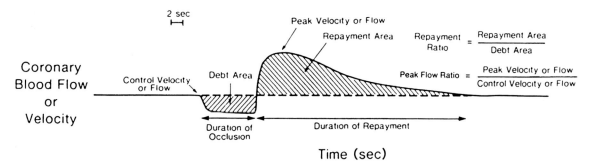

Figure 6–3. Hyperemic flow response after a brief period of coronary occlusion. Coronary blood flow, or flow velocity, is shown on the vertical axis; time is shown on the horizontal axis. After release of a 10-second coronary occlusion, hyperemic flow occurs, with peak velocity occurring by 4 seconds. The area under the flow velocity curve is termed the *repayment area.* (From Marcus ML: The Coronary Circulation in Health and Disease. New York, McGraw-Hill, 1983, p 75.)

P_{CO_2}, and declining pH,[21] as well as by circulating adenosine.[22, 23] Adenosine is a potent coronary vasodilator that is present in the normal heart. Left ventricular myocardial content of adenosine is increased promptly after 5 to 15 seconds of occlusion of the left coronary artery. In isolated perfused hearts a strong correlation is observed between coronary flow, adenosine release, and myocardial adenosine content.[23]

Reactive Hyperemia

Reactive hyperemia is a prompt, marked increase in coronary blood flow occurring in response to myocardial ischemia induced by coronary occlusion, immediately after release of the occlusion (Fig. 6–3).[24] For occlusion intervals of 5 to 180 seconds, the magnitude of the increase in flow is proportional to the duration of occlusion. Peak flow is achieved within 15 seconds of release of occlusion. The duration of the hyperemic response in animal models parallels the duration of occlusion. The *oxygen flow debt* is defined as the product of preocclusion coronary blood flow and the duration of occlusion; the debt is repaid two to four times basal levels by reactive hyperemia.[24] Coronary sinus oxygen content decreases transiently immediately on release of coronary arterial occlusion and then increases to levels close to those of arterial blood, eventually returning to control prehyperemia venous oxygen content.[25]

Adenosine appears to play a prominent role in the induction of reactive hyperemia. Although it is not the sole mediator of metabolic regulation of coronary resistance, adenosine appears to play a more important role than potassium, calcium, changes in osmolarity,[26] or prostaglandins.[27] Adenosine has been investigated as a clinically useful agent in the evaluation of coronary vasodilator reserve[28] because it

is (1) a potent vasodilator, (2) readily diffusible across cell membranes, (3) rapidly inactivated by deamination in blood or tissue and taken up or incorporated into nucleotides, (4) present in normal myocardium and increases rapidly with inadequate oxygen supply or increased oxygen need, (5) concentrated in myocardium under different physiologic conditions such as to induce predictable increases of coronary blood flow, and (6) unaccompanied by tachyphylaxis.

In animal models, the hyperemic response is attenuated in proportion to the severity of a stenosis within the coronary artery (Fig. 6–4).[29]

Autoregulation and Coronary Flow Reserve

Coronary flow reserve may be defined as the ability to maximally increase coronary blood flow over basal flow in response to demand.[30]

Physiologically, coronary arterial pressure and flow are maintained in a steady-state relationship by the process of autoregulation,[30] by which coronary flow can increase four to ten times basal level in response to demands such as exercise. With reduction of coronary arterial luminal cross-sectional area, the ability to augment coronary flow in response to demand becomes limited. The relationship between coronary pressure and flow in a normal heart is shown in Figure 6–5. With stable, unchanging myocardial metabolic oxygen demands, autoregulation maintains physiologic, relatively constant coronary blood flow over a wide range of coronary perfusion pressures.

Coronary flow reserve, defined as the ratio of flow during vasodilation to basal flow (under normal conditions), is normally about 5. In patients with atherosclerotic stenoses of differing severity in the epicardial coronary arteries, coronary flow reserve is generally reduced as a result

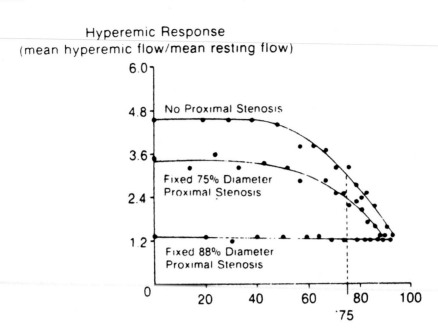

Hyperemic Response
(mean hyperemic flow/mean resting flow)

Percent Diameter Distal Stenosis

Figure 6–4. Limitation of the hyperemic response by coronary stenosis at various levels of percent diameter of distal artery stenosis in animal models. Coronary flow reserve begins to decline at approximately 60% diameter distal stenosis in normal vessels and at 50% distal stenosis in vessels with 75% diameter proximal stenosis. Coronary hyperemic flow response does not increase in vessels with proximal stenosis greater than 88% diameter. (From Gould KL, Lipscomb K, Hamilton GW: Physiologic basis for assessing critical coronary stenosis. Am J Cardiol 1974; 33:87–94. *Reprinted with permission from American Journal of Cardiology.*)

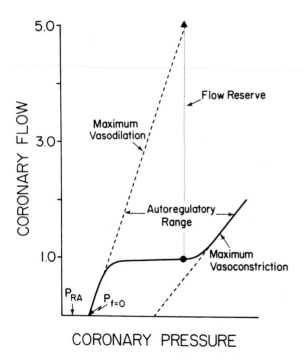

Figure 6–5. Relationship between coronary flow and coronary pressure in a normal coronary artery. The solid line represents physiologic autoregulation of flow in response to changes in pressure. The range of coronary pressure over which autoregulation is able to maintain "normal" flow is shown between the slope representing maximal vasodilation to the slope representing maximal vasoconstriction. Coronary reserve is thus determined by the difference between flow (on the "autoregulatory" graph) and the corresponding intercept in the maximal vasodilatory graph for a given pressure. $P_{f=0}$, pressure at zero flow; P_{RA}, right atrial pressure. (Reproduced with permission from Klocke FJ: Measurements of coronary flow reserve: Defining pathophysiology versus making decisions about patient care. Circulation 1987; 76:1183–1189. Copyright 1987 American Heart Association.)

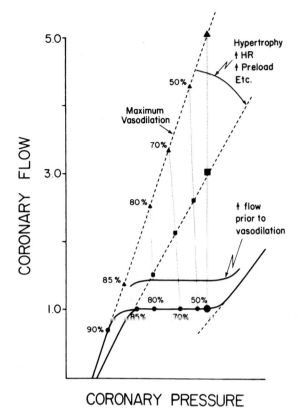

Figure 6-6. In patients with coronary artery disease, the line of maximal coronary vasodilatation is shifted downward and to the right, and this is influenced by factors such as hypertrophy, heart rate, and preload. In patients with significant coronary artery stenoses, the coronary flow reserve intercept on the line of maximal vasodilation is likewise decreased until resting coronary flow is reduced with stenoses less than 85% diameter narrowing. HR, heart rate. (Reproduced with permission from Klocke FJ: Measurements of coronary flow reserve: Defining pathophysiology versus making decisions about patient care. Circulation 1987; 76:1183–1189. Copyright 1987 American Heart Association.)

of an interplay of various complex factors (Fig. 6–6). The relationship between transstenotic pressure gradient and percentage of diameter narrowing in coronary arteries is nonlinear— disproportionately increasing gradients are observed as the stenosis exceeds 70% of luminal diameter. When luminal diameter is narrowed more than 90%, autoregulatory reserve is exhausted and normal levels of basal flow can no longer be maintained.[29] Thus, although the ratio of hyperemic to basal flow (coronary flow reserve) is about 5 in normal coronary arteries, maximal augmentation of flow is constrained in atherosclerotic vessels by flow-limiting stenoses. Thus, coronary flow reserve is reduced in these vessels. Accordingly, assessment of coronary flow reserve has been used to quantitate the physiologic consequence of coronary arterial stenosis. In animals without coronary atherosclerosis, this hypothetical model functions well. However, in humans, atherosclerosis, with its diffuse coronary involvement, introduces both theoretic and practical problems.

Determinants of Coronary Flow Reserve

Coronary flow reserve, as measured clinically, is determined by three principal factors: (1)

coronary arterial pressure, (2) flow before vasodilation, and (3) the position of the pressure-flow relationship during maximal vasodilation (see Fig. 6–5).[29, 30] During maximal vasodilation, modest changes in aortic (proximal coronary) pressure may induce significant changes in flow even in a normal coronary artery. In a diseased artery, relatively small dynamic changes in severity of stenosis (active vasoconstriction) superimposed on a fixed stenosis (e.g., increasing diameter stenosis from 80% to 85%), may produce significant changes in flow reserve (see Fig. 6–6).

Reduction in the diameter of the distal vessel occurring because of the passive collapse of the vessel in response to a decrease in intraluminal pressure during vasodilation may also substantially alter measured flow reserve. Several vasodilators,[31] including papaverine,[32] have been reported to produce occasional increases in stenotic resistance, consistent with passive collapse of a stenosis.[33]

Interpretation of changes in coronary flow reserve, as the ratio of two parameters, each of which is individually subject to various determinants, must take into account the potential influence of all of these determinants. For example, basal coronary flow before vasodilation (the denominator of the flow reserve equation) varies with metabolic demands of the myocardium. Following transient ischemia such as that occurring in association with coronary angioplasty, "basal" flow is usually increased above true basal flow measured before the ischemic intervention. Such an increase in basal flow reduces the calculated flow reserve even in the absence of a change in maximal coronary flow during maximal vasodilation. Because currently available Doppler techniques (see later) do not measure absolute flow, changes in basal flow may be difficult to identify. The coronary pressure-flow relationship during maximal vasodilation may vary on either a short-term or long-term basis. Chronic reduction of maximal flow during vasodilation commonly occurs in association with myocardial hypertrophy or infarction.[34] Reduced coronary reserve attributable to hypertrophy has been reported in hypertensive patients with normal coronary arteries and a 30% increase in left ventricular mass. Hypertrophy occurring in association with valvular and congenital anomalies may produce similar alterations in coronary vasodilator reserve.[34]

The pressure-flow relation during maximal vasodilation may be altered in conjunction with changes in hemodynamic factors, especially heart rate, contractility and preload, and blood viscosity. Alteration of coronary flow reserve in association with changes in these variables has not been comprehensively examined in patients.

MEASUREMENT OF MYOCARDIAL BLOOD FLOW

Currently, myocardial blood flow can be measured in humans with the use of the six techniques listed in Table 6–1. Only those techniques applicable in the cardiac catheterization laboratory are reviewed here.

Coronary Sinus Thermodilution Technique

The thermodilution technique, which is based on the widely used "cold" indicator-dilution method for measurement of cardiac output, involves cannulation of the coronary sinus with an end-hole catheter equipped with thermistors located at 1 cm from the distal tip and 4 to 6 cm proximal to the tip. A thermistor mounted at the end-hole of the catheter measures the temperature of infused solution. Room-temperature saline is infused at a specified rate with use of an infusion pump and becomes admixed with coronary sinus or great cardiac venous blood flowing retrogradely over the catheter. The change in temperature of blood flowing over the thermistor is proportional to the indicator (saline) infusion rate and the coronary sinus blood flow.

The coronary sinus thermodilution technique has been validated in animal models and, to a lesser extent, in humans.[2, 35] However, a precise, consistent correlation between coronary sinus flow measured in this manner and coronary arterial flow in humans with coronary artery disease has not been confirmed. Measurement of vein graft flow with use of cuff-type electromagnetic flow probes during bypass surgery has been suggested as a standard by which the technique might be validated.[36] Under these conditions, however, even the electromagnetic flow probe may be difficult to calibrate accurately. Difficulties encountered in validation of the thermodilution technique in the clinical situation are compounded by the potential for movement of the thermistors within the coronary sinus. It has been shown that the exact

Table 6–1. **Methods Used to Measure Myocardial Blood Flow**

Technique	Environment
Coronary sinus thermodilution	Cardiac catheterization laboratory, cardiac care unit
Gas clearance	Cardiac catheterization laboratory
Inert gas	
Radioactive gas	
Videodensitometric angiography	Cardiac catheterization laboratory
Radionuclide techniques	Cardiac catheterization laboratory
Nuclear medicine	
Positron emission tomography	Radiology suite
Noninvasive imaging	Radiology suite
Ultrasfast computed tomography	
Magnetic resonance imaging	
Flow probes	
Electromagnetic probe	Operating suite
Doppler probe	Cardiac catheterization laboratory

position and orientation of the thermistors relative to the ostia of the cardiac veins do not remain constant within the coronary sinus, despite fixation of the catheter and fluoroscopic confirmation of stable catheter position by comparison with known landmarks. Accurate measurement of coronary blood flow may also be adversely affected by the known variability of the pattern of venous drainage from the left ventricle and the presence of collateral flow that may not be detected angiographically. Patterns of coronary venous drainage may also be altered in the presence of severe coronary atherosclerosis, ischemia, or myocardial infarction, when the physiologic contribution of drainage from such vascular beds may be disproportionate.[17]

Additional limitations of this technique include (1) an inability to measure phasic coronary flow or rapid changes in mean flow because of the venous transit time and variation in coronary sinus dimensions; (2) an inability to measure blood flow from the right ventricle because of the variability of the patterns of venous drainage, which may frequently avoid the coronary sinus altogether; (3) an inability to detect changes in transmural distribution of myocardial perfusion; and (4) a provision of only an approximate estimate of regional left ventricular blood flow, because a large but indeterminate proportion of the left ventricular myocardium is drained by the distal coronary veins, whose anatomy is highly variable.

In general, the coronary sinus thermodilution technique should be considered adequate to detect only large changes ($\pm 30\%$) in great cardiac vein flow in patients with normal coronary arteries. In the presence of coronary artery disease the reliability of the technique is questionable.

Catheterization of the Coronary Sinus

When evaluating coronary blood flow and metabolism in humans, the coronary sinus is cannulated to (1) determine myocardial oxygen extraction and lactate production, (2) collect transmyocardial catecholamines or other metabolites, and (3) measure coronary sinus blood flow by thermodilution.

Coronary sinus thermodilution catheters are of two types. An 8-French catheter (Wilton-Webster, Altadena, CA) is constructed of woven Dacron and is equipped with three thermistors, one located at the distal tip, the second 1 cm proximal to the distal tip, and the third 4 to 5 cm proximal to the tip. The distal tip tapers to 5-French and is preshaped to a semilunar curve of 7 cm in diameter. The diameter of the central lumen is 1 mm; it will accept a 0.018-inch guide wire to aid in the manipulation of the catheter deep into the coronary sinus. The catheter is equipped with two pacing electrodes located 4 and 5 cm distal to the proximal tip.

The other available catheter (Elecath, Rahway, NJ) is composed of extruded polyvinylchloride. This catheter has a larger central lumen, is less stiff, and is preformed to a milder distal curve. It is also equipped with three thermistors; pacing electrodes are optional.

The Wilton-Webster catheter has the advantage of easier introduction via a brachial vein, but the small central lumen makes sampling of blood difficult. Conversely, the large central lumen of the Elecath catheter permits easy sampling, but in general the catheter is too soft to be inserted via the brachial route; the internal jugular vein approach is preferred.

In practice, coronary sinus thermodilution catheters are generally introduced by cutdown or percutaneous puncture of the left brachial vein, and the catheter is advanced under fluoroscopy in the posteroanterior projection into the right atrium. The tip of the catheter is directed medially toward the coronary sinus, and its position is assessed by small injections of radiographic contrast medium. Occurrence of ventricular ectopy indicates that the catheter has entered the right ventricle. If so, it is withdrawn and redirected posteriorly toward the ostium of the coronary sinus located at the inferior and posterior aspect of the tricuspid valve annulus. Difficulty with coronary sinus cannulation may be encountered if the right atrium is enlarged or if the heart is rotated by thoracic deformity or ventricular enlargement. Cardiac perforation is a risk of injudicious manipulation of the catheter in the right atrial appendage, against the lateral wall of the right atrium, or in the right ventricular apex.

Once the coronary sinus has been entered, catheter position is confirmed by repeated injections of radiographic contrast medium. The external end of the catheter is secured at the site of entry into the brachial vein, precluding movement of the catheter and thus minimizing the possibility of error introduced into flow measurements by thermistor position changes. When the catheter in introduced through a cutdown, the arm is fixed in a stable position; a sterile rubber band wrapped around the brachial vein may help maintain stable positioning of the catheter within the vein. If repeated sampling from the coronary sinus is required, a second catheter may be introduced via another vein for that purpose. After the catheter position is properly stabilized, pacing wires are

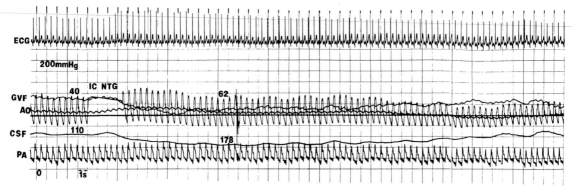

Figure 6–7. Representative example of coronary sinus thermodilution flow signals during the administration of 200 µg of intracoronary nitroglycerin (IC NTG). ECG *(top)* is the electrocardiogram. GVF, great cardiac vein flow; Ao, aortic pressure; CSF, coronary sinus flow; PA, pulmonary artery pressure. GVF at baseline is 40 mL/min. By 15 seconds after IC NTG, GVF increases to 62 mL/min. CSF increases from 110 to 178 mL/min, and this precedes the significant fall in aortic pressure on recirculation of IC NTG to the systemic circulation. (Increase in flow is indicated by downward deflection of the signal. The direction of deflection can be reversed for convenience if preferred.)

attached if required, and the central lumen of the catheter is connected to an injector system by means of a long, relatively stiff plastic tube. Either a controlled-infusion pump (Harvard pump) or a radiographic contrast medium power injector may be used. The relatively large volume of infusate required may necessitate multiple changes of the injector syringe of the Harvard pump, limiting the usefulness of this device. Our preference is to use a Medrad Mark IV radiographic injector (Medrad Company, Pittsburg, PA) loaded with room-temperature 5% dextrose in water and set to infuse at a rate of 40 mL/min. This instrument provides accuracy of ±2 mL/min of the desired flow rate. The electrical connections of the thermistors are completed. The recorder is calibrated for baseline body temperature so that introduction of room-temperature saline will induce a specific deflection of the electrical signal from the thermistor. This deflection is proportional to coronary blood flow, computed as[35]

$$F_b \text{ (ml/min)} = F_i \left(\frac{S_i \times C_i}{S_b \times C_b} \right) \left(\frac{T_b \times T_i}{T_b \times T_m} - 1 \right)$$

where F_b is the volume of blood (i.e., blood flow) and F_i is the volume of indicator (milliliters) participating in the process of heat exchange and mixing during a certain interval; T_b is the temperature of blood, T_i is the temperature of indicator, and T_m is the temperature of blood and indicator mixed (degrees Centigrade); S_b in the density of blood, S_i is the density of indicator (grams per centimeter cubed); C_b is the specific heat of blood, C_i is the specific heat of indicator (calories per gram per degree Centigrade). When 5% dextrose or normal saline is used as the indicator,

$$(S_i \cdot C_i) \div (S_b \cdot C_b) = 1.08$$

An example of the analog signal from a thermodilution coronary sinus flow catheter is illustrated (Fig. 6–7).

Gas Clearance Methods

Assessment of left ventricular myocardial perfusion by means of inert gas clearance techniques is based on an approach introduced by Kety and Schmidt[37] in 1945 for measurement of cerebral blood flow. The original Kety-Schmidt technique was modified for measurement of coronary blood flow by Eckenhoff and associates.[38] Inert gases (including helium, argon, nitrous oxide, and hydrogen) are, in effect, diffusible indicators, and their use is based on the diffusible indicator principle: the integrated difference between gas concentration in the arterial and coronary sinus blood is proportional to coronary flow per unit weight.[39] Use of this technique requires that the indicator (gas) is physiologically inert and its partition coefficient is known[1]; helium and argon are ideal because they are minimally soluble and are virtually eliminated in one lung passage, avoiding the complexities of recirculation.[2] The venous blood collection must be representative of the entire tissue region being evaluated[3]; coronary blood flow must be stable throughout the period of evaluation[4]; and the total difference in concentration of the indicator gas between coronary sinus and arterial blood must be quantitated until tissue saturation or desaturation is virtually complete.[40]

Operationally, the inert gas indicator may be inhaled or injected directly into the left atrium or ventricle or directly into the coronary arterial circulation. Quantitation of clearance of the indicator has been performed by various means, most effectively with gas chromatography, for assessment of changes in arterial and coronary sinus concentrations of the inert gases. Although use of nonradioactive gas clearance techniques has been validated under various conditions including low flow rates, the evaluation requires prolonged measurements (5 to 30 minutes), during which time coronary flow must remain constant. Coronary sinus flow represents venous drainage from the left ventricle predominantly, but assessment of transmural distribution of perfusion is not feasible.

Improved spatial resolution of myocardial perfusion has been reported with the use of xenon 133.[41, 42] Nevertheless, although the xenon 133 clearance technique allows estimation of blood flow per gram of myocardium in specific regions of the left ventricle, the right ventricle, and right atrium, the technique has several important limitations. Xenon 133 must be introduced directly into the coronary arteries, necessitating coronary cannulation. The correct approach to the computation of flow from washout curves is unclear; both fast and slow components of the washout curves have been used to compute flow rates. Necessary equipment is relatively expensive, including multicrystal gamma cameras and sophisticated computers. Accuracy of the technique is limited at lower flow rates (<200 mL/100 gm of myocardium); accuracy at high flow rates (>200 mL/100 gm) is also questionable.[42] The time constant of measurements is relatively long (seconds to minutes), whereas the time course of acute myocardial ischemia and interventions that modify coronary flow in humans is frequently brief, limiting the usefulness of the technique in dynamic situations. Thus, the gas clearance technique cannot be used in patient studies in which abrupt changes in coronary flow are expected. Repeated measurements are not possible, because xenon 133 is highly soluble in fat as well as cardiac muscle; thus, accumulation of the isotope in fat can detract from the validity of the washout. Again, the technique does not provide for measurement of transmural distribution of perfusion. Because of the theoretic and practical limitations mentioned, the inert gas and the xenon 133 clearance techniques are now used relatively infrequently in clinical practice.

In practice, xenon 133 is dissolved in 5 to 10 mL of normal saline and connected with a stopcock and flush syringe to the coronary catheter previously positioned in the coronary ostium and cleared of radiographic contrast medium.

With the patient supine on the catheterization table, a gamma camera is positioned over the patient's chest to record uptake of xenon 133 and the time course of washout of radioactivity. The patient's expired air is collected and vented outside the catheterization laboratory (and preferably the facility) to reduce airborne radioactive contamination. Scintigraphic data representing myocardial uptake of xenon 133, and its subsequent washout are processed by the computer to provide a quantitative estimate of myocardial perfusion.[41]

Videodensitometric Angiographic Techniques

Computer-based determination of the contrast transit time from one locus in the coronary arterial tree to another, using videodensitometry, is a nongeometric method used to analyze coronary flow velocity from coronary arteriograms.[43-47] The technique involves measurement of the attenuation of x-ray through a contrast-filled coronary artery. By analysis of its computer-enhanced radiopacity, the volume of contrast agent in the vessel is estimated. The leading edge of the contrast column is used to compute flow rate through the coronary artery. Volumetric coronary blood flow is then computed as the product of flow velocity and cross-sectional area of the vessel. Videodensitometry is not dependent on exact definition of vessel edges and is theoretically free from assumptions regarding the shape of the coronary artery lumen (see Chapter 10 for further discussion of videodensitometric techniques in assessment of myocardial perfusion).

In practice, videodensitometric evaluation of coronary angiograms involves specification of the arterial region of interest on a digitally analyzed and enhanced image of the coronary arteriograms on a computer matrix. The segment of artery specified in the region of interest must be parallel to the image intensifier, without overlap of other vessels. Standard coronary angiographic catheters are used to inject contrast medium, usually with a power injector (3 to 5 mL over a 3 second period from the right coronary artery and 7 to 9 mL over a 3-second period for the left coronary artery). Left or right anterior oblique angiographic views are used to display the arterial segments of interest. Nitroglycerin (200 µg sublingual or intracoronary) may be given before coronary angiography to obtain maximum vasodilation. Angiograms are obtained in multiple single-plane projections, usually with a 5-, 6-, or 7-inch image intensifier recording at film speeds of 60 frames/sec. Well-opacified end-diastolic angiographic frames showing the arterial region of interest are selected for analysis and digitized on a cineprojector. The image is projected through a sophisticated optical lens system into a high-quality video camera, and digitization of the images into the memory of a minicomputer is achieved with appropriate software. The digitized images are subsequently displayed on a video monitor. Flow velocity is then computed, with appropriate operator interaction.

Although coronary flow velocity estimated with use of videodensitometric techniques has been reported to correlate well with that estimated by other techniques, including Doppler catheters,[48] videodensitometric techniques are subject to several major limitations. Variables influencing the accuracy of measurements include the technique of the coronary arterial contrast medium injection, the hyperemic effects of contrast material itself, and the complexity and uncertainties of the algorithms used for the digital subtraction process and for computation of transit time. The relatively small caliber of the coronary arteries, together with their complex three-dimensional anatomy with multiple branch points, seriously limits the accuracy of videodensitometric assessment of contrast transit time, particularly at high flow rates. Neither absolute coronary blood flow nor transmural distribution of flow can be assessed.

In many studies reporting results of videodensitometric analysis of coronary flow, radiographic contrast medium has been used as the coronary vasodilator for determination of coronary flow reserve. Both ionic and nonionic contrast media are intermediate-strength coronary vasodilators, less potent than papaverine and adenosine but equally or more potent than intracoronary nitroglycerin.[49, 50] However, the dose-response relationship varies between patients, and the duration of peak hyperemic flow in response to contrast medium may be brief. Thus, peak flow may be missed when a "slow" technique, such as videodensitometry, is used.

In patients, coronary flow reserve computed by this technique has been reported to be in the range of 2, whereas external or intracoronary Doppler techniques indicate peak flow velocity of four to five times basal flow. Other results indicate that measured flow reserve is increased if intracoronary papaverine is used as the vasodilator rather than radiographic contrast medium.

Measurement of Coronary Flow Velocity with Doppler Devices

Doppler techniques provide accurate, continuous recordings of coronary flow velocity with a time constant measured in milliseconds. The technique has been extensively validated by comparison with changes in coronary flow assessed by timed coronary sinus measurements by the use of labeled microspheres, and with electromagnetic flow probes.[51, 52] Coronary blood flow velocity so recorded accurately reflects changes in absolute coronary volume flow.[51-55]

Flow velocity reserve and quantitative characteristics of reactive hyperemia are assessed most reliably in normal vessels that perfuse normal myocardium. Flow reserve in humans as measured with the Doppler technique in normal coronary arteries supplying a normal ventricle ranges from three and one-half to five times resting flow. These values are similar in awake and anesthetized patients undergoing open heart surgery and appear to be independent of age, gender, and the absence of superimposed atherosclerotic disease. The physiologic significance of a single coronary stenosis as assessed by analysis of Doppler velocity flow reserve has been evaluated, but the actual relationship between flow reserve and quantitative measures of severity of stenosis has not been fully delineated owing to a variety of complex interacting factors.[56-58] Nevertheless, study of translesional flow dynamics, using a Doppler guide wire, has shown significant promise for defining hemodynamic significance of a given coronary stenosis.[59]

Theory and Technique of Doppler Ultrasonography for Use in Measurement of Coronary Blood Flow Velocity

In 1843 Johann Doppler described the relationship between the shift in frequency of sound waves reflected from a moving object and its velocity.[60] The Doppler frequency shift is proportional to the velocity of the moving object relative to the position of the transmitter. The relationship between the Doppler frequency shift and the velocity of the moving object may be expressed as

$$V = (c \times f_d) \div (2f_o \times \cos \theta)$$

where V is the velocity of the object (meters per second); c is the velocity of sound in the medium; f_d is the frequency shift in kilohertz (difference between transmitted and received frequencies); $2f_o$ is twice the transmitter frequency; and $\cos \theta$ is the cosine of the angle θ between the ultrasound beam and the direction of flow.

Modern ultrasonic flowmeters use piezo-electric crystals to emit and receive ultrasound waves and thus to detect the Doppler shift described in the formula just defined. Catheters that are equipped with tip-mounted crystals (transmission frequency of 20 MHz) that function as ultrasound transmitters and receivers are available. If the angle between the crystal and the column of moving blood is known precisely, the velocity of blood flow can be computed. The characteristics of the flow velocity signal are determined by the shape of the velocity profile across the diameter of the artery, the angle of incidence of the ultrasound beam relative to the plane of the flow stream, and the position of the sample volume relative to a stenosis. Flow velocity can be converted to volume flow, provided that the cross-sectional area (CSA) of the vessel is constant, and the time-velocity integral (TVI) of the Doppler signal is known (flow = heart rate $\times$ CSA $\times$ TVI).[53] With use of pulsed ultrasound, the Doppler signal can be range-gated and directed toward a sample volume of red blood cells located within the artery at selected distances (optimally, 2 to 5 mm) from the transducer tip. Range-gating eliminates extraneous signals generated by the vascular walls and enables sampling of velocity signals within the intravascular wave front at small incremental distances from the crystal so that the maximum velocity may be detected.

Catheters equipped with Doppler crystals for assessment of coronary flow velocity were initially developed in 1974.[51] However, these catheters were too large (8-French) to be introduced subselectively into the coronary arteries; their use in patients with coronary artery disease was accordingly limited. In addition, seating and stability of the catheter's Doppler tip in the coronary ostia were suboptimal.

Modern Doppler catheters suitable for subselective introduction into the coronary arteries evolved from the Doppler suction cup catheter developed by investigators at the University of Iowa for use during open heart surgery.[52] These catheters, designed for introduction over 0.014-inch percutaneous transluminal coronary angioplasty (PTCA) balloon guide wires through wide-lumen angioplasty guide catheters, can be used to measure coronary flow velocity in individual coronary arteries of awake patients during cardiac catheterization.

Validation of Doppler Catheter Measurements

Catheter-induced obstruction of the coronary artery, although theoretically possible, has been shown to be of no physiologic importance. In fact, the CSA of the catheter is 0.8 mm[2], which is less than 10% to 15% of the CSA of a 3-mm diameter vessel. Studies in calves, with epicardial coronary arterial dimensions similar to those in humans, have shown identical peak coronary hyperemic responses with the catheter present within the artery and withdrawn from it.[54]

Measurements of coronary flow velocity with use of epicardial suction Doppler devices have been shown to correlate highly with simultaneous measurements timed to coronary sinus efflux.[52] Likewise, flow velocities measured with the intracoronary Doppler catheter correlate highly with those obtained with the epicardial Doppler technique over a wide range of flows (50 to 600 mL/min). Provided the technical limitations described in the following section are accepted, the intracoronary Doppler catheter appears to be remarkably reliable for the safe, accurate, reproducible, and repeatable measurement of coronary flow velocity in patients.

Technique of Intracoronary Flow Velocity Measurement

In practice, intracoronary flow velocity may be measured with use of 3-French Doppler catheters (Millar Instruments, Houston, TX; NuMed, Inc., Hopkinton, NY). A single 20-MHz piezoelectric crystal is mounted at the tip[55] or side[54] of the catheter. The side-mounted crystal emits an ultrasound beam at an angle 30 to 45 degrees from the longitudinal axis of the catheter.

The performance of the end-mounted versus side-mounted small Doppler catheters has been examined in models in vitro.[61] Comparison of indices of turbulence and recorded flow velocities in this model indicates that both catheters perform well ($r = 0.992$). With softer J-tipped wires such as those used clinically, the end-mounted catheter performed slightly less well because of contact with the vessel wall, whereas measurements with the side-mounted Doppler catheter were within 6% of ideal estimated flow velocity. In vivo, however, these relative merits may be balanced. The end-mounted catheters record similar signals on repeated insertion for serial measurements, whereas the angle of incidence of the side-mounted crystal may not be identical on repeated insertions. Both catheters have been demonstrated to measure flow velocity accurately and reproducibly.[61]

The Doppler catheter may be introduced into the coronary artery via a standard 8-French angioplasty guide catheter (left or right) positioned in the respective coronary ostium. The Doppler catheter is loaded onto a standard 0.012- to 0.014-inch angioplasty guide wire (Hi-

Torque Floppy II, Advanced Cardiovascular Systems, Inc., Temecula, CA). The guide wire is advanced and positioned well beyond the coronary lesion in a manner identical to that used for introduction of a PTCA balloon catheter. The Doppler catheter is then advanced over the guide wire and positioned immediately proximal (<0.5 cm) to the stenosis. If measurements are to be made in a normal artery, the tip of the Doppler catheter is positioned in a proximal segment distal to the origin of any major branch.

If coronary flow velocity reserve is to be assessed in conjunction with PTCA, the Doppler catheter is introduced into the artery first, and flow velocity measurements are made before and after intracoronary administration of a vasodilator (such as papaverine or adenosine). Coronary balloon dilation is then performed, followed by repeated assessment of flow velocity reserve. Use of a long (300-cm), 0.014-inch exchange guide wire facilitates introduction of the PTCA balloon and reintroduction of the Doppler catheter, obviating the need to cross the stenosis with the guide wire multiple times. The precise location of the Doppler catheter is re-

corded on videotape to facilitate identical placement of the catheter when flow velocity measurements are repeated after angioplasty.

Doppler velocity and hemodynamic signals are displayed and recorded on a photographic multichannel oscillographic recorder. Before introduction of the catheter, mean and phasic Doppler velocity signals are calibrated against an arbitrary internal signal of 0 to 100 cm/sec generated by the velocimeter.

Before introduction of the Doppler catheter, 5000 IU of heparin is administered intravenously. The handling characteristics of both types of 3-French Doppler catheters are similar to those of first-generation PTCA balloon catheters. Once the Doppler catheter has been advanced through the guiding catheter, its position and orientation may need adjustment to obtain an optimal flow velocity signal. Advancing the guide wire, backing out the guide catheter, or rotating the Doppler catheter may be necessary. The velocimeter range-gate is then adjusted in 0.5-mm increments until a maximal phasic signal is obtained with the use of fast oscilloscopic sweep speed (100 cm/sec) to ensure that the diastolic velocity profile is optimal.

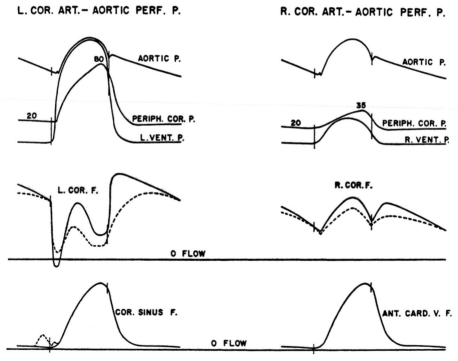

Figure 6–8. Ideal physiologic tracings of left and right coronary artery (COR ART) flow velocity (from an experimental animal preparation). Aortic perfusion pressure (PERF P), peripheral coronary pressure (PERIPH COR P), left ventricular pressure (L VENT P), with simultaneous left coronary flow (L COR F), and coronary sinus blood flow (COR SINUS F), are identified. Anterior cardiac vein flow (ANT CARD V F) is also shown on the bottom. Broken curves represent alterations that may be observed in patients. (From Best CH, Taylor NB [eds]: The Physiological Basis of Medical Practice. Baltimore, Williams & Wilkins, 1966, p 817.)

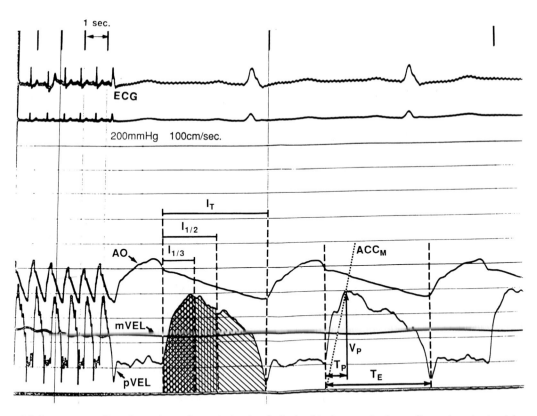

Figure 6–9. Intracoronary Doppler catheter flow velocity signal obtained in humans in the cardiac catheterization laboratory. Measurements made (see text) include diastolic flow velocity integral (I_T), one-half diastolic flow velocity integral ($I_{1/2}$), one-third flow velocity integral ($I_{1/3}$), aortic pressure (AO), mean velocity (mVEL), phasic velocity (pVEL), time to peak (T_P), velocity at peak (V_P), total time of diastolic flow (T_E), and mean acceleration time (ACC_M). ECG, electrocardiogram. (From Kern MJ, Deligonul U, Vandormael M, et al: Impaired coronary vasodilator reserve in the immediate postcoronary angioplasty period: Analysis of coronary artery flow velocity indexes and regional cardiac venous efflux. Reprinted with permission from the American College of Cardiology [Journal of the American College of Cardiology, 1989; 13:860–872.])

Once optimal Doppler signals have been obtained, hyperemia is stimulated pharmacologically. Filling and flushing the guide catheter with the selected drug deliver the agent nonselectively to the coronary circulation, although streaming effects generally concentrate the flow of the bolus in the direction of the intracoronary catheter. Although careful ostial seating of the guiding catheter is required for the drug to be reliably delivered into the coronary artery, removal of the guiding catheter immediately before the recording of flow velocity may be necessary to preclude damping of flow. Alternatively, the vasodilator drug may be administered directly through the Doppler catheter after careful positioning of the catheter in the coronary artery and removal of the guide wire. This method is theoretically preferable, because it ensures localization of the full dose to the artery under examination. However, the Doppler catheter should not be manipulated without the guide wire in place because the risk of vascular trauma may be higher. Also, repeated crossing of the stenosis with the guide wire may stimulate vasospasm, plaque activation, or thrombosis.

Coronary Velocity Signal Analysis

In our laboratory phasic and mean coronary flow velocity signals are recorded at both 10 and 100 mm/sec paper speed and are digitized with use of an off-line microcomputer system (Figs. 6–8 and 6–9). For reliable analysis, flow velocity signals should be stable and reproducible, with clearly demarcated phasic waveform configurations.

The diastolic flow velocity integral (DFVi) derived from the area below the flow velocity waveform between the aortic dicrotic notch and the systolic aortic upstroke (see Fig. 6–9) is computed. Absolute flow may then be estimated from the product of flow velocity integral, heart rate, and CSA of the normal proximal vessel segment.[53]

CSA of the vessel can be estimated by several techniques. Most simply the diameter of the vessel is measured at the site of the Doppler catheter tip from the coronary cineangiogram, corrected for magnification by use of the shaft of the guiding catheter as a known reference diameter. Assuming a circular diameter, the CSA of the vessel is then calculated from the radius (r), according to the standard formula

$$CSA = \pi \cdot r^2$$

To compensate for the noncircular profile of some vessels, diameters may be measured from two orthogonal views of the artery. If an intervention produces coronary vasodilation, diameters must be derived from angiograms before and after vasodilation.

The total time of diastolic flow velocity (T_E), time to peak maximal velocity (T_p), and first one third ($I_{1/3}$) and one half ($I_{1/2}$) of the total DFVi may be measured. Coronary artery resistance index (CVR_I) may be computed as the ratio of mean arterial pressure to mean coronary flow velocity. Coronary vasodilation reserve may be calculated in the following ways: (1) the ratio of peak hyperemic flow velocity to mean flow velocity may be calculated or (2) vasodilatory reserve may be normalized for changing pressure during hyperemia, computed as

Hyperemic mean velocity/MAP_{peak} ÷

Basal mean velocity/MAP_{basal}

where MAP_{peak} is mean arterial pressure at peak flow and MAP_{basal} is mean arterial pressure at basal flow.

Drugs Used to Assess Coronary Vasodilator Reserve

Various stimuli have been used to induce coronary vasodilation and hyperemia for the derivation of coronary vasodilator reserve (Table 6–2). In the operating room, coronary occlusion-release produces ischemic hyperemia. Hyperemia may be achieved with use of dipyridamole administered intravenously, papaverine administered by intracoronary injection, or adenosine given either intravenously or directly into the coronary artery.[63] Repeated measurements of coronary vasodilator reserve require the use of short-acting, nontoxic maximal vasodilators. In

Table 6–2. **Stimuli Used in Measurement of Coronary Vasodilator Reserve**

Intraoperative coronary occlusion
Contrast media
Nitroglycerin
Papaverine
Adenosine
Dipyridamole

patients with coronary atherosclerosis, papaverine induces brief, maximal arteriolar vasodilation and a marked increase in coronary blood flow.[32, 49, 50, 55] Intracoronary papaverine, as compared with intravenous dipyridamole or radiographic contrast media, has the advantage of inducing maximal vasodilation of very short duration, usually less than 3 minutes. When injected directly into normal coronary arteries, papaverine increases coronary flow velocity by an average of 5.2 ± 0.6 (mean ± SEM) times basal flow velocity. The vasodilator effects of papaverine, in standard 3- to 12-mg doses, are prompt and brief, with maximal hyperemia occurring 28 ± 4 seconds after intracoronary injection and returning to baseline within 128 ± 15 seconds.[32, 49] Its short duration of action and lack of major effects on systemic hemodynamics make papaverine an excellent vasodilator for these studies. Papaverine-induced prolongation of the electrocardiographic (ECG) QT interval, however, is frequent. Rare but potentially serious transient ventricular arrhythmias after intracoronary injection of papaverine have been reported, although they have proved treatable, either medically or with direct-current cardioversion.[64]

Adenosine, traditionally regarded as the physiologic coronary vasodilator,[23] may also be suitable for measurement of coronary flow velocity reserve in patients. Although intravenous administration of adenosine in animals produces marked hypotension and reflex tachycardia,[65] intracoronary administration, in appropriate dosage, has been reported to produce maximal coronary vasodilation with fewer systemic effects. It may indeed be superior to papaverine, because of an even shorter duration of vasodilation and lack of associated QT prolongation.[66] However, highly variable individual dose-response relationships, angina-like chest pain,[66] and occasional transient bradycardia and asystole may limit clinical application of this agent.[67]

Intravenous dipyridamole may also produce maximal coronary vasodilation, increasing blood flow velocity up to five times basal levels. However, time to peak flow after dipyridamole is prolonged (6 to 10 minutes), and vasodilator activity is apparent for more than 20 minutes, making the agent unsuitable for studies in which repeated measurements are necessary.[68] Neither intracoronary nitroglycerin nor contrast media (ionic, low osmolar, or nonionic) induce maximal hyperemia.

Limitations of the Doppler Catheter Technique

Disadvantages of the intracoronary Doppler catheter technique are few—measurement of relative rather than absolute flow velocity and the inability to compute absolute coronary volume flow constitute the two major drawbacks. When the technique is performed in conjunction with quantitative angiography for measurement of coronary arterial dimensions, however, volume flow can be estimated. As with most clinical techniques for measurement of flow, transmural distribution of flow cannot be assessed. Practical difficulties may be encountered in the presence of very proximal coronary arterial stenoses or vessels having side branches in the region under examination. Reproducible serial measurement of coronary flow velocity requires that (1) the CSA of the vessel being interrogated remain fixed, (2) the velocity profile across the vessel not be significantly distorted by atherosclerotic disease, and (3) the angle between the plane of the ultrasonic beam and sample volume remain constant.

Although the risks of intracoronary instrumentation include arterial spasm, intimal dissection, and vessel perforation, the incidence of complications of Doppler coronary catheterization is low in experienced hands. Nevertheless, because of the risk of vascular trauma, some investigators have recommended that only patients undergoing PTCA be subjected to subselective coronary instrumentation.[67]

Interpretation of coronary flow reserve requires consideration of the several factors that may affect either the numerator or the denominator of the flow reserve ratio. Hemodynamic factors (including changing distal arterial pressure, heart rate, or left ventricular end-diastolic pressure), altered contractility, and changes in vascular myogenic tone all can influence reactive and pharmacologic hyperemia.[63, 69, 70] Anatomic factors such as previous myocardial infarction, scarring, regional (ischemic) dysfunction (e.g., hypokinesis), and myocardial hypertrophy may affect vasodilator reserve. Factors related to the vasodilator (or its vehicle), including dose, osmolality, oxygen content, and chemical composition, as well as specific drug effects on the function of normal or abnormal endothelium, may also modify coronary hyperemic responses.[70] Administration of the vasodilator via the guiding catheter may result in delivery of an incomplete, inhomogeneous concentration of the drug to the vessel of interest. Suboptimal doses of papaverine may not elicit maximal hyperemia. Although doses as high as 12 to 14 mg of papaverine have been suggested,[32] a dose of 10 mg is generally considered sufficient to achieve maximal vasodilation.

Attention to catheter positioning with careful avoidance of large side branches (>12%

diameter of the major vessel) is required; if measurements are to be performed before and after angioplasty, placement of the catheter tip at identical intravascular loci is required on each occasion.

Complications of Coronary Vasodilator Reserve Measurements

Measurement of coronary vasodilator reserve with use of the subselective Doppler catheter has three obvious disadvantages: (1) the procedure takes time, which on occasion may not be affordable, particularly during complex angioplasty; (2) intracoronary instrumentation is required, with its inherent risks, including spasm, vascular trauma (especially dissection or perforation), local thrombosis, and plaque disruption; and (3) administration of a potent vasodilator is required.

Papaverine has been administered via the intracoronary route to many hundreds of patients with angiographically normal coronary arteries, to those with coronary atherosclerosis, and to those with angiographically normal coronary arteries after heterotopic cardiac transplantation. Papaverine reduces systemic arterial blood systolic and diastolic pressure by 6% to 10%, with similar increases in heart rate. QT and QTc intervals are significantly prolonged (18% to 27%) after intracoronary papaverine in patients with normal angiograms and in those with coronary artery disease. In this laboratory, the average (absolute) increases in QT interval in normal subjects and pre-PTCA and post-PTCA patients were 89 ± 64, 120 ± 76, and 95 ± 82 msec, respectively (P = NS).[71] Papaverine-induced changes in QT interval do not appear to correlate with any clinical, hemodynamic, or intracoronary flow velocity variables used in the measurement of coronary vasodilator reserve.

One report cited two episodes of ventricular tachycardia in more than 300 patients studied with doses of less than 12 mg of intracoronary papaverine.[64] In this laboratory, three cases of serious arrhythmia (two torsades de pointes, one marked sinus bradycardia with escape bigeminy) have been observed after intracoronary administration of papaverine (Fig. 6–10). No significant factors predisposing to either prolongation of QT intervals or to serious arrhythmias have been identified,[71] and no correlation between coronary flow reserve responses and changes in QTc interval has been found in normal subjects or in patients undergoing PTCA, either before or after the procedure.

Papaverine-induced arrhythmias are probably idiosyncratic in nature. For unknown rea-

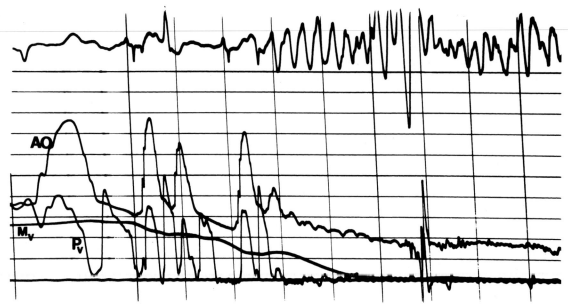

Figure 6–10. Coronary flow velocity (mean [M$_V$] and phasic [P$_V$] velocities) and aortic pressure (AO) after intracoronary papaverine. Torsades de pointes is documented on the electrocardiogram *(top)*. Mean coronary flow velocity before the arrhythmia is measured at 28 cm/sec. After the onset of torsades de pointes both AO and M$_V$ fell to zero. This patient required immediate direct-current cardioversion, which was successful with no complications. (From Kern MJ, Deligonul U, Serota H, et al: Ventricular arrhythmia due to intracoronary papaverine: Analysis of QT intervals and coronary vasodilatory reserve. Cathet Cardiovasc Diagn 1990; 19:229–236. Copyright 1990 John Wiley & Sons, Inc. Reprinted by permission of John Wiley & Sons, Inc.)

sons, ventricular arrhythmias have been documented to occur in women with normal coronary arteries[64] with no preceding QT interval prolongation. Papaverine causes prominent T wave depression in most species; mixtures of papaverine and ionic contrast media have additive ECG effects.[72] In the reported instances of serious arrhythmia, papaverine was administered in close temporal proximity to injection of ionic contrast media.[64] Although meglumine ioxaglate (Hexabrix) and papaverine hydrochloride may precipitate on contact in vitro,[73] no adverse clinical effects of this combination have been reported. Residual repolarization abnormalities attributable to contrast media may have an additive effect on papaverine-induced electrocardiographic abnormalities, and possibly, on the induction of arrhythmias. Thus, T wave and QT interval changes should be allowed to resolve before papaverine is administered. Because of their propensity to arrhythmia, patients with prolonged baseline QT intervals at rest should probably not be given papaverine.

Measurement of coronary vasodilator reserve with use of intracoronary catheters should be performed only by personnel thoroughly experienced in angioplasty techniques. Appropriately skilled personnel and proper equipment

to deal with life-threatening arrhythmias must be immediately available.

Special Instrumentation Used to Assess Coronary Flow Velocity

Judkins-style Doppler Catheter

The major limitation to the widespread use of intracoronary velocity techniques is the requirement for instrumentation of the coronary artery with an angioplasty guide wire and small-diameter catheter that must enter and traverse the coronary lumen. To facilitate more rapid and safe measurement of coronary flow velocity in patients while circumventing the need for intracoronary instrumentation and the limitations of earlier nonselective flow velocity catheters, we developed a Judkins-style Doppler-tipped angiographic catheter. This catheter permits measurement of flow velocity and coronary vasodilator reserve with results comparable with those achieved with use of the intracoronary Doppler catheter. It should facilitate measurement of flow velocity and vasodilator reserve in large populations of patients without focal coronary atherosclerotic disease, such as those who have undergone heterotopic cardiac transplantation and those with nonischemic cardiomyopathy, valvular heart disease, or syndrome X.

The Judkins-style Doppler-tipped catheter is an 8-French double-lumen extrusion of standard polyvinylchloride equipped with a 20-MHz Doppler velocity crystal positioned in the caudal portion of the distal tip (Fig. 6–11). The catheter is identical in shape and handling characteristics to the standard Judkins diagnostic catheter, although the distal tip is slightly less tapered. The technique for insertion of the Judkins-style Doppler catheter is identical to that for standard Judkins left coronary diagnostic catheters: The catheter is introduced via Seldinger technique over an 0.038-inch J-tipped safety guide wire and passed to the aortic root. After selective intubation of the left main coronary artery, injection of contrast material through the catheter lumen allows identification of the position and axial angulation of the catheter within the coronary ostium. When properly seated and range-gated (2 to 4 mm from the tip), the velocity signal is identical in timing, duration, and waveform to that obtained with the intracoronary Doppler catheter at the same location (Fig. 6–12). In our laboratory, coronary flow velocity data have been acquired without complications in more than

85% of patients in whom studies have been attempted with use of either the Judkins-style Doppler or the intracoronary Doppler catheter.

In a validation study in 19 patients with chest pain but no coronary artery disease, flow velocity recordings obtained with both the Judkins-style Doppler and the 3-French intracoronary DC-101 catheters were compared. Although the resting mean velocities recorded with the Judkins-style catheter were similar (13.7 ± 7.9 versus 9.6 ± 6.5 cm/sec, respectively), the hyperemic flow velocities recorded by the Judkins-style Doppler catheter were higher than those obtained with the intracoronary catheter (mean velocity 40.5 ± 18. 2 versus 31.7 ± 14. 2 cm/sec; $P < 0.05$). The relative changes from control to maximal hyperemic flow velocity were, however, similar (244% ± 144% versus 272% ± 119%, $P = $ NS) (Fig. 6–13). In addition, although peak velocities were higher, calculated values for coronary vasodilator reserve obtained with the two techniques were nearly identical (3.33 ± 1.36 versus 3.72 ± 1.20 units; $P = $ NS). There was strong correlation between the two measures ($r = 0.801$, $P < 0.001$). In six patients, changes in coronary flow velocity measured by the two catheters during respiratory maneuvers were virtually identical.

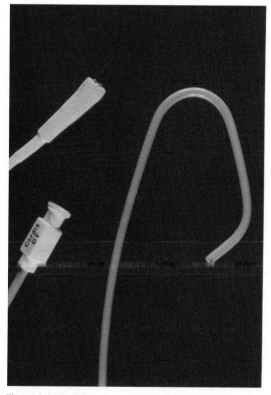
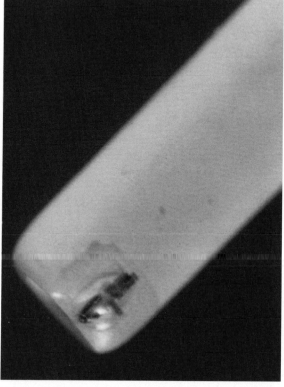

Figure 6–11. Judkins-Doppler–tipped angiographic catheter *(left)* demonstrating the crystal embedded in the wall of the Judkins catheter *(right)*.

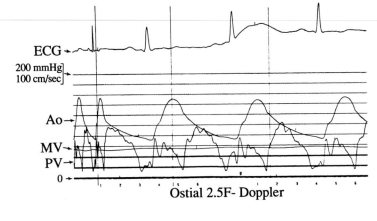

ECG
200 mmHg
100 cm/sec
Ao
MV
PV
0
Ostial 2.5F- Doppler

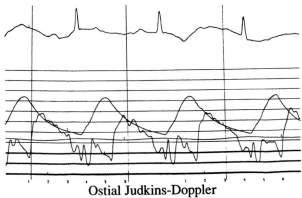

Ostial Judkins-Doppler

Figure 6–12. Comparison of flow velocity recordings obtained with 2.5-French Doppler (PC 101) and Judkins-style Doppler catheters at the left main ostial location. ECG, electrocardiogram; Ao, aortic pressure; MV, mean velocity; PV, phasic velocity. These two waveforms exhibit almost identical systolic and diastolic components. Derived indexes, including diastolic flow velocity integrals, and duration of diastole are similar.

The Doppler Guide Wire

More recently, to facilitate measurements of flow velocity in the smaller, more distal coronary arteries, an "ultrasonic guide wire" has been developed.[74–76] The Doppler Flowire (Cardiometrics Mountain View, CA) is a 175-cm-long, 0.018-inch steerable guide wire with an ultrasonic 12-MHz transducer mounted at its tip. The guide wire can be advanced through the lumen of a coaxial catheter and across a stenosis. The transducer generates a uniform beam of pulsed Doppler ultrasound encompassing the entire segment of the vessel, both proximal and distal to the stenosis. Volume flow can be calculated by use of the angiographically derived vessel diameters. Unlike other Doppler systems, this device samples flow velocity in the entire vessel and averages all of the "focal flow rates"; the conventional Doppler catheter measures flow velocity only at the catheter tip. Velocity signals are processed by fast Fourier transform. The Doppler spectrum is digitized, and the following parameters are calculated: peak diastolic velocity, peak systolic velocity, mean velocity or the time average of the spectral peak velocity waveform throughout the cardiac cycle,

integral of both the diastolic and systolic velocities, and the first one-third and first one-half flow fractions (Fig. 6–14).

As with all Doppler-based devices, the Flowire must be positioned as nearly parallel as possible to the direction of blood flow to detect accurately peak velocities. This requirement becomes more difficult to meet in tortuous arteries. However, careful repositioning and attention to the audio output of the spectral signals usually allow optimal transducer placement.

Impedance Catheters and Impedance Guide Wires

Interpretation of changes in coronary flow velocity reserve must take into account the several variables that may alter basal or peak flow velocity. For example, augmented basal flow velocity (induced pharmacologically or by ischemia, as during PTCA) may reduce the flow reserve ratio in the absence of changes in vasodilator capacity. Endothelial injury sustained during PTCA may also result in falsely lowered flow velocity reserve. To circumvent these variables, impedance catheters and guide wires that directly

CVR (units)

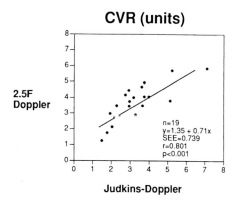

2.5F
Doppler

Judkins-Doppler

Mean Velocity (cm/sec)

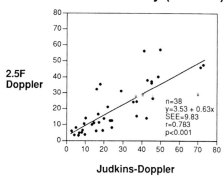

2.5F
Doppler

Judkins-Doppler

DFVI (units)

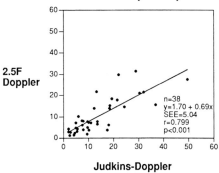

2.5F
Doppler

Judkins-Doppler

Figure 6–13. Coronary vascular resistance (CVR), mean flow velocity, and diastolic flow velocity integral (DFVI) measured with 2.5-French intracoronary Doppler (vertical axis) and the Judkins-style Doppler (horizontal axis) catheters. Highly significant correlations are documented between the two recordings.

measure absolute coronary flow have been developed.[77, 78] These instruments use electrical impedance technology, employing algorithms based on the Stewart-Hamilton indicator-dilution principle. The instrument comprises a balloon catheter incorporating a third lumen that terminates just proximal to the balloon (Fig. 6–15). Indicator (5% dextrose in water) is injected over 3 to 6 seconds through the third

lumen. Two pairs of microelectrodes located distal to the balloon detect changes in impedance induced by hypotonicity of the glucose solution relative to blood (Fig. 6–16).

Absolute coronary blood flow is inversely proportional to the integral of the impedance curve

$$Flow = K_S \cdot I \div A$$

where K_S is the "sensitivity constant" (slope of relationship of impedance to the concentration of dextrose 5% in water); I is the amount of dextrose 5% in water indicator; and A is the area under the first-pass transit (impedance) curve.

This technique allows measurement of absolute coronary flow at the site of indicator injection, that is, immediately proximal to the balloon. The measurement is unaffected by distal branching of the parent coronary artery, assuming (as has been shown to be the case) that adequate mixing of indicator with blood occurs between the point of injection and the microelectrodes. Placement of the balloon across a stenosis, however, may cause sufficient luminal obstruction to significantly limit flow (particularly during hyperemia), precluding use of this instrument for measurement of translesional flow.

To obviate this constraint, an 0.014-inch impedance guide wire equipped with a 2-mm electrode gap located several centimeters proximal to its tip has been developed.[78] In practice, a standard over-the-wire PTCA balloon is placed proximal to the stenosis, and the impedance guide wire is advanced through the balloon and across the stenosis. The indicator solution (5% dextrose in water) is then injected through the tip of the balloon catheter, inducing a measurable change in electrical impedance at the site of the microelectrodes located distal to the stenosis, and translesional absolute flow is measured.

Use of the impedance balloon catheter and guide wire systems has been extensively validated in vitro, in animal models, and in patients undergoing coronary angioplasty. Excellent correlations were obtained between absolute flow measured in canine coronary arteries by the impedance catheter and that measured by the electromagnetic flowmeter.

The advantage of the impedance technology is that it can be used to measure absolute coronary flow directly. Particular advantages of the impedance guide wire system include (1) its potential for use with any "over-the-wire" PTCA balloon catheters, (2) its extremely small CSA,

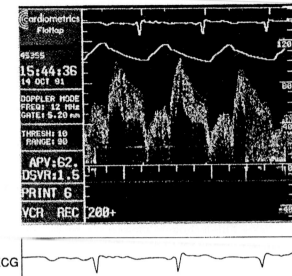

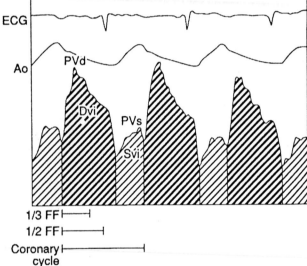

Figure 6–14. Intracoronary velocity spectrum recorded with a Doppler guide wire *(upper)* and schematic representation of the digitized spectral profile *(lower)*. ECG, electrocardiogram; Ao, aortic pressure; PVd = peak diastolic velocity; Dvi, diastolic velocity integral; PVs, peak systolic velocity; Svi, systolic velocity integral; 1/3 FF, first third of flow fraction; 1/2 FF, first half of flow fraction. (From Ofili EO, Kern MJ, Labovitz AJ, et al: Analysis of coronary blood flow velocity dynamics in angiographically normal and stenosed arteries before and after endolumen enlargement by angioplasty. Reprinted with permission from the American College of Cardiology [Journal of the American College of Cardiology, 1993; 21:308–316.])

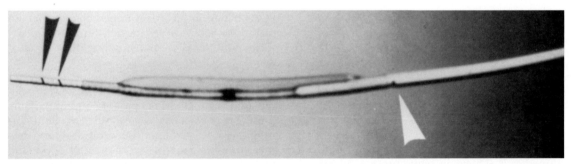

Figure 6–15. Impedance angioplasty balloon catheter designed for assessment of absolute coronary blood flow. The *white arrowhead* points to the side-hole through which the indicator (5 mL of 5% dextrose in water) is injected over a 3- to 6-second interval. This hypotonic indicator induces an increase in impedance measured at the distal electrode pair *(black arrowheads)*. The change in impedance is registered as an impedance curve; absolute coronary blood flow is derived from the inverse of the area under the impedance curve. (From Vogel RA, Martin LW: Transcatheter coronary artery diagnostic techniques. Tex Heart Inst J 1989; 16:195–203.)

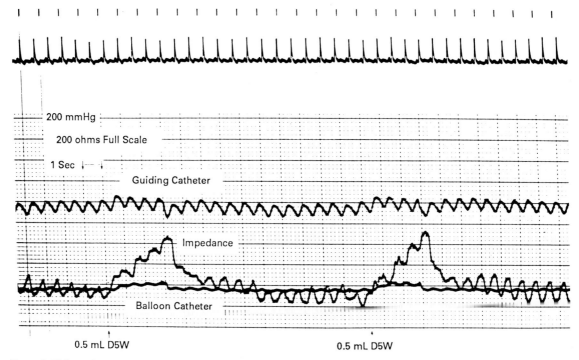

Figure 6–16. Impedance curves produced in a patient by the impedance angioplasty catheter during left anterior descending coronary artery dilation. Absolute coronary blood flow is inversely proportional to the area under the impedance curve, analogous to measurement of cardiac output by the indicator-dilution principle. (From Vogel RA, Martin LW: Transcatheter coronary artery diagnostic techniques. Tex Heart Inst J 1989; 16:195–203.)

which allows placement of the wire across a stenosis without compromise of flow, even during hyperemia, and (3) the fact that it allows measurement of flow through very proximal stenoses.

CLINICAL APPLICATION OF MEASUREMENTS OF CORONARY BLOOD FLOW

Measurement of coronary flow in patients is of particular interest in two areas: (1) determination of coronary vasomotor responses and (2) assessment of myocardial utilization of oxygen, metabolites, and other biochemical moieties in response to maneuvers designed to alter myocardial metabolism or ventricular function.

In the last decade, coronary flow has been evaluated in the cardiac catheterization laboratory in a number of clinical situations, including (1) before and after coronary angioplasty, (2) after bypass graft surgery, (3) assessment of coronary flow reserve, (4) myocardial function as a function of coronary reserve, and (5) ischemia testing. Routine clinical assessment of coronary flow and flow (velocity) reserve has yet to be proven of value. However, intracoronary Dopp-

ler techniques for measurement of coronary blood flow have expanded significantly our understanding of the pathophysiology of coronary artery disease and its sequelae and has set the stage for future developments.

Coronary Flow Velocity Measurements by Doppler Catheter with PTCA

Neither angiography (whether assessed visually or by computer-based quantitative techniques) nor measurement of the residual coronary translesional pressure gradient permits consistently accurate confirmation of the success of an angioplastic or atherectomic technique. Immediately after PTCA, quantitative and subjective angiographic assessments are often complicated by both intimal dissection and the accumulation of mural thrombi; the result is a hazy, distorted radiographic appearance. The accuracy of residual translesional pressure gradients is compromised by an inadequate frequency response with all except those measured by micromanometer pressure wires, as well as by the unpredictable and dynamic influence of distal collateral flow. Furthermore, a second lumen for measurement of translesional gradients is not available in the newer "low-profile" PTCA balloon catheters.

Coronary flow velocity reserve in response to a pharmacologic vasodilator has been investigated as a clinically useful predictor of the success of angioplasty.[78–85] Although coronary vasodilator reserve has been accepted as a reliable predictor of the physiologic severity of coronary stenoses[29, 30, 82] and as a measure of the efficacy of mechanical revascularization,[47, 58, 82] it has been found to remain depressed immediately after dilation in many patients after clinically successful PTCA (Fig. 6–17).[62, 79, 82–85] In contrast, coronary reserve assessed by either intracoronary Doppler catheter measurement[80] or digital radiographic techniques[82] has been shown to be normalized in most patients (in the absence of significant restenosis) at 7.5 months after the procedure. Thus, coronary flow velocity reserve, measured immediately after the balloon dilation, may not reflect the long-term success of the procedure.

Factors Responsible for Lack of Normalization of Coronary Flow Reserve After PTCA

Persistently abnormal flow reserve immediately after PTCA may be attributable to failure to reset autoregulatory homeostasis of epicardial and small precapillary arterioles,[86, 87] altered vasoreactivity due to damage to vascular smooth muscle,[88, 89] and inhibition or release of endothelial vasoactive or neurohumoral factors at

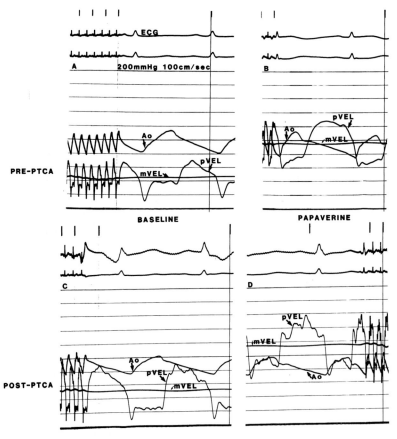

Figure 6–17. Coronary flow velocity measured before (baseline, *left panels*) and after *(right panels)* papaverine in patients undergoing successful coronary angioplasty. The upper panels show the pre-percutaneous transluminal coronary angioplasty (PTCA) mean (mVEL) and phasic (pVEL) coronary flow velocity and aortic pressure (Ao) recordings. mVEL of 22 cm/sec was recorded at baseline, increasing to 46 cm/sec during papaverine. Coronary flow reserve ratio of 2.01 was calculated. After angioplasty *(lower panels)* baseline mVEL was 26 cm/sec; peak hyperemic flow velocity after papaverine was 46 cm/sec. Coronary vasodilator reserve of 1.9 was calculated. Note that the configuration of the flow velocity waveforms during the hyperemic period in the postangioplasty period differ, with a brisker upstroke. The significance of coronary Doppler velocity waveforms in this setting has not been examined. (From Kern MJ, Deligonul U, Vandormael M, et al: Impaired coronary vasodilator reserve in the immediate postcoronary angioplasty period: Analysis of coronary artery flow velocity indexes and regional cardiac venous efflux. Reprinted with permission from the American College of Cardiology [Journal of the American College of Cardiology, 1989; 13:860–872.])

the site of vascular injury.[90–94] Platelet activation and release of platelet-mediated vasoactive products[95] at the site of endothelial damage may also play a role. Vascular smooth muscle hyperreactivity has been noted in atherosclerotic plaques and has been associated with enhanced vasoconstriction.[93, 94, 96]

Dilation of epicardial coronary arteries may also occur independently via flow-mediated, endothelium-dependent vasodilation.[92] Endothelial dysfunction may account for the inability of the atherosclerotic arterial segments to respond appropriately to vasodilator stimulation.[6]

Velocity and Flow Measurements Using a Doppler Guide Wire During PTCA

Although coronary flow reserve measurements have been inconsistent after PTCA, the Doppler ultrasound guide wire system has allowed predilation and postdilation analyses of blood velocity patterns, both proximal and distal to the site of stenosis. These studies have revealed that predilation phasic velocity measurements distal to a stenosis are different from normal vessels and, after PTCA, tend to normalize.[83] In 38 patients undergoing coronary angioplasty, significant improvement in mean time of average peak velocity was noted in distal coronary arteries after angioplasty (before 19 ± 12 cm/sec; after 35 ± 16 cm/sec; $P <0.01$). Increases in the proximal average peak velocity after angioplasty were less remarkable (before 34 ± 18 cm/sec; after 41 ± 14 cm/sec; $P <0.04$). Also, before PTCA mean diastolic to systolic velocity ratio measured distal to a significant stenosis was decreased compared with that in normal vessels (1.3 ± 0.5 versus 1.8 ± 0.5, $P <0.01$). After angioplasty, the abnormal distal phasic velocity patterns generally returned to normal, with a significant increase in the mean diastolic to systolic velocity ratio (1.3 ± 0.5 versus 1.9 ± 0.6; $P <0.01$) (Fig. 6–18). In contrast proximal to the stenosis, the phasic velocity patterns did not change after PTCA.[83]

Measurement of Coronary Flow Velocity Reserve by Digital Angiography

Coronary flow reserve computed from digitized coronary angiograms has been shown to be a reproducible, convenient technique for assessment of the functional significance of coronary artery obstruction.[97–99] Limitations of digital coronary angiography for measurement of coronary flow velocity include the need for precise reduplication of angiographic projections and of the timing and duration of contrast injections. Also, correlation of coronary flow reserve by digital angiography with lesion severity may be confounded by imprecise edge detection after coronary angioplasty in view of the disruption of the arterial intima and media, producing a hazy silhouette. Moreover, quantitative coronary angiography may not be sufficiently sensitive to detect diffuse, nonfocal coronary artery disease; that is, substantial intimal atherosclerosis resulting in diffuse obstruction may involve the entire length of an epicardial artery even though angiographic depiction of luminal contours may suggest only minimal lesions.[100] The diffuse nature of atherosclerosis, which is frequently not recognizable angiographically, may explain why minimal residual stenoses are sometimes associated with impaired coronary flow reserve.

Coronary Flow Reserve After Coronary Saphenous Vein Bypass Grafting

Coronary bypass surgery may restore coronary flow reserve to normal status. In one study in which Doppler catheters were used, coronary flow velocity was measured in 24 patients with 35 bypass grafts perfusing angiographically normal vessels, and in 13 patients with normal coronary vessels and normal myocardium.[58] Coronary flow reserve (5.0 ± 0.4) was recorded in 17 bypass grafts with uncompromised anastomoses perfusing normal myocardium, which was comparable with that in normal arteries (5.1 ± 0.6) even though the CSA of the native vessels was 40% smaller. Flow reserve in grafts supplying hypertrophied or infarcted myocardium was significantly reduced (2.7 ± 0.3). Thus, myocardial revascularization with vein grafts restored maximal coronary flow reserve to normal, provided the graft and coronary artery were not stenotic and the myocardium perfused was normal. The diffuse nature of atherosclerosis in these patients did not appear to impair maximal coronary flow reserve significantly when vessels were successfully bypassed.

Coronary Flow Reserve and Left Ventricular Functional Responses: A Test for Ischemia?

Pharmacologically induced coronary hyperemia may provoke new left ventricular wall motion abnormalities in regions supplied by critically stenosed coronary arteries in some patients,[101–109] whereas in others myocardial regions supplied by coronary arteries with similar or nearly identical stenoses may demonstrate either normal or hypercontractile response patterns.[101]

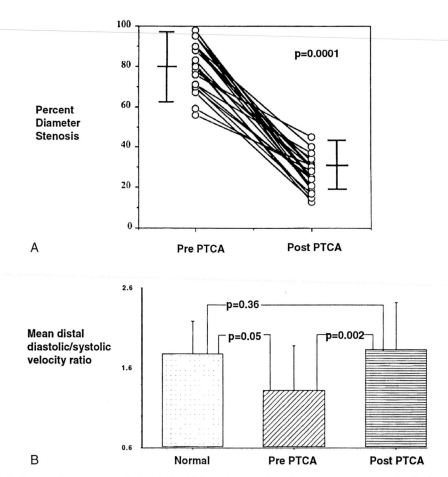

Figure 6–18. *A,* Percent diameter stenosis (vertical axis) in patients undergoing percutaneous transluminal coronary angioplasty (PTCA) and in whom Doppler guide wire flow velocity tracings, proximal and distal to the stenosis, were recorded before and after the dilation. *B,* Mean distal diastolic:systolic velocity ratio for normal subjects and for patients subjected to PTCA (see text for details). (*A* and *B* from Segal J, Kern MJ, Scott NA, et al: Alterations of phasic coronary artery flow velocity in humans during percutaneous coronary angioplasty. Reprinted with permission from the American College of Cardiology [Journal of the American College of Cardiology, 1992; 20:276–286.])

Such differences in left ventricular functional responses have been attributed to differing regional coronary vasodilator reserve. Proposed mechanisms include transmural coronary steal with redistribution of perfusion from subendocardium to subepicardium and increases in relative coronary stenosis gradient owing to an increase in coronary flow with reduction of distal perfusion pressure.[110]

To demonstrate the effects of coronary hyperemia on left ventricular functional responses,[111] 32 patients with single-vessel coronary artery disease and no angiographic collateral vessels were studied; 14 patients (group 1) underwent diagnostic coronary angiography and subsequent angioplasty. In this group, coronary vasodilator reserve was measured with an intracoronary Doppler catheter during papaverine-induced hyperemia. Left ventricular contractility was simultaneously assessed by two-dimen-

sional echocardiography. Another 13 patients (group 2) with angiographic single-vessel coronary disease received dipyridamole and underwent echocardiographic evaluation of the left ventricular functional response before coronary angioplasty. Coronary vasodilator reserve was not measured in this group. Coronary hyperemia induced with intravenous dipyridamole produced effects similar to that with papaverine on the augmentation of coronary blood flow[68, 101] and velocity.[32]

Coronary Flow Epicardial Blood and Coronary Steal

Regional blood flow maldistribution ("coronary steal") has been suggested as a cause of angina in some patients who receive vasodilating drugs.[30, 33, 112] The anatomic basis of coronary steal is usually coronary collateral vessels that exhibit varying, and occasionally adverse, responses to pharmacologic interventions with vasoactive drugs.[30, 33] Coronary collateral steal is a frequently incriminated but rarely documented cause of ischemia occurring in conjunction with administration of vasodilating agents. Such a case was represented in our laboratory by a 62-year-old woman who underwent repetitive coronary angiography and measurement of epicardial coronary flow velocity before and after papaverine, followed by nitroglycerin. The coronary arteriogram revealed mild proximal left anterior descending (LAD) stenosis, severe stenosis of a large diagonal branch, and mild right coronary artery disease. Extensive retrograde filling of the diagonal branch via collaterals from the distal left anterior descending was visualized along with moderate hypokinesis of the left ventricular lateral segment.

After 10 mg of intracoronary papaverine

was administered, the patient developed typical angina. Left coronary arteriography showed a marked decrease in retrograde collateral flow to the diagonal, with slow antegrade flow through this vessel (Fig. 6–19). Nitroglycerin, 200 μg intracoronary, was given, with complete relief of angina within 4 minutes. New electrocardiographic deep T wave inversion, which occurred after papaverine, was normalized after nitroglycerin administration. Repeat angiography (Fig. 6–19B) showed the restoration of prominent collateral filling of the diagonal branch (Fig. 6–19C). On repeat papaverine challenge, the chest pain and steal phenomenon were reproduced. Doppler flow velocity data after papaverine and nitroglycerin demonstrated no differences in resting levels. Left coronary flow velocity data were similar after papaverine and nitroglycerin, despite significant differences in the direction of collateral flow.

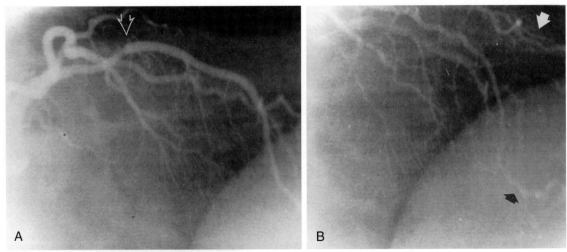

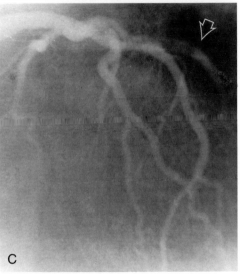

Figure 6–19. *A,* Angiographic coronary steal. Coronary angiogram (right anterior oblique projection) demonstrating patent left anterior descending, but totally occluded or subtotally occluded, large first diagonal coronary artery *(arrowhead). B,* Distal retrograde filling of the diagonal branch from the collateral *(black arrowhead)* that fills upward toward the distal diagonal branch *(white arrowhead)* on a late frame of the coronary cineangiogram. *C,* Antegrade filling of the large diagonal branch showing intraluminal thrombus *(arrowhead)* during chest pain. After nitroglycerin this branch was not opacified antegradely but was seen opacified retrogradely, consistent with a steal phenomenon produced by papaverine despite similar epicardial flow velocities. (*A* through *C* from Gudipati CV, Kern MJ, Aguirre FV, et al: Papaverine-induced chest pain due to coronary vascular steal: Demonstration with angiographic and intracoronary flow velocity measurements. Am Heart J 1989; 118[2]:404–407.)

Papaverine decreased retrograde collateral flow and produced angina; nitroglycerin increased the collateral flow and relieved angina.

One possible mechanism to explain coronary steal after papaverine administration is vasodilation and increased distal coronary flow with decreased distal left anterior descending pressure and thus decreased collateral pressure to the diagonal. Regional myocardial ischemia was then produced by coronary blood flow redistribution (steal) away from the distal diagonal territory. Nitroglycerin, acting on the resistance vessels, restored collateral flow and reversed the papaverine-induced steal phenomenon. In our patient, both nitroglycerin and papaverine increased left coronary flow (velocity) but had markedly different effects on small vessels and the collateral supply. This example illustrates the difficulties that may be encountered when evaluating coronary flow reserve with papaverine and other vasodilators in patients with regions dependent on collateral flow.

Human Coronary Stenosis Hemodynamics and Flow Velocity

Numerous studies have shown substantial intraobserver and interobserver variability in the estimation of coronary stenosis by visual interpretation of coronary arteriograms. Physiologic severity of stenosis depends on the length and the absolute diameter of the stenosis as well as relative (percentage of) narrowing, which is the most common clinical method for expressing severity of obstruction. Although fluid dynamic equations applied to quantitative coronary angiograms have been shown to accurately predict pressure-gradient flow characteristics of arterial stenoses in vitro,[113] in flexible arteries in vivo where stenoses are irregular, eccentric, tapering and altered by vasomotor tone, the assumptions on which such equations are based may not apply.

The functional and physiologic approaches to assessment of severity of coronary stenosis severity by measurement of coronary flow reserve have not gained wide acceptance for several reasons primarily related to the dependence of vasodilation reserve on several uncontrolled physiologic variables in addition to stenosis severity. Thus, flow reserve of a coronary artery containing a fixed stenosis is dependent on the basal physiologic conditions; the size and vasoreactivity of the distal coronary bed, metabolic properties; flow to infarcted, scarred, or hypertrophic myocardium; and other variables not readily discernible.

Recently, the most promising approach to validation of lesion severity has been the application of the Doppler guide wire, with spectral flow velocity data obtained both proximal and distal to the area of stenosis.[114] In 84 patients with coronary artery disease (lesions ranging from 28% to 99% diameter narrowing), a strong correlation was demonstrated between translesional pressure gradients and the ratios of the proximal to distal total flow velocity integrals ($r = 0.8$, $P < 0.001$), with a weaker relationship between quantitative angiography and pressure gradients ($r = 0.6$, $P < 0.001$). In lesions of intermediate severity (50% to 70% diameter narrowing by angiography), there was a poor correlation between translesional pressure gradients and angiographic severity ($r = 0.2$, $P =$ NS), but the flow velocity ratios continued to have a strong correlation ($r = 0.8$, $P < 0.001$). Currently, study of the translesional velocity relationships appears to provide the most reliable approach for assessment of hemodynamic significance in lesions of ambiguous severity by angiography.

REFERENCES

1. Marcus ML: Autoregulation in the coronary circulation. *In* Marcus ML (ed): The Coronary Circulation in Health and Disease. New York, McGraw-Hill, 1983, pp 93–109.
2. Pepine CJ, Mehta J, Webster WW, et al: In vivo validation of a thermodilution method to determine regional left ventricular blood flow in patients with coronary disease. Circulation 1978; 58:795–802.
3. Neufeld HN, Wagenvoort CA, Edwards JE: Coronary arteries in fetuses, infants, juveniles, and young adults. Lab Invest 1962; 11A:837–844.
4. MacAlpin RM, Abassi AS, Grollman JH, et al: Human coronary artery size during life. Diagn Radiol 1973; 108:567–576.
5. Roberts WC: Major anomalies of coronary arterial origin seen in adulthood. Am Heart J 1986; 111:941–963.
6. Ludmer PL, Selwyn AP, Shook TL, et al: Paradoxical vasoconstriction induced by acetylcholine in atherosclerotic coronary arteries. N Engl J Med 1986; 315:1046–1051.
7. Fish DR, Nabel EG, Selwyn AP, et al: Responses of coronary arteries of cardiac transplant patients to acetylcholine. J Clin Invest 1988; 81:21–31.
8. Werns SW, Walton JA, Hsia HH, et al: Evidence of endothelial dysfunction in angiographically normal coronary arteries of patients with coronary artery disease. Circulation 1989; 79:287–291.
9. Chilian WM, Bohling BA, Marcus ML: Capacitance function of epicardial coronary arteries. Federation Proceedings 1981; 40(2133):603.
10. Wusten B, Buss D, Deist H, et al: Dilatory capacity of the coronary circulation and its correlation to the arterial vasculature in the canine left ventricle. Basic Res Cardiol 1977; 72:636.
11. Christensen GC, Campeti FD: Anatomic and functional studies of the coronary circulation in the dog and pig. Am J Vet Res 1959; 20:18.
12. Berne RM, Rubio R: Coronary circulation. *In* Berne RM (ed): Handbook of Physiology, vol 1, section 2:

Cardiovascular System. Bethesda, MD, American Physiologic Society 1979, p 873.

13. Lund DD, Tomanek RJ: Myocardial morphology in spontaneous hypertensive and aortic constricted rats. Am J Anat 1978; 152:141.

14. Rakusan K: Quantitative morphology of capillaries of the heart: Number of capillaries in animal and human hearts under normal and pathologic conditions. Methods Arch Exp Pathol 1971; 5:272.

15. Gregg DE, Shipley RE: Studies of the venous drainage of the heart. Am J Physiol 1947; 151:13.

16. Rayford CR, Khouri EM, Lewis FB, et al: Evaluation of use of left coronary artery inflow and O$_2$ content of coronary sinus blood as a measure of left ventricular metabolism. J Appl Physiol 1959; 14:817.

17. Cohen MV, Matsuki T, Downey JM: Pressure-flow characteristics and nutritional capacity of coronary veins in dogs. Am J Physiol 1988; 255:H834–H846.

18. Young MA, Knight DR, Vatner SF: Autonomic control of large coronary arteries and resistance vessels. Prog Cardiovasc Dis 1987; 30:211–234.

19. Chilian WM, Eastham CL, Layne SM, et al: Small-vessel phenomenon in the coronary microcirculation: Phasic intramyocardial perfusion and coronary microvascular dynamics. Prog Cardiovasc Dis 1988; 31:17–38.

20. Belloni FL: The local control of coronary blood flow. Cardiovasc Res 1979; 13:63–85.

21. Braunwald E: Control of myocardial oxygen consumption: Physiologic and clinical considerations. Am J Cardiol 1971; 27:416.

22. Olsson RA, Snow JA, Gentry MK: Adenosine metabolism in canine myocardial reactive hyperemia. Circ Res 1978; 42:358.

23. Berne RM: The role of adenosine in the regulation of coronary blood flow. Circ Res 1980; 47:807–813.

24. Olsson RA: Myocardial reactive hyperemia. Circ Res 1975; 37:263.

25. Ruiter JH, Spaan JAE, Laird JD: Transient oxygen uptake during myocardial reactive hyperemia in the dog. Am J Physiol 1978; 235:H87.

26. Scott JB, Radawski D: Role of hyperosmolarity in the genesis of active and reactive hyperemia. Circ Res 1971; 28–29(Suppl I):26.

27. Dusting GJ, Moncada S, Vane JR: Prostaglandins—their intermediates and precursors: Cardiovascular actions and regulatory roles in normal and abnormal circulatory systems. Prog Cardiovasc Dis 1979; 21: 405.

28. Wilson RF, Wyche K, Christensen BV, et al: Effects of adenosine on human coronary arterial circulation. Circulation 1990; 82:1595–1606.

29. Gould KL, Lipscomb K, Hamilton GW: Physiologic basis for assessing critical coronary stenosis. Am J Cardiol 1974; 33:87–94.

30. Klocke FJ: Measurements of coronary flow reserve: Defining pathophysiology versus making decisions about patient care. Circulation 1987; 76:1183–1189.

31. Fam WM, McGregor M: Effect of coronary vasodilator drugs on retrograde flow in areas of chronic myocardial ischemia. Circ Res 1964; 15:355–365.

32. Wilson RF, White CW: Intracoronary papaverine: An ideal coronary vasodilator for studies of the coronary circulation in conscious humans. Circulation 1986; 72:444–451.

33. Becker LC: Conditions for vasodilator-induced coronary steal in experimental myocardial ischemia. Circulation 1978; 57:1103–1110.

34. Marcus ML: Effects of cardiac hypertrophy on the coronary circulation. In Marcus ML (ed): The Coronary Circulation in Health and Disease. New York, McGraw-Hill, 1983, p 285.

35. Ganz W, Tamura K, Marcus HS, et al: Measurement of coronary sinus blood flow by continuous thermodilution in man. Circulation 1971; 44:181–195.

36. VanDevanter SH, Mills RM, Lesch M: Thermodilution measurement of coronary sinus blood flow during cardiopulmonary bypass. Surg Forum 1975; 26:225.

37. Kety SS, Schmidt CF: The determination of cerebral blood flow in man by the use of nitrous oxide in low concentrations. Am J Physiol 1945; 143:53.

38. Eckenhoff JE, Hafkenschiel JH, Harmel MH, et al: Measurement of coronary blood flow by the nitrous oxide method. Am J Physiol 1948; 152:356.

39. Klocke FJ, Bunnel IL, Greene DG, et al: Average coronary blood flow per unit weight of left ventricle in patients with and without coronary artery disease. Circulation 1974; 50:547.

40. Marcus ML: Methods of measuring coronary blood flow. In Marcus ML (ed): The Coronary Circulation in Health and Disease. New York, McGraw-Hill, 1983, p 40.

41. Cannon PJ, Dell RB, Dwyer EM Jr: Measurement of regional myocardial perfusion in man with ^{133}Xenon and a scintillation camera. J Clin Invest 1972; 51:964–977.

42. Engel HJ: Assessment of regional myocardial blood flow by the precordial xenon 133 clearance technique. In Schaper W (ed): Pathophysiology of Myocardial Perfusion. Amsterdam, Elsevier-North Holland, 1979, p 58.

43. Collins SM, Skorton DJ, Harrison DG, et al: Quantitative computer-based videodensitometry and the physiological significance of a coronary stenosis: 1982 computers in cardiology. Long Beach, CA, IEEE Computer Society, 1982, pp 219–222.

44. Sanz ML, Mancini GBJ, LeFree MT, et al: Variability of quantitative digital subtraction coronary angiography before and after percutaneous transluminal coronary angioplasty. Am J Cardiol 1987; 60:55–60.

45. Demer L, Gould KL, Kirkeeide R: Assessing stenosis severity: Coronary flow reserve, collateral function, quantitative coronary arteriography, positron imaging, and digital subtraction angiography: A review and analysis. Prog Cardiovasc Dis 1988; 30:307–322.

46. Kirkeeide RL, Gould KL, Parsel L: Assessment of coronary stenoses by myocardial perfusion imaging during pharmacologic coronary vasodilation. Part VII: Validation of coronary flow reserve as a single integrated functional measure of stenosis severity reflecting all its geometric coronary dimensions. J Am Coll Cardiol 1986; 7:103–113.

47. Bates, ER, Aueron FM, Legrand V, et al: Comparative long-term effects of coronary artery bypass graft surgery and percutaneous transluminal coronary angioplasty on regional coronary flow reserve. Circulation 1985; 72:833–839.

48. Ikeda H, Koga Y, Utsu F, et al: Quantitative evaluation of regional myocardial blood flow by videodensitometric analysis of digital subtraction coronary arteriography in humans. J Am Coll Cardiol 1986; 8:809–816.

49. Zijlstra F, Serruys PW, Hugenholtz PG: The ideal coronary vasodilator for investigating coronary flow reserve: A study of timing, magnitude, reproducibility, and safety of the coronary hyperemic response after intracoronary papaverine. Cathet Cardiovasc Diagn 1986; 12:298–303.

50. Hodgson JM, Williams DO: Superiority of intracoronary papaverine to radiographic contrast for measuring coronary flow reserve in patients with ischemic heart disease. Am Heart J 1987; 114:704–710.

51. Cole JS, Hartley CJ: The pulsed Doppler coronary artery catheter: Preliminary report of a new technique

for measuring rapid changes in coronary artery flow velocity in man. Circulation 1977; 56:18–25.

52. Marcus ML, Wright C, Doty D, et al: Measurements of coronary velocity and reactive hyperemia in the coronary circulation of humans. Circ Res 1981; 49:877–891.

53. Hatle L, Angelsen B: Flow velocity and volumetric principles. *In* Doppler Ultrasound in Cardiology: Physical Principles and Clinical Applications, 2nd ed. Philadelphia, Lea & Febiger, 1985, p 14.

54. Wilson RF, Laughlin DE, Ackell PH, et al: Transluminal, subselective measurement of coronary artery blood flow velocity and vasodilator reserve in man. Circulation 1985; 72:82–92.

55. Sibley DH, Millar HD, Hartley CJ, et al: Subselective measurement of coronary blood flow velocity using a steerable Doppler catheter. J Am Coll Cardiol 1986; 8:1332–1340.

56. Wilson RF, Marcus ML, White CW: Prediction of the physiologic significance of coronary arterial lesions by quantitative lesion geometry in patients with limited coronary artery disease. Circulation 1987; 75:723–732.

57. Zijlstra F, Van Ommeren J, Reiber JHC, et al: Does the quantitative assessment of coronary artery dimensions predict the physiologic significance of a coronary stenosis? Circulation 1987; 75:1154–1161.

58. Wilson RF, White CW: Does coronary artery bypass surgery restore normal maximal coronary flow reserve? Circulation 1987; 76:563–571.

59. Donohue TJ, Kern MJ, Aguirre FV, et al: Assessing the hemodynamic significance of coronary artery stenoses: Analyis of translesional pressure-flow velocity relations in patients. J Am Coll Cardiol 1993; 22:449–458.

60. Doppler CJ: Uber das farbige Licht der Dopplesterne: Abhandlungen der Koniglichen Bohmischen Gesellschaft der Wissenschaften. 1842; 2:465.

61. Hangiandreou NJ, Toggart EJ, Mistretta CA: Investigation of the performance of two types of the Doppler catheter in vitro. Cathet Cardiovasc Diagn 1989; 18:108–117.

62. Kern MJ, Deligonul U, Vandormael M, et al: Impaired coronary vasodilator reserve in the immediate postcoronary angioplasty period: Analysis of coronary artery flow velocity indexes and regional cardiac venous efflux. J Am Coll Cardiol 1989; 13:860–872.

63. Warltier DC, Gross GJ, Brooks HL: Pharmacologic-versus ischemia-induced coronary artery vasodilation. Am J Physiol 1981; 240:H767–H774.

64. Wilson, RF, White CW: Serious ventricular dysrhythmias after intracoronary papaverine. Am J Cardiol 1988; 62:378–388.

65. Rembert JC, Boyd LM, Watkinson WP, et al: Effect of adenosine on transmural myocardial blood flow distribution in the awake dog. Am J Physiol 1980; 239:H7.

66. Sylven C, Jonzon B, Edlund A: Angina pectoris–like pain provoked by IV bolus of adenosine: Relationship to coronary sinus blood flow, heart rate, and blood pressure in healthy volunteers. Eur Heart J 1989; 10:48–54.

67. Zijlstra F, Juilliere Y, Serruys PW, et al: Value and limitations of intracoronary adenosine for the assessment of coronary flow reserve. Cathet Cardiovasc Diagn 1988; 15:76–80.

68. Marchant E, Pichard A, Rodriguez JA, et al: Acute effect of systemic versus intracoronary dipyridamole on coronary circulation. Am J Cardiol 1986; 57:1401–1404.

69. Marcus ML, Wilson RF, White CW: Methods of measurement of myocardial blood flow in patients: A critical review. Circulation 1987; 76:245–253.

70. Emanuelsson H, Holmberg S, Selin K, et al: Factors that modify the flow response to intracoronary injections. Circulation 1985; 72:287–291.

71. Kern MJ, Deligonul U, Serota H, et al: Ventricular arrhythmia due to intracoronary papaverine: Analysis of QT intervals and coronary vasodilatory reserve. Cathet Cardiovasc Diagn 1990; 19: 229–236.

72. Bookstein JJ, Higgins CB: Comparative efficacy of coronary vasodilatory methods. Invest Radiol 1977; 12:121–127.

73. Pilla TJ, Beshany SE, Shields JB: Incompatibility of Hexabrix and papaverine. Am J Radiol 1986; 146:1300–1301.

74. Doucette JW, Corl PD, Payne HM, et al: Validation of a Doppler guide wire for intravascular measurement of coronary artery flow velocity. Circulation 1992; 85:1899–1911.

75. Segal J, Kern MJ, Scott NA, et al: Alterations of phasic coronary artery flow velocity in man during percutaneous coronary angioplaty. J Am Coll Cardiol 1992; 20:276–286.

76. Ofili EO, Kern MJ, Labovitz AJ, et al: Analysis of coronary blood flow velocity dynamics in angiographically normal and stenosed arteries before and after endolumen enlargement by angioplasty. J Am Coll Cardiol 1993; 21: 308–316.

77. Martin LW, Johnson RA, Scott H, et al: Impedence measurement of absolute coronary blood flow using an angioplasty catheter: A validation study. Am Heart J 1991; 121:745–752.

78. Vogel RA, Martin LW: Transcatheter coronary artery diagnostic techniques. Tex Heart Inst J 1989; 16: 195–203.

79. Hoffman JIE: Maximal coronary flow and the concept of coronary vascular reserve. Circulation 1984; 70: 153–159.

80. Wilson RF, Johnson MR, Marcus ML, et al: The effect of coronary angioplasty on coronary flow reserve. Circulation 1988; 77:873–885.

81. O'Neill WW, Walton JA, Bates ER, et al: Criteria for successful coronary angioplasty as assessed by alterations in coronary vasodilatory reserve. J Am Coll Cardiol 1984; 3:1382–1390.

82. Zijlstra F, Reiber JC, Juilliere Y, et al: Normalization of coronary flow reserve by percutaneous transluminal coronary angioplasty. Am J Cardiol 1988; 61:55–60.

83. Segal J, Kern MJ, Scott NA, et al: Alterations of phasic coronary artery flow velocity in humans during percutaneous coronary angioplasty. J Am Coll Cardiol 1992; 20:276–286.

84. Serruys PW, Di Mario C, Meneveau N, et al: Intracoronary pressure and flow velocity with sensor-tip guide wires: A new methodologic approach for assesment of coronary hemodynamics before and after coronary interventions. Am J Cardiol 1993; 71:41D–53D.

85. Anderson HV, Kirkeeide RL, Stuart Y, et al: Coronary artery flow monitoring following coronary interventions. Am J Cardiol 1993; 71:62D–69D.

86. Hintze TH, Vatner SF: Reactive dilation of large coronary arteries in conscious dogs. Circ Res 1984; 54: 50–57.

87. Macho P, Hintze TH, Vatner SF: Regulation of large coronary arteries by increases in myocardial metabolic demand in the conscious dog. Circ Res 1981; 49: 594–599.

88. Soward AL, Essed CE, Serruys PW: Coronary arterial findings after accidental death immediately after successful percutaneous transluminal coronary angioplasty. Am J Cardiol 1985; 56:794–795.

89. Waller BF: Early and late morphologic changes in human coronary arteries after percutaneous translumi-

nal coronary angioplasty. Clin Cardiol 1983; 6: 363–372.

90. Holtz J, Forstermann U, Pohl U, et al: Flow-dependent endothelial-mediated dilation of epicardial arteries in the conscious dog: Effects of cyclooxygenase inhibition. J Cardiovasc Pharmacol 1984; 6:1161–1169.

91. Bates ER, McGillem MJ, Beals TF, et al: Effect of angioplasty-induced endothelial denudation compared with medial injury on regional coronary blood flow. Circulation 1987; 76:710–716.

92. Busse R, Trogisch G, Bassange E: The role of the endothelium and the local control of vascular tone. Basic Res Cardiol 1985; 85:475–490.

93. Henry PD, Yokoyama M: Supersensitivity of atherosclerotic rabbit aorta to ergonovine: Mediation by a serotoninergic mechanism. J Clin Invest 1980; 66:306–313.

94. Yokoyama M, Akita H, Mizutani T, et al: Hyperreactivity of coronary arterial smooth muscles in response to ergonovine from rabbits with hereditary hyperlipidemia. Circ Res 1983; 53:63–71.

95. Folts, JD, Crowell EB Jr, Rowe GG: Platelet aggregation in partially obstructed vessels and its elimination with aspirin. Circulation 1976; 54:365–370.

96. Barger AC, Beeuwkes R, Lainey LL, et al: Hypothesis: Vasa vasorum and neovascularization of human coronary arteries—a possible role in the pathophysiology of atherosclerosis. N Engl J Med 1984; 310:175–177.

97. Zijlstra F, den Boer A, Reiber JHC, et al: Assessment of immediate and long-term functional results of percutaneous transluminal coronary angioplasty. Circulation 1988; 78:15–24.

98. Pijls NH, Uijen GJ, Hoevelaken A, et al: Mean transit time for the assessment of myocardial perfusion by videodensitometry. Circulation 1990: 81:1331–1340.

99. Pijls NH, Aengevaeren WR, Uijen GJ, et al: Concept of maximal flow ratio for immediate evaluation of percutaneous transluminal coronary angioplasty result by videodensitometry. Circulation 1991; 83:854–865.

100. Schwartz JN, Kong Y, Hackell DB, et al: Comparison of angiographic and postmortem findings in patients with coronary artery disease. Am J Cardiol 1975; 36:174–178.

101. Picano E, Simonetti I, Masini M, et al: Transient myocardial dysfunction during pharmacologic vasodilation as an index of reduced coronary reserve: A coronary hemodynamic and echocardiographic study. J Am Coll Cardiol 1986; 8:84–90.

102. Picano E, Distante A, Masini M, et al: Dipyridamole echocardiography test in effort angina pectoris. Am J Cardiol 1985; 56:452–456.

103. Labovitz AJ, Pearson AC, Chaitman BR: Doppler and two-dimensional echocardiographic assessment of left ventricular function before and after intravenous dipyridamole stress testing for detection of coronary artery disease. Am J Cardiol 1988; 62:1180–1185.

104. White CW, Wright CB, Doty DB, et al: Does visual interpretation of the coronary arteriogram predict the physiologic importance of the coronary stenosis? N Engl J Med 1984; 310:819–824.

105. Legrand V, Mancini GBJ, Bates ER, et al: Comparative study of coronary flow reserve, coronary anatomy, and results of radionuclide exercise tests in patients with coronary artery disease. J Am Coll Cardiol 1986; 8:1022–1032.

106. Margonato A, Chierchia S, Cianflone E, et al: Limitations of dipyridamole-echocardiography in effort angina pectoris. Am J Cardiol 1987; 59:225–230.

107. Picano E, Morales MA, Distante A, et al: Dipyridamole-echocardiography test in angina at rest: Noninvasive assessment of coronary stenosis underlying spasm. Am Heart J 1986; 111:688–691.

108. Picano E, Lattanzi F, Masini M, et al: Comparison of the high-dose dipyridamole-echocardiography test and exercise two-dimensional echocardiography for diagnosis of coronary artery disease. Am J Cardiol 1987; 59:539–542.

109. Distante A, Picano E, Moscarelli E, et al: Echocardiographic versus hemodynamic monitoring during attacks of variant angina pectoris. Am J Cardiol 1985; 55:1319–1322.

110. Gould KL: Noninvasive assessment of coronary stenosis by myocardial perfusion imaging during pharmacologic coronary vasodilatation. Part I: Physiologic basis and experimental validation. Am J Cardiol 1978; 41:267–276.

111. Kern MJ, Pearson AC, Labovitz AJ, et al: Effects of pharmacologic coronary hyperemia on echocardiographic left ventricular function in patients with single-vessel coronary artery disease. J Am Coll Cardiol 1989; 13:1042–1051.

112. Gudipati CV, Kern MJ, Aguirre FV, et al: Papaverine-induced chest pain due to coronary vascular steal: Demonstration with angiographic and intracoronary flow velocity measurements. Am Heart J 1989; 118:404–407.

113. Gould KL, Kelley KO, Bolson EL: Experimental validation of quantitative coronary arteriography for determining pressure-flow characteristics of coronary stenosis. Circulation 1982; 66:930–937.

114. Donohue TJ, Kern MJ, Aguirre FV, et al: Assessing the hemodynamic significance of coronary artery stenoses: Analysis of translesional pressure-flow relations in patients. J Am Coll Cardiol 1993; 22:449–458.

Chapter 7

Radiographic Angiocardiography
Equipment and Contrast Agents

KIRK L. PETERSON

A fundamental function of a cardiac cathe terization procedure is to define accurately the pathologic anatomy of congenital or acquired heart disease. Also, on-line or real-time viewing is required for safe manipulation of catheters into and through the complex structures of the heart and vascular tree. Beginning with the first cardiac catheterization in humans,[1] a radiographic system has served as the imaging modality best suited for these functions. Iodinated contrast medium, delivered either selectively or nonselectively into the circulation, later developed as an indispensable adjunctive tool in improving image definition and revealing the internal dimensions and structure of the chambers and blood vessels of the heart (see Chapter 1).

This chapter is intended to acquaint the inquiring cardiologist with the elements and function of a radiographic installation in a catheterization laboratory. Also reviewed are the common types of radiographic contrast agents used in cardiac angiography. The chapter is not aimed to be an encyclopedic treatment of the technology of cardiac angiography; the reader is referred to other sources for in-depth coverage of the topic.[2, 3]

Cardiac Angiography Equipment

For any given plane of view, a basic catheterization laboratory x-ray installation consists of a generator and an x-ray tube and image intensifier mounted, respectively, on either end of a gantry that can be rotated approximately 180 degrees around the thorax while the patient is lying on a translucent x-ray table. Most laboratories have only one plane of view or gantry available; however, for study of congenital heart disease and some acquired lesions, a biplane installation is required,[4] and films are then taken near simultaneously in orthogonal views using alternate x-ray pulsing (Fig. 7–1).

The basic radiographic system is integrated with a number of other components (Fig. 7–2), including a video camera that can relay a fluoroscopic or cineangiographic image to a television monitor and also to an archiving device such as a videotape or videodisk recorder (some systems digitize an image in near real-time, store the data on a high-capacity disk or tape, and redisplay either the original or processed image on a digital television monitor); a film recording system that in most laboratories includes a 35mm cinecamera but that may also incorporate spot-film or large-film changers; and a film processing and display facility, which may also be incorporated into an off-line image processing system.

Generators

The generator transforms energy into a form that is suitable for x-ray production. The power supply that energizes the x-ray tube(s) is generally 3-phase, 12-pulse and has an output of 80 to 100 kW. For example, the relatively low line voltage supplied to the laboratory (240 V) must be amplified or transformed to 25,000 to 150,000 V to create high-quality radiographs. The stepped-up voltage coming out of the transformer must also be converted from alternating current to direct current. This is also performed within the generator using rectifier circuits. By pulsing the electrical voltage and combining the pulses as if they were three separate circuits, each out of phase temporally with the other (3-phase), an output voltage is produced that is close to the peak of each individual pulse. While pulsing the system at 12 pulses per cycle for each phase, the output varies ("ripples") mini-

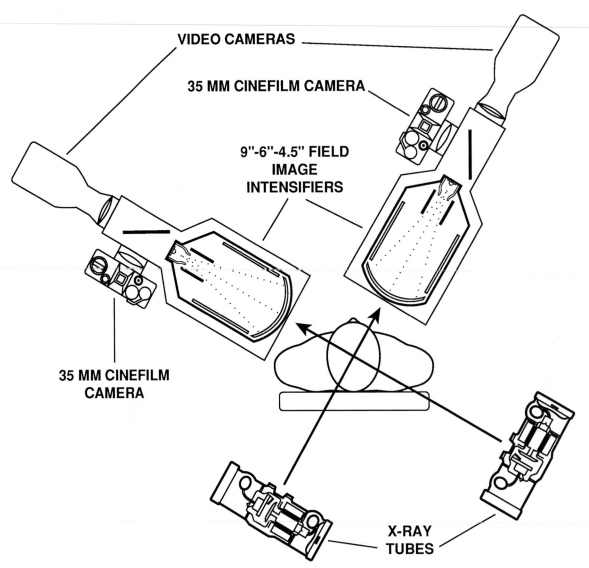

VIDEO CAMERAS

35 MM CINEFILM CAMERA

9"-6"-4.5" FIELD IMAGE INTENSIFIERS

35 MM CINEFILM CAMERA

X-RAY TUBES

Figure 7–1. Schematic of two orthogonal x-ray systems positioned around a patient lying supine on a cardiac catheterization table. The imaging components for each plane are mounted on supporting structures (gantries) that can be rotated from left to right as well as toward the the patient's feet and head. The x-ray tubes are positioned usually beneath the table, whereas the image intensifier, video cameras, and 35mm cinefilm cameras are mounted at the opposite end of the respective gantries. Most laboratories have image intensifiers that can be switched between variably sized fields of view (e.g., 9-inch, 6-inch, and 4.5-inch).

mally (<4%) and approximates a constant output potential.

Through the generator, the automatic brightness control system (or, occasionally, a human operator using manual controls) adjusts three parameters: (1) kilovoltage; (2) tube current in milliamperes; and (3) exposure time in milliseconds. Ideally, potential is released to the x-ray tube by secondary switching where the tube is switched on and off at the high-voltage side of a transformer or at the x-ray tube itself.[4] Secondary switching, as opposed to primary switching (where the tube is turned on or off by closing or opening the primary transformer winding), does not produce preexposure or postexposure soft radiation from charge stored in the capacitance of the high-voltage cables. Such generators produce a near square wave voltage output, which is optimal for pulsed-mode fluoroscopy and minimal-dose cineangiography.

Coordination of the pulses of x-ray exposure with the cinecamera(s), filming at 30 to 60 frames/sec, is essential. This function is handled by a cinepulse system that modulates the x-ray photon flow emanating out of the x-ray tube by controlling the duration of each expo-

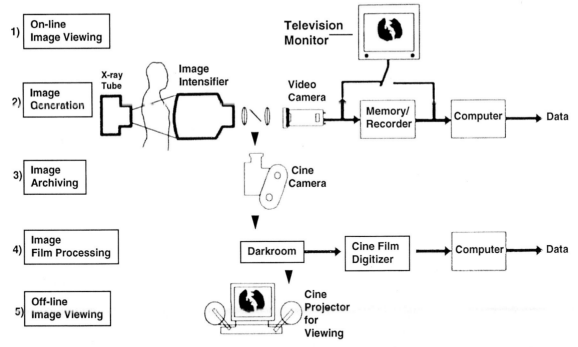

Figure 7–2. Diagram of the major components and their sequencing in a cardiac catheterization laboratory for on-line image viewing, acquisition (generation), film archiving and processing, and off-line viewing. Most laboratories continue to depend on 35-mm cinefilm for high-resolution viewing and permanent archiving of acquired angiographic images; however, digitally processed fluoroscopic images, stored on high-capacity CD-ROM disks, may, in time, become the dominant and standard storage modality for catheterization laboratories in the United States.[5] (From Guggenheim N: The angiographic equipment. *In* Three-dimensional reconstruction of the coronary tree from angiographic images and coronary blood flow measurement [Doctor of Science Thesis No. 2492]. Presented to the Faculty of Sciences, University of Geneva, Geneva, Switzerland, 1991, pp 51–56.)

sure. Generally, in the adult an exposure time of 5 to 8 msec, and for children 2 to 4 msec, is used while the voltage output is maintained at 70 to 90 kV for adults and 60 to 80 kV for children.

X-ray Tubes

An x-ray tube is fundamentally a high-voltage diode sealed in a vacuum enclosed by glass or aluminum; electrons are given off from a heated element in the cathode and accelerated toward the anode by the high voltage produced by the generator (Fig. 7–3). As the electrons impact the anode, approximately 1% of their energy generates x-rays; the remainder of the energy is converted primarily into heat. Thus, modern tubes must have the capacity for considerable heat dissipation. At a minimum, the storage capacities of the anode and the tube housing should be 1 million and 1.75 million heat units, respectively. All modern systems have monitoring devices and digital read-outs of heat build-up, and function is automatically suspended when a target amount is reached. Although the most recently designed x-ray tubes

are effective for limiting heat accumulation, even in the face of increased use with interventional cardiology procedures, they exhibit a finite life span and constitute one of the most expensive components of a catheterization laboratory to be maintained.

The anode of an x-ray tube is a large disk, approximately 15 to 22 cm in diameter, which revolves at 3,000 to 10,000 revolutions per minute. This rotation serves to distribute heat over a much larger area than the effective target area. As shown in Figure 7–3, the anode surface is angulated at approximately 100 degrees to the incident electron beam coming from the cathode. The area of projection of the electron beam on the surface of the anode is known as the *focal spot*. The angulation of the anode surface serves to increase the width of the annulus to about five times that of the apparent focus (1 × 1 mm²). If the target angle is more shallow, a smaller surface area for heat dissipation results, and there is more absorption of x-rays within the anode mass (the "heel effect"). This, in turn, results in reduced radiation intensity on the anode side of the field and reduced field coverage.

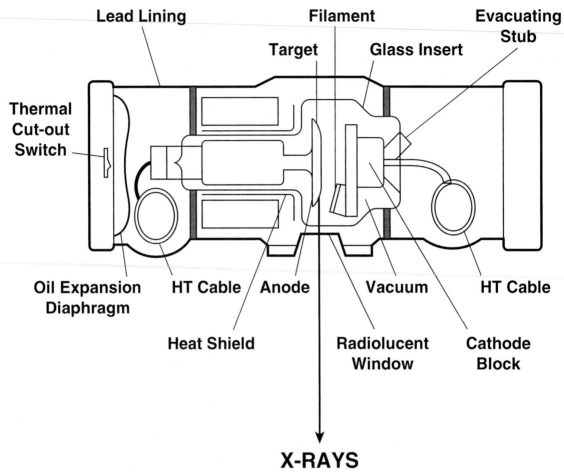

Lead Lining   Filament   Evacuating Stub

Target   Glass Insert

Thermal Cut-out Switch

Oil Expansion Diaphragm   HT Cable   Anode   Vacuum   HT Cable

Heat Shield   Radiolucent Window   Cathode Block

X-RAYS

Figure 7–3. Diagram of basic design of a rotating-anode x-ray tube. The cathode emits an electron beam of variable size that impacts on the rotating anode that, in turn, converts the beam into x-rays and heat. See text for other technical details.

The x-ray tube focal spot size has a significant influence on ultimate image resolution. The smaller the focal spot size, the better the resolution but the greater the radiation needed to provide penetration of biologic tissue and the greater the heat production. Thus, many systems allow a variable focal spot size; for highly angulated views and long source-to-image distances, a focal spot of 1 to 1.2 mm is preferred. Conversely, with more conventional views and shorter source-to-image distances, a smaller focal spot of 0.6 to 0.7 mm can be used.

Collimators

A collimator serves to reduce x-ray scatter and minimize off-focus radiation. Image quality is thereby improved, and radiation to the operator is minimized. Some x-ray tubes have collimators that extend directly into the recess of the tube housing and significantly impact on scatter emanating from the anode. A lead diaphragm can also be used at the tube port opening and sized to cover everything except the maximum field size that will be used. A contoured filter can also be placed over the portions of the field that are radiolucent, for example, the lungs, and thus serve to limit oversaturation or bright spots on the television monitor, videotape, and cinefilm images (see later discussion).

Spectrum of the X-ray Beam

The spectrum of energy (kiloelectron volt) of photons entering the patient depends on the anode target material, on the potential applied to the x-ray tube, and on any filters applied before reaching the patient. For photons with energies less than 10 keV, virtually all are attenuated by the tissue; between 10 keV and 25 keV, penetration increases rapidly and progressively; finally, above 40 keV penetration continues to increase but much more gradually. Because low-energy photons contribute nothing to image

information, aluminum and copper filters are used, generally, to screen out low-energy photons that would otherwise be absorbed in the patient's tissue. Regulations have been established that require minimally acceptable penetration for various types of filters at variable levels of kilovoltage.

Primary and Scatter Radiation and Use of Grids

Once filtered radiation enters human tissue, some photons pass directly through with no tissue interaction ("primary radiation") and convey a relief image on the receptor positioned on the other side (usually the image intensifier). However, some radiation interacts with tissue and scatters; some of this scatter then reaches the image intensifier and serves to degrade its quality. Special grids have been devised and mounted in front of the image intensifier to remove a portion of the scattered radiation. The grid is usually constructed of alternate strips of an x-ray–absorbing material (e.g., lead) and a relatively nonabsorbent interspace substance such as aluminum, carbon, and fiber. The interspaces of the grid are angled so as to be aligned with a specific point in space; under ideal conditions, this point of focus should coincide with the focal spot of the x-ray tube or the source of the primary radiation. This focusing allows primary radiation to pass through unaltered, whereas scattered radiation, which leaves the patient's body in a different direction, encounters the absorbent strips and is obstructed from passing through. The efficiency of a grid is determined by the dimensions of the lead strips, usually 2 to 5 mm, and the width of its interspaces, usually 0.25 to 0.4 mm. The ratio of these two dimensions, the "grid ratio," ranges generally from 5:1 to 16:1. Grids with higher ratios eliminate more scattered radiation but increase the radiation exposure to the patient and the x-ray tube loading. The amount of scatter radiation that passes a grid is typically less than 10%, but primary radiation is also significantly reduced by approximately 40% at the same time.

Image Intensifier and Television Chain

For an object to become visible as an x-ray image, it must have either a physical density or chemical composition different from its surrounding tissue. Thus, as radiation is transmitted through biologic tissue, there is variable absorption of the transmitted radiation, causing shadows of commensurate darkness on a recep-

tor surface. A number of factors, including radiation penetration, scatter, degree of filtering, and receptor characteristics, interact to bring about the ultimate contrast on the receptor surface.

In the cardiac catheterization laboratory, the immediate receptor on which the x-ray image is displayed is the image intensifier, a high-gain vacuum device that converts the relief image at its input phosphor into a focused, luminous image at its output (Fig. 7–4). Most modern image intensifiers have a thin phosphor layer, usually cesium iodide, that serves to convert the transmitted x-ray photons into light photons. A thin metal photocathode, positioned just behind the input phosphor, picks up the light photons and responds by emitting electrons. The electrons are then accelerated and focused on the output phosphor where the bright, minimized image, corresponding to the x-ray distribution on the input phosphor, is projected. Because of electronic focusing requirements, the surface of the input phosphor is convex; this creates some distortion of the projected image, particularly at the periphery referred to as *pincushion distortion*. If precise measurements of image dimensions are desired, one can correct for this distortion by using a rectilinear array of wires as a calibration grid (see Chapter 8).

A mirror near the output phosphor allows simultaneous reflection of the image both to a video camera and a 35mm cinefilm camera. In some laboratories a single-radiograph or serial-radiograph spot film camera (e.g., 120mm film) is also mounted and focused on the image conveyed by the output phosphor.

One of the major advantages of the modern image intensifier is its capacity to convey either a continuous or pulsed fluoroscopic image, even with relatively low levels of radiation. The video camera mounted on the image intensifier is then used to display on a television monitor a continuous x-ray image that picks up cardiac motion and allows visual monitoring of the insertion and manipulation of cardiac catheters. The image can be archived on a videotape or videodisk recorder that, in turn, can be used for instant replay of previously recorded sequences. "Road map" images can also be stored or superimposed on real-time images as references for therapeutic interventional procedures.

The magnification factor of the image intensifier can be changed by altering the voltage of the electrons that focus the electron image on the output phosphor. Also, in some image intensifiers the input image area can be reduced. As an image is magnified, however, in-

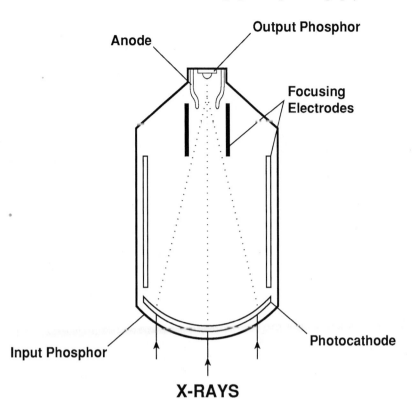

Figure 7–4. Diagram of the basic components of the image intensifier. After transmission through biologic tissue, x-rays create a relief image on the input phosphor layer, usually cesium iodide, that serves to convert x-ray photons into light photons. The photocathode picks up the light photons and emits electrons that are focused on the output phosphor on the opposite end. A partially reflective mirror picks up the generated image from the output phosphor and conveys it to a 35mm cinecamera and video camera. See text for further details.

creased radiation is necessary to achieve a high-contrast image that, consequently, leads to increased scatter radiation and a reduction in the signal-to-noise ratio. Most fluoroscopic systems in cardiac catheterization laboratories allow two or three fields of view (e.g., a 9-inch, 6-inch, and 4.5-inch diameter image). When maximum field of view is the primary requirement, the large field mode would be used; if image detail is sought (e.g., examining the struts of an implanted vascular stent), then the small field mode might be desirable.

Video Cameras and the Television Chain

The video camera tube serves to convert the light image coming off the input phosphor into an electronic signal. Fluoroscopic systems in catheterization laboratories generally are outfitted with either Vidicon or Plumicon tubes, pick-up tubes that are smaller and less complex than those used in commercial broadcast television systems. The most important difference between the Vidicon and Plumicon tubes is their image persistence, or lag. The Vidicon has an antimony trisulphide photoconductor, and its response is relatively slow; therefore, it is well suited for imaging of stationary organs. The Plumicon, by contrast, has a lead mono-oxide photoconductor and exhibits negligible lag or

persistence of the image. It also exhibits a superior signal-to-noise ratio and spatial resolution. Thus, it is particularly well suited for imaging of moving organs such as the heart. Saticon tubes are similar to Plumicon tubes, show some superior performance characteristics, and are now being installed in some laboratories.

The typical video camera tube is cylindrical; it is approximately 15 cm in length and has a diameter of approximately 25 mm. Images are projected onto the input screen by a focusing lens; the other end of the pick-up tube houses a heated cathode and other electrodes that form an electron gun. An electron beam is shot down the length of the evacuated tube and strikes the screen surface on which the input image has been focused. Synchronized electrical signals, one applied horizontally and one vertically, cause the electron beam to be swept over the surface of the input screen. In the United States a standard 525-line video system is used, where the beam begins in the upper left-hand corner and scans horizontally across the image to the right, whereupon it is redirected quickly back to the left hand side and deflected downward by approximately one beam width. A top-to-bottom sequential scan is completed in 1/60 second, forming one video field. A second scan, again completed in 1/60 second, is begun at the top of the image field,

INTERLACED SCAN

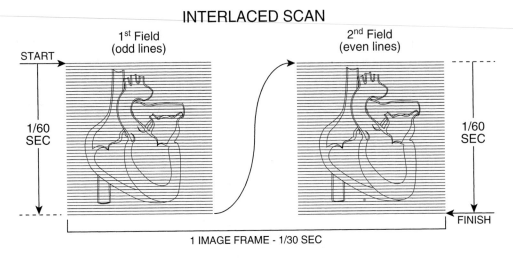

1st Field
(odd lines)

2nd Field
(even lines)

START

1/60
SEC

1/60
SEC

FINISH

1 IMAGE FRAME - 1/30 SEC

PROGRESSIVE SCAN
(all lines)

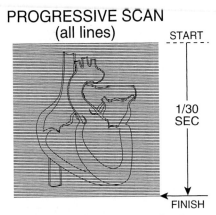

START

1/30
SEC

FINISH

Figure 7–5. Schematic diagram demonstrating the difference between an interlaced or combined television image *(upper)* and one displayed in a progressive fashion *(lower)*. The latter mode of display eliminates motion artifacts that might arise from the combination of two fields, taken sequentially at 1/60th of a second, into a single frame displayed at 1/30th of a second.

but this time the beam is displaced downward approximately one beam width with respect to the first set, forming a second video field. These two fields, forming 1/30 second of information, are interlaced or combined (Fig. 7–5, *upper*). When a videotape recording device is played back at 30 frames/sec, the human eye cannot appreciate significant flicker, although the image is not as continuous as might be appreciated at 60 frames/sec. In some modern angiocardiographic installations, video camera scanning and display of the fluoroscopic image is progressive, that is, there is sequential scanning of all raster lines at 60 fields/sec (Fig. 7–5, *lower*). This eliminates motion artifacts that might be the result of two fields, taken at different times, being combined into one single frame.

Spatial resolution in a television image is limited by both vertical and horizontal blur. Image quality is usually best if these two factors are approximately equal. On a television image,

vertical spatial resolution is a function of the finite size of the electron beam and the number of scan lines. When an anatomic structure is oriented at a slight angle to the horizontal scan lines, the object will appear wider because of the blur. The actual width of a scan line, w, is related to the number of scan lines and the vertical field of view, FOV. A final factor that determines vertical blur is the magnification factor related to the actual size of the image, for example, a coronary artery with a diameter of 3 to 4 mm. Ultimately,

$$B_v = 1.4 \cdot FOV/n \cdot m$$

where B_v is vertical blur, FOV is the image diameter in the plane of the object, n is the number of scan lines in the object, and m is the magnification factor. Vertical blur can be decreased by augmenting the number of scan lines used to form the video image, and, in fact, 1024-line television systems have now been implemented in many catheterization laboratory radiographic installations.

Horizontal blur is a function of the response time of the circuitry through which the video signal passes between the camera and the picture. This response time is normally described as a frequency bandwidth in units of megahertz (1000 cycles/sec). To optimize image quality, the circuit designer seeks to set the frequency response so as to equalize horizontal and vertical blur values.

Operators in the cardiac catheterization laboratory witness their catheter manipulations and contrast agent injections on a television monitor. In this component, an electron gun, similar to that in the video camera, produces a beam that scans the surface of the monitor while synchronized with the electron beam of the video camera. If unsynchronized, the image is either distorted horizontally or rolls in a vertical direction. Signals sent from the video camera tube control the brightness of the monitor beam along each point of its scan lines. Thus, the brightness of an element or spot on the monitor is determined by the brightness of the corresponding point on the camera tube screen. On the television monitor contrast and brightness controls can be used to optimize the gray scale difference between bright and dark areas of the total image. If the brightness level (which affects all picture elements) is augmented too much and reaches a preset maximum, an "oversaturation" of parts of the image occurs and contrast medium will decrease between dark and bright regions. It is the gray scale levels (ultimately determined by voltage levels) along each scan line that can be quantitated by digital processing and that serves as the basis for digital angiography (see Chapter 10).

Cameras, Film, and Associated Optical Systems

The transfer of the image from the output phosphor of the image intensifier to the cinefilm or spot-film camera is accomplished via a collimator, an image distributor, and a beam-splitting mirror. This latter structure allows a partial pass-through of the image to the video camera while reflecting the same image into the aperture of the camera(s). A lens behind the aperture focuses the image onto the film surface. The aperture controls the size (diameter) of the lens that is, in turn, an important factor in the efficiency of the lens. The relative lens area (efficiency) is customarily expressed as an f number; the smaller the lens area the higher the f num-

Table 7–1. Relation Between f Number and Efficiency of an Optical Lens

f Number	Efficiency (Relative Lens Area)
16	1
11	2
8	4
5.6	8
4	16
2.8	32
2.0	64
1.4	128
1.0	256

ber, and vice versa (Table 7–1). The lens efficiency or relative lens area is calculated as:

$$\text{Lens area} = \tfrac{1}{4}f^2$$

where the f number equals the focal length of the lens divided by the diameter of the lens.

Once the image passes through the camera aperture, it is focused onto the film surface by the intervening lens. The size of the image frame is determined by the camera lens, which is especially chosen depending on the type of film used (e.g., 35mm or 120mm) and the desired framing. The standard 35mm cinefilm has an image area of 25 × 18 mm, and the circular output of the image intensifier is projected onto this rectangular surface. Most laboratories choose to underframe the image so that the full circle recorded by the video camera is seen on the cinefilm. However, occasionally, the film image is overframed, in which case the operator must be careful to keep the diagnostic area of interest near the center of the fluoroscopic image on the television system; otherwise, important pathoanatomic information may be lost.

35mm Cinefilm

Over the last 35 years the primary archival medium for cardiac angiographic studies has been 35mm cinefilm recorded at either 30 or 60 frames/sec. This medium largely replaced the use of either single-plane or biplane serial film changers with exposure rates of 2 to 12 frames/sec. In some laboratories a spot-film changer (70 mm to 105 mm) was added to a radiographic system to provide a hard copy that could be carried into the clinic, patient chart, or operating theater. Cinefilm lacks the spatial resolution of radiographs taken with film changers, but the added temporal resolution and dynamic display have significant advantages for study of an organ that is constantly in motion. In time the combination of high-resolution fluoroscopy and digital processing and storage may make cinefilm obsolete[5]; however, most catheterization laboratories continue to depend on the 35mm cinefilm format.

The optical density (D) or darkening as light is transmitted onto cinefilm is defined by

$$D = \log[I_o/I] = \log[1/T]$$

where I_o and I are the intensities of light before and after passage through the film; T is the film transmittance $[I_o/I]$. The relation between the log of exposure and the optical density, D, forms a sigmoid-shaped curve known as the *Hurter-Driffield* (H-D) *curve* (Fig. 7–6). The precise profile of this curve is dependent on the film emulsion and the processing conditions. Contrast, at any exposure value, is determined by the slope of the curve. Only a portion of the middle of this relation is linear and forms the latitude of the film. The maximum slope in this region is referred to as the *gamma* (γ) of the film. Ideally, all of the exposure of a cardiac angiocardiogram should be within this range, although this is uncommonly attainable. However, if an image is exposed so that it falls on the lower left part of the curve (the "toe"), then little contrast material is transferred onto the image. Reduced ability to manifest contrast agent is also present if the image is exposed along the upper right (the "shoulder") of the curve. Inadequate or excessive exposure can result from two general conditions: (1) an incorrect exposure setting of the radiographic equipment (kilovolts, milliamperes, and exposure interval) or (2) an anatomic structure that produces a spectrum of exposure values that exceed the latitude range of the film.

Standard Projections for Cardiac and Coronary Angiography

Because various structures of the heart are situated and course in complex angles to either the anterior or lateral projection of the thorax, it is highly desirable to have an angulation capability for the x-ray gantry. As shown in Figure 7–7, a standard nomenclature has been developed for describing the projection in which a cardiac image is recorded. Except when positioned in the straight lateral projection, the x-ray tube is essentially always inferior to, and the image intensifier superior to, the horizontal plane of the patient. If the image intensifier is rotated toward the feet (and x-ray tube toward the head), the position of the gantry is said to be caudal. Conversely, if the image intensifier is angulated toward the head, the position is labeled as cranial. The actual degrees of rotation (e.g., 30, 60, or 75 degrees) from the direct anteroposterior position can also be used to describe explicitly the amount of rotation, either caudal or cranial. Similarly, the x-ray gantry can be rotated toward either the patient's left or right side; if the image intensifier is rotated toward the left, 30 degrees from the plane of the table and 60 degrees from the anteroposterior plane through the patient, then it is said to

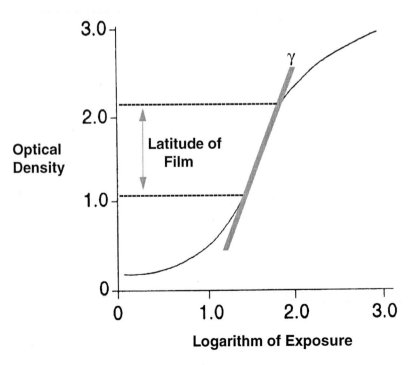

Figure 7–6. The Hurter-Driffield (H-D), or characteristic, sigmoid-shaped curve for film optical density versus the logarithm of exposure. Film contrast is determined by the slope of this curve; note that differences in contrast are linear only over the mid-portion of the relation, also known as the *latitude* of the film. The maximum slope in the latitude region is referred to as the γ of the film.

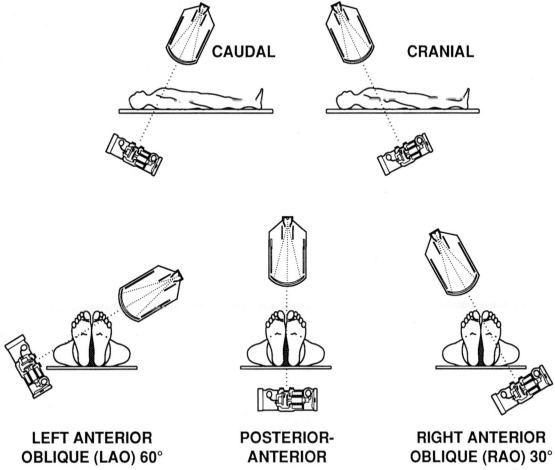

CAUDAL

CRANIAL

LEFT ANTERIOR OBLIQUE (LAO) 60°

POSTERIOR-ANTERIOR

RIGHT ANTERIOR OBLIQUE (RAO) 30°

Figure 7–7. Standard nomenclature used for description of the projection of image acquisition (x-ray gantry angulation). Note in the upper panel that *caudal* and *cranial* refer to the position of the image intensifier above, not the x-ray tube below, the patient. Also note in the lower panel that oblique views are described, as viewed from the feet, by an anterior polar coordinate system with 0 degrees at the top through 90 degrees left at the level of the x-ray table at the patient's left side, and 0 degrees at the top through 90 degrees right at the level of the x-ray table at the patient's right side. See text for further details.

be positioned in the left anterior oblique (LAO) 60-degree position (Fig. 7–7, *lower*). Or the gantry can be rotated toward the patient's right; if it is 30 degrees from the anteroposterior plane, it is said to be positioned in the right anterior oblique 30-degree position. Because most modern x-ray installations for cardiac catheterization can be rotated in any direction in three-dimensional space around an isocenter, there can be combinations of these labels (e.g., LAO 60 degrees or caudal 30 degrees). Most cinefilm runs during coronary angiography are recorded with the x-ray gantry in complex angles in order to properly visualize coronary obstructions in a plane parallel to the course of the vessel. In fact, the accuracy of our assessment of the severity of a coronary obstruction is dependent on the operator choosing appropriate projections for visualization (see Chapter 9).

Angiography Radiation Exposure to Patients and Health Personnel

Not to be ignored is the repetitive and accumulative radiation exposure sustained by patients, cardiologists, nurses, and technologists while in the cardiac angiography suite.[6] The unit of radiation dose commonly in use is the gray (Gy), with 1 Gy corresponding to 1 joule of energy absorbed per kilogram of material (Table 7–2). The older unit, the rad, is equal to 1/100th of a gray. Occasionally, because types of ionizing radiation other than x-rays are quantitated, an equivalent dose (H) in sievert (Sv) is calculated, whereby

$$H = w_R \cdot D$$

where H is the equivalent dose in sieverts, w_R is

Table 7–2. **Radiation Units Relevant to Interventional Cardiologists**

Radiation Measure	Traditional Unit	New International Unit
Quantity or dose (energy/mass)	rad; 1 rad = 0.01 Gy	Gray (Gy); 1 Gy = 1 J kg^{-1}; 1 Gy = 100 rads
Equivalent dose (H); see text	rem; 1 rem = 0.01 Sv	Sievert (Sv); 1 Sv = 100 rems
Exposure (X); X = charge/mass of air	Roentgen (R); 1 R = 2.58 × 10^{-4} coulombs (C) of charge kg^{-1} of air	Coulombs kg^{-1}

Modified from Johns PC, Renaud L: Radiation risk associated with PTCA. Primary Cardiology 1994; 20:27–31.

a weighting factor, and D is the dose in gray or rads. One sievert is equivalent to 100 rems (an old equivalent dose unit). For photon and electron beams (those encountered in x-ray exposure), 1 Gy is equivalent to 1 Sv. Although specific tissue radiosensitivity is variable, an exposure to irradiation is quantitated in roentgens (R). To an accuracy of about 20%, an x-ray beam exposure of 1 R gives a soft tissue absorption of about 1 rad (0.01 Gy).

As an example, during percutaneous transluminal coronary angioplasty (PTCA) a patient's skin entrance exposure per procedure has been calculated as approximately 124 R, of which about 70% is related to cineangiography and the rest to fluoroscopy.[7] Specific organ exposure dosages, on the average, are 93 mGy to the lungs, 49 mGy to the breast, 23 mGy to the bone marrow, and 10 mGy to the thyroid. An effective dose to the whole body of 20 mSv has been estimated from these data with an attendant cancer mortality risk of approximately 1 in 1000.[8] Patients undergoing PTCA are exposed commonly to other procedures, including myocardial scintigraphy, isotopic ventriculography, and diagnostic coronary angiography, that may increase further their radiation exposure. For example, one who receives a radioisotopic myocardial perfusion scan at rest and exercise, a diagnostic angiogram, and a subsequent PTCA would incur a total effect dose of approximately 48 mSv, and the aggregate cancer mortality risk would be about 1.9 × 10^{-3}.[6] This overall risk, therefore, should be factored into any comparison of interventional treatment with either surgical revascularization or medical therapy only.

Obviously, the net radiation exposure to in-room personnel (cardiologists, nurses, and technologists) depends on the total number of procedures performed per year, their average duration, and the fluoroscopy and cineangiography etiquette of the operator. Protective lead aprons and neck collars, as well as lead-penetrated eyeglasses, should be required and monitored in all laboratories. Moreover, detector badge surveillance is mandatory; excessive exposure for any given operator requires withdrawal of his or her privilege to perform catheterization procedures until corrective action is taken.

Radiographic Contrast Agents in Angiocardiography

During cardiac angiography, injection of iodinated contrast agent is essential for delineation of the anatomic relation of an individual cardiac structure to its neighbors, visualization of intracardiac shunts, assessment of the motion and size of ventricular and atrial chambers, and evaluation of the pathoanatomic changes in the coronary and pulmonary vessels.

High-osmolar, Ionic Contrast Agents

The commonly used iodinated, high-osmolar contrast agents (Hypaque-76 and Renografin-76), first formulated in the 1950s, are solutions of sodium or meglumine salts (diatrizoate with or without citrate). They have three iodine atoms for every two osmotically active particles and are referred to, therefore, as the 1.5 ratio ionic agents (Table 7–3). Their osmolality (approximately 1600 to 2000 mOsm/kg) is nearly 5.8 times that of plasma, and their sodium concentration varies between 160 and 190 mEq/L. This range of sodium concentration has been established as optimal for minimizing cardiac electrophysiologic changes during coronary arteriography.[9] Despite some bothersome side effects, the 1.5 ratio, nonionic agents are optimally radiopaque and enhance diagnostic images, and for many years their clinical benefit outweighed their risk and side effects.

High-osmolar, ionic contrast agents have been noted to have measurable hemodynamic and electrophysiologic effects during their administration.[10–12] All have a negative inotropic effect on the myocardium as evidenced by a depression of peak maximum rate of tension development. Moreover, the osmotic load of the usual dose (24 to 60 mL over 3 seconds) causes expansion of the circulating blood volume and an increase in the left ventricular end-diastolic

Table 7–3. **Commonly Used Iodinated Contrast Agents in Cardiac Angiography**

Product Category	Proprietary Name	Generic Constituent	Ratio of Iodine to Osmotically Active Particles	Calcium Chelation	Anticoagulant Effect
High-osmolar, ionic	Renografin-76	Diatrizoate and citrate	1.5	(+)	(+++)
High-osmolar, ionic	Hypaque-76	Diatrizoate only	1.5	(−)	(+++)
Low-osmolar, ionic	Hexabrix	Ioxaglate	3.0	(−)	(+++)
Low-osmolar, nonionic	Isovue	Iopamidol	3.0	(−)	(+)
Low-osmolar, nonionic	Omnipaque	Iohexol	3.0	(−)	(+)
Low-osmolar, nonionic	Optiray	Ioversol	3.0	(−)	(+)

(+) = present; (+++) = strongly present; (−) = absent.

volume and pressure. At the same time, these agents are vasodilators, and they cause a decrease in both systemic and coronary arterial vascular resistance. These vasodilatory effects are transient and disappear approximately 60 seconds after administration of the contrast agent.

Electrophysiologic perturbations are also prominent in the pharmacologic effects of high-osmolar, ionic contrast agents. Injection of one of these agents into the coronary artery that supplies the sinoatrial node causes a distinct depression of sinus automaticity that is transient and reversed by vagolytic maneuvers or drugs. Similarly, when contrast agent is injected into the coronary artery supplying the atrioventricular (AV) node, there is a depression of conductivity manifested by increasing AV nodal block (first, second, or third degree) that is again transient. Preadministration of atropine significantly protects against this response. There are also notable effects on repolarization associated with injection of these agents. The QT interval on the electrocardiogram is prolonged, irrespective of the route of administration. With coronary artery injections, there are also prominent, yet transitory, ST-T wave changes, reflecting effects on myocardial repolarization.

After exposure to these agents, depression of renal function, manifested by a transient reduction in the creatinine clearance and elevation of both the serum blood urea nitrogen and creatinine, has been noted. The pathogenesis of contrast agent–induced nephropathy is not well understood; medullary ischemia associated with a decrease in renal blood flow and hypoxia has been suggested as a possible mechanism.[13] Patients with preexistent diabetes mellitus, renal insufficiency, or renal insufficiency associated with a prerenal cause (low cardiac output) are particularly prone to elevate their serum creatinine level after an exposure to a 1.5 ratio ionic contrast agent. Less certain risk factors include a prior history of a contrast agent–induced episode of renal failure, a coexistent diagnosis of

multiple myeloma, or dehydration. Seldom do any of these high-risk or medium-risk patients go on to need temporary or chronic dialysis. Laboratory signs of worsening of renal function usually appears within 24 to 48 hours, and the associated oliguria can last 2 to 5 days. A return to baseline function is most often observed within 10 to 14 days.[14]

In an effort to maintain renal blood flow and inhibit kidney ischemia, preprocedure saline hydration, with or without an infusion of mannitol or furosemide immediately preceding the administration of the contrast agent, have been suggested as potentially useful prophylactic measures. Mannitol or furosemide administration, or both, is intended to minimize tubular oxygen demand by limiting sodium reabsorption. Recently, a randomized trial comparing hydration alone and hydration with either mannitol or furosemide as adjunctive measures was reported in patients with preexistent renal dysfunction.[15] It was found that hydration with 0.45% saline provided better protection than did hydration with 0.45% saline plus mannitol or furosemide. Furosemide was associated with a significantly greater increase in the serum creatinine concentration at 24 hours even in the patients who gained weight. It was postulated that the diuretic, given before the administration of the radiocontrast agent, may have caused systemic or renal hemodynamic changes that potentiated those of the contrast agents themselves. Thus, based on this most recent evidence, high-risk patients undergoing contrast angiography, and particularly those with diabetic nephropathy, are best pretreated with simple hydration. Limiting the amount of contrast agent given and avoidance of multiple procedures also are desirable measures to limit a given patient's risk.

The most serious, life-threatening side effect, although rare (approximately 1 in 1000 patients), is an anaphylactoid reaction, characterized by variable degrees of urticaria, angioedema, laryngeal edema, bronchospasm, arteriolar vasodilation, increased capillary permeability, and profound hypotension. The full-blown reaction mimics that of immunoglobin E–mediated anaphylaxis. However, in the case of an anaphylactoid reaction to contrast medium, no IgE antibody has been isolated. The reaction does not depend on the amount of contrast agent used, and it may occur with a patient's first exposure to the agent. Pretreatment with relatively high doses of corticosteroids can reduce significantly the incidence of repeat reactions in patients known to be allergic to a given contrast agent.[16] Lasser and associates[16] recommend a regimen of methylprednisolone given 12 hours, and then again 2 hours, before contrast agent administration. Because of the massive release of histamine during an anaphylactoid reaction, we also pretreat with 50 mg of diphenhydramine before any cardiac angiography procedure.

Low-osmolar, Ionic and Nonionic Contrast Agents

The low-osmolar, nonionic contrast agents were developed primarily in Europe in the 1980s and were first approved for use in the United States in 1985 (see Table 7–3). They exhibit the same radiopacity as high-osmolar agents, yet their osmolalities are in the range of 600 to 900 mOsm/kg. The nonionic monomers (e.g., iopamidol) in this group have eliminated the sodium and meglumine ions yet maintained three iodine atoms per molecule. All the members of this class have less negative inotropic effect on the myocardium; are less potent vasodilators; exhibit less effect on the left ventricular end-diastolic volume and pressure; and, based on a meta-analysis of available comparative studies, are perhaps less prone to worsen renal function.[12] They also have much less potential for causing sinus bradycardia and AV block during selective coronary angiography.

The low osmolar, non-ionic agents are widely acknowledged to reduce the most common nonsevere side effects such as nausea, vomiting, heat sensation, urticaria, and itching (Table 7–4).[17] However, significant controversy has developed over the benefit of nonionic agents in relation to their much higher cost (ratio of 20:1 in cost compared with ionic agents). Barrett and associates[18] have reported that the frequency of severe reactions, such as prolonged hypotension, pulmonary edema, and cardiac arrest, occurred 3.6 times more frequently in a high-osmolality (Renografin-76) than in a low-osmolality cohort of patients. A nearly contemporaneous study, however, reported by

Table 7–4. Incidence of the Common Side Effects with Ionic and Nonionic Iodinated Contrast Agents

Side Effect	Ionic (%)	Nonionic (%)
Nausea	4.6	1.0
Vomiting	1.8	0.4
Heat sensation	2.3	0.9
Urticaria	3.2	0.5
Itching	3.0	0.5

Modified from Katayama H, Yamaguchi K, Kozuka T, et al: Adverse reactions to ionic and nonionic contrast media: A report from the Japanese Committee on the Safety of Contrast Media. Radiology 1990; 175:621–628.

Steinberg and colleagues,[19] found no difference between high-osmolality (Hypaque-76) and low-osmolality groups. This difference has been attributed, possibly, to the strong calcium-chelating effect of the citrate in Renografin-76 as opposed to its absence in Hypaque-76. However, the study by Barrett and associates also appeared to include a more severely ill patient population.[20] Most laboratories are acknowledging the greater cost of the nonionic, low-osmolality agents by restricting their use to only those patients considered to be at higher risk for a contrast agent reaction.

Effects of Contrast Agents on Coagulation

Issues have recently been raised as to differing effects of the various classes of contrast agents on the coagulation system. These issues have become ever more relevant to the cardiologist as increasing numbers of catheterization procedures are performed for therapeutic reasons. All contrast agents are known to have an anticoagulant effect manifested by their ability to prolong the activated partial thromboplastin time. This property appears to be independent of the osmolar state; however, ionic, as compared with nonionic, agents appear to be more potent anticoagulants (see Table 7–3). As compared with nonionic agents, ionic agents demonstrate greater prolongation of the activated partial thromboplastin time and show greater inhibition of clot formation in glass or plastic syringes.

There appear to be some differences in platelet activation between high-osmolar and low-osmolar contrast agents. A recent study by Chronos and associates[21] used immunolabeling and flow cytometry to assess in vitro the effects of various contrast agents on platelet activation. Control blood, mixed with saline, demonstrated approximately 2% platelet activation. Hexabrix, an ionic, low-osmolar agent, activated 3% of platelets, an insignificant value compared with the control blood. However, Omnipaque, a nonionic, low-osmolar agent showed 60% to 80% platelet activation by 1 minute. These ex vivo observations would suggest that the nonionic agents, as compared with ionic agents and irrespective of osmolarity, have a strong propensity to cause platelet activation, the earliest step in arterial thrombotic occlusion. In separate analyses, these same authors reported that blood drawn from patients pretreated with aspirin and heparin and subsequently exposed in vitro to Omnipaque showed significant platelet activation, whereas Hexabrix showed no change from control.

The comparative risk of an ionic (Renografin-76) and a nonionic agent during PTCA was assessed by Gasperetti and coworkers[22] in a randomized patient investigation. Patients with a recent myocardial infarction or unstable angina (conditions known to be associated with intracoronary thrombus) were found to more commonly develop new thrombus if a nonionic agent was used for coronary opacification. No studies are available that compare high-osmolar and low-osmolar ionic agents and their effect on the acute thrombotic complications of PTCA.

REFERENCES

1. Forssmann W: Die sondierung des rechten herzens. Klin Wochenschr, 1929; 8:2085–2087.
2. Sprawls P Jr: Physical Principles of Medical Imaging. Rockville, MD, Aspen, 1987, pp 1–310
3. Hirshfeld JW Jr: Radiographic contrast agents. In Marcus ML, Schelbert HR, Skorton DJ, Wolf GL (eds): Cardiac Imaging: A Companion to Braunwald's Heart Disease. Philadelphia, WB Saunders, 1991, pp 162–181.
4. ACC/AHA Guidelines for Cardiac Catheterization and Cardiac Catheterization Laboratories: American College of Cardiology/American Heart Association Ad Hoc Task Force On Cardiac Catheterization [CJ Pepine, MD, Chairman]. J Am Coll Cardiol 1991; 18:1149–1182.
5. American College of Cardiology Cardiac Catheterization Committee, Nissen SE, Pepine CJ, Bashore TM, et al: Cardiac angiography without cine film: Erecting a "Tower of Babel" in the cardiac catheterization laboratory. J Am Coll Cardiol 1994; 24:834–837.
6. Johns PC, Renaud L: Radiation risk associated with PTCA. Prim Cardiol 1994; 20:27–31.
7. Pattee JL, Johns PC, Chambers RJ: Radiation risk to patients from transluminal coronary angioplasty. J Am Coll Cardiol 1993; 22:1044–1051.
8. International Commission on Radiological Protection Publication 60: 1990 Recommendations of the International Commission on Radiological Protection. Oxford, Pergamon Press, 1991, p 24.
9. Hirshfield JW Jr, Wieland J, Davis CA, et al: Hemodynamic and electrocardiographic effects of ioversol during cardiac angiography comparison with diatrizoate. Invest Radiol 1989; 24:138.
10. Higgins CB, Sovak M, Schmidt WS, et al: Direct myocardial effects of intracoronary administration of new contrast materials with low osmolality. Invest Radiol 1980; 15:39.
11. Higgins CB, Gerber KH, Mattrtey RF, et al: Evaluation of the hemodynamic effects of intravenous administration of ionic and nonionic contrast materials. Radiology 1983; 142:681.
12. Hirshfield JW Jr: Cardiovascular effects of iodinated contrast agents. Am J Cardiol 1990; 66:9F–17F.
13. Heyman SN, Brezis M, Epstein FH, et al: Early renal medullary hypoxic injury from radiocontrast and indomethacin. Kidney Int 1991; 40:632–642.
14. Coggins CH, Fang LST: Acute renal failure associated with antibiotics, anesthetic agents, and radiographic contrast agents. In Brenner BM, Lazarus JM (eds): Acute Renal Failure. Philadelphia, WB Saunders, 1983, pp 283–320.
15. Solomon R, Werner C, Mann D, et al: Effects of saline, mannitol, and furosemide on acute decreases in renal function induced by radiocontrast agents. N Engl J Med 1994; 331:1416–1420.
16. Lasser EC, Berry CC, Talner LB, et al: Pretreatment with corticosteroids to alleviate reactions to intravenous contrast material. N Engl J Med 1987; 317:845.
17. Katayama H, Yamaguchi K, Kozuka T, et al: Adverse reactions to ionic and nonionic contrast media: A report from the Japanese Committee on the Safety of Contrast Media. Radiology 1990; 175:621–628.
18. Barrett BJ, Parfrey PS, Vavasour HM, et al: A comparison of nonionic, low-osmolality radiocontrast agents with ionic, high-osmolality agents during cardiac catheterization. N Engl J Med 1992; 326:431–436.
19. Steinberg EP, Moore RD, Powe NR, et al: Safety and cost effectiveness of high-osmolality as compared with low-osmolality contrast in patients undergoing cardiac angiography. N Engl J Med 1992; 326:425–430.
20. Hirshfield JW Jr: Low-osmolality contrast agents—who needs them? N Engl J Med 1992; 326:482–484.
21. Chronos NAF, Goodall AH, Wilson DJ, et al: Profound platelet degranulation is an important side effect of some types of contrast media used in interventional cardiology. Circulation 1993; 88(part I):2035–2044.
22. Gasperetti CM, Feldman MD, Burwell LR, et al: Influence of contrast media on thrombus formation during coronary angioplasty. J Am Coll Cardiol 1991; 18:443–450.

Chapter 8

Left and Right Contrast Ventriculography
Methods for Quantitation of Volume and Mass

VALMIK BHARGAVA

In the assessment of adult and pediatric heart disease, left ventricular volume, ejection fraction, and myocardial mass are recognized as important determinants of prognosis and quality of life. In the cardiac catheterization laboratory, iodinated contrast left ventriculography is the imaging modality commonly employed to quantitate these important pathophysiologic parameters. Projected areas of the ventricular cavity, long-axis dimensions, and wall thickness are measured and then used to calculate chamber volumes based on geometric models, the percentage of change in volume between end-diastole and end-systole (ejection fraction), and the volume and weight of the muscle surrounding the cavity (myocardial mass). Frame-by-frame measurements of left ventricular volume and wall thickness, when combined with simultaneous left ventricular pressure determinations, also permit estimation of wall stress and chamber or myocardial compliance (see Chapters 11, 12, and 18).

VOLUME ESTIMATION

Contrast left ventriculograms are acquired customarily at 30 or 60 images per second and recorded on cinefilm or videotape. However, in digital cardiac catheterization laboratories the images also may be digitized on-line for analysis (see Chapter 10).

Selective Ventriculography

Ventriculography is performed by injecting 8 to 25 mL/sec of contrast medium over 1.5 to 4 seconds into the left ventricle. The total dose of contrast agent is based on patient conditions; for example, patients with renal failure or a small ventricular chamber receive a smaller amount (8 to 12 mL over 3 seconds); those with a large end-diastolic volume or high cardiac output receive a larger dose (36 to 60 mL over 3 seconds). For single-plane angiography, the images are usually acquired in the 30-degree right anterior oblique (RAO) projection[1, 2] and for biplane angiography either in the anteroposterior (AP) and lateral (LAT) projections[3] (Fig. 8–1) or in the 30-degree RAO–60-degree left anterior oblique (LAO) projections.[4] To avoid the myocardial-depressant and volume-loading effects of iodinated contrast agents it is recommended that left ventriculography be performed before coronary angiography,[5] although some authors disagree with this practice.[6]

Optimal positioning of the catheter tip in the ventricular cavity is crucial to achieving high-quality visualization of the dynamic anatomic changes of the left ventricle during systole and diastole. The catheter should be placed freely within the cavity, because ectopic, extrasystolic, and postextrasystolic beats cannot be used for proper assessment of baseline left ventricular function. The catheter tip should be away from the ventricular apex where the risk of stimulating arrhythmias by contrast agent injection is reduced. Also, the catheter tip should be placed near the middle of the cavity to avoid catheter recoil into the aorta during power injection of the contrast agent while still opacifying the entire cavity. Use of a pigtail catheter is preferable to reduce the direct impact of the contrast jet on the endocardium and to reduce the chance of arrhythmias. In those patients who have horizontally oriented hearts,

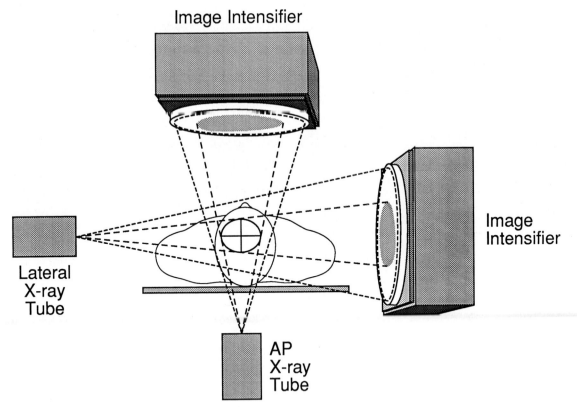

Figure 8–1. Schematic diagram showing the biplane radiographic imaging setup.

the use of an angled pigtail catheter to position the tip in the middle of the ventricular chamber is advocated. Test doses of contrast medium should be kept low to avoid their depressant effect.[5, 7] Although more expensive, nonionic contrast agents are more commonly selected over ionic agents because of their minimal effect on myocardial function and greater patient tolerance (see Chapter 7). Preferably, biplane angiograms should not be performed with two successive injections, because the second angiogram may manifest depressed function from the immediately previous contrast agent injection.[8]

Intravenous Injection

The left ventricle also can be visualized by injecting contrast agent into the vena cava, right atrium, right ventricle, or pulmonary artery (i.e., venous, or right side of the heart). This technique has the advantage of avoiding extrasystoles due to myocardial irritation by the catheter itself or from the velocity jets as contrast agent exits the catheter. It may also permit estimation of right ventricular function if the contrast agent is injected into the vena cava, right atrium, or right ventricle. If only left ventricular function needs evaluation, this approach provides a less invasive alternative. Pulmonary artery injection of contrast medium sometimes causes the patient to cough and experience undesirable motion; this can be minimized significantly by use of nonionic contrast agent injected into the right or left pulmonary artery.

With right-sided injections the left ventricular cavity edges are not as well delineated as with direct injection of contrast agent, owing to dilution of contrast agent by the time it appears in the left ventricular cavity. Ideally, the contrast agent should be injected at a rapid rate so as to yield a relatively high degree of opacification within the left ventricle. In patients with low cardiac output, the washout of the contrast agent from the right side of the heart may be slow, making isolated (with no contrast agent in the right heart) opacification and visualization of the left cavity difficult. Venous injection of a contrast agent to opacify the left ventricle is useful especially when a videodensitometric technique for the evaluation of ejection fraction is needed.[9] With the use of videodensitometry, it is important that no other simultaneously opacified chamber, such as the atria, right ventricle, and aorta, overlap with the left ventricular cavity; therefore, a 30-degree RAO projection is commonly employed.

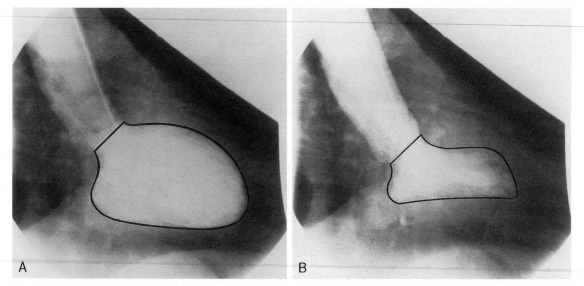

Figure 8–2. *A,* Left ventricular end-diastolic image. *B,* Left ventricular end-systolic image. The cavity silhouettes are shown in *A* and *B.*

It is better to visualize the right ventricular cavity by indirect injection of the contrast medium into the right atrium or the inferior vena cava; this reduces the likelihood of premature ventricular contractions and artifactual tricuspid regurgitation.[10, 11]

Mathematic Models

Geometric methods for estimation of left ventricular volume assume that the left ventricular shape is that of an ellipsoid.[3] Although the shape of the left ventricular cavity is complicated by the presence of the papillary muscles, its relatively convex, or football-shaped, geometry permits the use of simplified mathematic models. Alternatively, other more complex mathematic models have been used, for example, Simpson's rule.[12] For calculating ventricular cavity volume, end-diastolic and end-systolic frames are selected, and the opacified ventricular cavity silhouettes are traced (Fig. 8–2). End-diastolic and end-systolic consecutive frames (from the same beat) are selected by choosing the largest and the subsequent smallest visualized silhouettes, respectively. Usually, the beat for analysis is selected from the first three[13] to six[14] opacified sinus beats, preferably an earlier beat. Tracing of the silhouettes should be done by including the outermost edge of the visible contrast agent, that is, including the papillary muscle and trabeculation, and the left ventricular inflow tract.[1, 8, 15] The aortic valve plane is drawn from the inferior aspect of the sinuses of Valsalva. The long axis in the AP and RAO projection is drawn from the mid-aortic valve point to the apex, and for LAT or LAO view the longest axis.

Assuming that the x-ray projection of the opacified left ventricle is an ellipse, the volume, V, with major (L) and minor axes (a and b) is given by the following[3]:

$$V = \frac{4}{3} \cdot \Pi \cdot \frac{L}{2} \cdot \frac{a}{2} \cdot \frac{b}{2} = \Pi \cdot \frac{L \cdot a \cdot b}{6} \quad (1)$$

Projection of the ellipsoid in the two orthogonal planes are ellipses with areas of $\Pi \cdot L \cdot a/4$, and $\Pi \cdot L \cdot b/4$. Because a and b cannot be measured accurately, the projected areas (A_{RAO} and A_{LAO}) and long axis as projected in the two planes (L_{RAO} and L_{LAO}) are used to calculate the minor axes (area/length method) as follows[3]:

$$a = \frac{4 \cdot A_{RAO}}{\Pi \cdot L_{RAO}} \quad (2)$$

$$b = \frac{4 \cdot A_{LAO}}{\Pi \cdot L_{LAO}} \quad (3)$$

Substituting the values of a and b from Equations 2 and 3 into Equation 1 yields

$$V = \frac{\Pi \cdot 4 \cdot A_{RAO} \cdot 4 \cdot A_{LAO} \cdot L_{MAX}}{6 \cdot \Pi \cdot L_{RAO} \cdot \Pi \cdot L_{LAO}}$$

$$= \frac{0.849 \cdot A_{RAO} \cdot A_{LAO}}{L_{MIN}} \quad (4)$$

where L_{MIN} and L_{MAX} are minimum and maximum values of L_{RAO} and L_{LAO}. In the biplane formula for volume estimation L_{MIN} should be measured accurately, because L_{MAX} cancels out of the numerator and the denominator; this is usually from the LAO projection. As is evident, Equation 4 is valid for any two *orthogonal* views, even though I have used RAO and LAO subscripts, as long as at least one view projects the long axis reasonably parallel to the image plane. This formula has been shown empirically to be useful in other semiorthogonal views.[16] When this formula is used for single-plane analysis, assume that a equals b; that is, Equation 4 can be rewritten as

$$V = \frac{8 \cdot A_{RAO}^2}{3 \cdot \Pi \cdot L_{RAO}} = \frac{0.849 \cdot A_{RAO}^2}{L_{RAO}} \qquad (5)$$

For both single-plane and biplane left ventricular volume estimation, these formulas have been shown to be valid when the shape of the ventricle deviates from the assumed uniform ellipsoid (Fig. 8–3).[17]

Regression Equations

Both single-plane and biplane methods tend to overestimate the true left ventricular volume when compared with the left ventricular volume of postmortem casts,[1, 3, 18] but the single-plane method overestimates more than the biplane one.[18, 19] Volume overestimation is the result of inclusion of papillary muscles and trabeculation, which are included in the silhouette but do not contribute to the cavity volume. Thus, linear regression equations have been derived[3, 18, 20–25] relating measured (actual) cast volumes, V_{ACT}, and angiographically calculated volumes,

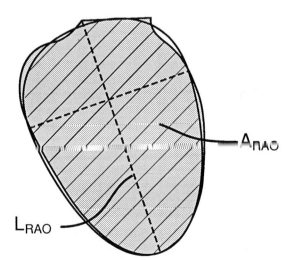

Figure 8–3. Schematic diagram showing how an asymmetric ellipsoid model of the ventricular silhouette approximates the projected area. (For details, see reference 17.)

V_{ANG}. These relationships are available for adult single-plane, and biplane as well as pediatric single-plane angiogram. A biplane regression equation has been shown to be valid for both the paired 30-degree RAO–60-degree LAO or AP-LAT projections. Each linear regression equation is given by:

$$V_{ACT} = m \cdot V_{ANG} + c \qquad (6)$$

where m and c are constants. Values of m and c are listed in Table 8–1.

Magnification Correction

The ventricular silhouette is usually recorded on cine or videoimage or in digital format. During acquisition, the image is first formed on the image intensifier; from there it is transferred to the film or the video camera and is finally displayed on the cine projector or the video monitor. To correct for magnification, a calibration grid consisting of 1-cm squares is located at the mid-level of the ventricle and its images are acquired on the same media, that is, film or videotape or in digital format.[2] The positioning of the grid at the mid-ventricular level is of critical importance,[25] because if the grid is placed erroneously by 2.5 cm (1 inch), the volumes will be off by 5% to 10%, and if the error in locating the grid is 5 cm (2 inches), then volumes may be miscalculated by as much as 25% to 40%.

To locate the grid at the mid-level of the ventricle, the following technique is suggested: Under fluoroscopy, in an orthogonal x-ray projection, a radiopaque object (e.g., a hemostat) is moved onto the chest of the patient to overlap with the catheter located in the mid-ventricular cavity, and this point is marked on the chest. The distance of this point from the image intensifier in the imaging projection is measured along with the source-to–image intensifier distance; later, a calibration grid is located at these settings and imaged. The magnification correction factor is calculated as the ratio of the actual area and its projection. The square root of this value is the linear correction factor used; that is, calculated volume is multiplied by the cube of the linear correction factor.

The size and region of the calibration grid used should be chosen to overlap with the ventricular silhouette (Fig. 8–4). This is important because the peripheral region of the image intensifier has pincushion distortion, and in so doing the calibration grid accounts for this pincushion distortion.[8] Pincushion distortion, without correction, may contribute 6% to 20% of the calculated volume.[32] A spherical ball is also

Table 8–1. Relationship Between Single-plane Versus Biplane and Actual Versus Estimated Left Ventricular Volume*

Investigator	Projection	Slope (m)	Intercept (c)	r	n	SEE	Age: Relationship
Greene et al[1]	RAO	1.0	0.0	0.988	18	—	Adult: RAO vs. biplane
Kasser and Kennedy[2]	RAO	0.787	7.8	0.972	32	20	Adult: RAO vs. biplane
Kennedy et al[21]	RAO	0.81	1.9	0.97	30	24	Adult: RAO vs. biplane
Sandler and Dodge[20]	AP	0.951	−3.0	0.99	55	15	Adult: AP vs. biplane
Kennedy et al[21]	AP	1.00	9.6	0.97	30	24	Adult: AP vs. biplane
Sandler et al[26]	AP	0.73	−15.0	—	15	25	Adult: AP vs. biplane
Wynne et al[18]	RAO	0.938	−5.7	0.99	11	5.5	Adult: V_{ACT} vs. RAO
Arcilla et al[10]	AP-LAT	0.992	−0.78	0.96	27	9.1	Adult: V_{ACT} vs. biplane
Rackley et al[27]	AP-LAT	0.926	10.2	—	97	15	Adult: V_{ACT} vs. biplane
Dodge, Sandler et al[3, 22,28]	AP-LAT	0.928	−3.8	0.995	84	8.2	Adult: V_{ACT} vs. biplane
Goerke et al[29]	AP-LAT	0.813	−13.2	0.97	60	—	Adult: V_{ACT} vs. biplane
Wynne et al[18]	RAO-LAO	0.989	−8.1	0.99	11	8	Adult V_{ACT} vs. biplane
Formanek et al[30]	Biplane	0.7–0.83	0	0.97–0.999	9–13	1.8–5.8	Adult: V_{ACT} vs. biplane
Ino et al[31]	RAO-LAO	0.77	−0.3	0.97	13	3.5	Children: V_{ACT} vs. biplane
Graham et al[23]	AP-LAT	0.974	−3.1	0.99	89	3	Children: V_{ACT} vs. biplane >15 mL
Graham et al[23]	AP-LAT	0.733	0.0	0.98	71	0.7	Children: V_{ACT} vs. biplane <15 mL
Fisher et al[24]	AP-LAT	0.412	−1.32	0.92	32	10.1	Children: $V_{ACT\text{-}ED}$ vs. biplane
Fisher et al[24]	AP-LAT	1.00	−1.24	0.86	31	5.8	Children: $V_{ACT\text{-}ES}$ vs. biplane
Ino et al[31]	AP-LAT	0.84	−0.3	0.96	13	3.9	Children: V_{ACT} vs. biplane

*Coefficients of linear regression from various studies relating (1) single-plane left ventricular volumes to those derived by biplane method and (2) actual (V_{ACT}) left ventricular volume to angiographic (V_{ANG}) estimates ($V_{ACT} = m·V_{ANG} + c$), for single-plane and biplane in adults and children. Correlation coefficient (r), number of casts or data points used for calculation (n), and SEE (standard error of estimate [mL] are also tabulated. $V_{ACT\text{-}ED}$, actual end-diastolic left ventricular volume; $V_{ACT\text{-}ES}$, actual end-systolic left ventricular volume.

Note: The independent (V_{ANG}) and dependent (V_{ACT}) variables in this table are presented with consistency, although they may have been published in a converse fashion in the original publication; if so, the slopes (m) and intercepts (c) were recomputed from the original equation published.

sometimes used for calibration. The advantage of using a centimeter grid is that when digitizing the area of the grid, one need only connect the intersection points on the grid, which are easy to draw. However, digitizing a circular region is time consuming and results in a polygon rather than a circle, leading to underestimation of the digitized grid area.

Sample worksheets used in our institution for calculation of single-plane and biplane left ventricular volumes are shown in Figures 8–5 and 8–6.

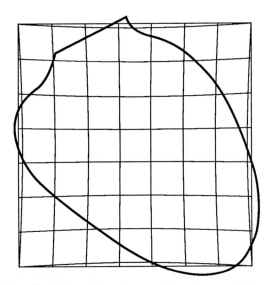

Figure 8–4. Projected centimeter grid superimposed with the ventricular diastolic silhouette. Note that the selection of the 7 × 7-cm grid overlaps with the left ventricular silhouette.

EJECTION FRACTION

Volumetric Calculation

Ejection fraction, EF, is the ratio of stroke volume, V_{STROKE}, and end-diastolic volume, V_{ED}, where V_{STROKE} is the difference between the end-diastolic and end-systolic, V_{ES}, volume. That is,

$$EF = \frac{V_{ED} - V_{ES}}{V_{ED}} = \frac{V_{STROKE}}{V_{ED}} \quad (7)$$

When single-plane analysis is used alone for calculation of ejection fraction, it is unnecessary to know or correct for magnification, because it cancels from both the numerator and the denominator. When biplane images are used to

Name: _____   Date: _____   Age: _____ years   Angiographic Heart Rate (HR): _____ beats/min   BSA: _____ m²

			Units	Variable	End-diastolic	End-systolic
1	Length of long axis from mid-aortic valve plane to apex		cm	L_d, L_s		
2	Area of ventricular silhouette		cm²	A_d, A_s		
3	LV calculated volume ($0.8488 \cdot A^2/L$)		mL	V_{cd}, V_{cs}		
4	Actual area of grid		cm²	A_{ACT}		
5	Measured or planimetered area of grid		cm²	A_{MEA}		
6	Linear correction factor $(A_{ACT}/A_{MEA})^{1/2}$			CF		
7	LV volume corrected for magnification ($V_c CF^3$)		mL	V_{ed}, V_{es}		
8	LV volume corrected by regression equation ($0.81 \cdot V_e + 1.9$)		mL	V_D, V_S		
9	Indexed volumes (V_D/BSA, V_S/BSA)		mL/m²	V_{DI}, V_{SI}		
10	Indexed stroke volume ($V_{DI} - V_{SI}$)		mL/m²	V_{STROKE}		
11	Ejection fraction $[(V_D - V_S)/V_D]$			EF		
12	Cardiac index (HR $\cdot$ $V_{STROKE/1000}$)		L/min/m²	CI		
13	Cardiac output (CI $\cdot$ BSA)		L/min	CO		

Figure 8-5. Thirty-degree RAO single-plane left ventricular volume calculation worksheet.

Name: _____

Date: _____

Age: _____ yrs

Angiographic Heart Rate (HR): _____ beats/min

BSA: _____ m²

		Variable	Units	End-diastolic		End-systolic	
				RAO	LAO	RAO	LAO
1	Actual area of grid	$A_{ACT,R}$; $A_{ACT,L}$	cm²				
2	Measured or planimetered area of grid	$A_{MEA,R}$; $A_{MEA,L}$	cm²				
3	Area correction factor (A_{ACT}/A_{MEA})	CF_{RAO}^2, CF_{LAO}^2					
4	Linear correction factor ($A_{ACT}/A_{MEA})^{1/2}$	CF_{RAO}; CF_{LAO}					
5	Length of long axis	$L_{1RAO,ED}$ $L_{1LAO,ED}$ $L_{1RAO,ES}$ $L_{1LAO,ES}$	cm				
6	Long axis corrected for magnification ($L_1 \cdot CF$)	$L_{RAO,ED}$ $L_{LAO,ED}$ $L_{RAO,ES}$ $L_{LAO,ES}$	cm				
7	Area of left ventricular silhouette	$A_{1RAO,ED}$ $A_{1LAO,ED}$ $A_{1RAO,ES}$ $A_{1LAO,ES}$	cm²				
8	Area corrected for magnification ($A_1 \cdot CF^2$)	$A_{RAO,ED}$ $A_{LAO,ED}$ $A_{RAO,ES}$ $A_{LAO,ES}$	cm²				
9	Minimum of RAO and LAO long axes (usually LAO)	$L_{MIN,ED}$ $L_{MIN,ES}$	cm				
10	Calculated ventricular volume ($0.8488 \cdot A_{RAO} \cdot A_{LAO})/L_{MIN}$)	V_{1ED} V_{1ES}	mL				
11	Volume corrected by regression equation $V = 0.989 \cdot V_1 - 8.1$	V_{ED} V_{ES}	mL				
12	Indexed volumes (V/BSA)	V_{EDI} V_{ESI}	mL/m²				
13	Indexed stroke volume ($V_{EDI} - V_{ESI}$)	V_{STROKE}	mL/m²				
14	Cardiac index ($V_{STROKE} \cdot HR/1000$)	CI	L/min/m²				
15	Cardiac output (CI $\cdot$ BSA)	CO	L/min				
16	Ejection fraction ($V_{ED} - V_{ES})/V_{ED}$)	EF					

Figure 8–6. Thirty-degree RAO-60-degree LAO biplane left ventricular volume calculation worksheet.

Note: This work sheet is also suitable for an AP/LAT biplane calculation if RAO is replaced by AP and LAO by LAT and the regression equation used is $V = 0.928\ V_1 - 3.8$ for adults and $V = 0.85\ V_1$ for children.

calculate ejection fraction, it is essential that the magnification correction be known in both planes. The ratio of ejection fraction divided by ejection time is defined as the mean normalized ejection rate. End-systolic frame selection is crucial to estimating ejection fraction accurately. When the end-systolic frame is chosen at the closure of the aortic valve, the end-systolic volume is smaller, the stroke volume is larger, and the ejection fraction is larger than when the mitral valve opening is used.[33] This is the result of the changes in projected end-systolic silhouette area even though the volume has not changed during the isovolumetric interval between aortic valve closure and mitral valve opening.

Videodensitometric Calculation

Use of densitometry permits the calculation of left[9, 19, 34-37], and right[34, 38] ventricular ejection fraction with no geometric assumptions.[39, 40] This technique is useful with digital systems only. Ideally, correction for scatter and veiling glare (a lead marker is placed in the image field, and the average brightness in a region under the lead marker is calculated and subtracted from each pixel [picture element] value) or other technique[41] is essential, along with logarithmic transformation of video intensities; otherwise, ejection fraction may be erroneously underestimated compared with geometrically calculated values. Videodensitometric estimation of ejection fraction requires image acquisition at constant radiographic technique, that is, constant kilovolt (peak) and milliampere. Images initially are digitized using a linear scale and corrected for scatter and veiling glare, and its values are logarithmically transformed. A region of interest over the ventricular silhouette is drawn, and in this region average videodensity is calculated at both end-diastole, V_D, and end-systole, V_S. This region should include ventricular silhouettes both at end-systole and end-diastole but exclude the aortic and mitral valves. Average videodensity over a background, V_B, region of interest is calculated from the systolic image. This horseshoe shaped background region encompasses the ejection shell but excludes the systolic ventricular silhouette.[9] Ejection fraction is calculated as:

$$EF = \frac{(V_S - V_D)}{(V_B - V_D)} \quad (8)$$

Equation 8 is valid for estimating both left and right ventricular ejection fractions. The videodensity technique requires that iodinated contrast media be mixed uniformly in blood; that is, the contrast agent should be injected in the vena cava for right ventricular function estimation and in the venous side, right heart, or pulmonary artery for left ventricular estimation. When used for right ventricular function assessment, the contrast agent should be injected in the right atrium or inferior vena cava.

Regurgitant Fraction

In patients with mitral or aortic regurgitation the forward stroke volume, SV_F, is calculated by dividing the cardiac output (determined by Fick or green dye or thermodilution technique, when tricuspid regurgitation is absent) by the heart rate. Regurgitant fraction, RF, is defined as:

$$RF = \frac{(SV_A - SV_F)}{SV_A} \quad (9)$$

where SV_A is the angiographic stroke volume. This assumes that heart rates during both ventriculography and either the Fick or thermodilution cardiac output estimation are similar; if this is not true, then stroke volumes are replaced by angiographic and forward cardiac outputs. Angiographic cardiac output is calculated as the product of angiographic stroke volume and the corresponding heart rate. Angiographic cardiac output is accurate in the absence of mitral or aortic regurgitation.

Regurgitant fraction is imprecise because each term in the equation is likely to have some error; this has been shown by estimating forward stroke volume by two different methods, that is, Fick and thermodilution, with poor agreement between the regurgitant fractions thus derived.[42] The regurgitant fractions for mitral and aortic valves cannot be separately estimated if both valves are incompetent.

LEFT VENTRICULAR MASS

Left ventricular mass (LV_{MASS}) using the area/length method[43] is calculated from the following equation:

$$LV_{MASS} = 1.05 \cdot (\text{left ventricular myocardial volume}) \quad (10)$$

$$LV_{MASS} = 1.05 \cdot (V_{C+M} - V_C) \quad (11)$$

where 1.05 is the specific gravity of the heart muscle, V_{C+M} is the volume of the cavity and the left ventricular myocardium, and V_C is the

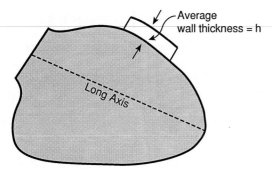

Figure 8–7. Left ventricular end-diastolic silhouette along with a segment of wall drawn used to estimate average wall thickness, calculated by dividing the area by the length of the myocardial segment.

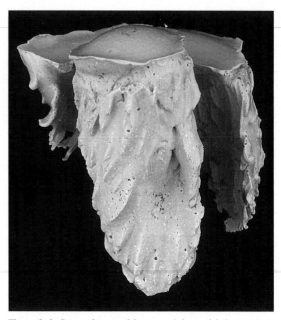

Figure 8–8. Casts of normal human right and left ventricles. Note that the right ventricle (shown posteriorly) is concave in shape and wraps around the left ventricle (shown anteriorly). Note also the significant trabecular appendages that complicate the assessment of right ventricular volume.

ventricular cavity volume. In Equation 11, end-diastolic volume is used for V_C; the V_{C+M} at end-diastole is calculated by incrementing both minor and major axes by twice the wall thickness (2h). Thus, the equation for cavity plus left ventricular wall volume is the following:

$$V_{C+M} = \Pi \cdot \frac{(L + 2h) \cdot (a + 2h) \cdot (b + 2h)}{6} \quad (12)$$

where, L is the long axis and a and b are the minor axes. Left ventricular myocardial mass estimation can be derived from biplane or single-plane projection. In any event the cavity volume is calculated and corrected by an appropriate regression equation to account for papillary muscles and trabeculation.

The wall thickness (h) can be measured usually in the AP[43] or 30-degree RAO[21] projection by averaging the wall thickness over a 3- to 4-cm segment of the lower anterolateral part of the left ventricle, being careful to avoid papillary muscle (Fig. 8–7). If the wall thickness is not well visualized in the contrast ventriculogram, then echocardiography can be used to measure wall thickness. For biplane analysis, Equation 12 can be written as:

$$V_{C+M} = \frac{\Pi}{6} \cdot (L + 2 \cdot h)$$
$$\cdot \left(\frac{4 \cdot A_{RAO}}{\Pi \cdot L_{RAO}} + 2 \cdot h \right) \cdot \left(\frac{4 \cdot A_{LAO}}{\Pi \cdot L_{LAO}} + 2 \cdot h \right) \quad (13)$$

This technique has been validated by comparison with postmortem hearts.[43, 44] Various regression equations are used to estimate the ventricular mass based on calculated values, from single-plane AP and 30-degree RAO and relating single-plane AP or 30-degree RAO to bi-

Table 8–2. **Relationship Between Actual and Estimated Versus Single-Plane and Biplane Left Ventricular Mass***

Investigator	Slope (m)	Intercept (c)	Projection	r	n	SEE	Relationship
Kennedy et al[21]	1.000	9.6	AP	0.92	30	53	Single Plane
Kennedy et al[21]	0.809	1.9	30-degree RAO	0.92	30	42	Single Plane
Rackley et al[27]	1.01	11.1	AP-LAT	—	23	23	Biplane
Kennedy et al[44]	1.04	−6.5	AP-LAT	0.97	26	32	Biplane
Kennedy et al[21]	0.83	53.0	AP	0.97	30	24	AP-single to Biplane
Kennedy et al[21]	0.90	15.0	30-degree RAO	0.97	30	24	RAO-single to Biplane

*Slope (m) and intercept (c) of linear regression ($M_{ACT} = m \cdot M_{ANG} + c$) between actual or true (M_{ACT}) and angiographically estimated (M_{ANG}) left ventricular mass and relationship between single-plane and biplane angiographically derived left ventricular mass. See Table 8–1 for additional abbreviations.

Note: The independent (M_{ANG}) and dependent (M_{ACT}) variables in this table are presented with consistency, although they may have been published in a converse fashion in the original publication; if so, the slopes and intercepts were recomputed from the equation published.

plane estimates of mass. The slope, m, and intercept, c, are given in Table 8–2.

RIGHT VENTRICULAR VOLUMES

Compared with the convex left ventricular cavity, the right ventricular cavity is a concave chamber that wraps around the left ventricle and has an abundance of trabeculation (Fig. 8–8). The concavity of this chamber depends on the relative size of the left ventricle and the position of the septum. Because of the cavity's unusual shape several models have been proposed for calculation of right ventricular volume, including the area/length method[45] parallelepiped,[10] prism,[10] pyramid,[46, 47] hemi-elliptical cylinders,[48] and the Simpson's rule.[11, 49–51] Biplane right ventricular angiography is commonly performed using AP-LAT views[11, 52–56]; however, some investigators prefer the 30 degree RAO,[48, 57] although biplane estimates are more reliable.[57] Most of the angiographic validation studies were done with ventricular casts that were all oriented in the same projection. When imaging a patient in the single-plane RAO projection, the fact that the heart is oriented differently in different people must be taken into account. Thus, a major limitation of this technique is its sensitivity to slight changes

in projection owing to differences in heart orientation within the thorax. Even a small angle change (± 10 degrees) leads to a significant volume deviation.[58]

Table 8–3 gives the results of linear regression between angiographically measured right ventricular volumes and actual volumes. Briefly, with Simpson's rule the chamber is assumed to consist of slices or disks whose diameter in each orthogonal plane is given by D, with subscripts A for AP or RAO projection and L for LAT or LAO projection. Subscripts o and e refer to the odd and even slice number. Thickness of the slice is denoted by h. Right ventricular volume, V (Fig. 8–9),[11, 29, 30, 49, 50, 59–65] is given by:

$$V = \frac{\Pi}{4} \cdot h \cdot \left(\sum_{o=1}^{n-1} D_{Ao} \cdot D_{Lo} + \frac{1}{2} \sum_{e=2}^{n} D_{Ae} \cdot D_{Le} \right) \quad (14)$$

Normal Range

The mean and standard deviations for left ventricular volumes, ejection fraction, and left ventricular mass for normal subjects are given in Table 8–4. Wall thickness for normal subjects is reported to be 10.9 $\pm$ 2.0 mm (SD) and 8.5 $\pm$ 0.5 mm (SEM).[66] The normal ratio of left ventricular mass to end-diastolic volume is about 1.

Table 8–3. Regression Analysis Between Angiographically Measured Right Ventricular Volumes and Actual Volumes*

Investigator	Method	Slope (m)	Intercept (c)	r	SEE	n
Graham et al[50]	Simpson's rule	0.649	0	0.992	6.73	26
Gentzler et al[49]	Simpson's rule	0.749	0	0.99	3.70	12
Fisher et al[11]	Simpson's rule	0.71	-1.15	0.97	3.77	48
Lange et al[60]	Simpson's rule	0.53	0	—	2.9–22.6	22
Goerke et al[29]	Simpson's rule	0.709	-7.1	0.953	—	30
Shimazaki et al[61]	Simpson's rule	0.76	1.5	0.98	12.4	10
Slutsky et al[62]	Simpson's rule	1.052	—	0.95	5.0	25
Dubel et al[63]	Simpson's rule	0.44	19.8	0.90	—	50
Formanek et al[30]	Simpson's rule	0.48–0.71	0	0.86–0.95	4.1–12.9	23
Pietras et al[64]	Simpson's rule	0.93	-8.8	0.96	6.8	19
Ino et al[65]	Simpson's rule	0.53	1.2	0.96	3.3	30
Mullins et al[68]	Simpson's rule	0.83	4.09	0.94	3.06	19
Mullins et al[69]	Simpson's rule	0.78	2.45	0.97	5.0	11
Arcilla et al[10]	Area/length	0.898	2.80	0.96	5.01	69
Graham et al[50]	Area/length	0.680	0	0.989	8.03	26
Arcilla et al[10]	Parallelepiped	0.739	4.08	0.95	9.15	36
Arcilla et al[10]	Parallelepiped	0.762	2.81	0.96	5.01	69
Graham et al[50]	Two-chamber	0.712	0	0.988	8.77	26
Fisher et al[11]	Prism	1.16	-1.04	0.98	2.94	48
Ferlinz et al[47]	Pyramid	0.893	3.862	0.99	5.7	9
Boak et al[48]	Hemi-elliptical	0.97	-5.5	0.995	4.7	7

*V_{ANG} = m $\cdot V_{ACT}$ + c, where V_{ANG} is the angiographically measured volume and V_{ACT} is the actual volume of the right ventricle. Note that Slope (m) is less than unity, which suggests an overestimation of right ventricular volume by all methods. See Table 8–1 for additional abbreviations.

Note: The independent (V_{ACT}) and dependent (V_{ANG}) variables in this table are presented with consistency, although they may have been published in a converse fashion in the original publication; if so, the slopes and intercepts were recomputed from the equation published.

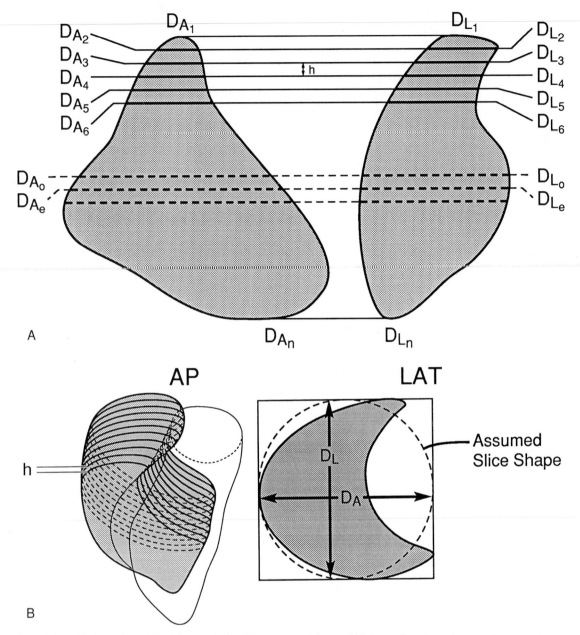

Figure 8–9. *A,* Biplane (AP, LAT) right ventricular silhouettes and the equithickness slices from the two planes are shown (h, anterior wall thickness in centimeters). Diameters D_{A1}, D_{A2}, . . . D_{Ao}, D_{Ae}, . . . D_{An} from the AP projection and D_{L1}, D_{L2}, . . . D_{Lo}, D_{Le}, . . . D_{Ln} from the LAT projection are shown. Subscripts o and e refer to the odd and even slice numbers, respectively (see text for details). *B, Left,* A stack of right ventricular slices is depicted. *Right,* The actual geometry as compared with the assumed elliptical shape for a slice is shown.

Reproducibility of Left Ventricular Global Parameters

Left ventricular end-diastolic volume can be measured reproducibly (intraobserver and interobserver variability) with an error of less than 3 mL/m² (<2% of control value), end-systolic volume less than 2 mL/m² (<2%), stroke volume less than 2 mL/m² (<2%), ejection frac-

tion less than 2% (<4%), and left ventricular mass less than 6 gm/m² (<4%).[67]

In Table 8–5 the normal right ventricular end-diastolic and end-systolic volumes (normalized by body surface area) are given. Simpson's method is the most commonly used for estimating right ventricular volume. The right ventricular end-diastolic volume is known to be somewhat larger than the left ventricular volume.[11,]

Table 8-4. Normal Values for Normalized Left Ventricular End-diastolic Volume Index (EDVI), Normalized End-systolic Volume (ESVI), Ejection Fraction (EF), and Normalized Left Ventricular Mass*

Investigator (Method of Tabulation)	Projection	No. of Patients†	Age Group	EDVI (mL/m²)	ESVI (mL/m²)	EF	Mass (gm/m²)	Left Ventricular Mass/EDV
Kennedy et al[70] (SD)	AP-LAT	16: vol; 22: mass	Adult	70 ± 20	24 ± 10	67 ± 8	92 ± 16	1.39 ± 0.41
Kennedy et al[71] (SD)	AP-LAT	50: vol & mass	Adult	71 ± 16	26 ± 8	63 ± 9	93 ± 18	—
Herman and Bartle[72] (SEM)	AP-LAT	6: vol	Adult	71 ± 8	30 ± 4	58 ± 2	—	—
Hood et al[66] (SEM)	AP-LAT	6: vol & mass	Adult	79 ± 4	28 ± 2	67 ± 3	93 ± 8	—
Arvidsson[73] (SD)	AP-LAT	16: vol	Adult	57 ± 18	15 ± 7	74 ± 11	—	—
Dodge et al[74]	AP-LAT	14: EF	Adult	—	—	64	—	—
Peterson et al[75] (SEM)	AP-LAT	22: vol	Adult	59 ± 4	14 ± 2	76 ± 2	—	—
Toma et al[76] (SD)	AP-LAT	8: vol	Adult	74 ± 13	20 ± 9	73 ± 8	—	—
Sanmarco et al[77] (SD)	Biplane	20: EDVI	Adult	80 ± 10	—	60–70	—	—
Wynne et al[18] (SD)	RAO-LAO	17: vol	Adult	72 ± 15	20 ± 8	72 ± 8	—	—
Pietras et al[78] (SD)	RAO-LAO	17: vol	Adult	70 ± 12	22 ± 5	68 ± 7	—	—
Thuring et al[79] (SD)	RAO-LAO	7: vol & mass	Adult women	73 ± 12	26 ± 7	65 ± 7	80 ± 15	—
Thuring et al[79] (SD)	RAO-LAO	18: vol & mass	Adult men	95 ± 15	35 ± 6	63 ± 4	96 ± 16	—
Thuring et al[79] (SD)	Single plane	18: vol & mass	Adult men	99 ± 15	33 ± 6	66 ± 4	98 ± 19	—
Thuring et al[79] (SD)	Single plane	7: vol & mass	Adult women	78 ± 14	24 ± 5	70 ± 7	84 ± 17	—
Rousseau et al[80] (SD)	Single plane	17: vol & mass	Adult	93 ± 18	27 ± 9	72 ± 6	93 ± 27	—
Falsetti et al[81] (SD)	Single plane	5: vol	Adult	104 ± 17	31 ± 9	70 ± 7	—	—
Huber et al[82] (SD)	Single plane	13: vol & mass	Adult	81 ± 15	—	70 ± 7	81 ± 18	1.02 ± 0.16
Schwarz et al[83] (SEM)	Single plane	10: vol & mass	Adult	77 ± 7	—	69 ± 2	73 ± 5	—
Miller and Swan[84] (SD)	AP-LAT	9: vol	Child 9 wk–14 yr	88 ± 11	32 ± 7	64 ± 6	—	—
Graham et al[23] (SD)	AP-LAT	37: vol & mass	Child >2 yr	73 ± 11	—	63 ± 5	86 ± 11	—
Graham et al[23] (SD)	AP-LAT	19: vol & mss	Child <2 yr	42 ± 10	—	68 ± 5	96 ± 11	—
Sano et al[89] (SD)	AP-LAT	20: vol & mass	Child	70 ± 17	23 ± 5	67 ± 3	66 ± 19	0.94 ± 0.13
Nakazawa et al[55] (SD)	AP-LAT	42: EF	Child	—	—	63 ± 1	—	—

*Based on data from all normal adults, average left ventricular EDVI[18, 66, 70–73, 75–83] is 75 mL/m², left ventricular ESVI[18, 66, 70–73, 75, 76, 78–81] is 24 mL/m², EF[18, 66, 70–83] is 68%, and left ventricular mass[66, 70, 71, 79, 80, 82, 83] is 90 gm/m².

†Number of patients studied, vol: for assessing left ventricular volume, mass: for assessing left ventricular mass; SD and SEM after name of investigator indicates whether standard deviation or standard error of the mean respectively, are tabulated.

Table 8-5. Normalized Right Ventricular End-diastolic (EDVI) and End-systolic (ESVI) Volumes and Ejection Fraction (EF)*

Investigator	Method	Age	n	EDVI (mL/m²)	ESVI (mL/m²)	EF
Unterberg et al[86]	RAO-LAO Simpson's rule	Adults	14	97 ± 19	41 ± 13	58 ± 8
Reddington et al[59]	RAO-LAO Simpson's rule	Adults	10	64 ± 13	—	62 ± 6
Gentzler et al[49]	RAO-LAO Simpson's rule	Adults	9	81 ± 13	39 ± 9	51 ± 8
Boak et al[48]	RAO-LAO Simpson's rule	Adults	8	72 ± 7	—	58 ± 3
Karsch et al[87]	RAO-LAO Simpson's rule	Adults	7	83 ± 6	36 ± 30	56 ± 3
Pietras et al[78]	RAO-LAO Simpson's rule	Adults	17	76 ± 14	33 ± 8	57 ± 4
Ferlinz et al[47]	RAO-LAO Pyramid method	Adults	6	76 ± 11	26 ± 6	66 ± 6
Ferlinz[88]	Pyramid method	Adults	10	74 ± 16	26 ± 6	—
Ferlinz[88]	Area/length method: pyramid method	Adults	10	69 ± 13	22 ± 5	68 ± 6
Thilenius et al[56]	Area/length: parallelepiped biplane	Infants <13 mo	7	64 ± 6	31 ± 5	52 ± 4
Thilenius et al[56]	Area/length: parallelepiped biplane	Children >13 mo	9	78 ± 16	30 ± 6	61 ± 4
Graham et al[50]	AP-LAT area/length & two chamber	Children > 1 yr	9	70 ± 13	25 ± 8	64 ± 9
Fisher et al[11]	AP-LAT prism method	Children >1 yr to adults 21 yr	70	64 ± 15	25 ± 7	61 ± 7
Fisher et al[11]	AP-LAT Simpson's rule	Children >1 yr to adults 21 yr	70	64 ± 15	25 ± 8	61 ± 8
Fisher et al[11]	AP-LAT Simpson's rule	Infants <1 yr	7	60 ± 15	—	—
Nakazawa et al[55]	AP-LAT Simpson's rule	Infants 1 d to children 16 yr	42	—	—	61 ± 1
Graham et al[50]	AP-LAT Simpson's rule	Infants <1 yr	7	39 ± 8	13	66 ± 7
Lange et al[58]	AP-LAT	Infants 1 mo to children 16 yr	100	—	—	63 ± 7
Carlsson et al[89]	AP-LAT	Children	4	69 ± 11	26 ± 5	62 ± 5

Note: Based on the normal values from all adults, average right ventricular EDVI[47–49, 59, 78, 86–88] is 80.1 mL/m², right ventricular ESVI[47, 49, 78, 86–88] is 26.1 mL/m², and right ventricular EF[47–49, 59, 78, 86–88] is 59%.

n, number of normal subjects included; mean values (±SD) are tabulated.

[58, 78, 89] Graham and associates[23, 50] did not observe this difference, possibly because of nonsimultaneous volume measurements in a given subject. Because the stroke volume for the left and right ventricles is the same, the right ventricular ejection fraction is lower than the left. Based on all unmatched nonsimultaneous published data available on normal subjects (see Tables 8–4 and 8–5),[18, 47 49, 59, 66, 70 83, 86 88] it is noted that the average left ventricular and right ventricular end-diastolic volumes are 75 and 80.1 mL/m², respectively, and the left ventricular and right ventricular ejection fractions are 68% versus 59%. The left and right ventricular stroke volumes are 51 and 54 mL/m², respectively. When the right ventricular volume is assumed to be 54 mL/m² (to match that for the left ventricular maintaining the end-diastolic volume), the right ventricular ejection fraction (64%) is still lower than that of the left ventricle. These data are in agreement with what is known (that the normalized left ventricular end-diastolic volume index is smaller than the right ventricular volume index and that the left ventricular ejection fraction is larger than the right) but remains undocumented conclusively.

REFERENCES

1. Greene DG, Carlisle R, Grant C, Bunnell IL: Estimation of left ventricular volume by one-plane cineangiography. Circulation 1967; 35:61–69.
2. Kasser IS, Kennedy JW: Measurement of left ventricular volumes in man by single-plane cineangiography. Invest Radiol 1969; 4:83–90.
3. Dodge HT, Sandler H, Ballew DW, Lord JD Jr: The use of biplane angiocardiography for the measurement of left ventricular volume in man. Am Heart J 1960; 60:762–776.
4. Rogers WJ, Smith R, Hood WP Jr, et al: Effect of filming projection and interobserver variability on angiographic biplane left ventricular volume determination. Circulation 1979; 59:96–104.
5. Baron MG: Angiographic determination of ejection fraction in coronary artery disease. Am J Cardiol 1973; 31:803–804.
6. Stern L, Firth BG, Dehmer GJ, et al: Effect of selective coronary angiography on left ventricular volumes and ejection fraction in man. Am J Cardiol 1980; 46;827–831.
7. Rahimtoola SH, Duffy JP, Swan HJC: Ventricular performance after angiocardiography. Circulation 1967; 35:70–78.
8. Gault JH: Angiographic estimation of left ventricular volume. Cathet Cardiovasc Diagn 1975; 1:7–16.
9. Chappuis FP, Widmann TF, Nicod P, Peterson KL: Densitometric regional ejection fraction—a new three-dimensional index of regional left ventricular function: Comparison with geometric methods. J Am Coll Cardiol 1988; 11:72–82.
10. Arcilla RA, Tsai P, Thilenius OG, Ranniger K: Angiographic method for volume estimation of right and left ventricles. Chest 1971; 60:446–454.
11. Fisher EA, DuBrow IW, Hastreiter AR: Right ventricular volume in congenital heart disease. Am J Cardiol 1975; 36:67–75.
12. Chapman CB, Baker O, Reynolds J, Bonte FJ: Use of biplane cinefluorography for the measurement of left ventricular volume. Circulation 1958; 18:1105–1117.
13. Carleton RA: Changes in left ventricular volumes during angiocardiography. Am J Cardiol 1971; 27:460–463.
14. Vine DL, Hegg TD, Dodge HT, et al: Immediate effect of contrast medium injection on left ventricular volumes and ejection fraction: A study using radio-opaque epicardial markers. Circulation 1977; 56:379–384.
15. Rackley CE: Quantitative evaluation of left ventricular function by radiographic techniques. Circulation 1976; 54:862–879.
16. Rogers WJ, Smith LR, Bream PR, et al: Quantitative axial oblique contrast left ventriculography: Validation of the method by demonstrating improved visualization of regional wall motion and mitral valve function with accurate volume determinations. Am Heart J 1982; 103:185–194.
17. Bhargava V, Shabetai R: Non-uniformity of the LV ellipsoid: Implications for area-length volume calculations. IEEE Comput Cardiol 1979, pp 351–354.
18. Wynne J, Green LH, Mann T, et al: Estimation of left ventricular volumes in man from cineangiograms filmed in oblique projections. Am J Cardiol 1978; 41:726–732.
19. Bursch JH, Ritman EL, Sturm RE, Wood EH: Videodensitometric determination of left ventricular ejection fraction and filling characteristics. Ann Biomed Eng 1975; 3:62–71.
20. Sandler H, Dodge HT: The use of single-plane angiocardiograms for the calculation of left ventricular volume in man. Am Heart J 1968; 75:325–334.
21. Kennedy JW, Trenholme SE, Kasser IS: Left ventricular volume and mass from single plane cineangiocardiogram: A comparison of anteroposterior and right oblique methods. Am Heart J 1970; 80:343–352.
22. Sandler H, Dodge HT, Hay RE, Rackley CE: Quantitation of valvular insufficiency in man by angiocardiography. Am Heart J 1963; 65:501–513.
23. Graham TP Jr, Jarmakani JM, Canent RV Jr, Morrow MN: Left heart volume estimation in infancy and childhood: Reevaluation of methodology and normal values. Circulation 1971; 43:895–904.
24. Fisher EA, Eckner FAO, DuBrow IW, Hastreiter AR: Correlation of angiographic and autopsy left ventricular dimensions in children. Circulation 1978; 58:739–746.
25. Cascade PN, Wajszczuk WJ, Kerin NZ, et al: Determination and importance of the magnification factor in the calculation of left ventricular volume: Development of a simple, accurate method. Cathet Cardiovasc Diagn 1978; 4:391–398.
26. Sandler H, Hawley RR, Dodge HT, Baxley WA: Calculation of left ventricular volume from single-plane (AP) angiocardiogram. J Clin Invest 1965; 44:1094–1095.
27. Rackley CE, Dodge HT, Coble YD, Hay RE: A method for determining left ventricular mass in man. Circulation 1964; 29:666–671.
28. Dodge HT, Sandler H, Baxley WA, Hawley RR: Usefulness and limitations of radiographic methods for determining left ventricular volume. Am J Cardiol 1966; 18:10–29.
29. Goerke RJ, Carlsson E: Calculation of right and left cardiac ventricular volumes: Method using standard computer equipment and biplane angiocardiograms. Invest Radiol 1967; 2:360–367.
30. Formanek A, Schey HM, Ekstrand KE, et al: Single versus biplane right and left ventricular volumetry: Cast

and clinical study. Cathet Cardiovasc Diagn 1984;
10:137–156.

31. Ino T, Benson LN, Mikalian H, et al: Correlation of left
ventricular angiographic casts and biplane left ventricular volumetry in infants and children. Am J Cardiol
1988; 61:441–445.

32. Bonard P, Tremblay G, LeBlanc AR, et al: A new
method for precise and complete correction of distortion on cincangiographic image: Its effect on left ventricular measurements. Cathet Cardiovasc Diagn 1978;
4:111–126.

33. Marier DL, Gibson DG: Limitations of two-frame
method for displaying regional left ventricular wall motion in man. Br Heart J 1980; 44:555–559.

34. Detrano R, MacIntyre WJ, Salcedo EE, et al: Videodensitometric ejection fraction from intravenous digital subtraction left ventriculograms: Correlation with conventional
direct contrast and radionuclide ventriculography. Radiology 1985; 155:19–23.

35. Nissen SE, Elion JL, Grayburn P, et al: Determination
of left ventricular ejection fraction by computer densitometric analysis of digital subtraction angiography: Experimental validation and correlation with area-length
methods. Am J Cardiol 1987; 59:675–680.

36. Tobis J, Nalcioglu O, Siebert A, et al: Measurement of
left ventricular ejection fraction by videodensitometric
analysis of digital subtraction angiograms. Am J Cardiol
1983; 52:871–875.

37. Chappuis F, Widmann T, Guth B, et al: Quantitative
assessment of regional left ventricular ejection fraction
by densitometric analysis of intravenous digital subtraction ventriculograms: Correlation with myocardial systolic shortening in dogs. Circulation 1988; 77:457–477.

38. Nissen SE, Friedman BJ, Waters J, et al: Right ventricular ejection fraction by videodensitometry of intravenous digital subtraction angiograms: Experimental validation and initial clinical trials. J Am Coll Cardiol
1984; 3:589.

39. Trenholm BG, Winter DA, Mymir D, Lansdown EL:
Computer determination of left ventricular volume using videodensitometry. Med Biol Engineering 1972;
10:163–173.

40. Bursch JH, Heintzen PH, Simon R: Videodensitometric
studies by a new method of quantitating the amount of
contrast medium. Eur J Cardiol 1974; 1:437–466.

41. Shaw CG, Ergun DL, Myerowitz PD, et al: A technique
of scatter and glare correction of videodensitometric
studies in digital subtraction videoangiography. Radiology 1982; 142:209–213.

42. Krayenbuehl HP, Ritter M, Hess OM, Hirzel H: The
use of invasive techniques, angiography, and indicator
dilution for quantification of valvular regurgitations.
Eur Heart J 1987; 8(Suppl C):1–9.

43. Rackley CE, Dodge HT, Coble YD, Hay RE: A method
for determining left ventricular mass in man. Circulation 1964; 29:666–671.

44. Kennedy JW, Reichenbach DD, Baxley WA, Dodge HT:
Left ventricular mass: A comparison of angiographic
measurements with autopsy weight. Am J Cardiol 1967;
19:221–223.

45. Milnor WR, Jose AD: Distortion of indicator-dilution
curves by sampling system. J Appl Physiol 1960; 15:
177–180.

46. Ferlinz J: Right ventricular function in adult cardiovascular disease. Prog Cardiovasc Dis 1982; 25:225–267.

47. Ferlinz J, Gorlin R, Cohn PF, Herman MV: Right ventricular performance in patients with coronary artery
disease. Circulation 1975; 52:608–615.

48. Boak JG, Bove AA, Kreulen T, Spann JF: A geometric
basis for calculation of right ventricular volume in man.
Cathet Cardiovasc Diagn 1977; 3:217–230.

49. Gentzler RD II, Briselli MF, Gault JH: Angiographic
estimation of right ventricular volume in man. Circulation 1974; 50:324–330.

50. Graham TP, Jarmarkani MM, Atwood GF, Canent RV
Jr: Right ventricular volume determinations in children:
Normal values and observations with volume or pres-
sure overload. Circulation 1973; 47:144–153.

51. Horn V, Mullins CB, Saffer SI, et al: A comparison of
mathematical models for estimating right ventricular
volumes in animals and man. Clin Cardiol 1979; 2:
341–347.

52. Graham TP, Atwood GF, Boucek RJ Jr, et al: Right
ventricular volume characteristics in ventricular septal
defect. Circulation 1976; 54:800–804.

53. Graham TP, Cordell D, Atwood GF, et al: Right ventricular volume characteristics before and after palliative
reparative operation in tetralogy of Fallot. Circulation
1976; 54:417–423.

54. Nakazawa M, Jarmakani JM, Gyepes MT, et al: Pre and
postoperative ventricular function in infants and children with right ventricular volume overload. Circulation
1977; 55:479–484.

55. Nakazawa M, Marks RA, Isabel-Jones J, Jarmakani JM:
Right and left ventricular volume characteristics in children with pulmonary stenosis and intact ventricular
septum. Circulation 1976; 53:884–890.

56. Thilenius OG, Arcilla RA: Angiographic right and left
ventricular volume determination in normal infants and
children. Pediatr Res 1974; 8:67–74.

57. Slutsky RA, Bhargava V, Dittrich H, Costello D: Comparison of single plane and biplane contrast analyses of
right ventricular function and size. Am Heart J 1982;
104:100–104.

58. Lange PE, Omnasch D, Farr FL, Heintzen PH: Angiocardiographic right ventricular volume determination:
Accuracy as determined from human casts and clinical
application. Eur J Cardiol 1978; 8:477–501.

59. Reddington AN, Gray HH, Hodson ME, et al: Characterization of the normal right ventricular pressure-volume relation by biplane angiography and simultaneous
micromanometer pressure measurements. Br Heart J
1988; 59:23–30.

60. Lange PE, Omnasch D, Farr FL, et al: Analysis of left
and right ventricular size and shape, as determined
from human casts: Description of the methods and its
validation. Eur J Cardiol 1978; 8:431–448.

61. Shimazaki Y, Kawashima Y, Mori T, et al: Angiographic
volume estimation of right ventricle: Re-evaluation of
the previous methods. Chest 1980; 77:390–395.

62. Slutsky R, Bhargava V, Dittrich H, Costello D: Comparison of single-plane and biplane contrast analyses of
right ventricular function and size. Am Heart J 1982;
104:100–104.

63. Dubel HP, Romaniuk P, Tschapek A: Investigation of
human right ventricular cast specimens. Cardiovasc Intervent Radiol 1982; 5:296–303.

64. Pietras RJ, Kondos GT, Kaplan D: Quantitative validation of cineangiographic biplane axial oblique right
ventricular volume measurement. Am Heart J 1987;
113:321–325.

65. Ino T, Benson LN, Mikalian H, et al: Correlation of
right ventricular volume using axial angulated ventriculography to known right ventricular cast volumes in
infants and children with congenital heart disease. Am
J Cardiol 1988; 61:161–165.

66. Hood WP Jr, Rackley CE, Rolett EL: Wall stress in the
normal and hypertrophied human left ventricle. Am J
Cardiol 1968; 22:550–558.

67. Rigaud M, Hardy A, Castadot M, et al: Variability and
reproducibility of quantitative left ventricular angiography. Cathet Cardiovasc Diagn 1989; 18:8–15.

68. Mullins CB, Jones DC: A computerized approach to a new model for measurement of right ventricular volume. Clin Res 1969; 17:18.

69. Mullins CB, Jones DC, Freeborn WA: Comparison of models for measurement of right ventricular volume. Clin Res 1970; 18:321.

70. Kennedy JW, Baxley WA, Figley MM, et al: Quantitative angiocardiography. Part I: The normal left ventricle in man. Circulation 1966; 34:272–278.

71. Kennedy JW, Doces JG, Stewart DK: Left ventricular function before and following surgical treatment of mitral valve disease. Am Heart J 1979; 97:592–598.

72. Herman HJ, Bartle SH: Left ventricular volumes by angiocardiography: Comparison of methods and simplification of techniques. Cardiovasc Res 1968; 2:404–414.

73. Arvidsson H: Angiographic determination of left ventricular volume. Acta Radiol 1961; 56:321–339.

74. Dodge HT, Hay RE, Sandler H: An angiographic method for directly determining left ventricular stroke volume in man. Circ Res 1962; 11:739–745.

75. Peterson KL, Skloven D, Ludbrook P, et al: Comparison of isovolumic and ejection phase indices of myocardial performance in man. Circulation 1974; 49:1088–1101.

76. Toma Y, Matsuda Y, Moritani K, et al: Left atrial filling in normal human subjects: Relation between left atrial contraction and left atrial early filling. Cardiovasc Res 1987; 21:255–259.

77. Sanmarco ME, Bartle SH: Left ventricular volume determination: Comparison of angiographic and thermal washout techniques. Circulation 1964; 29(Suppl 3): 151–152.

78. Pietras RJ, Kondos GT, Kaplan D, Lam W: Comparative angiographic right and left ventricular volumes. Am Heart J 1985; 109:321–326.

79. Thuring VC, Hess OM, Marakami T, et al: Normalwerte der linksventrikularen funktion: Biplane angiographic, unter berucksichtigung geschlechtsspezifischer unterschiede. Fortschr Rontgenstr 1989; 150:562–568.

80. Rousseau MF, Pouleur H, Charlier AA, Brasseur LA: Assessment of left ventricular relaxation in patients with valvular regurgitation. Am J Cardiol 1982; 50: 1028–1036.

81. Falsetti HL, Mates RE, Greene DG, Bunnel IL: V_{MAX} as an index of contractile state in man. Circulation 1971; 43:467–479.

82. Huber D, Grimm J, Koch R, Krayenbuehl HP: Determinants of ejection performance in aortic stenosis. Circulation 1981; 64:126–134.

83. Schwarz F, Flameng W, Langebartels F, et al: Impaired left ventricular function in chronic aortic valve disease: Survival and function after replacement by Björk-Shiley prosthesis. Circulation 1976; 60:48–58.

84. Miller GAH, Swan HJC: Effect of chronic pressure and volume overload on left heart volumes in subjects with congenital heart disease. Circulation 1964; 30:205–216.

85. Sano T, Ogawa M, Taniguchi K, et al: Angiographic assessment of left ventricular volume, afterload, and contractile state in normal children. Am J Cardiol 1990; 65:1021–1025.

86. Unterberg R, Plesak L, Voelker W, Karsck KR: Quantitative segmentale wandfunktionsanalyse der rechten kammer bei herzgesunden. Z Kardiol 1988; 77:120–124.

87. Karsch KR, Scheufler S, Blanke H, Rentrop KP: The right ventricle at rest and during exercise. Part I: Pump function of the normal right ventricle. Z Kardiol 1979; 68:485–490.

88. Ferlinz J: Measurement of right ventricular volumes in man from single-plane cineangiograms: A comparison to the biplane approach. Am Heart J 1977; 94:87–90.

89. Carlsson E, Keene RJ, Lee P, Goerke RJ: Angiographic stroke volume correlation of the two cardiac ventricles in man. Invest Radiol 1971; 6:44–51.

Chapter 9

Coronary Angiography
Methods, Quantitation, and Comparison with Other Imaging Modalities

RICHARD W. SMALLING

Cardiac catheterization and coronary angiography remain the comparative standard for the diagnosis and assessment of coronary artery disease and its severity. In a recent report of the Registry of the Society for Cardiac Angiography and Interventions (SCA&I)[1] of almost 80,000 patients who underwent cardiac catheterization and were entered into the registry, 83% of the procedures were performed primarily to evaluate coronary artery disease. Of these, most were males (64%), and most were older than 60 years of age (59%). Twenty percent of these procedures were performed on an outpatient basis, and only 2.4% were performed on an emergency basis. In this cohort of patients, coronary arteriography demonstrated significant coronary disease in 74% of patients, with 7% having significant left main coronary artery disease. Because routine stress testing has a sensitivity of only 60% and a false-positive rate as high as 40%, some have advocated that coronary angiography is the most appropriate first step in the evaluation of a middle-aged man with chest pain.[2]

HISTORICAL PERSPECTIVES

Coronary arteriography began as an accident, in the hands of Dr. Mason Sones, on October 30, 1958. During an injection of 40 mL of 90% of diatrizoate (Hypaque-M, 90%) into the sinus of Valsalva, the catheter inadvertently advanced into the right coronary artery, where approximately 30 mL of contrast agent entered that vessel selectively.[3] After an initial period of asystole, the patient was instructed to cough; he developed sinus bradycardia and then recovered. Dr. Sones then developed a special cathe-

ter, fabricated by United States Catheter, Inc., which consisted of a 2.7-mm shaft (8-French), with a tip tapering within 5 cm of the end to 1.6 mm (5-French). The tip of the catheter was open, and there were four side-holes within 7 mm of the distal end (Fig. 9–1). With this device, he was able to enter both coronary arteries in 954 of the initial 1020 patients who were studied with the primary intention of performing coronary arteriography. Subsequently, Dr. Melvin Judkins, a radiologist, developed percutaneous coronary catheters after studying percutaneous angiographic techniques in Sweden under Olsson and Boijsen. In 1967, Dr. Judkins developed the Judkins right and left coronary

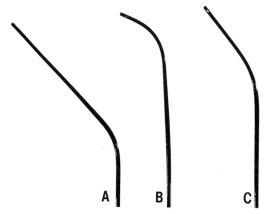

Figure 9–1. Sones coronary angiography catheters. These catheters feature a taper from 7- to 8-French to 5-French at the tip, and they have side-holes in addition to an end-hole, as illustrated. **A,** Long-tip Sones catheter for angiography in patients with dilated ascending aortas. **B,** Positrol Sones catheter for patients with narrow ascending aortas (may also be used with coronary bypass grafts and right coronary angiography). **C,** Standard-curve Sones catheter used for most patients.

159

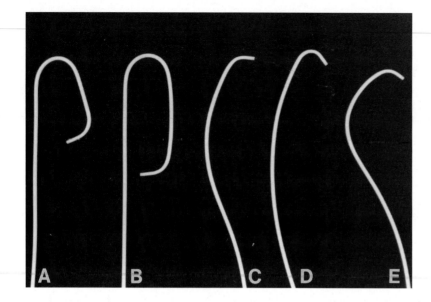

Figure 9–2. Judkins catheters. **A,** Judkins left, 4 cm catheter: the side-arm is 4 cm long from the primary to the secondary curve, allowing for cannulation of most left coronary arteries. **B,** Judkins left, 6 cm catheter: this catheter is designed for cannulating left coronary arteries in patients with dilated ascending aortas. The side-arm is 6 cm long. **C,** Standard Judkins right catheter (also available in various curves for dilated aortas). **D,** Internal mammary catheter. **E,** Left coronary bypass catheter.

catheters, which are now used in most coronary diagnostic procedures. The original Judkins catheters were also 8-French catheters reinforced with wire braid and tapered to 5-French at the tip (Fig. 9–2). The curves were more complicated than the Sones catheter and came in various sizes designed to accommodate different-sized aortic arches.[4]

CLINICAL INDICATIONS

The American College of Cardiology, with the American Heart Association Task Force on the Assessment of Diagnostic and Therapeutic Cardiovascular Procedures Subcommittee on Coronary Angiography, has published guidelines for performance of coronary angiography.[5] Three classifications are described as follows:

Class 1—represents conditions for which there is general agreement that coronary angiography is justified

Class 2—represents conditions for which coronary angiography is frequently performed, but there is a divergence of opinion with respect to its justification in terms of value and appropriateness

Class 3—represents conditions for which there is general agreement that coronary angiography is not justified

ASYMPTOMATIC PATIENTS. Candidates for coronary angiography, adhering to class 1 criteria, are those with evidence of high risk on noninvasive testing including ST depression at heart rates less than 120 beats/min, abnormal blood pressure response to exercise, or exercise induced ventricular tachycardia. Additional patients considered class 1 are those with abnormal thallium scans, fall in radionuclide ejection fraction during exercise, development of wall motion abnormalities during exercise, or at risk whose occupation involves the safety of others, such as airline pilots, bus drivers, and air traffic controllers. Class 3 patients represent those who have not had appropriate noninvasive testing, who are asymptomatic after bypass surgery or angioplasty, and are without evidence of ischemia.

SYMPTOMATIC PATIENTS. Class 1 patients have angina pectoris that has been inadequately responsive to medical treatment, angioplasty, thrombolytic therapy, or coronary artery bypass surgery. Also included are those with unstable angina pectoris, or those with angina pectoris who have high risk on noninvasive testing.

PATIENTS WITH ATYPICAL CHEST PAIN OF UNCERTAIN ORIGIN. Class 1 patients include those with electrocardiographic or radionuclide stress tests that indicate a high risk of coronary disease, when coronary artery spasm is suspected, or when there are associated symptoms or signs of abnormal left ventricular function or failure. Class 3 patients include those without objective signs of ischemia, who have had an earlier, technically satisfactory, normal coronary angiogram for the same chest pain.

ACUTE MYOCARDIAL INFARCTION. Patients presenting with evolving myocardial infarction undergo coronary angiography if they are considered candidates for emergency percutaneous transluminal coronary angioplasty. Typically, these are patients presenting with large anterior myocardial infarction within 6 hours after onset of chest pain or those with anterior or inferior myocardial infarction who have contraindications to thrombolytic therapy.

Patients who have completed their myocardial infarction, as long as 8 weeks after the infarction, could be considered class 1 candidates in the presence of (1) angina pectoris occurring at rest or with minimal activity, (2) evidence of myocardial ischemia on laboratory testing, (3) development of heart failure during the evolving phase with a left ventricular ejection fraction less than 45%, and (4) a non–Q wave myocardial infarction. Class 3 patients include the (1) presence of advanced physiologic age and (2) coexisting disease judged to be primarily responsible for the patient's prognosis (such as terminal cancer).

CONTRAINDICATIONS

Contraindications to coronary angiography must be considered relative, particularly in emergency situations. Recent evidence has suggested that emergency coronary arteriography and angioplasty in the setting of acute myocardial infarction may be as efficacious as, or perhaps superior to, thrombolytic therapy[6] (see Chapter 27). The Joint Task Force has suggested the following relative contraindications: (1) recent stroke (within 1 month); (2) progressive renal insufficiency; (3) active gastrointestinal bleeding; (4) fever that may be due to infection; (5) active infection; (6) short life expectancy due to other illnesses such as cancer and severe pulmonary, hepatic, or renal disease; (7) severe anemia; (8) severe uncontrolled systemic hypertension; (9) severe electrolyte imbalance; (10) severe systemic or psychological illness in which prognosis is doubtful or behavior is unpredictable, producing undue risk of cardiac catheterization; (11) very advanced physiologic age; and (12) patient refusal to consider definitive treatment such as angioplasty, bypass surgery, and valve replacement. Many of these conditions may be temporary or reversible, allowing relatively safe catheterization when the condition is corrected.

APPROPRIATE INDICATIONS FOR OUTPATIENT CORONARY ANGIOGRAPHY

The Ad Hoc Committee on Outpatient Catheterization for the SCA&I recently published guidelines for the selection of patients appropriate for outpatient catheterization and angiographic procedures,[7] as described in the following:

PATIENTS APPROPRIATE FOR OUTPATIENT CATHETERIZATION

1. Patients with stable angina pectoris
2. Asymptomatic patients following an uncomplicated myocardial infarction
3. Clinically stable patients with suspicion of coronary artery disease

PATIENTS NOT SUITABLE CANDIDATES FOR OUTPATIENT CATHETERIZATION

1. Patients with unstable, accelerated, crescendo, or preinfarction angina pectoris
2. Patients with ventricular ectopy requiring antiarrhythmic prophylaxis
3. Patients with uncompensated congestive heart failure or hypokalemia requiring treatment
4. Patients with severe aortic stenosis
5. Patients with suspicion of left main coronary artery disease
6. Patients with known bleeding disorders
7. Metabolically unstable patients who need care and observation for intercurrent disease
8. Patients with other serious medical conditions that would impact their postprocedural care
9. Patients who are emotionally labile

TECHNICAL PERFORMANCE OF CORONARY ANGIOGRAPHY

Percutaneous or Retrograde Femoral Approach

The Judkins approach is the most commonly used method for diagnostic coronary angiography. In my laboratory, both inguinal regions are prepped with antiseptic solution and draped, in the event that access is unsuccessful in one side or if further interventions are indicated (such as intra-aortic balloon placement). The femoral region is then anesthetized with 1% lidocaine, both superficially and deep, posterior to the femoral vein in an attempt to anesthetize the periosteum. The femoral artery is then punctured, using an 18-gauge thin-walled needle. On brisk return of arterial blood, a 0.035-inch tapered, movable core J-wire is then inserted through the 18-gauge needle and advanced into the iliofemoral vessels. Free wire motion is critical at this juncture. If the wire does not move freely up the iliofemoral vessels, then maneuvers need to be undertaken to determine the cause of the problem. Assuming free wire passage, a 6-French arterial introducer sheath is then placed over the wire. The wire and dilator are removed and the sheath is flushed with heparinized saline. Some centers do not routinely heparinize patients for diagnostic arteriography; however, my colleagues and I have chosen to reduce the heparin dosage from 5000 to 3000 U and not to employ protamine reversal. Other centers administer 5000 U of heparin with or without protamine reversal after termination of the procedure. Next, a 100-cm-long, 6-French Judkins left coronary catheter is preloaded with a 0.035-inch tapered, movable core J-wire and advanced through the sheath to the aortic arch and left in position above the sinus of Valsalva. The wire is then removed, and the catheter is aspirated, checking to make sure that the aspirate does not contain a plaque or thrombus. If a plaque or thrombus is encountered, then the catheter is aspirated until clear and is gently flushed. The Judkins catheter is then advanced, as in Figure 9–3, into the left main ostium while pressure is being continuously monitored through the lumen via a three-way manifold attached to the catheter. Before entering the left coronary ostium, the catheter is filled with contrast agent using an angiographic syringe attached to the three-way manifold. The purpose of the three-way manifold is to provide a pressure-monitoring port and supplies of contrast medium and heparinized saline flush. If the catheter fails to engage the left coronary ostium, gentle clockwise torquing accompanied by subtle advancement and retraction of the catheter usually causes it to engage appropriately. Patients with small aortic arches may be difficult to engage with a standard Judkins left, 4 cm catheter. In this instance, the catheter continually advances into the sinus of Valsalva and does not retract into the coronary ostium. This situation can be remedied by switching to a shorter-armed Judkins left coro-

nary catheter, such as a left, 3.5 cm version. Alternatively, in patients with large dilated ascending aortas, a larger Judkins catheter is necessary (typically, an FL5, or occasionally an FL6) for extremely dilated aortas (see Fig. 9–2). The left anterior oblique (LAO) projection is usually used to engage the left coronary ostium (60-degree LAO). In patients with difficult coronary ostia, visualization in the orthogonal projection (30-degree right anterior oblique [RAO]) is helpful. If the patients have short left main vessels, clockwise torquing is effective to direct the catheter toward the left anterior descending (LAD), with the catheter outside the left main ostium. Once the left main is engaged with the tip of the catheter, however, counterclockwise torquing is necessary to direct the catheter tip toward the LAD vessel. The opposite maneuvers are effective for engaging the circumflex vessel.

The Judkins right coronary catheter is advanced in similar fashion to the Judkins left coronary catheter to the level superior to the sinus of Valsalva. With clockwise rotation, the Judkins right coronary catheter tends to advance and rotate anteriorly (Fig. 9–4). Therefore, to successfully engage the right coronary ostium, it is necessary to position the Judkins right coronary catheter approximately 2 cm superior to the right coronary ostium before application of clockwise torque. Once the right coronary catheter descends and engages the ostium, slight counterclockwise torque (particularly when using 6-French catheters) tends to stabilize the catheter position for arteriograms. The right coronary artery is most easily engaged using the 45-degree LAO view. Pressure should be monitored carefully when engaging both coronary arteries, but the right coronary artery is particularly prone to wedging. In other words, the catheter may inadvertently advance into the conus branch or, occasionally, more distally into the right coronary artery, effectively occluding coronary blood flow. This results in very low pressure (coronary wedge pressure) being re-

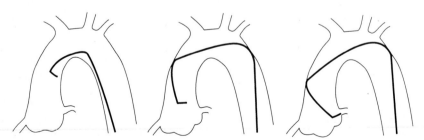

Figure 9–3. Judkins left technique for cannulation of the left main coronary artery. The catheter is advanced in profile in the LAO projection. As the catheter rounds the ascending aorta, it tends to engage the left main coronary artery, as illustrated.

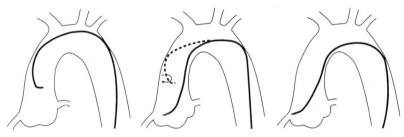

Figure 9–4. Cannulation of the right coronary artery with the Judkins right catheter. The Judkins right catheter is placed in profile in the LAO projection and advanced to the aortic cusp. It is then retracted approximately 2 to 3 cm above the coronary ostium, and clockwise torque is applied. The catheter will then advance on its own and rotate laterally to engage the right coronary artery orifice.

corded from the catheter. Gentle counterclockwise torque generally "dewedges" the catheter, allowing safe arteriography.

In most patients, Judkins-type catheters allow rapid cannulation of the coronary ostia, with minimal manipulation. One of the drawbacks, however, is the requisite catheter exchange.

Amplatz Technique

Another retrograde femoral technique was perfected by Amplatz and colleagues.[8] The Amplatz curve is similar to that achieved by the Sones catheter, which has been advanced and looped in the coronary sinus (Fig. 9–5). The catheter is advanced retrograde around the arch, as with the Judkins technique. The tip of the catheter is then positioned medial in the LAO projection facing the general direction of the left coronary ostium. The catheter is advanced with fluoroscopic and pressure monitoring. The tip then rises up the left sinus of Valsalva. As the tip

engages the coronary ostium, the catheter is withdrawn, further elevating the tip parallel to the left main coronary artery (Fig. 9–6). To engage the right coronary artery, clockwise torque is applied to the catheter while it is gently withdrawn. Once the catheter is disengaged, it is rotated laterally (clockwise) toward the right coronary ostium. It is then once again advanced until the right coronary ostium is engaged. Occasionally, it is necessary to use an Amplatz catheter with a smaller arm to engage the right coronary artery. The short tip, or modified right coronary Amplatz catheter (see Fig. 9–5), is useful for right coronary arteries with superior takeoffs, as well as for engaging coronary artery bypass grafts.

Single-catheter Femoral Technique

Schoonmaker and King[9] developed a multipurpose catheter, similar in shape to a Sones catheter, with more length (see Fig. 9–5), designed for single-catheter coronary angiography. The

Figure 9–5. Amplatz and multipurpose catheters. **A,** Left Amplatz II is a standard catheter for cannulating the left coronary artery in most patients. **B,** Left Amplatz III catheter has an enlarged loop for cannulation of the left coronary artery in patients with dilated ascending aortas. **C,** Modified right Amplatz catheter for cannulation of right coronary arteries, as well as coronary artery bypass grafts. **D,** Multipurpose catheter with a tapered tip, end-hole, and sideholes, similar to the Sones catheters.

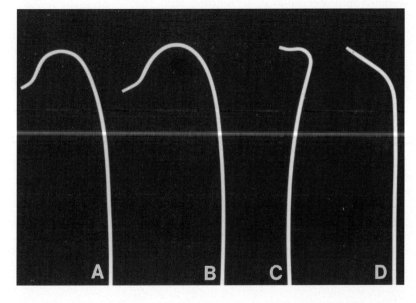

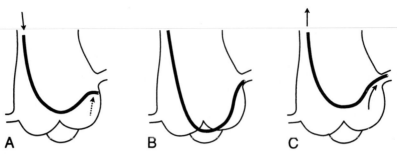

Figure 9–6. Technique of cannulation of the left coronary artery using the left Amplatz catheter. The catheter is placed in profile in the LAO projection. It is advanced into the left coronary cusp elevating the tip *(A* and *B)* and retracted, which then advances the tip into the left main coronary artery *(C)*. Gentle clockwise and counterclockwise rotation may be necessary, similar to the Sones technique.

catheter is advanced in a manner similar to the Judkins technique, around the aortic arch. Once the tip is in the region of the sinus of Valsalva, it is torqued so that its tip lies medial in the LAO projection and is advanced, forming a loop. The loop is then gradually advanced and withdrawn repetitively, with gentle torque being applied, to seek out the left coronary ostium, using a technique similar to Sones catheterization. After arteriography of the left system is achieved, clockwise torque with gradual withdrawal causes the catheter to rotate toward the right coronary ostium, allowing for visualization of that vessel. Some angiographers use this catheter for ventriculography as well, but it is an extremely arrhythmogenic catheter, allowing for rapid efflux of contrast agent out the end-hole, which often results in ventricular tachycardia during left ventriculography.

Retrograde Brachial (Sones) Technique

Sones, whose original technique for coronary angiography necessitated a cutdown onto the brachial artery and vein, accomplished this aseptically using local anesthesia. The brachial artery is dissected from the adjacent structures using blunt dissection. A small transverse arteriotomy is performed while the vessel is controlled using Silastic ligatures (Liga-Loops). In our laboratory, my colleagues and I routinely instill 1000 U of heparin into the distal brachial vessel and systemically heparinize using an additional 4000 to 5000 U before passage of the catheter. The Sones catheter has a tapered tip, starting out as 7- to 8-French and tapering to 5-French. It has one end-hole and four proximal side-holes, as previously described (see Fig. 9–1). The catheter is advanced through the brachiocephalic vessels using pressure and fluoroscopic control. Occasionally, difficulties are encountered in advancing the catheter owing to the tortuosity of the brachiocephalic vessels. A number of geo-

metric manipulations of the shoulder and neck have been devised to obviate these problems. However, the most straightforward approach is to simply use a 0.035-inch tapered core J-wire, which should negotiate even the most tortuous vessels. The initial passage of the catheter should be performed in the anteroposterior (AP) projection. However, as the catheter reaches the ascending aorta, the patient should be positioned in the LAO projection for cannulation of the coronary vessels. There are several modifications of the Sones catheter to allow for cannulation of patients with narrow or wide aortas (see Fig. 9–1). In general, the catheter tip is advanced in the medial direction toward the left coronary ostium. This tip usually impacts the aortic valve cusp, and with continued advancement of the catheter, prolapses upward, forming a loop. The loop is then withdrawn and torqued simultaneously clockwise and counterclockwise as necessary to engage the coronary ostium. Once the coronary ostium is engaged, the catheter is gently withdrawn, which further advances it into the left main coronary artery (Fig. 9–7). After coronary angiography of the left system is achieved, clockwise torque on the catheter with a gentle withdrawal motion allows it to orient itself toward the right coronary ostium (Fig. 9–8). Similar maneuvers can then be used to engage the right coronary ostium for filming of the right coronary artery. The Sones catheter can also be used for ventriculography, but again it is an end-hole catheter and is prone to be highly arrhythmogenic. Once coronary angiography and ventriculography have been performed, the catheter is withdrawn, and the arteriotomy site is then allowed to backbleed slightly to eliminate any possible thrombus.

The arteriotomy may be closed in several ways. I prefer a continuous running closure, which is a standard vascular surgery technique using 6-0 Prolene sutures. This results in minimal compromise of the arterial lumen, and as

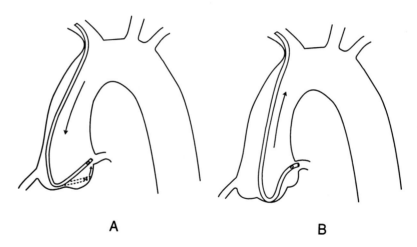

Figure 9–7. Catheterization of the left coronary artery, using the Sones technique. The catheter is advanced into the left coronary cusp, and with further forward pressure the tip tends to prolapse superiorly, as illustrated in *A*. Once the tip is superior to or near the left main coronary artery, gentle retraction of the catheter shaft tends to advance the catheter into position, forming the "cobra head," as illustrated in *B*.

the artery expands, with restoration of blood pressure within it, the suture line is pulled tighter, further ensuring minimal bleeding. Figure of eight stitches, as well as purse-string closures, are also used by some operators. Both of these techniques produce an obligate stenosis of the vessel, and the incidence of need for re-repair of these arteriotomy closures is high. The Sones technique is useful in patients with advanced aortoiliac disease, which precludes the retrograde femoral approach but requires far greater skill and training to successfully perform the procedure.

Percutaneous Retrograde Brachial Approach

Over time, the number of centers training cardiologists in the performance of the Sones technique has declined. A newer approach for retrograde brachial catheterization uses a percutaneous entry.[10] The brachial artery can be entered under local anesthesia using an 18-gauge thin-walled needle and standard J-tipped guide wire. Although some have used 7-French side-arm sheaths, most clinicians have switched to 6-French sheaths for the percutaneous brachial approach. After placement of the sheath,

5000 U of heparin is administered. Although 7-French sheaths accommodate a standard Sones catheter, smaller, 6-French Judkins catheters can also be used, (more easily from the left arm) or 6-French Amplatz catheters from either the left or right arm. After successful completion of the procedure, the heparin is reversed with protamine, and the sheath is removed, allowing for brief bleeding after sheath removal. Pressure is held for 10 to 15 minutes to the degree that does not completely obliterate the radial pulse. After 15 minutes of pressure holding, if no further bleeding occurs, the arm is immobilized for 4 hours on an armboard. The percutaneous approach allows operators not trained in the Sones technique to perform brachial catheterization using regular Judkins or Amplatz catheters.

Left Internal Mammary Angiography

The left internal mammary vessel is engaged using an internal mammary catheter, which is similar to the Judkins right coronary catheter, with a more angulated primary curve (see Fig. 9–5). In the AP projection the catheter is advanced over the wire into the aortic arch. The left subclavian vessel is engaged by counter-

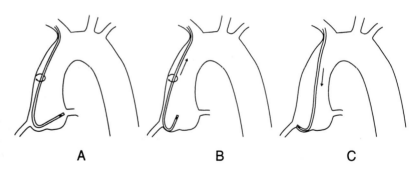

Figure 9–8. Cannulation of the right coronary artery with the Sones catheter. After successful cannulation of the left coronary artery, the catheter is torqued clockwise (*A*) and retracted slowly (*B*). The tip will rotate laterally where it then can be readvanced into the right coronary orifice (*C*).

A   B   C

clockwise torquing in the AP projection. As the tip engages the left subclavian vessel, the tapered, movable core J-guide is advanced antegrade through the subclavian artery. The catheter is then advanced approximately one half the distance between the sternum and the shoulder, over the wire, and the wire is removed. After aspiration and flushing, contrast agent is injected into the catheter to confirm its position. The catheter is then gently withdrawn with slight counterclockwise torque, rotating the tip anteriorly (Fig. 9–9). Repeated small contrast injections are necessary to determine the exact position of the ostium of the internal mammary vessel. It is best to use nonionic contrast agents when doing internal mammary injections, owing to the obligate pain associated with these injections using ionic contrast agents. The right internal mammary vessel can be engaged in a similar fashion using the innominate artery and employing clockwise torquing once within the vessel rather than counterclockwise torquing to rotate the tip anteriorly.

Aortocoronary Bypass Grafts

Aortocoronary bypass grafts can frequently be engaged using the Judkins right coronary catheter. After performing right coronary arteriography, the catheter tip is rotated counterclockwise and withdrawn up the ascending aorta using a rapid advance-and-retreat technique with gentle clockwise torquing. The tip is seen to engage the coronary artery bypass graft ostium (Fig.

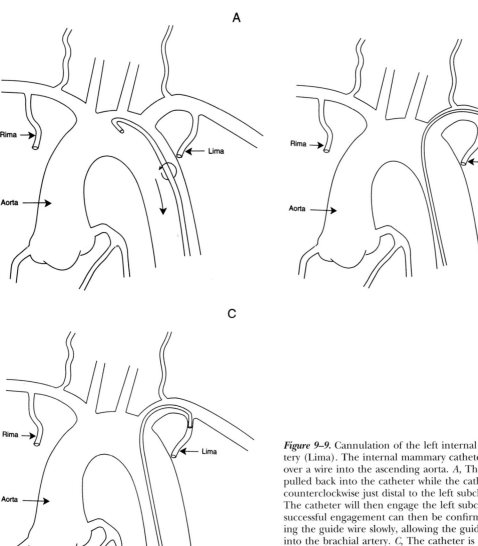

Figure 9–9. Cannulation of the left internal mammary artery (Lima). The internal mammary catheter is advanced over a wire into the ascending aorta. *A,* The wire is then pulled back into the catheter while the catheter is rotated counterclockwise just distal to the left subclavian origin. The catheter will then engage the left subclavian. *B,* The successful engagement can then be confirmed by advancing the guide wire slowly, allowing the guide wire to track into the brachial artery. *C,* The catheter is then advanced over the wire into the brachial artery. The wire is removed and the catheter is retracted and torqued counterclockwise to engage the internal mammary vessel.

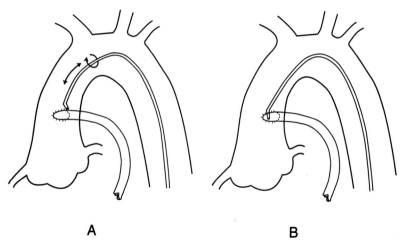

A   B

Figure 9–10. Cannulation of bypass grafts. Most bypass grafts can be engaged with the right Judkins coronary catheter, as illustrated. Occasionally, left-sided coronary artery bypass grafts require a left coronary artery bypass catheter, or modified right Amplatz catheter. The right coronary artery bypass grafts are most easily engaged with the multipurpose catheter. *A,* The right Judkins catheter is positioned in profile in the LAO projection in the vicinity of the bypass grafts, superior to the origin of the native right coronary artery. Gentle clockwise torque is applied to the catheter, as it is advanced and retracted. *B,* The catheter tip slowly rotates anteriorly, and with advancement and retraction engages the ostium of the bypass graft. Engagement is visualized on fluoroscopy when the catheter tip ceases to move. The correct position is then confirmed by a test injection of contrast medium.

9–10). Once the tip is firmly engaged, contrast injection confirms the presence within the graft, and graft angiography can be achieved. Right coronary artery bypass grafts are most easily engaged using the multipurpose catheter. With the tip of the multipurpose catheter in the ascending aorta, it is torqued gently clockwise, withdrawn, and advanced until it engages the right coronary artery bypass ostium. Care should be taken, at this point, to ensure that the catheter does not advance aggressively down the bypass graft, particularly if the graft is old and diffusely diseased. There are specially designed coronary artery bypass graft catheters that are similar to the Judkins right coronary catheter, with a more accentuated primary curve (left coronary artery bypass catheter; see Fig. 9–2). Additionally, internal mammary catheters can be used for bypass graft injections, as well as modified Amplatz catheters, as stated previously. Coronary artery bypass grafts are most easily engaged in the LAO projection, although some operators are comfortable in the RAO projection as well.

ANGIOGRAPHIC ANATOMY

The left coronary artery most commonly comprises two major branches: the LAD and the circumflex vessels. In approximately 10% of patients, an additional branch that arises at the junction of the LAD and circumflex is called

the *ramus intermedius branch*. The LAD vessel courses along the anterolateral aspect of the left ventricle and gives rise to septal perforator branches, which feed the superior two thirds of the interventricular septum; the diagonal branches that feed the anterolateral surface of the heart emanate from the LAD as well. The main branches of the circumflex vessel are called *obtuse marginal branches,* supplying the left lateral aspect of the heart. In 10% of patients, the circumflex vessel supplies the posterior intraventricular septum and posterior left ventricular wall. In this minority of patients, the circumflex is termed the *dominant vessel.* A view useful for a good overview of the LAD vessel is the LAO cranial view (Fig. 9–11*A*). This view allows the separation of the diagonal vessels from the LAD. The advent of C-arm radiographic stands has revolutionized coronary arteriography, allowing multiple, complex views, particularly in biplane installations. In biplane operations, an ideal initial view is the 60-degree LAO with 20 to 30 degrees of cranial angulation, combined with a 30-degree RAO with 20 to 30 degrees of caudal angulation. These orthogonal views adequately image the entire left coronary system in most patients (Fig. 9–12; see also Fig. 9–11). Occasionally, there is some question about the anatomy of the proximal LAD and diagonal vessels. A very steep 45-degree cranial, 45-degree LAO view in most instances clearly delineates the LAD/diagonal anatomy. The single best view for the circumflex

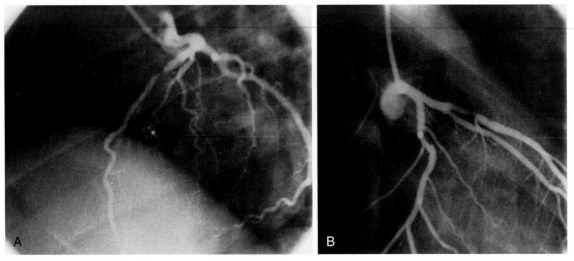

Figure 9–11. A, LAO cranial view of a discrete proximal concentric stenosis of the left anterior descending coronary artery. B, RAO caudal view of the same lesion.

vessel and its branches is the RAO 30 degrees with caudal (20- to 30-degree) angulation (Fig. 9–13; see also Fig. 9–12B) Occasionally, when there are questions regarding the anatomy of the bifurcation of the LAD and circumflex vessels, then the LAO caudal view (the so-called spleen or spider view) will effectively "look up under" the bifurcation of the LAD and circumflex vessels. Additional useful views include the AP and lateral views. The AP view with perhaps slight RAO angulation is probably the best one for visualizing the left main vessel (Fig. 9–14).[11] The AP view with 30 degrees of cranial and perhaps slight LAO angulation is an excellent view for separating the septal perforators and diagonal vessels from the LAD proper in its

proximal and mid-portions. The lateral view with perhaps slight cranial angulation also is useful for the mid and distal LAD as well as the proximal portion of the circumflex vessel.

Right Coronary Artery

The right coronary artery supplies the sinus node artery in its proximal portion in approximately 50% of patients. Between 85% and 90% of patients have dominant right coronary arteries, which means that the right coronary artery supplies the atrioventricular nodal artery and the posterior descending coronary artery. Occasionally, large right coronary arteries also supply the left posterior aspect of the left ventricle with

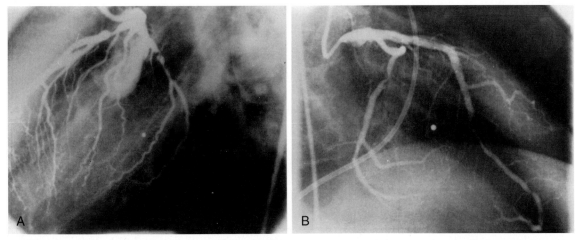

Figure 9–12. A, LAO cranial view of an eccentric stenosis of the left anterior descending coronary artery and serial stenoses of the left circumflex vessel. B, RAO caudal view demonstrating a long tubular mid-left anterior descending coronary artery stenosis in addition to an eccentric, possibly ulcerated lesion of the left circumflex vessel.

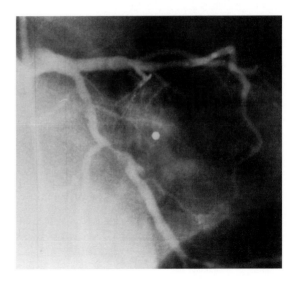

Figure 9–13. RAO caudal view demonstrating a complex and ulcerated lesion of the left circumflex with possible thrombus distal to a critical stenosis.

so-called right posterolateral branches. Other significant branches that arise from the right coronary artery include the conus branch and the acute marginal branches, which supply blood to the right ventricle proper.

The right coronary artery is typically visualized in the 45-degree RAO and 45-degree LAO projections. The most useful view is the 45-degree LAO view, which adequately delineates the anatomy in most patients (see Fig. 9–25*B*). Occasionally, bifurcation lesions at the crux or junction of the right coronary artery and posterior descending vessels require some cranial angulation to better visualize the bifurcation.

Developmental Abnormalities

Congenital coronary artery anomalies are rare. Yamanaka and Hobbs[12] evaluated 126,595 patients undergoing coronary arteriography at the Cleveland Clinic. In this population the inci-

dence of coronary anomalies was 1.33%. Most of these were anomalies of origin and distribution. As illustrated by Table 9–1, more than half of the anomalies were represented by either a separate origin of the LAD and circumflex vessels, *in the left sinus of Valsalva,* or origin of the circumflex from the right sinus of Valsalva or the right coronary artery. Although these cases may represent an increased technical difficulty in coronary arteriography, they have no significant clinical implications. The most serious coronary anomaly is the origin of a coronary artery from the pulmonary artery rather than from the aorta. Again, as illustrated by Table 9–1, this is exceedingly rare, occurring in only 13 patients (fewer than 0.01%). A rare but potentially serious coronary anomaly is illustrated by Figure 9–15, in which the left main vessel courses between the pulmonary artery and the aorta. It is believed that the slitlike left main channel becomes compromised by pressure between the

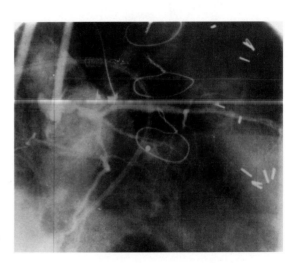

Figure 9–14. Discrete eccentric stenosis of the left main coronary artery in the shallow RAO (AP) projection.

Table 9–1. Incidence of Coronary Artery Anomalies in a Study by Yamanaka and Hobbs[12]

	No.	Incidence (%)	Anomalies (%)
Benign			
Separate origin of LAD and CX in LSV	513	0.41	30.4
CX from RSV or RCA	467	0.37	27.7
Coronary artery from PSV			
LMT from PSV	1	0.0008	0.06
RCA from PSV	4	0.003	0.24
Anomalous origin from ascending aorta			
LMT from aorta	16	0.013	0.95
RCA from aorta	188	0.15	11.2
Absent CX ("superdominant RCA")	4	0.003	0.24
Intercoronary communication	3	0.002	0.18
Small coronary artery fistulas	163	0.12	9.7
Total	**1359**	**1.07**	**80.6**
Potentially Serious			
Coronary artery origin from pulmonary artery			
LMT from pulmonary artery	10	0.008	0.59
LAD from pulmonary artery	1	0.0008	0.06
RCA from pulmonary artery	2	0.002	0.12
Coronary origin from opposite aortic sinus			
LMT from RSV	22	0.017	1.3
LAD from RSV	38	0.03	2.3
RCA from LSV	136	0.107	8.1
Single coronary artery			
R-I	1	0.0008	0.06
R-II	19	0.015	1.1
R-III	5	0.004	0.30
L-I	20	0.016	1.2
L-II	11	0.009	0.65
Multiple or large-sized fistulas	62	0.05	3.7
Total	**327**	**0.26**	**19.4**

LAD, left anterior descending; CX, circumflex; RCA, right coronary artery; LMT, left main trunk; LSV, left sinus of Valsalva; RSV, right sinus of Valsalva; PSV, posterior sinus of Valsalva; R-I, R-II, R-III, L-I, L-II, see Figs. 9–15 to 9–19.

Adapted from Yamanaka O, Hobbs RE: Coronary artery anomalies in 126,595 patients undergoing coronary arteriography. Cathet Cardiovasc Diagn 1990; 21:28–40. Copyright © 1990, John Wiley & Sons, Inc. Reprinted by permission of John Wiley & Sons, Inc.

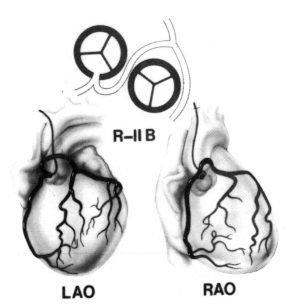

Figure 9–15. Ectopic origin of the left coronary artery from the right ("between" type, R-IIB). The right coronary artery gives rise to an ectopic origin of the left main coronary artery, which then passes between the aorta and the pulmonary artery before its bifurcation into the LAD and circumflex. (From Yamanaka O, Hobbs RE: Coronary artery anomalies in 126,595 patients undergoing coronary arteriography. Cathet Cardiovasc Diagn 1990; 21:28–40. Copyright © 1990, John Wiley & Sons, Inc. Reprinted by permission of John Wiley & Sons, Inc.)

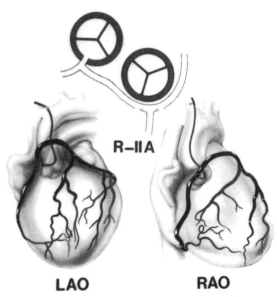

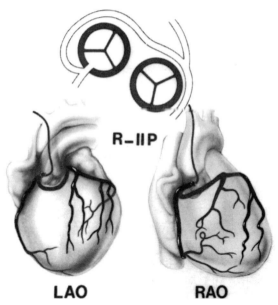

Figure 9–16. Ectopic origin of the left main coronary artery of the "anterior" type, R-IIA. (From Yamanaka O, Hobbs RE: Coronary artery anomalies in 126,595 patients undergoing coronary arteriography. Cathet Cardiovasc Diagn 1990; 21:28–40. Copyright © 1990, John Wiley & Sons, Inc. Reprinted by permission of John Wiley & Sons, Inc.)

Figure 9–17. Ectopic origin of the left main coronary artery in the "posterior" position, R-IIP. The left main coronary artery courses posteriorly to the aorta and pulmonary artery. (From Yamanaka O, Hobbs RE: Coronary artery anomalies in 126,595 patients undergoing coronary arteriography. Cathet Cardiovasc Diagn 1990; 21:28–40. Copyright © 1990, John Wiley & Sons, Inc. Reprinted by permission of John Wiley & Sons, Inc.)

great vessels and predisposes these patients to sudden coronary events or sudden death. Coronary artery bypass surgery has been used in these patients effectively. The coronary anomalies arising from the right sinus of Valsalva are classified as to whether the vessels pass in front of the aorta and pulmonary artery (Fig. 9–16), posterior to the aorta and pulmonary artery (Fig. 9–17), or between them. The final classification of coronary anomalies (aside from atrioventricular fistulas) describes the origin of a single coronary artery from either the right or left sinus of Valsalva (Figs. 9–18 and 9–19).

Pathologic Lesions and Patterns

SINGLE-VESSEL DISEASE. As illustrated by Figure 9–11, the prototypic single-vessel single-cor-

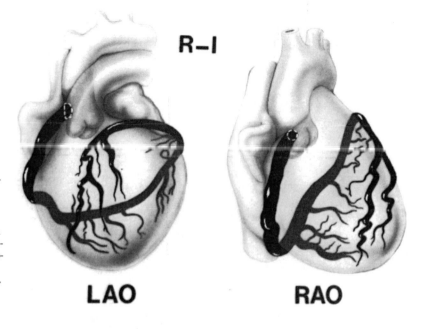

Figure 9–18. Anomalous origin of the entire coronary artery system from the right coronary ostium, R-I. (From Yamanaka O, Hobbs RE: Coronary artery anomalies in 126,595 patients undergoing coronary arteriography. Cathet Cardiovasc Diagn 1990; 21:28–40. Copyright © 1990, John Wiley & Sons, Inc. Reprinted by permission of John Wiley & Sons, Inc.)

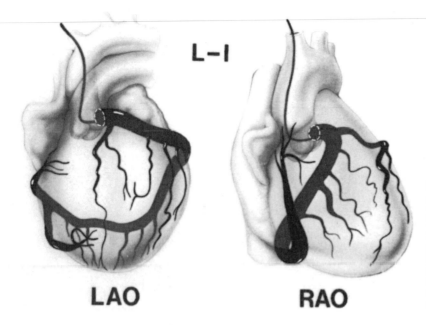

L-I

LAO   RAO

Figure 9–19. Anomalous origin of a single coronary artery from the left coronary ostium, L-I. (From Yamanaka O, Hobbs RE: Coronary artery anomalies in 126,595 patients undergoing coronary arteriography. Cathet Cardiovasc Diagn 1990; 21:28–40. Copyright © 1990, John Wiley & Sons, Inc. Reprinted by permission of John Wiley & Sons, Inc.)

onary lesion is concentric and discrete, as illustrated in this proximal lesion of the LAD coronary artery. The margins are well circumscribed, and the lesion is less than 2.5 cm in length; the remaining vessels in this patient are essentially normal. This is an ideal lesion for treatment with coronary angioplasty. Figure 9–20 illustrates a right coronary stenosis, which is also discrete and concentric, in the proximal portion of an adequately sized right coronary artery. There was no distal disease, and the remaining vessels are relatively normal. In con-

trast, however, Figure 9–14 illustrates a 60% eccentric stenosis of the left main coronary artery in a patient with prior coronary artery bypass surgery. Such a lesion in the patient with previously untreated remaining vessels represents an extreme hazard without revascularization.

MULTIVESSEL DISEASE. Ascending the ladder of complexity, Figures 9–12 and 9–21 illustrate two patients with multivessel disease. Figure 9–12*A* depicts a patient with a relatively discrete but eccentric proximal LAD stenosis (as seen in this LAO cranial view), as well as an eccentric high-grade stenosis of the left circumflex vessel, with continuing tubular stenoses of the circumflex distal to the proximal stenosis. When occlusions of native coronary arteries are encountered, one must search for the presence of collaterals to the occluded vessel. As illustrated by Figure 9–21*A*, the native LAD coronary artery is totally occluded in its very proximal portion. The circumflex vessel remains patent; however, the first obtuse marginal branch of the circumflex has a long stenosis. Injection of the right coronary artery, as revealed in Figure 9–21*B*, illustrates prominent collateral vessels to the distal LAD vessels via the intraventricular septum.

UNSTABLE LESIONS. Plaque rupture is often associated with ulceration as well as thrombus formation. Figure 9–13 illustrates a left circumflex vessel with a tight stenosis and filling defect distal to the stenosis. Immediately adjacent to the filling defect on the contralateral side of the vessel is an area of ulceration that is ill

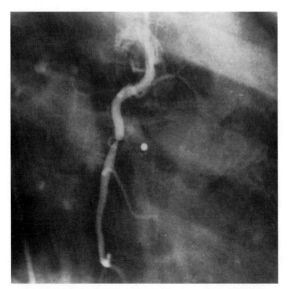

Figure 9–20. Discrete concentric stenosis of the mid-portion of the right coronary artery in the RAO projection.

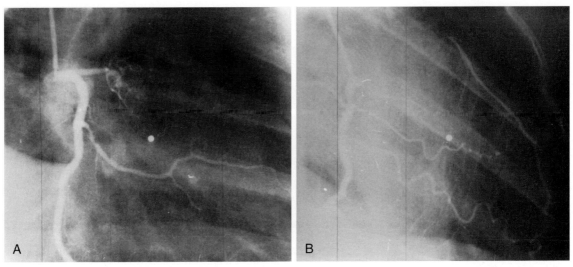

Figure 9–21. *A,* RAO caudal view of the left coronary artery demonstrating total occlusion of the proximal left anterior descending and a complex lesion of the origin of the first obtuse marginal branch of the circumflex vessel. *B,* RAO projection of the right coronary artery demonstrating collaterals filling the left anterior descending vessel via the transapical pathway as well as through the intraventricular septum.

defined and presumably associated with thrombus. Figure 9–22 illustrates a right coronary artery with a critical stenosis in its mid-portion, with multiple irregularities both proximal and distal to the stenosis, consistent with ulceration. The natural progression of unstable plaques is to produce thrombi, which subsequently may occlude the vessel. Figure 9–23 demonstrates a patient with prior bypass, with a right coronary artery containing two discrete areas of thrombus, distal to a critical stenosis. The natural progression of such thrombotic lesions is to total occlusion, as illustrated by Figure 9–24. In this figure, the LAD vessel has multiple areas of thrombus in its proximal portion, followed by a total occlusion in its mid-portion (Fig. 9–24*A*).

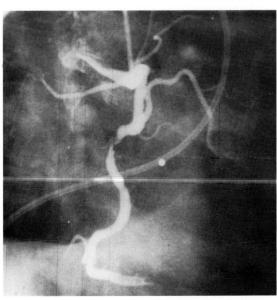

Figure 9–22. RAO view of the right coronary artery demonstrating a critical stenosis with ulceration distal to the most severe portion.

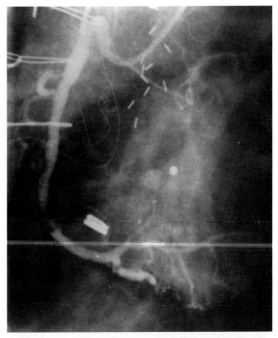

Figure 9–23. LAO view of the right coronary artery in a patient with prior bypass surgery, demonstrating a middle to distal critical stenosis of the right coronary artery with thrombi beyond the distal stenosis, seen as filling defects in the column of contrast medium.

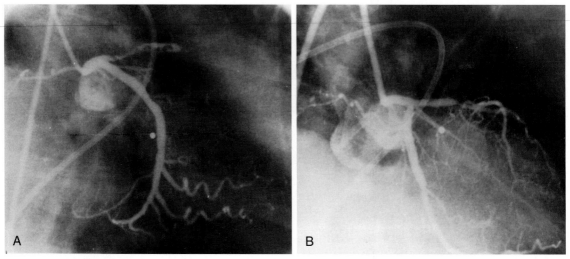

Figure 9–24. *A,* RAO caudal view of the left coronary artery demonstrating a thrombus proximal to a total occlusion of the left anterior descending vessel. *B,* The same vessel after administration of intracoronary urokinase. The thrombus is now resolved, and a critical stenosis of the LAD remains.

After administration of intravenous recombinant tissue plasminogen activator, the thrombi are dissolved and patency is restored to the distal vessel (Fig. 9–24*B*). A more dramatic example of this phenomenon is illustrated by Figure 9–25. Here, a right coronary artery is totally occluded in its mid-portion (Fig. 9–25*A*). Direct coronary angioplasty was applied, which effectively restored patency. However, dilation of the distal stenosis in the artery was accompanied by dissection, as illustrated by Figure 9–25*B*. Despite the extraluminal contrast agent, the vessel

remained patent and the patient had an uneventful recovery.

COMPLICATIONS OF CARDIAC CATHETERIZATION WITH CORONARY ANGIOGRAPHY

A report from the 1991 Registry of the SCA&I, in a total of more than 92,000 patients, suggested that death occurred in diagnostic catheterization in 0.11% of cases. Myocardial in-

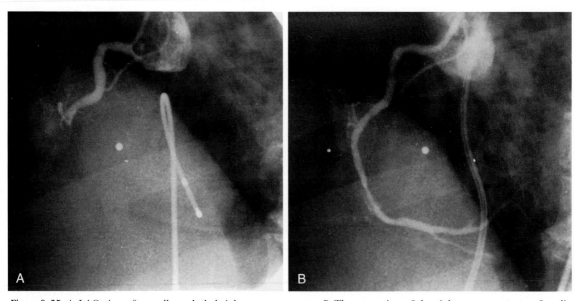

Figure 9–25. *A,* LAO view of a totally occluded right coronary artery. *B,* The same view of the right coronary artery after direct angioplasty for acute myocardial infarction. A stenosis is visualized proximal to the crux of the vessel, which has been successfully dilated with coronary angioplasty. Dissection lines are apparent medial and lateral to the area of the stenosis.

farction was less frequent at 0.06%, whereas neurologic events occurred in 0.05%. Factors identified that contributed to complications were diabetes in 13%, hypertension in 31%, and impaired renal function in 2.3% of patients with complications. Twenty-six percent of patients with complications had unstable angina, whereas 6.2% had congestive heart failure. Thus, diagnostic coronary arteriography appears to be a safe procedure in the hands of skilled operators.[1] There is a trend toward performing diagnostic coronary arteriography without heparin, particularly in the outpatient setting. Although I routinely use 3000 U of heparin in such patients, anecdotal reports from laboratories that do not use heparin suggest this approach may be favorable, with a decreased incidence of groin hematomas and bleeding complications after the procedure.

ESSENTIALS OF QUANTITATIVE ANGIOGRAPHY

Visual Assessment of Severity of Stenosis

Several major problems exist regarding the visual assessment of coronary arteriograms. The first problem is the variability in interpretation. A number of studies have demonstrated that the variability of different, experienced angiographers' interpretations of assessment of the critical lesion are often no better than a coin toss.[13–17] Disagreement about the number of vessels with a major stenosis (70% or greater) occurs in more than 30% of patients.[15] Rather than reporting the percent diameter stenosis, most angiographers are "calibrated" to report the percent area stenosis, which actually may be a better physiologic indicator of stenosis severity.[17] A second serious consideration is that of the correct method for assessing stenosis severity. White and colleagues[16] have demonstrated that the percent stenosis did not correlate with physiologic measurement of reactive hyperemia in humans. Gould and associates[18] have demonstrated that the increase in coronary blood flow after a period of ischemia (so-called reactive hyperemia) is blunted by increasing severity of stenoses. Normal coronary flow reserves should be between three and five times resting blood flow in the absence of hypertrophy, prior infarction, anemia, or other hypermetabolic conditions. The variability of estimating stenosis severity by percent stenosis can be reduced significantly by substituting a hemodynamic assessment of the stenosis severity that incorporates the stenosis length, the entrance and exit

diameters of the stenosis, as well as the percent area stenosis. This has been termed the *stenosis flow reserve* by Gould and coworkers.[18] The stenosis flow reserve has been incorporated into several on-line digital imaging systems and can be used for decision making regarding stenosis severity at the time of diagnostic catheterization. However, in the setting of multiple, less severe, but sequential stenoses, calculations regarding stenosis severity are less reliable. It has become apparent that the extent of the disease estimated by angiography is significantly underestimated by angiography alone when compared with intravascular ultrasonographic assessment. Long, diffuse narrowing of the vessels may be just as important as tight, discrete stenoses. How then should we assess coronary arteriograms objectively for decision making?

Manual Quantitation

The easiest method to attempt quantitated stenosis severity is the use of manual or digital calipers. Kalbfleisch and associates[19] analyzed 155 lesions using a hand-held caliper system and compared this with results obtained from a computerized quantitative coronary arteriographic system. They found that the caliper method underestimated severe stenoses and overestimated less severe stenoses and that the reproducibility of the caliper technique was very poor.[19] Given that the percentage of diameter stenosis is, in itself, a poor estimation of stenosis severity, the caliper technique does not seem to be useful for the critical analysis of stenosis severity.

Manual Tracing

A slightly more sophisticated technique employs manual tracing of the arteriograms in biplane views and digitizing of the traced images with calculation of orthogonal vessel diameters along a center line of the superimposed vessel images.[20] The system corrects for pin cushion distortion and x-ray beam divergence; however, it is slow, labor intensive, and unsuitable for on-line assessment of lesion severity. Additionally, reliance on the visual assessment of the lesion boundary renders a great potential for observer bias.

The next most logical step is to detect vessel boundaries and subsequently identify stenoses automatically using digital techniques. Once the visual information is converted into a two-dimensional numeric representation, automated edge detection techniques can be used. Typically, the region of interest is identified by an operator and a center line is created within the vessel lumen along its midline. Next, perpendicular lines are constructed along this center line that are then interrogated by the border detection algorithms of an individual analysis system.[21] Typically, border detection algorithms use both density gradient criteria as well as threshold criteria. In other words, the absolute value of the gray level of information is used in addition to the rate of change in that gray level. An a priori understanding of the physics of a given x-ray system allows for optimization of the edge detection system such that vessels may be quantitated down to 0.1 to 0.2 mm in diameter.[21] Such algorithms can be incorporated in the system for on-line assessment of lesion severity. Serruys and colleagues recently compared the on-line assessment using the Philips DCI System with their own cardiovascular angiographic analysis system (CAAS). They found that the on-line digital analysis of coronary arteriograms was excellent and correlated well with off-line analysis.[22]

One of the major difficulties with border detection techniques in the assessment of stenosis severity arises in irregular stenoses or in stenoses previously subjected to coronary angioplasty. In this situation, the internal dimensions of the stenosis have been significantly modified by the angioplasty technique. Thus, although the borders may be significantly enhanced, the overall lumen may be enhanced to a much lesser degree. For instance, dissection lines can occur, which will push the detected boundary outside the true boundary of the lumen. In such situations a densitometric approach may be better.[23, 24] The densitometric approach identifies the borders of the vessel using standard border detection techniques and then integrates the density of the gray level information between the borders. Given a known absorbance of x-ray energy by a given volume of contrast medium, one can calculate the volume of the vessel in a given cross section, and thus calculate regional areas from the densitometric information. Although controversy exists regarding the accuracy of this technique, it is probably superior to border detection in irregular stenoses, ulcerated lesions, lesions containing thrombus, and lesions immediately after angioplasty.

Beyond Geometric X-ray Analysis

TRANSLESIONAL PRESSURE-FLOW RELATIONSHIPS. During the early days of coronary angioplasty, translesional gradients were routinely measured to assess the efficacy of the dilation. Because of the bulky nature of these dilation catheters, the gradients were often subject to question, and a number of investigators published a poor correlation between pressure gradient responses and actual stenosis severity. Recently, several devices have become available, at least on an investigational basis, that may change the way we look at the functional significance of vessels in the catheterization laboratory. Velocity measurements use an 0.018-inch intracoronary Doppler-tip angioplasty guide wire, whereas pressure measurements were achieved with either an 0.018-inch pressure monitoring wire or a 2.2-French infusion catheter.[25, 26] Donohue and colleagues[26] have demonstrated that the ratio of the velocity distal to a stenosis divided by the velocity proximal to the stenosis is a sensitive indicator of stenosis severity and correlates well with transstenotic pressure gradient information. In contrast, however, the percentage of diameter stenosis compared with translesional pressure gradients correlated poorly in severe or moderate lesions.

TREE ANALYSIS. As stated previously, diffuse disease often impacts coronary flow reserve and is difficult to quantify. Seiler and colleagues[27] have proposed a new type of analysis that measures the lengths of the coronary segments, which when summed, correlate nicely with the mass of myocardium supplied by a given vessel. Knowing the mass of the myocardium supplied by a given vessel and the length then allows one to calculate the area of vessel at any given point necessary for supplying the requisite amount of blood to that region. This method allows one to calculate the true flow reserve even in the presence of diffuse disease. Thus, the quantitation of coronary artery disease continues to be in evolution with the miniaturization of intravascular ultrasonographic technologies, as well as the development of intracoronary angioscopy techniques. Further refined analysis methodologies will continue to evolve for at least the short term.

INTRAVASCULAR ULTRASONOGRAPHY AND CORONARY ANGIOSCOPY COMPARED WITH ANGIOGRAPHY

Although coronary angiography is the gold standard for evaluating coronary stenoses, other techniques are certainly complementary. It has been shown that intravascular ultrasonography identifies potentially significant coronary disease in vessels that appear angiographically to be mildly diseased in a significant number of patients.[28] To demonstrate this point, Figure

9–26 illustrates the case of a 42-year-old man who was admitted to a hospital with an acute myocardial infarction. The patient developed ventricular tachycardia and fibrillation and was found to have an anterior myocardial infarction, which was treated successfully with thrombolytic therapy. He was transferred to our hospital for cardiac catheterization, which revealed a hazy area in the origin of his LAD coronary artery that appeared to be noncritical by both visual observation and quantitative angiography (Fig. 9–26A). Because of the hazy nature of the origin, it was feared that the lesion was highly eccentric, and this resulted in evaluation using intravascular ultrasonography. As illustrated by

Figure 9–26B, the intravascular ultrasonographic probe partially occluded the LAD vessel, suggesting that it was indeed significantly stenosed. Ultrasonographic images obtained from the proximal LAD, just distal to the stenosis, as illustrated by Figure 9–26C, demonstrated that the LAD was approximately 4.8 to 5 mm in diameter. Pullback of the ultrasonographic catheter demonstrated a highly eccentric plaque, with some calcification and a minimal lumen diameter of approximately 2.5 to 2.7 mm (Fig. 9–26D). The ultrasonographic imaging demonstrated that the lesion was exactly perpendicular to the origin of the circumflex vessel and therefore it was treated with directional

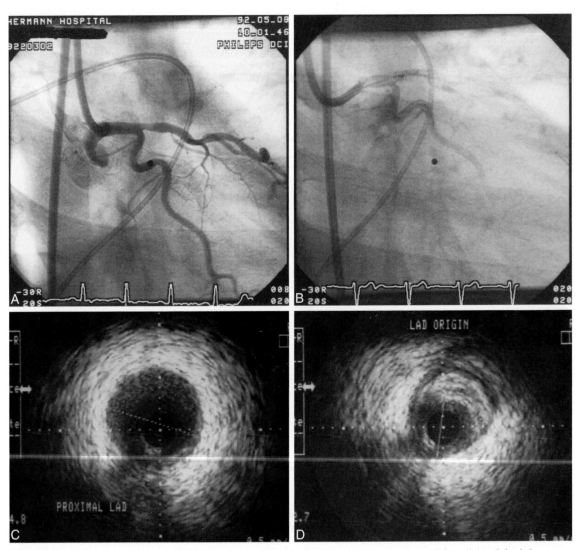

Figure 9–26. A, RAO caudal view of a left coronary artery demonstrating a hazy appearance of the origin of the left anterior descending coronary artery. B, Passage of a 4.3-French ultrasound catheter totally occludes the left anterior descending vessel, suggesting that it is significantly stenosed. C, Intravascular ultrasonography of the proximal LAD distal to the hazy area demonstrating an internal lumen diameter of 4.8 mm. D, An eccentric stenosis of the proximal LAD visualized by intravascular ultrasonography with a minimal lumen diameter of 2.7 mm in the presence of eccentric plaque.

Illustration continued on following page

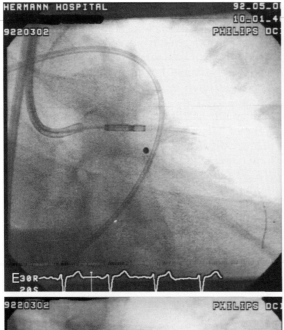

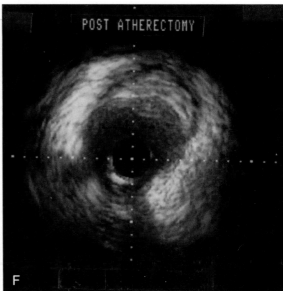

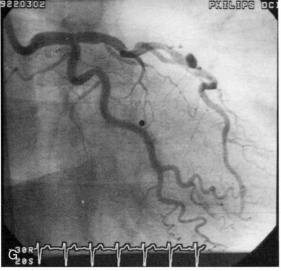

Figure 9–26 Continued E, Directional atherectomy of the eccentric plaque. *F,* Intravascular ultrasonography of the stenosis after atherectomy demonstrating a scalloped appearance of the plaque with an increased lumen of almost 4.5 mm. *G,* RAO caudal projection of the same vessel after atherectomy demonstrating an improved lumen.

atherectomy, as illustrated by Figure 9–26*E.* The eccentric plaque was removed effectively by the atherectomy, and the lumen was enlarged to 4 mm, as illustrated by Figure 9–26*F.* Postprocedural arteriography demonstrated improvement of the lumen (Fig. 9–26*G*), with no residual haziness, and the patient had no subsequent clinical events.

My colleagues and I have recently compared 19 patients treated with interventional procedures for obstructive coronary disease, using intravascular ultrasonography, angioscopy, and coronary angiography in all patients. As illustrated by Table 9–2, intravascular ultrasonography was highly effective in detecting intralesional calcium, whereas angioscopy was

Table 9–2. Comparison of Stenosis Features as Assessed by Angiography, Intravascular Ultrasonography, and Angioscopy in 19 Patients After Coronary Interventions

	Dissection	Ruptured Plaque	Intraluminal Flap	Clot	Intralesional Calcium
Intravascular ultrasonography	1	0	1	0	14
Angioscopy	0	10	11	6	0
Angiography	4	0	0	1	1

more sensitive for detecting ruptured plaque, intraluminal flaps, and thrombus. Angiography, on the other hand, seemed to be more sensitive for detecting dissection but was highly insensitive at detecting other stenosis features. As these devices become more user friendly, it is likely that their use will be a routine feature of analysis and treatment of complex coronary lesions. We suspect that intravascular ultrasonographic imaging may in fact become the gold standard for evaluation of coronary disease, both after coronary interventions and in the case of borderline stenoses.

REFERENCES

1. Johnson LW, Krone R, The Registry Committee of the Society for Cardiac Angiography and Interventions: Cardiac catheterization 1991: A report of the Registry of the Society for Cardiac Angiography and Interventions (SCA&I). Cathet Cardiovasc Diagn 1993; 28:219–220.
2. Statson WB, Fineberg HV: Coronary artery disease: What is a reasonable diagnostic strategy? Ann Intern Med 1981; 95:385–386.
3. Geddes LA, Geddes LE: The Catheter Introducers. Chicago, Mobium Press, 1993, pp 39–40.
4. Geddes LA, Geddes LE: The Catheter Introducers. Chicago, Mobium Press, 1993, pp 46–50.
5. Ross J Jr, Brandenburg RO, Dinsmore RE, et al: Guidelines for coronary angiography: A report of the American College of Cardiology/American Heart Association Task Force on Assessment of Diagnostic and Therapeutic Cardiovascular Procedures (Subcommittee on Coronary Angiography). J Am Coll Cardiol 1987; 10:35–50.
6. Grines CL, Browne KF, Marco J, et al: A comparison of immediate angioplasty with thrombolytic therapy for acute myocardial infarction. N Engl J Med 1993; 328:673–679.
7. Clark DA, Moscovich MD, Vetrovec GW, Wexler L: Guidelines for the performance of outpatient catheterization and angiographic procedures. Cathet Cardiovasc Diagn 1992; 27:5–7.
8. Amplatz K, Formanek G, Stanger P, Wilson W: Mechanics of selective coronary catheterization via femoral approach. Radiology 1967; 89:1040.
9. Schoonmaker FW, King SB: Coronary arteriography by the single-catheter percutaneous femoral technique: Experience in 6800 cases. Circulation 1974; 50:735.
10. Cohen M, Rentrop KP, Cohen BM: Safety and efficacy of percutaneous entry of the brachial artery versus cutdown and arteriotomy for left-sided cardiac catheterization. Am J Cardiol 1986; 57:682–684.
11. Nath PH, Valasquez G, Castaned-Zuniga WR, et al: An essential flow in coronary arteriography. Circulation 1979; 60:101–106.
12. Yamanaka O, Hobbs RE: Coronary artery anomalies in 126,595 patients undergoing coronary arteriography. Cathet Cardiovasc Diagn 1990; 21:28–40.
13. Detre KM, Wright E, Murphy ML, Takaro T: Observer agreement in evaluating coronary angiograms. Circulation 1975; 52:979–986.
14. Zir LM, Miller SW, Dinsmore RE, et al: Interobserver variability in coronary angiography. Circulation 1976; 53:627–632.
15. DeRouen TA, Murray JA, Owen W: Variability in the analysis of coronary arteriograms. Circulation 1977; 55:324–328.
16. White CW, Wright CB, Doty DB, et al: Does visual interpretation of the coronary arteriogram predict the physiologic importance of a coronary stenosis? N Engl J Med 1984; 310:819–824.
17. Fleming RM, Kirkeeide RL, Smalling RW, Gould KL: Patterns in visual interpretation of coronary arteriograms as detected by quantitative coronary arteriography. J Am Coll Cardiol 1991; 18:945–951.
18. Gould KL, Kirkeeide RL, Buchi M: Coronary flow reserve as a physiologic measure of stenosis severity. J Am Coll Cardiol 1990; 15:459–474.
19. Kalbfleisch SJ, McGillen MJ, Pinto IMG, et al: Comparison of automated quantitative coronary angiography with caliper measurements of percent diameter stenosis. Am J Cardiol 1990; 65:1181–1184.
20. Brown BG, Bolson E, Frimer M, Dodge HT: Quantitative coronary arteriography: Estimation of dimensions, hemodynamic resistance, and atheroma mass of coronary artery lesions using the arteriogram and digital computation. Circulation 1977; 55:329–337.
21. Kirkeeide RL, Fung MS, Smalling RW, Gould KL: Automated evaluation of vessel diameter from arteriograms. IEEE Comput Cardiol 1982; 215–218.
22. Haase J, Nugteren SK, van Swijndregt EM, et al: Digital geometric measurements in comparison to cinefilm analysis of coronary artery dimensions. Cathet Cardiovasc Diagn 1993; 28:283–290.
23. Smalling RW: Can the immediate efficacy of coronary angioplasty be adequately assessed? J Am Coll Cardiol 1987; 10:261–263.
24. Serruys PW, Reiber JHC, Wijns W, et al: Assessment of percutaneous transluminal coronary angioplasty by quantitative coronary angiography: Diameter versus densitometric area measurements. Am J Cardiol 1984; 54:482–488.
25. Di Mario C, de Feyter PJ, Slager CJ, et al: Intracoronary blood flow velocity and transstenotic pressure gradient using SensorTip pressure and Doppler guide wires: A new technology for the assessment of stenosis severity in the catheterization laboratory. Cathet Cardiovasc Diagn 1993; 28:311–319.
26. Donohue TJ, Kern MJ, Aguirre FV, et al: Assessing the hemodynamic significance of coronary artery stenoses: Analysis of translesional pressure-flow velocity relations in patients. J Am Coll Cardiol 1993; 22:449–458.
27. Seiler C, Kirkeeide RL, Gould KL: Measurement from arteriograms of regional myocardial bed size distal to any point in the coronary vascular tree for assessing anatomic area at risk. J Am Coll Cardiol 1993; 21:783–797.
28. Porter TR, Sears T, Xie F, et al: Intravascular ultrasound study of angiographically mildly diseased coronary arteries. J Am Coll Cardiol 1993; 22:1858–1865.

Chapter 10

Digital Cardiac Angiography

G. B. JOHN MANCINI

Digital angiography is commonly available in most modern cardiac catheterization laboratories and is now integrated into routine practice. Although most research efforts have focused on powerful and innovative quantitation of images, dominant interest is in using the image enhancement capabilities of this technology to assist qualitative, visual assessment and to expedite routine daily catheterization procedures. A decade ago, during prominence of the "noninvasive" era in cardiology, digital angiography was seen as a way to make even catheterization laboratories less invasive. Although this effort met with disappointing results, the current invasive era of thrombolysis and angioplasty is a more viable and fruitful environment for the application of digital angiographic methods. Image manipulation, enhancement, and quantitation are of immediate practical need when performing angioplasty. The ability to roam over a digital image in a zoom mode is particularly useful for delineating complex lesions, partially obstructing thrombi, or dissections. Roadmapping, by simple or sophisticated means, is used to expedite angioplasty balloon placement. Use of on-line coronary quantitation to assist in selecting an optimal balloon size is common in several laboratories. In addition, numerous unresolved issues relating to thrombolysis and mechanical recanalization create many research applications. Accordingly, this chapter serves to summarize the proven and potential uses of digital angiography.

INSTRUMENTATION AND PHYSICAL PRINCIPLES

Many of the initial investigations in digital angiography used general-function computer equipment and off-line analysis of images initially recorded on videotape and later digitized for processing and quantitation. Modern systems have evolved to provide direct, on-line image acquisition onto large-capacity hard disk drives, thereby avoiding the image degradation caused by digitization of video images. Biplane digital acquisitions and electrocardiograph (ECG)-gated studies are now also possible with most modern systems. Long-term archiving and retrieval, however, continue to be substantive problems that are compounded by incompatibilities from system to system. Previous inadequacies in long-term storage capacity have been overcome by the more widespread use of optical disks. Digital tape devices are also currently being evaluated to fit this role. However, the familiarity and ease of handling of film-based patient studies have encouraged some manufacturers to also allow for simultaneous recording of both film and digital images.[1] This obviates issues of long-term digital storage and compatibility.

Brennecke[2] and Kruger[3] provided a comprehensive summary of the principles of physics that affect the quality of digital angiographic images. The final quality of a digital image is the result of the complex interaction between both physical and technical parameters of a sophisticated imaging chain. The simple function of this chain is to convert x-ray energy to light energy that can be recorded and displayed. The x-rays are affected, however, by characteristics of the x-ray generator and x-ray tube, the patient, the image intensifier, and the video camera. The signal is then subject to the performance characteristics of the digitization system. Finally, the specific image processing method affects the image quality. Therefore, enhancement or degradation of overall image quality can occur at any point along this chain.

The essential components of image quality relevant to cardiac catheterization include the spatial, temporal, and contrast resolution of the image. The spatial resolution of the digital image is partially determined by the image matrix size. The matrix size is defined by the number of pixels per line and the number of lines per image. In clinical applications, this size is generally 256 × 256 for ventricular or aortographic studies and 512 × 512 for coronary or graft studies. Whether the latter applications definitely require 1024 × 1024 image matrices is not totally resolved. This is largely because there appear to be greater limitations to achievable resolution inherent in the other components of the imaging chain listed earlier.[4, 5]

Temporal resolution has two components: the number of images obtained per second and the pulse width of the x-rays used to create the images. Ventriculography can be adequately performed at a frame rate of 30 per second. Arteriography does not require as high a frame rate (a rate of 10 to 15 per second may be sufficient), but because of the rapid motion of the arteries, a small radiographic pulse width is required to avoid image blurring. For this same reason, progressive scanning is required for arteriography, that will minimize the edge blurring caused by the use of standard, interlaced video scanning.

Contrast resolution can be defined by two components: the signal-to-noise ratio and object conspicuity. The signal-to-noise ratio can be shown to be a function of pixel area, the specific tissue absorption, the concentration of contrast material, the thickness of the contrast-laden object, and the square root of the x-ray dose.[2] Consequently, to maintain a constant signal-to-noise ratio, halving of the contrast dose must be compensated by a fourfold increase in radiation dose. Similarly, an increase in matrix size that makes the area of each pixel smaller must be paralleled by an increase in x-ray dose.

Object conspicuity is a function of the ratio between iodine and noniodine signals in an image. The noniodine signals consist of both random noise and structured noise (such as ribs and diaphragm). Subtraction removes structured noise and increases the conspicuity of iodine signals against the backdrop of random noise. This conspicuity can be further enhanced by expanding the resulting small-intensity range to the full dynamic range of the system (typically 256 shades of gray). Random noise can be altered by various averaging and filtering algorithms that can profoundly alter image interpretation. For example, visual analysis of digital images may be facilitated by edge-enhancement algorithms[6, 7] whereas these same algorithms may adversely affect the precision and accuracy of automated edge-detection algorithms used for quantitative arteriography.[8] In contrast, averaging algorithms that smooth out background noise may enhance the performance of edge-detection programs.[8]

Image digitization is accomplished by sampling the video signal with an electronic gate followed by quantitation of the video intensity into 256 (or 1024) gray levels and spatial encoding of these values. Modern digital angiographic systems provide real-time digitization and storage of the video signal onto large hard disks. These data can be retrieved rapidly for image processing as well as for subjective and quantitative analysis. Long-term archival is performed on floppy disks, hard disks, magnetic tape, optical disks, videotapes, or digital tapes. Combinations of these are extremely common. Incompatibility of these media from system to system is rapidly becoming intolerable as more laboratories are equipped with digital systems. As a consequence, there is now a growing tendency to go back to more general computer hardware that can be configured for digital angiography but updated easily and interfaced to image networks. Continual insistence on this type of flexibility and compatibility by clinical users may finally foster some uniformity in the manufacturing field. Such uniformity would also foster greater use of digital angiography and total elimination of cinefilm requirements.

IMAGE PROCESSING METHODS

Digital angiography provides powerful options for either suppressing or subtracting elements of an image devoid of diagnostic content. Subtraction can be performed with respect to one of several physical variables: time, energy, or depth.[9, 10] In cardiac applications, the most common forms are mask-mode subtraction and time-interval difference methods. Both are forms of temporal subtraction that depend on the difference in opacification of objects of interest at different times after contrast injection. In mask-mode subtraction the digitized image frames during peak opacification are subtracted from single or averaged frames of the same area before the arrival of contrast media. Alternatively, the mask may be ECG-gated so that each frame of the precontrast and postcontrast phases is aligned with respect to the phase of the cardiac cycle. This process removes obscuring, noniodinated structures such as ribs and diaphragm, but the subtraction is effective only in the absence of patient motion. Otherwise, misregistration artifacts result. The method is most used in ventriculographic applications or in applications designed to demonstrate bypass graft patency, or myocardial perfusion. These studies are not as severely affected by slight degrees of misregistration. Studies of coronary morphology, however, are best performed without sub-traction because some degree of misregistration is extremely common and will cause errors in edge detection.

Time-interval difference methods give a display of the motion of iodinated structures or the motion of an iodine bolus. This results from subtraction of iodinated images obtained at specified time intervals (such as once per R-R interval and every-other-frame). This effectively eliminates all stationary portions of the field of view. If the time interval is brief, then effects of motion misregistration are also minimized. Imaging of myocardial perfusion,[11] wall thickness[12] and wall motion abnormalities[13] are a few applications that use time-interval difference techniques.

Other subtraction methods are quite uncommon.[9, 10] A method of particular promise, however, is the dual-energy subtraction method proposed by Van Lysel and associates.[14] This method is akin to the older K-edge subtraction methods where two energy levels of x-rays, one above and one below the K-edge of iodine, were used in alternate frames and then subtracted from one another to effectively remove soft tissue components that account for most misregistration artifacts.[9] In the newer application proposed by van Lysel and associates, the x-ray kilovolts (peak) are both above the K-edge of iodine, which allows a greater beam flux and hence a higher signal-to-noise ratio in the final images. The most striking effect of this technique is the virtual elimination of misregistration artifacts, the single most important day-to-day cause of image degradation. This factor alone probably outweighs some of the drawbacks of the approach, which include a 30% to 40% decrement in iodine signal relative to standard mask-mode techniques, an increase in image noise, a decrement in framing rate, and an increase in x-ray exposure per image frame. Although the technique is not commercially available, the diagnostic content of images obtained by this method even in the face of patient motion is excellent and will likely promote continued development and commercialization of the technique.

ARCHIVING OF DIGITAL IMAGES

The issues of matrix size and usable resolution impact directly on a major, unsettled problem in this field: archiving and retrieval of digital data. A comprehensive discussion of this issue is provided by Cox and Dwyer.[15] Typically, a complete coronary examination might entail a

minimum of five or six coronary arteriograms, each lasting 5 to 10 seconds. Thus, at 30 frames/sec and using a 512×512 (8 bit) matrix, this yields about 500 megabytes of data. In a laboratory performing 1000 cases per year, the archival load would be in the 500-gigabyte range. Four times this amount would result by using 1024×1024 matrices. These demands may be minimized by using lower or staggered acquisition frame rates,[16] data compression,[15] spatial multiplexing,[17] or adaptive differential pulse code modulation.[14] Optical disks, digital tapes, or both, appear to be the most promising methods for long-term digital archival demands of this magnitude. Long-term stability of these media has not been tested, and the possible need for routine updating of images archived on these media has been raised.[17] Some existing laboratories use videotapes for long-term storage at the expense of both short-term and long-term degradation of image quality. Some digital technologies (such as computed tomography [CT] and magnetic resonance imaging) record the digital images on film. Although this appears counterproductive to the goal of eliminating the costs of film, the advisability of incurring the current costs of completely digital storage remains a serious question that is not nearly resolved.[18] The attractiveness of simultaneous storage onto digital disk and cineimaging is therefore evident at this time.[1, 14] An alternative is the provision of simultaneous digital media and video recording. This would obviate the use of film and the time needed to develop it. This archival method would be at a reasonable cost and widely compatible. Because postprocessing of video images might be less than optimal, the angiographer may need to make a decision about the likelihood of this need and use both digital media and videotape for long-term archiving in selected cases. Simultaneous digital recording onto disk and digital tape is yet another attractive alternative that is being evaluated.[19]

CONTRAST AND VASODILATOR INJECTION

In typical cardiac catheterization practice, the general tenet for contrast injection can be summarized as follows: Give enough contrast agent at a rapid enough rate to maximize diagnostic yield and minimize the need to repeat studies. This approach generally holds true for digital applications, but it is important to understand several unique factors related to contrast agent injection for specialized applications. For example, patient discomfort that may cause motion and contrast-induced arrhythmias should be avoided because many digital applications involve subtraction or meticulous timing of events that cannot be optimally performed in the presence of arrhythmias or misregistration artifacts. Newer agents that are either nonionic or of lower osmolarity are generally favored. The costs of such agents continue to mandate their use only on a selective basis. Intravenous ventriculography is facilitated by maximizing the difference in contrast density between the mask phase (precontrast) and the contrast phase. Theoretically, an intravenous contrast injection that gives a high peak iodine concentration in a narrow or compact bolus should be ideal for purposes of subtraction. Such a situation allows selection of mask and contrast phases that are close in time, resulting in maximal contrast enhancement while the possibility of misregistration is minimized. Applications in the coronary circulation mandate even greater attention to the details of contrast agent injection. For example, one method of coronary flow reserve calculation (see later) depends on virtual displacement of blood by contrast material. High doses at high flow rates are necessary.[20] The exact amount of contrast injection is not critical in this application. In contrast, the indicator-dilution approach used by some groups predicates use of precisely measured boluses of contrast agent that must be injected subselectively and in such a way that reflux into other coronary beds or the aorta does not occur.[21]

Aside from these factors, contrast material itself is used as an indicator in several digital applications, but it is not ideal in this function because it perturbs blood flow. These perturbations have been characterized in detail—they consist of two and sometimes three distinct phases. If the catheter is partially obstructing, a transient increase in blood flow is noted at the onset of injection. This effect is likely of mechanical origin and results from the transmission of the injection pressure head into the coronary circulation. This is followed by a fall in blood flow that is directly proportional to the amount of contrast agent injected. The nadir of this fall occurs early if the contrast agent is injected rapidly or late if the agent is injected slowly. The cause of this phase of diminished blood flow is multifactorial and is related to the effects of the media on red blood cell deformability as well as the intrinsic viscosity of the agents. The dominant factor appears to be due to the effect of hyperosmolarity on red blood cell shape and deformability, which in turn result in an increase in blood viscosity. Membrane

binding of contrast agents also contributes to this effect. The last phase after contrast injection is that of hyperemia. This phase is of variable magnitude, depending on the dose and type of agent, and of variable duration. It appears to be a consequence of both the hyperosmolarity of the agent as well as its secondary effects on hemodynamics, contractility, and induction of frank ischemia. The use of a power injector can ensure that these complex effects remain as systematic as possible because both dose and rate of injection can be controlled (Fig. 10–1).[22, 23] The hyperemia induced by contrast agents is generally not maximal because dilators such as adenosine and papaverine can induce much greater hyperemic responses.

Other special considerations in the evaluation of coronary dynamics are the potential deleterious effects of coronary dilators and the interaction of coronary dilators with contrast agents. Intracoronary papaverine in doses between 8 and 12 mg is currently the agent of choice for the assessment of coronary flow reserve by selective angiographic methods. Bookstein and Higgins[24] have shown in dogs that the coronary hyperemic response after a bolus injection of papaverine into a coronary artery is of the same magnitude as after a 15-second occlusion of the coronary artery. Hodgson and Williams[25] compared induction of hyperemia in humans administered papaverine and hyperosmolar contrast media and showed a twofold greater hyperemic response after papaverine. Wilson and White[26] assessed doses of 4, 8, 12, and 16 mg of intracoronary papaverine and demonstrated a maximal hyperemic response after 8 mg in most left coronary arteries and after 12 mg in all left coronary arteries. In the right coronary artery, the equivalent doses were 6 and 8 mg, respectively. The onset of maximal vasodilation after papaverine injection was around 16 seconds. It peaked and was maintained for 49 seconds on average, and the effects had nearly dissipated completely by approximately 128 seconds (Fig. 10–2). Zijlstra and colleagues[27] demonstrated excellent reproducibility of the coronary hyperemic response after administration of intracoronary papaverine. The maximal hyperemic response occurred between 24 and 37 seconds after injection, and the effects completely dissipated within 5 minutes, thus allowing repeated assessments of coronary blood flow reserve.

Intracoronary injection of papaverine appears to be a safe procedure. It is recommended that doses not exceed 12 mg for the left coronary system or 8 mg for the right coronary system. Practitioners should be aware of tran-

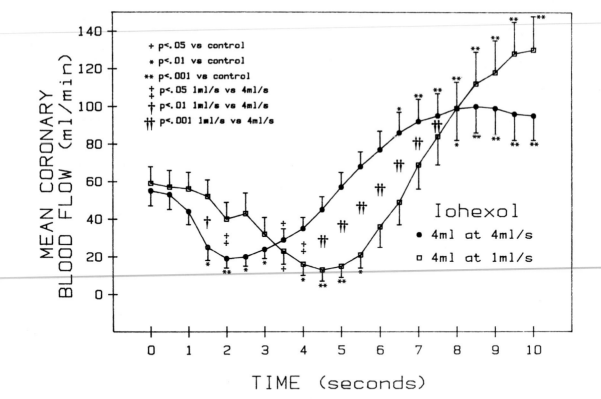

Figure 10–1. The effects of a rapid (4 mL/sec) and slow (1 mL/sec) injection of contrast material (iohexol) into the coronary artery are illustrated. The nadir occurs earlier with the more rapid injection. Hyperemia occurs subsequently and is maximal at 8 to 10 seconds. (Adapted with permission from Friedman HZ, DeBoe SF, McGillem M, Mancini GBJ: The immediate effects of iohexol on coronary blood flow and myocardial function. Circulation 1986; 74:1416–1423. Copyright 1986 American Heart Association.)

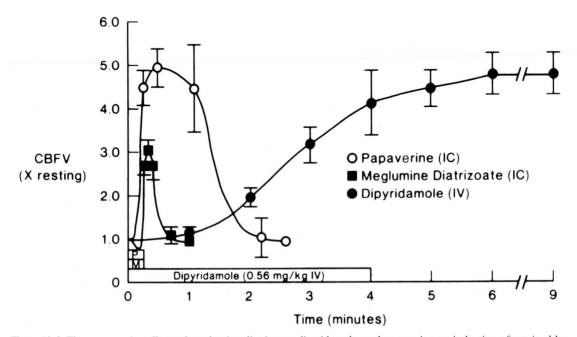

Figure 10–2. The comparative effects of meglumine diatrizoate, dipyridamole, and papaverine on induction of maximal hyperemia are illustrated. Note the submaximal hyperemia induced by the contrast agent relative to the prompt and maximal response to papaverine. CBFV, cerebral blood flow volume. (Reproduced with permission from Wilson RF, White CW: Intracoronary papaverine: An ideal coronary vasodilator for studies of the coronary circulation in conscious humans. Circulation 1986; 73:444–451. Copyright 1986 American Heart Association.)

sient ST-T changes, QT prolongation, and U wave appearance. Anecdotal reports of ventricular tachycardia and fibrillation as well as enhancement of stimulated ventricular arrhythmias have been published.[28, 29] These effects on myocardial repolarization may not be the result of subendocardial ischemia or "coronary steal" because they have been seen in normal subjects. In more than 300 cases, Wilson and White[30] demonstrated only two instances of serious ventricular dysrhythmias, and one instance occurred in a patient with normal coronary arteries.

Some contrast materials may interact with papaverine to form a potentially toxic precipitate.[31] This has not been noted with nonionic contrast material.[32] However, papaverine should not be routinely flushed into the coronary artery with solutions other than normal saline or other physiologic solutions unless drug incompatibilities have been deliberately examined and excluded.[31, 32] Adenosine is also available and is often used in preference to papaverine for assessing coronary vascular dynamics.

VENTRICULAR FUNCTION

Intravenous Ventriculography

Most of the early cardiac applications of digital angiography focused on the potential of the technique to obtain relatively noninvasive ventriculograms by intravenous contrast injection performed on an outpatient basis and in conjunction with exercise. Many groups have shown the comparability of this approach to direct ventriculography. Applications in determining ventricular volumes, ejection fractions, wall motion, and the effects of atrial pacing or exercise all show excellent results.[33–35] The advantages are that (1) arterial puncture is not required, (2) arrhythmias are not present during the left ventricular phase of contrast transit, and (3) contrast material is homogeneously dispersed and therefore the images are more readily amenable to videodensitometric analyses.

There are, however, many practical problems that far outweigh these advantages and that have diminished the enthusiasm for widespread use of the method. The chance of misregistration artifact increases because of the duration of time between the onset of intravenous contrast injection and the time of optimal left ventricular images. Moreover, large amounts of contrast agent are required to obtain adequate levophase ventriculograms. Therefore, total contrast dose can accumulate quickly and limits

the number of repeated studies that can be performed. The need for repeated injection is frequent owing to misregistration that occurs commonly with intravenous studies. Many of these concerns will dissipate when dual-energy subtraction methods become commercially available. High doses of contrast material, however, would still make the method unsuitable for use in patients with poor cardiac output, hemodynamic instability, or renal dysfunction. Injection of contrast material into peripheral veins may also lead to contrast extravasation. More central injection (subclavian vein, superior vena cava, right atrium, or pulmonary artery) leads to increased time for instrumentation and detracts from the relatively noninvasive aspect of the procedure. Finally, the availability of small-gauge catheters used in outpatient cardiac catheterization diminishes concerns about arterial puncture in most patients.

Direct Ventriculography

Direct ventriculography using low doses of contrast material is a popular application of digital angiography. This method yields diagnostically accurate images suitable for volume, ejection fraction, and wall motion analyses. Numerous laboratories have validated the use of this technique.[36] Moreover, the technique is safer in hemodynamically compromised patients because small doses of contrast agents can be used. More comprehensive study of patients is achieved by repeating ventriculography to assess orthogonal views and the effects of pacing or exercise or to calculate end-systolic pressure-volume relations.[37] These can be obtained without inordinate increases in contrast usage.

Wall Thickness and Myocardial Mass

Wall thickness and myocardial mass can be measured by radiographic means. This is time consuming and not always possible owing to poor visualization of the epicardial heart border. Digital images subjected to enhancement methods can alleviate both of these problems. Radtke and coworkers[38] developed a modified time-interval-difference image-processing method capable of demonstrating the myocardial wall so that thickening, mass, and infarct size can be measured. Grob and associates[39] also demonstrated the usefulness of digital angiography for this purpose. This laboratory has studied the method of Radtke and coworkers (Fig. 10–3) as well as simpler image-processing methods for extracting wall thickness information. Software was developed as an extension of the centerline

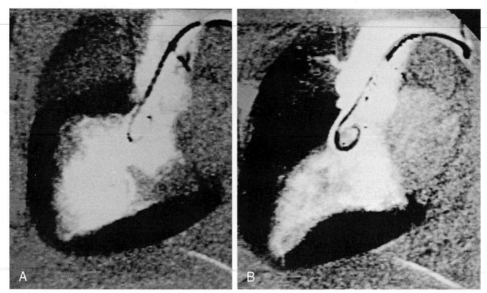

Figure 10–3. End-diastolic *(A)* and end-systolic *(B)* images of a canine heart in the left posterior oblique projection. Both endocardial and epicardial boundaries are evident and amenable to derivation of wall thickening or mass measurements.

method of wall motion analysis. This system of measuring thickening was better than wall motion methods for measuring infarct size.[40] The method was also extended to measure myocardial mass.[41] Overestimation of wall thickening is known to occur when radiographic techniques are used to measure wall thickening. This is most problematic in hypertrophic ventricles and is a result of contrast extrusion from between trabeculae at end-systole. As a result, the ratio of measures of mass from end-diastolic and end-systolic images, which should ideally give a ratio of one, generally yields a ratio of less than one. This ratio, however, can be used to uniformly rescale wall thickening values to minimize overestimation.[41]

Wall Motion Analysis

Specific methods of wall motion quantitation are discussed in Chapters 11 and 19. However, the image-processing methods of digital angiography can also be used to help visually emphasize areas of regional dysfunction. For example, by subtracting end-diastolic and end-systolic frames of a left ventricular study, an "ejection shell" image can be generated that provides a single-frame summary of overall wall motion.[42] Another application, that of phase analysis, involves encoding of the temporal characteristics of the videodensity changes in each pixel making up a ventricular study. This method gives an indication of the asynchrony of contraction induced by wall motion abnormalities.[43] Per-

haps the greatest contribution of digital angiography to wall motion assessment is the potential to automate this tedious process by applications of real-time edge-detection algorithms. If properly constructed, these algorithms can take into account the three basic features used intuitively by clinicians to assess regional function (such as motion and coordination of motion and shape), thereby making the programs robust and accurate. In an interactive way, these features can be used to derive edges and to quantitate or interpret the diagnostic content of the images. Such methods, akin to machine vision and artificial intelligence applications used in industry, are only in their infancy in cardiology but hold great promise for the future.[44]

VALVULAR DISEASE

Digital angiography has been evaluated for the study of valvular regurgitation. Bursch and Heintzen[45] have delineated several specific methods for using the videodensity and geometric image data in the calculation of regurgitant fractions (Fig. 10–4). Grayburn and colleagues[46] validated a method for calculating regurgitant fraction in dogs with aortic insufficiency. Regurgitant fraction obtained by digital time-intensity analysis was compared with that obtained by electromagnetic flow probes. Results showed good agreement over a broad range of regurgitation. Klein and coworkers[47] demonstrated that the ratio of the density of areas of interest over the left ventricle

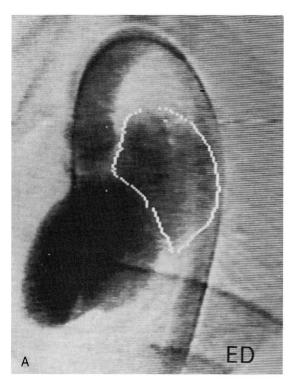 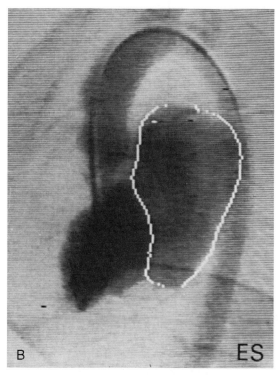

A   ED

B   ES

Figure 10–4. End-diastolic (ED) *(A)* and end-systolic (ES) *(B)* ventricular phases in a patient with mitral regurgitation. The atrium is outlined in each image, and the densitometric intensity values are quantitated to determine the regurgitant fraction. (*A* and *B* from Bursch JH, Heintzen PH: The role of digital subtraction angiography in congenital and valvular disease. *In* Mancini GBJ [ed]: Cardiac Applications of Digital Angiography. New York, Raven Press, 1988, pp 199–218.)

and the aorta at the end of injection correlated well with clinical angiographic grading of the severity of aortic regurgitation in patients.

EVALUATION OF GRAFT PATENCY

Before the availability of interventions such as angioplasty, there were limited options in a postbypass patient experiencing recurrent chest pain (such as graft revisions). Thus, methods to define graft patency alone were once highly desirable. The evaluation of graft patency by digital methods has met with some success by both the intravenous and direct arterial methods.[48] However, the performance of cine-CT is generally regarded as better than that of digital angiography. Even so, neither technique provides details of the anastomoses or the location of stenoses, and mere patency information is insufficient for the modern-day assessment of postbypass patients because mechanical recanalization of stenotic grafts is now possible. Accordingly, the most common use of digital angiography in the evaluation of such patients is as a screening procedure at the time of cardiac catheterization. The method is used to locate the ostia of the grafts when implanted markers

are absent. This is performed as a low-contrast-dose aortogram (20 to 30 mL of contrast agent) that can be used as a "roadmap" to expedite direct cannulation of the grafts or to prevent wastage of time and contrast material in seeking grafts that are actually occluded.

QUANTITATIVE CORONARY ANGIOGRAPHY

Techniques

Reiber[49] has extensively reviewed quantitative coronary arteriographic systems. Three broad categories can be defined: film-based, digital-based, and both film- and digital-based systems. The third system is particularly attractive, and its description is emphasized in this chapter. It allows the greatest flexibility in image handling. Both immediate and delayed analyses are accommodated. Films from other institutions can be analyzed, as can digital images if converted into compatible formats. If digital angiograms are obtained, then studies can be facilitated by obviating the laborious and time-consuming steps of film development and digitization. Applications in videodensitometry can be pursued more easily and without the intervening effects of film type and development methods. Perfusion imaging is also easier. Finally, until the optimal digital system is derived and as long as the existing digital systems remain marginally compatible, a combined system is a safe investment for investigators and clinicians interested in quantitative arteriography.

The parameters determined by each of the different systems are quite variable. The most common parameters include minimum diameter, reference diameter, and percentage of diameter of stenosis (percent diameter stenosis). The next most common parameters are densitometrically determined percent area stenosis and minimum area. Only a few algorithms give measures of lesion length, area (or mass) of atherosclerosis, symmetry of lesions, and calculations of theoretic, transstenotic pressure gradients or coronary flow reserve. Algorithms providing the simple geometric parameters of minimum di-

ameter and percent stenosis meet the greatest needs of clinicians and researchers. Minimum diameter measurements are also highly reproducible.[49-51] Such limited capabilities, however, severely impede the ability to quantitate more sophisticated and potentially more prognostically important parameters. This is underscored by burgeoning evidence relating the roughness of lesions to unstable angina[52] and the relation between functional measures of coronary stenosis and clinical outcome.[53] Aside from flexibility and ease of use, the most important criteria for judging specific systems relate to validation studies and actual in vivo or clinical performance. The development of the University of Michigan system is profoundly influenced by this philosophy, and extensive validation efforts have been performed (Figs. 10–5 and 10–6). However, as emphasized by Reiber[49] and Herrington and associates,[54] validation of different systems is quite variable, and the parameters in the reports are

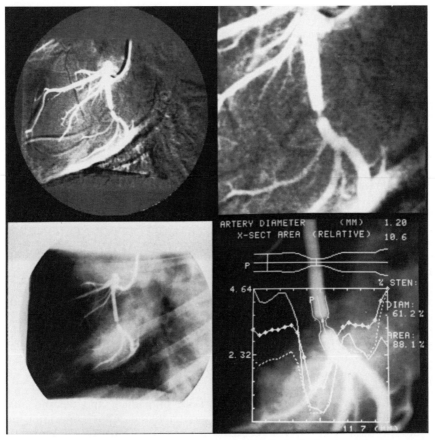

Figure 10–5. Coronary arteriograms obtained in a dog with a stenosing cylinder in the circumflex artery. The upper panels are mask-mode subtracted; the lower panels are original digital images. The right-hand panels are magnified by a factor of 4. Quantitation is shown in the overlay in the bottom right panel. Separate curves plot diameter, geometric area, and videodensitometric profiles against lesion length (abscissa). (Reproduced with permission from Mancini GBJ, Simon SB, McGillem MJ, et al: Automated quantitative coronary arteriography: Morphologic and physiologic validation in vivo of a rapid digital angiographic method. Circulation 1987; 75:452–460. Copyright 1987 American Heart Association.)

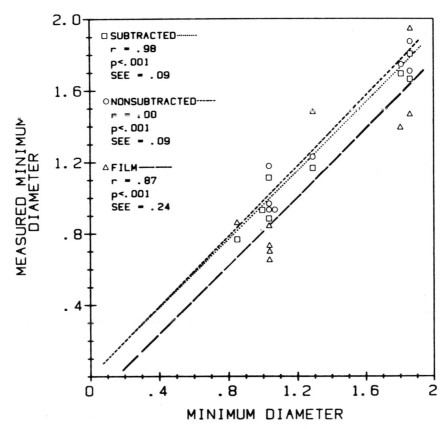

Figure 10–6. Actual (abscissa) versus measured (ordinate) diameter of stenosis in millimeters. All image types (film, digital subtracted, digital nonsubtracted) are shown. (Reproduced with permission from Mancini GBJ, Simon SB, McGillem MJ, et al: Automated quantitative coronary arteriography: Morphologic and physiologic validation in vivo of a rapid digital angiographic method. Circulation 1987; 75:452–460. Copyright 1987 American Heart Association.)

disparate enough to make head-to-head comparisons almost impossible.

Parameters

Percent Diameter Stenosis

Percent diameter stenosis is the most commonly used clinical parameter. Although conceptually simple, diffuse atherosclerosis may invalidate the accuracy of the reference segment, thereby causing an underestimation of hemodynamic severity. The presence of obvious or subtle proximal ectasia also adds ambiguity to the validity of the reference measurement.[55] Moreover, the reproducibility of the measurement is largely dependent on the specific method of deriving the reference segment value. Measures made at a single point are difficult to reproduce except in the most uniform of prestenotic, arterial segments. Measures averaged over longer lengths overcome some of this variability. Another approach is to statistically determine the reference dimension as some percentile of the diameter measurements obtained over specified lengths of the prestenotic and poststenotic areas. This method gives an interpolation of edges intended to estimate the original luminal diameter before occurrence of the atherosclerotic process. The percent diameter stenosis is then calculated from the minimum diameter and the interpolated normal diameter at this specific point. This approach is less user dependent, but it is only applicable if the distal segment is free of disease and if branches are adequately handled by the edge-detection algorithm.[49]

Geometric Calculation of Minimum Area and Percent Area Stenosis

Stenoses are seldom of simple geometric configuration. Single-plane analyses are applied to the view showing the most stenotic aspect of the lesion. To calculate percent area stenosis by geometric means, another view is used to determine the major axis of the stenosis on the presumption that it is elliptical. There are several difficulties with this approach. An elliptical configuration is an approximation or assumption. Truly orthogonal views are difficult to obtain, especially without foreshortening or overlap of other vessels. Spears and associates[56] have shown that one must examine many views to be certain that the true minor and major axes of an ellipse are identified. Almost all of the errors affecting quantitation (such as motion blurring and limited resolution) tend to cause overestimations of diameters. This systematic error is then compounded in the biplane calculation. The maximal stenosis in each view is presumed to be located at the same area, and this may also be erroneous. Consequently, biplane analyses of lesions may be quite difficult. Some groups use biplane images and average the results from each view. This still leads to a systematic increase in stenotic area or a decrease in percent stenosis compared with single-plane analyses. Therefore, for most clinical and research purposes, the single view, obtained from *many*, showing the most severe narrowing should probably be used for quantitative purposes. As a result, serial or comparative studies must be performed in the same angiographic projection. For assessment of progression of coronary disease, Ellis and coworkers[51] have shown that the best variability characteristics are achieved with minimum diameter measures and mean diameter measures. The latter showed the smaller standard deviation.

Videodensitometric Calculation of Minimum Area and Percent Area Stenosis

The pitfalls in determining minimum area and percent area stenosis outlined in the previous section provide strong impetus for developing accurate videodensitometric methods that provide rotationally invariant results. Such methods, however, are currently not robust enough for use in practice, although meticulous research applications are feasible. Digital angiography is particularly suited to this application because the complex image preprocessing required to linearize the relation between contrast depth and x-ray transmission can be easily implemented. Such applications, however, are few, and there are residual limitations of current techniques.

Wiesel and associates[57] evaluated a combined geometric and videodensitometric approach for measuring stenoses created in dogs. They used edge detection applied to the normal segment and videodensitometry applied to the stenosis to determine the absolute luminal cross-sectional area. Relatively few stenoses were imaged, and the minority were truly irregular.

There was a moderate correlation between known lesion area and the combined edge detection–videodensity approach ($r = 0.76$; SE = 0.71 mm^2; absolute area deviation = 0.65 mm^2).

Tobis and coworkers[58] studied 19 patients before and after percutaneous transluminal coronary angioplasty (PTCA). They compared geometric and videodensitometric stenosis measurements obtained from digital angiograms. Although intimal tears and dissections are expected to make edge-detection methods inaccurate after angioplasty, in fact, the mean stenosis measurements by either technique were the same. Interobserver variability was similar in each method. Since videodensitometry should, in theory, provide a rotationally invariant assessment of percent stenosis, they also compared results from orthogonal views of single lesions. Although the densitometry showed a good correlation of results, the edge-detection methodology was no worse. There was, therefore, no apparent added value of densitometry in this clinical application.

Sanz and colleagues[50] analyzed 13 consecutively acquired, unselected, biplane digital subtraction angiograms before and after PTCA. In both instances measures of absolute diameter showed less interobserver variability than densitometry or percent automated diameter stenosis measurements. In these routinely acquired clinical images, relative videodensitometric cross-sectional area correlated poorly with images from the orthogonal view.

Skelton and coworkers[59] undertook a large clinical study of 100 discrete lesions in 45 patients. Comparisons were made among direct on-line digital, ECG-gated digital subtraction and digitized cinefilm images. Videodensitometric percent area stenosis data showed correlation coefficients among the different modalities between 0.80 to 0.89. These correlations were less and the apparent variability was greater than for similar comparisons of geometric measurements. No real gold standard was available to evaluate the significance of these results, but the investigators pointed out that many more factors contribute to nonlinearity of contrast concentration of cineangiograms than of on-line digital images. Other experience suggests that the inferior relation between film-derived and on-line digital-derived videodensitometric measurements is a result of larger errors in the film-derived data.[4, 60, 61]

Katritsis and coworkers[62] studied 73 lesions in 63 patients who had undergone coronary angioplasty. Digital subtraction coronary angiograms were analyzed with an automated border-detecting computer program capable of simultaneous geometric and densitometric cross-sectional area estimation. They showed good agreement between geometric and densitometric percent area stenoses on the pre-PTCA digital angiograms. After PTCA, however, important discrepancies existed. Densitometric evaluation demonstrated a significantly greater mean coefficient of variation between different views after PTCA but not before. This degree of variation was much larger than noted for geometric evaluations on the same views. The results are similar to those demonstrated by Sanz and associates,[50] except that the deficiencies in densitometry from different views was limited only to the post-PTCA analyses. Although the distortion of the vessel lumen after angioplasty is assumed to render geometric methods potentially inaccurate, the altered geometry after angioplasty cannot fully explain the results of Katritsis and coworkers[62] because no excess variability was noted for geometric measurements before or after angioplasty. The authors postulated that distortion of the vessel as a result of angioplasty may have interfered with the mixing of contrast medium and blood, hence invalidating any assumptions about uniform dye distribution and thereby also invalidating densitometry measurements. Further studies are required to more fully elucidate these practical problems.

Johnson and associates[63] have compared intraluminal echocardiography with quantitative arteriography to assist in validation of area measurements by videodensitometry. Integrated optical density correlated well with echocardio-graphically determined cross-sectional area measurements when both circular and complex lesions were studied in nonforeshortened views. This is important confirmatory evidence of the potential of videodensitometry in clinical practice. It is an innovative and direct method of validating the accuracy of the procedure.

These results, although generally promising, are quite different from the excellent results noted almost routinely in phantom studies or in studies using highly selected images demonstrating optimal background conditions, meticulous density calibrations to ensure linearity, and absence of foreshortening of either normal or stenotic segments. In biplane images, one must be confident that the long axis of the lesion and normal segments is parallel to the image-intensifier planes and perpendicular to the x-ray beams. This "triple orthogonality" can be achieved in new-generation catheterization laboratories,[64] and the process can be automated substantially in digital catheterization laboratories[65] (Fig. 10–7). At this point, it is believed that the role of videodensitometry should be in rapid calculation of relative cross-sectional areas in a single view, and if repeated studies are anticipated, then the same view must be used to avoid large errors due to potential differences in foreshortening, background, veiling glare, and scatter. Accordingly, substantially increased efforts are required before robust methods are devised that will allow for successful and rapid clinical application of videodensi-

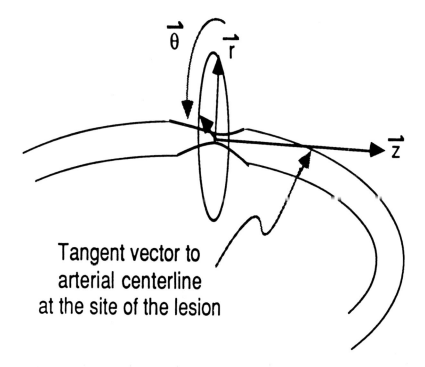

Figure 10–7. Schematic representation of the optimal orientation of a lesion within an imaging plane to achieve "triple orthogonality," a prerequisite for accurate geometric and videodensitometric quantitation. The long axis of the lesion is in the direction of Z and remains so throughout the revolution described by r and θ. Gantries of a biplane system should be located on the circle through the lesion defined by the coordinate system shown to provide optimal images. (From Sitomer J, LeFree MT, Anselmo EG, et al: Computer image–guided gantry positioning for optimization of quantitative coronary arteriography. Am J Card Imaging 1989; 3:191–198.)

tometric techniques even with on-line digital images.

Integrated Indices of Stenosis Severity

The goal of the approach of integrated indices of stenosis severity (lesion resistance and theoretic "stenosis" flow reserve) is to help translate morphologic features into physiologic variables that demonstrate the hemodynamic significance of the lesions. These attempts allow comparisons of the theoretic, physiologic significance of different lesions under standardized conditions. Consequently, the calculations are based on assumed and fixed values of flow, driving pressure, distal pressure, and blood viscosity. They disregard potential differences in the status of the perfusion bed (such as hypertrophy) or distal vasculature. The most extensive of these approaches is the component analysis model proposed by Kirkeeide and colleagues[66] in which measures of normal and stenotic vessel area as well as length and entrance and exit angles can be combined to calculate a theoretic flow reserve (stenosis flow reserve). This approach is attractive because actual measures of flow reserve are subject to numerous factors that can make the interpretation of single measures ambiguous.[67–69] The caveat is that one must recognize the theoretic nature of the predictions that are designed only for comparing stenoses by taking into account all of their important morphologic characteristics. The component analysis method, for example, determines a totally normal theoretic flow reserve in a patient with mild morphologic coronary disease and aortic stenosis, whereas an actual measure of flow reserve may well show substantive impairment in such a patient.[70] Therefore, the derived measures of stenosis flow reserve are likely to be of prognostic importance only to the extent that the underlying presumptions mimic the true, prevailing parameters in an individual patient.

Comparability of Film and Digital Coronary Angiograms

Controversy exists regarding the suitability of digital images as replacement for film. Tobis and coworkers[71] reported a study in which different observers independently identified and measured focal coronary narrowings using digital subtraction angiograms and standard 35mm cineangiograms. The digital angiograms consisted of a $512 \times 512 \times 8$-bit pixel matrix. Owing to rapid evolution of digital hardware and software at that time, the study was undertaken in two parts. In phase 1 of the study, 38 patients (35 with interpretable studies without misregistration artifacts) were studied with continuous fluoroscopic exposures and an interlaced camera readout of 30 frames/sec. Images were subjected to subtraction using a blurred mask and then converted back to videotape. Two observers analyzed both these images with manually operated calipers. Results within 10% were considered equivalent; otherwise, results from the digital images were described as overestimating or underestimating the cineangiographic results used as the reference standard. The results agreed within 10% in 76% of cases. Underestimation by the digital technique occurred in 18% and overestimation in 6% of cases. Although these results were quite favorable, it was believed that the overall quality of film was better because the image acquisition parameters and processing methods resulted in substantial noise in the video images.

In phase 2, 19 patients were studied with more advanced techniques. Pulsed radiographic mode and a progressive scan camera were used. In addition, only a single-frame mask was used, and the observers were allowed to use an edge-enhancement algorithm and a $\times 4$ magnification algorithm. Four observers quantitated the paired cineangiograms and digital angiograms, again using hand-held calipers. The results showed no significant difference in the mean percent diameter narrowing (53% $\pm$ 31% versus 52% $\pm$ 31%, digital versus film, respectively). No difference in variability of measurements between the two methods could be detected. In two patients, unsubtracted images were used because of excessive subtraction artifact. It was apparent that even when the digital images were suboptimally processed by older methodologies, the digitally based quantitations compared quite favorably to the film-based results. This study suggested, however, that at least in some patients, misregistration continued to be a problem and that fluoroscopic exposure levels and interlaced camera readout were not optimal for digital applications in coronary quantitation.

Bray and associates[72] analyzed 32 lesions in 15 patients using the technique of high-pass temporal filtration digital subtraction. An interlaced camera readout and radiographic exposure levels were used. A $480 \times 792 \times 8$-bit image matrix and a framing rate of 30 Hz were used. Standard 35mm cineangiograms were acquired simultaneously. Three observers using calipers analyzed the image sets, and the overall results demonstrated a correlation coefficient of 0.73 with an SEE of 9.1% diameter stenosis. The average severity (49% for film images and 47%

for digital images) and the variability of the measurements (average standard deviation for film of 6.6% and for digital of 7.7%) were indistinguishable. Twenty-eight percent of measurements were more than 10% different between methods, and 5% were more than 20% different. This variability was substantially reduced when multiple observations were averaged and then compared. Thus, for routine quantitation, this study was unable to demonstrate any striking loss of clinical information when digital imaging was compared with cineangiography. The study also confirms the merits of radiographic exposure levels. The authors suggest that progressive camera readout for such applications would improve results further.

Vas and colleagues[73] analyzed 36 coronary stenoses by three methods: visual interpretation of a single cineangiographic image, visual interpretation of a digital angiographic image ($512 \times 512 \times 8$-bit matrix, nonenhanced, nonfiltered, and nonmagnified), and quantitation using a digital caliper system ($\times 2$ magnification). Radiographic exposure levels were used, but the use of progressive or interlaced readout was not mentioned. No differences in the average percent diameter stenosis measurements were found (visual film analysis = 59.1% ± 22.7%; visual digital analysis = 60.8% ± 25.6%; caliper quantitation = 55.5% ± 21.3%). Overall image quality was judged to be at least as good as the film. Results demonstrated no significant adverse effects on the perception and quantification of stenoses. Overall, the digital calipers improved intraobserver and interobserver reproducibility. Visual interpretation of both film and digital images overestimated the caliper results, especially in the 50% to 75% diameter stenosis range. The mean standard deviations of visual film analysis (12.6%) and digital analysis (10.7%) were equal but higher than for caliper analysis (3.8%). When the four angiographers used the caliper method, they agreed within 10% diameter stenosis on all readings, whereas substantially poorer agreement occurred with visual interpretation, irrespective of the type of image. Thus, using an improved electronic caliper method, nonsubtracted images, and radiographic exposure levels, digital images were comparable with film images in providing quantitative information.

Goldberg and coworkers[74] studied a total of 77 patients with mask mode, $512 \times 512 \times 8$-bit, 30-frame/sec digital angiography using boosted fluoroscopy (i.e., the tube current was between fluoroscopic levels and full radiographic levels and ranged between 10 and 30 mA). Single views were compared with standard cineangiog-

raphy in 27 patients (95 arteries). Two angiograms agreed with visual assessment within one grade of severity in 84% of cases, including comparisons of normal segments. Multiple-view digital angiograms were compared in 50 patients (144 arteries), and visual agreement within one grade occurred in 90%, including normal segments. The film images were acquired using magnification mode, whereas digital images were acquired in a 9-inch mode so that the entire coronary tree could be seen without panning to avoid misregistration artifact during subtraction. Use of the 9-inch mode has the effect of yielding a larger pixel size in the digital images, but despite this bias, the comparisons were quite favorable. Moreover, the investigators noted that 95% of collateralized vessels on film images were also noted on the digital angiograms. The grading of the collateral vessels agreed in 81% of instances with the cine assessment. As in the other studies, misregistration in several cases precluded analysis. Because only boosted fluorography was used, the authors believed that mask subtraction was mandatory to provide sufficient contrast resolution. One can conclude from this study that for practical purposes, the visual interpretation of coronary stenoses is quite comparable whether film or digital imaging is used.

Skelton and associates[59] examined the effects of digital image acquisition mode and subtraction techniques on the quantitation of coronary stenosis involving 100 discrete lesions in 45 patients. Each lesion was assessed from direct on-line digital, ECG-gated digital subtraction and digitized cinefilm images. Geometric measures of percent diameter stenosis and minimum lesion diameter showed correlations between 0.90 and 0.98, with slopes between 0.93 and 1.00. Thus, the measurements were not strongly affected by image-acquisition mode or by ECG-gated digital subtraction. These geometrically derived results were superior to similar comparisons using videodensitometric techniques.

Gurley and colleagues[1] recently compared unprocessed digital angiograms and conventional cineangiograms for the diagnosis and quantification of coronary stenoses in both phantoms and clinical subjects. In contrast with the prior study, this group used unmagnified, 512×512 digital images and caliper quantification of the stenoses. The effects of image subtraction were not assessed, and absolute minimum diameter measurements were not made. Additionally, the two images were acquired simultaneously such that 85% of the image-intensifier light intensity was used to expose film, and only 15% of the light intensity was used to generate the digital image. Even under these conditions, phantom studies showed no differences in performance between digital and film imaging. In analysis of patient images, the overall interobserver variability was also equivalent. However, the authors noted that digital evaluation of percent stenosis in patients generally overestimated film results and that this overestimation was progressively more severe with milder lesions, lesions in vessels less than 2 mm in diameter, and branch stenoses. This study underscores the need for each laboratory to ascertain the equivalence of the two imaging techniques under the specific or likely conditions of use. For the most part, the lack of automated quantitation, the failure to use image magnification, and the diminution in light source for the generation of digital images were strong biases against the digital imaging technique.

The reviewed studies suggest that analysis of digital- and film-based coronary angiograms is essentially equivalent when several factors are taken into account. In my experience, subtracted images yield results of equivalent precision but with slightly higher interobserver and intraobserver variability even when gross misregistration is not evident. This increase is believed to be due to increased image noise and the potential presence of subtraction artifacts in mask mode processed arteriograms. Therefore, my laboratory does not recommend clinical use of subtraction techniques for coronary arteriography.

Although film-based radiography has a high theoretic resolution, attainment of this in clinical circumstances is prevented by several factors. The difference in attenuation coefficients between iodinated contrast medium and tissue is not great and may perturb edge detection in areas with significant variations in background density. The usual measurement of the resolving power of a system by using tungsten wires or lead strips does not truly reflect the much poorer object contrast in coronary angiograms. Moreover, the usable spatial resolution of film, considering the physical properties of cesium iodide image intensifiers, the effects of the main objective lens in the image distributor and the cinecamera optics, is markedly deteriorated from the theoretic intrinsic resolution of cinefilm. The usable spatial resolution of film is approached by that of a high-quality video pickup tube. A second major factor is that the automated edge-detection scheme used in the investigation by my colleagues and myself was optimized for the noise frequency of digital images. It should also be recognized that the reported investigations used different imaging systems, film types, and processing methods. Different processing systems and film types may alter the accuracy compared with digital images. Thus, the small differences shown in some studies may not apply under all circumstances and in all laboratories, as evidenced by the work of Skelton and colleagues[59] and Gurley and associates.[1] Moreover, in spite of these differences, the relation between commonly measured parameters of coronary stenosis and reactive hyperemia have been shown to be equivalent among modalities, suggesting that no major differences of physiologic importance are present.[75]

All of the studies described earlier used digital images with a matrix density no greater than 512×512. Meticulous studies using a matrix density of 1024×1024 have failed to demonstrate any substantive improvement in quantitative accuracy when used in currently available x-ray systems.[4, 5]

The following summarizes the information in this section:

1. A definite advantage of film-based imaging over digital imaging using a 512×512 matrix size when fully automated quantitation is performed has not been shown.

2. A definite advantage of 1024×1024 digital image matrix size has not been shown.

3. Subtracted images in clinical subjects are vulnerable to misregistration artifacts and cannot be recommended for quantitative analyses.

4. Because nearly all sources of error (motion unsharpness, limited spatial resolution, oblique orientation of the vessel with respect to the x-ray beam, geometric magnification) serve to cause overestimates in actual luminal dimensions, and because truly orthogonal views are difficult to achieve clinically, a strong case can be made for assessing minimal luminal diameters in a view showing the lesion to its best advantage.

5. When serial studies are anticipated, the view must be reproduced as closely as possible.

6. Radiographic exposure levels and progressive scan readout are needed to maximize signal-to-noise ratios and minimize motion blurring.

7. Full contrast doses are needed so that opacification is optimal.

8. Framing rates not less than 10 Hz are required to provide a sufficient number of frames for delineation of lesions.

9. The catheter and stenosis should be as close as possible to the central portion of the image field to reduce the effects of pin-cushion

distortion when quantitation is to be undertaken.

10. Fully automated and quantitative programs applied to magnified digital images yield results that are comparable to film-based analyses.

CORONARY FLOW RESERVE

Methods

The methods proposed for the measurement of coronary flow reserve can be categorized by the theory on which they are based. There are five basic methods based on analysis: (1) transit time[76, 77]; (2) indicator-dilution curves[21]; (3) washout curves[78]; (4) transfer functions[79]; and (5) combined appearance, time, and density curves.[80] A comprehensive comparison of these techniques can be found in other work.[81] This section concentrates on the method based on appearance, time, and density data because the bulk of the clinical applications has been undertaken with it.

This approach was developed empirically at the University of Michigan in two distinct stages. The first phase explored the concept that appearance of contrast agent in the myocardium was inversely proportional to flow.[11] It is an outgrowth of the transit time method, but it avoided the disadvantage of requiring potentially inaccurate geometric calculations of arterial segments. Additionally, it was geared toward measurement of relative, not absolute, flow; did not require high temporal resolution or precise dosages of contrast; and did not require subselective injection of contrast medium. Finally, the early phase of contrast washin was analyzed to avoid the potential problems inherent in washout analyses that may coincide with the time when flow has been substantially perturbed by contrast material. The results with this early approach showed good correlation with measures of coronary sinus and great cardiac vein flow in patients in whom variations in flow were induced with atrial pacing.[82] Some degree of underestimation of flow ratios was noted. This underestimation was substantial in the second phase of study, which involved studies of animals and alteration of coronary flow by papaverine or contrast material instead of atrial pacing.[80] Hodgson and coworkers[80] highlighted the potential importance of the density information in helping to rectify the problem of underestimation. In addition, to compensate for uncertainties in timing due to the limited temporal resolution of the images (one per cycle), ECG-gated contrast injections were used and appearance times were assigned as 0.5, 1.5, 2.5, and so forth, for each consecutive cardiac cycle after contrast injection. Whenever heart rate stability could not be maintained by atrial pacing, then cycle length appearance times were converted to absolute seconds. Using these empiric approaches, Hodgson and coworkers[80] demonstrated a marked improvement over the previous method based solely on appearance times. A strong linear correlation with simultaneously measured electromagnetic flow was demonstrated in the animal model. These results have been confirmed and further refined by Cusma and associates.[20] More recent validation studies using tracer-labeled microspheres show that although the imaging method does correlate with true perfusion measures, some underestimation of high-flow states and significant variability can occur.[83] Thus, the method is most suitable for applications wherein large serial differences are expected[84] or wherein large differences between populations are expected (such as patients with or without positive exercise tests) (Fig. 10–8; see also the color section).[53]

Comparisons with Stress Testing and Quantitative Arteriography

Legrand and coworkers[53] undertook a comparative study of flow reserve, quantitative percent stenosis, and exercise test measurements in patients with coronary disease. Two broad groups were investigated—those with and those without prior infarction, collateralized zones, or both. In patients without prior infarction or collateral vessels, a rough correlation between percent stenosis measurement and flow reserve values was found. There was strong concordance among exercise-induced regional wall motion abnormalities or thallium defects, percent diameter stenosis greater than 50% in the artery serving that region, and flow reserve values of less than 2 measured by contrast-induced hyperemia and digital angiography. Strongest concordance was noted with very severe (>75%) and very mild (<25%) stenoses. The clinical diagnostic value of the flow reserve and exercise test results was greatest in determining the functional significance of the intermediate grade lesions, especially when single-vessel disease was present. In the presence of multivessel disease, the exercise test results tended to reflect congruity only with the vascular bed showing the most severely depressed flow reserve, percent stenosis, or both.

In the setting of prior infarction, collateral

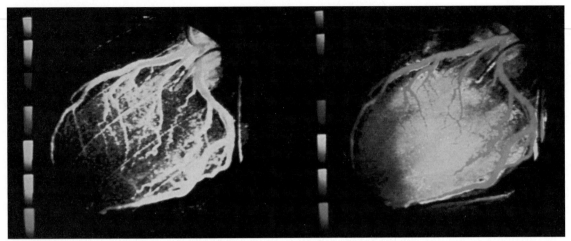

Figure 10–8. Color-coded and intensity-modulated parametric image from a patient with normal coronary flow reserve. Colors encode temporal characteristics of the contrast medium bolus (contrast medium appearance in first cycle = red, second cycle = yellow, etc.). Intensity reflects the amount of contrast medium (and flow) in the myocardium. The left panel depicts flow at rest. The right panel was obtained after intracoronary injection of papaverine to induce maximal hyperemia. (See also color section.)

flow, or both, there was a significant relation between abnormal exercise test results and stenoses greater than 50%. Coronary flow reserve measurements, however, tended to be extremely low and therefore less well correlated with percent diameter stenosis. Moreover, the exercise-induced regional abnormalities were associated with lower flow reserve values (<1.3) than in the group without infarction or collaterals.

These studies underscore the value of coronary flow reserve measurements in assessing the true significance of moderate stenoses and the caution required when evaluating the meaning of isolated flow reserve measurements in the presence of prior infarction or collateralization.

Hodgson and coworkers[84] determined flow reserve before and after angioplasty in 20 patients with single-vessel disease. Using papaverine as the hyperemic stimulus, they demonstrated a doubling of the flow reserve value after the procedure that was of a similar magnitude in adjacent, nonstenotic, and nondilated arteries. The flow reserve in these arteries, however, was decidedly less than that measured by the same technique in totally normal subjects. This finding may result from the presence of unrecognized coronary disease in angiographically normal coronary arteries of patients with focal lesions in other beds.

Bates and Mancini and others[85–87] used digital angiography to assess the adequacy of bypass grafts soon and late after surgery. Immediate and sustained improvements were measured that were equivalent to results achieved by angioplasty, but flow reserve measurements were

still depressed relative to normal values. It possibly reflects residual, diffuse atherosclerosis, alterations of adrenergic tone, arteriolar intimal thickening and fibrosis, or chronic microembolization of platelet aggregates. Hodgson and colleagues[88] compared the flow reserve of sequential internal mammary bypass grafts with that of sequential and single saphenous vein grafts. All results were comparable but, overall, the values achieved were less than flow reserve values typical of totally normal patients, a finding similar to that of Bates and colleagues.

CONCLUSIONS

This chapter summarizes the methods of digital angiography that are used in modern-day cardiology practice and those that are being refined for potential daily use. Whether digital methods will ultimately usurp the traditional film-based angiographic methods remains to be determined, but clinical needs, technologic advances, and sophistication in therapeutic options within the catheterization laboratory appear to be causing an inexorable, but slow, movement in that direction.

REFERENCES

1. Gurley JC, Nissen SE, Booth DC, et al: Comparison of simultaneously performed digital- and film-based angiography in assessment of coronary artery disease. Circulation 1988; 78:1411.
2. Brennecke R: Physics and instrumentation for digital angiocardiography. *In* Mancini GBJ (ed): Clinical Appli-

Digital Cardiac Angiography   **197**

cations of Cardiac Digital Angiography. New York, Raven Press, 1988, pp 3–18.

3. Kruger RA: A comparative summary of image processing methods in digital angiography. *In* Mancini GBJ (ed): Clinical Applications of Cardiac Digital Angiography. New York, Raven Press, 1988, pp 19–36.

4. LeFree MT, Simon SB, Mancini GBJ, et al: A comparison of 35mm cinefilm and digital radiographic image recording: Implications for quantitative arteriography. Invest Radiol 1988; 73:176–183.

5. Gomes AS, Papin PJ, Mankovich NJ, Lois JF: Digital subtraction angiography: A comparison of 512^2 and 1024^2 imaging. AJR Am J Roentgenol 1986; 146:853–858.

6. Whiting JS, Eigler NL, Pfaff JM, et al: Improved angiographic detection of coronary morphology in spatially filtered images [abstract]. Circulation 1988; 80:II-356.

7. Gurley JC, Nissen SE, Haynie D, et al: Does computer-based edge enhancement alter the interpretation of digital coronary arteriograms? J Am Coll Cardiol 1990; 15:83A.

8. Kavanaugh K, Pinto IMF, McGillem MJ, et al: The effects of video frame averaging, smoothing, and edge enhancement algorithms on the accuracy and precision of quantitative coronary arteriography. Int J Card Imaging 1990; 5:233–239.

9. Riederer SJ, Kruger RA: Intravenous digital subtraction: A summary of recent developments. Radiology 1983; 147:633–638.

10. Mancini GBJ, Higgins CB: Digital subtraction angiography: A review of cardiac applications. Prog Cardiovasc Dis 1985; 18:111.

11. Vogel R, LeFree M, Bates E, et al: Application of digital techniques to selective coronary arteriography: Use of myocardial contrast appearance time to measure coronary flow reserve. Am Heart J 1984; 107:153–164.

12. Mancini GBJ, McGillem MJ, Pinto IMF, et al: Validation of a new method for measuring wall thickening and myocardial mass from digital angiograms. Circulation 1988; 78:II-64.

13. Birchler B, Hess OM, Murakami T, et al: Comparison of intravenous digital subtraction cineangiography with conventional contrast ventriculography for the determination of the left ventricular volume at rest and during exercise. Am Heart J 1985; 6:497.

14. Van Lysel MS, Ergun DL, Miller WP, et al: Cardiac digital angiography and dual-energy subtraction imaging: Current and future trends. Am J Card Imaging 1987; 1:254–266.

15. Cox GG, Dwyer SJ: Archiving digital formatted image data. *In* Mancini GBJ (ed): Clinical Applications of Cardiac Digital Angiography. New York, Raven Press, 1988, pp 37–54.

16. Weiss M, Bellotti J, Whiting J, et al: Staggered acquisition: Improved coronary angiographic images at lower x-ray dose. Circulation 1983; 70(Suppl II):II-325.

17. Brennecke R: Digital imaging systems for coronary angiography. *In* Reiber JHC, Serruys PW (eds): New Developments in Quantitative Coronary Arteriography. Dordrecht, The Netherlands, Kluwer Academic, 1988, pp 1–12.

18. Don C: The future of radiography: Cassetteless or filmless? J Can Assoc Radiol 1988; 39:83–90.

19. Gurley JC, Nissen SE, Booth DC, et al: Cine-film replacement: Application of real-time digital cassette tape to coronary arteriography. J Am Coll Cardiol 1990; 15:83A.

20. Cusma JT, Toggart EJ, Folts JD, et al: Digital subtraction angiographic imaging of coronary flow reserve. Circulation 1987; 75:461–472.

21. Nissen SE, Elion JL, Booth DC, et al: Value and limitations of computer analysis of digital subtraction angiog-

raphy in the assessment of coronary flow reserve. Circulation 1986; 73:562–571.

22. Friedman HZ, DeBoe SF, McGillem M, Mancini GBJ: The immediate effects of iohexol on coronary blood flow and myocardial function. Circulation 1986; 74:1416–1423.

23. Friedman HZ, DeBoe SF, McGillem MJ, Mancini GBJ: Immediate effects of graded ionic and nonionic contrast injections on coronary blood flow and myocardial function: Implications for digital coronary angiography. Invest Radiol 1987; 22:722–727.

24. Bookstein JJ, Higgins CB: Comparative efficacy of coronary vasodilatory methods. Invest Radiol 1977; 12:121–128.

25. Hodgson JM, Williams DO: Superiority of intracoronary papaverine to radiographic contrast for measuring coronary flow reserve in patients with ischemic heart disease. Circulation 1985; 72:III-453.

26. Wilson RF, White CW: Intracoronary papaverine: An ideal coronary vasodilator for studies of the coronary circulation in conscious humans. Circulation 1986; 73:444–451.

27. Zijlstra F, Serruys PW, Hugenholtz PG: Papaverine: The ideal coronary vasodilator for investigating coronary flow reserve? A study of timing, magnitude, reproducibility and safety of the coronary hyperemic response after intracoronary papaverine. Cathet Cardiovasc Diag 1986; 12:298–303.

28. Lindner E, Katz LN: Papaverine hydrochloride and ventricular fibrillation. Am J Physiol 1941; 133:155.

29. Mahomed Y, Moorthy SS, Brown JW, King RD: ECG changes with papaverine injection into coronary artery bypass grafts. Anesthesiology 1984; 61:350.

30. Wilson RF, White CW: Serious ventricular dysrhythmias after intracoronary papaverine. Am J Cardiol 1988; 62:1301–1302.

31. Pilla TJ, Beshany SE, Shields JB: Incompatibility of Hexabrix and papaverine. AJR Am J Roentgenol 1986; 146:1300–1301.

32. Mancini GBJ, McGillem MJ: Papaverine as a coronary vasodilator. AJR Am J Roentgenol 1986; 147:1095–1096.

33. Norris SL, Slutsky RA, Mancini GBJ, et al: Comparison of digital intravenous ventriculography with direct left ventriculography for quantitation of left ventricular volumes and ejection fractions. Am J Cardiol 1983; 51:1399–1403.

34. Mancini GBJ, Norris SL, Peterson KL, et al: Quantitative assessment of segmental wall motion abnormalities at rest and after atrial pacing using digital intravenous ventriculography. J Am Coll Cardiol 1983; 2:70–76.

35. Goldberg HL, Moses JW, Borer JS, et al: Exercise left ventriculography utilizing intravenous digital angiography. J Am Coll Cardiol 1983; 2:1092–1098.

36. Mancini GBJ, Hodgson JM, Legrand V, et al: Quantitative assessment of global and regional ventricular function with low-contrast dose digital subtraction ventriculography. Chest 1985; 87:598–602.

37. Starling MR, Mancini GBJ: The end systolic pressure volume relationship: Current concepts and the role of imaging in its calculation. *In* Mancini GBJ (ed): Cardiac Applications of Digital Angiography. New York, Raven Press, 1988, pp 143–168.

38. Radtke W, Bürsch JH, Brennecke R, et al: Assessment of left ventricular muscle volume by digital angiocardiography. Invest Radiol 1983; 18:149–154.

39. Grob D, Hess OM, Monrad E, et al: Determination of left ventricular wall thickness and muscle mass by intravenous digital subtraction angiocardiography: Validation of the method. Eur Heart J 1988; 9:73–86.

40. McGillem MJ, Mancini GBJ, DeBoe SF, Buda AJ: Modification of the centerline method for assessment of

echocardiographic wall thickening and motion: A comparison with areas of risk. J Am Coll Cardiol 1988; 11:861–866.

41. McGillem MJ, Pinto IMF, Mancini GBJ: Determination of wall thickening and myocardial mass by digital ventriculography. Am J Card Imaging 1989; 3:244–252.

42. Gerber KH, Slutsky RA, Ashburn WL, et al: Detection and assessment of severity of regional ischemic left ventricular dysfunction by digital fluoroscopy. Am Heart J 1982; 104:27–35.

43. Lyons J, Norell M, Gardner J, et al: Phase and amplitude analysis of exercise digital left ventriculograms in patients with coronary disease. Br Heart J 1989; 62: 102–111.

44. Tehrani S, Weymouth TE, Mancini GBJ: Knowledge-guided left ventricular boundary detection. Proceedings of Applications of Artificial Intelligence VII. SPIE Technical Symposium on Aerospace Sensing, Orlando, 1989, pp 503–514.

45. Bursch JH, Heintzen PH: The role of digital subtraction angiography in congenital and valvular disease. In Mancini GBJ (ed): Cardiac Applications of Digital Angiography. New York, Raven Press, 1988, pp 199–218.

46. Grayburn PA, Smith MD, Harrison MR, et al: Quantitation of aortic regurgitation by computer analysis of digital subtraction angiography. J Am Coll Cardiol 1987; 10:1122–1127.

47. Klein LW, Agarwal JB, Stets G, et al: Videodensitometric quantitation of aortic regurgitation by digital subtraction aortography using a computer-based method analyzing time-density curves. Am J Cardiol 1986; 58:753–756.

48. Lupon-Roses J, Montana J, Domingo E, et al: Venous digital angioradiography: An accurate and useful technique for assessing coronary bypass graft patency. Eur Heart J 1986; 7:979–986.

49. Reiber JHC: Morphologic and densitometric quantitation of coronary stenoses: An overview of existing quantitation techniques. In Reiber JHC, Serruys PW (eds): New Developments in Quantitative Coronary Arteriography. Dordrecht, The Netherlands, Kluwer Academic, 1988, pp 34–88.

50. Sanz ML, Mancini GBJ, LeFree MT, et al: Variability of quantitative digital subtraction coronary angiography before and after percutaneous transluminal coronary angioplasty. Am J Cardiol 1987; 60:55–60.

51. Ellis S, Sanders W, Goulet C, et al: Optimal detection of the progression of coronary artery disease: Comparison of methods suitable for risk factor interventions trials. Circulation 1986; 74:1235–1242.

52. Ambrose JA, Hjemdahl-Monsen CE: Arteriographic anatomy and mechanisms of myocardial ischemia in unstable angina. J Am Coll Cardiol 1987; 9:1397–1402.

53. Legrand V, Mancini GBJ, Bates ER, et al: Comparative study of coronary flow reserve, coronary anatomy, and results of radionuclide exercise tests in patients with coronary artery disease. J Am Coll Cardiol 1986; 8:1022.

54. Herrington DM, Walford GA, Pearson TA: Issues of validation in quantitative coronary angiography. In Reiber JHC, Serruys PW (eds): New Developments in Quantitative Coronary Arteriography. Dordrecht, The Netherlands, Kluwer Academic, 1988, pp 34–88.

55. Glasgov S, Weisenberg E, Zarins CK, et al: Compensatory enlargement of human atherosclerotic coronary arteries. N Engl J Med 1987; 316:1371–1375.

56. Spears JR, Sandor T, Baim DS, et al: The minimum error in estimating coronary luminal cross-sectional area from cineangiographic diameter measurements. Cathet Cardiovasc Diag 1983; 9:119–128.

57. Wiesel J, Grunwald AM, Tobiasz C, et al: Quantitation of absolute area of a coronary arterial stenosis: Experimental validation with a preparation in vivo. Circulation 1986; 74:1099–1106.

58. Tobis J, Nalcioglu O, Johnston WD, et al: Videodensitometric determination of minimum coronary artery luminal diameter before and after angioplasty. Am J Cardiol 1987; 59:38–44.

59. Skelton TN, Kisslo KB, Bashore TM: Comparison of coronary stenosis quantitation results from on-line digital and digitized cinefilm images. Am J Cardiol 1988; 62:381–386.

60. LeFree MT, Mulvancy JA, Vogel RA: Image corrections for digital radiographic geometric and videodensitometric distortions [abstract]. Radiology 1985; 157:36.

61. LeFree MT, Simon SB, Lewis RJ, et al: Digital radiographic coronary artery quantitation. In Proceedings of the IEEE Computer Society, Computers in Cardiology. Long Beach, CA, IEEE Computer Society, 1987, pp 99–102.

62. Katritsis D, Lythall DA, Anderson MH, et al: Assessment of coronary angioplasty by an automated digital angiographic method. Am Heart J 1988; 116:1181–1187.

63. Johnson MR, McPherson DD, Fleagle SR, et al: Videodensitometric analysis of human coronary stenoses: Validation in vivo by intraoperative high-frequency epicardial echocardiography. Circulation 1988; 77:328–336.

64. Wollschlager H, Zeiher AM, Bonzel T, et al: Optimal biplane imaging of coronary segments with computed exact triple orthogonal projections. Proceedings of the Second International Symposium on Coronary Arteriography, Dordrecht, The Netherlands, Martinus Nijhoff, June 1987, p 19.

65. Sitomer J, LeFree MT, Anselmo EG, et al: Computer image-guided gantry positioning for optimization of quantitative coronary arteriography. Am J Card Imaging 1989; 3:191–198.

66. Kirkeeide RL, Gould KL, Parsel L: Assessment of coronary stenoses by myocardial perfusion imaging during pharmacologic coronary vasodilation. Part VII: Validation of coronary flow reserve as a single integrated functional measure of stenosis severity reflecting all its geometric dimensions. J Am Coll Cardiol 1986; 7: 103–113.

67. Hoffman JIE: Maximal coronary flow and the concept of coronary vascular reserve. Circulation 1984; 70: 153–159.

68. Klocke FJ: Measurements of coronary flow reserve: Defining pathophysiology versus making decisions about patient care. Circulation 1987; 76:1183–1189.

69. Sibley D, Bulle T, Baxley W, et al: Acute changes in blood flow velocity with successful coronary angioplasty [abstract]. Circulation 1986; 74:II-193.

70. Marcus ML, Doty DB, Hiratzka LF, et al: Decreased coronary reserve—a mechanism for angina pectoris in patients with aortic stenosis and normal coronary arteries. N Engl J Med 1982; 307:1362–1367.

71. Tobis J, Nalcioglu O, Iseri L, et al: Detection and quantitation of coronary artery stenosis from digital subtraction angiograms compared with 35 millimeter film cineangiograms. Am J Cardiol 1984; 54:489–496.

72. Bray BE, Anderson FL, Hardin CW, et al: Digital subtraction coronary angiography using high-pass temporal filtration: A comparison with cineangiography. Cathet Cardiovasc Diagn 1985; 11:17–24.

73. Vas R, Eigler N, Miyazono C, et al: Digital quantification eliminates intraobserver and interobserver viability in the evaluation of coronary artery stenosis. Am J Cardiol 1985; 56:718–723.

74. Goldberg HL, Moses JW, Fisher J, et al: Diagnostic accuracy of coronary angiography utilizing computer-based digital subtraction methods: Comparison to conventional cineangiography. Chest 1986; 90:793–797.

75. Mancini GBJ, Simon SB, McGillem MJ, et al: Automated quantitative coronary arteriography: Morphologic and physiologic validation in vivo of a rapid digital angiographic method. Circulation 1987; 75:452–460.

76. Rutishauser W, Bussman W-D, Noseda G, et al: Blood flow measurement through single coronary arteries by roentgen densitometry. Part I: A comparison of flow measured by radiologic techniques applicable in the intact organism and by electromagnetic flowmeter. AJR Am J Roentgenol 1970; 109:12–20.

77. Rutishauser W, Noseda G, Bussman WD: Blood flow measurements through single coronary arteries by roentgen densitometry. Part II: Right coronary artery flow in conscious man. AJR Am J Roentgenol 1970; 109:21–24.

78. Whiting JS, Drury JK, Pfaff JM, et al: Digital angiographic measurement of radiographic contrast material kinetics for estimation of myocardial perfusion. Circulation 1986; 73:789–798.

79. Eigler NL, Pfaff JM, Whiting JS, et al: Digital angiographic transfer function analysis of regional myocardial perfusion: Measurement system and coronary contrast transit linearity. *In* Heintzen PH, Bursch JH (eds): Progress in Digital Angiocardiography. Dordrecht, The Netherlands, Kluwer Academic, 1988, p 265.

80. Hodgson JM, Legrand V, Bates ER, et al: Validation in dogs of a rapid digital angiographic technique to measure relative coronary blood flow during routine cardiac catheterization. Am J Cardiol 1985; 55:188–193.

81. Mancini GBJ: Applications of digital angiography to the coronary circulation. *In* Marcus ML (ed): Cardiac Imaging: Principles and Practice. Philadelphia, WB Saunders, 1991, pp 310–347.

82. Vogel RA, Bates ER, O'Neill WW, et al: Coronary flow reserve measured during cardiac catheterization. Arch Intern Med 1984; 144:1772–1777.

83. Hess OM, Mancini GBJ, Pinto IMF, et al: Microsphere validation of a digital angiographic method for measuring coronary flow reserve. Circulation 1990; 82:1138–1444.

84. Hodgson JM, Riley RS, Most AS, Williams DO: Assessment of coronary flow reserve using digital angiography before and after successful percutaneous transluminal coronary angioplasty. Am J Cardiol 1987; 60:61–65.

85. Bates ER, Aueron FM, LeGrand V, et al: Comparative long-term effects of coronary artery bypass graft surgery and percutaneous transluminal coronary angioplasty on regional coronary flow reserve. Circulation 1985; 72: 833–839.

86. Bates ER, Mancini GBJ: Digital radiographic assessment of coronary angioplasty and bypass graft revascularization results. *In* Mancini GBJ (ed): Cardiac Applications of Digital Angiography. New York, Raven Press, 1988, p 291.

87. Bates ER, Vogel RA, LeFree MT, et al: The chronic coronary flow reserve provided by saphenous vein bypass grafts as determined by digital coronary radiography. Am Heart J 1984; 108:462–468.

88. Hodgson JM, Singh AK, Drew TM, et al: Coronary flow reserve provided by sequential internal mammary artery grafts. J Am Coll Cardiol 1986; 7:32–37.

Chapter 11

Assessment of Systolic Left Ventricular Function

HANS P. KRAYENBÜHL*
OTTO M. HESS

The term *ventricular function* is related to the function of the heart as a pump, whereas the term *myocardial function* is related more specifically to the function of the heart as a muscle. The ejection performance of the left ventricle is dependent on loading conditions (preload and afterload), synchronicity of contraction, and myocardial contractility. Heart rate as an additional determinant should be mentioned, although its mechanism of influencing ventricular performance is not a primary one but rather consists in altering both preload (filling of the ventricle) and intrinsic inotropic state (myocardial contractility). *Preload* is defined as the extent of muscle fiber stretch existing before systole. Clinical measures of preload are left ventricular end-diastolic pressure or volume and, more precisely, end-diastolic wall stress. *Afterload* is the load that muscle fibers within the ventricular wall have to sustain during ventricular ejection. The most simple measure of left ventricular afterload is systolic or mean aortic pressure. Afterload is, however, much better approximated by systolic wall stress, which is a function of ventricular pressure, size, and wall thickness. Impairment of synchronicity of left ventricular contraction occurs under pathologic conditions, such as in left bundle branch block, massive left ventricular hypertrophy, and ischemia. Contractility, or inotropic state, reflects the level of intrinsic contractile function of the myocardium with respect to the property both to shorten and to develop force. Hence, in cardiac muscle physiology contractility has been assessed by the maximal intrinsic velocity of shortening of the contractile units at zero load or by the maximal force they develop at isometric conditions (no external fiber shortening).

*Hans P. Krayenbühl died in July 1993.

These basic quantities of ventricular contractility cannot be determined in humans. There are, however, hemodynamic variables that are related to one or the other of the basic contractile properties of cardiac muscle; from an empiric point of view, they have given insight into the contractile quality of the myocardium (i.e., myocardial function). None of these variables of left ventricular systolic function that are discussed subsequently reflects solely and exclusively myocardial contractility, but they are always to some extent influenced by the actual loading conditions. Thus, there is no ideal measure available for quantifying contractility in humans.[1]

STANDARD HEMODYNAMICS

The classic measures of left ventricular pumping performance include cardiac output, stroke volume, stroke work (mean systolic blood pressure × stroke volume), and stroke power (stroke work/ejection time). As single parameters they yield only little information with respect to ventricular contractility, although severe reduction is generally associated with depressed contractile function.[2] The usefulness of these measures of external performance is enhanced when they are related to an estimate of end-diastolic fiber stretch (end-diastolic pressure, volume, or stress). When at least two pairs of data points are available, a ventricular function curve can be constructed, the steepness of which represents an approximation of the level of left ventricular contractile function. Maneuvers that allow the determination of pairs of data different from control measurements include isometric and dynamic exercise; acute volume loading by leg raising or infusion of fluid; acute pressure

201

loading by pharmacologic agents such as angiotensin, methoxamine, and phenylephrine; and
acute reduction of preload by caval obstruction.
The slope of the linear relationship between
stroke work and end-diastolic volume (the preload recruitable stroke work),* has been found,
in conscious dogs, to be responsive to alterations in inotropic state.[3] An increase in slope
indicates an increase in contractility and vice
versa. In patients with heart failure an inconsistent degree of linearity of individual stroke work
versus left ventricular end-diastolic volume relations has been described.[4]

Interpatient as well as intrapatient comparisons of left ventricular contractility based on
ventricular function curves are, however, not
devoid of the following problems:

1. Afterload (blood pressure) affects the
magnitude of stroke work and therefore the
position of left ventricular function curves, independently of differences or changes in contractility.

2. Interpatient differences of left ventricular compliance and the occurrence of intrapatient shifts of the left ventricular pressure-volume relationship consequent to changes in
right ventricular filling pressure or coronary
perfusion pressure during interventions that
change preload and afterload make substitution
of end-diastolic pressure for end-diastolic volume or fiber length invalid.[5]

3. The need to determine several hemodynamic data points renders the construction of
ventricular function curves impractical for routine purposes.

4. In the intact circulation the construction
of an ideal ventricular function curve (change
in preload without a change in contractility) is
rarely obtained because the pharmacologic
agent or maneuver used influences, per se, myo-

*SW = PRSW (EDV − Vw), where SW = stroke work,
PRSW = preload recruitable SW, EDV = left ventricular
end-diastolic volume, and Vw = left ventricular volume at
zero SW.

cardial contractility either by directly acting on
the myocardium or by altering the autonomic
nervous outflow to the heart via reflexes.

5. In the presence of mitral or aortic regurgitation, or both, estimation of the total left ventricular stroke volume by standard techniques
for cardiac output determination (by indicator-
dilution or Fick technique) is not feasible.

EJECTION PHASE PARAMETERS: VOLUMETRIC AND DIMENSIONAL VARIABLES

Global Ejection Performance

Left Ventricular Ejection Fraction

Ejection fraction (EF) is the most commonly
used measure of left ventricular ejection performance because of its prognostic value; it is expressed in percentages. The magnitude of EF
does not directly reflect myocardial contractility
because it is dependent on preload, afterload,
synchronicity of contraction, and heart rate. In
normal subjects an excessive rise in afterload
may reduce EF to a value of 50% or slightly less.
A more severely reduced EF (≤ 45%) can be
considered as an indicator of depressed myocardial function, regardless of the cardiac disorder
and loading conditions present.

When localized contraction disturbances
are present, values of EF obtained from single-
plane right anterior oblique (RAO) cineangiograms may differ substantially from those
obtained from biplane angiograms. Hence, biplane cineangiography is the preferred method
for left ventricular volumetry and determination of EF. Table 11–1 gives an overview of EF
values by biplane techniques in normal subjects.

In many laboratories EF is calculated from
uncalibrated biplane cineangiograms. A more
correct determination includes, however, the
separate calculation of angiographic left ventricular end-diastolic and end-systolic volumes with
respective individual corrections by regression
equation from cast studies.[11]

Table 11–1. **Angiographic Left Ventricular Ejection Fraction in Normal Subjects**

Author	n	Age (yr)	Angiographic Projection	Technique of Calculation	Ejection Fraction (%)		
					Mean	*SD*	*Range*
Kennedy et al[6]	16	16–68	Biplane (AP/LAT)	Area-length	67	8	56–78
Moraski et al[7]	15	33–59	Biplane (AP/LAT)	Area-length	55	4	50–64
Peterson et al[8]	22	31–59	Biplane (AP/LAT)	Area-length	76	9	59–88
Gould et al[9]	12		Biplane (AP/LAT)	Area-length	58	6	—
Toma et al[10]	8	24–64	Biplane (AP/LAT)	Area-length	73	8	61–82
Wynne et al[11]	17	34–59	Biplane (RAO/LAO)	Area-length	72	8	59–85
Eichhorn et al[12]	10	19–51	Biplane (RAO/LAO)	Area-length	69	6	62–83
Thüring et al[13]	25	20–67	Biplane (RAO/LAO)	Area-length	64	5	58–76

Table 11–2. **Angiographic Mean Normalized Systolic Ejection Rate (MNSER) in Normal Subjects**

Author	n	Age (yr)	MNSER (EDV/sec)		
			Mean	*SD*	*Range*
Peterson et al[8]	22	31–59	3.32	0.84	1.90–5.10
Johnson et al[14]	10	42–62	2.29	0.17	2.07–2.65
Ensslen et al[15]	10	36–58	2.25	0.25	—
Brunner et al[16]	94	16–63	2.40	—	2.00–3.24
Schwarz et al[17]	10	—	2.36	0.28	—
Huber et al[18]	13	19–48	2.59	0.36	2.08–3.19

EDV, end-diastolic ventricular pressure.

Subtle abnormalities of left ventricular emptying in patients with still-normal global EF may be assessed from a reduced volume ejected in early systole. In normal subjects the volume changes for the first, second, and third thirds (in percentage of stroke volume) have been reported to be 44% ± 3%, 33% ± 2%, and 21% ± 3%, respectively.[14]

Mean Normalized Systolic Ejection Rate

The mean normalized systolic ejection rate (MNSER) is obtained as EF/left ventricular ejection time; it is expressed as end-diastolic volumes per second. Hence, it is an index of velocity of global left ventricular emptying. Normal values are summarized in Table 11–2.

MNSER has been shown to separate patients with normal from those with diseased left ventricular myocardium.[8] A slight depression of MNSER can occur in patients with normal EF but prolonged ejection time such as in aortic stenosis or mitral insufficiency, including, in this situation, the "isovolumetric" contraction time from end-diastole to aortic valve opening. Conversely, in left heart failure with an abnormally short left ventricular ejection time, EF is likely to be more severely depressed than MNSER.[14]

Regional Contraction Performance

Regional Shortening

It is generally recognized that visual evaluation of cineangiograms may miss subtle abnormalities of regional wall motion and that quantitative techniques are necessary. There is, however, controversy about which quantitative method for evaluation of end-diastolic and end-systolic images is the most valid. The system used for comparison is important for the definition of a localized contraction disorder. Those who believe that movement of the heart per se within the thoracic cavity significantly influences the position of the left ventricular silhouettes in the projection under study superimpose the end-diastolic and the end-systolic images. Either the long axes and the mid-points of the aortic valve[19] or the long axes and the axes bisecting the long axes perpendicularly[20, 21] are superimposed. When the heart's motion in the chest is minimal, markers outside the heart (either the ribs and the diaphragm[22] or external lead markers alone)[23] or in combination with an internal landmark such as the diaphragm can be used for comparing the end-diastolic and end-systolic ventricular silhouettes.[24] According to the reference system used and the specific axis system applied, the extent of axis shortening in normal subjects varies.

Because of this variability, each catheterization laboratory must establish its own control values of regional shortening in an adequate number of normal subjects. Figures 11–1 and 11–2 illustrate our normal values of 25 subjects in the RAO and LAO projection with a simple system of three transverse axes after quadrisection of the long ventricular axis and with a radial system consisting of 25 axes inscribed from the contour of the ventricular silhouettes to the mid-point of the long ventricular axis after superposition of the end-diastolic and end-systolic images.[13] With both axes systems the variability of regional shortening was largest in the basal septal portion in the LAO projection. However, variability was consistently smaller with the radial than with the orthogonal axes system. Figure 11–3 depicts regional wall motion with the use of the centerline technique in the RAO projection.[25] The units of regional shortening are not in percentage of end-diastolic axis dimensions but in percentage of ventricular end-diastolic perimeter. With this technique variability is highest at the apex. Realignment of end-diastolic and end-systolic ventricular silhouettes increased rather than decreased variability at the apex.[25]

Regional Velocity of Fiber Shortening

The only regional velocity of fiber shortening that is of some practical importance is the mean velocity of endocardial circumferential fiber shortening (Vcf) at the equator of the ventricu-

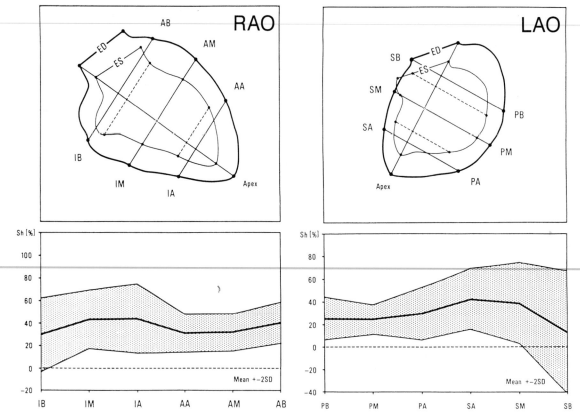

Figure 11–1. Regional systolic shortening in an orthogonal axes system (RAO and LAO projection). The orthogonal transverse axes were inscribed by quadrisection of the long ventricular axes extending from the mitral-aortic junction to the apex. In the lower panels the normal range of shortening for the six hemiaxes in the RAO and LAO projection is presented. The data were obtained from 24 control subjects with a mean age of 46 years.[13] AB, anterobasal; AM, anteromedial; AA, anteroapical; IA, inferoapical; IM, inferomedial; IB, inferobasal; SB, septobasal; SM, septomedial; SA, septoapical; PA, posteroapical; PM, posteromedial; PB, posterobasal; Sh, percentage regional hemiaxis shortening; ED, end-diastolic left ventricular silhouette; ES, end-systolic left ventricular silhouette.

lar ellipsoid in the RAO or AP projection (mean Vcf in circumferences per second). Mean Vcf is obtained as

$$(\text{MED} - \text{MES})/\text{ET} \cdot \text{MED} \qquad (1)$$

where MED and MES are left ventricular transverse diameter at the minor equator in end-diastole and end-systole, respectively, and ET is left ventricular ejection time. In myocardial and valvular disease mean Vcf has been used tacitly as a measure of global left ventricular perfor-

mance, although this quantity is, in a strict sense, a regional function parameter. Values of mean Vcf reported in normal subjects are summarized in Table 11–3.

PRESSURE-DERIVED INDICES OF LEFT VENTRICULAR CONTRACTILE FUNCTION

In analogy to the mechanics of the isometrically contracting isolated cardiac muscle, various ve-

Table 11–3. Angiographic Mean Velocity of Circumferential Fiber Shortening (mean Vcf) at the Equator of the Left Ventricular Ellipsoid

Author	n	Age (yr)	Mean Vcf (circ⁻¹/sec) in Normal Subjects		
			Mean	SD	Range
Karliner et al[26]	13		1.50	0.28	1.23–2.03
Peterson et al[8]	22	31–59	1.83	0.55	1.10–3.16
Johnson et al[14]	10	42–62	1.30	0.15	1.07–1.63
Brunner et al[16]	34	18–63	1.43	—	1.00–1.92
Ensslen et al[15]	10	36–58	1.22	0.19	—

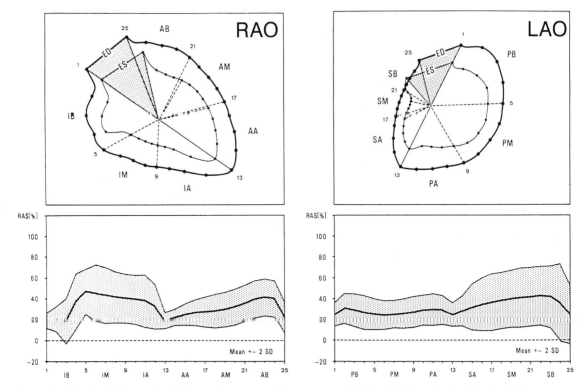

Figure 11–2. Regional left ventricular shortening in a radial axes system (RAO and LAO projection). In the RAO projection 13 inferior and 12 anterior radial axes were inscribed. The aortic area was not incorporated into the analysis. The inferior axes were drawn in steps of angles of 15 degrees; the anterior axes were inscribed at identical angles at less than 15 degrees. In the LAO projection 13 radial axes were inscribed for the posterior and inferior regions (in steps of 15 degrees) and 12 axes for the septal region (equal steps of less than 15 degrees). The lower panels show the normal ranges of regional axis shortening (RAS) in the RAO and LAO projection obtained from 24 control subjects.[13] See Figure 11–1 legend for abbreviations.

Figure 11–3. Centerline technique for the assessment of regional shortening in the RAO projection. *A,* The end-diastolic and end-systolic silhouettes are presented, and the mid-points of shortening of 100 chords are inscribed in a clockwise fashion from the anterior portion of the aortic valve to the mitral-aortic junction. *B,* The extent of regional shortening from end-diastole to end-systole in the 100 chords is shown. *C,* The shortening fraction normalized for end-diastolic perimeter of 64 control subjects is shown. (*A* through *C* adapted from Sheehan FA, Stewart DK, Dodge HT, et al: Variability in the measurement of regional left ventricular wall motion from contrast angiograms. Circulation 1983; 68:550–559.)

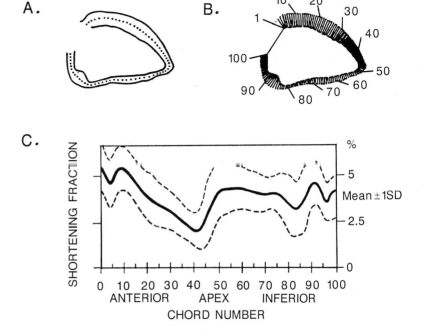

locity indices have been derived from high-fidelity pressure measurements during the iso-volumetric phase of left ventricular systole (isovolumetric indices). Although none of these indices indicates basic muscle contractility in a strict sense, because of several methodologic limitations and assumptions, they have shown empiric usefulness in helping to distinguish a "good" from a "bad" heart.[27]

Maximal Rate of Rise of Left Ventricular Pressure

Maximal rate of rise of left ventricular pressure (maxdP/dt) is easily measured at catheterization by continuous electronic differentiation of the left ventricular high-fidelity pressure tracing (Fig. 11–4). MaxdP/dt not only is dependent on the inotropic state but also is influenced by preload,[28, 29] heart rate,[29] and muscle mass.[30–32] When maxdP/dt falls into the early part of the ejection phase, its value is underestimated. This occurs when diastolic aortic pressure is low, such as in chronic aortic insufficiency. Table 11–4 presents values of maxdP/dt obtained in normal subjects at rest.

To be used as an index of contractility maxdP/dt has been normalized for left ventricular end-diastolic circumference.[33] This normalized quantity showed stability during acute preloading and afterloading in humans with good sensitivity to inotropic interventions. Another possibility is to construct an isovolumetric ventricular function curve by plotting maxdP/dt versus end-diastolic volume.[28] Although the slope of this relation is a sensitive load-independent measure of inotropic state, the construction of the curve is tedious because of the need to determine two or more data points at one given contractile state.

Peak Measured Velocity of Shortening and Extrapolated Maximal Velocity of Shortening of the Contractile Elements

Peak measured velocity of shortening ($\dot{V}$pm) and extrapolated maximal velocity of shortening ($\dot{V}$max) of the contractile elements are derived from isovolumetric pressure-velocity curves. Using a two-component model for heart muscle, and assuming that there is no fiber shortening during the isovolumetric phase of systole, the velocity of shortening of the contractile elements is calculated as[34, 35]

$$\dot{V}_{CE} = (dP/dt)/k \cdot P + c \qquad (2)$$

where P is left ventricular high-fidelity pressure, k is the stiffness constant, and c is the intercept of the diagram of active stiffness versus load. Because c has been shown to be small in experiments on isolated cat papillary muscle[36] and more recently in the left ventricular myocardium of humans,[37] it is neglected for the calculation of $\dot{V}$ce. For k, the numeral 28 as found in the cat papillary muscle[38] has generally been used. The assumption of an uniform value of k is, however, not ideal when one deals with interpatient comparisons. Thus, k was recently

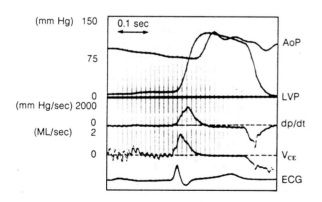
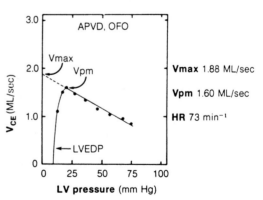

Vmax was obtained by straight-line extrapolation.

AoP = aortic pressure; APVD = anomalous pulmonary venous drainage; dp/dt = first derivative of LVP;
ECG = electrocardiogram; HR = heart rate; LVEDP = left ventricular end-diastolic pressure; LVP = left ventricular pressure;
ML = muscle lengths; OFO = open foramen ovale; V_{CE} = instantaneous velocity of shortening of contractile elements in muscle
lengths per second; Vmax = extrapolated maximal velocity of shortening; Vpm = peak measured velocity of shortening

Figure 11–4. Left ventricular high-fidelity pressure tracing and corresponding pressure-velocity curve in a patient with anomalous pulmonary venous drainage and normal left ventricular function. (From Krayenbühl HP, Hess OM, Turina J: Assessment of left ventricular function. Cardiovasc Med 1978; 3:883–910.)

Table 11–4. Isovolumic Contractile Indices in Normal Subjects

Author	n	Age (yr)	HR (beats/min)	maxdP/dt (mm Hg/sec)	Vpm (ML/sec)	Vmax (ML/sec)
Krayenbühl et al[31]	25	28 (15–55)	72 ± 14 (49–107)	1670 ± 320 (980–2340)	1.47 ± 0.19 (1.14–1.96)	1.86 ± 0.26 (1.47–2.39)
Peterson et al[8]	22	47 (31–59)	77 ± 14 (48–107)	1661 ± 324 (1146–2265)	1.57 ± 0.30 (1.15–2.15)	1.87 ± 0.37 (1.32–2.93)
Quinones et al[33]	9	37 (18–52)	88 ± 11 (58–100)	1508 ± 245 (1350–2144)	—	—
Fifer et al[30]	7	48 (37–53)	73 ± 10 (50–81)	1386 ± 383 (963–2278)	—	—

Ranges are in parentheses.
HR, heart rate; see text for other abbreviations.

calculated in individual patients[37] according to the formula[39]:

$$k \ (circ^{-1}) = 0.87 \ (maxdS/dt)/Sp \cdot \dot{V}_{cfSp} \quad (3)$$

where S is left ventricular meridional wall stress, Sp is peak systolic wall stress, circ is circumferences, and $\dot{V}_{cfSp}$ is normalized mid-wall circumferential fiber shortening velocity at peak stress.

This calculation assumes that in an isovolumetric beat dS/dt at a systolic wall stress identical to peak systolic wall stress of the corresponding auxotonic (ejecting) beat amounts to 87% of maxdS/dt. This percentage value had been derived by comparing isovolumetric and ejecting beats in patients during open heart surgery.[37] In control subjects k as determined by Equation 3 was 15 ± 1 (SD) $circ^{-1}$. In patients with left ventricular hypertrophy from aortic stenosis, k was 14 ± 3 $circ^{-1}$. Thus, the findings in humans paralleled those in animals where hypertrophy as the consequence of chronic mechanical overload was not associated with altered active stiffness.[40–45]

The left panel of Figure 11–4 shows the continuous tracing of left ventricular dp/dt and (dp/dt)/pressure (P). Taking into account a k value of 28 $circ^{-1}$ (dp/dt)/P was labeled $\dot{V}ce$ and expressed in muscle lengths (MLs) per second. The right panel presents the plot between $\dot{V}ce$ and left ventricular pressure. Its descending limb was extrapolated to zero left ventricular pressure. The extrapolated value on the $\dot{V}ce$ axis corresponds to "total pressure" Vmax. Owing to many assumptions Vmax determined in this way has to be taken as an index of Vmax rather than a true unloaded velocity of contractile element shortening. Table 11–4 gives an overview on values of Vpm and total pressure $\dot{V}$max obtained in normal subjects.

Comparison Between Isovolumetric and Ejection Phase Indices

Between the two types of contractile measures fair but not close correlations have been de-scribed. The correlations may vary according to the underlying heart disease. In patients with coronary artery disease total pressure $\dot{V}$max and peak measured velocity of contractile element shortening correlated with left ventricular EF with a r value of 0.76 and 0.78, respectively.[44] In patients with aortic stenosis the correlations between the two aforementioned isovolumetric indices and MNSER showed r values of 0.50 and 0.53, respectively.[16]

VARIABLES INCLUDING LEFT VENTRICULAR VOLUMETRIC AND DIMENSIONAL AS WELL AS PRESSURE MEASUREMENTS

Maximal Time-Varying Elastance and the Slope of the End-Systolic Pressure-Volume Relationship (end-systolic elastance)

When isochronic, instantaneous pressure-volume data points of differently loaded beats are subjected to linear regression analysis, slopes of varying steepness are obtained.[46] These slopes are termed *time-varying elastance* (E[t]) and

$$E(t) = P(t)/\dot{V}(t) - \dot{V}_0(t) \quad (4)$$

$\dot{V}_0$ is the extrapolated volume at zero pressure for a set of isochronic pressure-volume coordinates, P is pressure, and $\dot{V}$ is volume. The maximum slope is called *maximal time-varying elastance* (Emax), and its occurrence in time has been used to define end-systole. When from each of the differently loaded beats an end-systolic point defined as the maximal ratio $(P/\dot{V} - \dot{V}_0)$ is chosen regardless of timing and linear regression analysis is applied to the entire set of points, a slope is obtained which is termed *end-systolic elastance* (Ees).[47] Both Emax and Ees have been used as indices of inotropic state. Generally, there is disparity between Emax and

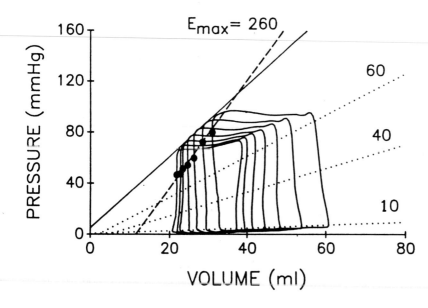

Figure 11–5. Maximal time-varying elastance (E_{max}) and end-systolic elastance in a closed-chest dog. The volumes were obtained by conductance catheter. The E (t) relations are shown at 4 time points: 10, 40, 60 *(dotted lines)* and 260 msec after the onset of systole *(dashed line)*. This last line indicates the slope of E_{max}. The solid line shows the end-systolic elastance. This slope is clearly less steep than E_{max}. (From Kass DA, Maughan WL: From "Emax" to pressure-volume relations: A broader view. Circulation 1988; 77:1203–1212.)

Ees, with individual values for Ees being lower than those of Emax (Fig. 11–5).[47]

Approximations of "true" end-systolic elastance are obtained from the linear regressions of systemic arterial dicrotic notch pressure and simultaneous left ventricular volume, left ventricular pressure and volume at the time of peak negative dP/dt, minimal left ventricular volume and simultaneous left ventricular pressure, systemic arterial dicrotic notch pressure and minimal left ventricular volume, and peak left ventricular or systemic arterial pressure and minimal left ventricular volume.[4] The slopes of these end-systolic pressure-volume relations correlate variably with "true" Ees[4] or Emax.[48] Table

11–5 provides estimates of Emax and Ees in normal subjects or in patients with normal left ventricular function.

There are several problems with the assessment of the end-systolic elastance. The determination of only two or three data pairs of pressure-volume coordinates, as usually done in humans, may be insufficient for a statistically adequate regression analysis. The necessary changes in loading conditions to obtain Ees may alter contractile state, less in patients with compromised than in those with preserved left ventricular function. The end-systolic pressure-volume relationship may be nonlinear outside the range of commonly observed levels of left

Table 11–5. Slopes of End-systolic Pressure-volume Relationships in Patients with Normal LV Function

Author	Type of Elastance	Data Points Used	Intervention	Slope	Comments
Grossman et al[49]	Ees	Aortic dicrotic notch pressure, minimal LV volume	IV nitroprusside; IV methoxamine; buccal erithrityl-tetranitrate	4.9 mm Hg/mL/m² (1.9–7.0)	6 mitral regurgitation 1 atypical chest pain
Mehmel et al[50]	Ees	Aortic dicrotic notch pressure, minimal LV volume	After propranolol and IV atropine; sublingual ISDN; IV methoxamine	2.6 mm Hg/mL (0.6–6.35)	11 CAD
McKay et al[51]	Emax	Maximal slope from isochronic pressure-volume data	On β-blockers or after IV atropine; IV nitroglycerin; IV nitroprusside; IV phenylephrine	4.7 mm Hg/mL/m² (2.6–7.7)	5 normal subjects
Starling et al[48]	Emax	Maximal slope from isochronic pressure-volume data	IV methoxamine; IV nitroprusside	5.5 mm Hg/mL (3.4–6.7)	10 atypical chest pain

LV, left ventricular; see text for other abbreviations.

ventricular end-systolic pressure, and hence linear extrapolation to determine $\dot{V}_0$ may be in error. The way by which loading conditions are changed to obtain several end-systolic pressure-volume coordinates may, by itself, have an influence on Ees. In the experimental animal an increase in end-systolic pressure with constant end-diastolic volume led to a greater Ees than an increase of end-systolic pressure associated with an increased end-diastolic volume and stroke volume.[52] Furthermore, Ees and Emax are dependent on ventricular size[53-55] and mass,[48, 56] and for a precise assessment of contractile state in animals and patients, standardization of elastance appears advisable when end-diastolic volume or mass differ considerably among individuals.

Assessment of end-systolic elastance by the calculation of the left ventricular systolic pressure/end-systolic volume[57] ratio is inadequate because it is assumed erroneously that the true end-systolic pressure-volume relationship has a volume intercept of zero. This "index" of Ees should not be used.

In patients with chronic pressure or volume overload, or both, with myocardial hypertrophy and chamber dilation, end-systolic load is more adequately assessed by the calculation of wall stress than only by left ventricular pressure.[58, 59] The use of end-systolic stress instead of pressure can prevent an incorrect evaluation of inotropic state, which can occur in concentric hypertrophy from aortic stenosis based on Ees.[59] To avoid load manipulations for the construction of the end-systolic stress-volume relationship, stress-volume relations have been assessed in one cardiac cycle from peak stress down to end-systolic stress.[60] This relationship is fairly linear, but its slope is flatter than that of the true end-systolic stress-volume relationship.

Left Ventricular Wall Stress

In the hypertrophied heart ventricular preload and afterload should be expressed by the corresponding wall stresses rather than by end-diastolic or systolic left ventricular pressure because not only pressure but also the actual chamber size and wall thickness determines the load to which each unit of the wall cross-section is exposed. For the calculation of left ventricular wall stress, thin-walled and thick-walled models have been proposed.

With the thin-walled model of Sandler and Dodge[61]:

$$\text{Circumferential stress} = \frac{P \cdot b}{h} \left[1 - \frac{b^3}{a^2 (2b + h)} \right] \quad (5)$$

With the thick-walled model of Falsetti[62]:

$$\text{Circumferential stress} = \frac{P \cdot 2b}{4h} \cdot \frac{(4a^2 - 2b^2)}{(2a^2 - 2b \cdot h)} \quad (6)$$

In both formulas[61, 62] P is left ventricular pressure; h is left ventricular wall thickness; b is endocardial minor (transverse) semiaxis; and a is endocardial major (long) semiaxis.

With the thick-walled model of Mirsky[63]:

$$\text{Circumferential stress} = \frac{P \cdot b}{h} \cdot \left(1 - \frac{h}{2b} - \frac{b^2}{2a^2} \right) \quad (7)$$

Note that in Mirsky's formula, b is *mid-wall* minor semiaxis and a is *mid-wall* major semiaxis. P and h are as just defined.

In Table 11–6 values for end-diastolic and systolic circumferential wall stress, as found in control subjects, are presented.

The inverse relationship between *ventricular systolic shortening* (expressed by the EF or percentage of endocardial or mid-wall circumferen-

Table 11–6. **Systolic and End-diastolic Circumferential Wall Stress in Control Subjects**

	Author	Peak systolic (k dyne/cm²)	Mean systolic (k dyne/cm²)	End-systolic (k dyne/cm²)	End-diastolic (k dyne/cm²)
Thin-walled model (Sandler and Dodge)	Hood et al[64]	327 ± 24*	—	—	30 ± 4*
	Gaasch et al[65]	377 (312–446)	—	—	26 (13–34)
	Gould et al[9]	358 ± 74†	—	—	—
	Huber et al[18]	368 (275–451)	—	—	34 (15–57)
	Pouleur et al[60]	375 ± 60†	—	215 ± 79†	—
Thick-walled model (Falsetti)	Schwarz et al[17]	293 ± 19*	—	—	31 (14–54)
	Huber et al[18]	341 (250–425)	—	—	—
Thick-walled model (Mirsky)	Gunther et al[66]	—	277 (240–294)	—	36 (25–44)
	Wisenbaugh et al[67]	256 ± 16†	188 ± 10†	124 ± 20†	36 ± 11†
	Corin et al[68]	348 ± 44†	267 ± 30†	162 ± 19†	36 ± 11†

*Standard error (SE).
†Standard deviation (SD).
Ranges are in parentheses.

tial fiber shortening) and *afterload* in terms of peak systolic, mean systolic, or end-systolic circumferential wall stress is an excellent means to characterize left ventricular contractile state.[18, 66, 68-70] When contractility is depressed, the systolic shortening-stress relation is shifted downward with respect to the range of the inverse relationship found in normal subjects.[66, 68-71] It is important that the control range of the shortening-stress relationship encompass coordinates not only at a normal but also an increased wall stress, comparable with the stress found in chronic left ventricular overload. Control data at high wall stress can be obtained by elevating acutely left ventricular pressure by methoxamine or angiotensin II. In normal subjects EF does not fall below 50% during massive increase of systolic wall stress.[48] The systolic shortening-afterload relationship is influenced to a certain extent by the preload. The coordinates of patients with normal contractility but enhanced preload should be displaced to the right. Absence of this rightward shift was observed in patients with chronic mitral regurgitation and normal EF but increased end-dia-

stolic wall stress and hence was indicative of mild depression of left ventricular contractility.[68]

Another way to assess minute differences in left ventricular contractility in patients with normal EF is to plot left ventricular preload (in terms of end-diastolic wall stress) versus a measure of systolic isovolumetric performance, that is, maxdP/dt. We have found that in 27% of patients with aortic stenosis having a normal left ventricular EF, the relationship between maxdP/dt and end-diastolic stress was shifted rightward to the control range,[72] indicating that left ventricular contractility was slightly depressed. In these patients EF was maintained within normal limits by the mobilization of preload reserve (Fig. 11-6).

ACUTE STRESS TESTING AND LEFT VENTRICULAR FUNCTION

Isometric and dynamic exercises have been used to place an additional pressure or combined volume and pressure load on the left ventricle for assessing its contractile reserve. The tradi-

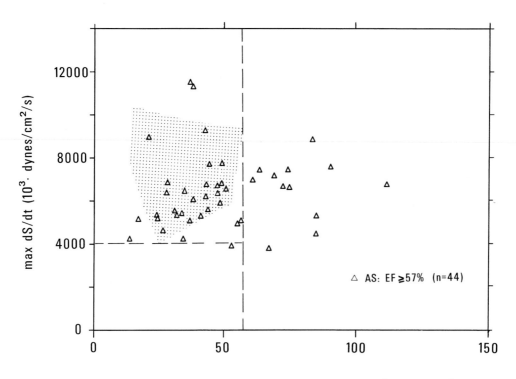

Figure 11-6. Relationship between maximal rate of rise of left ventricular circumferential wall stress (maxdS/dt) and end-diastolic wall stress in 44 patients with aortic stenosis (AS) and an ejection fraction (EF) ≧57%. The shaded area encompasses the values found in 23 control subjects. Thus, the upper left quadrant defines the normal relationship between maxdS/dt and end-diastolic stress. In 12 patients the relationship was shifted to the right. Hence, left ventricular myocardial contractility appeared to be mildly depressed in these patients. Mobilization of preload reserve allowed maintenance of EF within normal limits.

Table 11–7. **Left Ventricular Angiographic Data at Rest and During Supine Exercise (91 W) in 9 Control Subjects***

	HR (beats/min)	EDVI (mL/m²)	ESVI (mL/m²)	SVI (mL/m²)	EF (%)
Rest	69	92	33	59	64
Exercise	118	96	29	67	70
P	<0.001	NS	<0.05	<0.01	<0.01

*Mean age of control subjects is 49 years.
HR, heart rate; EDVI, end-diastolic volume index; ESVI, end-systolic volume index; SVI, stroke volume index; EF, ejection fraction.

tional way is to construct a ventricular function curve by relating stroke work to left ventricular end-diastolic pressure or pulmonary wedge pressure.[1, 73, 74] Similarly, an isovolumetric contractile index, $\dot{V}pm$ or total pressure $\dot{V}max$, has been plotted versus left ventricular end-diastolic pressure.[75] In all these function diagrams the specific reaction to exercise is mediated not only by the level of systolic contractile reserve but also by the passive diastolic properties of the left ventricular chamber. Diastolic chamber abnormalities may become manifest during dynamic exercise when systolic performance is still well preserved.[76]

Cineangiography with simultaneous high-fidelity pressure measurements has been shown to be a powerful technique for detecting exercise-induced abnormalities of left ventricular global and regional systolic function,[77] relaxation, filling, and passive diastolic properties.[78] In Table 11–7 left ventricular angiographic volumetric data obtained during supine exercise in control subjects are presented.[79] With modern digital subtraction techniques accurate left ventricular volumes may also be obtained during exercise after contrast agent injection into the superior vena cava.[80]

REFERENCES

1. Amende I, Krayenbühl HP, Rutishauser W, Wirz P: Left ventricular dynamics during handgrip. Br Heart J 1972; 34:688–695.
2. Parmley WW, Tomoda H, Diamond G, et al: Dissociation between indices of pump performance and contractility in patients with coronary artery disease and acute myocardial infarction. Chest 1976; 67:141–146.
3. Glower DD, Spratt JA, Snow ND, et al: Linearity of the Frank-Starling relationship in the intact heart: The concept of preload recruitable stroke work. Circulation 1985; 71:994–1009.
4. Aroney CN, Herrmann HC, Semigran MJ, et al: Linearity of the left ventricular end-systolic pressure-volume relation in patients with severe heart failure. J Am Coll Cardiol 1989; 14:127–134.
5. Glantz SA, Parmley WW: Factors which affect the diastolic pressure volume curve [editorial]. Circ Res 1978; 42:171–180.
6. Kennedy JW, Baxley WA, Figley MM, et al: Quantitative

7. Moraski RE, Russell RO Jr, Smith McK, Rackley CE: Left ventricular function in patients with and without myocardial infarction and one, two or three vessel coronary artery disease. Am J Cardiol 1975; 35:1–10.
8. Peterson KL, Skloven D, Ludbrook P, et al: Comparison of isovolumic and ejection phase indices of myocardial performance in man. Circulation 1974; 49:1088–1101.
9. Gould KL, Kennedy JW, Frimer M, et al: Analysis of wall dynamics and directional components of left ventricular contraction in man. Am J Cardiol 1976; 38:322–331.
10. Toma Y, Matsuda Y, Moritani K, et al: Left atrial filling in normal human subjects: Relation between left atrial contraction and left atrial early filling. Cardiovasc Res 1987; 21:255–259.
11. Wynne J, Green LH, Mann T, et al: Estimation of left ventricular volumes in man from biplane cineangiograms filmed in oblique projections. Am J Cardiol 1978; 41:726–732.
12. Eichhorn P, Grimm J, Koch R, et al: Left ventricular relaxation in patients with left ventricular hypertrophy secondary to aortic valve disease. Circulation 1982; 65:1394–1404.
13. Thuering CH, Hess OM, Murakami T, et al: Normalwerte der linksventrikularen Funktion: Biplane Angiokardiographie, unter Berucksichtigung geschlechtsspezifischer Unterschiede. Fortschr Rontgenstr 1989; 150:562–568.
14. Johnson LL, Ellis K, Schmidt D, et al: Volume ejected in early systole: A sensitive index of left ventricular performance in coronary artery disease. Circulation 1975; 52:378–389.
15. Ensslen R, Schwarz F, Thormann J, Schlepper M: Left ventricular ejection and ejection reserve during isoproterenol infusion in hypertrophic obstructive cardiomyopathy. Z Kardiol 1977; 66:633–640.
16. Brunner HH, Steiger U, Goebel NHJ, Krayenbühl HP: Left ventricular contractile function in aortic stenosis evaluated by isovolumic and ejection phase indexes. Am Heart J 1977; 93:147–159.
17. Schwarz F, Flameng W, Langebartels F, et al: Impaired left ventricular function in chronic aortic valve disease: Survival and function after replacement by Björk-Shiley prosthesis. Circulation 1979; 60:48–58.
18. Huber D, Grimm J, Koch R, Krayenbühl HP: Determinants of ejection performance in aortic stenosis. Circulation 1981; 64:126–134.
19. Herman MV, Heinle RA, Klein MD, Gorlin R: Localized disorders in myocardial contraction: Asynergy and its role in congestive failure. N Engl J Med 1967; 277:222–232.
20. Hamilton GW, Murray JA, Kennedy JW: Quantitative angiocardiography in ischemic heart disease: The spectrum of abnormal left ventricular function and the role of abnormally contracting segments. Circulation 1972; 45:1065–1080.

21. Krayenbühl HP, Schoenbeck M, Rutishauser W, Wirz P: Abnormal segmental contraction velocity in coronary artery disease produced by isometric exercise and atrial pacing. Am J Cardiol 1975; 35:785–794.

22. Shubrooks SJ Jr, Zir LM, Dinsmore RE, Harthorne JW: Left ventricular wall motion response to intravenous propranolol. Circulation 1975; 52:124–129.

23. Kitamura S, Kay JH, Krohn BG, et al: Geometric and functional abnormalities of the left ventricle with a chronic localized noncontractile area. Am J Cardiol 1973; 31:701–707.

24. Chaitman BR, Bristow JD, Rahimtoola SH: Left ventricular wall motion assessed by using fixed external reference systems. Circulation 1973; 48:1043–1054.

25. Sheehan FA, Stewart DK, Dodge HT, et al: Variability in the measurement of regional left ventricular wall motion from contrast angiograms. Circulation 1983; 68:550–559.

26. Karliner JS, Gault JH, Eckberg D, et al: Mean velocity of fiber shortening: A simplified measure of left ventricular myocardial contractility. Circulation 1971; 44:323–333.

27. Brutsaert DL, Sonnenblick EH: Cardiac muscle mechanics in the evaluation of myocardial contractility and pump function: Problems, concepts, and directions. Progr Cardiovasc Dis 1973; 16:337–361.

28. Little WC: The left ventricular dP/dtmax end-diastolic volume relation in closed-chest dogs. Circ Res 1985; 56:808–815.

29. Wallace AK, Skinner NS, Mitchell JH: Hemodynamic determinants of the maximal rate of rise of left ventricular pressure. Am J Physiol 1963; 205:30–36.

30. Fifer MA, Gunther S, Grossman W, et al: Myocardial contractile function in aortic stenosis as determined from the rate of stress development during isovolumic systole. Am J Cardiol 1979; 44:1318–1325.

31. Krayenbühl HP, Rutishauser W, Wirz P, et al: High-fidelity left ventricular pressure measurements for the assessment of cardiac contractility in man. Am J Cardiol 1973; 31:415–427.

32. Mason DT: Usefulness and limitations of the rate of rise of intraventricular pressure (dp/dt) in the evaluation of myocardial contractility in man. Am J Cardiol 1969; 23:516–527.

33. Quinones MA, Gaasch WH, Alexander JK: Influence of acute changes in preload, afterload, contractile state, and heart rate on ejection and isovolumic indices of myocardial contractility in man. Circulation 1976; 53:293–302.

34. Mason DT, Spann JF Jr, Zelis R: Quantification of the contractile state of the intact human heart. Am J Cardiol 1970; 26:248–257.

35. Sonnenblick EH, Parmley WW, Urschel CW: The contractile state of the heart as expressed by force-velocity relations. Am J Cardiol 1969; 23:488–503.

36. Yeatman LA Jr, Parmley WW, Urschel CW, Sonnenblick EH: Dynamics of contractile elements in isometric contractions of cardiac muscle. Am J Physiol 1971; 220:534–542.

37. Ritter M, Hess OM, Murakami T, et al: Left ventricular systolic series elastic properties in aortic stenosis before and after valve replacement. Cardiovasc Res 1988; 22:759–767.

38. Sonnenblick EH: Series elastic and contractile elements in heart muscle: Changes in muscle length. Am J Physiol 1964; 207:1330–1338.

39. Forward SA, McIntyre KM, Lipana JG, Levine HJ: Active stiffness of the intact canine left ventricle: With observations on the effect of acute and chronic myocardial infarction. Circ Res 1966; 19:970–979.

40. Parmley WW, Spann JF Jr, Taylor RR, Sonnenblick EH: The series elasticity of cardiac muscle in hyperthyroidism, ventricular hypertrophy, and heart failure. Proc Soc Exptl Biol Med 1968; 127:606–609.

41. Grossman W, Haynes F, Paraskos JA, et al: Alterations in preload and myocardial mechanics in the dog and in man. Circ Res 1972; 31:83–94.

42. Mason DT, Spann JF Jr, Zelis R, Amsterdam EA: Alterations of hemodynamics and myocardial mechanics in patients with congestive heart failure. Progr Cardiovasc Dis 1970; 12:507–557.

43. Falsetti HL, Mates RE, Greene DG, Bunnell IL: Vmax as an index of contractile state in man. Circulation 1971; 43:467–479.

44. Rogers WJ, Russell RO Jr, Moraski RE, et al: Comparison of indices of muscle and pump performance in patients with coronary artery disease. Cathet Cardiovasc Diagn 1975; 1:17–34.

45. Graham TP Jr, Jarmakani JM, Canent RV Jr, Anderson PAW: Evaluation of left ventricular contractile state in childhood: Normal values and observations with a pressure overload. Circulation 1971; 44:1043–1052.

46. Suga H, Sagawa K: Instantaneous pressure-volume relationships and their ratio in the excised, supported canine left ventricle. Circ Res 1974; 35:117–126.

47. Kass DA, Maughan WL: From "Emax" to pressure-volume relations: A broader view. Circulation 1988; 77:1203–1212.

48. Starling MR, Walsh RA, Dell'Italia LJ, et al: The relationship of various measures of end-systole to left ventricular maximum time-varying elastance in man. Circulation 1987; 76:32–43.

49. Grossman W, Braunwald E, Mann T, et al: Contractile state of the left ventricle in man as evaluated from end-systolic pressure-volume relations. Circulation 1977; 56:845–852.

50. Mehmel HC, Stockins B, Ruffmann K, et al: The linearity of the end-systolic pressure-volume relationship in man and its sensitivity for assessment of left ventricular function. Circulation 1981; 63:1216–1222.

51. McKay RG, Aroesty JM, Heller GV, et al: Assessment of the end-systolic pressure-volume relationship in human beings with the use of a time-varying elastance model. Circulation 1986; 74:97–104.

52. Baan J, Van der Velde ET: Sensitivity of left ventricular end-systolic pressure-volume relation to type of loading interventions in dogs. Circ Res 1988; 62:1247–1258.

53. Berko B, Gaasch WH, Tanigawa N, et al: Disparity between ejection and end-systolic indexes of left ventricular contractility in mitral regurgitation. Circulation 1987; 75:1310–1319.

54. Hsia HH, Starling MR: Is standardization of left ventricular chamber elastance necessary? Circulation 1990; 81:1826–1836.

55. Nakano K, Sugawara M, Ishihara W, et al: Myocardial stiffness derived from end-systolic wall stress and logarithm of reciprocal of wall thickness. Circulation 1990; 82:1352–1361.

56. Belcher P, Boerboom L, Oliger G: Standardization of end-systolic pressure-volume relation in the dog. Am J Physiol 1985; 249:H547–H554.

57. Nivatpumin T, Katz S, Scheuer K: Peak left ventricular systolic pressure/end-systolic volume ratio: A sensitive detector of left ventricular disease. Am J Cardiol 1979; 43:969–974.

58. Reichek N, Wilson J, St J Sutton M, et al: Non-invasive determination of left ventricular end-systolic stress: Validation of the method and initial application. Circulation 1982; 65:99–108.

59. Shroff SG, Weber KT, Janicki JS: End-systolic relations: Their usefulness and limitations in assessing left ventricular contractile state. Int J Cardiol 1984; 5:253–259.

60. Pouleur H, Rousseau MF, van Eyll C, et al: Assessment of left ventricular contractility from late systolic stress-volume relations. Circulation 1982; 65:1204–1212.

61. Sandler H, Dodge HT: Left ventricular tension and stress in man. Circ Res 1963; 13:91–104.

62. Falsetti HL, Mates RE, Grant C, et al: Left ventricular wall stress calculated from one-plane cineangiography. Circ Res 1970; 26:71–83.

63. Mirsky I: Left ventricular stress in the intact human heart. Biophys J 1969; 9:189–208.

64. Hood WP Jr, Rackley CE, Rolett EL: Wall stress in the normal and hypertrophied human left ventricle. Am J Cardiol 1968; 22:550–558.

65. Gaasch WH, Battle WE, Oboler AA, et al: Left ventricular stress and compliance in man: With special reference to normalized ventricular function curves. Circulation 1972; 45:746–762.

66. Gunther S, Grossman W: Determinants of ventricular function in pressure-overload hypertrophy in man. Circulation 1979; 59:679–688.

67. Wisenbaugh T, Spann JF, Carabello BA: Differences in myocardial performance and load between patients with similar amounts of chronic aortic versus chronic mitral regurgitation. J Am Coll Cardiol 1984; 3:916–923.

68. Corin WJ, Monrad ES, Murakami T, et al: The relationship of afterload to ejection performance in chronic mitral regurgitation. Circulation 1987; 76:59–67.

69. Taniguchi K, Nakano S, Kawashima Y, et al: Left ventricular ejection performance, wall stress, and contractile state in aortic regurgitation before and after valve replacement. Circulation 1990; 82:798–807.

70. Wisenbaugh T, Booth D, de Maria A, et al: Relationship of contractile state to ejection performance in patients with chronic aortic valve disease. Circulation 1986; 73:47–53.

71. Krayenbühl HP, Hess OM, Schneider J, Turina M: Physiologic or pathologic hypertrophy. Eur Heart J 1983; 4(Suppl A):29–34.

72. Krayenbühl HP, Hess OM, Ritter M, et al: Left ventricular systolic function in aortic stenosis. Eur Heart J 1988; 9(Suppl E):19–23.

73. Helfant RH, de Villa MA, Meister SG: Effect of sustained isometric handgrip exercise on left ventricular performance. Circulation 1971; 44:982–993.

74. Ross J Jr, Gault JH, Mason DT, et al: Left ventricular performance during muscular exercise in patients with and without cardiac dysfunction. Circulation 1966: 34:597–608.

75. Krayenbühl HP, Grimm J, Turina M, Senning A: Assessment of left ventricular function in aortic valve disease by isometric exercise. Circ Res 1981; 48(Suppl I):149–155.

76. Monrad ES, Hess OM, Murakami T, et al: Abnormal exercise hemodynamics in patients with normal systolic function late after aortic valve replacement. Circulation 1988; 77:613–624.

77. Carroll JD, Hess OM, Studer NP, et al: Systolic function during exercise in patients with coronary artery disease. J Am Coll Cardiol 1983; 2:206–216.

78. Carroll JD, Hess OM, Hirzel HO, Krayenbühl HP: Exercise-induced ischemia: The influence of altered relaxation on early diastolic pressures. Circulation 1983; 67:521–528.

79. Nonogi H, Hess OM, Ritter M, Krayenbühl HP: Diastolic properties of the normal left ventricle during supine exercise. Br Heart J 1988; 60:30–38.

80. Birchler B, Hess OM, Murakami T, et al: Comparison of intravenous digital subtraction cineangiocardiography with conventional contrast ventriculography for the determination of the left ventricular volume at rest and during exercise. Eur Heart J 1985; 6:497–509.

Chapter 12

Assessment of Diastolic Left Ventricular Function

OTTO M. HESS

DEFINITIONS

According to the classic definition,[1] diastole starts when the mitral valve opens and blood enters the left ventricle, and it ends with the onset of systolic contraction when the mitral valve closes. The clinical definition of diastole includes isovolumic relaxation as well and, hence, diastole commences at end-ejection, when the aortic valve closes (Fig. 12–1). However, relaxation is an active adenosine triphosphate–consuming process and belongs, strictly speaking, to systole. The definition of Brutsaert and associates[1] assumes that diastole starts with the true passive filling phase, which begins after completion of rapid filling. For the purpose of this chapter, the clinical definition of diastole is used, which is familiar to most cardiologists and is most widely used in the literature.

TERMINOLOGY

The relevant terms that are used in the chapter are the following:

1. *Stress* is defined as force per cross-sectional area (grams or dynes per square centimeter).

2. *Strain* (ϵ) is a dimensionless quantity and represents the change in length of a material in percentage or fraction of its initial length. Two definitions are used clinically: Lagrangian strain and natural strain.

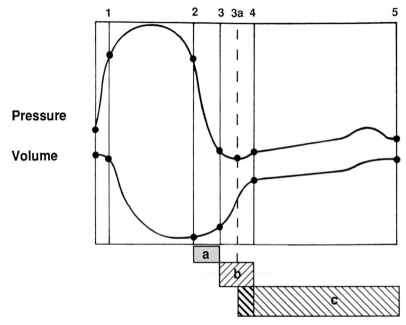

Figure 12–1. Schematic representation of the left ventricular pressure and volume curve. The points represent the following: point 1, aortic valve opening; point 2, aortic valve closure (equals end-systole); point 3, mitral valve opening; point 3a, the lowest diastolic pressure; point 4, the end of rapid diastolic filling; and point 5, end-diastole. The isovolumic relaxation (a) extends from end-systole to mitral valve opening, the rapid filling phase (b) from mitral valve opening to the point where the high rate of filling decreases suddenly, and passive diastolic filling (c) from the lowest diastolic pressure to end-diastole.

3. *Lagrangian strain* (ϵ) is defined as

$$\epsilon = (1 - l_0)/l_0$$

where l is equal to the instantaneous length and l_0 represents the reference length at a common (small) preload.

4. *Natural strain* (ϵ) is defined as

$$\epsilon = \ln(l/l_0)$$

5. *Elasticity* describes the property of a material to return to its initial length after the distending force is removed.

6. *Distensibility* is defined as the change in volume relative to a change in pressure (dV/dP); this term is often synonymous with the term *compliance.*

7. *Stiffness* is the reciprocal of distensibility and is defined as the change in pressure relative to the change in volume (dP/dV). *Ventricular stiffness* represents the global changes of the ventricle, whereas *myocardial stiffness* represents the changes of the myocardium itself. Ventricular properties are defined by the pressure-volume and myocardial properties by the stress-strain relationship.

8. *Creep* is the time-dependent elongation of a material held at a constant stress.

9. *Stress relaxation* is the time-dependent decrease in stress of a material held at a constant elongation.

10. *Viscoelasticity* is the property of a material that depends not only on the change in length (strain) but also on the rate of change in length (strain rate).

PHYSIOLOGY OF LEFT VENTRICULAR DIASTOLIC FUNCTION

Relaxation

Isovolumic relaxation starts with aortic valve closure, which often precedes the occurrence of peak negative dP/dt, and ends with mitral valve opening (see Fig. 12–1). The onset and rate of relaxation are governed by a variety of factors,[1, 2] such as load, inactivation, and synchronicity. When the afterload is increased during systolic contraction, the onset of relaxation is delayed and the rate is diminished.[3] Peak systolic pressure, end-systolic dimensions, coronary filling (stretching of muscle fibers), and deformation energy (elastic recoil) are the main determinants of relaxation load. Inactivation (inotropic state) and synchronicity of relaxation are major determinants of the rate of relaxation.[1, 3, 4]

Several indices have been used for quantita-

tion of relaxation, such as peak negative dP/dt, the time constant of isovolumic pressure or stress decay,[5–7] and the pressure half-time.[8] It should be realized that these indices are dependent on load, inactivation, and uniformity of relaxation.

Early Diastolic Filling

The rapid filling phase extends from mitral valve opening to the point at which the rate of filling decreases suddenly (see Fig. 12–1). There are essentially four mechanisms that govern rate and extent of rapid diastolic filling: (1) internal and external restoring forces (elastic recoil), which influence diastolic suction and hence early diastolic filling[9, 10]; (2) rate of relaxation, which is dependent on inotropic state and uniformity of relaxation; (3) driving pressure, which corresponds to the pressure gradient between the left atrium and left ventricle; and (4) passive diastolic stiffness of the left ventricle.

The rate of rapid filling has been determined invasively through frame-by-frame evaluation of left ventricular angiograms and noninvasively by Doppler echocardiography. Peak filling rate as well as the filling rate during the first half of diastole have been used as a measure of rapid diastolic filling.[11, 12]

Passive Diastolic Function

Passive diastolic function is characterized by the pressure-volume (chamber properties) and stress-strain (muscle properties) relationships of the left ventricle during the passive diastolic filling period, which extends from the end of early rapid diastolic filling to end-diastole (see Fig. 12–1). Some authors also have included the short filling phase from the lowest diastolic pressure to the end of the rapid filling phase.[13–16] This may be legitimate under some instances but may not be in others because relaxation may not be complete at the lowest diastolic pressure, especially when it is delayed, such as in patients with myocardial hypertrophy. Viscous forces are important determinants during early diastolic filling and may cause deviations from a true monoexponential pressure-volume relationship during high flow states such as exercise or pacing-induced tachycardia.[5, 15–17] According to Weisfeldt and coworkers,[18] relaxation is 97% complete at 3.5 times the time constant of isovolumic pressure decay after aortic valve closure. In control subjects, we have found that at the lowest diastolic pressure, 3.9 time constants had elapsed, whereas in patients with hypertrophic cardiomyopathy, only 2.4 time constants had elapsed; thus, relaxation is far from being com-

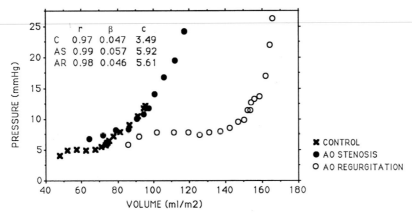

Figure 12–2. Pressure-volume relationship in a control patient (C), a patient with aortic stenosis (AS), and one with aortic regurgitation (AR). The pressure-volume curve is shifted to the right of the control curve in the patient with aortic (AO) regurgitation but is similar in the patient with aortic stenosis and the control patient. The calculated slope (β) of the pressure-volume curve (equals the constant of chamber stiffness) is slightly increased in aortic stenosis (0.057) but normal in aortic regurgitation (0. 046). The correlation coefficient (r) of the linear regression between the natural logarithm of left ventricular pressure and volume (see Table 12–3) is high in all three patients (>0.97). (See p. 218 for a description of curve parameters, using a monoexponential asymptote.)

plete in hypertrophic cardiomyopathy at the time when passive diastolic filling commences.[4]

Chamber Properties

Chamber properties are reflected by the diastolic pressure-volume or pressure-circumference relationship. The steepness of the exponential left ventricular pressure-volume curve represents the constant of chamber stiffness (β) (Fig. 12–2). A variety of factors determine the steepness and position of the pressure-volume curve and hence chamber stiffness (Table 12–1). Intrinsic properties of the left ventricle such as myocardial structure (collagen network), volume/mass ratio, and coronary perfusion as well as extrinsic factors such as ventricular interaction and pericardial constraint, play a major role as determinants of chamber properties.

Muscle Properties

Muscle properties are reflected by the diastolic stress-strain relationship. The steepness of the

Table 12–1. Determinants of Passive Left Ventricular Diastolic Function

Intrinsic Factors	Extrinsic Factors
Elastic properties	Ventricular interaction
Viscous properties	Pericardium
Inertia	Vascular volume
Wall thickness and geometry	(= erectile effect)
Myocardial structure	Intrathoracic pressure
Elastic recoil and relaxation	
Coronary perfusion	
Temperature, osmolarity	

exponential left ventricular stress-strain relationship represents the constant of muscle stiffness (β) (Fig. 12–3). A variety of factors influence the steepness of the stress-strain curve. Because strain is normalized to a common preload (e.g., zero wall stress), the position of the stress-strain relationship is similar in different patients (e.g., strain is zero when wall stress is zero). The basic determinants of muscle stiffness are structural properties such as the collagen network; furthermore, the volume/mass ratio, coronary vascular volume, and perfusion as well as temperature[8, 19–21] are all determinants of muscle stiffness (see Table 12–1).

MATHEMATIC EVALUATION

Isovolumic Relaxation

The most commonly used index for quantitation of isovolumic relaxation is the time constant of isovolumic pressure decay (T; msec), which has been shown to be exponential under most circumstances[7] but may deviate from a true monoexponential pressure decay in aortic regurgitation[22] or during acute myocardial ischemia.[23] Originally, Weiss and coworkers[7] determined the time constant T from a logarithmic pressure-time relation that assumes that the asymptote of pressure decay is zero and does not take baseline shifts into account.[23] However, it has been shown in the open-chest dog[9, 10] that left ventricular pressure in the transiently nonfilling working heart declines to values below zero. Therefore, most authors have used a logarithmic pressure-time relationship with as-

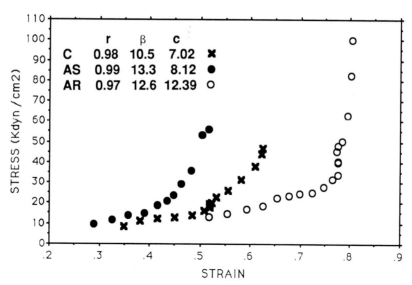

Figure 12–3. Stress-strain relationship in the same three patients as in Figure 12–2. The slope of the stress-strain relationship (β) represents the constant of myocardial stiffness, which is increased in both aortic stenosis (13.3) and aortic regurgitation (12.6) when compared with the control patient (10.5). The stress-strain curve is shifted to the left of the control patient in aortic stenosis and to the right of the control curve in aortic regurgitation. The correlation coefficient (r) of the linear regression between the natural logarithm of left ventricular stress and strain (see Table 12–3) is high in all three patients (>0.97). See Figure 12–2 for abbreviations and key.

ymptote. The time constant has been determined from several different models, including the derivative model, which is based on the relationship between instantaneous negative dP/dt and pressure during the phase of isovolumic relaxation and which is independent of baseline shifts (Fig. 12–4). The equation used to describe left ventricular pressure decay during isovolumic relaxation is[7]

$$P = Ae^{-\alpha t} + P_b$$

where P is left ventricular pressure (mm Hg),

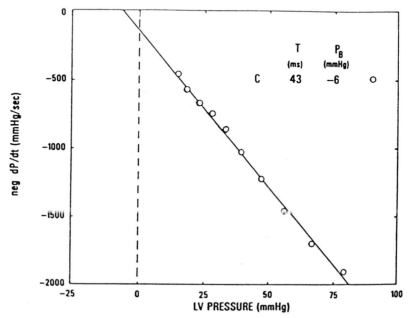

Figure 12–4. Determination of the time constant (T) of left ventricular pressure decay from the linear relationship between left ventricular (LV) pressure and negative dP/dt during isovolumic relaxation, which is defined as the time interval between peak negative dP/dt and mitral valve opening. The time constant (T) is 43 msec in this control patient, and the intercept (P_B) is −6 mm Hg.

A is left ventricular pressure at peak negative dP/dt (mm Hg), e is the base of the natural logarithm, α is the slope of the pressure-time relationship (1/sec), t is time (sec), and P_b is the pressure asymptote (mm Hg). The time constant is, according to Weiss,[7] defined as:

$$T = -1/\alpha$$

Calculation of the time constant includes different techniques such as the derivative method and the nonlinear curve–fitting or polynomial curve–fitting procedure.[8, 19] The derivative method assumes a linear relationship between negative dP/dt and left ventricular pressure during isovolumic relaxation in the presence of a monoexponential pressure decay:

$$dP/dt = \alpha(P - P_b)$$

or $\quad dP/dt = -1/T(P - P_b)$

or $\quad T = -(P - P_b)/dP/dt$

A sample calculation is given in Table 12–2, and a representative plot of negative dP/dt versus left ventricular pressure is shown in Figure 12–4. The normal value for the time constant of relaxation (n = 10) using the derivative model is 41 ± 12 msec.[15]

Early Diastolic Filling

Left ventricular diastolic filling from invasive data has been obtained angiographically from frame-by-frame analyses using instantaneous filling rates at 20 msec intervals.[11, 12] To minimize error due to random noise in the left ventricular volume-time curve, angiographic data are filtered with a fifth-grade moving average.[12] Diastolic filling rates are calculated as:

$$FR = V (t + 0.02) - V(t - 0.02)/0.04$$

where FR is the filling rate (mL/s), V is the left ventricular volume (mL), and t is time (sec). The greatest values occurring in the first and second halves of diastole are termed *early* and *late peak filling rates*, respectively (Fig. 12–5). The diastolic filling time interval from the beginning of diastolic filling to end-diastole can be divided into a first and second half, and the ratio of the volume increase during the first (%V1) and second (%V2) halves of diastole has been used as a measure of early and late diastolic filling (see Fig. 12–5). Normal values for peak filling rate (n = 6) are 483 ± 111 mL/sec during early diastole and 321 ± 102 mL/sec during late diastole; %V1 amounted to 65% ± 10 and %V2 to 35%.[12]

More recently, Doppler echocardiography has been used noninvasively to determine diastolic filling. However, this technique allows measurement of diastolic flow velocity and not absolute filling rates in milliliters per second. Thus, peak flow velocity during early (E-wave) and late (A-wave) diastolic filling as well as the E/A-wave ratio have been used as measures of diastolic filling.

Passive Diastolic Function

Chamber Properties

Calculation of chamber stiffness has been performed by plotting left ventricular diastolic filling pressure against left ventricular diastolic volume or midwall circumference[8, 13–15, 19] from the lowest diastolic pressure to end-diastole including[13–15, 25, 26] or excluding[27] the early rapid filling phase (see Fig. 12–2). The diastolic pressure-volume or pressure-dimension relationship is curvilinear and has been fit to a variety of nonlinear equations,[5, 13–15, 27] most of which are based on an exponential relationship:

$P = \alpha e^{\beta V}$ $\qquad$ (elastic model)
$P = \alpha e^{\beta V} + \zeta dV/dt$ $\quad$ (viscoelastic model)
$P = \alpha e^{\beta V} + c$ $\qquad$ (asymptote model)

Mathematic evaluation has been carried out by a nonlinear curve–fitting procedure[5, 14, 15, 28] or by a linear regression analysis using an iteration

Table 12–2. **Calculation of the Time Constant of Isovolumic Relaxation Using the Derivative Method**

Basic function: dP/dt = α (P – P_b) T = –1/α	
dP/dt	**Pressure**
−1799	63
−1654	56
−1498	50
−1346	44
−1208	38
−1025	31
−895	26
−798	21
−736	18
−654	14
Calculated linear regression:	dP/dt = −23.8 · P − 299
	T = 42 msec
	P_b = −12.5 mm Hg
	r = 0.9994

dP/dt, first derivative of left ventricular pressure (mm Hg/sec); α, slope of the dP/dt versus P relationship (1/sec); P, left ventricular pressure (mm Hg); T, time constant of left ventricular pressure decay (msec); P_b, pressure intercept at dP/dt = 0 (mm Hg); r, correlation coefficient. A linear regression equation was used for calculation of the slope α and intercept P_b.

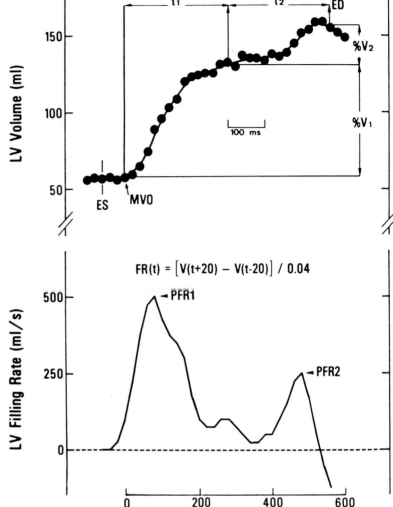

Figure 12–5. Left ventricular (LV) diastolic filling in a control patient. LV volumes *(upper)* were determined angiographically every 20 msec. Instantaneous LV filling rates *(lower)* and peak filling rates during early diastole (PFR1) and during atrial contraction (PFR2) are indicated. The volume increase from mitral valve opening (MVO) to end-diastole (ED) was determined and divided into a first (t_1) and a second (t_2) half. Percent volume increase during the first $(\%V_1)$ and second $(\%V_2)$ half of diastole are used as a measure of early and late diastolic filling. ES, end-systole. ms, milliseconds. (From Murakami M, Hess OM, Gage JE, et al: Diastolic filling dynamics in patients with aortic stenosis. Circulation 1986; 73: 1162–1174.)

procedure.[29, 30] The exponential equation with two variables (P, V) and three constants (e.g., α, β, c) can be transformed into a linear equation:

$$\ln(P - c) = \ln\alpha + \beta V$$

which can be solved by an iteration procedure, assuming given values for the c constant and by gradually changing c until the best curve fit with the highest correlation coefficient (r) is achieved (see later). These iterations can be performed easily on a personal computer.[8, 19] The constant α represents the intercept; the constant β (constant of chamber stiffness), the slope or steepness of the pressure-volume relationship; the constant ζ, the viscous constant; and c, the asymptote. *Normal values* (n = 9) for the constant of chamber stiffness β are 0.029 ±

0.011 mL^{-1} and for the c constant, 0.2 ± 4.5 mm Hg.[15]

The elastic model has been used by several authors over many years, but this model does not describe the true pressure-volume relationship sufficiently because it does not correct for baseline changes or viscous influences. More recently, viscoelastic models[11, 16, 00] or asymptote models[27, 30] have been used to correct for changes in passive elastic properties caused by viscous influences[4, 5, 14, 28] or by acute baseline changes due to acute myocardial ischemia or alterations in preload and afterload.[27, 30, 31]

Muscle Properties

Calculation of left ventricular myocardial stiffness has been achieved by plotting instantaneous left ventricular diastolic wall stress against left ventricular midwall strain[8, 13, 17, 27, 28] from the lowest diastolic pressure to end-diastole[14, 15] or from the end of the rapid filling phase to the peak of the a-wave.[27] Various equations have been used to calculate left ventricular meridional, circumferential, or radial wall stress using thin-wall and thick-wall models.[32] Left ventricular midwall strain has been determined from the Lagrangian or natural strain definition (see earlier), which are both dependent on the reference length at a wall stress of 0 kdyn/cm². Zero wall stress can be obtained in only a minority of patients and, thus, an extrapolation procedure has to be used to determine the reference muscle length at a common wall stress of 1 kdyn/cm² or 1 gm/cm² (approximately 0.8 mm Hg). The reference length at a wall stress of 1 kdyn/cm² (L_1) can be obtained from the diastolic wall stress-midwall length relationship:

$$S = \alpha e^{\beta L} + c$$

where
$$L_1 = -\ln\alpha/\beta$$

L_1 is used instead of l_0 for calculation of left ventricular midwall strain (ϵ) either due to the Lagrangian or the natural strain definition. *Normal values* for L_1 (n = 9) are 14.5 ± 2.8 cm.[30] Following determination of diastolic wall stress and midwall strain (see Fig. 12–3), curve fitting is performed using the same three exponential equations as for the pressure-volume relationship:

$$S = \alpha^* e^{\beta^*\epsilon} \quad \text{(elastic model)}$$
$$S = \alpha^* e^{\beta^*\epsilon} + \zeta^* E/dt \quad \text{(viscoelastic model)}$$
$$S = \alpha^* e^{\beta^*\epsilon} + c^* \quad \text{(asymptote model)}$$

The mathematic evaluation can be carried out by a nonlinear curve–fitting procedure[5, 14, 15] or by a linear regression analysis using an iteration procedure as shown in Table 12–3. The constant α^* represents the intercept; the constant β^*, the slope or steepness of the stress-strain relationship (constant of myocardial stiffness); the constant ζ^*, the viscous constant; and c^*, the asymptote. *Normal values* for the constant of muscle stiffness β^* are 14.4 ± 7.1 (n = 9), and for the c^* constant they are 1.1 ± 5.8 kdyn/cm².[30]

The constant of myocardial stiffness represents the mechanical properties of the heart muscle itself. The higher the constant, the stiffer the muscle. The most appropriate model to use in the presence of high strain rates (dE/dt) is the viscoelastic model, or in the presence of baseline shifts, (e.g., acute ischemia, pressure

Table 12–3. Calculation of the Constant of Myocardial Stiffness (Asymptote Model) Using an Iteration Procedure

Basic function:	$S = \alpha^* e^{\beta^*\epsilon} + c^*$	(1)
or	$\ln(S - c^*) = \ln\alpha^* + \beta^*\epsilon$	(2)

Equation (2) is used as a linear regression analysis for calculation of α^* and β^*. The constant c^* is iterated until the correlation coefficent (r) of the linear regression between $\ln(S - c^*)$ and $\ln\alpha^* + \beta^*\epsilon$ is maximal. Iteration is started at a c^* value, which is equal to the lowest diastolic stress ($c^* = 11.2$ gm/cm²) and then changed in steps of 1 and 0.1 gm/cm²:

	r	β*	c*
Iteration steps for	0.9554	10.0	11.1
$c^* = 1.0$ gm/cm²:	⇒ 0.9847	5.5	10.1
	0.9823	3.7	9.1
Iteration steps for	0.9847	6.0	10.3
$c^* = 0.1$ gm/cm²:	⇒ 0.9848	5.7	10.2
	0.9847	5.5	10.1

The final result is $\beta^* = 5.7$, $c^* = 10.2$ gm/cm², and the correlation coefficent for the stress-strain relationship is 0.9848.

S, left ventricular wall stress (gm/cm²); α^*, elastic constant (gm/cm²); e, base of the natural logarithm; β^*, constant of myocardial stiffness; ϵ, left ventricular midwall strain; c^*, asymptote (gm/cm²). For determination of strain, the reference length L_1 must be calculated by an iteration procedure (see Passive Diastolic Function in text). Then, in a second step, α^*, β^*, and c^* are determined, as shown in this table.

overload hypertrophy, drug interventions) the asymptote model is most appropriate.[27]

DETERMINANTS OF LEFT VENTRICULAR DIASTOLIC FUNCTION

Relaxation

The onset and rate of relaxation are influenced by a variety of factors such as load, inactivation and uniformity of load. These three factors are the main determinants of isovolumic relaxation.[1]

Loading Conditions

Experimentally, it has been shown that when the left ventricle faces an additional load early during contraction (i.e., a contraction load), the onset of relaxation will be delayed and the rate of relaxation will be diminished.[1, 25, 33] If the load is added during the late phase of ejection (i.e., a relaxation load), relaxation will be accelerated.[33] Early and late systolic pressure, the degree of end-systolic deformation, coronary filling and intramyocardial turgor (myocardial fiber stretch), and ventricular dimensions are

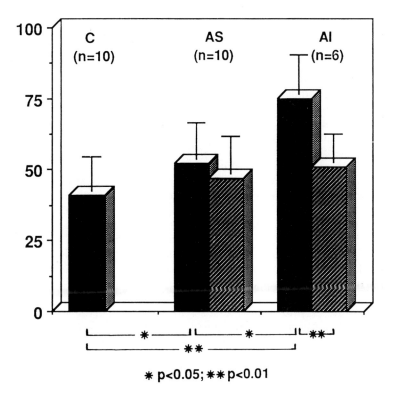

TIME CONSTANT OF ISOVOLUMIC RELAXATION

Figure 12–6. Time constant of left ventricular pressure decay (T) in controls (C) and patients with aortic stenosis (AS) and aortic insufficiency (AI) before *(dark bars)* and after *(hatched bars)* successful aortic valve replacement. Relaxation is prolonged preoperatively in both chronic pressure and volume overload but is normalized after successful valve replacement. Thus, regression of myocardial hypertrophy seems to be associated with an improvement in the rate of relaxation, although the influence of altered loading conditions might have played a role in the prolongation of the time constant of relaxation before operation. (From Hess OM, Felder L, Krayenbuchl HP: Diastolic function in valvular heart disease. Herz 1991; 16:124-129.)

some of the major determinants of the loading conditions for relaxation. An increase in left ventricular peak systolic pressure, mean aortic pressure, or left ventricular end-systolic pressure is generally accompanied by an increase in T.[4, 33] An increase in preload has, however, no effect on T, as shown by Zile and coworkers.[34] Prolongation of T occurs regularly with severe myocardial hypertrophy. In patients with aortic stenosis (T = 52 msec) or aortic insufficiency (T = 75 msec), the time constant is significantly prolonged[22] compared with controls (T = 41 msec; Fig. 12–6). This prolongation of T is probably due to left ventricular hypertrophy and the increase in afterload. Successful aortic valve replacement is associated with a normalization of relaxation in aortic stenosis (T = 17 msec) and a significant reduction of the time constant in aortic regurgitation (T = 51 msec); parallel to the decrease in T, left ventricular muscle mass decreased by 37% in aortic stenosis and by 30% in aortic regurgitation. It is of interest that prolongation of T occurs in patients with severe myocardial hypertrophy even before indices of left ventricular systolic function, such as isovolumic contractile indices or ejection fraction, are decreased.[22]

Inactivation

A change in inotropic state usually is accompanied by a change in relaxation. An increase in inotropic state is associated with an augmentation in the speed of relaxation (= decrease in the time constant T) and vice versa. However, it is important to know that maneuvers with a similar inotropic action on systolic function do not necessarily have the same effect on T: catecholamines lead to a decrease in T, whereas T is increased in the postextrasystolic beats.[35] In the latter case, the reduced inactivation is the result of the intracellular calcium accumulation, which is responsible for the potentiation of systolic contraction but offsets the accelerating effect on relaxation.

Synchronicity

Prolongation of relaxation occurs with left ventricular asynchrony due to abnormal activation in the presence of a bundle branch block, asymmetric distribution of myocardial hypertrophy, or regional wall motion abnormalities during myocardial ischemia. Asynchrony and increased end-systolic volume in patients with acute myocardial ischemia are important factors that are responsible for the rate and also the extent of pressure decay. The myocardium may never be completely relaxed between systolic contractions, especially when diastole is brief, such as during exercise. The presence of a large akinetic area (e.g., an infarcted region) or ischemic zone may impair the rate of relaxation because inhomogeneous relaxation is responsible for the temporal disruption of the relaxation process. This disruption of the relaxation process may cause an abnormal interaction among different regions of the left ventricle. The ischemic zone may show passive contractions after systolic elongation during the preceding cardiac cycle (e.g., late systolic shortening), which results in regional dyssynchrony.[36] Some authors have used a biexponential model for the calculation of the time constant because left ventricular pressure fall during isovolumic relaxation showed a flat early and a steep late portion during myocardial ischemia.[23] Therefore, two time constants have been calculated, a first one (T_1) during the 40 msec immediately after peak negative dP/dt and a second one (T_2) during the remaining isovolumic relaxation period. T_2 is considered to represent the true time constant of relaxation, whereas T_1 is characteristic of the early relaxation phase with different relaxation rates in different left ventricular regions. T_1 was found to be 55 ± 8 msec and T_2 was 44 ± 7 msec under resting conditions in 14 patients with coronary artery disease; both time constants increased significantly to 79 ± 17 msec (T_1) and to 51 ± 8 msec (T_2) during a 20-second occlusion (percutaneous transluminal coronary angioplasty) of one major coronary artery.[31]

Early Diastolic Filling

Left ventricular filling is a dynamic process involving active and passive properties of the atrium and the ventricle.[10] The rate of left ventricular pressure decay and the atrioventricular pressure gradient are the major determinants of early diastolic filling, whereas the diastolic stiffness of the left ventricle becomes increasingly more important during the later phase of diastolic filling. The atrioventricular pressure difference is determined by several factors, such as the elastic recoil, the rate of left ventricular pressure decay, left atrial pressure at the time of mitral valve opening, filling time, and stroke volume.

Elastic Recoil (Restoring Forces)

The normal left ventricle contracts to a volume smaller than its elastic equilibrium and then rebounds by an elastic recoil to cause negative left ventricular pressure and, thus, ventricular diastolic suction. Extensive systolic cavity reduction to a small end-systolic volume produces internal and external restoring forces that enhance early diastolic filling. It has been shown in the transiently nonfilling left ventricle that left ventricular pressure falls to negative values.[9] The negative intraventricular pressure sucks blood from the left atrium into the left ventricle and enables the ventricle to fill rapidly. A loss of elastic recoil such as during acute myocardial ischemia is associated with an impairment of early diastolic filling and is counterregulated by an increase in left atrial driving pressure.[37] Quantification of elastic recoil under clinical conditions is difficult, but some authors have used the end-systolic volume as a measure of elastic recoil; the smaller the volume, the larger the elastic recoil and vice versa. The elastic recoil plays an important role in early diastolic filling in the normal left ventricle, especially during physical exercise, when the diastolic filling time interval is shortened. The minimum diastolic pressure decreases during exercise (Fig. 12–7) as a result of the enhanced diastolic restoring forces and the increased speed of relaxation.[17] A loss of elastic recoil can be observed with the occurrence of regional asynchrony in patients with exercise-induced ischemia.[38]

Relaxation

The rate of relaxation is an important determinant of early diastolic pressures and filling rates. Delayed and incomplete relaxation may postpone the onset of diastolic filling. Myocardial hypertrophy,[22] acute ischemia, and pacing-induced asynergy[37, 38] prolong relaxation and, hence, influence early diastolic filling. A forceful ventricular contraction with enhanced elastic recoil can partially compensate for delayed relaxation such as seen in patients with hypertrophic cardiomyopathy. However, in most patients, elastic recoil and the rate of relaxation are reduced in parallel, such as during myocardial ischemia or in patients with systolic pump failure. Inflow obstructions in patients with mitral stenosis or constrictive pericarditis are associated with negative early diastolic pressures as a sign of diastolic suction.

The term *complete* or *incomplete diastolic relaxation* has become popular in recent years.[18, 39, 40] The completeness of relaxation has been assessed from the number of time constants (T) that have elapsed between end-systole and the lowest diastolic pressure. According to Weiss and coworkers,[7] left ventricular relaxation is

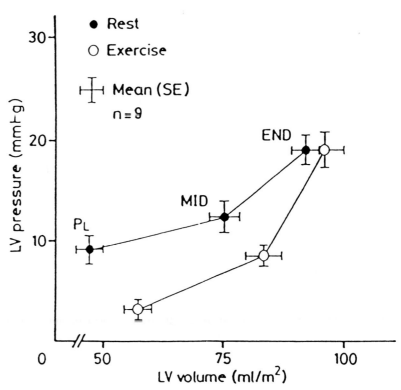

Figure 12–7. Left ventricular pressure-volume relationship in nine control patients at rest *(closed symbols)* and during submaximal bicycle exercise *(open symbols)*. Data of the nine patients are averaged at the lowest diastolic pressure (PL), at mid-diastole (MID) as well as end-diastole (END). There is a downward displacement of the pressure-volume curve during exercise that is most pronounced during early and mid-diastole. Thus, the left ventricle is able to reduce the lowest diastolic filling pressure under exercise conditions by enhancing elastic recoil and increasing the rate of relaxation. At the same time, the pressure-volume curve becomes steeper during exercise probably owing to the higher filling rates with an increased viscous resistance. (From Nonogi H, Hess OM, Ritter M, Krayenbühl HP: Diastolic properties of the normal left ventricle during supine exercise. Br Heart J 1988; 60:30–38.)

complete to 97% when 3.5 time constants have elapsed (see earlier). This ratio amounted to 3.9 in controls and was significantly reduced to 2.4 (*P*<.05 versus controls) in patients with hypertrophic cardiomyopathy.[4]

Driving Pressure

The atrioventricular pressure gradient is a major determinant of early diastolic filling.[10] At a constant left atrial pressure, an acceleration of left ventricular pressure decay augments early diastolic filling and vice versa. A decrease in left ventricular filling is, however, compensated by an increase in left atrial driving pressure. Filling may be even enhanced when diastolic pressure is increased, such as is seen in patients with severe aortic stenosis.[12] In patients with acute myocardial ischemia, a reduction in early diastolic filling can be often seen because elastic recoil is diminished and left ventricular relaxation is delayed. However, normal filling rates were observed at rest and during dynamic exercise in patients with coronary artery disease and exercise-induced ischemia[37] mainly due to the sizable increase in filling pressure. The increase in driving pressure compensated completely for the loss of elastic recoil and delayed relaxation during exercise-induced ischemia. A potentially important factor that has not been studied in

the past is that the atrioventricular pressure gradient reflects also the properties of the atrium.[9, 10]

Passive Elastic Properties

The passive elastic properties influence early diastolic filling in a complex way: At the beginning of diastolic filling, the heart is small and the operating stiffness is low, but at end-diastole, the heart is filled and operating stiffness is high. Thus, the influence of the passive elastic properties on diastolic filling varies from early to late diastole, or in other words, the inflow resistance increases during diastolic filling. Ventricular chamber size, muscle mass, and structural alterations play an important role as determinants for the passive elastic properties, and as a consequence, also influence diastolic filling. In general terms, the bigger the heart, the higher the filling pressure; or the thicker the wall, the larger operating stiffness becomes and, thus, the smaller diastolic filling is. Changes in passive elastic properties and alterations in filling can be observed primarily in patients with severely dilated hearts or with stiff ventricles, such as in hypertrophic cardiomyopathy.

Passive Diastolic Function

For practical purposes, it is important to distinguish between ventricular and myocardial properties. Ventricular passive elastic properties are directly related to the symptoms of the patient, whereas the myocardial properties reflect the functional status of the heart muscle itself and may or may not be influenced by the organ as a whole. Many authors believe that the passive elastic properties of the myocardium represent the structural properties of the heart muscle and, thus, might ultimately influence clinical course and prognosis.

Viscoelasticity

The heart is a viscoelastic organ; viscous forces retard deformation and are proportional to the velocity gradient between different myocardial layers. The following two phenomena have been associated with the viscoelastic nature of the heart: the *creep phenomenon* (i.e., elongation of the muscle under a constant load) and *stress relaxation* (i.e., decrease in stress with time when the muscle is held at a constant length). These two phenomena have been observed in the papillary muscle and also in the experimental animal. Viscous effects have been observed during rapid length changes, such as during early diastolic filling and during atrial contraction.[16, 28, 41] Under conditions induced by exercise, a downward shift of the left ventricular diastolic pressure-volume relationship was observed in normal subjects (see Fig. 12–7). This downward shift was most prominent during early diastole and was thought to be due to the enhanced elastic recoil and the increased rate of relaxation (see earlier). The increase in slope of the diastolic pressure-volume relationship during exercise is probably due to an increased viscous resistance caused by the rapid inflow with high diastolic lengthening rates.[17] Viscous effects were also observed in patients with severe myocardial hypertrophy and enlarged left ventricles due to aortic valve disease.[14, 15] Increased viscous forces were mainly seen during early diastolic filling, whereas viscous forces were minimal during late diastolic filling. Corrections for these viscous effects were performed by a mathematic procedure using a viscous term (see Mathematic Evaluation Section earlier).

Myocardial Structure and Volume/Mass Ratio

The basic determinant for the passive elastic properties of the left ventricle is myocardial structure. The composition of the heart muscle with its muscular and collagen fractions and the collagen network with the perimysial and endomysial fibers, as well as the struts and strands between the single cardiac fibers, are probably the main determinants of the mechanical properties of the heart muscle itself. Weber[42] has shown that a rearrangement of the collagen network caused by a change in size and geometry of the left ventricle is associated with a change in its elastic properties. The volume/mass ratio has been used[8, 13, 19, 26] as a simple clinical parameter for the assessment of the geometry of the left ventricle and the type of hypertrophy (eccentric versus concentric). A high volume/mass ratio (e.g., eccentric hypertrophy) has been associated with a low chamber stiffness of the left ventricle, and a low volume/mass ratio has been associated with a high chamber stiffness of the left ventricle. In an attempt to include myocardial structure as well, Hess and coworkers[15] have substituted muscle mass with fibrous mass (i.e., muscle mass multiplied by percent interstitial fibrosis; gm/m^2) and used the reciprocal of the volume/fibrous mass ratio as a measure for left ventricular geometry and structure.[15] These authors observed a good exponential relationship between the volume/fibrous mass ratio and the constant of myocardial stiffness in patients with aortic valve disease. Interstitial fibrosis (i.e., nonmuscular interstitial space) also correlated with the constant of myocardial stiffness (Fig. 12–8), that is, the more interstitial fibrosis is present, the stiffer the myocardium becomes. Similar observations have been made in the experimental animal.[24, 43]

Ventricular Interaction and the Pericardium

Interactions between cardiac chambers have been reported in the intact animal and in humans.[44–46] Filling of the right chamber caused an upward shift of the left ventricular diastolic pressure-volume curve, which was thought to be due to an increase in intrapericardial pressure or other factors such as septal displacement, increased septal stiffness, and stretching of common fibers within the interventricular septum.[47] Acute volume loading of the heart with the pericardium intact shifts the entire left ventricular pressure-volume curve upward[45] because of a rise in intrapericardial pressure. Nitroprusside infusion shifts the pressure-volume curve downward, accompanied by a drop in intrapericardial pressure. These acute shifts of the diastolic pressure-volume curve were abolished when the experiments were repeated after removal of the pericardium.[45] Thus, an intact pericardium plays an important role in ventricular interaction, but the magnitude of the displacement of the diastolic pressure-volume curve is different when the left ventricle and left atrium (pressure

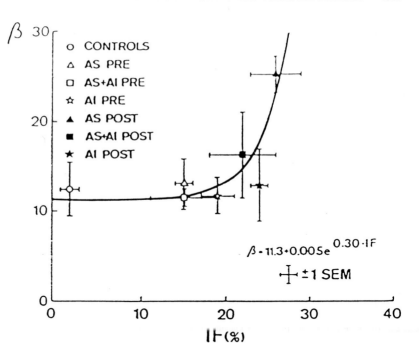

Figure 12–8. Correlation between interstitial fibrosis (IF) and constant of myocardial stiffness (β) in controls, patients with aortic stenosis (AS), combined valve lesions (AS+AI), and aortic insufficiency (AI) before and after successful valve replacement. There is an exponential relationship between these two parameters, indicating that myocardial structure or interstitial tissue is a major determinant of the passive elastic properties in patients with aortic valve disease. Thus, myocardial stiffness tends to increase when fibrosis is larger than 20%. (From Hess OM, Ritter M, Schneider J, et al: Diastolic function in aortic valve disease: Techniques of evaluation and pre-/postoperative changes. Herz 1984; 9:288–296.)

loading) or when all four chambers (volume loading by fluid infusion) are distended at the same time.

The upward shift of the diastolic pressure-volume relationship during acute ischemia[38] is a complex interplay of different mechanisms, including ventricular interaction, loss of elastic recoil, delayed and incomplete relaxation, Frank-Starling mechanism, and erectile effect (see later). As an indirect measure of intrapericardial pressure, the *right atrial pressure* can be used in the absence of significant right-sided heart disease.[48]

Erectile Effect

Salisbury and coworkers have shown that an increase in intramyocardial blood volume is associated with an upward shift of the diastolic pressure-volume curve.[49] This effect was explained by an increase in myocardial turgor, which was thought to be responsible for the increase in myocardial stiffness (i.e., erectile effect). In a more recent study, however, Templeton and coworkers[20] were not able to confirm this observation. It seems clear that the intramyocardial turgor has some effect on the passive elastic properties of the left ventricle, but these effects seem to be small and differences in the diastolic stiffness difficult to obtain.

EFFECT OF EXERCISE ON DIASTOLIC FUNCTION

The effect of dynamic exercise on left ventricular function has been analyzed by many authors

and many techniques. Attention has been focused mainly on the systolic performance, but little is known about the diastolic function during exercise.

Diastolic Function in Controls

Nonogi and coworkers[17] have studied left ventricular diastolic function at rest and during supine bicycle exercise (mean workload 91 watts) in 9 normal subjects. They observed a fall in end-systolic volume, a decrease in the time constant of left ventricular isovolumic pressure decay, and a drop in the lowest diastolic pressure. Peak and mean filling rates increased by 71% and 142%, respectively, during exercise, whereas the diastolic pressure-volume relationship (see Fig. 12–7) showed a downward displacement with a significant increase in slope (dP/dV) from 0.22 to 0.40 mm Hg/mL/m². End-diastolic pressure and volume, however, remained unchanged. These results show that elastic recoil is enhanced, and left ventricular relaxation is faster during exercise than at rest. These two phenomena probably are responsible for the decrease in early diastolic pressure (see Fig. 12–7). The increase in diastolic chamber stiffness (ΔP/ΔV) from rest to exercise is probably related to an increased viscous resistance caused by the high diastolic lengthening rates.

Diastolic Function in Aortic Valve Disease

The effect of exercise on diastolic function was evaluated in patients late after successful valve replacement (10 ± 2 years) in the presence of a normal systolic function.[50] Twenty patients were studied at rest and during supine bicycle exercise (mean workload 112 watts); 14 patients had a normal increase in mean wedge pressure during exercise (<20 mm Hg; mean value 16 mm Hg), but six showed an abnormal rise to 33 mm Hg while end-diastolic volume remained unchanged. This derangement of diastolic function became evident only during exercise and may reflect irreversible structural changes that are not severe enough to affect systolic function as well. Thus, diastolic dysfunction might precede systolic dysfunction and might help identify patients with an already advanced stage of valvular heart disease.

REFERENCES

1. Brutsaert D, Rademakers FE, Sys SU: Triple control of relaxation: Implications in cardiac disease. Circulation 1984; 69:190–196.
2. Kumada T, Karliner JS, Pouleur H, et al: Effects of coronary occlusion on early ventricular diastolic events in conscious dogs. Am J Physiol 1979; 237:H542–H549.
3. Gaasch WH, Blaustein AS, Andrias CW, et al: Myocardial relaxation. Part II: Hemodynamic determinants of rate of left ventricular isovolumic pressure decline. Am J Physiol 1980; 239:H1–H6.
4. Krayenbühl HP: Diastolic ventricular function: A short overview. Cardiologia 1988; 33:15–20.
5. Hess OM, Osakada G, Lavelle JF, et al: Diastolic myocardial wall stiffness and ventricular relaxation during partial and complete coronary occlusions in the conscious dog. Circ Res 1983; 52:387–400.
6. Pouleur H, Rousseau MF, van Eyll C, Charlier AA: Assessment of regional left ventricular relaxation in patients with coronary artery disease: Importance of geometric factors and changes in wall thickness. Circulation 1984; 69:696–702.
7. Weiss JL, Frederiksen JW, Weisfeldt ML: Hemodynamic determinants of the time-course of fall in canine left ventricular pressure. J Clin Invest 1976; 58:751–760.
8. Mirsky I: Assessment of diastolic function: Suggested methods and future considerations. Circulation 1984; 69:836–841.
9. Yellin EL, Hori M, Yoran C, et al: Left ventricular relaxation in the filling and non-filling intact canine heart. Am J Physiol 1986; 250:H620–H629.
10. Yellin EL, Nikolic S, Frater RWM: Left ventricular filling dynamics and diastolic function. Cardiovasc Dis 1990; 32:247–271.
11. Murakami M, Hess OM, Krayenbühl HP: Left ventricular function before and after diltiazem in patients with coronary artery disease. J Am Coll Cardiol 1985; 5:723–730.
12. Murakami M, Hess OM, Gage JE, et al: Diastolic filling dynamics in patients with aortic stenosis. Circulation 1986; 73:1162–1174.
13. Gaasch WH, Battle WE, Oboler AA, et al: Left ventricular stress and compliance in man: With special reference to normalized ventricular function curves. Circulation 1972; 45:746–762.
14. Hess OM, Grimm J, Krayenbühl HP: Diastolic simple elastic and viscoelastic properties of the left ventricle in man. Circulation 1979; 59:1178–1187.
15. Hess OM, Ritter M, Schneider J, et al: Diastolic stiffness and myocardial structure in aortic valve disease before and after valve replacement. Circulation 1984; 69:855–865.
16. Pouleur H, Karliner JS, LeWinter MM, Covell JW: Diastolic viscous properties of the intact canine left ventricle. Circ Res 1979; 45:410–419.
17. Nonogi H, Hess OM, Ritter M, Krayenbühl HP: Diastolic properties of the normal left ventricle during supine exercise. Br Heart J 1988; 60:30–38.
18. Weisfeldt ML, Frederiksen JW, Yin FCP, Weiss JL: Evidence of incomplete left ventricular relaxation in the dog: Prediction from the time constant for isovolumic pressure fall. J Clin Invest 1978; 62:1296–1302.
19. Mirsky I, Pasipoularides A: Clinical assessment of diastolic function. Prog Cardiovasc Dis 1990; 32:291–318.
20. Templeton GH, Ecker RR, Mitchell JH: Left ventricular stiffness during diastole and systole: The influence of changes in volume and inotropic state. Cardiovasc Res 1972; 6:95.
21. Templeton GH, Wildenthal K, Willerson JT, Reardon EC: Influence of temperature on the mechanical properties of cardiac muscle. Circ Res 1974; 34:624–634.
22. Eichhorn P, Grimm J, Koch R, et al: Left ventricular relaxation in patients with left ventricular hypertrophy secondary to aortic valve disease. Circulation 1982; 65:1395–1404.
23. Brower RW, Meij S, Serruys PW: A model of asynchronous left ventricular relaxation predicting the bi-exponential pressure decay. Cardiovasc Res 1983; 17:482–488.
24. Holubarsch C, Holubarsch T, Jacob R, et al: Passive elastic properties of myocardium in different models and stages of hypertrophy: A study comparing mechanical, chemical, and morphometric parameters. Perspec Cardiovasc Res 1983; 7:323–336.
25. Hori M, Inoue M, Kitakaze M, et al: Loading sequence is a major determinant of afterload-dependent relaxation in intact canine heart. Am J Physiol 1985; 249:H747–H754.
26. Gaasch WH, Levine HJ, Quinones MA, Alexander JK: Left ventricular compliance: Mechanisms and clinical implications. Am J Cardiol 1976; 38:645–653.
27. Peterson KL, Tsuji J, Johnson A, et al: Diastolic left ventricular pressure-volume and stress-strain relations in patients with valvular aortic stenosis and left ventricular hypertrophy. Circulation 1978; 58:77–90.
28. Rankin JS, Arentzen CE, McHale PA, et al: Viscoelastic properties of the diastolic left ventricle in the conscious dog. Circ Res 1977; 41:37–45.
29. Bortone AS, Hess OM, Chiddo A, et al: Functional and structural abnormalities in patients with dilated cardiomyopathy. J Am Coll Cardiol 1989; 14:613–623.
30. Corin WJ, Murakami M, Monrad SE, et al: Left ventricular passive diastolic properties in chronic mitral regurgitation. Circulation 1991; 83:797–807.
31. Serruys PW, Wijns W, Piscione F, et al: Ejection, filling, and diastasis during transluminal occlusion in man: Consideration on global and regional left ventricular function. In Grossman W, Lorell BH (eds.): Diastolic Relaxation of the Heart. Boston-Dordrecht-Lancaster, Martinus Nijhoff Publishing, 1988, pp 255–279.
32. Huisman RM, Sipkema P, Westerhof N, Elzinga G: Comparison of models used to calculate left ventricular wall force. Med Biol Comput 1980; 18:133–144.
33. Gaasch WH, Carroll JD, Blaustein AS, Bing OHL: Myocardial relaxation: Effects of preload on the time course of isovolumetric relaxation. Circulation 1986; 73:1037–1041.
34. Zile MR, Conrad CH, Gaasch WH, et al: Preload does not affect relaxation rate in normal, hypoxic, or hyper-

trophic myocardium. Am J Physiol 1990; 258: H191–H197.

35. Carroll JD, Widmer R, Hess OM, et al: Left ventricular isovolumic pressure decay and diastolic mechanics after postextrasystolic potentiation and during exercise. Am J Cardiol 1983; 51:583–590.

36. Tennant R, Wiggers CJ: The effect of coronary occlusion on myocardial contraction. Am J Physiol 1935; 112:351–361.

37. Carroll JD, Hess OM, Hirzel HO, Krayenbühl HP: Dynamics of left ventricular filling at rest and during exercise. Circulation 1983; 68:59–67.

38. Carroll JD, Hess OM, Hirzel HO, et al: Left ventricular systolic and diastolic function in coronary artery disease: Effects of revascularization on exercise-induced ischemia. Circulation 1985; 72:119–129.

39. Carroll JD, Lang RM, Neumann AL, et al: The differential effects of positive inotropic and vasodilator therapy on diastolic properties in patients with congestive cardiomyopathy. Circulation 1986; 74:815–825.

40. Lorell BH, Paulus WJ, Grossman W, et al: Improved diastolic function and systolic performance in hypertrophic cardiomyopathy after nifedipine. N Engl J Med 1980; 303:801–803.

41. Noble MIM: The diastolic viscous properties of cat papillary muscle. Circ Res 1977; 40:288–292.

42. Weber K: Cardiac interstitium in health and disease: The fibrillar collagen network. J Am Coll Cardiol 1985; 5:811–826.

43. Motz W, Strauer BE: Left ventricular function and collagen content after regression of hypertensive hypertrophy. Circulation 1989; 13:43–50.

44. Hess OM, Bhargava V, Ross J Jr, Shabetai R: The role of the pericardium in interactions between the cardiac chambers. Am Heart J 1983; 106:1377–1383.

45. Shirato K, Shabetai R, Bhargava V, et al: Alteration of the left ventricular diastolic pressure-segment length relation produced by the pericardium: Effects of cardiac distension and afterload reduction in conscious dogs. Circulation 1978; 57:1191–1198.

46. Taylor RR, Covell JW, Sonnenblick EH, Ross J Jr: Dependence of ventricular distensibility on filling of the opposite ventricle. Am J Physiol 1967; 213:711–718.

47. Ross J Jr: Acute displacement of the diastolic pressure-volume curve of the left ventricle: Role of the pericardium and the right ventricle. Circulation 1979; 59: 32–37.

48. Tyberg JV, Taichman GC, Smith ER, et al: The relation between pericardial pressure and right atrial pressure: An intraoperative study. Circulation 1986; 73:428–432.

49. Salisbury PF, Cross CE, Rieben PA: Distensibility and water content of heart muscle before and after injury. Circ Res 1960; 8:788.

50. Monrad ES, Hess OM, Murakami M, et al: Abnormal exercise hemodynamics in patients with normal systolic function late after aortic valve replacement. Circulation 1988; 77:613–624.

Chapter 13

Assessment of Right Ventricular Function

MARVIN A. KONSTAM
JAMES E. UDELSON

Assessment of right ventricular (RV) function has several documented applications.[1-3] In the setting of acute or chronic ischemic heart disease, documentation of RV systolic dysfunction may indicate the presence of RV ischemia or infarction.[4-6] In severe pulmonary hypertension, RV systolic function usually is impaired due to abnormal systolic load. Indices of RV performance have been found to correlate roughly with pulmonary artery pressure in patients with valvular or congenital disease, left ventricular failure, or primary pulmonary or pulmonary vascular disease.[7-14] In the setting of an acute ventricular septal defect, RV systolic function has been found to be a major predictor of survival following surgical repair.[15] Likewise, in patients with congenital heart disease, assessment of RV systolic performance may provide important physiologic insight and may help guide therapy and predict surgical outcomes.[13, 14, 16] Altered RV function may represent the explanation for continued functional impairment following repair of congenital anomalies such as atrial and ventricular septal defects, transposition of the great arteries, pulmonic stenosis, and tetralogy of Fallot.[17-19] When RV systolic functional impairment occurs in the presence of normal loading conditions, such an abnormality may be due to coronary artery obstructive disease, right coronary artery thrombosis or spasm, preferential involvement of the right ventricle with a myopathic process, or RV dysplasia. Assessment of RV function in conjunction with exercise may augment the physiologic information gained. An abnormal exercise response (decrease or no change in ejection fraction) has been described in the presence of right coronary artery disease[4-6] or in pulmonary hypertension.[20, 21] In the former circumstance, ejection fraction is presumed to

decrease because of an inability to increase contractility in response to augmented systolic load. In the setting of pulmonary hypertension, pulmonary vascular recruitment is near maximum at rest. During exercise, pulmonary vascular resistance fails to decrease, pulmonary artery pressure increases further, and the right ventricle succumbs to its excessive load.

In the setting of left-sided heart failure, RV systolic function has been found to correlate with survival,[22, 23] as well as with functional status.[24] The relation between RV function and survival is likely to be complex. RV dysfunction is a marker of excessive systolic load and, therefore, of increased left-sided heart filling pressure or pulmonary vascular pathology, or both. Alternatively, RV dysfunction may indicate involvement of the right ventricle with the primary ischemic or myopathic process that induced left-sided heart failure. Thus, RV systolic failure may be an indicator of severe hemodynamic derangement, carrying a poor prognosis, or it may contribute primarily to accelerated clinical deterioration. These two mechanisms are likely to coexist. Patients in whom RV function is preserved tend to have relatively normal functional capacity.[24] However, such patients may be prone to develop rapid-onset pulmonary edema, even in the absence of active myocardial ischemia.[25] In contrast, RV dilatation and systolic failure are generally accompanied by a clinical syndrome of functional incapacity and systemic venous congestion but are rarely associated with rapid-onset pulmonary edema, because the dilated, compliant right ventricle tends to buffer abrupt changes in intravascular volume.

RV volume and systolic function are strongly influenced by pharmacologic interventions that alter systolic and diastolic load. Drug therapy in congestive heart failure has little demonstrable effect on left ventricular ejection fraction. In contrast, RV function may be improved by, and may be used to monitor, vasodilator therapy.[26–29] Agents with inotropic action also have been observed to improve RV systolic function,[7, 28, 30] although these effects may be predominantly the result of reduced RV systolic load.

TECHNIQUES

A variety of techniques are available for assessing RV systolic performance in the cardiac catheterization laboratory. These include (1) contrast ventriculography, employing conventional cineangiography; (2) digital angiography; (3) indicator-dilution volumetrics, including the thermodilution technique; and (4) impedance volumetrics. In addition, RV function may be assessed by the noninvasive imaging modalities of radionuclide ventriculography, echocardiography, magnetic resonance imaging, and computerized tomography.

The configuration of the right ventricle makes functional assessment, which is based on volumetrics, inherently more difficult and less precise than the corresponding measurements for the left ventricle. The RV shape is complex and does not readily lend itself to any simple geometric approximation. Unlike the left ventricle, the right ventricle comprises anatomically (and embryologic) distinct inflow (sinus) and outflow (conus) portions. These two portions of the right ventricle are separated by the crista supraventricularis.[31] Mechanical systole proceeds from the inflow to the outflow regions, with contraction of the inflow region normally preceding that of the outflow region by 25 to 50 milliseconds.[32] Attempts at geometric approximation of RV volume are further confounded by the coarse myocardial trabeculations of the RV free wall and right side of the interventricular septum (Fig. 13–1). A large muscle bundle, known as the moderator band, extends from the inferior aspect of the interventricular septum to the free wall, where it attaches to the anterior papillary muscle. More than the left ventricle, the right ventricle changes its shape substantially from diastole to systole and under conditions of pressure and volume overload. The pattern of contraction of the normal right ventricle may be likened to movement of the sides of a bellows, with two approximately parallel (but in the case of the right ventricle, curved rather than flat) walls moving toward and away from each other, rather than concentric movement toward a common central axis. However, in the volume-overloaded right ventricle, this pattern may be substantially altered because the interventricular septum becomes

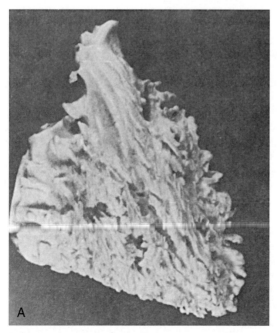 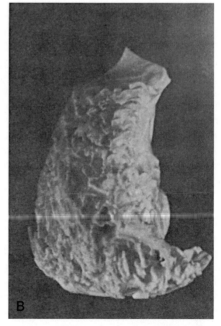

Figure 13–1. Latex cast of a human right ventricle in right anterior oblique *(A)* and left anterior oblique *(B)* positions, showing the characteristic irregular chamber contour and coarse trabeculation. (*A* and *B* copyrighted and reprinted with the permission of Clinical Cardiology Publishing Co., Inc., and/or the Foundation for Advances in Medicine and Science (FMS), Box 832, Mahwah, New Jersey 07430, USA.)

concave toward the RV cavity during diastole and systolic contraction is more concentric. These inherent difficulties must be considered when interpreting clinical or investigational studies directed at assessing RV function.

Difficulties in RV volumetric measurement and variability in methodologies have resulted in disagreement regarding normal RV ejection fraction. Estimates of the lower limits of normal for RV ejection fraction have ranged from approximately 0.40 to 0.50.

Cine Right Ventriculography

Conventional right ventriculography is performed using cineradiographic imaging during chamber opacification by injection of radiographic contrast media into the vena cava, right atrium, or right ventricle. Generally, contrast media is injected via a catheter with multiple side holes, such as a pigtail, Eppendorf, or Berman (balloon-tipped with side holes) catheter, in volumes of 25 to 45 mL in adults or 1 to 1.5 mL/kg in infants and children.[33, 34] Typical injection rates begin at 4 to 5 mL/sec in infants and range from 15 to 25 mL/sec in adults. The total dose and injection rate for contrast medium must be based on the nature of the underlying pathology, with higher doses and injection rates required in the presence of RV volume overload. Final selection of dose and injection rate is made following inspection of the appearance of the ventricle during a test injection. When the injection is made directly into the right ventricle, the catheter tip should be in the direction of the apex, not the outflow tract. Failure to observe this precaution often results in grossly inadequate opacification of the RV inflow region and inadequate assessment of tricuspid regurgitation.

Measurement of ejection fraction requires that images be obtained at near-maximal (diastolic) and near-minimal (systolic) RV volumes. The filming rate necessary to achieve this goal depends on the heart rate. For clinical measurement of ejection fraction, filming at a rate of 15 frames per cardiac cycle is sufficient for approximating minimal and maximal volumes. Filming below this rate may result in underestimation of ejection fraction. Filming at rates of 30 to 40 frames per cardiac cycle is necessary to assess time-dependent indices of ventricular systolic and diastolic performance, such as ejection and filling rates, and to construct volume curves through the cardiac cycle.

In contrast to the left ventricle, the complexity of the shape of the right ventricle obviates adequate estimates of RV volume from single-plane ventriculography. Biplane ventriculography generally is performed in either (1) posteroanterior and lateral projections or (2) right-anterior-oblique and left-anterior-oblique projections. Visualization of the right ventricle in the posteroanterior or left-anterior-oblique view is optimized by cranially angulating the radiographic beam approximately 15 to 20 degrees to reduce foreshortening of the RV cavity and improve separation of the RV outflow tract from the pulmonary artery.

One of two approaches may be employed for estimation of RV volume (Fig. 13–2): (1) assumption of a geometric approximation of the overall RV shape, and (2) use of Simpson's rule (see also Chapter 8). Several models may be employed for approximating the overall RV shape including (1) a combination of an ellipsoidal body and a cylindrical outflow tract[34]; (2) a pyramid[35]; (3) a prism, with rectangular frontal and lateral planes and a triangular horizontal plane[33]; and (4) a prolate ellipsoid.[36] The dimensions of these various models generally are derived from biplane ventriculograms. The methodology of Simpson's rule entails dividing the ventricle into a series of thin slices, presuming the shape of each slice, calculating its volume accordingly, and summing the various volumes. This technique probably provides for more accurate volumetric estimation. Using Simpson's rule, each cross-sectional RV slice has been likened in shape to either an ellipse,[33, 34, 36, 37] a triangle,[36] or a rectangle.[33] Good agreement between radiographic geometric calculations and direct volumetric measurement has been found with application of these techniques to postmortem radiopaque RV casts.[33-37] Because RV configuration changes substantially through the cardiac cycle and with differences in distension pressure, it is questionable whether postmortem cast findings are applicable to end-systolic volume or to end-diastolic volume in the setting of altered loading conditions. Nevertheless, Simpson's rule analysis probably provides reasonably accurate estimation of RV volumes in vivo.

Right ventriculography is relatively safe and carries less risk than left-sided heart catheterization with left ventriculography. Uncommon complications include right-sided heart perforation with cardiac tamponade, pulmonary embolism, and right bundle branch block. Pulmonary embolism due to catheter-derived thrombus is rarely clinically relevant. Right bundle branch block generally is self-limited. However, it occurs with sufficient frequency to warrant rapid accessibility to ventricular pacing in patients with a baseline left bundle branch block. Ven-

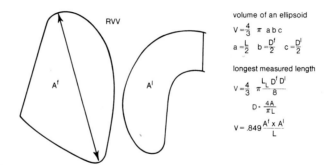

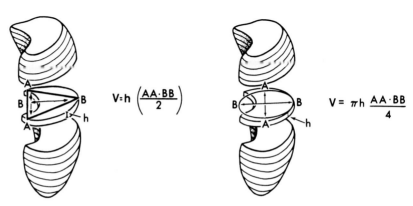

Figure 13-2. Schematics and formulas for two approaches employed for contrast ventriculographic estimation of right ventricular volume (RVV). *Upper,* Calculations are based on assuming RV shape to be that of a prolate ellipsoid, with a, b, and c the three perpendicular hemiaxes. L_L = longest measured length *(arrow)*; D^f and D^l are minor dimensions, as viewed in anteroposterior and lateral projections, respectively; A^f and A^l are planimetered areas in anteroposterior and lateral projections, respectively. *Lower,* Calculations are based on triangular *(left)* and elliptical *(right)* modifications of Simpson's rule. (Copyrighted and reprinted with the permission of Clinical Cardiology Publishing Co., Inc., and/or the Foundation for Advances in Medicine and Science (FMS), Box 832, Mahwah, New Jersey 07430, USA.)

tricular arrhythmias occur almost universally during RV catheterization but rarely result in sustained ventricular tachycardia. In addition to the usual potential adverse effects of intravascular administration of contrast media, abrupt hemodynamic deterioration may occur following right-sided heart contrast media administration in patients with severe pulmonary hypertension. In such patients, right ventriculography either should be avoided or performed using reduced volumes of contrast media.

Digital Ventriculography

With digital angiography,[38, 39] imaging is performed using a television camera that is interfaced to a computer, which acquires and stores the images on a digital matrix. Digital imaging may be employed to reduce the degree of invasiveness of right ventriculography and for facilitating automated volume calculation by either geometric or densitometric approaches. Following acquisition, images may be processed using techniques such as image subtraction, back-

ground subtraction, contrast enhancement, and edge enhancement to improve image quality. Adequate images for volumetric and functional analysis may be performed using injection of smaller amounts of contrast media or with injection of contrast material into a peripheral or central vein. These advantages reduce the invasive nature of RV contrast injection.

In addition to conventional geometric volumetric analysis, as described earlier, digital computerized imaging permits estimation of RV volume by densitometry. The density of contrast media within the RV cavity (calculated as image density in the region of the right ventricle during passage of the contrast bolus, minus image density prior to contrast injection) is directly proportional to RV volume during any portion of the cardiac cycle. The technique is most suitable to estimating relative changes in RV volume and thereby calculating the ejection fraction. The accuracy of absolute volume estimates is more questionable. Densitometric analysis offers the advantage of not relying on geometric assumptions. Errors may result from inaccurate identification of RV boundaries, particularly if chamber overlap exists, or from inaccurate estimation of so-called background density; that is, image density that is not contributed by the contrast media bolus. Because relative volumes are estimated by integrating the image density over the entire RV region, only a single projection is needed. Densitometric volume analysis is best performed in the right-anterior-oblique projection, confining measurements to the time prior to entrance of significant amounts of contrast media into the pulmonary circulation. This projection minimizes RV–right atrial chamber overlap, permitting accurate measurements following central or peripheral venous contrast administration or in the setting of tricuspid regurgitation.

With digital imaging, the capabilities of the computer limit the rate of information acquisition, resulting in a trade-off between acquisition rate and the information content of each image. The matrix size is an expression of the number of picture elements composing each image and is a limitation of the ultimate image resolution. For example, a matrix size of 256×256 indicates that each image comprises 256 rows, each row containing 256 picture elements. A matrix size of 256×256 is usually adequate for ventriculography, although the improved resolution afforded by matrix sizes of 512×512 or even 1024×1024 may be needed for adequate definition of small blood vessels during angiography. For a given computer system, the greater the number of picture elements or the greater the information content (the so-called gray scale) of each picture element, the slower will be the limit of image acquisition. Adequate frame rates for ventricular functional analysis are discussed earlier under cineventriculography. Thus, during vascular imaging, one might reduce the framing rate in order to achieve optimal image resolution, whereas during ventriculography, one might sacrifice resolution in order to achieve adequate framing rate for functional analysis.

Thermodilution Volumetrics

RV ejection fraction may be derived from analysis of the high-frequency components of the time-concentration curve generated downstream following RV or right atrial indicator injection.[40–43] Temperature generally is the most convenient indicator, with calculations derived from the thermodilution curve. Until recently, ventriculography and noninvasive imaging had replaced thermodilution RV ejection fraction measurement because of issues of accuracy and ease of study performance. However,

in recent years, there has been resurgence of interest in thermodilution RV ejection fraction measurement because of availability of combination injection-thermistor catheters, which possess a temperature-frequency response fast enough to accurately plot events during each cardiac cycle. This catheter permits RV ejection fraction measurement without ventriculography during right-sided heart catheterization or in the intensive care unit, and it facilitates repeated measurement following intervention, such as drug therapy.

Figure 13–3 illustrates time-temperature curves (decrease in temperature denoted by an upward deflection), with temperature sampled in the pulmonary artery following RV injection of a bolus of cold saline. The left side is a normal curve, and the right side illustrates a curve generated from a patient with heart failure. Each horizontal step represents a diastolic plateau, with rapid changes in temperature occurring during RV systole. The ratio of the heights of each pair of successive steps (e.g., step 2 / step 1; step 3 / step 2) is constant and represents the fraction of RV end-diastolic volume remaining following systole (residual fraction (RF); end-systolic volume/end-diastolic volume). Ejection fraction (EF) is calculated as $1 - RF$. If stroke volume (SV) is calculated by thermodilution or other techniques, then RV end-diastolic (ED) and end-systolic (ES) volumes (V) may also be calculated: $EDV = SV/EF$; $ESV = EDV - SV$.

Several limitations of this technique must be stated. First, as seen in Figure 13–3, with markedly reduced stroke volume and RV ejection fraction, the distinction among successive steps may become blurred, resulting in inaccuracies in ejection fraction estimation. Second, the technique is not likely to be accurate in the presence of a significant degree of tricuspid regurgitation. Third, inadequate bolus mixing may result in inaccuracies in ejection fraction measurement.[42] With recognition of these shortcomings, thermodilution RV ejection fraction measurement is a clinically useful technique in selected circumstances.

Impedance Volumetrics

Changes in ventricular volume may be estimated by examining changes in the impedance to electrical flow imposed by intraventricular blood. This technique is facilitated by the greater electrical resistivity of myocardial tissue compared with that of blood. This concept has been employed in studying left ventricular and, to a lesser extent, RV function[44] by use of an

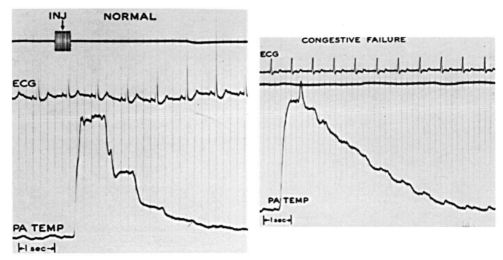

Figure 13–3. Time-temperature (TEMP) curves, with temperature sampled in the pulmonary artery (PA) following right ventricular injection (INJ) of a bolus of cold saline. A decrease in temperature is denoted by an upward deflection. *Left,* Normal curve. *Right,* Curve generated from a patient with heart failure and reduced right ventricular systolic function. (From Rapaport E, Wong M, Ferguson RE, et al: Right ventricular volumes in patients with and without heart failure. Circulation 1965; 31:531–541.)

impedance catheter. For a cylindric volume, V, of length L, the resistance, R, between the two ends of the cylinder may be expressed by the formula,

$$R = \frac{\rho L^2}{V}$$

where ρ is the resistivity of blood. The impedance catheter is positioned along the long axis of the ventricle. A constant electrical current is applied across electrodes at either end of the ventricle, and instantaneous voltage is measured between electrode pairs positioned along the catheter length. Instantaneous impedance is derived and used to calculate relative ventricular volumes. Figure 13–4 shows simultaneous RV pressure and impedance-derived volume measurements before and during a Valsalva maneuver.

Several factors limit the accuracy of impedance volumetric measurements. Among these factors are the following: First, the assumption that the myocardium does not contribute to conductance within the ventricle is not completely correct. Second, the resistivity is not necessarily constant but varies with several factors, including temperature, hematocrit, and blood velocity. Third, differences in catheter position result in varying locations of the catheter electrodes within the ventricle, and these differences may alter volume measurements. Fourth, the geometric assumptions employed to estimate volume may not be accurate in the case of the irregularly shaped right ventricle.

CONCEPTS OF RIGHT VENTRICULAR FUNCTIONAL ASSESSMENT

For either the right or the left ventricle, the ejection fraction (or any volume- or dimension-based index) is a measure of the performance of the ventricle as a pump coupled to a circulation. Changes in the load imposed by that circulation are reflected in measures of ejection performance. Ejection fraction is more readily altered by changes in loading conditions in the normally thin-walled right ventricle than in the left ventricle, and loading factors must be considered before a depressed ejection fraction may be interpreted to reflect RV myocardial pathology. In the setting of valvular heart disease, obstructive lung disease, or left-sided heart failure, RV ejection fraction is strongly influenced by afterload and has been found to correlate roughly with pulmonary artery pressure.[7-14] Increased preload tends to augment RV ejection fraction. In patients with left-to-right shunting through an atrial septal defect, RV ejection fraction tends to remain normal even in the presence of moderate pulmonary hypertension.[14] Following repair of an atrial septal defect, RV ejection fraction often falls, paralleling the decrease in preload.[14] Attempts to distinguish a primary index of contractility have focused on the analogy between the tension-load relation of isolated cardiac muscle and the end-systolic pressure-volume relation of the intact ventricle, whether it is isolated or coupled to the circulation. For the isolated or coupled left ventricle, the relation between end-systolic pressure and

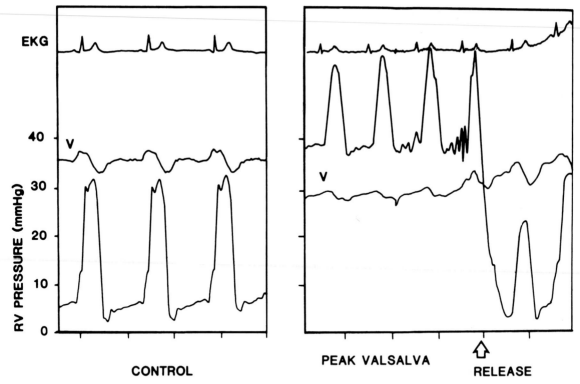

Figure 13–4. Simultaneous measurement of right ventricular (RV) pressure and impedance volume (V) with Valsalva maneuver. (From McKay RG, Spears JR, Aroesty JM, et al: Instantaneous measurement of left and right ventricular stroke volume and pressure-volume relationships with an impedance catheter. Circulation 1984; 69:703–710.)

end-systolic volume, when derived over a range of loading conditions, has been shown by many investigators to be linear over a physiologic range of load[45, 46] and responsive in predictable ways to positive or negative inotropic interventions.

Although recent findings have indicated that the ventricular end-systolic pressure-volume relation may not truly be linear at very high or low loads,[47] its slope is thought to be fairly independent of load within a physiologic range and represents a reasonable index of contractility. These concepts have facilitated the study of ventricular performance in situations such as valvular heart disease and cardiomyopathy, in which the ejection fraction is not always representative of the true state of myocardial function because of important alterations in preload and afterload.

Although most attention has focused on the development of these concepts for the left ventricle, studies have demonstrated that the RV end-systolic pressure-volume relation is also linear in the isolated preparation[48] (Fig. 13–5), as well as in humans either with normal RV function[49] or with heart failure and pulmonary hypertension.[26]

In order to construct an end-systolic pressure-volume relation for either the right or left ventricle, both pressure and volume data must be generated under multiple loading conditions. These multiple data points may be achieved by infusion of a pure vasoconstrictor (such as phenylephrine) or a pure vasodilator (such as nitroprusside or nitroglycerin). A micromanometer catheter is placed into the body of the right ventricle for high-fidelity pressure recording. RV volume is determined simultaneously by contrast ventriculography[50] or by radionuclide ventriculography.[7, 26, 27, 49]

In creating loops representing instantaneous pressure and volume throughout the cardiac cycle, the pressure-versus-time data may be digitized and averaged over several beats to minimize respiratory phasic influences. Volume-versus-time data are analyzed from a frame-by-frame contrast ventriculographic study or from a radionuclide time-activity curve. The pressure and volume data are aligned in time. These data are then displayed on an x axis (volume)–y axis (pressure) grid as pressure-volume loops. The end-systolic pressure-volume relation is derived by determining the pressure-volume coordinate at the time of end-systole (or an approxi-

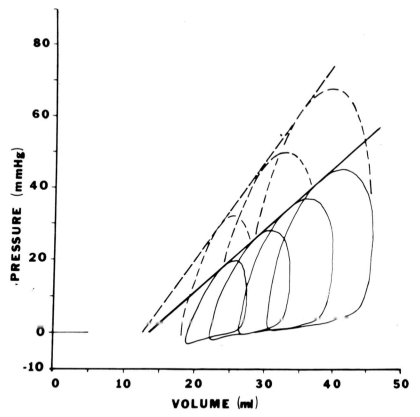

Figure 13–5. Ejecting right ventricular pressure-volume loops from a single isolated canine heart under baseline contractile state *(solid lines)* and during epinephrine infusion to augment contractility. (From Maughan WL, Shoukas AA, Sagawa K, Weisfeldt ML: Instantaneous pressure-volume relationship of the canine right ventricle. Circ Res 1979; 44:309–315.)

mation) for each loading condition and by performing linear regression analysis using the selected end-systolic data points. The slope of this relation represents ventricular systolic stiffness and is a load-independent index of ventricular contractility.

In some studies, the pulmonary artery dicrotic notch pressure has been taken as an estimate of RV end-systolic pressure and has been combined with volume data under variable loading conditions to derive a systolic pressure-volume relation. For both the normal[49] and myopathic ventricle,[26, 27] this technique yields a linear relation between pressure and volume, the position of which is dependent on the inotropic state (Fig. 13–6).[7, 49, 51] For example, the RV end-systolic pressure volume relation has been found to shift to the left with infusion of dobutamine.[49]

In a study from our laboratory,[27] the end-systolic pressure-volume relation was derived for both the left and right ventricles in patients with congestive heart failure secondary to dilated cardiomyopathy. In general, the slopes were of lesser magnitude for the right ventricle

than for the left ventricle (Fig. 13–7). This finding indicates that changes in end-systolic pressure more strongly influence the extent of RV emptying than the extent of left ventricular emptying[27]; that is, the right ventricle operates at a lesser degree of systolic stiffness or contractility than the left ventricle. The reasons for this difference may relate to differences in wall thickness, in the geometric efficiency of tension development, or in the temporal efficiency between the two ventricles, because, as noted previously, mechanical systole occurs 25 to 50 ms earlier in the inflow compared with the outflow region of the right ventricle.

A clinical correlate to these findings has been demonstrated by investigating the effects of amrinone, a positively inotropic, vasodilating phosphodiesterase inhibitor, on RV and left ventricular performance in patients with congestive heart failure.[28] Stroke volume improved similarly in both ventricles. This change was accompanied by a large decrease in pulmonary artery end-systolic pressure and a shift of the RV end-systolic pressure-volume point along the pressure-volume line generated during nitroprus-

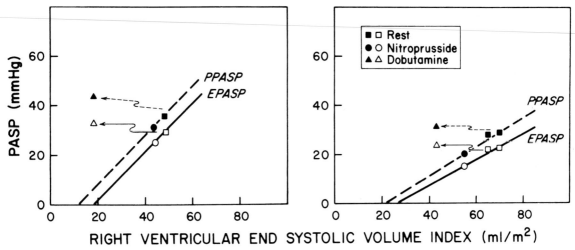

Figure 13–6. Relationships of pulmonary artery peak-systolic pressure (PPASP) and end-systolic pressure (EPASP) versus right ventricular end-systolic volume in two patients with obstructive pulmonary disease. A dobutamine-induced increase in right ventricular contractility is accompanied by shifts in the pressure-volume relations, as indicated by a reduction in right ventricular volume below the level anticipated for a given systolic pressure in the baseline state. (From Brent BN, Berger HJ, Matthay RA, et al: Physiologic correlates of right ventricular ejection fraction in chronic obstructive pulmonary disease: A combined radionuclide and hemodynamic study. Am J Cardiol 1982; 50:255–262.)

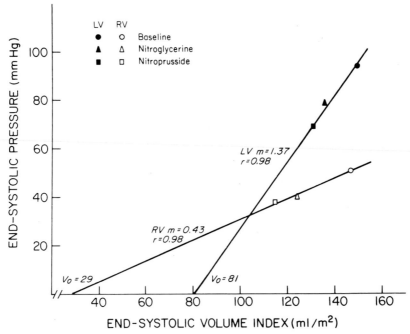

Figure 13–7. Comparison of left ventricular (LV) and right ventricular (RV) end-systolic pressure-volume relations (group mean data with linear regression lines) derived from 10 patients with biventricular failure due to healed myocardial infarction or dilated cardiomyopathy. Pulmonary or systemic arterial end-systolic (dicrotic notch) pressures are plotted against radionuclide-derived RV or LV end-systolic volumes, respectively, at baseline and during infusion of nitroprusside and nitroglycerine. The shallower slope of the RV relation indicates lesser RV systolic stiffness compared with the left ventricle. That is, identical changes in systolic pressure effect greater changes in systolic performance for the right ventricle than for the left ventricle. m, slope; r, correlation coefficient; V_0, volume-axis intercept. (From Konstam MA, Levine HJ: Effects of afterload and preload on right ventricular systolic performance. *In* Konstam MA, Isner JM: The Right Ventricle. Dordrecht, Kluwer Academic, 1988, p 27.)

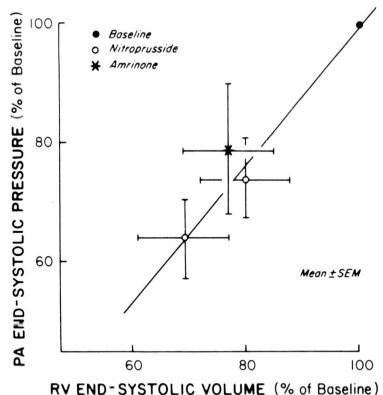

Figure 13–8. Relation of pulmonary artery (PA) end-systolic pressure versus right ventricular (RV) end-systolic volume (group means) in nine patients with left ventricular systolic dysfunction related to healed myocardial infarction or dilated cardiomyopathy. The effect of amrinone on RV systolic performance is predominantly explainable on the basis of reduced RV afterload. There is a lack of demonstrable shift of the amrinone pressure-volume point from the regression line formed by data derived at baseline and during nitroprusside infusion. (From Konstam MA, Cohen SR, Salem DN, et al: Amrinone effect on right ventricular function: Predominance of afterload reduction. Circulation 1986; 74:359–366.)

side infusion, indicating that the increment in stroke volume could be accounted for by reduced afterload in the pulmonary bed (Fig. 13–8). Thus, the low systolic stiffness of the right ventricle results in an overshadowing of changes in contractile state by changes in systolic load.

SUMMARY

Assessment of systolic function is rendered less exact for the right ventricle compared with the left ventricle because of the complex structure of the right ventricle. Nevertheless, considerable insight into RV function may be achieved through application of contrast ventriculography, digital subtraction angiography, or thermodilution or impedance volumetrics, as well as through application of a variety of noninvasive imaging modalities. These techniques have been widely applied and have yielded clinically relevant information in myocardial, coronary, congenital, and acquired valvular heart disease and in cor pulmonale.

The strong influence of loading conditions on parameters of RV systolic performance must be considered when interpreting ejection fraction measurements. The concepts of end-sys-

tolic pressure-volume analysis, developed for the left ventricle, may be applied to investigate the right ventricle as well and permit examination of systolic performance independent of load.

REFERENCES

1. Cohen M, Fuster V: What do we gain from the analysis of right ventricular function? J Am Coll Cardiol 1984; 3:1082–1084.
2. Goldman ME: Emerging importance of the right ventricle. J Am Coll Cardiol 1985; 5:925–927.
3. Ferlinz J: Right ventricular function in adult cardiovascular disease. Prog Cardiovasc Dis 1982; 25:225–267.
4. Johnson LL, McCarthy DM, Sciacca R, Cannon PJ: Right ventricular ejection fraction during exercise in patients with coronary artery disease. Circulation 1979; 60:1284.
5. Maddahi J, Berman DS, Matsuoka DT, et al: Right ventricular ejection fraction during exercise in normal subjects and in coronary artery disease patients: Assessment by multiple-gated equilibrium scintigraphy. Circulation 1980; 62:133.
6. Brown KA, Okada RD, Boucher CA, et al: Right ventricular ejection fraction response to exercise in patients with coronary artery disease: Influence of both right coronary artery disease and exercise-induced changes in right ventricular afterload. J Am Coll Cardiol 1984; 3:895–901.
7. Brent BN, Berger HJ, Matthay RA, et al: Physiologic correlates of right ventricular ejection fraction in chronic obstructive pulmonary disease: A combined radionuclide and hemodynamic study. Am J Cardiol 1982; 50:255–262.

8. Iskandrian AS, Hakki AH, Ren BF, et al: Correlation among right ventricular preload, afterload and ejection fraction in mitral valve disease: Radionuclide, echocardiographic and hemodynamic evaluation. J Am Coll Cardiol 1984; 6:1403–1411.

9. Morrison D, Goldman S, Wright AL, et al: The effect of pulmonary hypertension on systolic function of the right ventricle. Chest 1983; 84:248–257.

10. Winzelberg GC, Boucher CA, Pohost GM, et al: Right ventricular function in aortic and mitral valve disease. Chest 1981; 79:520–528.

11. Korr KS, Gandsman EJ, Winkler ML, et al: Hemodynamic correlates of right ventricular ejection fraction measured with gated radionuclide angiography. Am J Cardiol 1982; 49:71–77.

12. Berger HJ, Matthay RA, Loke J, et al: Cardiac performance with quantitative radionuclide angiocardiography: Right ventricular ejection fraction with reference to findings in chronic obstructive pulmonary disease. Am J Cardiol 1978; 41:897–905.

13. Yabek SM, Berman W, Dillon T: Right ventricular contractile function in children with congenital heart disease. Am J Cardiol 1984; 53:899–901.

14. Konstam MA, Idoine J, Wynne J, et al: Right ventricular function in pulmonary hypertensive adults with and without atrial septal defects. Am J Cardiol 1983; 51:1144–1148.

15. Radford MJ, Johnson RA, Daggett WM Jr, et al: Ventricular septal rupture: A review of clinical and physiologic features and an analysis of survival. Circulation 1981; 64:545–53.

16. Baker EJ, Shubao C, Clarke SEM, et al: Radionuclide measurement of right ventricular function in atrial septal defect, ventricular septal defect and complete transposition of the great arteries. Am J Cardiol 1986; 57:1142–1146.

17. Ninomiya K, Duncan WJ, Cook DH, et al: Right ventricular ejection fraction and volumes after mustard repair: Correlation of two dimensional echocardiograms and cineangiograms. Am J Cardiol 1981; 48:317–324.

18. Graham TP: Ventricular performance in adults after operation for congenital heart disease. Am J Cardiol 1982; 50:612–620.

19. Peterson RJ, Franch RH, Fajman WA, Jones RH: Comparison of cardiac function in surgically corrected and congenitally corrected transposition of the great arteries. J Thorac Cardiovasc Surg 1988; 96:227–236.

20. Cohen M, Horowitz, Machac J, et al: Response of the right ventricle to exercise in isolated mitral stenosis. Am J Cardiol 1985; 55:1054–1058.

21. Matthay RA, Berger HJ, Davies RA, et al: Right and left ventricular exercise performance in chronic obstructive pulmonary disease: Radionuclide assessment. Ann Intern Med 1980; 93:234.

22. Polak JF, Holman BL, Wynne J, Colucci WS: Right ventricular ejection fraction: An indicator of increased mortality in patients with congestive heart failure associated with coronary artery disease. J Am Coll Cardiol 1983; 2:217–224.

23. Brill DM, Konstam MA, Vivino PG, et al: Importance of right ventricular systolic function as an independent predictor of mortality in patients with congestive heart failure. Circulation 1989; 80:II-649.

24. Baker BJ, Wilen MM, Boyd CM, et al: Relation of right ventricular ejection fraction to exercise capacity in chronic left ventricular failure. Am J Cardiol 1984; 54:596.

25. Brill DM, Konstam MA, Vivino PG, et al: Rapid-onset pulmonary edema in patients with left ventricular systolic dysfunction: A syndrome related to right ventricular ejection fraction. J Am Coll Cardiol 1989; 13:179A.

26. Konstam MA, Salem DN, Isner JM, et al: Vasodilator effect on right ventricular function in congestive heart failure and pulmonary hypertension: End-systolic pressure-volume relation. Am J Cardiol 1984; 54:132–136.

27. Konstam MA, Cohen SR, Salem DN, et al: Comparison of left and right ventricular end-systolic pressure-volume relations in congestive heart failure. J Am Coll Cardiol 1985; 5:1326–1334.

28. Konstam MA, Cohen SR, Salem DN, et al: Amrinone effect on right ventricular function: Predominance of afterload reduction. Circulation 1986; 74:359–366.

29. Brent BN, Berger HJ, Matthay RA, et al: Contrasting acute effects of vasodilators (nitroglycerin, nitroprusside, and hydralazine) on right ventricular performance in patients with chronic obstructive pulmonary disease and pulmonary hypertension: A combined radionuclide-hemodynamic study. Am J Cardiol 1983; 51:1682–1689.

30. Brill DM, Konstam MA, Metherall J, et al: Acute and chronic response to oral enoximone in severe congestive heart failure: Sustained hemodynamic improvement and preferential effect on right ventricular systolic performance. J Am Coll Cardiol 1989; 13:101A.

31. James TN: Anatomy of the crista supraventricularis: Its importance for understanding right ventricular function, right ventricular infarction and related conditions. J Am Coll Cardiol 1985; 6:1083–1095.

32. Hurford WE, Zapol WM: The right ventricle and critical illness: A review of anatomy, physiology, and clinical evaluation of its function. Intensive Care Med 1988; 14:448–457.

33. Fisher EA, DuBrow IW, Hastreiter AR: Right ventricular volume in congenital heart disease. Am J Cardiol 1975; 36:67–75.

34. Graham TP, Jarmakani JM, Atwood GF, Canent RV: Right ventricular volume determinations in children: Normal values and observations with volume or pressure overload. Circulation 1973; 47:144–153.

35. Ferlinz J, Gorlin R, Cohn PF, Herman MV: Right ventricular performance in patients with coronary artery disease. Circulation 1975; 52:608–615.

36. Horn V, Mullins CB, Saffer SI, et al: A comparison of mathematical models for estimating right ventricular volumes in animals and man. Clin Cardiol 1979; 2:341–347.

37. Gentzler RD, Briselli MF, Gault JH: Angiographic estimation of right ventricular volume in man. Circulation 1974; 50:324–330.

38. Lange PE, Budach W, Radtke W, et al: Right ventricular imaging with digital subtraction angiocardiography using intraventricular contrast injection. Am J Cardiol 1984; 54:839–842.

39. Cohen M, Monsen C, Francis X, et al: Comparison of single plane videodensitometry-based right ventricular ejection fraction in right and left anterior oblique views to biplane geometry-based right ventricular ejection fraction. J Am Coll Cardiol 1987; 10:150–155.

40. Rapaport E, Wong M, Ferguson RE, et al: Right ventricular volumes in patients with and without heart failure. Circulation 1965; 31:531–541.

41. Dhainaut J, Brunet F, Monsallier JF, et al: Bedside evaluation of right ventricular performance using a rapid computerized thermodilution method. Crit Care Med 1987; 15:148–152.

42. Morrison DA, Stovall R, Sensecqua J, Friefeld G: Thermodilution measurement of the right ventricular ejection fraction. Cathet Cardiovasc Diagn 1987; 13:167–173.

43. Voelker W, Gruber HP, Ickrath O, et al: Determination of right ventricular ejection fraction by thermodilution

technique—a comparison to biplane cineventriculography. Intensive Care Med 1988; 14:461–466.

44. McKay RG, Spears JR, Aroesty JM, et al: Instantaneous measurement of left and right ventricular stroke volume and pressure-volume relationships with an impedance catheter. Circulation 1984; 69:703–710.

45. Sagawa K: The end-systolic pressure-volume relations of the ventricle: Definition, modifications, and clinical use [editorial]. Circulation 1981; 63:1223–1227.

46. Grossman W, Braunwald E, Mann T, et al: Contractile state of the left ventricle in man as evaluated from end-systolic pressure-volume relations. Circulation 1977; 56:845–852.

47. Kass DA, Beyar R, Lankford E, et al: Influence of contractile state on curvilinearity of in situ endsystolic pressure-volume relations. Circulation 1989; 79:167–178.

48. Maughan WL, Shoukas AA, Sagawa K, Weisfeldt ML: Instantaneous pressure-volume relationship of the canine right ventricle. Circ Res 1979; 44:309–315.

49. Brown KA, Ditchey RV: Human right ventricular pressure-volume relation defined by maximal elastance. Circulation 1988; 78:81–91.

50. Dell'Italia LJ, Walsh RA: Right ventricular diastolic pressure-volume relations and regional dimensions during acute alterations in loading conditions. Circulation 1988; 77:1276–1282.

51. Eichhorn EJ, Konstam MA, Weiland DS, et al: Differential effects of milrinone and dobutamine on right ventricular preload, afterload and systolic performance in congestive heart failure secondary to ischemic or idiopathic dilated cardiomyopathy. Am J Cardiol 1987; 60:1329–1333.

Chapter 14

Coronary Angioscopy

C. TODD SHERMAN

Even though the introduction of fiberoptic instruments to medicine has been relatively recent, its impact on many subspecialties has been prodigious. Modern-day practices of orthopedics, gastroenterology, pulmonology, gynecology, and otolaryngology, to name a few, depend on fiberoptic examinations. Because of obstacles inherent in the cardiovascular system however, routine use of fiberoptics in this subspeciality remains forthcoming. Nevertheless, investigators performing intraluminal angioscopy (fiberoptic examination of the inside of blood vessels) with currently available rudimentary devices have successfully displayed images that foretell a bright future for this technique. It has been touted as the means by which we might assess a lesion's intimal morphology to decide on appropriate therapy, inspect the luminal aspect of surgical anastomoses to improve acute graft closure rates, better aim laser energy at atherosclerotic plaque to lessen perforation rates, assess the performance of atherectomy devices to facilitate removal of plaque while preserving vascular integrity, and quantify the cross-sectional area of a stenosis.

Since its first use as a rigid, large-caliber, cumbersome device to more recent times, vascular endoscopy has not yet completely lived up to these auspicious expectations. The reasons for this are mostly technical, because the information already gained from successful angioscopy has been shown to be both valuable and unique. Despite some clever solutions, these technical problems continue to impede the acceptance of angioscopy as a common diagnostic technique.[1, 2] Nevertheless, a substantial amount of clinically relevant information has been obtained from angioscopy of autopsy specimens, from animal models, and from patient's vessels at the time of catheterization and during surgery.

THE COMPONENTS OF AN ANGIOSCOPY SYSTEM

An appreciation of the complexity of angioscopy begins with consideration for the multiple components that comprise the angioscopy system, each of which performs a unique function: the inherently dark vascular target is first transformed by the illumination system; the distal lens cap creates a suitable image of the target; the fiberoptic waveguide transmits this image from the target's remote site; and the proximal viewing lens transforms the image into presentable format for eyepiece, camera, or video viewing. As with any integrated multicomponent system, its overall performance is derived from both the qualities of the individual elements and the interfaces linking them.

The Fiber

Central to any angioscopy system is the fiber, a glass rod that has been drawn out to be a long, very thin, flexible cable. When this glass fiber is coated with a material of different refractory index, an optical insulator called *cladding*, it can transmit light around curves. This seemingly impossible phenomenon is explained by the principle of total internal reflection and refraction (Fig. 14–1). Light traveling through a curved fiber is reflected almost an infinite number of times, appearing to bend. The specific compositions of the fiber and its cladding determine the efficiency and fidelity of light transmission through it. The fiber's diameter determines the size of a picture element (pixel), which, in turn, influences picture resolution.

The Fiber Bundle

The manner in which individual fibers are packaged into a bundle greatly affects image quality. A single fiber is a conduit for a single point of light; the fiber bundle, transmitting light point by point, creates an image similar to that of a newspaper's photo. Because each fiber represents a single pixel, the optimal bundle design would be very dense, housing the greatest number of the smallest diameter fibers. Although

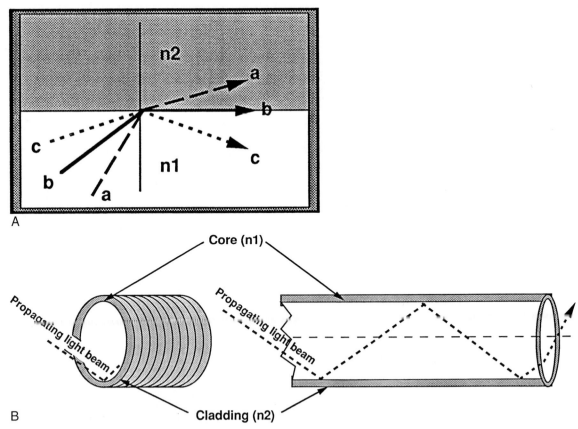

Figure 14–1. *A,* By Snell's law, at the interface of two media (n1 and n2), a light beam is refracted (a) when the incident angle is less than the critical angle (b). It is reflected back into the incident media (c) when it is greater than the critical angle. *B,* A light beam, repeatedly reflected at the interface between fiber core and cladding (total internal reflection), is transmitted through flexible fiberoptics.

limiting the amount of bundle dead space is essential to image resolution, this should not occur at the expense of increased fiber-to-fiber interference. This interference, called *cross-talk,* occurs when transmitted wavelengths leak to adjacent element fibers or pixels, causing distortion.

For medical applications, the most commonly used bundle is fused. Thousands of individually clad fibers are bunched, heated, and drawn out, a process that simultaneously elongates the bundle, thins the fibers, and fuses them into a bundle by coalescence of the cladding. A fiberoptic bundle made this way can achieve a very small diameter and maximum resolution by minimizing the area incapable of imaging (dead space), and can be easily incorporated into a catheter suited for medical use. While flexibility of the catheter (an important feature when imaging coronary arteries) is not sacrificed, fidelity of the fiber geometric arrangement is also ensured. *Coherence* refers to a bundle whose fiber arrangement is retained from one end to the other, providing faithful reproduction of the transmitted image, pixel by pixel.

In a nonfused bundle, individually clad fibers can slide over neighboring fibers, imparting greater flexibility to the bundle as a whole. Unfused bundles are much larger in diameter than fused bundles of equal pixel number. Dead space is larger, but fiber cross-talk is less of a problem. Such scopes can retain image coherency by locking the fibers' positions at each end of the device.

Initial angioscopes used bunches of 12-μ fibers. Standard technology now uses 3000 fibers of 2-μ diameter to produce a 0.6-mm diameter scope. In the near future, we can expect devices of similar outer diameter housing 6000 fibers of 1.5-μ diameter. Because resolving power increases linearly with decreasing pixel size, we can expect improved detail from future fused-bundle angioscopes. The limit to resolution, assessed by the ability to differentiate line-pairs, depends on the size of the fiber (pixel size) and packing density (Fig. 14–2). Because each fiber carries only one color at a time, to

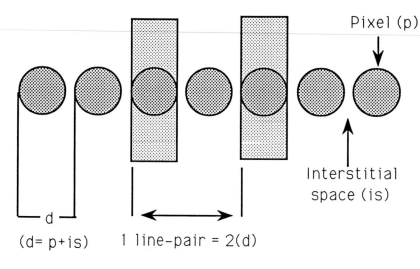

$$\text{resolution (line-pairs/mm)} = 1/(2d)$$

Figure 14–2. Determinants of fiber resolution, showing angioscopic resolution, assessed by the ability to differentiate line-pairs per millimeter, depends on pixel size (p) and packing density or interstitial space (is).

distinguish individual lines that are a single pixel in width, at least one pixel must separate them. For fibers whose diameters are typically 2 μ, spaced 0.2 μ apart, the theoretic limit to resolution (line-pair resolution = 1/[mm distance between pixel centers × 2]; the imaging bundle shown in Figure 14–3) is 227 line-pairs/mm (1/[0.0022 × 2]). Cross-talk distortion reduces the theoretic resolution to about 200 line-pairs/mm.

Distal Lens Cap

Another important aspect of the angioscopy system is the presentation of an image to the fiberoptic bundle. This is accomplished through

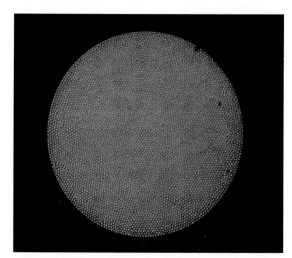

Figure 14–3. Cross-sectional view of imaging bundle, magnified to display pixel and dead space geometry.

a lens mounted on the distal tip of the scope by special adhesives. Currently, the lens system best suited for this application is the gradient index (GRIN) lens (Fig. 14–4). This lens is unlike a conventional spherical-type lens typically found in corrective lenses and cameras, which refracts light only at its surface interface. The GRIN lens is a cylinder of glass that is capable of bending light along its entire length. Subtle alterations in the lens' composition determines its index profile. The degree of refraction depends on this index and the length of lens traversed by the light beam. The focal length of a GRIN lens is altered by modifying its material, and thus its index profile, or by changing its length. Because this type of lens is easily miniaturized (Fig. 14–5) and surface curvature is not critical, it is well suited to be mounted on the tip of a fiberoptic bundle.

The most important qualities of the angioscope's lens are its field of view, numeric aperture, depth of field, and resolving power. The optimal lens affords the widest perspective possible (a large field of view) with the greatest clarity and least amount of distortion and illumination requirements. When the intent is imaging a coronary artery whose caliber varies from 1 to 4 mm, a 60-degree field of view is the most versatile. Under these circumstances, pincushion distortion (distortion created by nonlinear radial magnification) is tolerable and requirements for illumination can be met without unwieldy technical adaptations. The GRIN lens also has a relatively long depth of field, allowing objects several millimeters apart to be in focus simultaneously. This affords a larger

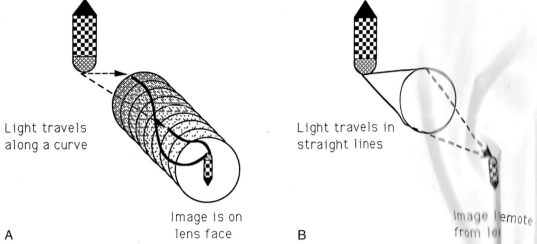

Light travels along a curve

Image is on lens face

A

Light travels in straight lines

Image remote from lens

B

Figure 14–4. Comparison of the GRIN lens *(A)* and spheric lens *(B)* systems. The GRIN lens is more suitable for mounting on the tip of miniaturized angioscopes. (See text for details.)

area for diagnostic examination at any single scope position, which, in turn, assists in the difficult chore of establishing perspective. Ultimately, the function of this lens is to reduce a coronary image (which may be as large as 4 mm in diameter) and focus it on the angioscope's 0.18-mm imaging bundle. There can be substantial loss of resolution in this process. Because the magnification factor of such lenses increases linearly with distance, objects just 3 mm from the lens are reduced in size by a power of 10. Thus, an angioscope capable of resolving 200 line-pairs/mm at near contact discerns only 20 line-pairs at 3-mm distance. Diagnostic images of objects whose dimensions are as small as 75 μ are obtainable.

The Coupler

The coupler is the first step in the transfer of the image from the fiberoptic to the viewing monitor (Fig. 14–6). The coupler rectifies the image relayed by the fiber bundle and focuses it on the camera's sensor surface. Over-magnification of the bundle's image emphasizes its dot composition or so-called pixelization, distracting the eye from optimal interpretation of the image. With appropriate selection, the magnifying lenses, camera, and monitor will not further limit the resolution of the system. The coupler lens can be selected to magnify a fiber's 2-μ pixel image 7.5 times to a 15-μ image. Because the pixel size of a typical $\frac{1}{2}$-inch charged

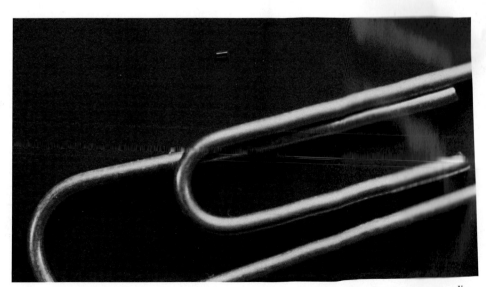

Figure 14–5. Demonstration of the relatively small size of the GRIN lens in relation to a paper clip.

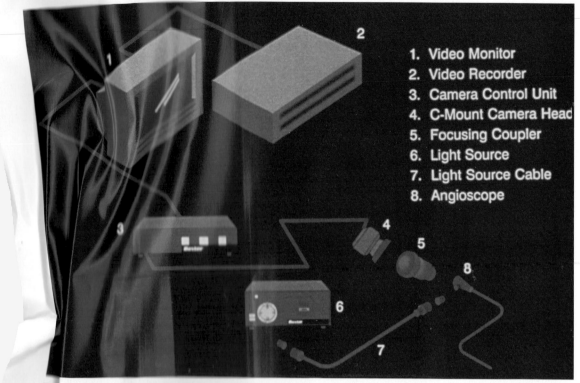

1. Video Monitor
2. Video Recorder
3. Camera Control Unit
4. C-Mount Camera Head
5. Focusing Coupler
6. Light Source
7. Light Source Cable
8. Angioscope

Fig. 6. A typical videoscopy system. A xenon arc lamp transmits high-intensity white light via the light source cable (7) to angioscope (8). The focusing coupler (5) remagnifies the image relayed by the fiber bundle in the angioscope and uses it on the sensor surface of the video camera (4). A video monitor (1) and video tape recorder (2) can then be used to display and archive the image, respectively.

coupled device (CCD) video camera is 12 μ, resolution is not further compromised. In a typical system, the image from a 0.2-mm bundle is magnified 330 times to become a 66-mm display on a 13-inch (330-mm) monitor.

The Camera

Owing to their very small size and excellent performance, solid state cameras constructed with CCD sensors have dominated almost all medical applications. More than 330 horizontal lines of resolution ensures image clarity. Fast shuttering capability prevents the white out of light reflected off the vessel lumen. Their standard National Television Standards Committee (NTSC) output allows easy connection (see Fig. 14–6) to all state-of-the-art hardware, including monitors, video recorders, digital frame grabbers, and computerized image processors. The ½-inch camera format has excellent resolving power, light sensitivity, and magnification that does not accentuate the image's pixels. The camera, which fits in the palm of a hand, can be sterilized or easily placed within a sterile plastic sheath. The images can then be viewed

in real time on a high-resolution television monitor while they are being recorded simultaneously on video tape, allowing more critical review after the procedure. Alternatively, images can be viewed through a hand-held optical lens or a still camera, although this approach is somewhat less convenient.

Illumination

The goal of angioscopy is to view an artery that is normally well-hidden from light. Thus, the angioscopy system must provide its own source of illumination. A high-pressure xenon arc lamp, which radiates uniformly over the visible spectra, is most concordant with both human vision and camera technology. Its near-pure white light output contributes to color fidelity. This source is connected by a flexible fiberoptic cable to the proximal angioscope, where it couples with special fibers integrated into the angioscope (see Fig. 14–6). These noncoherent fibers, typically 125 μ in diameter and arranged concentrically around the imaging bundle, guide light distally to the viewing field with minor attenuation in the visible spectra. The efficient channeling of light from the source to the targeted arterial segment decreases wattage requirements and reduces tissue exposure to heat.

The Catheter

For intravascular use, fiber bundles are packaged within a jacket of polyvinylchloride or polyethylene. Although this may be all that is required for an intraoperative angioscope catheter, further sophistication and refinements

are necessary for percutaneous use in the cardiac catheterization laboratory. Angioscope catheters designed for this use appear outwardly similar to typical balloon angioplasty catheters. The Baxter Imagecath (Baxter-Edwards LIS Division, Irvine, CA), typical of the new generation of scopes, is a flexible triple-lumen catheter of 4.5-French (1.5 mm) outer diameter (Fig. 14–7). It is capable of monorail tracking over a conventional 0.014-inch angioplasty guide wire, distal irrigation with rates up to 0.75 mL/sec, and has a proximal occlusion balloon to facili-

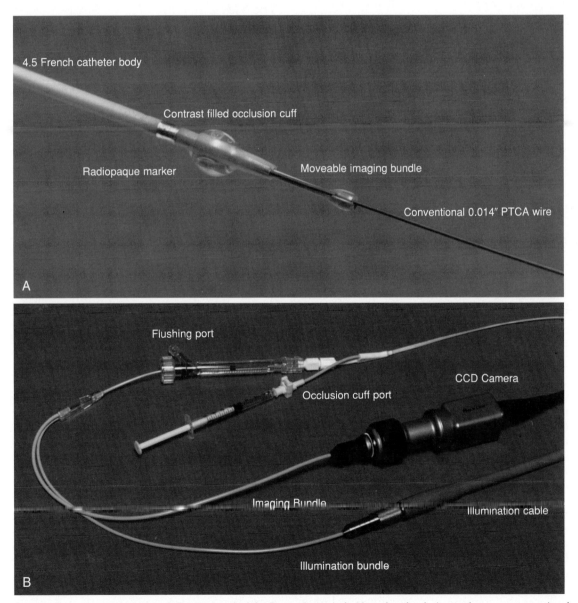

Figure 14–7. A, A magnified view of the distal end of the Baxter Imagecath. Note that the device tracks over a conventional 0.014-inch guide wire and also occludes proximal flow with an inflatable cuff that is proximal to the movable imaging bundle. B, Proximal end of the Baxter Imagecath system. Note the ports for inflation of the occlusion cuff and for flushing of saline into the field of view; combined use of these features allows a blood-free field for illumination.

tate a bloodless viewing field. A unique feature of this device allows independent movement of the imaging bundle through the bloodless field that is created by active flushing and a stationary inflated cuff. The balloon cuff's material is compliant, designed to occlude varying caliber arteries up to 4 mm. It operates at very low inflation pressures to avoid vessel trauma or an angioplasty effect.

Although individual fibers can be bent into loops of a few millimeters in diameter before snapping, bundled fibers encased in a plastic jacket are less flexible. It is the distal tip of the angioscopic catheter, where all the fibers are fused and the rigid lens attached, that exhibits the most inflexibility. Nevertheless, angioscope catheters with bending diameters of less than 1 cm, like the 4.5-French Imagecath, are commercially available (see Fig. 14–7).

Although early angioscopes were simple illumination and imaging waveguides, they were considered costly prototypes to be cherished. These devices, resterilized using ethylene oxide gas, were reused until broken fibers made their images uninterpretable. Separate disposable catheters were used to deliver the fiberoptics to the coronary site and to create a suitable bloodless field. With the benefits of lower costs for fiberoptics and mass production, sterile angioscopes are now packaged for single use only.

As with any catheter in a curved vessel, the angioscope will hug a coronary artery's outer edge, impeding visualization. To align the scope coaxial to the vessel, a number of methods have been attempted to steer the scope. An inflatable occlusion cuff, designed primarily to stop antegrade flow, can push a catheter off the obscuring wall. Alternatively, the angioscope can be advanced over a guide wire with a preshaped spiral segment, directing it away from its otherwise natural course. True steering ability, similar to that already incorporated into larger-caliber fiberoptic devices such as bronchoscopes, awaits further miniaturization.

Creating a visual field unoccupied by blood is essential when performing angioscopy because the presence of even small amounts prevents quality imaging. This goal, which is relatively easy to achieve during intraoperative angioscopy, required creative catheter engineering for percutaneous coronary angioscopy. Early attempts to use solely an infusion of transparent fluid to overcome blood flow at the target site were often unsuccessful. Equally ineffective was the sole use of a proximal occlusion balloon. The methods combined, however, consistently created the desired effect. Inflation of a proximal, low-pressure, compliant balloon

greatly reduces antegrade flow without incurring all the risks attendant to inflation of a typical angioplasty balloon. Then, an initial bolus of normal saline at body temperature, infused distal to the balloon, overcomes any remaining antegrade and collateral blood flow. Once the field is clear, a lower rate of infusion will maintain the effect. Although it is possible to perform such an infusion by hand, a roller-pump or injector (MedRad, Pittsburgh, PA) can infuse preprogrammed quantities and rates at the touch of a foot pedal.

The Video System

Images are displayed on a high-resolution color television monitor. Digitization of an acquired image may enhance color and, by interpolation, ameliorate the pixelization of the image. Such manipulations may add to the aesthetics of an image but cannot increase its information content or diagnostic quality

THE DEVELOPMENT OF ANGIOSCOPY: A HISTORICAL PERSPECTIVE

Vascular endoscopy was considered only a curiosity when my colleagues and I published our findings from intraoperative coronary angioscopy in 1987.[3] The fiberoptic devices used in this study were simple adaptations of designs intended for use in other medical disciplines with quite different requirements and specifications. Nevertheless, the results from this study established angioscopy as a serious and valuable diagnostic tool.

A summary of the results of our study is shown in Tables 14–1 and 14–2. At the time of bypass surgery, we examined multiple coronary arteries. When study patients presented with an acute coronary syndrome, the angioscopic examination always included the lesion considered responsible for the abrupt change in symp-

Table 14–1. **Sensitivity of Angiography for Detecting Complex Plaques and Thrombi Among Patients with Stable and Unstable Coronary Artery Disease**

	Complex Plaque		Thrombus	
	Present	*Absent*	*Present*	*Absent*
Angioscopy	4	22	7	22
Angiography	1/4	22/22	1/7	22/22

From Sherman CT, Litvack F, Grundfest WS, et al: Coronary angioscopy in patients with unstable angina pectoris. N Engl J Med 1986; 315:913.

Table 14–2. **Frequency of Complex Plaque and Thrombus Among Patients with Stable and Unstable Coronary Artery Disease**

	Complex Plaque	Thrombus
Patients with Unstable Ischemia	4/10	7/10
Accelerated	3/3	0/3
Rest	1/7	7/7
Patients with Stable Disease	0/17	0/17

From Sherman CT, Litvack F, Grundfest WS, et al: Coronary angioscopy in patients with unstable angina pectoris. N Engl J Med 1986; 315:913.

toms. In patients with a stable clinical history and thus without an identifiable culprit lesion, we included in the examination as many arteries and segments as possible. The angioscopic images were readily categorized into three types that correlated well with the patients' clinical history. In those patients with a history of worsening angina associated with stress or exertion, angioscopy revealed the culprit coronary lesion to be an ulcerated plaque. If symptoms included spontaneous angina at rest, then angioscopy showed the culprit lesion to have obstructive thrombus as part of the lesion, presumably superimposed on an ulcerated plaque. By comparison, in patients with stable symptoms, all the examined lesions were smooth surfaced, noncomplex, and without thrombus, although they were often severely obstructive. Conventional angiography usually could not allow these qualitative details of plaque morphology to be discerned.

With the help of angioscopy, we have come to realize that contrast coronary angiography, which is considered the gold standard test, often fails to detect subtle yet crucial coronary morphology. Further, the two-dimensional view of coronary obstructions offered by angiography probably fails to reveal the true physiologic significance of a blockage.[4] Angioscopy offers a unique vantage point (i.e., from within the vessel) to assess the cross-sectional area of a stenosis. Despite these prospects, percutaneous coronary angioscopy was unrealistic until recently, when fiberoptic technology, fueled by the telecommunications industry, developed ultrathin, flexible fibers. Reflecting these constraints, most early published data are from either peripheral vascular or intraoperative angioscopy, in which fiberoptic design requirements were less rigorous.

Percutaneous angioscopy of the peripheral vasculature is much less challenging than percutaneous coronary angioscopy. The relatively straight course of peripheral vessels allows easy passage of the angioscopy catheter compared with the serpentine, small-caliber coronary arteries. The coronary arteries supply the pumping heart, which is in constant motion and critically dependent on its continuous blood flow. This is in stark contrast to the status of the peripheral arteries. When coronary blood flow is disturbed, angina, arrhythmias, myocardial infarction, and death can result. Thus, unlike peripheral angioscopy, the duration of the procedure, the amount of instrumentation, and the volume of flush are all critical issues in percutaneous coronary angioscopy.

Comparing the techniques of intraoperative and percutaneous coronary angioscopy reveals further disparity. When the heart is arrested and the patient is on bypass pump, the surgeon can perform angioscopy in an unhurried fashion with less concern for provoking ischemia. The target vessel is dissected out and its blood flow controlled. The scope is placed directly into the surgeon's arteriotomy, adjacent to the lesion to be examined. Both the scope and vessel can be manipulated by the surgeon's hand. Because the heart is not beating and is bathed in cardioplegia, ischemia is not a critical issue.

THE RATIONALE TO PURSUE PERCUTANEOUS CORONARY ANGIOSCOPY

With all the difficulties inherent in percutaneous angioscopy, medical investigators continue to aggressively pursue the technique and encourage engineers to produce more refined devices. The potential targets for visualization are numerous (Table 14–3). This approach offers to validate the findings of intraoperative coronary angioscopy, in which it was found that unstable ischemia often results from unstable, complex, intimal pathology. Similar discoveries may occur in patients with related syndromes. Patients with clinical syndromes whose etiology is poorly understood and do not require surgery can also be examined and their coronary etiology exposed. Such patients include those without coronary artery disease who suffered sudden

Table 14–3. Dimensions and Characteristics of Potential Targets for Coronary Angioscopy

Target Structure	Size Range (mm)	Unique Surface Qualities
Arterial lumen	1–4	Color can be white, yellow, or red
Anastomoses	1–4	Sutures can be 0.003 mm
Plaque details	0.3–1.0	Ulcerated, hemorrhage, & smooth surface
Dissection and flaps	0.3–1.0	Transverse, longitudinal, double-lumen
Thrombus	0.3–4.0	Color can be red/brown/white, depending on age & composition

cardiac death or those with documented vasospasm.

Percutaneous coronary angioscopy also offers the potential for live visual monitoring of coronary interventions such as balloon and laser angioplasty, atherectomy, rotational ablation, stent placement, and thrombolysis. Qualitative imaging of a coronary's inner surface may disclose why some lesions abruptly close after balloon dilation, reveal the stimuli for restenosis, or clarify when thrombolysis is indicated. Intravascular angioscopic imaging may accurately aim a laser beam to reduce perforations, direct an atherectomy blade to enhance debulking of atheroma, or aid placement of a coronary stent.

In 1985, Spears[5] and his collaborators first described the results of percutaneous coronary angioscopy in humans, which was performed while patients were in the cardiac catheterization laboratory. Over the next 3 years, Japanese investigators were pioneers in percutaneous angioscopy.[6–8] In their studies, angioscopes of outer dimensions ranging from 1.8 to 0.75 mm were advanced from the carotid, brachial, and femoral arteries to the coronary arteries of humans, dogs, pigs, and sheep. Diverse coronary morphologies have been visualized, including atheromatous plaques, thrombi, intimal damage after balloon angioplasty, thrombolysis, and collateral blood flow.

Early results from a 1991 multicenter trial using the Baxter Imagecath for percutaneous coronary angioscopy have shown an overall success rate of 81% (Table 14–4). Thus far, the results have been tabulated from examinations of 135 lesions in 65 patients before and after balloon angioplasty, atherectomy, and stent placement, as well as in orthotopic transplant patients. An average of 2.1 sites (ranging from 1 to 2.4 sites) were targeted per patient, each site examination lasting an average of 13.8 minutes (ranging from 8.4 to 30 minutes). Success rates were excellent for the circumflex and right coronary arteries (94% and 91%, respectively), whereas left anterior descending (LAD) examinations were less productive (63% success rate). Examinations of the mid and distal segments of all vessels were very successful (86% and 89%, respectively), whereas proximal segments proved more difficult (66% success rate). Excluding the area that proved least successful, the proximal LAD (56% success), the success rate for proximal lesions was 81%. Saphenous vein grafts, which were well represented in this study, proved relatively easy to image (24 out of 26 [92%]).

The results from Japanese investigators, using a similar over-the-wire angioscope and similar percutaneous techniques, were less encouraging. For reasons that are unclear, the results compiled from three research groups[6–8] were very different from those achieved with the Baxter Imagecath. Their overall success rate was 66% (190 out of 288 target lesions), and the success rates for individual coronary arteries varied little (LAD, 69%; circumflex, 67%; right, 58%).

IMPORTANT FINDINGS RESULTING FROM THE USE OF ANGIOSCOPY

An Adjunct to Intraoperative Angiography

It is not surprising that the first practical use for angioscopy was described with intraoperative viewing of the peripheral vasculature. Vascular surgeons confirmed that the information derived from angioscopy is unique, complementary to angiography, and clinically relevant when performed with their procedures.[9] Leery that the data derived from angiography alone are sufficient to detect important, remediable vascular lesions, Baxter and associates,[9] in a prospective study, compared intraoperative angioscopy with arteriography following femoral-distal bypass. They concluded that completion angiography, the current standard, is only 67% sensitive and 95% specific at detecting technical mishaps that contribute to early graft closure after femoral-distal bypass graft surgery. Angioscopy was 100% sensitive and 100% specific for detecting these abnormalities. In a study by Segalowitz and colleagues,[10] surgeons often elected

Table 14–4. **Angioscopic Success Rates by Target Vessel and Location: Experience with the Imagecath and Others**

Vessel	Location			Total	Others
	Proximal	*Mid*	*Distal*		
LAD	14/25 (56%)	13/20 (65%)	3/3 (100%)	30/48 (63%)	123/177 (69%)
Circumflex	2/2 (100%)	12/12 (100%)	3/4 (94%)	17/18 (94%)	18/27 (67%)
RCA	11/14 (79%)	26/27 (96%)	2/2 (100%)	39/43 (91%)	49/84 (58%)
SVG	—	—	—	24/26 (92%)	—
Total	27/41 (66%)	51/59 (86%)	8/9 (89%)	110/135 (81%)	190/288 (66%)
Total less LAD	13/16 (81%)	38/39 (97%)	5/6 (83%)	80/87 (92%)	67/111 (60%)

LAD, left anterior descending coronary artery; RCA, right coronary artery; SVG, saphenous vein graft.

not to perform completion angiography based on angioscopic data. Graft patency was 94% in their study. These authors' experience is not unique.[11, 12] With widespread use of angioscopy in the future, causes of graft failure might be reduced (Table 14–5), and the need for intraoperative arteriography might be limited to only those patients in whom documentation of distal runoff is needed, greatly aiding patients who are sensitive to dye and fluid volume (e.g., those with renal insufficiency or congestive heart failure).

Although intraoperative coronary angioscopy is well recognized as being superior to angiography at detecting a significant amount of intraluminal pathology,[13] it has yet to find its clinical niche. It has been speculated that angioscopic inspection of the internal aspect

Table 14–5. **Angioscopic Findings Correlating with Graft Failure**

	Angioscopic Findings
Vein graft	Competent valve leaflets (unlysed/partially lysed), unligated tributaries (AV fistula), vein recanalization (webs/strands), thrombus (organized, platelet, fresh), mural sclerosis, intimal hyperplasia, sclerotic shortened valve leaflets, valvulotome-induced 'injury,' residual thrombus after thrombolysis, atherosclerotic degeneration.
Anastomosis	Intimal flaps, distorted or small apex, irregular anastomosis, thrombus (oragnized, platelet, fresh), arterial/venous wall pathologic condition.
Artery	Intimal flaps/dissections, thrombus (organized, platelet, fresh), occlusive disease, plaque characteristics.

AV, arteriovenous
From Miller A, Jepsen SJ, Stonebridge PA, et al: New angioscopic findings in graft failure after infrainguinal bypass. Arch Surg 1990; 125:749–755. Copyright 1990, American Medical Association.

of anastomoses during coronary artery bypass surgery will improve acute graft failure rates, but to date corroborating data have not been found. Richens and associates[14] hinted at the potential of intraoperative coronary angioscopy when they described a patient needing mitral valve replacement. The preoperative angiogram was equivocal for the suspected diagnosis of left main dissection. Only by intraoperative angioscopic imaging was the need for coronary artery bypass surgery clearly identified.

Such cases might foreshadow angioscopy's routine use in determining qualitative aspects of coronary artery lesions. We are realizing that present-day diagnostic methods are poor at predicting the natural history or activity of a lesion. Nevertheless, it is rupture or ulceration of a plaque that causes dramatic changes in a patient's clinical course. Angioscopy seems best suited to determine a lesion's qualitative details, which may correlate to its predisposition to rupture or ulcerate. Although it is likely that an appropriate treatment plan will depend more on this type of data than the degree of stenosis, these crucial data remain lamentably unavailable.

Angioscopic Evaluation of Catheter Interventions

The dominance of balloon angioplasty has been challenged by a burgeoning number of new devices for vascular intervention. Angioscopy has been added to the list of tools used to interrogate the mechanism of action and efficacy of these devices. Avoiding the technical difficulties inherent in angioscopy performed in flowing blood streams, a number of autopsy studies have given us insight into the mechanism of these new devices as well as balloon angioplasty. These rudimentary studies have also hinted at the promise of live angioscopic monitoring of these devices during the procedure.

Ahn and coworkers[15] examined 30 ex situ human arteries and 39 in situ cadaveric arteries before and immediately after rotational endarterectomy with the Rotablator (Heart Technology, Bellevue, WA). The smooth, highly polished intraluminal surface depicted by angioscopy was corroborated by microscopy and angiography. Gehani and colleagues[16] used angioscopy to monitor the Kensey angioplasty device, a flexible polypropylene catheter with a rotating distal cam that creates a vortex of saline. Angioscopy helped confirm that the vortex of infused saline at the catheter's distal tip kept the rotating catheter central in the lumen. Similar to other such studies, angioscopy proved excellent at detecting post-procedure intimal flaps and thrombi but was inferior to conventional angiography for detecting perforations. Ebner and associates[17] performed angioscopy and angiography in autopsied aortic specimens before and after conventional balloon angioplasty. After successful dilation, angioscopy consistently revealed plaque compression, longitudinal tears, and detached plaque that did not encroach on the vessel's lumen. By comparison, transverse tears interfered with physiologic flow and were associated with histologic findings regularly noted in autopsied specimens after failed angioplasty. This phenomena increased in frequency as the ratio of balloon diameter to vessel diameter increased. Post-dilation angioscopy was routinely handicapped by turbidity created by vessel wall fragments suspended in the normally transparent flush solution. The prevalence of this turbidity suggests that plaque rupture and draining are common after both successful and failed balloon dilation. Angioscopic observations by White and coworkers[18] in five patients with restenosis support the accumulating evidence that such lesions differ morphologically from primary atherosclerosis. Although atherosclerosis usually appeared pigmented, angioscopy easily identified restenosis by its glistening white surface.

The Detection of Coronary Thrombus

Angioscopic investigations concerning thrombosis, the recognized culprit for most acute coronary syndromes, continue to yield insight into more successful treatment strategies. Ritchie and colleagues[19] used angioscopy to assess the efficacy of mechanical, pharmacologic, and combined techniques for removal of thrombus. They performed angiography and angioscopy in canine femoral arteries after a thrombotic occlusion was created using crush injury, clamp occlusion, and injection of thrombin. Not surprisingly, angioscopy was consistently more sensitive than angiography at detecting thrombus. But where angiography excelled at distinguishing subtotal from total thrombotic occlusion, angioscopy was deficient, revealing only large, red, convex masses. Because it was unable to visualize around the convex borders of a thrombus, angioscopy was inadequate at defining the full extent of such lesions. Angioscopy was also limited by the need for vigorous flushing, the rigidity of the instrument, and the lack of quantitative information. Mizuno and associates,[20] performing percutaneous coronary angioscopy in patients with acute coronary syndromes, observed that the thrombi invariably present at the culprit lesions appeared different according to the patient's clinical syndrome. Whereas those patients with acute myocardial infarction had the familiar red thrombi, those with unstable angina often had gray-colored thrombi, presumably owing to a predominance of platelets. However impressive, it remains unproved that the details of thrombus uniquely disclosed by in vivo angioscopy have true clinical utility.

Angioscopy-Assisted Laser Angioplasty

Because delivering laser energy and receiving angioscopic images both depend on fiberoptics, attempts to combine these technologies seem valid and warranted. White and coworkers[21] investigated the application of angioscopy for aiming and monitoring argon and Nd:YAG laser angioplasty in canine femoral and carotid arteries, and femoral, iliac, and jugular veins. The saline flush required for angioscopy absorbed and attenuated the Nd:YAG energy, impeding efficient ablation of tissue. They also performed intraoperative angioscopy in patients' atherosclerotic peripheral vessels before, during, and after thermal angioplasty with a metal-tipped laser probe. In 16 of the 24 patients (67%) in whom thermal angioplasty was attempted, the angioscope could not reach the targeted area because a preceding stenotic lesion prevented its passage. Adequate imaging depended on the vessel's caliber, which was optimal only when the lumen was patent and large enough to easily accommodate the scope but not so large as to render the visual field inconsequential. Despite these shortcomings, angioscopy effectively directed the laser procedure, keeping the probe out of side branches and false channels resulting from dissections. After the procedure, 88% of angioscopic examinations were successful, revealing thermal damage, mural thrombus, false channels, and intimal fragmentation with charring and flaps. The authors conclude that, at present, angioscopic assistance of laser angioplasty is practical only for patent atherosclerotic arteries in which disease is mild and stenoses are well localized. Angioscopy assistance seems very effective during the removal of venous valves, a procedure required for in situ bypass graft surgery. Although the qualitative information gained from angioscopy has definite value, it is doubtful whether the procedure would ever fully replace intraoperative angiography.

Fujisawa and coworkers[22] cleverly adapted an innovation promulgated by Shure and associates[23] for imaging pulmonary vascular lesions (see Chapter 15). They affixed an inflatable latex balloon to the distal tip of a large-bore, multichannel angioscope. The balloon, inflated with transparent saline, can be pressed against the targeted area, displacing opaque blood for visualization without need for saline flushing. Shure's group demonstrated that large-caliber vascular structures, like the main pulmonary artery, can be successfully imaged with this technique, where otherwise the magnitude of flush required would be prohibitive. Fujisawa's group approached their intended targets, which were surgically implanted masses in the canine right atrium and vena cava, from the internal jugular vein. Angioscopic visualization was excellent, with little distortion of color or anatomic detail. Laser energy was applied through the inflated balloon to the target via a fiberoptic bundle located in another channel of the catheter. As anticipated, the energy from the Nd:YAG laser used in this study could heat the saline, opacify the transparent latex, and often burst the balloon. Nevertheless, the right atrium's muscle bundles and the vena cava, azygos, and innominate venous systems were imaged in detail. This study demonstrated that angioscopic imaging is possible in large, blood-filled cardiac chambers without need of an irrigation system. Not only is fiberoptic imaging possible through an inflated balloon but laser energy can also be administered in very limited doses. Nevertheless, the drawbacks of this system are substantial. The instrument is unwieldy, requiring a large entry site incision. Its steering system is unsophisticated, and because it is not advanced over the wire, the potential to cause damage is appreciable. The clinical applications for the Nd:YAG laser also require further investigations.

Lee and colleagues[24] used Nd:YAG laser energy to recanalize a total occlusion of the superficial femoral artery after pretreatment with urokinase. The lumen was then enlarged using directional atherectomy. Although angioscopy was not performed simultaneously with either of the procedures, post-laser angioscopy revealed a new, heavily charred lumen. After atherectomy, angioscopy revealed a widely patent lumen disfigured by small "trenches and crevices." This brief report confirmed that angioscopy can distinguish atherosclerotic plaque, thrombi, and flaps but is unable to evaluate the length of a lesion or quantify its dimensions.

CARDIOSCOPY AND MYOCARDIAL ARCHITECTURE

Uchida and associates[25] were the first to image the cardiac chambers of living patients with percutaneous angioscopy. They maneuvered 9-French guide catheters with latex balloons secured to their distal tips to suspicious segments of the left ventricle during routine cardiac catheterization. Angioscopes were advanced within these catheters into the inflated balloons. When pressed against the myocardium, the fully inflated balloons created a bloodless viewing field. These investigators compared the endocardial color and trabeculae from patients with dilated cardiomyopathy and acute myocarditis with that of controls who had no appreciable heart disease (Table 14–6). They also documented signs of gross myocardial injury that would have been undetected without angioscopy. Despite the small number of patients and lack of histologic confirmation or compelling consistency, these results are intriguing. Endocardium that was either light yellow or blue-white and the presence of thickened trabeculae predicted the biopsy diagnosis of dilated cardiomyopathy. If endocardium was rose colored or the trabeculae were swollen, the patient had acute myocarditis on biopsy. Endocardium that was red, white, or light brown was never seen in normal controls, nor were punctate bleeding and surface thrombus. The novel technique employed in this study is, nevertheless, rudimentary. At present, the balloon-tipped catheter requires a 9-French arterial access, supplementary flush to create an adequate viewing field, and lidocaine because of the high incidence of ventricular ectopy. The high anterior wall and septum remain inaccessible for these catheters.

ANGIOSCOPY AND INTRAVASCULAR ULTRASOUND

Because angioscopy can provide visual images of only the superficial surfaces of a vessel while intravascular ultrasound can reveal transmural anatomic details, the two technologies may be complementary.[26] Kopchok and coworkers[27]

Table 14–6. **Angioscopic Findings in Patients with Two Cardiac Syndromes and Normal Controls**

		Control	Dilated Cardiomyopathy	Acute Myocarditis
Endocardial color		—	Light yellow	—
		—	White	White
	Brown		Brown/light brown	Brown/light brown
		—	Blue-white	—
		—	Red	Red
	Reddish brown		Reddish brown	Reddish brown
				Rose
Trabeculae	Systolic thickening		Thick	Swollen
Other		—	Thrombus	Bleeding, thrombus

From Uchida Y, Nakamura F, Oshima T, et al: Percutaneous fiberoptic angioscopy of the left ventricle in patients with dilated cardiomyopathy and acute myocarditis. Am Heart J 1990; 120:677–687.

combined these two imaging modalities during both in vitro and live canine angioplasty by passing an 0.8-mm angioscope through the central lumen of a 7.8-French (2.6-mm) ultrasound catheter. Although the instruments require further refinement, the data from angioscopy and ultrasound are unique and supplement each other. Together, they may help maximize the luminal diameter resulting from angioplasty while minimizing damage to the normal wall segments. Siegel and colleagues[28] confirmed these speculations when they compared these two intravascular imaging techniques with conventional angiography in two patients undergoing peripheral vascular angioplasty. They found striking differences in the diagnostic abilities of these tools. In one patient, angiography revealed a 4-cm-long 75% occlusive lesion, angioscopy demonstrated localized thrombus within this lesion, and ultrasound showed the entire arterial segment to be diffusely diseased and calcified. The second patient had a totally occluded superficial femoral artery, which was confirmed by all three modalities. After angioplasty, angiography showed a smooth 65% residual stenosis, but a severely disrupted intima was disclosed by angioscopy and ultrasound revealed a 3-cm subintimal dissection.

QUANTIFICATION

Modern diagnostics increasingly require an objective, quantitative assessment of arterial diameter, stenosis diameter, growth and regression of plaque and thrombus, and micromovements of small intraluminal particles. Because of angioscopy's known resolving power and its unique intravascular vantage point, it seems to be a good candidate to meet these needs. Unfortunately, perspective, which is a requirement for intravascular quantification, is not easily realized.

We are allowed visual perspective because our brain integrates simultaneous images obtained from each of our two eyes placed a few inches apart. It is by this same principle, called parallax, that early astronomers determined the moon's distance from earth and its dimensions. Such measurements are gathered either by simultaneous appraisals from telescopes located on different continents or at different times from a single telescope as it changes position during orbit. If the distance between imaging sites is known, calculating the change in an object's area from one site to the next will yield the object's absolute distance. From this approach, the object's actual dimensions are calculated from the magnification charts for the system. Applying parallax to measurements within a vessel requires either a scope with two separate image bundles or a single scope gathering images at multiple sites a known distance apart. Because the size of current binocular fiberoptic scopes prohibits their placement in a coronary artery, only the single-scope technique has been investigated.

Friedl and associates[29] used a single-image bundle scope to record an intravascular image from multiple sites under ideal circumstances. Each scope and lens was calibrated for its unique nonlinear magnification. It was assumed that there was no pincushion distortion and that all features were on a single plane perpendicular to the scope. After validating their system by measuring phantoms at random scope distances, they examined stenoses within cadaveric canine arteries created by ligatures. The position of the angioscope, mounted to a micropositioning stage, was precisely recorded as it gathered images from separate sites. The scope-to-object distance was calculated by measuring the image obtained at three sites that were a known distance apart. Compared with planimetry of the histologic specimen, angioscopy had an average error of 15% in this ideal setting. Unfortunately, objects of interest within a patient's vessel are far from the ideal, rarely lying on a single perpendicular plane. Furthermore, precise measurement of the scope's distal tip movement within a coronary artery is very inaccurate because it can only be estimated indirectly at the skin entry site. Between these sites, the scope has traversed 120 cm of sinuous coronary, central, and peripheral arteries, which makes meaningful measurements inconceivable.

Lee and colleagues[30] applied these principles during intraoperative angioscopy of coronary arteries in eight patients at the time of bypass surgery. Eleven diseased sites were imaged at known distances and then assessed manually with calipers. After the magnification characteristics of the lens was determined, absolute dimensions were calculated and compared with the angiographic worst view of the same lesion. The correlation coefficient was 0.9 ($P < .001$). The authors acknowledged that such precision is possible only under ideal circumstances in which lens-to-object distance can be accurately measured, imaging is straightforward, vessels are completely straight, and all system distortions are considered.

Some innovative researchers have attempted three-dimensional reconstruction of coronary arteries using established holographic techniques, but to date their work is rudimentary.[31, 32]

POTENTIAL COMPLICATIONS OF PERCUTANEOUS ANGIOSCOPY

Although the theoretic complications of angioscopy are many, in practice, their occurrence has been rare. The angioscope catheter and wire may directly damage the coronary endothelium during placement by tearing or perforating the arterial wall. Damage can also occur indirectly. During attempts to obtain a bloodless field, the flushing solution is infused at low volumes (2–4 mL/sec) but a high-pressure jet-stream can cause damage. An occlusion balloon cuff may be inflated proximal to the targeted arterial segment to help create a clear viewing field. From experience with balloon angioplasty, we know that even at low balloon pressures, arteries can respond unpredictably with dissection, spasm, thrombosis, and even reactive hyperplasia at a site previously considered normal.

When angioscopy is performed as intended to aid in the diagnoses of patients with heart disease, the risks are further amplified. The increased procedure time, the added fluid volume from flushing, and the periods of ischemia during imaging are all potentially more hazardous to this category of patients.

As with any new technology, one must expect breakdowns. Because the integrity of the multicomponent coronary angioscopy system depends on each high-tech element and their interfaces, the sources for mishap are many.

LIMITATIONS OF PERCUTANEOUS CORONARY ANGIOSCOPY

Despite angioscopy's laudable contributions to coronary artery imaging, the technique has noteworthy intrinsic limitations. A tight proximal stenosis or the natural funneling shape of a vessel will restrict the catheter's passage and thus the extent of distal vascular examinations. Although this limitation is shared by intravascular ultrasound, angioscopy is further hampered by its ability to examine only surface morphology and its critical dependence on illumination. Even with proper illumination, imaging can be clouded by even the smallest amount of blood or debris. Under the best circumstances, angioscopy's fiberoptic and lens system is subject to pincushion distortion and the lack of depth perception afforded by a its single "eye." Even discounting these impediments, angioscopic images are difficult to quantify and their interpretation remains subjective, influenced by operator experience and proficiency.

Angioscopy cannot be undertaken frivolously. Although its yield has demonstrated some clinical value, it is obtained at a very definite price. Because legitimate clinical indications for coronary angioscopy do not yet exist, it is still considered a nonreimbursable research tool. The potential harm and cost to a patient must be weighed against an unproven clinical benefit. The components are fragile, expensive, and require expert handling and care. For all these reasons, the procedure requires carefully conceived protocols, informed consent, and a team of physicians and technicians willing to devote energy, time, and finances to a research program.

FUTURE DIRECTIONS

Angioscopy's maturation from a mere curiosity to a powerful diagnostic tool depended on a convergence of forces. The recognition of the importance of thrombus and ulcerated plaque created a renewed regard for qualitative features of coronary pathology, which were poorly detected by conventional angiography. The success of percutaneous catheter techniques in treating atherosclerotic coronary artery disease motivated research into the use of related devices, like the angioscope. Advances in the miniaturization and production of flexible fiberoptics allowed the construction of practical fiberoptic catheters to then be tested.

At present, the motivations that initiated angioscopy research persist, strengthened by accumulated experience. Data have correlated the qualitative features of a coronary lesion with patients' clinical syndromes and the success of balloon angioplasty. Intracoronary thrombolysis, atherectomy devices, and lasers have successfully treated atherosclerotic coronary disease, but strict guidelines for their application may require more detailed information obtainable, in part, from angioscopy. It seems only natural that more precise diagnoses and monitoring abilities will be required. The safety, utility, and difficulties of angioscopy techniques, which have now been aptly demonstrated, have challenged industry to engineer a more steerable angioscope and improve optics and imaging.

The prospect of an angioscope whose size and flexibility rival a coronary angioplasty guide wire, whose imaging capabilities are excellent anywhere in the coronary arterial tree, and whose images reveal qualitative and quantitative details previously the sole domain of the pathologist seems only a fantasy. But just over a decade ago, it seemed fantasy that catheters would extend our therapeutic reach to the level we now take for granted. The possibility that our diagnostic reach should follow suit should now seem much less implausible.

REFERENCES

1. White RA: Indications for fiberoptic angioscopy and intraluminal ultrasound. Compr Ther 1990; 16:23–30.
2. Borgini L, Almgren CC: Peripheral vascular angioscopy. AORN J 1990; 52(30):543–550.
3. Sherman CT, Litvack F, Grundfest WS, et al: Coronary angioscopy in patients with unstable angina pectoris. N Engl J Med 1986; 315:913.
4. Marcus ML, Skorton DJ, Johnson MR, et al: Visual estimates of percent diameter coronary stenosis: 'A battered gold standard.' J Am Coll Cardiol 1988; 11:882–885.
5. Spears JR, Spokojny AM, Marais J: Coronary angioscopy during cardiac catheterization. J Am Coll Cardiol 1985; 6:93–97.
6. Arai T, Nakagawa M, Kiuchi K, et al: Visualization in human coronary arteries by 5F balloon catheter endoscope. In Abraham Katzir (ed): Optical Fibers in Medicine IV. Proc. SPIE 1067, 186–189, 1989.
7. Sakurada M, Mizuno K, Miyamota K, et al: Angioscopy by a new percutaneous transluminal coronary angioscope. In Abraham Katzir (ed): Optical Fibers in Medicine V. Proc. SPIE 1201, 63–68, 1990.
8. Inoue K, Kuwaki K, Ochiai H, et al: Percutaneous transluminal coronary angioscopy as the guiding therapy for intracoronary thrombolysis and angioplasty. In Vogel JHK, King SB III (eds): Interventional Cardiology: Future Directions. St. Louis, CV Mosby, 1989, p 1.
9. Baxter BT, Rizzo RJ, Finn WR, et al: A comparative study of intraoperative angioscopy and completion arteriography following femoral-distal bypass. Arch Surg 1990; 125:997–1002.
10. Segalowitz J, Grundfest WS, Treiman RL, et al: Angioscopy for intraoperative management of thromboembolectomy. Arch Surg 1990; 125:1357–1362.
11. Miller A, Jepsen SJ, Stonebridge PA, et al: New angioscopic findings in graft failure after infrainguinal bypass. Arch Surg 1990; 125:749–755.
12. LaMuraglia GM, Cambria RP, Brewster DC, Abbott WM: Angioscopy guided semiclosed technique for in situ bypass. J Vasc Surg 1990; 12:601–604.
13. Grundfest WS, Litvack F, Sherman T, et al: Delineation of peripheral and coronary detail by intraoperative angioscopy. Ann Surg 1985; 202:394–400.
14. Richens D, Renzulli A, Hilton CJ: Dissection of the left main coronary artery: Diagnosis by angioscopy. Ann Thorac Surg 1990; 49:469–470.
15. Ahn SS, Auth D, Marcus DR: Removal of focal atheromatous lesions by angioscopically guided high-speed rotary atherectomy. J Vasc Surg 1988; 7:292–300.
16. Gehani AA, Ball SG, Latif AB, et al: Experimental and clinical percutaneous angioscopy: Experience with dynamic angioplasty. Angiology 1990; 41:809–816.
17. Ebner H, Wex P, Dragojevic D: The mechanism of angioplasty: Endoscopic and morphometric investigations in an experimental model. Eur J Vasc Surg 1989; 3:543–547.
18. White CJ, Ramee SR, Mesa JE, Collins TJ: Percutaneous coronary angioscopy in patients with restenosis after coronary angioplasty. J Am Coll Cardiol 1991; 17:46B–49B.
19. Ritchie JL, Hansen DD, Johnson C, et al: Combined mechanical and chemical thrombolysis in a experimental animal model: Evaluation by angiography and angioscopy. Am Heart J 1990; 119:64–72.
20. Mizuno K, Satomura K, Miyamoto A, et al: Angioscopic evaluation of coronary artery thrombi in acute coronary syndromes. N Engl J Med 1992; 326:287–291.
21. White GH, White RA, Colman PD, Kopchok GE: Experimental and clinical applications of angioscopic guidance for laser angioplasty. Am J Surg 1989; 158:495–501.
22. Fujisawa T, Yamaguchi Y, Seto T, et al: Nd:YAG laser irradiation to intraluminal mass lesions of the superior vena cava under laser balloon angioscopy in an experimental canine model. Jpn J Surg 1990; 20:411–417.
23. Shure D, Gregoratos G, Moser KM: Fiberoptic angioscopy: Role in the diagnosis of chronic pulmonary arterial obstruction. Ann Intern Med 1985; 103:844.
24. Lee G, Morelli R, Long JB, et al: Combined laser-thermal and atherectomy treatment of peripheral arterial occlusion: Documentation by angioscopy and angiography. Am Heart J 1989; 118:1324–1327.
25. Uchida Y, Nakamura F, Oshima T, et al: Percutaneous fiberoptic angioscopy of the left ventricle in patients with dilated cardiomyopathy and acute myocarditis. Am Heart J 1990; 120:677–687.
26. White GH, Siegel SB, Colman PD, et al: Intraoperative coronary angioscopy: Development of practical techniques. Angiology 1990; 41:793–800.

27. Kopchok GE, White RA, Guthrie C, et al: Intravascular ultrasound: A new potential modality for angioplasty guidance. Angiology 1990; 41:785–792.

28. Siegel RJ, Chae JS, Forrester JS, Ruiz CE: Angiography, angioscopy, and ultrasound imaging before and after percutaneous balloon angioplasty. Am Heart J 1990; 120:1086–1090.

29. Friedl SE, Abela GS, Tomaru T, et al: Quantitative endovascular angioscopy. *In* Abraham Katzir (ed): Optical Fibers in Medicine IV, Proc. SPIE 1067, 197–202, 1989.

30. Lee G, Garcia JM, Corso PJ, et al: Correlation of coronary angioscopic to angiographic findings in coronary artery disease. Am J Cardiol 1986; 58:238–241.

31. von Bally G: Fiber optic holographic endoscopy. *In* Abraham Katzir (ed): Optical Fibers in Medicine V. Proc. SPIE 1201, 535–542, 1990.

32. Podbielska H, Friesem A: Endoscopic optical metrology—the possibilities of holographic interferometry. *In* Abraham Katzir (ed): Optical Fibers in Medicine V. Proc. SPIE 1201, 552–560, 1990.

Chapter 15

Pulmonary Angioscopy

DEBORAH SHURE
WILLIAM AUGER
KENNETH MOSER
KIRK L. PETERSON

Angioscopy has a long and interesting history beginning with the first attempt at cardioscopy, endoscopy of the heart chambers and valves, by Rhea and Walker in 1919.[1] Most of the work in angioscopy over the following 50 years focused on examination and manipulation of cardiac valves,[1-9] but as surgical techniques for open heart surgery and valve replacement became widespread, the limited interest in angioscopy died out until its recent revival.[10-13] This revival appears to have been spurred by a combination of advances in fiberoptics and advances in percutaneous approaches to problems that formerly remained in the domain of open surgery.

Over this time, one of the major problems of angioscopy has been that of visualization through the opaque medium of blood. This problem has been dealt with by a variety of creative techniques, which can be grouped into three basic approaches: flushing blood from the field of view, mechanical displacement of blood, and hemodilution. Hemodilution, filling the vessel with a transparent blood substitute, has been used exclusively in the coronary circuit[14] and would be practical only in such a small volume system of end arteries. Flushing blood with saline has been used successfully in angioscopy of peripheral vessels and coronary arteries, as well as for direct visualization of pulmonary vessels during cardiopulmonary bypass.[10-13, 15] Flushing techniques alone, in nonsurgical situations, have not been successful in large vascular beds or in the chambers of the heart, because the volume of fluid needed for adequate visualization leads to fluid overload.[9, 16] This consideration is particularly important in patients who may be hemodynamically compromised because of their underlying medical condition.

Mechanical displacement of blood by an optically clear device has been the most successful method of viewing valves,[7] congenital cardiac defects,[17-19] and major vessels.[19, 20] A variety of devices has been used to displace blood, including the lens itself,[1, 2] optical grade Lucite,[7] deformable plastics,[9] and balloons.[3, 9] Nonoperative applications have used either inflatable viewing balloons[16-24] or techniques combining both balloon technology and low-volume saline infusion.[25] Because of the nature of the pulmonary arterial bed and the frequently tenuous hemodynamic status of patients with pulmonary vascular disease, mechanical displacement using balloon techniques to transiently arrest blood flow has been our method of choice for pulmonary angioscopy.

Our experience in pulmonary angioscopy has evolved in large part from interest in the problems associated with the diagnosis of chronic pulmonary thromboemboli. Although acute pulmonary emboli are relatively easy to diagnose by conventional tests, including lung scans and angiography, chronic pulmonary emboli may be more difficult to diagnose. Because chronic thromboembolic obstruction of major pulmonary arteries is a surgically treatable cause of pulmonary hypertension,[26, 27] the diagnosis is a particularly important one to establish with certainty. In addition, because the location of the obstructing process is important in determining operability, it is also important to be able to ascertain the proximal extent of the process.[26, 27]

When acute emboli, which fill the lumen of a vessel, fail to resolve, they organize into fibrous material that becomes incorporated into the vessel wall and obstructs, or partially obstructs, the lumen. At this stage, they no longer present the classic angiographic image of acute thromboembolism but rather cause a variety of unusual images that may be misleading. The misleading nature of the angiogram is sometimes due to partial recanalization through an obstructed area and partly because angiograms are not as sensitive to wall abnormalities as to luminal abnormalities. With these problems in mind, we became interested in the diagnostic ability of angioscopy as a direct visualization technique to aid in the diagnosis of chronic pulmonary emboli and in determining operability.

EQUIPMENT AND METHODS

Angioscopes

Pulmonary angioscopy poses a different set of problems from angioscopy of the coronary bed or intraoperative angioscopy of peripheral vessels. The problems are created by the physical characteristics of the pulmonary arterial circulation and have influenced our choice of instruments and techniques. Relevant aspects of the pulmonary arterial bed are the wide variation in vessel size (particularly in patients with pulmonary hypertension), the degree of vessel branching through which the angioscope must be maneuvered for an adequate examination, the large volume of the bed, and in pathologic states, the presence of a greatly expanded bronchial collateral circulation that anastomoses with the pulmonary arteries at a precapillary level.[28] An additional consideration is the frequency of right ventricular failure in patients with severe pulmonary hypertension with the consequent danger of fluid overload. These considerations and the desire to achieve a preoperative rather than an intraoperative diagnosis have strongly affected our approach.

Although there has been some progress in catheter-based angioscopy systems,[21, 25] the desire to have an instrument that can be directed has stimulated the development of our current pulmonary angioscopes. Essentially, they are modifications of traditional medical fiberoptic endoscopes. They have evolved over the past 12 years to longer, narrower instruments that are suitable for passage from peripheral veins. The initial angioscope (Machida Corp., Norwood, NJ) was 4 mm in outside diameter with a 0.8-mm internal channel for balloon inflation.[23] Its bundle was 80 cm long. Distal tip deflection of 90 degrees was achieved from a lever in the proximal handle. The second prototype (Olympus Corp., Lake Success, NY) was longer and narrower (3.2 mm diameter, 120 cm long). The 36% decrease in cross-sectional area facilitated passage of the angioscope from the arm, neck, or groin.[29] Its inflation channel was 0.5 mm, and its distal tip deflected 180 degrees by a similar mechanism. The third prototype (Machida Corp., Oakwood, NJ) had a diameter of 3 mm (12% smaller cross-sectional area than the second prototype) and a 100-cm bundle with a 0.5-mm inflation channel and 70 degrees of distal tip deflection.[30] This angioscope had a modified tip of stainless steel with a lip at the top and bottom that provided a secure area to attach the balloon without damaging the covering of the fiber bundle. The fourth prototype was 120 cm long and 3 mm wide, and had 90 degrees of distal tip deflection. A slight tapering of the tip made secure balloon attachment

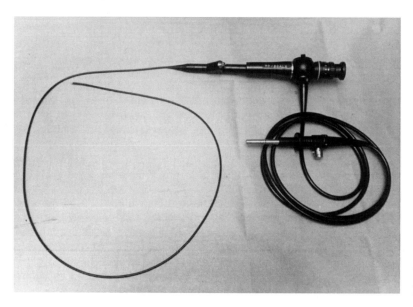

Figure 15–1. Olympus Angioscope. (Courtesy of Olympus Corporation, Lake Success, NY.)

more difficult than with previous models. The latest pulmonary angioscope, which is the one we use, is a modification of the second prototype (Fig. 15–1). Although its length and tip deflection remain the same, the external diameter is 3.0 mm and a spool-like, stainless steel tip has been added (Fig. 15–2). This modification provides the same security of balloon attachment as in the Machida instrument.

All prototypes used a disposable balloon attached to the distal tip. Two materials have been used for balloons: a polyurethane[31] and a thermoplastic elastomer.[30] Both are nonthrombogenic, as are the material used to secure the balloon to the angioscope (Teflon-coated nylon braided thread) and the covering of the angioscope bundle. The polyurethane balloon was transparent in its deflated state but was not optimally elastic. The thermoplastic elastomer balloon is adequately elastic but not transparent in its deflated state. It becomes transparent, however, with minimal inflation. All the balloons are inflated with carbon dioxide to avoid air embolism in case of balloon rupture. The balloons are capable of inflation from a resting diameter of 3 mm to 2 cm.

The balloon is secured to the tip by careful repetitive wrapping of thread, with the ends pulled underneath the wrapping to prevent unraveling (Fig. 15–3). The use of fine (6/0) braided thread as opposed to monofilament thread makes the wrapping considerably easier and more secure. This attachment, while tedious, has proved to be extremely secure. No balloon has detached from the angioscope in over 150 procedures in humans and animals.

Documentation

Some form of documentation of endoscopic findings is extremely important. Significant

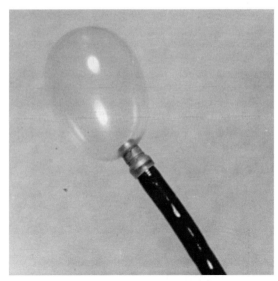

Figure 15–3. Inflated viewing balloon secured to distal tip of the angioscope with fine Teflon-coated nylon suture.

findings may not be fully appreciated on first viewing in the midst of a rapidly pulsating vascular bed. Although a 150-watt halogen light source is adequate for visualization through the angioscope itself, good photographic documentation usually requires at least a 300-watt xenon light source.

We have used both still photography and videotaping for documentation. For still photography, a 35-mm camera equipped with an endoscopic screen and an adapter for the angioscope head provides high-resolution images. An automatic winder (particularly equipped with a foot pedal) greatly facilitates the use of the camera. Multiple photographs ensure that important findings will be captured despite the motion of the system. The disadvantage to still photography is the length of the processing time; review of the procedure cannot be immediate.

Videotaping provides the advantage of immediate playback and review, although the resolution of the image is not as good as with 35-mm still photographs. Videotaping, however, provides an additional advantage of dynamic viewing. The use of newer, sterilizable solid state, so called chip, cameras makes videotaping more practical than formerly with the use of single- or triple-tube color cameras. The use of 3/4 tape (U-Matic format) or Super VHS videotape is advisable for the best quality recording. Although the key to good still photography is multiple shots, the secret to good videotaping is to focus for a sufficient length of time on each finding. Rapid movement of the angioscope makes adequate observation difficult.

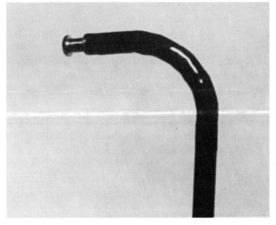

Figure 15–2. Distal end of the Olympus Angioscope, in flexion. (Courtesy of Olympus Corporation, Lake Success, NY.)

Another aspect of recording that deserves attention is documentation of location. With some systems, a character generator can be used to place a written record of the location of the angioscope on the videotape. We have found it useful to attach the fluoroscopic output to one channel of the video recorder to visually document the location of the tip of the angioscope during fluoroscopy. We then switch channels to record the angioscopic image.

Technique

The size and relatively difficult-to-maneuver prototype angioscopes of the past posed substantive limitations to venous access. With the larger angioscopes (3.2 mm external diameter or greater), a percutaneous approach in larger, hard-to-compress veins, such as the internal jugular, was avoided given the concerns of bleeding in patients with elevated central venous pressures. A venotomy to access an external jugular or antecubital vein, typically on the patient's right side, was the preferred method for insertion of the angioscope. The percutaneous femoral vein approach was attempted only when other vessels were occluded or too small to accommodate the angioscope, or when the flexibility characteristics of the angioscope warranted a straight approach from the groin. The smaller, more maneuverable pulmonary angioscopes in use at present allow greater latitude in central venous access. Using a segment of a 10-French catheter sheath to cover the balloon and distal tip of the angioscope, the instrument can be inserted easily through an 11-French vascular sheath placed in the internal jugular vein (again, preferably on the patient's right). Because the majority of angioscopic procedures are performed following right-sided heart catheterization and pulmonary angiography, vascular access for these other procedures (usually an 8-French sheath) is up-sized to the 11-French caliber. Applying torque to the angioscope has not been significantly impeded using this size for vascular access, and we have not experienced a major hemorrhagic complication with this technique, even in the setting of elevated central venous pressures. However, we have avoided this approach in patients with markedly abnormal clotting times.

Following insertion, under fluoroscopic guidance, the angioscope can be advanced to the right atrium without inflation of the balloon. With the tip of the instrument fully flexed, the tricuspid valve and right ventricular chamber are carefully traversed, allowing flexion to be released as the pulmonic valve is approached. Especially in the setting of right ventricular enlargement, balloon inflation during this latter maneuver may assist passage across the pulmonic valve. However, we have found that minimizing the number of balloon inflations during passage through the right heart chambers decreases the risk of pinhole ruptures in the balloon. Once in the main pulmonary artery, the use of intermittent fluoroscopy is also essential to ascertain the position of the tip of the angioscope. The balloon can be gently inflated until blood is just displaced and an image appears. Using both the image and the feel of resistance in the plunger of a CO_2-filled syringe, the operator can avoid overdistension of both the balloon and the vessel. Complete occlusion of the vessel is not always necessary for adequate visualization of the vascular wall. The balloon itself does not provide any significant resistance to moving the angioscope and usually has no adverse hemodynamic consequences when it is carefully inflated.[24, 32]

The use of distal tip deflection is important in both guiding the angioscope through branches and in increasing the view obtained. While lobar and sublobar vessels generally can be occluded (or mostly occluded) safely providing a good view of the vessel lumen and wall, occlusion of a left or right main pulmonary artery in a patient with significant pulmonary hypertension usually is not desirable.[24] In addition, patients with high pulmonary artery pressure may have extremely dilated main pulmonary arteries that cannot be adequately occluded. For visualization of these central arteries, the angioscope tip is flexed into the vessel wall, with the balloon inflated and moved along the wall. The angioscope can then be rotated to view other aspects of the wall.

Distal tip deflection is also important in viewing more peripheral lobar and sublobar vessels to compensate for the relatively narrow angle of view (usually 60 degrees) of thin fiber bundles. In these areas, small movement of the distal tip with the balloon inflated often brings into view additional branches or wall abnormalities that would be missed with a static angioscope tip.

Using these techniques of fluoroscopic guidance, balloon visualization, and distal tip deflection, a complete examination of pulmonary arteries to sublobar (segmental) branches can be carried out in a timely fashion. With one operator controlling the angioscope levers and balloon inflation and deflation, and another guiding the instrument, the angioscopic procedure can typically be accomplished within 15 minutes from the time of entry into the right ventricle. Although photographic or videotape documentation adds some additional time to the procedure, it is sufficiently important to be considered a necessary component. The procedure can take longer in cases with an unusually dilated right ventricle or unusually large and tortuous main pulmonary arteries. In the case of a dilated right ventricle, entry into the main pulmonary artery can be difficult. In the case of an unusually large and tortuous pulmonary artery, movement of the angioscope from left to right sides can be difficult.

ANIMAL STUDIES

In our initial study,[23] we demonstrated in a dog the ability of pulmonary angioscopy to detect acute, experimentally induced emboli. The angioscope consisted of a pediatric bronchoscope modified with a latex balloon attached with silk suture. Although the instrument allowed the operator to identify acute emboli, the material of the balloon and the attaching thread were thrombogenic.

In a subsequent study,[31] we compared angioscopic identification and localization of acute pulmonary emboli in an animal model with lung perfusion scanning. The results of autopsy data were used as the reference standard. Angioscopy was performed after embolization in the experimental animals, followed by four-view lung perfusion scans. The materials used in this study were nonthrombogenic. A set of control animals was used to ascertain if angioscopy itself could produce lung scan perfusion defects. In these animals, angioscopy was performed, followed by lung perfusion scanning without experimental embolization.

No scan defects were seen in the control animals, and no emboli were seen at angioscopy or autopsy indicating that angioscopy did not cause lung scan abnormalities or induce local thrombosis. Among the embolized dogs, 23 emboli were found at autopsy. Lung perfusion scanning detected 23 defects, but these defects did not correspond to the autopsy findings in all cases. In three dogs, disparities occurred. For example, a single lobar scan defect was noted by scan in a case in which three separate sublobar emboli were found at autopsy and by angioscopy. Angioscopy identified and correctly located 21 of 23 emboli, which were all the emboli within the range of the angioscope (4-mm diameter vessels). This study demonstrated the anatomic accuracy of the angioscopic technique.

In another study,[32] we examined the safety of the procedure by studying electrocardio-graphic, hemodynamic, and gas exchange findings in experimental animals. Angioscopy was performed in animals before and after pulmonary embolization. All the parameters were examined in various locations in the right side of the heart and pulmonary arteries with the angioscope balloon deflated and then inflated for 1 minute. No changes in hemodynamics or gas exchange were noted during angioscopy before embolization. After embolization, minor increases occurred in mean systemic pressure and cardiac output. These effects were unrelated to the location of the angioscope or the state of balloon inflation. A small number of arrhythmias, comparable to those seen during right-sided heart catheterization,[33] were observed under both the control and experimental conditions and were unrelated to angioscope position or balloon inflation.

CLINICAL TRIALS

Having established the capability and safety of pulmonary angioscopy in an animal model, we have been engaged in examining the clinical utility of this intervention. These efforts have been focused on the diagnosis of large-vessel, chronic pulmonary emboli because of the difficulty often encountered in establishing this diagnosis by conventional techniques and because of the therapeutic implications of establishing a diagnosis, as mentioned earlier. In this well-defined setting, it has been possible to clearly compare the outcome of conventional diagnostic techniques with that of angioscopy and to assess the effect of each method on therapeutic decisions.

Patients are candidates for pulmonary angioscopy if they have pulmonary hypertension and are suspected of having chronic pulmonary artery obstruction. Initial evaluative studies consist of chest radiographs, electrocardiogram, pulmonary function tests, arterial blood gas measurements, and lung ventilation and perfusion scans. In selected cases, particularly in those patients with unilateral main pulmonary artery obstruction, computerized tomography or magnetic resonance imaging, or both, have also been performed. If patients are still suspected of having chronic pulmonary artery obstruction (usually because of perfusion scan abnormalities) they undergo right-sided heart catheterization with hemodynamic measurements, followed by pulmonary angiography of the left and right sides. Although it was believed in the past that pulmonary angiography was risky in patients with significant pulmonary hypertension, the experience in these patients has been benign because of adherence to careful guidelines.[34] In cases in which a reasonable possibility of coronary disease or unrelated left ventricular dysfunction exists, left-sided heart catheterization, left ventriculography, and coronary angiography are also performed. Based on these studies, a decision is made about diagnosis and the surgical accessibility of the vascular abnormalities that are believed to be chronic thrombi. If diagnostic questions remain, angioscopy is then performed and an independent assessment is made of the diagnosis and operability of the lesions. For those patients who then go on to have their chronic thrombi surgically removed (through a pulmonary thromboendarterectomy), a correlation is made between the surgical results and the angiographic and angioscopic findings.

We have now performed pulmonary angioscopy according to this protocol in over 100 patients; some of the findings were reported previously.[24, 30, 35] In the course of these studies, we have found that chronic pulmonary emboli have endoscopic features that allow them to be distinguished from other causes of pulmonary artery obstruction. The normal pulmonary artery has a round or oval contour with a smooth, pale, glistening appearance to the intima and bright red blood filling the lumen (Fig. 15–4). The features of organized chronic emboli correspond to their anatomic sequelae, and consist of roughening and irregular contour of the vessel lumen (Fig. 15–5) due to partial recanalization,

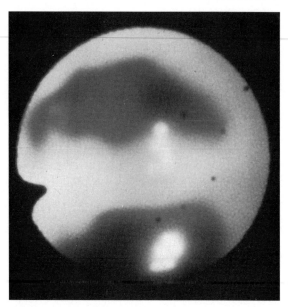

Figure 15–5. Roughening and irregularity of the contour of the pulmonary artery, believed to be secondary to partial recanalization, as visualized by the angioscope positioned just proximal to a bifurcation. (See also color section.)

pitting of the intimal surface (Fig. 15–6) due to intimal fibrosis, bands and webs through the lumen (Fig. 15–7) due to remnants of organized thrombi,[36] and pitted masses of chronic embolic material incorporated into the vessel wall (Fig. 15–8). (For Figs 15–4 through 15–8, see also the color section).

These findings are distinguishable from

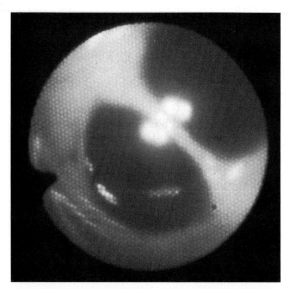

Figure 15–4. A normal pulmonary artery bifurcation as viewed through an angioscope; note the smooth, pale, glistening appearance of the intima; bright red blood fills the lumen. (See also color section.)

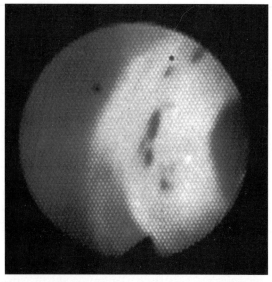

Figure 15–6. Pitting of the internal vessel surface, believed to be due to intimal fibrosis and organization of laminated clot. Blood in the lumen has been displaced by the inflated balloon at the tip of the angioscope. (See also color section.)

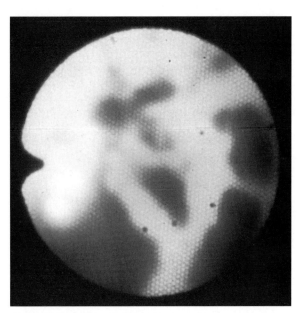

Figure 15–7. Bands and webs, remnants of an organized thromboembolic clot, as visualized through the angioscope. (See also color section.)

other causes of pulmonary artery obstruction and other wall abnormalities.[24, 30, 35] Using angioscopy, we have detected acute pulmonary emboli, extrinsic compression of a pulmonary artery, atherosclerotic plaques associated nonspecifically with pulmonary hypertension, and a fibrosarcoma of the pulmonary artery.

These results have been obtained without significant complications. Patients experience arrhythmias compatible with those that occur with right-sided heart catheterization, usually during passage through the right ventricle. Examination of the pulmonary arteries seldom causes hemodynamic consequence. One patient who had complete obstruction of the left pulmonary artery and narrowing of the right pulmonary vessel experienced transient hypotension when the angioscope was positioned in the nonoccluded pulmonary artery with the balloon inflated. This case illustrates the importance of avoiding occlusion of the main pulmonary arteries by using the tip deflection technique to view these central vessels.

In some cases, the results of angioscopy have had an impact on the suspected diagnosis. These changes included finding chronic emboli in cases of suspected agenesis and finding extrinsic vessel compression, tumor, and large protruding atherosclerotic plaque in cases of suspected chronic emboli. Just as significantly, angioscopy enables us to determine operability of patients with chronic pulmonary emboli in approximately 75% of cases, when the decision

could not be made with certainty based on the pulmonary angiogram.

To date, it appears that angioscopy is particularly useful in cases in which the diagnosis or the proximal extent of the chronic embolic process is not certain based on conventional tests or in cases in which the history or physical findings are not consistent with the angiographic findings. Conversely, angioscopy may not be necessary when the history and angiogram are consistent with the diagnosis of chronic thromboembolic obstruction and the proximal extent of the process is certain.

FUTURE CONSIDERATIONS

Although the results of our clinical experience have indicated a significant diagnostic role for pulmonary angioscopy, some equipment problems remain to be resolved. These include the diameter, flexibility, and sturdiness of the angioscope, as well as the method of balloon attachment.

The current instrument diameter of 3.0 mm is suitable for insertion through a catheter cannulating an internal jugular vein. However, a smaller diameter would further reduce the size of the vascular access sheath and facilitate passage to the pulmonary vessels. Because the size of the pulmonary arteries being examined is adequate to allow a decision about operability in the setting of chronic thromboembolic disease, a smaller diameter angioscope is not

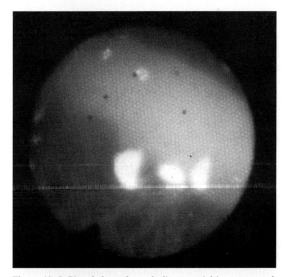

Figure 15–8. Pitted thromboembolic material incorporated into the vessel wall. White spots in the image represent reflected light off the inflated balloon at the tip of the angioscope. The small black dots are due to broken optical fibers that do not transmit light. (See also color section.)

needed for this reason. The limitation to a smaller diameter is the tip deflection mechanism rather than fiber bundle technology. In conventional medical endoscopes, the mechanism for tip deflection is so bulky that it prevents very small diameters from being achieved. An alternative tip deflection mechanism is needed if a smaller angioscope were to be constructed.

One possibility for a smaller angioscope is a catheter-based angioscope with a simpler deflection mechanism. Although a guide wire can be used in catheter-based angioscopes for placement of the device at present, this technique provides only for static placement of the angioscope without allowing for dynamic guidance or tip deflection to increase the field of view or examine the larger central arteries. Guiding balloon catheters have similar limitations.[21, 25]

A catheter-based system would also deal with other problems. Because of the fragility of glass fiber bundles, they need to be stiffened somewhat to limit breakage. This stiffness can create problems in passing the angioscope through a dilated right ventricle. Because tip deflection is practical in one plane at present, a catheter-based instrument could, if constructed correctly, provide the needed sturdiness to allow torquing the angioscope from the periphery in percutaneous procedures.

An additional advantage of a catheter-based instrument relates to balloon attachment. Although the current wrapping procedure is workable, it is not a commercially applicable technique. A bonded balloon would be feasible, but balloons have a limited life span and could not reasonably be attached to an expensive fiberoptic endoscope. A balloon could, however, be bonded to a disposable catheter with inexpensive fiberoptics incorporated in the bundle. The optics and proximal handle would be reusable. At present, disposable fiberoptic bundles exist but without distal viewing balloons or tip deflection mechanisms. Alternatively, other mechanisms for disposable balloon attachment such as a screw-on system to a conventional endoscope are possible, but they are more complex and would entail an increase in the instrument's diameter. These alternatives are being explored.

Future directions in the balloon visualization technique involve exploration of other applications. Its role in the diagnosis of acute pulmonary emboli in relation to lung perfusion scans and angiograms remains to be defined. Its usefulness in other pulmonary disorders requires further clarification prior to more widespread use.[21] It would also be an appropriate

technique for visualization of cardiac structures. Using Carlens' rigid angioscope,[17, 18] it was possible to detect atrial and ventricular septal defects and anomalous pulmonary venous return. Angioscopy would similarly appear to be a reasonable technique for visualization of valves.[20] Possible applications would include preoperative assessment of damaged porcine valves, detection of papillary muscle rupture, and assessment of valvulopathy. In the course of pulmonary angioscopy,[23, 24, 30, 35] we have found that valves, papillary muscle, coronary sinus, and the foramen ovale can be visualized. In all of these cases, the results of angioscopy will need to be compared with conventional techniques to establish its true role.

Another exciting possible future application is the combination of direct optical visualization with ultrasound imaging. Ultrasound imaging has become possible with catheter-based instrumentation.[37, 38] Because ultrasound is sensitive to depth but not to surface detail, the combination of optical visualization with the information of ultrasound imaging may prove useful in selected applications. Ultrasound technology incorporated into a good guidance system with distal tip deflection have the potential to greatly expand the information obtained from a single catheterization. Other possible applications include directed myocardial biopsy, laser use (already in intraoperative use in some vascular beds), and manipulation of surgical instruments from a percutaneous insertion site. The current proliferation of new technology may well make some of these applications possible in the near future.

REFERENCES

1. Cutler EC, Levine SA, Beck CS: The surgical treatment of mitral stenosis. Arch Surg 1924; 9:689–819.
2. Allen DS, Graham EA: Intracardiac surgery: A new method. JAMA 1922; 79:1028–1030.
3. Harken DE, Glidden EM: Experiments in intracardiac surgery. J Thorac Surg 1943; 12:566–572.
4. Brock RC: Pulmonary valvulotomy for the relief of congenital pulmonary stenosis. Br Med J 1948; 1:1121–1126.
5. Bailey CP, Glover RP, O'Neill TJE, Ramirez HPR: Experiences with the experimental surgical relief of aortic stenosis. J Thorac Surg 1950; 20:516–541.
6. Murray G: A cardioscope. Angiology 1950; 1:334–336.
7. Butterworth RF: A new operating cardioscope. J Thorac Surg 1951; 22:319–322.
8. Boulton HE, Bailey CP, Costas-Durieux J, Gemeinhardt W: Cardioscopy: Simple and practical. J Thorac Surg 1954; 27:323–329.
9. Sakakibara S, Iikawa T, Hattori J, Inomata K: Direct visual operation for aortic stenosis: Cardioscope studies. J Int Coll Surg 1958; 29:548–562.
10. Sherman CT, Litvak F, Grundfest W, et al: Coronary

angioscopy in patients with unstable angina pectoris. N Engl J Med 1986; 315:913–919.

11. Vollmar JF, Loeprecht H, Hutschenreiter S: Advances in vascular endoscopy. Thorac Cardiovasc Surgeon 1987; 35:334–341.

12. Van Stiegmann GV, Pearce WH, Bartle EJ, Rutherford RB: Flexible angioscopy seems faster and more specific than arteriography. Arch Surg 1987; 122:279–282.

13. McCowan TC, Ferris EJ: Percutaneous angioscopy for the radiologist. *In* White GH, White RA (eds.): Angioscopy: Vascular and Coronary Applications. Chicago, Year Book, 1989, pp 189–202.

14. Spears RJ, Marais HJ, Serur J, et al: In vivo coronary angioscopy. J Am Coll Cardiol 1983; 1:1311–1314.

15. Morshuis WJ, Jansen EW, Vincent JG, et al: Intraoperative fiberoptic angioscopy to evaluate the completeness of pulmonary embolectomy. J Cardiovasc Surg 1989; 30:630–634.

16. Dee P, Crosby I: Fiberoptic studies of the aortic valve in dogs. Br Heart J 1979; 39:459–461.

17. Carlens E, Silander T: Method for direct inspection of the right atrium: Experimental investigation in the dog. Surgery 1961; 49:622–624.

18. Carlens E, Silander T: Cardioscopy. J Cardiovasc Surg 1963; 4:512–515.

19. Tanabe T, Yokota A, Sugie S: Cardiovascular fiberoptic endoscopy: Development and clinical application. Surgery 1980; 87:375–379.

20. Gamble WJ, Innis RE: Experimental intracardiac visualization. N Engl J Med 1967; 277:1397–1403.

21. Kubo S, Fujita K, Nakatomi M: Angioscopic findings of the peripheral pulmonary arteries in patients with chronic pulmonary diseases. Nippon Kyobu Shikkan Gakkai Zasshi 1992; 30:2018–2022.

22. Lacombe P, Foster DW, Laborde F, et al: A new technique of pulmonary arterial angioscopy: Capnoangioscopy. An experimental study. Presse Med 1990; 19:1899–1901.

23. Moser KM, Shure D, Harrell JH II, Tulumello J: Angioscopic visualization of pulmonary emboli. Chest 1980; 77:198–201.

24. Shure D, Gregoratos G, Moser KM: Fiberoptic angioscopy: Role in the diagnosis of chronic pulmonary arterial obstruction. Ann Intern Med 1985; 103:844–850.

25. Uchida Y, Tomaru T, Kato S: Percutaneous pulmonary angioscopy using a guiding balloon catheter. Clin Cardiol 1988; 11:143–148.

26. Moser KM, Auger WR, Fedullo PE: Chronic major-vessel thromboembolic pulmonary hypertension. Circulation 1990; 81:1735–1743.

27. Jamieson SW, Auger WR, Fedullo PF, et al: Experience and results with 150 pulmonary thromboendarterectomy operations over a 29 month period. J Thorac Cardiovasc Surg 1993; 106.116–127.

28. Liebow AA, Hales MR, Bloomer WE, et al: Studies on the lung after ligation of the pulmonary artery. II. Anatomical changes. Am J Pathol 1950; 26:177–195.

29. Shure D, Moser KM, Peterson KL, Gregoratos G: Fiberoptic pulmonary angioscopy: A comparison of two prototype angioscopes. SPIE 1985; 576:32–34.

30. Shure D, Buchbinder M, Peterson KL: Pulmonary vascular angioscopy—current results. SPIE 1988; 906:82–86.

31. Shure D, Moser KM, Harrell JH II, Hartman MT: Identification of pulmonary emboli in the dog: Comparison of angioscopy and perfusion scanning. Circulation 1981; 64:618–621.

32. Shure D, Moser KM, Konopka RG: Hemodynamics and gas exchange during angioscopy in the dog. Angiology 1984; 35:97–103.

33. Swan HJC, Ganz W, Forrester J: Catheterization of the heart in man with use of a flowdirected balloon-tipped catheter. N Engl J Med 1970; 283:447.

34. Nicod P, Peterson K, Levine M, et al: Pulmonary angiography in severe chronic pulmonary hypertension. Ann Intern Med 1987; 107:565–568.

35. Shure D: Pulmonary Angioscopy. *In* White GH, White RA (eds): Angioscopy: Vascular and Coronary Applications. Chicago, Year Book, 1989, pp 177–188.

36. Peterson KL, Fred HL, Alexander JK: Pulmonary arterial webs: A new angiographic sign of previous thromboembolism. N Engl J Med 1967; 277:33–35.

37. Ricou F, Nicod PH, Moser KM, Peterson KL: Catheter-based intravascular ultrasound imaging of chronic thromboembolic pulmonary disease. Am J Cardiol 1991; 67:749–752.

38. Tapson VF, Davidson CJ, Gurbel PA, et al: Rapid and accurate diagnosis of pulmonary emboli in a canine model using intravascular ultrasound imaging. Chest 1991; 100:1410–1413.

Chapter 16

Myocardial Biopsy
Techniques, Indications, and Complications

HOWARD C. DITTRICH
RALPH SHABETAI

INDICATIONS

A number of developments are occurring in the field of cardiology that may, in the relatively near future, alter indications for endomyocardial biopsy in the diagnosis of myocarditis and its response to immunosuppressive therapy.[1] Current practice requires serial endomyocardial biopsies after cardiac transplantation and when following some patients who require large doses of anthrocycline antibiotics. However, investigations seeking less invasive and more economical means of following these patients are being actively pursued. Efforts to apply morphometry and other quantitative techniques to biopsy samples of the endomyocardium to provide prognostic information have not been uniformally successful but are still being developed. Finally, endomyocardial biopsy may well assume a more prominent role when the techniques of immunology and molecular biology, including in situ hybridization of viral nucleic acids and amplification, are more widely applied to the biopsy specimens.[2]

At the present time, there are five major and several as yet unestablished indications for endomyocardial biopsy (Table 16–1).

Myocarditis

It is often difficult or impossible to distinguish between acute viral myocarditis and the onset of idiopathic dilated cardiomyopathy by standard clinical and laboratory means. The presence of inflammatory cells, almost always lymphocytes, on endomyocardial biopsy material with associated myocardial cell necrosis is the accepted standard for the diagnosis of myocarditis. These findings are present in about 5% to 10% of patients undergoing endomyocardial biopsy within 3 months of the onset of unexplained heart failure,[3] but previous studies had reported a considerably greater frequency. Much of the disparity between these reports is related to the histologic criteria employed in making the diagnosis of myocarditis. Another potentially important reason for the wide variation in the reported frequency of myocarditis is the periodicity of enteroviral infections such as coxsackievirus B, a known cardiotrophic agent. Endomyocardial biopsy is performed primarily to distinguish between myocarditis and early dilated cardiomyopathy, and to assess the response to immunosuppressive treatment. Unfortunately, the therapeutically relevant diagnostic information obtained in this setting is low. The major goal of the myocarditis treatment trial sponsored by the National Heart-Lung and Blood Institute was to study the efficacy of immunosuppressive therapy in myocarditis. This trial has been completed and failed to prove the superiority of immunosuppressive treatment. However, the number of randomized patients was disappointingly small.

Differentiating Restrictive Cardiomyopathy from Constrictive Pericarditis

In many cases, it is relatively simple to tell the difference between constrictive pericarditis and restrictive cardiomyopathy; indeed the distinction can often be made on clinical and routine laboratory investigation. However, in other cases, the differential diagnosis can remain in doubt even after detailed imaging studies and cardiac catheterization. Typically, the history provides no definitive clues, the electrocardiogram shows only nonspecific changes, and chest radiography does not demonstrate calcification of the pericardium. In these cases, imaging stud-

Table 16–1. **Applications of Endomyocardial Biopsy**

Current Application
 Myocarditis—diagnosis and follow-up
 Differentiating constrictive pericarditis from restrictive
  cardiomyopathy
 Detection of systemic myocardial disorders
 Monitoring cardiac transplant rejection
 Monitoring anthracycline cardiotoxicity
Potential Application
 Diagnosis of myocardial inflammatory process in
  patients with life-threatening ventricular arrhythmias
 In situ hybridization of viral nucleic acid particles for
  definition of pathogenic cause of myocarditis

---

ies are often normal or equivocal, and cardiac catheterization shows only moderate pulmonary hypertension, normal systolic function of the left ventricle, and diastolic pressures of the two ventricles that are elevated and equal to each other. Although computed tomography and nuclear magnetic resonance have improved our ability to detect an abnormally thick pericardium, the diagnosis may still be elusive because pericardial thickness may be normal in some cases of constrictive pericarditis, especially that caused by visceral constriction. Likewise, echocardiography-Doppler findings said to be useful in making the differential diagnosis need to be tested in larger numbers of patients. Therefore, in a significant proportion of cases, endomyocardial biopsy is of great value. Before the introduction of endomyocardial biopsy, cases of this kind could be diagnosed only by exploratory thoracotomy or median sternotomy. Now, if endomyocardial biopsy shows extensive fibrosis, radiation injury, or another pathologic process, the patient can be spared exploratory operation, because the incidence of falsely excluding constrictive pericarditis is low.[4] In other words, if the endomyocardial biopsy does not reveal myocardial pathology, the diagnosis of constrictive pericarditis is very likely. Endomyocardial biopsy thus has significantly reduced the indications for exploratory operation to establish the cause of restrictive physiology.

Systemic Myocardial Disorders

Endomyocardial biopsy is performed when a diagnosis such as amyloidosis, hemochromatosis, sarcoidosis, radiation injury, abnormal storage disease, or idiopathic fibrosis is considered a reasonable possibility. Clearly, the diagnostic yield is greater in a process such as amyloidosis, which is diffuse, than in a focal process such as sarcoidosis.

 In most cardiac catheterization laboratories, detection of systemic myocardial disorders ranks low among the indications for endomyocardial biopsy, but in highly specialized centers to which large numbers of highly selected cases are referred, the yield is considerably higher.[5, 6]

 Endomyocardial biopsy for the diagnosis of systemic myocardial disorders is indicated for the circumstance in which reasonable clinical grounds for this cardiac diagnosis exist but proof that other organs are affected cannot be obtained. Endomyocardial biopsy for this indication is also sometimes carried out when proof of the systemic disorder affecting other organs already exists, together with suspicious signs of cardiac involvement, such as that found on echocardiography. In these instances, the procedure is often performed more to confirm a diagnosis than to make it, and therefore, it need not always be carried out.

Evaluation of Cardiac Transplant Recipients

In the early stages after successful cardiac transplantation, members of the cardiac transplantation team perform endomyocardial biopsy frequently to detect subclinical rejection and to assess the immunosuppressive regimen. Thereafter, endomyocardial biopsy is performed routinely and additionally whenever there is evidence suggestive of allograft rejection. Endomyocardial biopsies performed later in the postoperative course are sometimes performed by the cardiac transplantation team, but more often, they are performed by physicians and in laboratories not associated with the cardiac transplantation team. Because of the increasing frequency of combined heart-lung transplantation, it is important to recognize that endomyocardial biopsy cannot be relied on to predict pulmonary rejection.[7] An excellent review of endomyocardiac biopsy is that by Billingham.[8]

Anthracycline Cardiotoxicity

Irreversible cardiotoxicity may appear well before clinical heart failure in patients who have received more than 240 mg/M^2 of doxorubicin.[9] Therefore, when the oncologist wishes to push anthracycline dosage to the limit, the cardiologist may be asked to perform endomyocardial biopsy in the absence of heart failure or even evidence of ventricular dysfunction. Biopsy may be performed before starting treatment, or more commonly, when the conventional upper limit of dosage has been reached. Further dosing can then be guided by the biopsy findings.

Potential Applications

Endomyocardial biopsy has been performed in patients with life-threatening ventricular arrhythmias, but the results are still debatable. It has been claimed that histologic findings of myocarditis, endocardial fibrosis, or interstitial fibrosis are seen in the majority of patients with ventricular arrhythmias in whom cardiac anatomy and function are otherwise normal.[10, 11] No data are available, however, to suggest that treatment other than conventional antiarrhythmic therapy benefits these patients. The value of biopsy in this group of patients remains to be established, and we do not routinely advocate it when the only indication is arrhythmia.

An important percentage of patients with acquired immunodeficiency syndrome (AIDS) develop congestive heart failure, and in a small minority of these patients, cardiac failure is the presumed cause of death. Myocarditis has been identified in more than 50% of patients at postmortem examination, but the importance of this finding is not clear. Less often, myocarditis has been documented by endomyocardial bi-

opsy. Culture of tissue obtained by endomyocardial biopsy in patients with the human immunodeficiency virus (HIV) has yielded the virus in two AIDS patients with heart failure.[12, 13] At present, no evidence exists to support HIV as the direct cause of heart failure in the majority of patients with AIDS. In the future, increased use of in situ hybridization and polymerase chain reaction (PCR) of viral nucleic acid particles and new culture techniques should allow more accurate characterization of pathogenic causes of myocarditis.

TECHNIQUES

The most commonly practiced technique for endomyocardial biopsy is based on work begun at Stanford University in the early 1970s, where a highly satisfactory bioptome,[14] which replaced the original design of Sakakihara and Konno,[15] was developed (Fig. 16–1). By the year 1978, the Stanford group was able to report over 1300 procedures[16] without a fatality and in which the most serious complications was cardiac tampon-

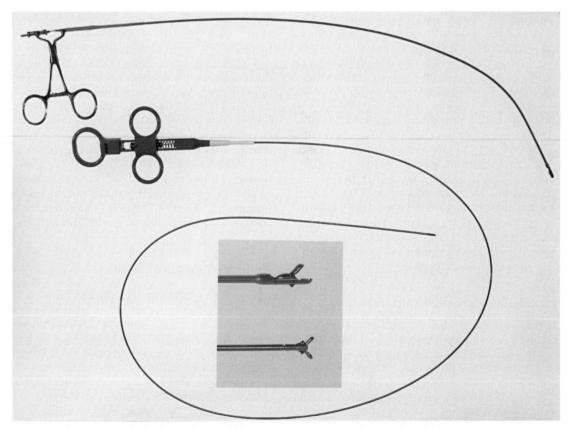

Figure 16–1. Shown on top is the shorter Stanford bioptome for right ventricular sampling via the internal jugular route. The longer, disposable Cordis bioptome, which is used for left ventricular biopsies, is also shown. The inset shows a close-up view of these two bioptomes. Note the larger Stanford bioptome jaws.

ade, which occurred in four patients, and the total complication rate was less than 1%. Fowles and Mason reviewed their own experience and those of others 6 years later.[17]

Before these developments, which made endomyocardial biopsy a safe and easy technique, more hazardous approaches such as sampling the myocardium with a Vim-Silverman needle through a thoracotomy[18] or percutaneously[19] had been tried, but not surprisingly, these techniques gained minimal acceptance.

Right Ventricular Biopsy— Stanford Technique

The Stanford (Caves) bioptome (see Fig. 16–1) is generally introduced percutaneously via the right internal jugular vein. The instrument is only 50 cm long, a feature that optimizes torque control and the operator's ability to know precisely the location of the cutting jaws. Although the instrument is sufficiently flexible to permit easy manipulation within the right-sided heart structures, the spatial orientation of the handle is uniformally the same as that of the cutting jaws. The jaws are large enough to routinely obtain samples 1 to 3 mm in diameter. One jaw is fixed, and the other can be opened and closed by the hemostat handle at the proximal end.

The anterior approach to the internal jugular vein is most commonly used. The two heads of the sternocleidomastoid muscle are identified. If necessary, the patient should be asked to raise the head to assist in this procedure. There should be no pillow under the head unless the patient is orthopneic and the venous pressure is elevated. The patient's head is turned to the left. The apex of a triangle formed at its base by the clavicle and 3 cm superiorly by its apex at the convergence of the two heads of the sternomastoid is identified. Local anesthesia and a skin puncture are performed at this site.

Infiltration with local anesthesia should be limited to the superficial tissues to avoid accumulation of fluid in the carotid sheath that envelops the internal jugular vein. The location of the vein should be explored with a small needle, such as one about 1 1/2 inches long and 21 gauge; longer needles are not necessary and may cause complications. The needle is directed inferiorly and tilted 30 to 45 degrees posteriorly and 10 to 20 degrees laterally. When blood can be easily sampled, a small incision is made and dilated, after which the exploring needle is replaced with an 18-gauge thin-walled needle, and then a #9 sheath equipped with a

diaphragm is introduced in a standard fashion into the vein. In order to avoid producing an air embolism, patients in whom venous pressure is not elevated should be asked to suspend respiration in the expiratory phase whenever the bioptome or catheters are being introduced or withdrawn via the sheath.

Standard right-sided heart catheterization is then carried out and particular note made of the magnitude and characteristics of the right atrial pressure pulse and of the fluoroscopic appearance of cardiac pulsations. Systemic heparinization is not employed at this stage. Thereafter, the bioptome is introduced through the sheath and advanced to the lower third of the atrium, with its tip directed laterally and the jaws remaining closed. Thereafter, the tip is rotated clockwise and the catheter is gently slid through the tricuspid valve. Gentle probing with the closed tip against the wall should induce ventricular extrasystoles, confirming that the bioptome is in the right ventricle, not in the coronary sinus (Fig. 16–2A). Correct placement can be confirmed by viewing the bioptome in the left anterior oblique projection (see Fig. 16–2B), which should demonstrate the tip directed posteriorly in the anterior ventricle. In some laboratories, two-dimensional echocardiography is also used to ascertain the position of the bioptome and identify any possible complications, most notably septal perforation.[20]

Once the operator is confident that the closed tip of the bioptome is in contact with the ventricular septum, the bioptome is withdrawn about 1 cm and the jaws are opened. The bioptome is readvanced to the ventricular septum and pressed against it moderately firmly. The jaws are then closed using two clicks of the hemostat handle. After a brief pause, the instrument is sharply but not forcefully withdrawn, a maneuver that usually engenders a premature ventricular depolarization in a successful biopsy. If the bioptome requires a strong tug to disengage from the septum, the jaws must be opened and the instrument gently backed away, because this sensation may indicate that a chorda tendinea or pericardium may be enclosed between the bioptome jaws. The jaws of the bioptome must remain closed until the instrument is withdrawn from the sheath. In patients being biopsied several years after cardiac transplantation, it may be necessary to biopsy sites in the right ventricle other than the septum to obtain readable samples.

After removing the sample from the jaws of the instrument, making sure that no fibrin, clot, or other tissue remains on the instrument, the procedure is repeated until sufficient biopsies

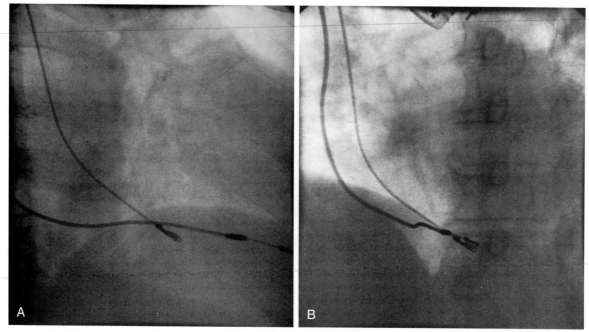

Figure 16–2. A, Cineangiographic frame in the right anterior oblique position obtained during right ventricular endomyo-cardial biopsy. A pacemaker lead is seen with its tip at the apex of the right ventricle. The tip of the bioptome has crossed the spine and is below the diaphragm against the interventricular septum, where the biopsy was taken. *B,* Left anterior oblique view of the bioptome position seen in *A.* Note that the bioptome is directed posteriorly but is in an anterior car-diac chamber (the right ventricle).

(usually four to seven) have been obtained. If the biopsy is to be followed by left-sided heart catheterization and coronary arteriography, heparin is given once it has been ascertained that the biopsy has been accomplished without cardiac perforation.

Transfer of Biopsy Material from the Bioptome to Specimen Containers

Under a good light, the operator fixes the tip of the bioptome with the jaws open so that the specimen can be removed without disrupting the tissue. It is essential not to use forceps or any other crushing instrument. A pair of small-gauge needles or a stream of saline can be used to remove the sample, or a part of it, from the hinge between the jaws. The development of contraction bands may be minimized if the tis-sue is allowed to relax in air, perhaps covered by a drop of saline, before being inserted into fixative.

Alternative Approaches

The posterior access to the internal jugular vein is less commonly employed for endomyocardial biopsy but may be adopted when the anterior

approach is relatively contraindicated, such as because of hematoma or infection from a re-cent cannulation of the internal jugular vein. The posterior route may also be preferred by physicians who have more experience with this approach.

Long Sheath Techniques

In some patients, it is not possible to carry out endomyocardial biopsy from the right internal jugular vein, and in others, it may be desired to biopsy the left ventricle. The left and right ventricles can be biopsied via the femoral artery and vein, respectively, but longer, more flexible bioptomes are then required. The left ventricle may also be biopsied via the transseptal route.[21] To facilitate maneuvering these bioptomes from the groin, a standard pigtail catheter inside a radiopaque sheath is introduced into the de-sired ventricle using standard Seldinger tech-nique.[21, 22] The sheath is long enough to reach the ventricle but shorter than the bioptome. When the pigtail catheter is properly positioned in the ventricle, the sheath is advanced through the tricuspid or aortic valve and the pigtail cath-eter is withdrawn.

Once the long sheath has been positioned satisfactorily in the ventricle, a bioptome can be passed down the sheath. Before doing so, the operator should ensure that blood flows back freely to be certain that the tip is free and that the sheath is not kinked. In general, flushing should not be undertaken because this maneuver may cause air embolism. Monitoring aortic or left ventricular pressure through a side port is possible but likely to give unsatisfactory damped waveforms.

A number of different bioptomes are suitable for introduction by the long sheath technique. Most commonly in the United States, either the longer, thinner version of the Stanford instrument or the Cordis modification of the King's bioptome is used (Fig. 16–3A and B). The latter has two movable jaws, which unless actively closed by the operator, naturally remain in the open position. After securing the biopsy,

the operator actively keeps the jaws in the closed position until the bioptome has been withdrawn. Until recently, this bioptome used to have the disadvantage of having smaller jaws; however, it also has the advantage that it is disposable, eliminating the careful maintenance procedures necessary for the Stanford instrument. At present, the Cordis bioptome has larger jaws (volume 5.3 mm³).

Operators who have little recent experience with cannulation from the neck but with plentiful experience cannulating the femoral vein may achieve better results and encounter fewer complications when they perform transfemoral venous endomyocardial biopsy.[23]

A bioptome equipped with a tip-deflecting device to facilitate passage from the femoral artery is available,[24] but we have not experi-

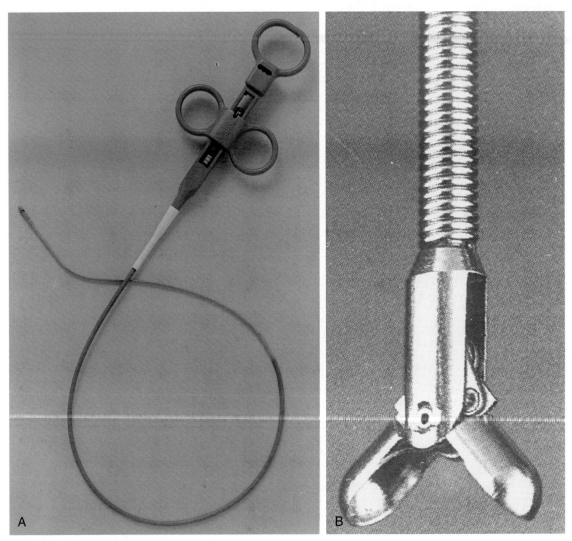

A   B

Figure 16–3. Disposable Cordis bioptome. *A,* The complete instrument, including the mechanism for closing the jaws, which is magnified in *B.*

enced enough difficulty when using the standard technique to feel the need for its use.

COMPLICATIONS AND RISKS

In the Stanford series of over 4000 cases, tamponade occurred in only 0.14% of patients, none of which required thoracotomy. Transient arrhythmia, atrial ventricular conduction block, or transient nerve palsies (recurrent laryngeal and phrenic) may be induced. A small risk of pneumothorax or air embolism is associated with jugular venous puncture. Previously, a 5.4% incidence of angiographically documented coronary artery to right ventricular fistula was reported in 74 heart transplant recipients at the time of annual coronary angiography,[25] and we have encountered one such case. The patient developed a continuous murmur and a 1 to 1.3 left-to-right shunt, which we elected not to treat. None of the fistulae were judged to be hemodynamically significant. A questionnaire listing complications worldwide from 6739 cases found an overall complication rate of 1.17%, including 28 perforations of the right side of the heart (0.42%) and two deaths (0.03%).[17] In a series of 2454 endomyocardial biopsies performed in 133 cardiac transplant recipients, 74 (30%) complications occurred, but most were associated with venous cannulation, not the biopsy itself.[25] Thus, in practiced hands, the procedure appears to be remarkably safe regardless of the technique employed.

REFERENCES

1. Mason JW, O'Connell JB: Clinical merit of endomyocardial biopsy. Circulation 1989; 79:971–979.
2. Kandolf R, Ameis D, Kirschner P, et al: In situ detection of enteroviral genomes in myocardial cells by nucleic acid hybridization: An approach to the diagnosis of viral heart disease. Proc Natl Acad Sci 1987; 84:6272–6276.
3. Chow L, Dittrich H, Shabetai R: Endomyocardial biopsy in patients with unexplained congestive heart failure. Ann Intern Med 1988; 109:535–539.
4. Schoenfeld MH, Supple EW, Dec WG, Fallon JT: Restrictive cardiomyopathy versus constrictive pericarditis: Role of endomyocardial biopsy in avoiding unnecessary thoracotomy. Circulation 1987; 75:1012–1017.
5. Nippoldt TB, Edwards WD, Holmes DR, et al: Right ventricular endomyocardial biopsy. Clinic Pathologic Correlates in 100 consecutive patients. Mayo Clin Proc 1982; 57:407–418.
6. Parillo JE, Aretz HT, Palacio I, et al: The results of endomyocardial biopsy can frequently be used to diagnose myocardial disease in patients with idiopathic heart failure. Circulation 1984; 69:93–101.
7. Clanville AR, Imoto E, Baldwin JC, et al: The role of right ventricular endomyocardial biopsy in the long-term management of heart-lung transplant recipients. J Heart Transplant 1987; 6:375–381.
8. Billingham M: Endomyocardial biopsy diagnosis of acute ejection in cardiac allografts. Prog Cardiovasc Dis 1990; 33:11–18.
9. Bristow MR, Mason JW, Billingham ME, Daniels JR: Doxorubicin cardiomyopathy, endomyocardial biopsy and cardiac catheterization. Ann Intern Med 1971; 88:168–175.
10. Sugrue DD, Holmes DR Jr, Gersh BJ, et al: Cardiac histologic findings in patients with life-threatening arrhythmias of unknown origin. J Am Coll Cardiol 1984; 4:952–957.
11. Strain JE, Grose RM, Factor SM, Fisher JD: Results of endomyocardial biopsy in patients with spontaneous ventricular tachycardia but without apparent structural heart disease. Circulation 1983; 68:1171–1181.
12. Calbrese LH, Proffitt MR, Yen-Lieberman B, et al: Congestive cardiomyopathy and illness related to the acquired immunodeficiency syndrome (AIDS) associated with isolation of retrovirus from myocardium. Ann Intern Med 1987; 107:691–692.
13. Dittrich H, Chow L, Denaro F, Spector S: Human immunodeficiency virus, coxsackievirus, and cardiomyopathy. Ann Intern Med 1988; 108:308–309.
14. Caves PK, Scholz WP, Dong E Jr, et al: New instrument for transvenous cardiac biopsy. Am J Cardiol 1974; 33:264.
15. Sakakibara S, Kono S: Endomyocardial biopsy. Jpn Heart J 1962; 3:537–543.
16. Mason JW: Techniques for right and left ventricular endomyocardial biopsy. Am J Cardiol 1978; 41:887–892.
17. Fowles RE, Mason JW: Role of cardiac biopsy in the diagnosis and management of cardiac disease. Prog Cardiovasc Dis 1984; 27:153–179.
18. Sutton DC, Sutton GC: Needle biopsy of human ventricular myocardium. Am Heart J 1960; 60:364–370.
19. Bullock RT, Murphy ML, Pearce MB: Intracardiac needle biopsy of the ventricular septum. Am J Cardiol 1965; 16:227–233.
20. Strachovsky G, Xeldis SM, Katz S, McNulty-Mackey M: Two dimensional echocardiographic monitoring during percutaneous endomyocardial biopsy. J Am Coll Cardiol 1985; 6:609–611.
21. Brooksby IAB, Jenkins BS, Davies MJ, et al: Left ventricular endomyocardial biopsy: Description and evaluation of the technique. Cathet Cardiovasc Diag 1977; 3:115–121.
22. Brooksby IAB, Swanton RH, Jenkins BS, Webb-Peploe MM: Long sheath technique for introduction of catheter tip manometer or endomyocardial bioptome into left or right heart. Br Heart J 1974; 36:908–912
23. Anderson JL, Marshall HW, Allison SR: The femoral venous approach to endomyocardial biopsy: Comparison with internal jugular and transarterial approaches. Am J Cardiol 1984; 53:833–837.
24. Kawai C, Kitaura Y: New endomyocardial biopsy catheter for the left ventricle. Am J Cardiol 1977; 40:63–65.
25. Henzlova MJ, Nath H, Bucy RP, et al: Coronary artery to right ventricle fistula in heart transplant recipients: A complication of endomyocardial biopsy. J Am Coll Cardiol 1989; 14:258–261.

Chapter 17

Myocardial Biopsy
Preparation and Interpretation

COLIN M. BLOOR
PARVIZ HAGHIGHI

ENDOMYOCARDIAL BIOPSY

General Features

Endomyocardial biopsies, often performed as independent diagnostic procedures during cardiac catheterization, evaluate the status of cardiac transplant patients or diagnose other patients with various cardiac diseases.[1, 2] Most biopsy studies focus on the light and electron microscopic features of the tissue; biochemical features of the tissue also may hold important clues to the diagnosis and therapy of certain diseases, such as dilated cardiomyopathy.[3] Thus, the future for endomyocardial biopsy looks promising.

Endomyocardial biopsies are very safe procedures. The reported incidence of complications is less than 1.5%.[4, 5] Thus far, deaths are not directly attributable to the biopsy procedure. These statistics show that endomyocardial biopsy is safer than renal or liver biopsies.[2]

This chapter is based on our experience at a University Medical Center and a Veterans Administration Hospital for the past decade. Most patients undergoing endomyocardial biopsy in these institutions had the clinical diagnosis of cardiomyopathy or myocarditis. The complications we observed were similar to those reported by others and included perforation of the right ventricular free wall, occasional arrhythmias, and infection.[1, 2] Similar complications occur in transplant patients; also, coronary artery–right ventricular fistula has been reported.[6, 7]

Tissue Procurement and Processing

The biopsy specimens obtained with the bioptome should be gently removed with a small needle. The use of forceps may cause a crush injury, which makes the tissue uninterpretable. The endomyocardial biopsy fragments are usually about 3 mm in maximum diameter. No further cutting is necessary for light microscopy processing. The size of individual biopsy fragments depends, to some extent, on the type of bioptome used. One should obtain a minimum of three fragments, but five fragments are preferable in all cases and between five and eight fragments in cases of suspected myocarditis. For example, with the Stanford bioptome in cardiac transplant cases, a 5% false-negative rate may be expected if three fragments are obtained. This false-negative rate decreases to 2% if one obtains four fragments.[8] On withdrawing the bioptome, we pick up the endomyocardial biopsy fragments from the bioptome and immediately transfer them to fixative. If the fragments float, this usually indicates that fat rather than muscle is present in the sample. We recommend that one use 10% neutral buffered formalin at room temperature for fixation for light microscopy and 2.5% glutaraldehyde for fixation for electron microscopy. To reduce sampling error, we cut the paraffin blocks for light microscopy at a thickness of 5 μ at four levels. We use hematoxylin-eosin stain on the first and last cuts and Masson trichrome stain to show fibrosis and the necrotic fibers to better advantage, and blank sections are done on the two sections in between. The gross description of the sample received should include the number of fragments and the presence of blood clots, fat, or unusual structures, such as those related to atrioventricular valves. Each slide should contain at least five tissue ribbons.

Some pathologists include iron stain in the routine stains to screen for hemochromatosis. Normally, no iron is present in the myofibers on Prussian blue reaction. For demonstration of amyloid, various authors have recommended a variety of stains (sulfated Alcian blue, Congo red, methyl or crystal violet, thioflavine T). Amyloid material may stain variably when using one stain. We use periodic acid–Schiff (PAS) stain to bring out sarcolemmal membrane, to accentuate the vessels (it may show excess positivity in diabetics), and to show the lipochrome pigment to advantage. On glutaraldehyde fixed material for electron microscopy, the thick (0.5-µ) sections stained, such as with toluidine blue, are used as a screening step. This method detects abnormalities before formal electron micrographs are available. Some tissue may be snap frozen in liquid nitrogen or isopentane and dry ice, and deep frozen at −70°C for possible future studies, such as immunofluorescence or other procedures. Antigens apparently are retained under such circumstances for several years. One usually prepares 5 to 10 blocks for electron microscopy. For evaluation of anthracycline cardiotoxicity, however, one submits the entire tissue sample for electron microscopy and examines a minimum of 10 blocks.

Artifacts and Limitations

In our experience, the appearance of contraction bands is the most frequent artifact in endomyocardial biopsies (Fig. 17–1). Contraction bands usually are not evidence for ischemic injury. Similarly when contraction bands occur, they may pull the adjacent sarcoplasm with them, thus creating apparent cytoplasmic vacuoles. These vacuoles should not be misinterpreted as myocytolysis (see Fig. 17–1). The edges of endomyocardial biopsy fragments may

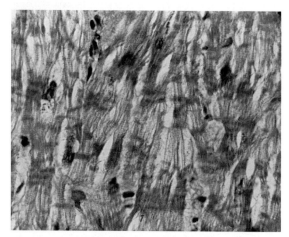

Figure 17–1. Contraction bands. These dense protein precipitates within the myocardial fibers cause the adjacent sarcoplasm to appear pale and "empty," simulating myocytolysis. Hematoxylin and eosin. ×160.

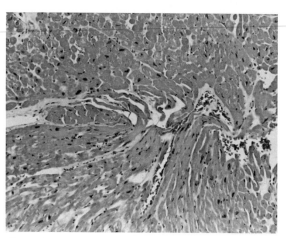

Figure 17–2. Artifact. In the center of the field is "pinching" artifact. This can cause prominent eosinophilia of the myofibers simulating necrosis. Other cytologic criteria of necrosis are absent. Hematoxylin and eosin. ×40.

be more eosinophilic than the center. These changes are not definitive evidence of myonecrosis. Trichrome stain may prove helpful in arriving at the correct diagnosis.

One should be cautious in diagnosing myofiber disarray, particularly if the biopsy does not include the deep interventricular septum, as is almost always the case. Consequently, one defers the diagnosis to the time of open biopsy taken during the correction of asymmetric septal hypertrophy. The normal trabeculae carnae of the right ventricular apex may show myofiber disarray. Crush artifacts commonly occur at the site of contact with the bioptome and may simulate necrosis (Fig. 17–2). Also, blood clots forming on the surface of myocardial fragments may cause confusion unless one finds evidence of organization in the clot (Fig. 17–3).

Endocardium may spuriously appear thickened if sections are tangentially sectioned. The myocardial interstitium normally has some mature collagen around blood vessels that may be misinterpreted as interstitial fibrosis. Excessive separation of myofiber bundles can occur without true interstitial edema. Telescoping of arterial walls may simulate vascular thrombosis or true arteriosclerosis. Interpretation of interstitial mononuclear cells can be a difficult problem (Fig. 17–4). This usually is due to either the plane of sectioning of myofibers (e.g., myofibers cut in cross-section are mistaken for lymphocytes) or the fact that normally mononuclear cells are present in the interstitium.

Myocardial Cells

Contraction bands are the most common artifacts. They resemble those seen in acute is-

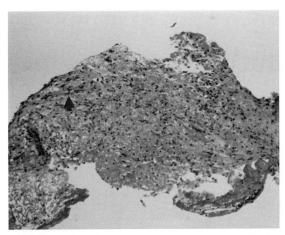

Figure 17–3. Organizing thrombus. Note the ingrowth of spindle-shaped fibroblasts *(arrowhead)* into the thrombus. Hematoxylin and eosin. ×40.

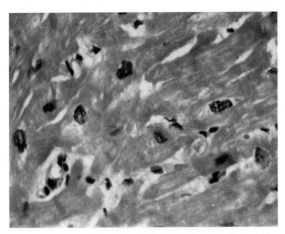

Figure 17–5. Myocardial hypertrophy. Note the enlarged, hyperchromatic nuclei of the myocardial fibers. Hematoxylin and eosin. ×160.

chemic injury, catecholamine-induced myocardial injury, and other disorders.[9] However, the biopsy procedure itself induces most contraction bands seen in the tissue.

The diameter of the myocardial cell is an index of hypertrophy and can be quantified. Occasionally in the dilated heart, the myocytes are stretched and appear normal in diameter. Thus, the appropriate criteria for hypertrophy are the presence of nuclear changes, such as enlargement, irregular shapes, and darker staining[10] (Fig. 17–5).

Myocardial Interstitium

Interstitial fibrosis may be a common finding in ischemic and hypertrophied hearts.[11, 12] The location of the collagen may be perivascular,

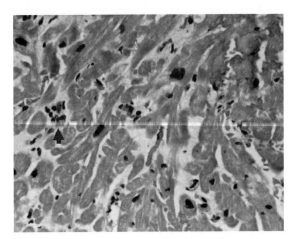

Figure 17–4. Interstitial mononuclear cells. These cell aggregates *(arrowhead)* should not be confused with myocarditis. Hematoxylin and eosin. ×100.

pericellular, or patchy.[13] When fibrosis is extensive, ischemia is usually the cause.

The identification of leukocytes in the interstitium is critical. Their presence suggests inflammatory diseases, such as myocarditis or transplant rejection. When leukocytes are at the margins of the biopsy tissue, they usually represent adherent blood elements of no significance.

Lymphocytes normally occupy the interstitium.[14–16] Data from biopsy and autopsy specimens show that the mean number of interstitial lymphocytes is less than 5 per high-power field.[17, 18] For this estimate, one should examine 10 high-power (×400) fields in the specimen. Lymphocyte counts exceeding these limits are indicative of disease, although some caution should be exercised recognizing the potential therapeutic implications of the diagnosis.[14]

Other features of concern within the interstitium are myocardial edema and small-vessel obstruction. Myocardial edema is difficult to evaluate in the biopsy specimen. Small vessels compressed by the procedure suggest that thrombotic occlusion is present. Elastic stains are very useful because they demonstrate whether artifact or a thrombotic process or intimal disease is present in the suspected vessels.

Endocardium

Normally, the endocardial thickness is greater in the left ventricle than in the right ventricle.[19] In biopsy specimens, the thickness of the endocardium may be difficult to assess because the plane of sectioning is critical. Occasionally, a segment of chordae tendinae of the tricuspid valve may be present. This appears as a thin

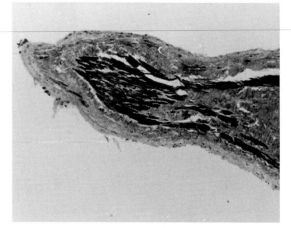

Figure 17–6. Papillary muscle fragment. Note the uniformly thick layer of subendocardial fibrous connective tissue. Masson trichrome. ×40.

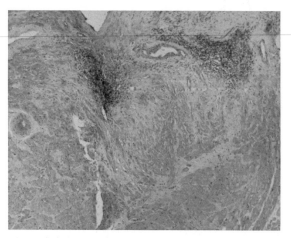

Figure 17–7. Previous biopsy site. Note the localized, subendocardial scar that traps myofibers. It contains patches of lymphocytic infiltrate and some thick-walled vessels. Periodic acid–Schiff (PAS). ×16.

chord of dense collagen. However, when chordal segments are present in the biopsy, valvular regurgitation rarely occurs. A portion of papillary muscle also may be present in the biopsy (Fig. 17–6).

Pericardium

To diagnose that the bioptome has perforated the myocardium, a distinct layer of mesothelial cells must be present.[1] Adipose tissue is observed in elderly or obese patients as a result of direct extension of epicardial fat into the myocardium.[20]

Biopsy of Previous Biopsy Site

On repeat biopsies, owing to the architecture of the right ventricle, the bioptome may sample from the same location.[1] The histologic features depend on the elapsed time since the previous biopsy. A recent site may show a crater in the endocardium with overlying mural thrombus. Later, inflammation occurs mimicking an acute rejection response. Subsequent stages show organization with granulation tissue. A healed site usually shows focal fibrosis and disarray of the underlying myocytes (Figs. 17–7 and 17–8).

ACUTE MYOCARDIAL DISEASE

The two major categories of acute myocardial disease observed in endomyocardial biopsy specimens are myocarditis and acute rejection of cardiac transplants. On some occasions, endomyocardial biopsy samples may show features of acute myocardial ischemic injury.

Myocarditis

This is a nonischemic inflammatory or immunologic disease involving the myocardium.[15, 21–23] Using the term primary implies an idiopathic etiology, whereas using the term secondary requires the identification of a specific causative agent. The clinical signs and symptoms of myocarditis are diverse, including unexplained heart failure, chest pain, and arrhythmias.[15–17, 21, 24–32]

Sampling error is the most common cause of false-negative tissue diagnoses.[15, 16] If one obtains five to eight biopsy samples, this possibility is minimal. False-positive diagnoses may result from misinterpretation of noninflammatory interstitial cells as lymphocytes. In most institutions, positive biopsy diagnoses of myocarditis

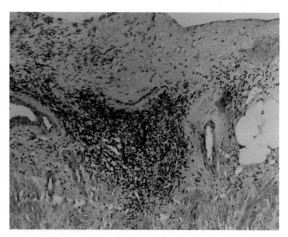

Figure 17–8. Previous biopsy site. On higher magnification a dense lymphocytic infiltrate lies within the subendocardial scar. Fat also is entrapped in the right portion of the field. PAS. ×40.

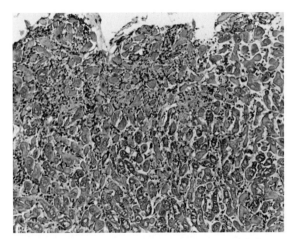

Figure 17–9. Myocarditis. Note the diffuse nature of the interstitial, inflammatory infiltrate. The endocardium is present at the upper border of the field. Masson trichrome. ×40.

in the presence of strong clinical signs still are a minority of cases.[33, 34]

The major histologic features of myocarditis include a leukocyte infiltrate and nonischemic injury (Figs. 17–9 and 17–10). The infiltrate is classified as mild, moderate, or severe, and as focal, confluent, or diffuse.[15, 35] One can adequately evaluate the intensity of the inflammatory process by endomyocardial biopsy as shown in Chagas' disease.[36] The nature of the infiltrate is also important in determining the etiology. Namely, is it lymphocytic, neutrophilic, mixed, eosinophilic, or giant cell? Myocarditis eventually heals by either resolution or organization with fibrosis.

Some forms of myocarditis are diagnosed with confidence. The presence of giant cells, granulomas, or groups of eosinophils are suffi-

ciently abnormal. However, when lymphocytes are present in low numbers or diffusely located, the diagnosis may be difficult. In these cases, one should use quantitative criteria. Other investigators have recommended that one determine the mean number of lymphocytes from counts in 10 to 20 high-power (×400) fields. For a diagnosis of myocarditis, the mean count should be more than 5 per high-power field.[17]

According to established criteria, one should diagnose the microscopic features of a patient's first biopsy as myocarditis, borderline myocarditis, or no myocarditis.[21] Only in subsequent biopsies should one describe the findings in reference to time, such as ongoing, healing, or healed myocarditis. In some diseases, endomyocardial biopsy may show continuous progression of the lesion from fiber destruction to fibrosis with compensatory hypertrophy.[37]

Some disorders may mimic myocarditis in biopsy specimens (Fig. 17–11). These include idiopathic dilated cardiomyopathy, acute myocardial infarct, and involvement of the myocardium by lymphoma. Separation of these entities depends on other clinical findings. Other histologic findings are useful in the diagnosis of an acute myocardial infarct. The myocyte necrosis observed in a myocardial infarct shows coagulative necrosis in the acute phase. In the healing phase, it has clusters of pigment-laden macrophages.

Cardiac Transplant Rejection

When acute rejection occurs in a cardiac transplant, an infiltration of lymphocytes occurs.[1, 38, 39] The changes are diffuse and are present in all regions of the myocardium. Other studies report that only 1 or 2 biopsy specimens are

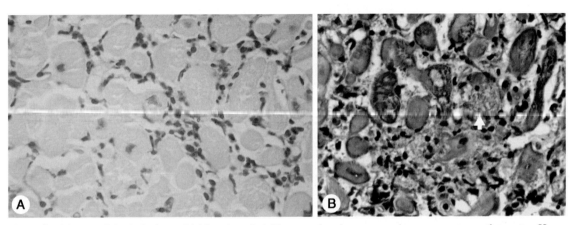

Figure 17–10. Myocarditis. *A,* An interstitial lymphocytic infiltrate and early myonecrosis are present near the center. Hematoxylin and eosin. ×100. *B,* On higher magnification necrotic myocardium *(arrowhead)* is surrounded by a mononuclear infiltrate. Masson trichrome. ×160.

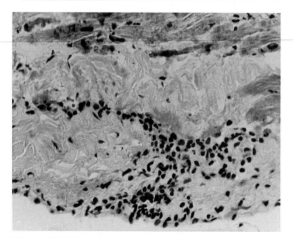

Figure 17–11. Lymphocytic aggregate within fibrous tissue. These cell aggregates may be confused with myocarditis. In this case other histologic criteria for myocarditis were absent. Hematoxylin and eosin. ×100.

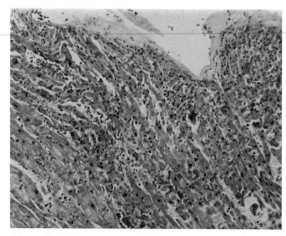

Figure 17–13. Acute myocardial ischemia. On higher magnification there is a severe inflammatory cell response in the subendocardial region. This may be confused with myocarditis. Hematoxylin and eosin. ×40.

needed to establish the diagnosis.[40, 41] Interstitial edema, perivascular karyorrhexis, and perivascular infiltrate are significant signs of early cardiac rejection before the development of myocyte necrosis.[42]

When acute rejection develops in patients receiving cyclosporine, it takes a longer time to resolve.[1, 39]

Because transplant patients are immunosuppressed and susceptible to infection, the heart may be involved with an infectious process.[1] Thus, one should look for specific infectious agents, such as a virus.

In extended management of transplant patients (longer than 6 months after transplantation), endomyocardial biopsy sometimes is performed only for specific indications rather than for surveillance.[43]

Acute Myocardial Ischemic Injury

On rare occasions, the endomyocardial biopsy samples may show features of acute myocardial ischemic injury. In these cases, there is a severe inflammatory cell response that may be confused with myocarditis. However, there often is an associated extravasation of erythrocytes into the interstitial spaces and myocytolysis. Contraction bands also are present (Figs. 17–12, 17–13, and 17–14).

CHRONIC MYOCARDIAL DISEASE

Chronic myocardial diseases diagnosed on endomyocardial biopsy are either idiopathic or

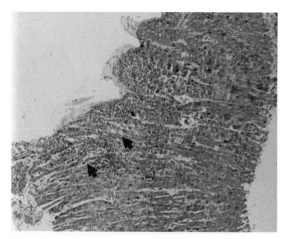

Figure 17–12. Acute myocardial ischemia. Note the overall increased cellularity of the subendocardial myocardium *(arrowheads)*. Hematoxylin and eosin. ×16.

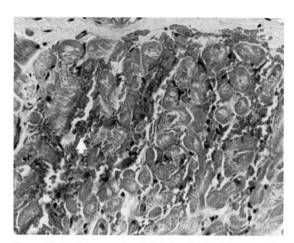

Figure 17–14. Acute myocardial ischemia. Higher magnification of the previous field shows erythrocytes *(arrowhead)* in the interstitium and the presence of myocytolysis. Hematoxylin and eosin. ×100.

secondary. The term idiopathic implies that the process results from a primary injury to the myocyte by an unknown etiologic agent. The term secondary implies that the lesion is a manifestation from other systemic disease.

In the idiopathic group are dilated cardiomyopathy, hypertrophic cardiomyopathy, and some cases of restrictive cardiomyopathy. The systemic myocardial diseases include sarcoidosis, neoplastic diseases, diseases resulting from chemotherapy (e.g., anthracycline), hemochromatosis, storage diseases, and inflammatory diseases.

Idiopathic Cardiomyopathies

Dilated Cardiomyopathy

The histologic features of idiopathic dilated cardiomyopathy are highly nonspecific and variable.[1, 2, 20, 44-59] There may be a high incidence of inflammatory infiltrates, such as lymphocytes, in dilated cardiomyopathy, but their presence does not imply an active myocarditis.[60] Most frequently one sees myocyte hypertrophy and interstitial fibrosis. The biopsy may even appear normal. Some investigators report that interobserver variability is high in reporting endomyocardial biopsy specimens from patients with dilated cardiomyopathy. Thus, quantitative and standardized methods are needed to increase diagnostic consistency.[61] Some,[57, 62, 63] but not all, studies show that quantitation of the loss of contractile elements correlates well with prognosis. Immunohistochemical studies on endomyocardial biopsy samples may be useful.[64] The biopsy features of idiopathic dilated cardiomyopathy are similar to those seen in cardiomyopathy triggered by other agents, such as alcoholic cardiomyopathy, postpartum cardiomyopathy, familial dilated cardiomyopathy, cardiomyopathy associated with Friedreich's ataxia, and Keshan cardiomyopathy associated with selenium deficiency.[65] Thus, owing to the nonspecificity of the histologic features, one should make the diagnosis of idiopathic dilated cardiomyopathy from biopsies only after excluding other ischemic, valvular, hypertensive, and toxic disorders. Also the clinical findings must be consistent. However, the high scores reported for postmyocarditis in dilated cardiomyopathy suggest a previous myocarditis is an important cause of this disease.[66]

Hypertrophic Cardiomyopathy

In this disorder, the most frequent findings seen on biopsy are myocyte hypertrophy and intersti-

tial fibrosis. The myofiber disarray usually occurs in the deeper regions of the ventricular septum, which is not routinely sampled by the bioptome.[35] Some investigators have tried to establish criteria to distinguish hypertrophic cardiomyopathy from other forms of heart disease.[67, 68] The accepted approach is not to diagnose hypertrophic cardiomyopathy from the biopsy specimen but to rule out other diseases that may mimic it. Other investigators report that quantitative measurements of endomyocardial biopsy specimens are useful in making this diagnosis.[69] Muscle fiber size, volume density of the interstitium, and the extent of fibrosis can be reasonably estimated on five samples.[70]

Restrictive Cardiomyopathy

The classic example of restrictive cardiomyopathy is involvement of the myocardium in primary amyloidosis. In this instance, cardiac biopsy is the diagnostic tool of choice.[71] If one suspects amyloidosis, one should perform additional tests using stains such as Congo red, sulfated Alcian blue, methyl violet, and thioflavine T. Most important is the performance of electron microscopy to show the characteristic fibrillar structure of the amyloid.[71] Amyloid may encircle and constrict individual myocytes, form amorphous interstitial masses, or be present in vascular and endocardial locations (Figs. 17–15 and 17–16A to C). In electron micrographs, the parallel and interlacing arrays of amyloid fibrils are clearly evident (see Fig. 17–16C). Immunohistochemical staining with antiserum to human prealbumin is useful in distinguishing between primary amyloidosis and senile amyloidosis.[72]

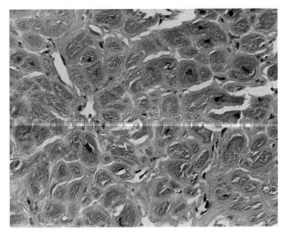

Figure 17–15. Amyloidosis (primary). The pericellular deposits of amyloid ring the myofibers. Hematoxylin and eosin. ×100.

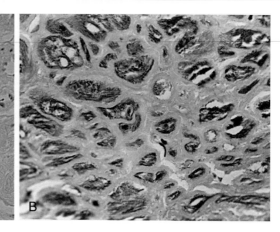

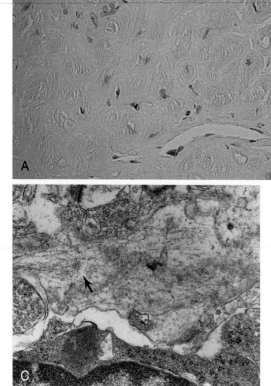

Figure 17–16. Amyloidosis (primary). *A,* The individual myofibers are encircled by pale eosinophilic rings of amyloid. Hematoxylin and eosin. ×100. *B,* On higher magnification the amyloid deposits have an amorphous appearance. Masson trichrome. ×160. *C,* Electron micrograph showing the parallel and interlacing arrays of amyloid fibers *(arrow)*. ×40,000.

This distinction is important because the treatment and prognosis of the two entities differ.

Also, one can diagnose other forms of restrictive cardiomyopathy, such as primary endocardial fibroelastosis, by endomyocardial biopsy.[73] Ultrastructural changes suggest that increased elastoplastic activity of smooth muscle cells occurs in the endocardium.[74]

Systemic Myocardial Diseases

Sarcoidosis

When sarcoidosis involves the heart, the clinical features are varied and include arrhythmias, ventricular aneurysms, chest pain, failure, mitral insufficiency, pericardial effusion, pericardial constriction, and tamponade.[75-80] If pulmonary

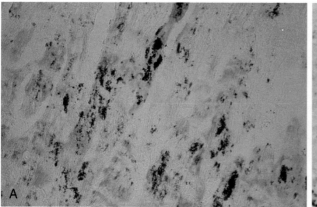

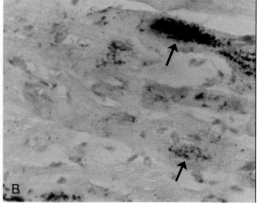

Figure 17–17. Hemochromatosis. *A,* Thick iron deposits, blue staining material, are within the cytoplasm of the myocardial fibers. Iron stain. ×40. *B,* Dense iron deposits are present within the myocardial fibers. Some deposits are in the perinuclear region *(arrows)* resembling lipofuchsin pigment. Iron stain. ×100.

involvement in sarcoidosis is severe, right ventricular hypertrophy may be present due to pulmonary hypertension.

The characteristic histologic features of cardiac sarcoidosis include granulomatous or giant cell myocarditis. In these cases, one must rule out an infectious etiology. Endomyocardial biopsies have been diagnostic in this disease.[81, 82]

Neoplastic Diseases

Metastatic neoplastic disease frequently involves the heart.[83] The most frequent metastatic tumors involving the heart include melanomas, lymphomas, and leukemia.[83–85] Other primary neoplastic lesions of the heart diagnosed by endomyocardial biopsy include intracardiac sarcoma.[86] If the initial clinical presentation shows cardiac manifestations, endomyocardial biopsy may be useful in establishing the primary diagnosis.

Anthracycline Cardiotoxicity

Dose-related cardiotoxicity limits the usefulness of antineoplastic anthracycline antibiotics, especially doxorubicin hydrochloride (Adriamycin), in the treatment of malignancies.[87, 88] When heart failure ensues, this toxicity has a 50% mortality.[87, 88] The use of serial endomyocardial biopsies is a reliable and accurate method to evaluate cardiotoxicity before cardiac failure occurs.[89]

The characteristic lesions seen on biopsy are dilation of the sarcotubules and loss of the contractile elements.[90–92] To be certain of the significance of these changes, one should do a reference biopsy before the onset of therapy.

Hemochromatosis

One can easily make this diagnosis with an iron stain because no stainable iron is normally present in the heart[93, 94] (Fig. 17–17). The iron deposits usually are near the nuclear poles. When extensive deposits are present, the iron may be present throughout the sarcoplasm. In advanced cases, it may result in fibrosis and restrictive or dilated cardiomyopathy.[95]

Storage Diseases

When one suspects glycogen storage disease, one fixes the biopsy specimens in absolute alcohol. Electron microscopy usually is needed because characteristic ultrastructural alterations are present. Cardiac involvement in storage diseases occurs in Fabry's disease,[96, 97] Gaucher's disease,[98] and glycogen storage disease.[99]

Inflammatory Diseases

One can identify specific infectious etiologies of myocardial disease on endomyocardial biopsy. Most frequently, these etiologies have included viral inclusions, fungi, and Toxoplasma organisms in the hearts of transplant patients or immunosuppressed patients.[1] Other inflammatory disorders identified on endomyocardial biopsy include Churg-Strauss syndrome,[100] acute rheumatic myocarditis,[101] Kawasaki disease,[102, 103] vasculitis,[104, 105] systemic lupus erythematosus,[106] rheumatoid arteritis,[107] and hypereosinophilic syndrome.[108]

REFERENCES

1. Billingham ME: The role of endomyocardial biopsy in the diagnosis and treatment of heart disease. In Silver MD (ed): Cardiovascular Pathology. New York, Churchill Livingstone, 1983, p 1205.
2. Edwards WD, Holmes DR Jr: Transvenous endomyocardial biopsy. In Brandenburg RO, Fuster V, Giuliani ER, McGoon DC (eds): Cardiology: Fundamentals and Practice. Chicago, Year Book Medical Publishers, 1987, p 506.
3. Unverferth DV, Baker PB: Value of endomyocardial biopsy. Am J Med 1986; 80:22–32.
4. Richardson PJ: Endomyocardial biopsy technique. In Bolte H (ed): Myocardial Biopsy: Diagnostic Significance. Berlin, Springer-Verlag, 1980, p 3.
5. Fowles RE, Mason JW: Myocardial biopsy [editorial]. Mayo Clin Proc 1982; 57:459.
6. Fitchett DH, Forbes C, Guerraty AJ: Repeated endomyocardial biopsy causing coronary arterial–right ventricular fistula after cardiac transplantation. Am J Cardiol 1988; 62:829–831.
7. Locke TJ, Furniss SS, McGregor CG: Coronary artery–right ventricular fistula after endomyocardial biopsy. Br Heart J 1988; 60:81–82.
8. Spiegelhalter DJ, Stovin PGI: Analysis of repeated biopsies following cardiac transplantation. Stat Med 1983; 2:33.
9. Karch SB, Billingham ME: Myocardial contraction bands revisited. Hum Pathol 1986; 17:9.
10. Edwards WD: Applied anatomy of the heart. In Brandenburg RO, Fuster V, Giuliani ER, McGoon DC (eds): Cardiology: Fundamentals and Practice. Chicago, Year Book Medical Publishers, 1987, p 47.
11. Moore GW, Hutchins GM, Bulkley BH, et al: Constituents of the human ventricular myocardium: Connective tissue hyperplasia accompanying muscular hypertrophy. Am Heart J 1980; 100:610.
12. Fuster V, Danielson MA, Robb RA, et al: Quantitation of left ventricular myocardial fiber hypertrophy and interstitial tissue in human hearts with chronically increased volume and pressure overload. Circulation 1977; 55:504.
13. Anderson KR, Sutton MG, Lie JT: Histopathological types of cardiac fibrosis in myocardial disease. J Pathol 1979; 128:79.
14. Tazelaar HD, Billingham ME: Myocardial lymphocytes:

Fact, fancy or myocarditis. Am J Cardiovasc Pathol 1987; 1:47–50.

15. Edwards WD: Myocarditis and endomyocardial biopsy. Cardiol Clin 1984; 2:647.

16. Edwards WD: Current problems in establishing quantitative histopathologic criteria for the diagnosis of lymphocytic myocarditis by endomyocardial biopsy. Heart Vessels 1985; 1(Suppl 1):138–142.

17. Edwards WD, Holmes DR Jr, Reeder GS: Diagnosis of active lymphocytic myocarditis by endomyocardial biopsy: Quantitative criteria for light microscopy. Mayo Clin Proc 1982; 57:419.

18. Foley DA, Edwards WD: Quantitation of leukocytes in endomyocardial tissue from 100 normal hearts at autopsy: Implications for diagnosis of myocarditis from biopsy specimens of living patients. Am J Cardiovasc Pathol 1988; 2:145.

19. Okada R: Clinicopathological study on the thickening of parietal endocardium in the adult heart. Jpn Heart J 1961; 2:220.

20. Edwards WD: Endomyocardial biopsy and cardiomyopathy. Cardiovasc Rev Rep 1983; 4:820.

21. Aretz HT, Billingham ME, Edwards WD, et al: Myocarditis: A histopathologic definition and classification. Am J Cardiovasc Pathol 1987; 1:3.

22. Jacobs B, Matsuda Y, Deodhar S, Shirey E: Cell-mediated cytotoxicity to cardiac cells of lymphocytes from patients with primary myocardial disease. Am J Clin Pathol 1979; 72:1.

23. Laufer A: Human and experimental myocarditis: The possible role of immune processes in pathogenesis. Isr J Med Sci 1975; 11:37.

24. Dec GW Jr, Palacios IF, Fallon JT, et al: Active myocarditis in the spectrum of acute dilated cardiomyopathies: Clinical features, histologic correlates and clinical outcome. N Engl J Med 1985; 312:885.

25. Fenoglio JJ Jr, Ursell PC, Kellogg CF, et al: Diagnosis and classification of myocarditis by endomyocardial biopsy. N Engl J Med 1983; 308:12.

26. Kereiakes DJ, Parmley WW: Myocarditis and cardiomyopathy. Am Heart J 1984; 108:1318.

27. Mason JW, Billingham ME, Ricci DR: Treatment of acute inflammatory myocarditis assisted by endomyocardial biopsy. Am J Cardiol 1980; 45:1037.

28. Parrillo JE, Aretz HT, Palacios I, et al: The results of transvenous endomyocardial biopsy can frequently be used to diagnose myocardial diseases in patients with idiopathic heart failure: Endomyocardial biopsies in 100 consecutive patients revealed a substantial incidence of myocarditis. Circulation 1984; 69:93.

29. Strain JE, Grose RM, Factor SM, Fisher JD: Results of endomyocardial biopsy in patients with spontaneous ventricular tachycardia but without apparent structural heart disease. Circulation 1983; 68:1171.

30. Subramanian R: The pathology of myocarditis and cardiomyopathy. In Robinson JA, O'Connell JB (eds): Myocarditis: Precursor of Cardiomyopathy. Lexington, MA, Collamore Press, 1983, p 129.

31. Vignola PA, Aonuma K, Swaye PS, et al: Lymphocytic myocarditis presenting as unexplained ventricular arrhythmias: Diagnosis with endomyocardial biopsy and response to immunosuppression. J Am Coll Cardiol 1984; 4:812.

32. Zee-Cheng CS, Tsai CC, Palmer DC, et al: High incidence of myocarditis by endomyocardial biopsy in patients with idiopathic congestive cardiomyopathy. J Am Coll Cardiol 1984; 3:63.

33. Chow LC, Dittrich HC, Shabetai R: Endomyocardial biopsy in patients with unexplained congestive heart failure. Ann Intern Med 1988; 109:535–539.

34. Lie JT: Myocarditis and endomyocardial biopsy in un-
explained heart failure: A diagnosis in search of a disease. Ann Intern Med 1988; 109:525–528.

35. Maron BJ, Roberts WC: Hypertrophic cardiomyopathy and cardiac muscle cell disorganization revisited: Relation between the two and significance. Am Heart J 1981; 102:95.

36. Higuchi ML, De Morais CF, Pereira Barretto AC, et al: The role of active myocarditis in the development of heart failure in chronic Chagas' disease: A study based on endomyocardial biopsies. Clin Cardiol 1987; 10:665–670.

37. Pereira Barretto AC, Mady C, Arteaga-Fernandez E, et al: Right ventricular endomyocardial biopsy in chronic Chagas' disease. Am Heart J 1986; 111:307–312.

38. Billingham ME: Diagnosis of cardiac rejection by endomyocardial biopsy. Heart Transplant 1981; 1:25.

39. Billingham ME: Endomyocardial biopsy detection of acute rejection in cardiac allograft recipients. Heart Vessels 1985; 1(Suppl 1):86–90.

40. Caves PK, Stinson EB, Billingham ME, et al: Diagnosis of human cardiac allograft rejection by serial cardiac biopsy. J Thorac Cardiovasc Surg 1973; 66:461.

41. Rose AG, Uys CJ, Losman JG, Barnard CN. Evaluation of endomyocardial biopsy in the diagnosis of cardiac rejection: A study using bioptome samples of formalin-fixed tissue. Transplantation 1978; 26:10.

42. Herskowitz A, Soule LM, Mellits ED, et al: Histologic predictors of acute cardiac rejection in human endomyocardial biopsies: A multivariate analysis. J Am Coll Cardiol 1987; 9:802–810.

43. Glanville AR, Imoto E, Baldwin JC, et al: The role of right ventricular endomyocardial biopsy in the long-term management of heart-lung transplant recipients. J Heart Transplant 1987; 6:357–361.

44. Baandrup U, Florio RA, Roters F, Olsen EGJ: Electron microscopic investigation of endomyocardial biopsy samples in hypertrophy and cardiomyopathy: A semiquantitative study in 48 patients. Circulation 1981; 63:1289.

45. Baandrup U, Olsen EGJ: Critical analysis of endomyocardial biopsies from patients suspected of having cardiomyopathy. I: Morphological and morphometric aspects. Br Heart J 1981; 45:475.

46. Breithardt G, Kuhn H, Knieriem H: Prognostic significance of endomyocardial biopsy in patients with congestive cardiomyopathy. In Kaltenbach M, Loogen F, Olsen EGJ (eds): Cardiomyopathy and Myocardial Biopsy. Berlin, Springer-Verlag, 1978, p 258.

47. Dick MR, Unverferth DV, Baba N: The pattern of myocardial degeneration in nonischemic congestive cardiomyopathy. Hum Pathol 1982; 13:740.

48. Fast JH, Kubat K, Vanhaelst UJGM, Stekhoven JHS: The usefulness of an endomyocardial biopsy in heart disease of unknown etiology. Int J Cardiol 1986; 11:317.

49. Ferrans VJ, Massumi RA, Shugoll GI, et al: Ultrastructural studies of myocardial biopsies in 45 patients with obstructive or congestive cardiomyopathy. Recent Adv Cardiac Struct Metab 1973; 2:231.

50. Fujita M, Neustein HB, Lurie PR: Transvascular endomyocardial biopsy in infants and small children: Myocardial findings in 10 cases of cardiomyopathy. Hum Pathol 1979; 10:15.

51. Keren A, Billingham ME, Weintraub D, et al: Mildly dilated congestive cardiomyopathy. Circulation 1985; 72:302

52. Kunkel B, Lapp H, Kober G, Kaltenbach M: Correlations between clinical and morphologic findings and natural history in congestive cardiomyopathy. In Kaltenbach M, Loogen F, Olsen EGJ (eds): Cardiomyopa-

thy and Myocardial Biopsy. Berlin, Springer-Verlag, 1978, p 271.

53. Lewis AB, Neustein HB, Takahashi M, Lurie PR: Findings on endomyocardial biopsy in infants and children with dilated cardiomyopathy. Am J Cardiol 1985; 55:143.

54. Nippoldt TB, Edwards WD, Holmes DR Jr, et al: Right ventricular endomyocardial biopsy: Clinicopathologic correlates in 100 consecutive patients. Mayo Clin Proc 1982; 57:407.

55. O'Connell JB, Costanzo-Nordin MR, Subramanian R, Robinson JA: Dilated cardiomyopathy: Emerging role of endomyocardial biopsy. Curr Probl Cardiol 1986; 11:450.

56. Rose AG, Beck W: Dilated (congestive) cardiomyopathy: A syndrome of severe cardiac dysfunction with remarkably few morphological features of myocardial damage. Histopathology 1985; 9:367.

57. Schwarz F, Mall G, Zebe H, et al: Quantitative morphologic findings of the myocardium in idiopathic dilated cardiomyopathy. Am J Cardiol 1983; 51:501.

58. Sekiguchi M: Electron microscopical observations of the myocardium in patients with idiopathic cardiomyopathy using endomyocardial biopsy. J Mol Cell Cardiol 1974; 6:111.

59. Unverferth BJ, Leier CV, Magorien RD, Unverferth DV. Differentiating characteristics of myocardial nuclei in cardiomyopathy. Hum Pathol 1983; 14:974.

60. Tazelaar HD, Billingham ME: Leukocytic infiltrates in idiopathic dilated cardiomyopathy: A source of confusion with active myocarditis. Am J Surg Pathol 1986; 10:405–412.

61. Shanes JG, Ghali J, Billingham ME, et al: Interobserver variability in the pathologic interpretation of endomyocardial biopsy results. Circulation 1987; 75:401–405.

62. Figulla HR, Rahlf G, Nieger M, et al: Spontaneous hemodynamic improvement or stabilization and associated biopsy findings in patients with congestive cardiomyopathy. Circulation 1985; 71:1095.

63. Schwarz F, Mall G, Zebe H, et al: Determinants of survival in patients with congestive cardiomyopathy: Quantitative morphologic findings and left ventricular hemodynamics. Circulation 1984; 70:923.

64. Deguchi H, Hayashi T, Kotaka M, et al: In situ analysis with monoclonal antibodies of lymphocyte subsets in myocardial biopsies from patients with dilated cardiomyopathy and idiopathic (viral) myocarditis. Jpn Circ J 1987; 51:1365–1372.

65. Edwards WD: Cardiomyopathies. Hum Pathol 1987; 18:625.

66. Hasumi M, Sekiguchi M, Yu ZX, et al: Analysis of histopathologic findings in cases with dilated cardiomyopathy with special reference to formulating diagnostic criteria on the possibility of postmyocarditic change. Jpn Circ J 1986; 50:1280–1287.

67. Nunoda S, Genda A, Sekiguchi M, Takeda R: Left ventricular endomyocardial biopsy findings in patients with essential hypertension and hypertrophic cardiomyopathy with special reference to the incidence of bizarre myocardial hypertrophy with disorganizations and biopsy score. Heart Vessels 1985; 1:170.

68. Van Noorden S, Olsen EGJ, Pearse AGE: Hypertrophic obstructive cardiomyopathy: A histological, histochemical and ultrastructural study of biopsy material. Cardiovasc Res 1971; 5:118.

69. Frenzel H, Schwartzkopff B, Reinecke P, et al: Evidence for muscle fiber hyperplasia in the septum of patients with hypertrophic obstructive cardiomyopathy (HOCM): Quantitative examination of endomyocar-

dial biopsies (EMCB) and myectomy specimens. Z Kardiol 1987; 76:14–19.

70. Schwartzkopff B, Uhre B, Ehle B, et al: Variability and reproducibility of morphologic findings in endomyocardial biopsies of patients with hypertrophic obstructive cardiomyopathy. Z Kardiol 1987; 76:26–32.

71. Pellikka PA, Holmes DRJ, Edwards WD, et al: Endomyocardial biopsy in 30 patients with primary amyloidosis and suspected cardiac involvement. Arch Intern Med 1988; 148:662–666.

72. Olson LJ, Gertz MA, Edwards WD, et al: Senile cardiac amyloidosis with myocardial dysfunction: Diagnosis by endomyocardial biopsy and immunohistochemistry. N Engl J Med 1987; 317:738–742.

73. Hashimoto T, Yano K, Matsumoto Y, Hashiba K: Contracted form of primary endocardial fibroelastosis in a young adult without congestive heart failure. Jpn Heart J 1988; 29:121–126.

74. Rosnowski A, Ruzyllo W: Ultrastructural aspects of endomyocardial biopsy in restrictive cardiomyopathy: evaluation of elastogenesis. Cor Vasa 1986; 28:67–72.

75. Lemery R, McGoon MD, Edwards WD: Cardiac sarcoidosis: A potentially treatable form of myocarditis. Mayo Clin Proc 1985; 60:549.

76. Lorell B, Alderman EL, Mason JW: Cardiac sarcoidosis: Diagnosis with endomyocardial biopsy and treatment with corticosteroids. Am J Cardiol 1978; 42:143.

77. Ratner SJ, Fenoglio JJ Jr, Ursell PC: Utility of endomyocardial biopsy in the diagnosis of cardiac sarcoidosis. Chest 1986; 90:528–533.

78. Roberts WC, McAllister HA Jr, Ferrans VJ: Sarcoidosis of the heart: A clinicopathologic study of 35 necroscopy patients (group I) and review of 78 previously described necropsy patients (group II). Am J Med 1977; 63:86.

79. Sekiguchi M, Numao Y, Imai M, et al: Clinical and histopathological profile of sarcoidosis of the heart and acute idiopathic myocarditis: Concepts through a study employing endomyocardial biopsy. I: Sarcoidosis. Jpn Circ J 1980; 44:249.

80. Silverman KJ, Hutchins GM, Bulkley BH: Cardiac sarcoid: A clinicopathologic study of 84 unselected patients with systemic sarcoidosis. Circulation 1978; 58:1204.

81. Fukuhara T, Morino M, Sakoda S, et al: Myocarditis with multinucleated giant cells detected in biopsy specimens. Clin Cardiol 1988; 11:341–344.

82. Valantine HA, Tazelaar HD, Macoviak J, et al: Cardiac sarcoidosis: Response to steroids and transplantation. J Heart Transplant 1987; 6:244–250.

83. Lammers RJ, Bloor CM: Pathology of cardiac tumors. *In* Kapoor AS (ed): Cancer and the Heart. New York, Springer-Verlag, 1986, pp 1–20.

84. Hanley PC, Shub C, Seward JB, Wold LE: Intracavitary cardiac melanoma diagnosed by endomyocardial left ventricular biopsy. Chest 1983; 84:195.

85. Johnston IDA, Popple AW: Right ventricular outflow tract obstruction secondary to small intestinal lymphoma. Br Heart J 1988; 19:599.

86. Hausheer FH, Josephson RA, Grochow LB, et al: Intracardiac sarcoma diagnosed by left ventricular endomyocardial biopsy. Chest 1987; 92:177–179.

87. Billingham ME: Some recent advances in cardiac pathology. Hum Pathol 1979; 10:367.

88. Bristow MR, Mason JW, Billingham ME, Daniels JR: Doxorubicin cardiomyopathy: Evaluation by phonocardiography, endomyocardial biopsy and cardiac catheterizaton. Ann Intern Med 1978; 88:168.

89. Mason JW, Bristow MR, Billingham ME, Daniels JR: Invasive and noninvasive methods of assessing Adriamycin cardiotoxic effects in man: Superiority of histo-

pathologic assessment using endomyocardial biopsy. Cancer Treat Rep 1978; 62:857.

90. Billingham ME, Mason JW, Bristow MR, Daniels JR: Anthracycline cardiomyopathy monitored by morphologic changes. Cancer Treat Rep 1978; 62:865.

91. Cambridge G, MacArthur CGC, Waterson AP, et al: Antiobodies to Coxsackie B viruses in congestive cardiomyopathy. Br Heart J 1979; 41:692.

92. Lefrak EA, Pitha J, Rosenheim S, Gottlieb JA: A clinicopathologic analysis of adriamycin cardiotoxicity. Cancer 1973; 32:302.

93. Baba Y, Konishi H, Yokoi Y, et al: [Cardiac hemochromatosis diagnosed by endomyocardial biopsy: The first case reported in Japan]. Nippon Naika Gakkai Zasshi 1987; 76:1547–1553.

94. Fitchett DH, Coltart DJ, Littler WA, et al: Cardiac involvement in secondary hemochromatosis: A catheter biopsy study and analysis of myocardium. Cardiovasc Res 1980; 14:719.

95. Cutler DJ, Isner JM, Bracey AW, et al: Hemochromatosis heart disease: An unemphasized cause of potentially reversible restrictive cardiomyopathy. Am J Med 1980; 69:923.

96. Broadbent JC, Edwards WD, Gordon H, et al: Fabry cardiomyopathy in the female confirmed by endomyocardial biopsy. Mayo Clin Proc 1981; 56:623.

97. Matsui S, Murakami E, Takekoshi N, et al: Cardiac manifestations of Fabry's disease: Report of a case with pulmonary regurgitation diagnosed on the basis of endomyocardial biopsy findings. Jpn Circ J 1977; 41:1023.

98. Edwards WD, Hurd HP II, Partin JR: Cardiac involvement by Gaucher's disease documented by right ventricular endomyocardial biopsy. Am J Cardiol 1983; 52:654.

99. Olson LJ, Reeder GS, Noller KL, et al: Cardiac involvement in glycogen storage disease. III: Morphologic and biochemical characterization with endomyocardial biopsy. Am J Cardiol 1984; 53:980.

100. Kim CH, Vlietstra RE, Edwards WD, et al: Steroid-responsive eosinophilic myocarditis: Diagnosis by endomyocardial biopsy. Am J Cardiol 1984; 53:1472.

101. Ursell PC, Albala A, Fenoglio JJ Jr: Diagnosis of acute rheumatic carditis by endomyocardial biopsy. Hum Pathol 1982; 13:677.

102. Yutani C, Okano K, Kamiya T, et al: Histopathological study on right endomyocardial biopsy of Kawasaki disease. Br Heart J 1980; 43:589.

103. Yutani C, Go S, Kamiya T, et al: Cardiac biopsy of Kawasaki disease. Arch Pathol Lab Med 1981; 105:470.

104. Kereiakes DJ, Ports TA, Finkbeiner W: Endomyocardial biopsy in Henoch-Schönlein purpura. Am Heart J 1984; 107:382.

105. Shanes JG, Lyons MF, Saffitz J, et al: Persistent endomyocardial biopsy-proven vasculitis following cure of endocarditis. Am Heart J 1984; 108:614.

106. Fairfax MJ, Osborn TG, Williams GA, et al: Endomyocardial biopsy in patients with systemic lupus erythematosus. J Rheumatol 1988; 15:593–596.

107. Slack JD, Waller B: Acute congestive heart failure due to the arteritis of rheumatoid arthritis: Early diagnosis by endomyocardial biopsy: A case report. Angiology 1986; 37:477–482.

108. Borgfeldt C, Hansen B, Manthorpe R: The hypereosinophilic syndrome: Report of a case with successful medical treatment following cardiac biopsy. Scand J Rheumatol 1988; 17:51–54.

DIAGNOSIS

Chapter 18

Catheterization and Angiography in Valvular Heart Disease

KIRK L. PETERSON

In the 1990s valvular heart disease remains worldwide a major human affliction that often requires diagnostic cardiac catheterization and angiography. The disease presents in either an isolated or multiple valve form and exhibits variable etiologic, pathologic, and pathophysiologic features. Individual valve dysfunction is related either to regurgitation (leakage) or stenosis (obstruction), or both, that in turn leads to morphologic and functional adaptations in the form of dilation and hypertrophy of the corresponding atrium and ventricle.

Noninvasive techniques, particularly two-dimensional echocardiography with Doppler velocity recordings and pseudocolor imaging, have significantly improved the cardiologist's acumen in detecting and quantifying the morphologic and pathophysiologic abnormalities of valvular heart disease. Nevertheless, cardiac catheterization and angiography remain important confirmatory diagnostic procedures in those patients for whom noninvasive studies are technically inadequate or the severity of the lesion remains ambiguous.

ETIOLOGY

Multiple Valve Disease

Despite a significant decline in the incidence of acute rheumatic fever over the antecedent 4 decades,[1-3] rheumatic heart disease remains the most common cause of multiple valve heart disease, with mitral, aortic, tricuspid, and pulmonic valvulitis occurring in a descending order of frequency. Rheumatic aortic valvulitis occurs uncommonly without simultaneous involvement of the mitral valve. Similarly, rheumatic lesions of right-sided valves are not observed unless there is concomitant involvement of the mitral

or aortic valve, or both. Acute or subacute infectious endocarditis, diseases of connective tissue (e.g., rheumatoid arthritis), Marfan's syndrome, and congenital hypoplasia or malformations can likewise, but less commonly, lead to multiple valvular dysfunction.

Isolated Valve Disease

MITRAL VALVE. Acquired, isolated mitral valve obstruction develops most often as a consequence of rheumatic valvulitis; uncommonly, it may be related to a left atrial tumor, thrombus, or degenerative calcification.[4] Congenital hypoplasia of the mitral valve or a supravalvular membrane (cor triatriatum) may be detected for the first time in adulthood and simulate the clinical presentation of acquired disease.

On postmortem examination the rheumatic mitral valve demonstrates thickening of the cusps with partial fusion of the commissures. There may be thickening and shortening of the chordae tendineae, and this geometric alteration of the supporting structures contributes to reduced leaflet motion. Late in the disease heavy calcification of the valve leaflets is seen that may or may not be associated with annular calcification as well.

A broad spectrum of disease processes leads to isolated (acute or chronic) mitral regurgitation,[4] although in some countries rheumatic valvulitis remains the predominant cause. Other primary causes to be considered include (1) rupture of one or more chordae tendineae due to bacterial endocarditis, trauma, connective tissue disease, or an idiopathic condition; (2) papillary muscle dysfunction (necrosis or fibrosis) secondary to coronary artery disease; (3) rupture of a papillary muscle secondary to acute myocardial infarction or trauma, associated with acute mitral insufficiency and a rapid hemodynamic deterioration; (4) collagen disorders; and (5) congenital or inheritable disorders, such as Marfan's syndrome, myxomatous transformation (mitral valve prolapse syndrome), endocardial cushion defects, and single papillary muscle with a "parachute" configuration. Mitral regurgitation may also occur as a consequence of obstructive hypertrophic cardiomyopathy or secondary to massive dilation of the left ventricle and mitral valve annulus in patients with advanced myocardial failure of whatever cause. Heavy, degenerative calcification of the mitral annulus is also believed to cause significant mitral regurgitation.

AORTIC VALVE. In more than one half of adult patients with isolated aortic stenosis, obstruction is related to degeneration, stiffening, and calcification of a bicuspid aortic valve, a congenital lesion estimated to occur in 1% of the population.[5-10] In the remainder, the valve is tricuspid but again deformed in the elderly by degenerative thickening and calcification. In a few patients, a rheumatic process may play a role, although such causation is difficult to prove.[6-8] Calcium deposition may extend into the aortic annulus and into the upper portion of the ventricular septum, causing disturbances of conduction across the atrioventricular node, bundle of His, or left bundle branch.

Isolated leakage of the aortic valve is caused primarily by diseases of the valve leaflets themselves or secondarily by dilation and disruption of the aortic annulus associated with primary diseases of the aortic root.[11] These latter disorders cause dilation of the root of the ascending aorta, which, in turn, leads to stretching of the aortic root annulus and loss of coaptation of the valve leaflets. Acute or subacute aortic valve leaflet disease is most commonly secondary to infective endocarditis, spontaneous prolapse, or traumatic rupture. Acute aortic insufficiency associated with aortic root disease is secondary to aortic dissection, chest trauma, or an acute aortitis as seen in infectious endocarditis. Solitary, chronic insufficiency of the aortic valve is most commonly congenital in origin but can be acquired secondary to a host of systemic or inheritable illnesses, including ankylosing spondylitis, rheumatoid arthritis, relapsing polychondritis, systemic lupus erythematosus, Marfan's syndrome, Hurler's syndrome, osteogenesis imperfecta, severe hypertension, or infectious endocarditis. Chronic insufficiency may also be found in association with the aortic root disease secondary to Marfan's syndrome, idiopathic annuloaortic ectasia, chronic aortitis secondary to syphilis, or aneurysms of the ascending aorta secondary to arteriosclerosis and aging. In some patients with a membranous ventricular septal defect, the aortic valve becomes incompetent secondary to prolapse of the right or noncoronary cusps down into the orifice of the defect. If encountered with concomitant involvement of the mitral valve, aortic regurgitation is most commonly rheumatic in origin.

TRICUSPID VALVE. As a solitary lesion, obstruction of the tricuspid valve is a rare disorder. It is usually secondary to a congenital malformation[12] but can also be acquired secondary to endomyocardial fibroelastosis, carcinoid heart disease, systemic lupus erythematosus, endocarditis, pacemaker lead–induced fibrosis, or constriction of the right-sided atrioventricular groove in association with adhesive or constrictive pericarditis.[13-18] Either primary or metastatic tumors in the right atrium can also lead to tricuspid valve obstruction and present with a similar clinical syndrome.[19-21] Because of its rarity as an isolated lesion yet relatively common occurrence with rheumatic involvement of left-sided valves, signs of tricuspid stenosis should prompt a careful search for concomitant dysfunction of the aortic or mitral valves.

Isolated tricuspid regurgitation is most commonly a functional lesion secondary to pulmonary hypertension and right ventricular dilation. Solitary dysfunction of the tricuspid valve may also be seen as a consequence of myxomatous change of the valve leaflets,[22] bacterial endocarditis (due to direct erosion of the valve leaflets or rupture of chordae tendineae), congenital displacement of the valve leaflets into the right ventricle (Epstein's anomaly), or traumatic avulsion of a valve leaflet or papillary muscle.

PULMONIC VALVE. Obstruction of the pulmonic valve essentially always occurs as a congenital, rather than an acquired, valvular lesion. Nevertheless, an intrapericardial tumor can compress the right ventricular outflow tract, causing a pressure gradient between the right ventricle and the pulmonary artery. Also, blood-borne metastatic tumors or thromboemboli, or primary right-sided heart tumors, may lodge or arise in the right ventricular outflow tract and cause pulmonic valve obstruction. Isolated pulmonic regurgitation may be acquired as a consequence of severe pulmonary hypertension with dilation of the pulmonic valve annulus. Although it more commonly involves the tricuspid valve, infectious endocarditis also may rupture or erode primarily the pulmonic valve leaflets, creating the clinical picture of isolated pulmonic regurgitation. Nevertheless, in the absence of infectious endocarditis or primary disease of the lungs with pulmonary hypertension, isolated pulmonic regurgitation is usually congenital in origin.

PATHOPHYSIOLOGY

GENERAL PRINCIPLES. The functional effects of stenosis or regurgitation, or both, of a heart valve should be understood primarily in terms of the resultant influences on intravascular and intracardiac pressures and flow, effects on the pulmonary vascular and systemic venous systems, and the acuteness or chronicity of a given lesion. Also to be considered are the tissue (muscle and collagen) and geometric adaptations that occur in the ventricular or atrial chamber most directly influenced by the volume or pressure overload. For example, a left ventricular volume overload causes chamber dilation and increased muscle mass but with maintenance of a normal end-diastolic mass-to-volume ratio (eccentric hypertrophy). In contrast, a left ventricular pressure overload is associated characteristically with little if any ventricular dilation until late in the course of the illness, and the compensatory increase in muscle mass is marked by an increase in the mass-to-volume ratio (concentric hypertrophy).

ESTIMATION OF SEVERITY OF VALVE STENOSIS BY THE GORLIN EQUATION. The primary method for detection of valve obstruction by cardiac catheterization has been the demonstration of a pressure gradient across the valve during transvalvular flow. Early in the history of cardiac catheterization, however, Gorlin and Gorlin[23] recognized the flow dependence of the pressure gradient. They turned to the physics of hydraulic behavior and formulated an equation for calculation of valve orifice size based on the Torricelli model for nonturbulent fluid through a planar orifice.[23, 24] The Gorlin equation was based on the following mathematic relations and postmortem or surgical observations:

$$Q = A \cdot V \cdot C_C \quad \text{or} \quad A = \frac{Q}{V \cdot C_C} \quad (1)$$

where A is the anatomic area of the valve, Q is the flow during the period that a given valve is open, V is the velocity of flow, C_C is a constant of orifice contraction relating functional to anatomic valve area, and

$$V = C_V \cdot \sqrt{2gh} \quad \text{or} \quad V = C_V \cdot \sqrt{1960 \cdot h} \quad (2)$$

where V is the average velocity of transvalvular flow, C_V is a second constant for viscous frictional losses, g is acceleration due to gravity (980 cm/s per s), and h is the mean pressure gradient across the valve in centimeters of water.

Then, by substituting and combining C_C, C_V, and 1.166 (the square root of the factor to change millimeters of mercury to centimeters of water) into a comprehensive constant, k, a more familiar form of the Gorlin equation is obtained, as follows

$$A = \frac{Q}{K \cdot 44.3 \sqrt{h}} \quad (3)$$

where A is area, Q is flow, k is the combined (C_C, C_V, and 1.166) constants and other empiric factors, and h is the mean pressure gradient, $\overline{dP}$, in millimeters of mercury during the period of transvalvular flow.

In their original publication, the Gorlins pointed out that Equation 3 was derived for a steady flow system rather than for the nonlinear, non-Newtonian, and pulsatile characteristics of the circulatory system of humans.[23, 24] Thus, mean flow (Q_{mean}) was used in the numerator of Equation 3. Other authors have since pointed out that if one is to calculate A_{mean} using Q_{mean}, then $\sqrt{\overline{dP}}$, rather than $\sqrt{\overline{dP}}$, is the valid term in the denominator.[25] Alternatively, to calculate the root mean square of area (A_{rms}), one could use the root mean square of flow, Q_{rms}, in the numerator, and $\sqrt{\overline{dP}}$ would then be the valid term in the denominator. In this latter case,

$$A_{rms} = \frac{Q_{rms}}{k \cdot 44.3 \cdot \sqrt{\overline{dP}}} \quad (4)$$

However, A_{rms} approximates A_{mean}, and Q_{rms} approximates Q_{mean}; if both are substituted in Equation 4, the traditional Gorlin equation is once again obtained.

In addition, in Equation 3, Q refers to the cardiac output divided by the number of seconds per minute occupied by transvalvular flow. Thus,

$$Q = \frac{CO \ (mL/min)}{DFP(s) \cdot HR \ (beats/min)} \quad (5)$$

for the mitral or tricuspid valve and

$$Q = \frac{CO \ (mL/min)}{SEP(s) \cdot HR \ (beats/min)} \quad (6)$$

for the aortic or pulmonic valve, where CO is cardiac output in milliliters per minute, DFP is diastolic filling period in seconds, HR is heart rate in beats per minute, and SEP is systolic ejection period in seconds.

Before the advent of left ventricular catheterization, the Gorlins applied their formula to patients with mitral stenosis. They assumed an end-diastolic pressure of 5 mm Hg, calculated a mitral valve gradient by using a pulmonary capillary wedge tracing for the left atrial pressure, and estimated diastolic flow per second by subtracting the systolic ejection period off an arterial pressure pulse from the RR interval of the electrocardiogram. This approach overestimated the actual diastolic filling period by including the isovolumetric relaxation and contraction periods. When the Gorlins used these algorithms in their initial 11 patients with mitral stenosis, they found that an empiric constant (C) of 0.7 should also be added to the denominator of their equation so that their calculated areas would best correlate with direct measurements of anatomic valve area on either postmortem or surgical specimens. Because they did not have comparable data for the other cardiac valves, an empiric constant of 1.0 was assumed for the application of the formula to aortic, tricuspid, or pulmonic stenosis. Subsequently, after measuring the diastolic filling period directly from simultaneous left ventricular and left atrial pressure pulses, the empiric constant of 0.7 for the mitral valve was revised to 0.85.[26] Thus, since the early 1970s, the most commonly used equations have been as follows:

$$A = \frac{CO/(DFP \cdot HR)}{0.85 \cdot k \cdot 44.3 \cdot \sqrt{\overline{dP}}} = \frac{CO/(DFP \cdot HR)}{k \cdot 37.7 \cdot \sqrt{\overline{dP}}} \quad (7)$$

for the mitral valve and

$$A = \frac{CO/(SFP \cdot HR)}{1.0 \cdot k \cdot 44.3 \cdot \sqrt{\overline{dP}}} = \frac{CO/(SFP \cdot HR)}{k \cdot 44.3 \cdot \sqrt{\overline{dP}}} \quad (8)$$

for the aortic, pulmonic, and tricuspid valves, where A is the anatomic valve orifice area, DFP is the diastolic filling period measured from the opening to the closing of the mitral or tricuspid valve, SFP is the systolic flow period measured from the opening to the closing of the aortic or pulmonic valve, HR is heart rate, k is the combined (C_C, C_V, and 1.166) constant, and $\overline{dP}$ is the average pressure gradient during the DFP or the SFP.

USE OF NOMOGRAM TO COMPUTE VALVE AREA. Once flow per diastolic or systolic second is calculated and the mean pressure gradient is

determined, the valve orifice area can then be readily estimated on a graphic nomogram (Fig. 18–1). In the example shown, a patient with a mean diastolic gradient across the mitral valve of 12 mm Hg, and a transvalvular mitral flow of 88 mL/diastolic second, is shown to have a calculated mitral valve area (using the Gorlin equation and an empiric constant of 37.7) of 0.65 cm^2. Note that if this same patient had exhibited an identical mean diastolic pressure gradient and transvalvular flow per second across the tricuspid valve, the calculated valve orifice area would be even lower at approximately 0.57 cm^2, a difference explained by the empiric constant of 1.0 for the tricuspid, as opposed to 0.85 for the mitral valve.

RELATION BETWEEN THE GORLIN AND CONTINUITY EQUATIONS FOR VALVE AREA. If one converts instantaneous velocity to a pressure gradient, using the simplified Bernoulli equation,[27] then the valve orifice area provided by Equation 3 is very close to that derived from the continuity equation, as used with Doppler two-dimensional echocardiography. Assuming a flat velocity profile, and for contiguous sites where the timing of the passage of blood is the same, then

$$Q_1 = A_1 V_1 \quad (9)$$

and

$$A_1 V_1 = A_2 V_2 \quad (10)$$

where Q_1 is instantaneous flow (milliliters per second), A_1 and A_2 are the cross-sectional areas (square centimeters) of the contiguous sites, and V_1 and V_2 are the instantaneous velocities of flow (centimeters per second) in the same areas. It follows from Equation 9 that

$$Q^2 = A^2 V^2 \quad or \quad A^2 = \frac{Q^2}{V^2} \quad (11)$$

and from the simplified Bernoulli equation,[27]

$$dP = 3.94 \cdot V^2 \quad (12)$$

Substituting in Equation 11,

$$A^2 = \frac{Q^2}{dP/3.94} \quad or \quad A = \frac{Q}{\sqrt{dP/1.98}} \quad (13)$$

Finally, to convert the result to square centimeters (the velocity, V, in the simplified Bernoulli equation is in meters per second), the denominator is multiplied by 100, giving

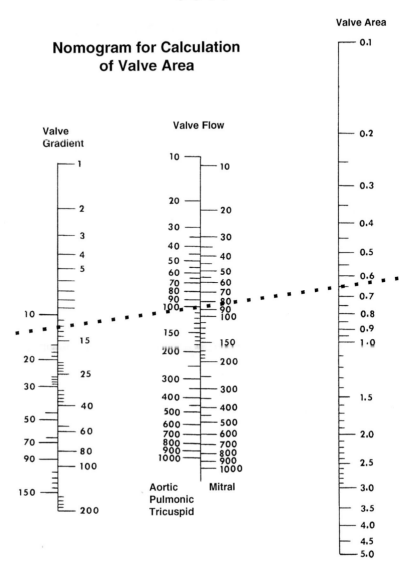

Nomogram for Calculation of Valve Area

Valve Gradient

Valve Flow

Valve Area

Aortic
Pulmonic
Tricuspid

Mitral

Figure 18–1. Valve area (right column, use of Gorlin's equation) calculated from a nomogram that relates the mean valve gradient to transvalvular flow per diastolic or systolic second. The middle column reflects the differing empiric constants for the mitral valve (0.85) versus that for the aortic, pulmonic, and tricuspid valves (1.0). (See text for details of calculation.)

$$A = \frac{Q}{50.4\sqrt{dP}} \qquad (14)$$

The fact that both the Gorlin and continuity equations are derived by the same hydraulic principles undoubtedly explains their strong correlation and near line of identity for estimation of the aortic valve orifice area. The correlation is less valid for the mitral valve where the Gorlin equation has been used with an empiric constant of 0.7 to 0.85 in the denominator.[25]

FLOW DEPENDENCE OF THE GORLIN FORMULA. Although the Gorlin equation remains a valuable index of severity of valve orifice stenosis, it has also been shown to be influenced significantly by the underlying flow conditions.[28–34] Controversy has risen over the ultimate source of the flow dependence of the equation; two

mechanisms appear possible. First, as flow increases, the force available to open the valve would also augment and potentially force the valve to open to a larger area. This mechanism would likely be demonstrated in milder degrees of valve stenosis where the leaflets would be less stiff and calcified. Second, alternatively, the equation may not be applicable under all flow and orifice area conditions; for example, the discharge constants may vary with changes in orifice size or Reynolds number, Re,[35–37] where

$$Re = V \cdot diameter \cdot \frac{\rho}{\mu} \qquad (15)$$

and ρ is blood density (grams per cm^3) and μ is blood viscosity (dynes per second per cm^2).

Cannon and colleagues, using a fixed orifice model in a pulse duplicator system, have demonstrated that the Gorlin formula constant varies directly and linearly with the square root of the mean pressure gradient.[31] They proposed accounting for this dependence by multiplying the constant k by the square root of the pressure gradient, or

$$A = \frac{Q}{k \cdot 44.3 \cdot \sqrt{\overline{dP}} \cdot \sqrt{\overline{dP}}} \quad \text{or} \quad A = \frac{Q}{k \cdot 44.3 \cdot \overline{dP}} \quad (16)$$

where the Q is the transvalvular flow, k is the traditional Gorlin combined constant, and $\overline{dP}$ is the average pressure gradient during the period of transvalvular flow. Cannon and colleagues reported that Equation 16 provided a high correlation ($r = 0.98$) with prosthetic valves of known orifice size installed in their hydraulic system.

If one ignores the constants k and 44.3, Equation 16 is very close mathematically to the inverse of valve resistance, an index defined as

$$R = \frac{\Delta P}{F} \quad (17)$$

where R is resistance, ΔP is the difference in mean pressure across any two points in a circulatory system, and F is the flow between these two points. Before the Gorlins published their formula, other authors had suggested that resistance be used as an index of the severity of valve stenosis.[38, 39] In a series of 40 patients with aortic stenosis, Ford and colleagues found that resistance varied inversely with calculated Gorlin area, but there was significant variation about the mean relation.[40] All of this variability was accounted for by variations in the pressure gradients at each value of calculated area. Moreover, in five published studies of a total of 83 valves, calculated area was found to change at least three times more than resistance when pressure gradient was varied.[41] Casale and associates also reported that increase in transvalvular flow in aortic stenosis, induced by an infusion of dobutamine, caused an increase in the calculated Gorlin area by 0.03 to 0.30 cm², whereas valve resistance did not change.[33] Therefore, there is some rationale for applying the concept of valve resistance, calculated from catheterization data, to quantify severity of valve obstruction. Further analyses, particularly in other valves beside the aortic, are needed before there is widespread application of the concept.

THE GORLIN FORMULA AND ITS DEPENDENCE ON CARDIAC OUTPUT. Calculation of valve orifice area is dependent implicitly on an accurate deter-

mination of transvalvular flow during either systolic ejection (aortic or pulmonic valve) or diastolic filling (mitral or tricuspid valve). Unfortunately, none of the presently available methods for measurement of transvalvular flow is optimally precise or accurate (see Chapter 5). Moreover, in a patient with a low-flow state, or in the presence of valvular regurgitation, determination of cardiac output by both the Fick and indicator dilution methods show differences of greater than 20% in a significant number of people.[42] Both in a low-output state, as well as with significant valve regurgitation where the monoexponential decay of indicator may be lost, the Fick technique is generally acknowledged to be the preferable method for determination of cardiac output. Scrupulous attention to the details of determining the oxygen consumption, however, is essential.

THE GORLIN FORMULA AND COINCIDENT VALVE REGURGITATION. Application of the Gorlin formula to any given cardiac valve is significantly limited when valve regurgitation is concomitantly present and the transvalvular antegrade flow is estimated by measurement of the cardiac output, because an unknown amount of blood is regurgitated and recrosses the valve during the subsequent cardiac cycle. In this circumstance, there is an underestimation of the transvalvular flow per second and a smaller orifice size is calculated than is actually present. Use of left ventricular angiography to estimate total stroke volume allows computation of a regurgitant volume; however, this approach is fraught with all the potential errors in measurement of both systemic cardiac output and left ventricular volume (see Chapters 5 and 8).

ESTIMATION OF SEVERITY OF VALVE REGURGITATION. Regurgitation through either an atrioventricular or semilunar valve is determined by the size of the valve orifice while incompetent, the time interval of regurgitation, and the total stroke volume of the ejecting ventricle. The stroke volume is, in turn, related to the adaptations in the ejecting ventricle to increased diastolic filling, that is, the compensatory increase in preload, the increase in size of the ejecting chamber, and the integrity of myocardial contractility.[43] Methods implemented in the cardiac catheterization laboratory to quantitate regurgitation have included indicator dilution techniques,[44-47] catheter-tip velocity transducers,[48] upstream sampling of xenon 133,[49] and, finally and most important, contrast angiography.[50-57] In the 1990s only the latter technique is used with regularity to assess severity of valve leakage. Contrast angiography, preferably when performed in a biplane mode, is also the primary mode for quantitating ventricular size and function (end-diastolic and end-systolic volumes) and total stroke volume (TSV) in the setting of atrioventricular or semilunar valve regurgitation (see Chapter 8). If net forward stroke volume (FSV) is calculated from either a Fick or an indicator dilution determination, one can then determine the regurgitant volume (RV) and regurgitant fraction (RF) per beat as,[50, 51]

$$RV = TSV - FSV \qquad (18)$$

and

$$RF = (TSV - FSV)/TSV \qquad (19)$$

As detailed in Table 18–1, semiquantitative criteria have been established that, when combined with clinical and noninvasive diagnostic features, serve to categorize the severity of a volume overload imposed by valve leakage.[57]

CAVEATS ABOUT SEMIQUANTITATIVE EVALUATION OF VALVE REGURGITATION. Although there is a general correspondence between contrast angiographic indices of regurgitation (regurgitant volume and regurgitant fraction) and the semiquantitative assessment of the leakage, there are many instances where the two approaches are at variance.[57] Such variance appears to be particularly notable in patients with 3+ or 4+ degrees of regurgitation and significant dilation of the left ventricle (Fig. 18–2). Thus, care should be exercised in using the semiquantitative method alone as a criterion for correction of the valve leakage.

It is also recognized that the stimulation of premature ventricular contractions during the course of either left or right ventricular contrast agent injection may significantly influence the presence and severity of valve regurgitation across the corresponding atrioventricular valve.

Special effort should be taken, therefore, to avoid premature contractions during the course of filming.

Tricuspid and pulmonic regurgitation, using the right atrium, right ventricle, and pulmonary artery as the index chambers, can also be assessed by similar criteria to those used for mitral and aortic regurgitation, respectively. However, the degree of regurgitation may be partially affected by the need to place a catheter through either the pulmonic or tricuspid orifice, with consequential holding open of one or more valve leaflets.

Finally, simultaneous filming of the contrast agent injection in orthogonal, biplane projections helps avoid the confounding effects of inadequate roentgenographic penetration of the cardiac chambers and valves under study.

HEMODYNAMIC AND ANGIOGRAPHIC STUDY OF INDIVIDUAL VALVE LESIONS

Mitral Stenosis

INDICATIONS. In patients with mitral stenosis, cardiac catheterization and angiography usually are performed before cardiac surgery even though the clinical features of the lesion are quite typical, and all noninvasive diagnostic information point to the presence of moderate to severe obstruction. In experienced hands the risk of morbidity or mortality during the procedure is quite small, and the data obtained certifies the relation between the patient's symptoms and objective measurements of the transvalvular pressure gradient, cardiac output, level of the pulmonary venous pressure, and the calculated valve orifice area. Some authors have argued, nevertheless, that an invasive investigation, in

Table 18–1. **Assessment of Severity of Valvular Regurgitation by Cine Contrast Angiography**

Grade of Severity	Regurgitant Fraction	Mitral Regurgitation	Aortic Regurgitation
0	0	No regurgitation	No regurgitation
1+	0.1–0.2	Contrast agent in LA only near mitral valve; clears in next diastole	Contrast agent in LV outflow tract only
2+	0.1–0.3	Regurgitation to mid LA but not progressive; contrast agent persists in LA on next diastole	Contrast agent in LV body; persists for up to 1 beat
3+	0.2–0.4	Contrast agent fills entire LA over 2 or 3 beats; LA density less than that in LV	Progressively fills entire LV cavity in 2 or 3 beats; LV density < ascending aorta
4+	0.4–0.8	Contrast agent fills into pulmonary veins on 1 beat; LA density ≥ LV	Contrast fills entire LV on 1 beat; LV density ≥ aorta

LA, left atrial; LV, left ventricular.

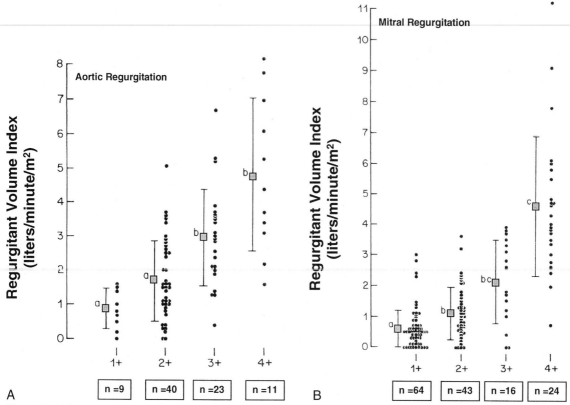

Figure 18–2. Plots relating regurgitant volume index to subjective determination of severity of aortic regurgitation *(A)* and mitral regurgitation *(B)* by selective contrast angiography. (Reprinted by permission of the publisher from Croft CH, Lipscomb K, Mathis K, et al: Limitations of qualitative angiographic grading in aortic or mitral regurgitation. American Journal of Cardiology 53:1593–1598. Copyright 1984 by Excerpta Medica Inc.)

the setting of definite clinical and echocardiographic signs of mitral stenosis, is superfluous and does not influence the ultimate operative result.[58, 59] Other authors have questioned whether some patients, without catheterization, will be scheduled for surgery before it is required.[60, 61] Moreover, in the United States, where many patients with mitral stenosis are middle aged or older, there is a need to determine coronary artery anatomy before proceeding with thoracotomy and cardiopulmonary bypass. Finally, preoperative catheterization and angiography provide baseline information for later evaluation if surgery is postponed or the results of valve surgery are not as salutary as expected.

TECHNICAL CONSIDERATIONS. Essential to the invasive investigation of mitral stenosis, either at rest or during exercise, are (1) measurement of an accurate cardiac output and (2) recording of an accurate phasic pressure gradient across the mitral valve. In most patients with mitral stenosis, a high-quality pulmonary capillary wedge tracing matches well with a direct left atrial pressure pulse.[62] If a resting pulmonary

capillary wedge tracing of high quality cannot be obtained, transseptal puncture of the left atrium can then be performed (see Chapter 2). It is also sound practice to record the pulmonary capillary wedge pressure in several loci of the pulmonary vasculature. This may help to rule out coincident and localized pulmonary venous obstruction as a source of the pressure gradient. Although equivalent to the left atrial pressure, the pulmonary capillary wedge tracing is usually delayed by 40 to 120 msec, with the peak of the v wave occurring after the downslope of the left ventricular pressure pulse. The peak a and v wave pressures on the pulmonary capillary wedge tracing are usually approximately 2 or 3 mm Hg less, and the troughs of the x and y descents approximately 2 or 3 mm Hg greater, than the same values on the direct left atrial pressure pulse (Fig. 18–3A); the mean pressures for both tracings, therefore, are generally equivalent. There is usually superior correspondence with the true left atrial pressure when an end-hole catheter (e.g., Cournand), positioned in the distal ramifications of the pulmonary vascular bed, as opposed to a balloon occlusion catheter, is used to record the pulmo-

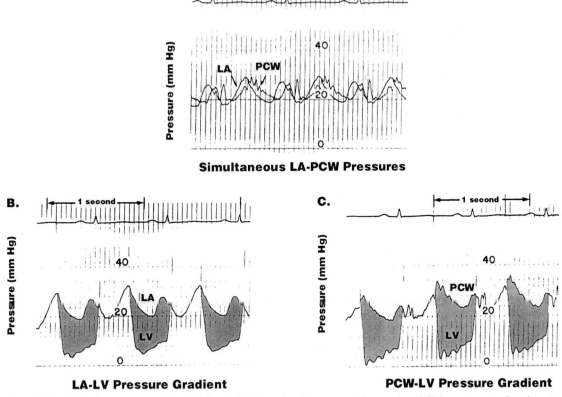

Figure 18–3. *A,* Simultaneous recording of left atrial (LA) and pulmonary capillary wedge (PCW) pressure tracings in a patient with mitral stenosis. Note the temporal delay of PCW versus LA and the slight inequality of a and v waves and the troughs of the *x* and *y* descents. *B,* Simultaneous registration of LA and left ventricular (LV) pressure pulses in a patient with mitral stenosis. *C,* Simultaneous registration of PCW and left ventricular pressure pulses in the same patient as in *B.* Note the change in the shape of the area of pressure gradient compared with direct LA-LV tracing. (See text for discussion.) (From Lange RA, Moore DM, Cigarroa RG, Hillis LD: Use of pulmonary capillary wedge pressure to assess severity of mitral stenosis: Is true left atrial pressure needed in this condition? J Am Coll Cardiol 1989; 13:825–829.)

nary capillary pressure. Before calculating the mean transvalvular pressure gradient from a pulmonary capillary wedge tracing, it is advisable to phase shift the latter tracing so that the peak of the v wave matches temporally the same pressure on the left ventricular pressure pulse (Fig. 18–3*B* and *C*).

PATHOPHYSIOLOGY. The fundamental abnormality of cardiac function in mitral stenosis is mechanical obstruction to emptying of the left atrium with development of a diastolic pressure gradient between the left atrium and ventricle (Fig. 18–4). With moderate to severe mitral stenosis, the overall profile of diastolic flow into the left ventricle is blunted so that distinct rapid-filling and slow-filling phases are no longer seen before atrial systole. The pressure difference between the left atrium and ventricle is relatively high during early diastole, declines slowly throughout mid and late diastole (delayed *y* descent), and then, if normal sinus

rhythm persists, the gradient again augments with atrial contraction (a wave). The height of the a wave depends on the integrity of left atrial contractility and the severity of valve obstruction. Provided there is mild to moderate valve obstruction of relatively short duration, atrial contractility remains normal, a relatively large a wave is generated, and adequate left ventricular diastolic filling is maintained. If the valve orifice area progressively narrows, impedance to filling increases, the left atrium dilates, its contractile function declines, and overall diastolic filling of the left ventricle is then compromised. If atrial fibrillation supervenes, left atrial contractile function disappears and the a wave can no longer be seen on the left atrial pressure pulse (Fig. 18–5); coincidentally, there is a reduction in diastolic left ventricular filling and the cardiac output. The height of the v wave during ventricular systole depends on the compliance of the left atrium, the rate and magnitude of

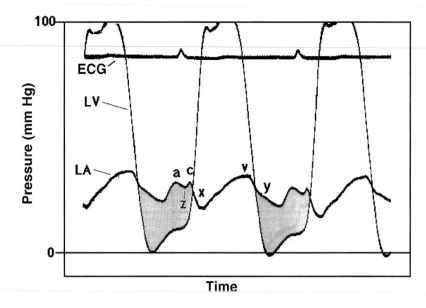

Figure 18–4. High-fidelity micromanometric tracings of left ventricular (LV) and left atrial (LA) pressures in a patient with pure, severe mitral stenosis. Note the pan-diastolic pressure gradient between the two chambers, and the characteristic delay in the y descent on the LA pressure pulse. The z point on the LA pressure pulse coincides with mitral valve closure and end-diastolic pressure on the LV pressure pulse,

left atrial filling, and the presence and magnitude of coincident mitral regurgitation.

RELATION BETWEEN TRANSMITRAL FLOW AND PRESSURE GRADIENT. Analysis of the relation between transmitral diastolic flow and the coincident pressure gradient, at various degrees of severity of mitral valve obstruction (as calculated by the Gorlin equation), facilitates understanding of the clinical manifestations of mitral stenosis. As shown in Figure 18–6, the normal mitral valve orifice is 4.0 to 6.0 cm², and large increases in diastolic flow, even at peak exercise, result in a minimal increase in the transvalvular pressure gradient. With moderate narrowing of the mitral orifice area (<1.5 cm²), the mean left atrial pressure may become mildly elevated at rest (>12 mm Hg,), but augments to 15 to 25 mm

Hg with physical exertion. However, as the valve orifice diminishes to 1.0 cm² or less, small increases in transmitral flow result in a relatively large increase in the pressure gradient. At this stage of the disease, the increased left atrial pressure during or immediately after physical exertion may lead to pulmonary edema (see Fig. 18–6).

EFFECT OF ASSOCIATED CONDITIONS. Other concurrent conditions or illnesses associated with an augmented cardiac output, such as pregnancy, thyrotoxicosis, and anemia, exaggerate the pressure gradient in mitral stenosis. In these circumstances, a measurement of the pressure gradient alone may give a misleading impression of the severity of mitral stenosis. For example, if the cardiac output is unusually high

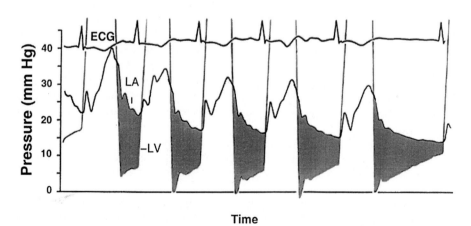

Figure 18–5. Fluid-filled catheter pressure recordings of left ventricular (LV) and left atrial (LA) pressure pulses in a patient with atrial fibrillation and severe mitral stenosis. There is no a wave on the LA pressure pulse. Note the reduction in the mean diastolic gradient as the RR interval lengthens. (See text for discussion.)

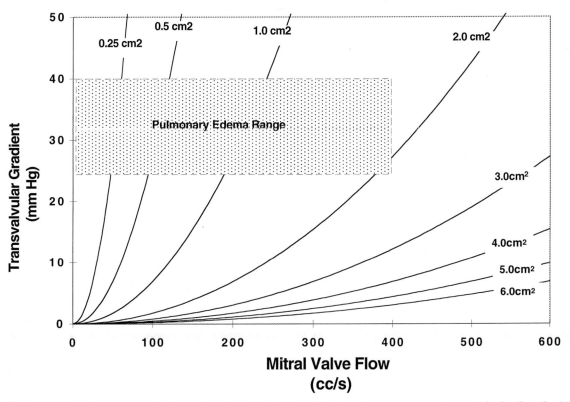

Figure 18–6. Plot of mean transvalvular gradient (vertical axis) in millimeters of mercury versus transmitral valve flow (horizontal axis) in milliliters per second for valve orifice areas of various sizes (isopleths from 0.25 to 6.0 cm²). Calculated valve orifice areas are based on Gorlin's equation with an empiric constant of 0.85. The shaded area indicates the range of valve orifice sizes and flow values over which a patient may exhibit pulmonary edema. (See text for discussion.)

(double the normal value), then for any given valve orifice size, the left atrial pressure will be markedly elevated (quadruple the value at a normal cardiac output). Conversely, if the cardiac output is low, a mild or moderate elevation of the left atrial pressure may belie the presence of severe stenosis (see Fig. 18–6).

EFFECT OF HEART RATE. Heart rate exerts an important influence on the pathophysiologic manifestations of mitral stenosis because diastolic flow per minute across the mitral valve depends not only on the valve orifice area and pressure gradient but also on the duration of diastole. Increased frequency of contraction occurs primarily at the expense of diastolic filling time, and the duration of left ventricular systole shortens only slightly. Thus, as the RR interval shortens in the patient with mitral stenosis, there is less time for the left atrial and ventricular pressures to equilibrate, and the mean left atrial pressure increases (see Fig. 18–5). An increase in heart rate with physical exertion, or during an atrial arrhythmia (e.g., atrial fibrillation) with a rapid ventricular response, often precipitates increased severity of symptoms.

PULMONARY VENOUS AND ARTERIAL HYPERTENSION AND RIGHT HEART FAILURE. In some patients with mitral stenosis, in whom the left atrial pressure rises slowly and gradually over a period of years, a left atrial mean pressure as high as 30 to 35 mm Hg can be tolerated without the development of extravasation of fluid into the intraalveolar space.[63] The speed with which lung fluid accumulates at any given pulmonary capillary pressure appears related primarily to lymphatic drainage capacity, which may vary from patient to patient, and to individual variations in alveloar-capillary barrier permeability, as well as interstitial oncotic and hydrostatic pressures.[64-66] In contrast, a relatively sudden increase in left atrial pressure, as might be provoked by exercise testing during the cardiac catheterization procedure, may induce a rapid accumulation of lung fluid with attendant pulmonary edema.

With persistent elevation of the left atrial pressure at rest, there is a coincident increase in the pulmonary arterial pressure, referable to two major factors: (1) retrograde transmission of the elevated pressures within the left atrium, pulmonary veins, and pulmonary capillaries and

(2) an increase in the pulmonary vascular resistance that, in most patients, appears totally reversible once the mitral valve obstruction is relieved.[67-69] In some patients reactive vasoconstriction is accompanied by morphologic changes (intimal proliferation and medial thickening in the walls of the small pulmonary arteries).[70] In time, worsening of the mitral valve obstruction, loss of left atrial contractile function, onset of atrial fibrillation, and an increasingly resistant pulmonary vascular bed all serve to reduce the cardiac output. There is then a limit to any further increase in left atrial pressure, which may even fall somewhat as the cardiac output becomes significantly diminished. In advanced, severe mitral stenosis, the pulmonary artery pressure may equal or exceed systemic arterial pressure, and the right ventricle is subjected to a sustained high pressure overload, eventually culminating in tricuspid regurgitation and right heart failure.

EXERCISE HEMODYNAMICS. Measurements during supine exercise of intracardiac and pulmonary pressures, as well as cardiac output and the arteriovenous oxygen difference, are particularly useful in quantifying the severity of stenosis in patients with equivocally severe valve obstruction. Or, in some patients there may be a discrepancy between the preprocedure symptoms and the resting hemodynamic measurements. For example, some patients with mild to moderate mitral stenosis become very symptomatic with physical exertion despite normal rest hemodynamic findings. Often, in this latter group, a significant elevation of the pulmonary capillary and pulmonary artery pressures occurs owing to very high heart rates and short diastolic filling intervals with exercise; or, these patients may develop an inappropriate increase in pulmonary vascular resistance as the left atrial pressure increases.[71]

Again, as can be deduced from Figure 18–6, in patients with a valve area of less than 1.0 cm², the transmitral gradient rises precipitously with the diastolic flow and heart rate increase brought about by exercise. Concomitantly, the left atrial, pulmonary capillary wedge, pulmonary artery, and right ventricular pressures elevate. During exertion these same patients exhibit a reduction in cardiac output relative to their increase in total body oxygen consumption, and an inappropriate widening of the arteriovenous oxygen difference.[72-74] Other pathophysiologic factors that may contribute to a reduced exercise capacity include (1) an increase in lung stiffness secondary to chronic pulmonary venous congestion and pulmonary

hemosiderosis[75, 76]; (2) left ventricular dysfunction secondary to reduced preload and contractile disturbances[77-86] (see later); and (3) right ventricular dysfunction secondary to a sustained pressure overload associated with pulmonary hypertension.[87]

FLUOROSCOPY. Visualization by fluoroscopy of the mitral valve annulus and apparatus, either in the right anterior oblique or cranially angulated left anterior oblique projection, yields important information as to the extent of valvular and perivalvular calcification, the mobility of the mitral valve leaflets, and the rigidity of the subvalvular apparatus. In rheumatic mitral stenosis nodular calcification is often distributed variably throughout the valve leaflets; in contrast, in degenerative calcific mitral stenosis of the elderly, the calcium is predominantly annular in distribution or may form a crescent at the base of the posterior leaflet. Extensive leaflet and subvalvular apparatus calcification limits successful valvuloplasty (either surgically or by percutaneous balloon dilation) and portends a need for prosthetic valve replacement.

LEFT VENTRICULOGRAPHY. Contrast cine left ventriculography is performed routinely at the time of cardiac catheterization to assess left ventricular contractility, mitral valve anatomy and pliability, and the presence or absence of mitral regurgitation.

A number of investigations have uncovered the presence of left ventricular dysfunction in the resting state in some, but not all, patients with mitral stenosis.[77-86] Potential causes of this dysfunction appear related to an immobilization of the posterolateral and posterobasal segments of the left ventricle by a rigid mitral valve annulus and valve, foci of myocardial fibrosis related to previous or ongoing rheumatic myocarditis, chronic underfilling of the chamber due to inflow obstruction, or an inordinately high end-systolic stress. Any one or more of these abnormalities can lead to reduction in the resting ejection fraction that is mild compared with the other hemodynamic alterations seen in mitral stenosis. Paradoxically, in some patients a higher than normal end-diastolic volume index has been found.[83, 85, 86]

The left ventricular contrast angiogram can also be helpful for defining mitral valve pathoanatomy and function. The motion of the mitral valve leaflets is usually best seen in profile in either a right anterior oblique or direct left lateral projection. With commissural fusion the normal M-shaped motion of the anterior leaflet is lost; instead, the fused anterior and posterior leaflets form a dome over the valve orifice that can be seen throughout diastole filling. The greater the calcification and commissural fusion, the greater the limitation of valve motion. In some patients, a negative contrast jet can be seen as inflow into the left ventricle is restricted by the narrowed central valve orifice. In many patients there is evidence of chordal fusion and shortening that contributes to the malfunctioning of the valve. Both chordal anatomy, as well as the presence or absence of valvular calcification, are weighed carefully by the surgeon in the decision about whether to perform a mitral valvulotomy (closed or open) or to implant a valve prosthesis.

Rarely, the contrast left ventriculogram visualizes and reveals unsuspected mitral valve obstruction due to a ball-valve tumor (e.g., a myxoma [Fig. 18–7]) or thrombus. Also, infrequently, a congenital deformation of the mitral valve is uncovered, as in the parachute mitral valve where large, redundant leaflets can be seen to dome and prolapse off a single papillary muscle at the base of the ventricle.

LEFT ATRIAL ANGIOGRAPHY. If a supravalvular membrane (cor triatriatum), with or without concomitant mitral valve obstruction, is suspected as a cause of reduced diastolic left ventricular filling, then contrast opacification of the left atrium is desirable. This can be accomplished directly via injection of contrast material through a transseptal catheter placed into the left atrium or indirectly by injection into a pulmonary artery catheter with filming over the left atrium during the levophase passage of the contrast agent.

SELECTIVE CORONARY ANGIOGRAPHY. This procedure is also performed in older patients (older than 40 years of age) or in younger patients with chest pain in order to uncover latent or occult coronary artery disease that is high-risk before a surgical or balloon valvuloplasty procedure. Occasionally, coronary angiography detects either a left atrial thrombus or tumor by visualizing neovascularization originating from an atrial branch off either the circumflex or right coronary arteries.

Mitral Regurgitation

INDICATIONS. Cardiac catheterization and angiography are performed in the patient with mitral regurgitation whenever its cause or severity remains ambiguous, or in the patient being considered for surgical valve repair or prosthetic valve replacement. On rare occasion a cardiologist confronts a young, symptomatic patient with severe and isolated mitral regurgitation, along with left atrial and left ventricular dilation demonstrable by two-dimensional echocardiography with color Doppler imaging, who can be safely referred for surgical therapy without a cardiac catheterization and left ventriculography being performed preoperatively.

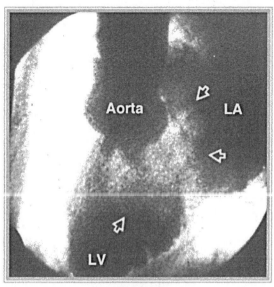
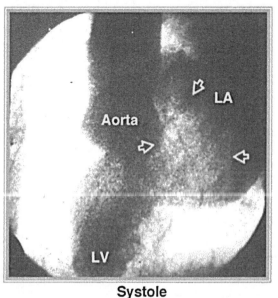

Diastole   Systole

Figure 18–7. Left ventriculogram of a patient with a left atrial myxoma attached to the interatrial septum. Note that during diastole the tumor mass *(arrows)* moves through the mitral valve, obstructing the orifice. During systole, it is ejected backward into the left atrium.

Both right and left heart pressure measurements, along with a cine left ventriculogram, should be performed during the procedure. In patients 40 years of age or older, or if coronary artery disease is suspected as a cause of the mitral regurgitation, selective coronary angiography should also be performed.

TECHNICAL CONSIDERATIONS. As in the study of mitral stenosis, particular attention should be paid to the quality and characteristics of the pulmonary capillary wedge, pulmonary artery, and left ventricular pressure pulses. Use of an end-hole catheter, wedged far into the periphery of the lung, rather than a proximal balloon occlusion catheter, provides a superior pulmonary capillary wedge tracing. In entering the left ventricle, the operator must be careful not to pass the catheter through chordal structures and cause iatrogenic mitral regurgitation. Simultaneous registration of the left ventricular and pulmonary capillary wedges tracing help assess the presence or absence of coexistent mitral stenosis.

PATHOPHYSIOLOGY. The fundamental abnormality of cardiac function in mitral regurgitation (insufficiency) is retrograde ejection of a portion of the left ventricular systolic stroke volume into the left atrium with augmentation of left ventricular filling during the rapid filling period of the subsequent diastole. Leakage of the mitral valve may commence as soon as the left ventricular pressure in early systole exceeds that in the left atrium and extend throughout systole until the left ventricular pressure falls below that in the left atrium; or, the leakage may occur only during the mid-portion and latter portions of systole. In either circumstance, a volume overload of varying degree is placed on the left ventricle, which must then undergo adaptive changes to maintain systemic cardiac output within normal limits.

An important pathophysiologic characteristic of mitral insufficiency relates to the relatively favorable loading conditions provided by the low-impedance pathway for blood to exit from the left ventricle. Because pressure in the left atrium is much lower than that in the aorta, with mitral regurgitation the average afterload or active tension in the wall of the left ventricular chamber tends to fall more abruptly than normal late in systole, and this effect favors increased shortening of the myocardial wall because of the inverse relation between force and fiber shortening (and velocity).[88] Also, myocardial oxygen consumption is little affected by the increased volume load imposed by mitral regurgitation. It is believed that these favorable loading conditions, as well as the minimal effect on myocardial oxygen consumption, explain the notable tolerance of patients for this lesion and their relatively prolonged clinical course.[89]

LEFT VENTRICULAR ADAPTATIONS. The left ventricular chamber size enlarges as a result of increased fiber stretch, replication of sarcomeres in both series and parallel, and possibly reorientation of myofiber alignment.[43] Thus, the left ventricle manifests a pattern of eccentric hypertrophy where the mass-to-volume ratio remains relatively normal. These adaptive changes allow delivery of a much larger than normal total stroke volume but with maintenance of a normal extent of shortening of each unit of the enlarged ventricular circumference.

Although the left ventricle uses the Frank-Starling mechanism (increased fiber stretch) to increase total stroke volume in mitral regurgitation, the increase in end-diastolic volume is out of proportion to the increase in end-diastolic pressure. In fact, the end-diastolic pressure in chronic mitral regurgitation may remain within normal limits despite large increases in end-diastolic volume.[90] This shift of the diastolic pressure-volume relation to the right allows the ventricle to generate large stroke volumes without subjecting the lungs to high pulmonary venous pressure.

With chronic, severe mitral regurgitation, myocardial contractility eventually becomes depressed and left ventricular function deteriorates despite the favorable outlet impedance conditions. This stage is marked by a reduction in the extent of shortening (low normal or reduced ejection fraction), an increase in the residual (end-systolic) volume of the ventricle, and a rise in the end-diastolic pressure into an abnormal range. Pulmonary venous and pulmonary arterial hypertension then develop, and the events in the right-sided heart parallel those described for mitral stenosis with pulmonary hypertension.

In contrast with the gradual evolution of left ventricular adaptations described for chronic, mitral regurgitation, acute mitral leakage, usually caused by a ruptured chordae tendineae, is associated with marked elevation of the left atrial pressure (as a consequence of a large v wave and high end-diastolic pressure in the left ventricle), pulmonary hypertension, and reduced cardiac output. Acute pulmonary edema may also develop in this setting.

LEFT ATRIAL ADAPTATIONS. With chronic mitral regurgitation the left atrium responds by progressive dilation with an associated increase in its capacitance and elasticity.[91] This change

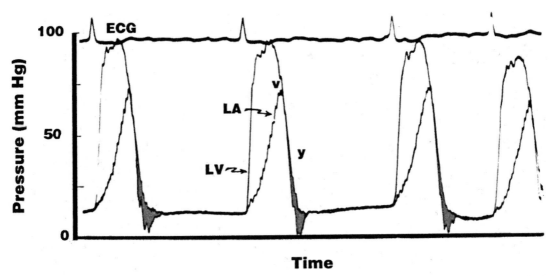

Figure 18–8. Left ventricular (LV) and left atrial (LA) pressure pulses in a patient with isolated, severe mitral regurgitation and atrial fibrillation. The a and c waves in the LA tracing are not evident, and the v wave is markedly accentuated to nearly 70 mm Hg. The LA *y* descent follows closely the decline in pressure in the LV. A small pressure gradient (gray area) is evident during the phase of rapid diastolic filling because of the large volume of antegrade flow across the valve. (From Peterson KL, Ross J Jr: Cardiac catheterization and angiography. *In* Braunwald E, Isselbacher K, Petersdorf R, et al [eds]: Harrison's Principles of Internal Medicine, 11th ed. New York, McGraw-Hill, 1987.)

in the size and material properties of the left atrial chamber allows the storage of a much larger percentage of the regurgitant volume and mitigates the elevation of the large v wave and left atrial mean pressure as seen in acute mitral regurgitation.

HEMODYNAMIC MEASUREMENTS. Pressure measurements either in the pulmonary arterial wedge or left atrial positions usually reveal an elevated v wave (>20 mm Hg peak value), followed by a relatively rapid *y* descent as the mitral valve opens and an excessive inflow of blood traverses the mitral valve (Fig. 18–8). There is not uncommonly a small pressure gradient across the mitral valve during early diastole, reflecting functional mitral stenosis in the presence of increased flow (see Fig. 18–8). If the mitral regurgitation is relatively acute and severe, a very large v wave is generated owing to the fact that the left atrium remains relatively normal sized and noncompliant and left ventricular shortening remains normal to supernormal (see Fig. 18–8). If the *v* wave is sufficiently large, it may be seen superimposed on the pulmonary artery pressure tracing. Conversely, in long-standing severe mitral regurgitation, the v wave may be extremely small owing to massive dilation of the left atrium and a significant increase in its capacitance.[92] When myocardial contractility becomes severely diminished, depression of the total stroke volume may also contribute to the lack of generation of a significantly elevated v wave.

The effective cardiac output depends on the severity of the regurgitant leak, the acuteness versus chronicity of the process, the adaptations of the left ventricle to the volume overload, and the maintenance of normal myocardial contractility. Generally, unless the mitral regurgitation is of acute onset, cardiac output remains normal at rest until relatively late in the natural history of the disease. Although there are inconsistent findings with exercise, the patient with mitral regurgitation generally manifests a subnormal increase in the cardiac output with exercise. One study analyzed the severity of regurgitation during exercise and found no change.[93]

EFFECT OF LOADING CONDITIONS. It is well recognized that the v wave height is very sensitive to loading conditions and the dynamic changes in the severity of mitral regurgitation.[94] For example, hand gripping, a physiologic intervention that increases systemic arterial pressure, augments heart rate and myocardial contractility, and increases in left ventricular end-diastolic volume cause the height of the v wave to markedly increase (Fig. 18–9). Conversely, administration of a pharmacologic agent that diminishes left ventricular afterload, such as nitroprusside or hydralazine, causes a significant reduction in the height and prominence of the v wave as the degree of mitral regurgitation diminishes.

LEFT VENTRICULOGRAPHY. The severity of mi-

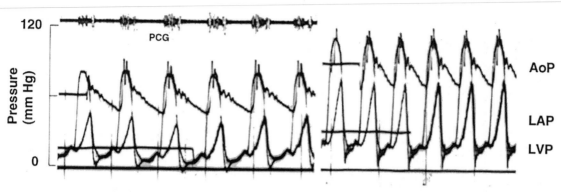

Figure 18–9. Pressure tracings in the aorta (AoP), left atrium (LAP), and left ventricle (LVP), along with a phonocardiogram (PCG) at rest and during hand-gripping intervention. The LAP and LVP tracings are recorded with micromanometric catheters. Note the marked increase in the v wave of the LAP tracing as the aortic pressure increases in response to the hand-gripping maneuver. (Courtesy of Prof. Hans Peter Krayenbuhl, Policlinic, Department of Medicine, University of Zurich.)

tral valve leakage is best estimated by use of selective left ventricular cineangiography (see Table 18–1). The density of contrast agent that enters the left atrium retrograde from the left ventricle can be appreciated; moreover, the size of the left atrium can be assessed and regurgitation of blood into the pulmonary veins can be observed. By measuring the total stroke volume of the left ventricle and subtracting from it the systemic stroke volume (calculated from heart rate and cardiac output measured by either Fick or indicator-dilution techniques), the amount of regurgitant flow into the left atrium can be quantitated (see earlier). When mitral regurgitation is severe, the regurgitant fraction of the total stroke volume may be well in excess of 0.50.

Left ventricular cineangiography, particularly in the right anterior oblique or lateral projections, allows visualization of the mitral valve anatomy and in some patients demonstration of a flail mitral valve leaflet, as seen in myxomatous degeneration of the mitral valve (Fig. 18–10).

Combined Mitral Stenosis and Insufficiency

Combined mitral stenosis and insufficiency is often associated with a heavily calcified valve that has limited leaflet mobility and a "fish-mouth" central orifice. Because systolic regurgitation augments antegrade flow during the subsequent diastole, a transvalvular pressure gradient can develop in patients with a relatively mild compromise of the mitral orifice area (approximately 2.0 cm²). Significant dilation of the left

atrium is seen owing to the combined pressure and volume overload on the chamber. Unless rheumatic myocarditis is still active, there is usually only mild to moderate dilation of the left ventricle, and myocardial failure is not as commonly observed as in patients with pure mitral regurgitation. It is of interest that combined (stenosis and regurgitation) lesion of the mitral valve confers a worse survival curve than an isolated lesion by itself.[95] The presence of pulmonary hypertension is also clearly associated with a worsened prognosis.[96]

HEMODYNAMIC MEASUREMENTS. In the setting of combined mitral stenosis and insufficiency, the pressure pulses from the left heart reveal an early and mid-diastolic gradient across the mitral valve, but if the diastolic filling period is sufficiently long, the left atrial and left ventricular pressures equilibrate during the period of slow ventricular filling (Fig. 18–11). The v wave is often dominant, reflecting the augmented systolic expansion and dilation of the left atrium. To estimate the orifice size of the mitral valve, true diastolic flow must be calculated as the sum of right ventricular stroke volume and the amount of retrograde regurgitation from the left ventricle on the previous systole. The amount of regurgitation is calculated as the difference between total left ventricular stroke volume (measured on a contrast left ventricular angiogram) and the stroke volume calculated from a Fick or indicator-dilution cardiac output and the resting heart rate.

Aortic Stenosis

INDICATIONS. Although noninvasive Doppler measurements have significantly helped the

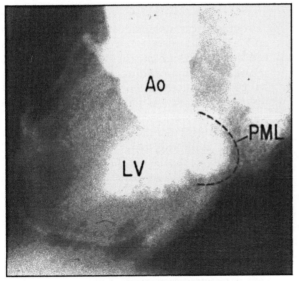 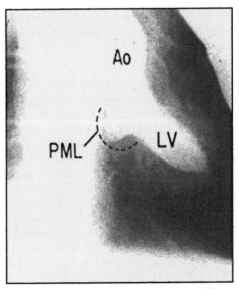

Left Anterior Oblique   **Right Anterior Oblique**

Figure 18–10. Left ventriculogram, end-systole, in the left anterior oblique and right anterior oblique projections in a patient with a flail posterior mitral leaflet (PML) secondary to a ruptured chordal structure. The dotted lines outline the extent of the posterior displacement of the leaflet at the end of ejection. Ao, aorta; LV, left ventricle.

quantification of the severity of valve obstruction in aortic stenosis, cardiac catheterization and angiography continue to be indicated in most patients with this diagnosis. Important information to be obtained by the invasive study are (1) confirmation of the severity of valve obstruction and determination of associated valve lesions such as mitral regurgitation, mitral stenosis, or aortic regurgitation; (2) the presence or absence of significant coronary artery disease that might require operative revascularization at the time of an aortic valve replacement or reconstruction; and (3) assessment of the left ventricular diastolic filling pressures as they reflect the compliance properties of the left ventricular chamber. It is also crucial in some

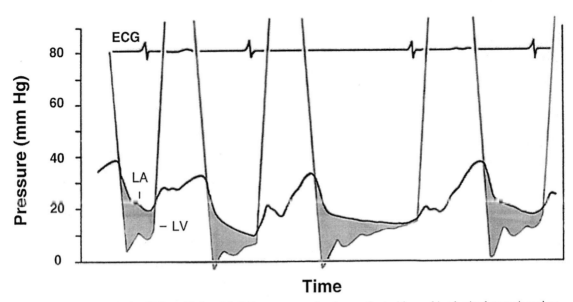

Figure 18–11. Left ventricular (LV) and left atrial (LA) pressure pulses in a patient with combined mitral stenosis and regurgitation. Note that the transvalvular gradient (gray area) disappears near the end of diastolic filling on beats with a long RR interval on the electrocardiogram (ECG). The patient is in atrial fibrillation and thus there is no a wave on the LA pressure pulse.

patients to document that the left ventricular outflow obstruction exists at the level of the aortic valve and not either below or above (see Chapters 21 and 25).

TECHNICAL CONSIDERATIONS. Most commonly, the aortic valve pressure gradient is recorded by use of a left ventricular catheter, placed retrograde across the aortic valve, that is then pulled back into the ascending aorta (Fig. 18–12). Provided the RR interval of all beats on the pullback remain the same, the left ventricular and ascending aortic tracings can then be superimposed (either manually or by computer processing) for calculation of the maximum and mean gradients. Pullback gradients can be confounded, however, by (1) improper registration of the left ventricular and ascending aortic pressure pulses; (2) presence of pulsus alternans (see Fig. 18–12); (3) stimulation of premature beats on the pullback; (4) effects of the respiratory cycle; and (5) a contribution of the cross section of the retrograde catheter itself to the severity of the aortic valve obstruction.

This effect of the retrograde catheter on the measurement of the aortic valve gradient is particularly notable in severe aortic stenosis, the so-called Carabello sign.[97] As shown in Figure 18–13, withdrawal of a retrograde catheter into the ascending aorta can lead to an immediate rise in the femoral artery pressure pulse, reflecting partial relief of the orifice obstruction. This sign is seen in more than 80% of patients with a valve orifice area smaller than 0.5 cm².

Alternatively to a pullback tracing, the operator can use two catheters, one placed either retrograde or transseptally into the left ventricle and a second placed retrograde into the ascending aorta, to measure simultaneous left ventricular and ascending aortic pressures (Fig. 18–14). A double-lumen pigtail catheter, with the holes placed on either side of the aortic valve, can also be used to register a simultaneous left ventricular–ascending aortic pressure gradient. With this latter approach, however, the operator must be careful that the ascending aortic luminal pressure is not excessively damped. This can be assessed by recording the ascending aortic pressure through both lumina before entering the left ventricle with the distal one.

The least desirable approach is to estimate the aortic valve pressure gradient by using a simultaneous registration of the left ventricular and femoral or brachial artery pressure pulses. These latter pressures are altered by the impedance characteristics of the arterial vascular tree, as discussed in Chapter 3. In 26 patients, Folland and colleagues studied the aortic valve left ventricular–ascending aortic gradient and compared it with the left ventricular–femoral artery pressure gradient, with and without realignment.[98] Without realignment there was a systematic overestimation, and with realignment an underestimation, of the left ventricular–ascending aortic gradient. With realignment the augmented peak systolic pressure serves to underestimate the gradient; without realignment, the inappropriate offset to the right (time delay in registration) serves to augment the gradient.

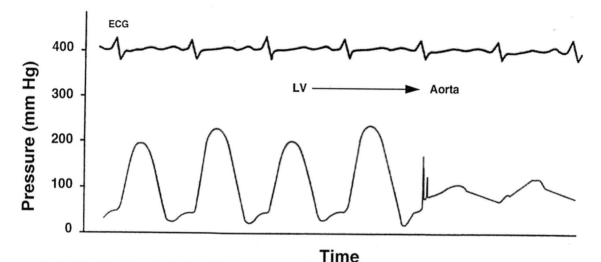

Figure 18–12. Pullback of a micromanometric catheter from the left ventricle (LV) across a stenotic aortic valve into the aorta. Note the nearly 100-mm Hg peak gradient that is demonstrated. Also note that the left ventricular pressure pulse exhibits pulsus alternans and a relatively "isometric" configuration.

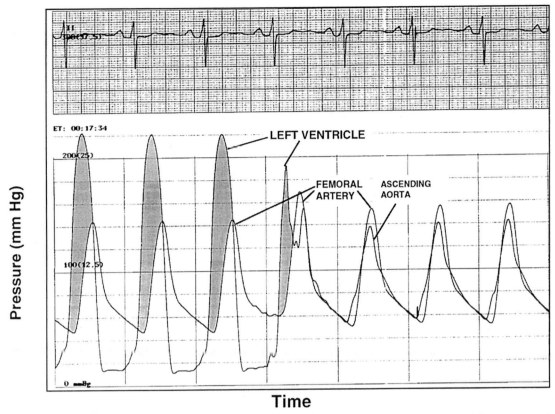

Figure 18–13. Demonstration of the augmentation of femoral artery systolic pressure as a catheter is withdrawn retrograde across a tightly stenotic aortic valve, reflecting partial relief of the orifice obstruction (so-called Carabello's sign). Note also the differences in the timing and configuration of the ascending aortic and femoral pressure pulses.

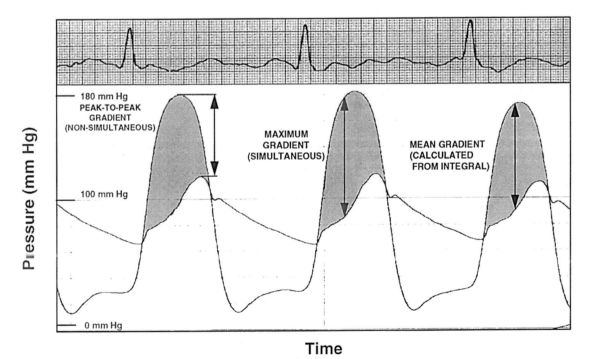

Figure 18–14. Simultaneous micromanometric pressures recorded on either side (left ventricle and ascending aorta) of a tightly stenotic aortic valve. The pressure gradient during systole is shaded gray. The tracing demonstrates the difference in definition of ''peak-to-peak,'' maximum, and mean pressure gradients. Note the delayed upstroke and the early anacrotic notch in the ascending aortic pressure pulse, which are findings typical of severe valvular aortic stenosis.

In cases where the valve orifice area is marginally severe (e.g., 0.7 to 1.0 cm²), the errors inherent in the left ventricular–femoral artery measurements can become crucial. Thus, we prefer the techniques of a pullback, or dual, simultaneous measurements of left ventricular and ascending aortic pressures, to estimate the valve orifice size.

Irrespective of the method for measuring the transvalvular gradient, it is important to perform a careful withdrawal of a catheter (preferably a single-holed or micromanometric catheter) from the body of the left ventricle into the aorta to certify that the pressure gradient exists at the level of the aortic valve and that neither obstructive hypertrophic cardiomyopathy nor a fixed subvalvular obstruction is coexistent and contributing to the pressure overload on the left ventricle.

In those patients with a high-velocity jet during systolic ejection there may be some difficulty in maintaining the selective seating of a coronary angiographic catheter in either the left or right coronary artery orifices. Alternatively, there may be significant poststenotic dilation of the ascending aorta that complicates reaching the coronary orifices with standard catheters. Use of a relatively stiff coronary angiographic catheter, with a longer tip-to-elbow length, usually allows selective engagement of the coronary orifices (see Chapter 9).

PATHOPHYSIOLOGY. The fundamental pathophysiologic abnormality created by aortic valve obstruction is the development of a pressure overload (gradient) during ejection between the left ventricle and the ascending aorta. At normal levels of cardiac output, the aortic valve orifice area must be reduced by more than 60% of its normal area for a significant pressure gradient to be produced. However, a murmur may be created by turbulent flow in the absence of a pressure gradient. As shown in Figure 18–15, by the Gorlin equation there is a nonlinear relation between the pressure and flow across the stenotic orifice, the orifice area being directly related to flow and inversely proportional to the square root of the pressure gradient. Thus, if the cardiac output is reduced by 30%, the pressure gradient will fall by about 50%, and the severity of the stenosis will be underestimated if the pressure gradient alone is relied on. With a normal cardiac output, mild aortic stenosis is associated with valve orifice calcula-

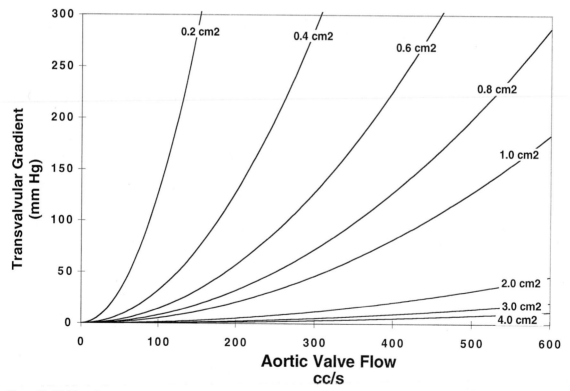

Figure 18–15. Plot of mean transvalvular gradient (vertical axis) in millimeters of mercury versus transaortic valve flow (horizontal axis) in milliliters per second for valve orifice areas of various sizes (isopleths from 0.2 to 4.0 cm²). Calculated valve orifice areas are based on Gorlin's equation with an empiric constant of 1.0. (See text for discussion.)

tions ranging between 1.0 and 1.5 cm^2 (normal area is equal to 2.5 to 4.0 cm^2). Moderate stenosis is present with a valve area of 0.7 to 1.0 cm^2. With severe stenosis, the valve orifice area usually is 0.5 cm^2 or less, and the transvalvular pressure gradient is often higher than 100 mm Hg.

The typical changes in the configuration of the ascending aortic pressure pulse, including a slow-rising upstroke, an early anacrotic notch, and a systolic shudder, are helpful signs for identifying significant aortic valve obstruction (see Fig. 18–14). Also, the more severe the aortic valve obstruction, the more likely that the left ventricular pressure pulse will take on an "isometric" configuration, that is, a relatively symmetric force generation and dissipation profile (see Figs. 18–12 and 18–14).

EFFECT OF HEART RATE CHANGES AND EXERCISE. In contradistinction to mitral stenosis, a decrease in heart rate, for any level of cardiac output, causes an increase in the transvalvular aortic gradient owing to an augmentation of stroke volume and the flow per systolic second.

A number of studies have evaluated the hemodynamic response to supine bicycle exercise in isolated aortic stenosis.[99–101] With muscular exercise and its attendant increase in heart rate, cardiac output is increased and diastole is primarily abbreviated; therefore, more time is available per minute for systolic ejection. Generally, systolic flow per second increases, and the gradient augments often to quite high levels. However, if the increase in ejection duration is proportional to the increase in flow, then the gradient may increase minimally. With exercise, there may be a mild increase in the calculated aortic valve area, suggesting either a further widening of the orifice or, more likely, a flow dependence of the constants in the Gorlin equation (see above).[29, 102]

MYOCARDIAL OXYGEN CONSUMPTION. As a consequence of the pressure load on the left ventricle and the increase in muscle mass, the oxygen demands of the left ventricular myocardium are augmented by aortic stenosis. Also, the reduction of the aortic valve orifice area can lead to a diminution of the diastolic pressure in the ascending aorta, and diastolic coronary perfusion pressure declines at a time when myocardial oxygen demand has been enhanced. Thus, it is understandable that angina pectoris is common in aortic stenosis even in the absence of coronary artery disease. Transient myocardial ischemia by the above mechanisms may also explain, at least in part, the development of serious ventricular arrhythmias and the in-

creased incidence of sudden death in this disorder. Similarly, arrhythmias, perhaps coupled with transient hypotension caused by momentary inability to maintain cardiac output (particularly during assumption of the upright posture) may explain the incidence of syncopal attacks that frequently characterize the clinical course of patients with aortic stenosis.

LEFT VENTRICULAR ADAPTATIONS. The early responses of the left ventricle to a significant pressure overload are not well documented in humans. However, in experimental constriction of the ascending aorta, the earliest physiologic response is an increase in the left ventricular end-diastolic volume and compensatory use of the Frank-Starling mechanism.[103] Blood is then forced across the narrowed valve at a higher velocity to maintain stroke volume within normal limits. With a chronic pressure overload, the left ventricle develops concentric hypertrophy, an increase in muscle mass brought about by enlargement of individual fibers as well as laying down of additional sarcomeres in parallel.[104] Thus, the ratio of left ventricular wall mass to chamber volume increases, a structural adaptation that serves to maintain the average force or tension in the ventricular wall at relatively normal levels, without substantial enlargement of the left ventricular cavity. Because wall stress (or force) is directly proportional to systolic pressure and chamber size but inversely related to wall thickness, concentric hypertrophy creates a condition where the increased pressure load is distributed over a larger number of muscle fibers.

LEFT VENTRICULAR DIASTOLIC PROPERTIES. The concentric pattern of hypertrophy seen in aortic stenosis leads to changes in the diastolic properties of the left ventricle.[105–107] The stiffness of the left ventricular chamber augments in response to the increased muscle mass as well as secondary to a variable increase in the intrinsic stiffness of individual muscle fibers. To fill the left ventricle during diastole, the left atrium develops a more forceful contraction, which serves to generate a more prominent presystolic pressure (a wave) in the left atrial and left ventricular pressure tracings and that elevates the end-diastolic pressure to near 20 mm Hg. However, an increase of the end-diastolic pressure by this mechanism does not indicate necessarily left ventricular myocardial failure, and the mean left atrial pressure may still be maintained at relatively normal levels.

DEPRESSED LEFT VENTRICULAR SYSTOLIC FUNCTION. With the passage of time, myocardial failure develops in aortic stenosis in response partly to the pressure overwork on the hypertrophied left ventricle and in response also to the development of myocardial fibrosis. Left ventricular dysfunction is marked by an increase in end-systolic volume, augmentation of the end-diastolic volume, and reduction of the stroke volume. There is also evidence, however, that reduced myocardial shortening may be related to an uncompensated elevation of equatorial wall stress, that is, an excessive afterload.[108–110] As shown in Figure 18–16, in 30 patients, 11 normal subjects and 19 with severe aortic stenosis, there was an inverse relation between the mean velocity of circumferential shortening (mean V_{cf}) at the mid-wall and the calculated mean stress at the mid-wall. The five aortic stenotic patients with the most significant reduction of mean V_{cf} demonstrated a concomitant reduction of isovolumetric peak dP/dt; the remaining 14 patients with isovolumetric peak dP/dt less than 1438 mm Hg per second exhibited reduced shortening but to a much lesser degree. The authors concluded from this analysis that an afterload excess may also contribute to reduced myocardial shortening in advanced aortic stenosis.[108] It may also explain the prompt improvement in left ventricular shortening that can be seen in the immediate period after aortic valve replacement.

Aortic stenosis with significant concentric hypertrophy is one of the conditions, along with hypertensive heart disease and hypertrophic cardiomyopathy, where endocardial measures of myocardial shortening may exaggerate a mean shortening rate at the mid-wall. As shown in Figure 18–17, for any particular endocardial value for V_{CF}, the corresponding mid-wall value is less in patients with aortic stenosis than in normal subjects.[108]

MEAN LEFT ATRIAL PRESSURE. In the natural

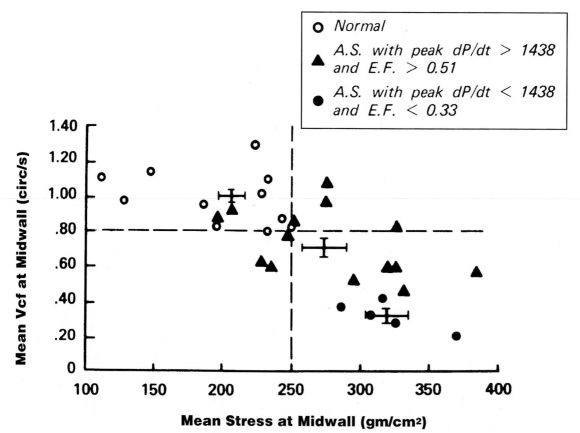

Figure 18–16. Plot of mean velocity of circumferential shortening (V_{cf}) at mid-wall (vertical axis) versus mean systolic stress at mid-wall (horizontal axis) in normal subjects, in patients with aortic stenosis (AS) with a normal ejection fraction and peak dP/dt, and in patients with aortic stenosis with a subnormal ejection fraction and peak dP/dt. The mean ± SE is shown for each group of patients. Analysis suggests that both myocardial failure *(closed circles)* and excess equatorial stress *(closed triangles)* are operative in depression of mid-wall V_{cf} in valvular aortic stenosis. (From Peterson KL: Instantaneous force-velocity-length relations of the left ventricle: Methods, limitations, and applications in humans. *In* Fishman AP [ed]: Heart Failure. Washington, Hemisphere, 1978, pp 121–132.)

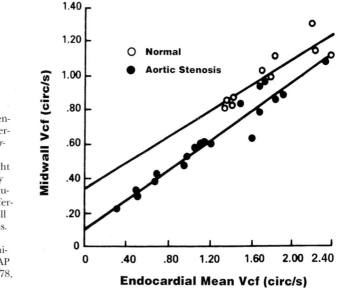

Figure 18–17. Plot of mid-wall (vertical axis) and endocardial (horizontal) mean velocities of circumferential fiber shortening in normal subjects *(open circles)* and patients with valvular aortic stenosis and left ventricular hypertrophy *(closed circles)*. A straight line was fitted to the data point for each group by the least-squares method. Note that for any particular endocardial value for mean velocity of circumferential shortening (V_{cf}), the corresponding mid-wall value is less in patients with valvular aortic stenosis. (From Peterson KL: Instantaneous force-velocity-length relations of the left ventricle: Methods, limitations, and applications in humans. *In* Fishman AP [ed]: Heart Failure. Washington, Hemisphere, 1978, pp 121–132.)

history of aortic stenosis, the left atrial pressure increases initially in response to a change in the diastolic properties of the left ventricle and then subsequently, as it dilates, secondary to a movement of the ventricle up its pressure-volume curve. Signs of pulmonary venous congestion ensue with the associated symptoms of orthopnea and exertional dyspnea. In the late stages of aortic stenosis, cardiac output may fall to such a low level that the murmur across the tightly stenotic aortic valve is nearly inaudible. At this stage, the patient is in grave danger of sudden death and the risk of investigating and surgically intervening on the patient increase substantially.

CARDIAC ARRHYTHMIAS. Atrial fibrillation is not as common as in mitral valve disease, but when it occurs, it is deleterious to overall cardiac function because of the loss of the left atrial contractile contribution to ventricular filling. Usually the onset of atrial fibrillation indicates that significant left atrial distension and dilation have occurred. If atrial fibrillation is present at the time of the heart catheterization, it is important to analyze multiple beats, of varying RR interval, to properly assess the severity of aortic valve obstruction. In a much smaller group of patients, particularly those in the sixth decade and beyond, complete heart block, or lesser degrees of atrioventricular block, can occur owing to dystrophic calcification in and around the specialized conduction system.

FLUOROSCOPY. Adult patients with aortic stenosis, particularly those older than 50 years of age, essentially always exhibits annular and

leaflet calcification by fluoroscopy.[111] In fact, if one cannot visualize a calcified aortic valve by fluoroscopy in this group, the diagnosis should be questioned. These same investigators reported that the extent of aortic valve calcification correlated with the peak aortic systolic gradient. With quite heavy calcification, it can be seen to extend into the mitral annulus, up the aortic root, and around the orifices of the coronary arteries. In younger patients with aortic stenosis, fluoroscopy is not particularly valuable.

LEFT VENTRICULAR AND ASCENDING AORTIC ANGIOGRAPHY. It is important to perform selective left ventricular angiography to document the functional status of the left ventricle and to exclude significant mitral regurgitation. Both the straight right anterior oblique and left anterior oblique projections with cranial angulation are useful for demonstrating the left ventricular outflow tract and for confirming that the aortic valve is the site of the obstruction. Oftentimes, the aortic valve is well visualized on this same injection and shows the typical characteristics of incomplete or absent opening during ejection (so-called doming), thickening, and calcification (Fig. 18–18). To minimize hemodynamic perturbations, we have found it useful to use low-osmolality contrast agents (see Chapter 7) for left ventriculography. In those patients in whom coexistent aortic regurgitation or abnormalities of aortic valve architecture (e.g., vegetations) are suspected, ascending aortography is also often revealing. This injection also assists in the choice of catheter size for performance of selective coronary angiography.

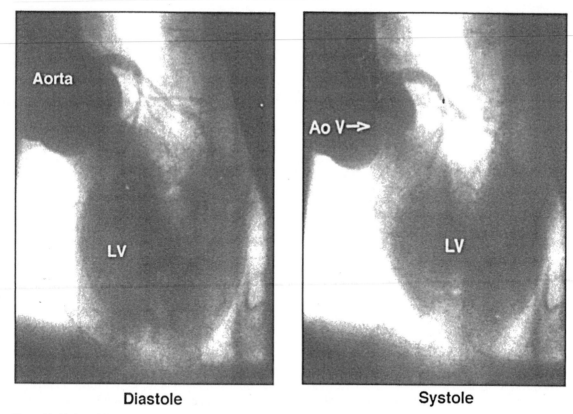

| Diastole | Systole |

Figure 18–18. Ascending cineaortogram, left anterior oblique projection, in a patient with combined aortic stenosis and insufficiency. Note the "doming" of the aortic valve (AoV) *(arrow)* during systole. LV, left ventricle.

SELECTIVE CORONARY ANGIOGRAPHY. In older patients (older than 40 years of age) or in any patient with symptoms of angina pectoris, it is imperative that selective coronary angiography be performed before surgery. Lack of appreciation of significant coronary artery lesions can lead to difficulty during surgical treatment, and coronary revascularization procedures are usually carried out at the time of the aortic valve replacement.

Aortic Regurgitation

INDICATIONS. Any patient being considered for aortic valve replacement for chronic aortic regurgitation should undergo cardiac catheterization and angiography before surgery. The status of left ventricular function, the severity of the valvular regurgitation, the presence or absence of associated lesions, and the anatomy of the coronary arterial tree all are assessed or confirmed during this procedure. Each of these factors influences the approach of the cardiac surgeon and provides important prognostic information to the patient and the physician.

Both right and left heart pressure measure-

ments, along with an ascending cineaortogram (as well as a selective left ventriculogram if the left ventricle is inadequately opacified during the aortogram) should be performed during the procedure. In patients that are older than 40 years of age, or if coronary artery disease is suspected as a coincident disease process, selective coronary angiography should also be performed.

In contrast, if the diagnosis of acute, severe aortic regurgitation is substantiated by clinical and echocardiographic findings, it may not be necessary to perform cardiac catheterization before referring the patient for surgical correction. The cardiologist must weigh the risk of subjecting a very ill patient to contrast angiography, with the associated volume load and delay in surgery, as opposed to the benefit of obtaining information that will be useful in applying the surgical procedure. The ascending aortogram may help visualize and locate a valve ring abscess, a ruptured sinus of Valsalva aneurysm, or multiple valve involvement in the setting of infectious endocarditis. Visualization of an aortic dissection, with its entry and exit sites, may be helpful to the surgeon in planning the surgical approach.

TECHNICAL CONSIDERATIONS. Generally, aortic regurgitation can be studied using only one left-sided catheter inserted retrograde by way of a peripheral artery. A right-sided catheter should also be inserted to assess the pulmonary artery and pulmonary capillary wedge pressures and for measurement of cardiac output. In patients in whom a vegetation is suspected to be located on the aortic valve, it is inadvisable to traverse the plane of the aortic valve into the left ventricle for fear of dislodging the vegetation.

PATHOPHYSIOLOGY. The fundamental defect in aortic regurgitation (insufficiency) is retrograde leakage of blood from the ascending aorta into the left ventricle during diastole due to incomplete coaptation of the aortic valve leaflets. This condition results in a diastolic volume overload (either acute or chronic) of the left ventricle and an augmentation of the amount of blood ejected into the ascending aorta during the following systole. In severe aortic regurgitation the amount of blood that regurgitates into the left ventricle may exceed 50% of the total stroke volume. The lower systolic pressure at which the aortic valve opens (due to the diastolic run-off on the previous beat) serves to facilitate ventricular unloading in early systole; however, this effect of lowered impedance is less favorable than in mitral regur-

gitation. The ultimate clinical manifestations of aortic regurgitation depend on the volume of blood leaked per beat, the acuteness or chronicity of the process, and the adaptation of the left ventricle to the valve leakage. If the regurgitation slowly worsens, the left ventricle has sufficient time to compensate for the volume overload, and signs of congestive heart failure are delayed, sometimes for many years.

ACUTE REGURGITATION. Acute aortic regurgitation precludes time necessary for myocardial adaptation, and the left ventricle moves quickly up its diastolic pressure-volume curve, causing a marked elevation of the left ventricular diastolic pressures and early closure of the mitral valve (Fig. 18–19).[112-114] There is minimal increase in the left ventricular end-diastolic volume or fiber length, and the total stroke volume cannot increase sufficiently to compensate for the regurgitant volume; thus, forward stroke volume and cardiac output fall. The high left ventricular diastolic pressures also serve to minimize the run-off into the left ventricle; therefore, the diastolic pressure in the aorta may remain near normal and the arterial pulse pressure increases little, if at all.

CHRONIC REGURGITATION. In chronic aortic regurgitation, the left ventricle adapts to the

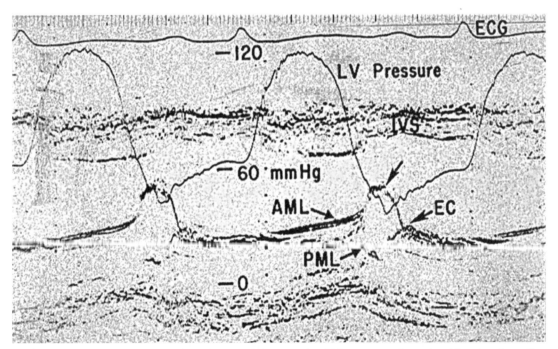

Figure 18–19. Simultaneous recording of a high-fidelity left ventricular (LV) pressure pulse and an M-mode echocardiogram in a patient with staphylococcal endocarditis and acute aortic insufficiency. Note the early closure (EC) of the mitral valve at the time that the anterior (AML) and posterior (PML) mitral leaflets coapt. Also note the very high LV diastolic pressures, including an end-diastolic pressure of 60 mm Hg.

volume overload by using the Frank-Starling mechanism (increased fiber stretch); however, eccentric hypertrophy with replication of sarcomeres in both series and parallel must also occur to explain the very large end-diastolic volume measurements seen in some patients (so-called cor bovinum). This compensatory mechanism allows the enlarged left ventricle to deliver a greater stroke volume while maintaining a normal extent of shortening for each unit of the enlarged chamber. However, myofiber slippage may also contribute to the increase in ventricular size.

The hemodynamic and afterload conditions in chronic aortic regurgitation resemble those for chronic mitral regurgitation, but with two important differences: (1) the total stroke volume is ejected into a high-impedance circuit (the aorta and systemic arteries), and because the total forward stroke volume is augmented, the left ventricular and aortic systolic pressures are elevated (usually ≥160 mm Hg with severe aortic regurgitation); and (2) because the aortic valve is incompetent, the diastolic pressure in the aorta falls to subnormal levels during diastole, thereby reducing the diastolic perfusion pressure across the coronary arterial bed (Fig. 18–20). Compromise of coronary blood flow occurs especially during periods of reduced peripheral systemic vascular resistance (such as with exercise) or slow heart rate (such as with sleep). Because eccentric myocardial hypertrophy is associated with a sizable increase in total myocardial oxygen demand, patients with aortic regurgitation are particularly prone to develop angina pectoris in the absence of coronary artery disease.

LEFT VENTRICULAR ADAPTATIONS. As with mitral regurgitation, chronic aortic regurgitation is associated with a shift to the right of the intrinsic pressure-volume curve of the left ventricle. Although end-diastolic volume increases twofold or threefold, the end-diastolic pressure remains relatively normal until late in the course of the illness when myocardial dysfunction supervenes. Thus, the lungs are spared the effects of elevation of the left atrial and pulmonary venous pressures, and the patient develops signs of pulmonary congestion only late in the course of the illness. However, if chronic aortic regurgitation becomes severe, marked by a negligible gradient at end-diastole between the aorta and the left ventricle, the patient becomes quite symptomatic. In some instances, preclosure of the mitral valve may also occur, leading to a dissociation between the rising left ventricular pressure and the left atrial pressure.

HEMODYNAMIC MEASUREMENTS. The intracardiac and large vessel pressure pulses reveal elevation of the systolic pressures in the left ventricle and aorta (see Fig. 18–20); a small pressure gradient may be noted across the aortic valve. A rapid upstroke and low diastolic pressure are also characteristic of the aortic pressure. Simultaneous recording of the left ventricular and a direct left atrial or pulmonary arterial wedge tracings can demonstrate a pressure gradient between the left ventricle and left atrium, occurring early in diastole and attributable to impaired opening of the anterior mitral leaflet. In chronic aortic regurgitation the left ventricular end-diastolic pressure is normal or only mildly elevated, provided myocardial function has re-

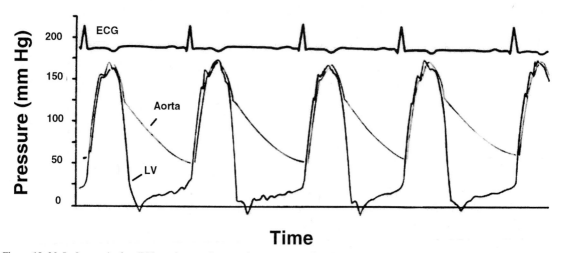

Figure 18–20. Left ventricular (LV) and ascending aortic pressure pulses in a patient with chronic aortic insufficiency. Note the widened systemic arterial pulse pressure, the low end-diastolic pressure in the aorta (50 mm Hg), and the moderate augmentation of aortic systolic pressure. (See text for discussion.)

mained normal. However, with acute aortic regurgitation, the left ventricle dilates rapidly, and the end-diastolic pressure elevates to levels of 40 to 50 mm Hg (see previous discussion under Pathophysiology about adaptive shifts in the intrinsic pressure-volume curve of the left ventricle).

EFFECTS OF HEART RATE AND EXERCISE. The response to exercise in patients with chronic aortic regurgitation has been studied and found to be quite heterogeneous.[115–118] Two factors, a drop in the systemic vascular resistance and an increase in heart rate with shortening of the diastolic filling period, serve to diminish the regurgitant fraction. Thus, the increase in cardiac output for any given degree of total body oxygen consumption may remain normal. The responses of the left ventricular end-diastolic and left atrial pressures to exercise are variable and tend not to correlate with either symptomatic status or the severity of the aortic regurgitation. For these reasons, exercise hemodynamic measurements are seldom sought in catheterization studies of aortic insufficiency.

ASCENDING ROOT AORTOGRAPHY AND LEFT VENTRICULOGRAPHY. In most patients supravalvular injection of contrast medium into the aortic root provides the best means of assessing the severity of aortic valve leakage (see Table 18–1). With severe regurgitation, the contrast agent opacifies equally the left ventricle and the aorta, and three or four beats are required before the contrast medium is cleared from the left ventricle. Left ventricular end-diastolic and end-systolic volumes and ejection fraction can be evaluated from this injection. In most patients who are surgical candidates, the end-diastolic volume is more than 150 mL/m² of body surface area. (The normal value is 90 mL/m²). The supravalvular ascending aortic injection is useful also for identification of associated disease of the aortic wall (e.g., aneurysmal dilation) and for morphologic study of the sinuses of Valsalva and the aortic valve leaflets. This injection is particularly valuable for the determination of the extent and size of an ascending aortic aneurysm (Fig. 18–21). In most instances, the presence or absence of a tricuspid, as opposed to bicuspid, aortic valve can be determined.

Combined Aortic Stenosis and Insufficiency

Severe aortic stenosis is often associated with a mild degree of aortic regurgitation; similarly, severe aortic regurgitation may exhibit a mild systolic pressure gradient across the valve. However, in some patients the aortic valve is both severely stenotic and insufficient, leading to significant, combined pressure and volume over-

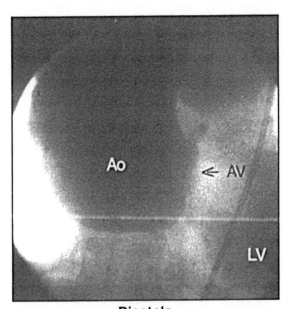
Diastole

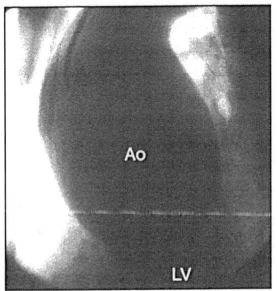
Later Cine Frame

Figure 18–21. Injection (left anterior oblique projection) of a large amount of contrast agent into the ascending aorta (Ao) in a patient with a very large ascending aortic aneurysm associated with aortic insufficiency. Note the size of the aneurysm relative to the size of the left ventricle (LV) on the diastolic frame. Panning upward *(right)* allows determination of the distal extent of the aneurysmal dilation. AV, aortic valve.

load on the left ventricle. The energy demands imposed by this combined lesion are generally greater than with either of the lesions in an isolated state. Because diastolic regurgitation augments systolic flow across the aortic valve on the following beat, a reduction in the aortic valve orifice area to 2.0 cm² can be associated with a gradient of 30 to 60 mm Hg between the left ventricle and the ascending aorta. The profile of the pressure gradient is notable for an early, mid, and late pressure difference but with maintenance of a relatively normal pulse pressure in the ascending aorta.

Both chamber dilation and increased wall thickness are seen, owing to the combined pressure and volume overload. The pattern of hypertrophy, therefore, is a combination of eccentric and concentric types with a tendency for the left ventricular diastolic filling pressures to be elevated because of an increase in the mass-to-volume ratio. With long-standing presence of the lesions, the left atrium dilates in response to the increased filling pressures in the left ventricles.

HEMODYNAMIC MEASUREMENTS. Patients with a combination of aortic lesions exhibit a pressure gradient between 30 and 100 mm Hg, depending on the relative importance of the valve obstruction as compared with its insufficiency. When the left ventricular myocardium fails, the amount of regurgitation diminishes because of a reduced pressure gradient between the aorta and the left ventricle. At the same time, the cardiac output usually diminishes, and the pressure gradient across the valve declines accordingly.

As with combined mitral stenosis and insufficiency, the true orifice size of the aortic valve cannot be determined unless the true systolic flow per second across the valve is estimated. Again, this is accomplished by quantitative left ventriculography where total stroke volume is measured as the difference between the end-diastolic and end-systolic volumes on a cineangiogram. The difference, then, between the total stroke volume and the systemic stroke volume, measured by the Fick or indicator-dilution technique, allows the computation of the total amount of regurgitation per beat and the regurgitant fraction per beat.

Tricuspid Stenosis

INDICATIONS. In patients with tricuspid stenosis cardiac catheterization and angiography are indicated whenever the obstruction is suspected to be severe by the clinical findings or by two-dimensional echocardiography with Doppler velocity recordings and pseudocolor imaging. It should be carefully looked for in all patients undergoing cardiac catheterization because of rheumatic heart disease. Also, in any patient undergoing catheterization in whom there has been a long-standing ventricular endocardial pacemaker lead across the tricuspid valve, a careful search should be made for a transvalvular gradient.

TECHNICAL CONSIDERATIONS. Because the valve gradient in tricuspid stenosis is generally relatively small, great care must be taken to ensure that the pressure recordings are well calibrated. Ideally, either two catheters should be used to record simultaneous right ventricular and right atrial pressures; alternatively, a double-lumen catheter can be used, with the individual lumina registering pressure from either side of the valve.

If a significant gradient is uncovered (e.g., >2 or 3 mm Hg), then the transducers should be switched, without recalibration, between the two measuring catheter sites to validate that the gradient is accurate and not artifactual.

PATHOPHYSIOLOGY. The fundamental abnormality of cardiac function in tricuspid stenosis is mechanical obstruction to right atrial emptying due to reduction in the tricuspid valve orifice size with development during diastole of a significant pressure gradient between the right atrium and ventricle. When compared with mitral stenosis and its effect on the lungs, a considerably lower pressure gradient (e.g., 3 or 4 mm Hg) is associated with symptoms and signs of congestion in the distribution of the systemic veins flowing into the right atrium. The normal tricuspid valve orifice area is 8 to 12 cm²; significant symptoms or signs of tricuspid stenosis may be seen when the valve orifice is compromised to 2 cm² or less (Fig. 18–22). As with mitral stenosis, the gradient across the valve is dependent on the diastolic filling period (or heart rate) and the diastolic flow per second or cardiac output. Thus, exercise is associated with a significant increase in the pressure gradient across the valve. There is a limit to which diastolic filling of the right ventricle can be maintained by the pumping action of skeletal muscle contraction, inspiratory suction, and atrial contraction. Thus, cardiac output tends to fall earlier in the clinical course of tricuspid stenosis than with a comparable severity of mitral stenosis.

HEMODYNAMIC MEASUREMENTS. Provided the patient remains in normal sinus rhythm, the

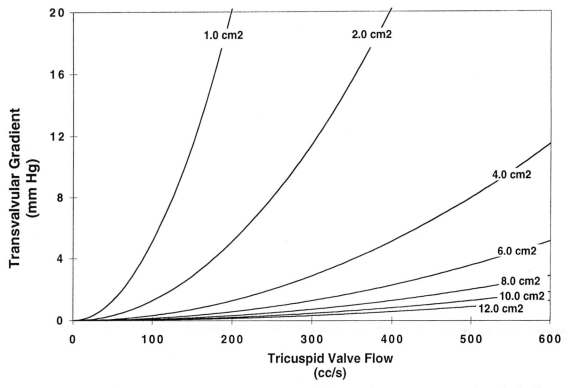

Figure 18–22. Plot of mean transvalvular gradient (vertical axis) in millimeters of mercury versus transtricuspid valve flow (horizontal axis) in milliliters per second for valve orifice areas of various sizes (isopleths from 1.0 to 12.0 cm²). Calculated valve orifice areas are based on Gorlin's equation with an empiric constant of 1.0. (See text for discussion.)

right atrial pressure pulse in tricuspid stenosis is characterized by an exaggerated a wave that results from a forceful right atrial contraction against the obstructed tricuspid valve (Fig. 18–23). As with mitral stenosis, there is slowing of the y descent and absence of diastasis between the right atrial and right ventricular pressure pulses. Heart rate and the RR interval influences the mean diastolic gradient as it does in mitral stenosis. These effects of heart rate are subtle, however, because in most instances the valve gradient is no more than 5 to 8 mm Hg.

At rest the cardiac output is usually low normal or reduced; during exercise the normal augmentation is significantly compromised, a finding that undoubtedly explains the common complaint of fatigue in these patients. In fact, whenever the pulmonary artery and pulmonary capillary wedge pressures do not increase even though severe mitral valve stenosis is suspected, then a careful search for right ventricular inlet obstruction, secondary to tricuspid stenosis, should be made.

The tricuspid valve may also become obstructed as part of the inflammatory and constrictive process around the atrioventricular rings in patients with constrictive pericarditis.

As shown in Figure 18–24, the pressure gradient is particularly apparent during early diastole; the pressure then equilibrates during mid and late diastole when there is little flow between the right atrium and ventricle.

Tricuspid Regurgitation

INDICATIONS. Cardiac catheterization for primary, isolated tricuspid regurgitation is seldom required, although hemodynamic and angiographic assessment is occasionally considered as a prelude to tricuspid valve surgery during the acute or convalescent phase of treatment for tricuspid valve endocarditis. Much more commonly, this lesion is studied as part of the hemodynamic investigation of a patient with unexplained pulmonary hypertension who is undergoing pulmonary angiography (see Chapter 23).

PATHOPHYSIOLOGY. The fundamental abnormality of cardiac function in tricuspid regurgitation is retrograde systolic ejection of a portion of the stroke volume into the right atrium, with augmentation on the subsequent diastole of the

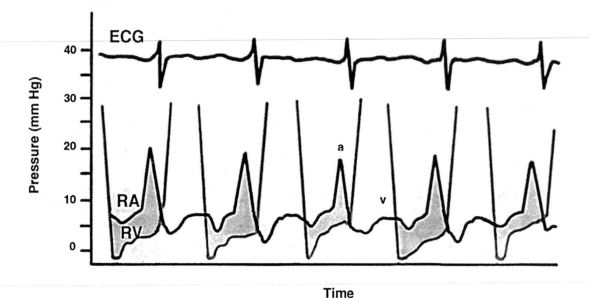

Figure 18–23. Right atrial (RA) and right ventricular (RV) pressure pulses in a patient with tricuspid stenosis. The transvalvular diastolic gradient is shaded in gray. Note the exaggerated a wave, the delayed y descent, and the lack of diastasis during diastole. (See text for discussion.)

amount of blood filling the right ventricle. In like fashion to mitral regurgitation, tricuspid regurgitation provides a low-impedance outlet for ventricular systolic ejection, explaining in part the tolerance of most patients for the presence of the lesion. In response to the volume load on the right ventricle and atrium, both chambers dilate and tend to displace the left

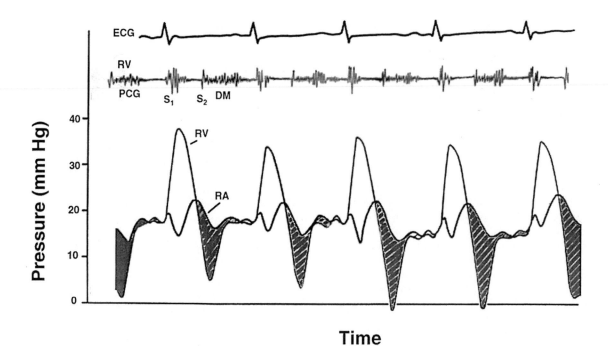

Figure 18–24. High-fidelity micromanometric right ventricular (RV) and right atrial (RA) pressure pulses in a patient with constrictive pericarditis and evidence of tricuspid valve obstruction to flow, particularly during early diastole. An intracardiac phonocardiogram (PCG) is also recorded from the inlet of the right ventricle. The shaded area displays the diastolic pressure gradient that is confined primarily to the period during which there is flow across the valve. The diastolic murmur (DM) also corresponds to the period of the pressure gradient.

ventricle in a posterior direction. With long-standing presence of the lesion, the filling pressures on the right side of the heart increase, and the resultant augmentation in systemic venous pressure leads to congestion of the viscera (liver, spleen, kidneys, small intestine, and large intestine), and an elevated hydrostatic pressure in both the upper and lower extremities. Finally, right ventricular myocardial function deteriorates, and the cardiac output becomes compromised at rest.

HEMODYNAMIC AND ANGIOGRAPHIC ASSESSMENT. At the time of right-sided heart catheterization, tricuspid regurgitation is detected by the presence of a large v wave in the right atrial pressure pulse; in severe forms of tricuspid leakage, the v wave may actually follow the contour of the right ventricular pressure pulse (so-called ventricularization), although the peak systolic pressure in the right atrium always remains less than that in the right ventricle (Fig. 18–25). The right atrial mean pressure may reach levels of 20 mm Hg. In end-stage right heart failure, the right ventricular diastolic pressures become markedly elevated and their phasic diastolic contour may be indistinguishable from that seen with constrictive pericarditis or a restrictive cardiomyopathy.

Cinefilming of a selective injection of contrast agent into the right ventricle serves to document the degree of dilation of the chamber, demonstrates regurgitation of dye into the right atrium, and, in some instances, certifies morphologic abnormalities of the tricuspid valve leaflets. For example, the right ventricular injection may demonstrate the downward displacement of the leaflet attachments of the tricuspid valve in Ebstein's anomaly. Metastatic or primary tumors within the right heart chambers can also be demonstrated.

Pulmonic Stenosis

Pulmonic stenosis is essentially always the result of a congenital lesion of the heart. Therefore, the important features of this lesion are considered in detail in Chapter 25.

Pulmonic Regurgitation

The basic cardiac defect in pulmonic regurgitation is retrograde leakage of blood from the main pulmonary artery into the right ventricle during diastole. Unless the pulmonary artery diastolic pressure is severely elevated, the driving force between the pulmonary artery and right ventricle is not large, and the regurgitant fraction of the stroke volume remains relatively small. Moreover, the right ventricle can tolerate a relatively large volume overload, and, thus, the patient with pulmonic regurgitation commonly exhibits no impairment of cardiac output either

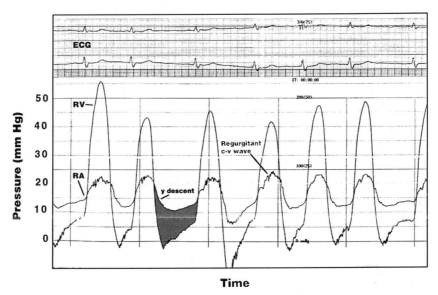

Time

Figure 18–25. Simultaneous right ventricular (RV) and right atrial (RA) micromanometer pressure pulses in a patient with severe, combined tricuspid regurgitation and stenosis, and atrial fibrillation. Note the early diastolic delay in the y descent, the early regurgitant c-v wave during systole, and the so-called ventricularization of the RA pressure pulse. Note also the shutter on the RA pressure pulse during systole due to tricuspid regurgitation and the high-frequency oscillations on the RV pressure pulse during diastole due to tricuspid valve stenosis. The shaded area represents the diastolic pressure gradient on a single beat.

at rest or during exercise. Also, the right ventricular end-diastolic and right atrial mean pressures are not elevated ordinarily unless there is an associated pressure overload on the right ventricle, or, the pulmonic regurgitation is severe and long-standing.

MULTIPLE VALVE LESIONS

Many patients, particularly those with rheumatic valvular disease, manifest significant dysfunction of two or more valves. The clinical recognition and analysis of the functional importance of multiple valve lesions is considerably more challenging than for isolated lesions, and specialized diagnostic tests (particularly cardiac catheterization and angiography) assume even greater importance in the evaluation of such patients for cardiac surgery. If one of the valve lesions is of greater severity, then clinical manifestations of the dysfunction of that valve tend to predominate. However, as a general axiom, if two valve lesions are of approximately equal severity, then the more proximal or upstream lesion in the heart predominates and may mask the severity of the downstream lesion. Finally, one valve lesion, by virtue of its underlying pathophysiology, often potentiates the severity of a second lesion. Chronic aortic incompetence causes significant left ventricular dilation that, in turn, worsens the severity of coexistent mitral regurgitation.

TECHNICAL CONSIDERATIONS. The presence of multiple valve lesions often complicates the approach to entering selected chambers and obtaining reliable hemodynamic data during cardiac catheterization. In the setting of both severe aortic and mitral stenosis, or in the setting of mechanical prostheses in both areas, entrance into the left ventricle may be problematic and require a percutaneous puncture of the apex of the left ventricle.[119, 120] Cardiac output determinations by the thermodilution technique, performed to determine transmitral or transaortic valve flow are confounded by the presence of a regurgitant lesion at the site of injection, such as tricuspid regurgitation. In this instance, much greater dependence should be placed on the determination of cardiac output by the Fick technique.

Performance of an adequate left ventriculogram may then be limited by the size of the needle or sheath that can be safely placed through the apex. Also, the combined effects of two lesions in series, such as aortic and mitral regurgitation, may undermine the adequacy of the delineation of the relevant pathoanatomy and pathophysiology by cineangiography. A larger amount of contrast medium then needs to be injected into the aortic root to visualize quantitatively the severity of both regurgitant lesions.

Combined Aortic and Mitral Valve Disease

AORTIC REGURGITATION AND MITRAL STENOSIS. Aortic regurgitation often occurs in association with mitral stenosis or combined mitral stenosis and insufficiency.[121, 122] If the mitral stenosis is quite severe and limiting left ventricular filling, the common attributes of aortic regurgitation may be diminished. The systemic arterial pulse pressure may not be as widened, the left ventricular volume may remain relatively normal, and ascending aortography may underestimate the severity of the aortic valve leakage.

AORTIC STENOSIS WITH MITRAL STENOSIS OR INSUFFICIENCY. The incidence of aortic stenosis in association with mitral valve disease has declined significantly as rheumatic heart disease has become less frequent in industrialized countries. In fact, the combination of severe aortic stenosis and significant mitral stenosis or regurgitation, both requiring prosthetic valve replacement, is relatively uncommon. Because mitral stenosis or regurgitation, or both, tend to reduce left ventricular output, the transaortic valvular pressure gradient may be significantly reduced with this combination. It is particularly important that one not depend on this gradient for surgical strategy and to calculate an actual aortic valve orifice area based on accurate determination of the mean pressure gradient and the cardiac output (see earlier).

AORTIC REGURGITATION WITH MITRAL REGURGITATION. If both the aortic and mitral valves are severely and chronically regurgitant, the left ventricular is subjected to a relatively massive volume overload. As with the isolated regurgitant lesions, such patients may exhibit a latent period of many years before significant symptoms appear. Nevertheless, the patient should be observed carefully for insidious worsening of symptoms and signs of left ventricular enlargement. Moreover, it is now believed important to intervene surgically before the left ventricle is excessively dilated and the ejection fraction is subnormal (see discussion of surgical management in the section on isolated mitral or isolated aortic regurgitation). Usually, the systemic arterial pressure pulse manifests a widened pulse pressure, although the peak systolic pressure may not be as high as in pure aortic insufficiency owing to the reduction of forward stroke volume by coexistent mitral regurgitation. If only severe aortic regurgitation is relieved at the time of cardiac surgery, the mitral regurgitation appears less important postoperatively owing to the reduction in left ventricular size. Unfortunately, cineangiography does not provide sufficient detail to make a preoperative decision about the need to either replace or reconstruct a regurgitant mitral valve in the setting of severe aortic insufficiency. The cardiac surgeon, keeping in mind that the mitral regurgitation will be less once the aortic leakage is no longer present, is forced to make an intraoperative decision about the need for mitral valve surgery.

Combined Tricuspid and Left-Sided Valve Lesions

Organic disease of the tricuspid valve occurs in association with mitral or aortic valve lesions in approximately 10% of patients with chronic rheumatic heart disease.[122]

In the patient with combined dysfunction of the aortic, mitral, and tricuspid valves, tricuspid valve surgery is performed (in addition to replacement of the aortic and mitral valves) provided there is evidence at cardiac catheterization of (1) tricuspid stenosis (valve area <2.0 cm^2); (2) combined severe tricuspid stenosis and insufficiency; (3) tricuspid insufficiency with only mild to moderate pulmonary hypertension (peak pulmonary artery systolic pressure <50 mm Hg); or (4) tricuspid insufficiency with severe pulmonary hypertension and right atrial mean pressure higher than 15 mm Hg. Generally in the last circumstance cited, right ventricular myocardial dysfunction is severe, and prompt, rather than gradual, relief of the tricuspid valve insufficiency is salutary for the patient's survival in the immediate postoperative period. Annuloplasty with insertion of a semiannular ring has also gained favor for palliation of tricuspid regurgitation secondary to pulmonary hypertension.

REFERENCES

1. Boudoulas H, Vavuranakis M, Wooley CF: Valvular heart disease: The influence of changing etiology on nosology. J Heart Valve Dis 1994; 3(5):516–526.
2. Taubert KA, Rowley AH, Shulman ST: Seven-year national survey of Kawasaki disease and acute rheumatic fever. Pediatr Infect Dis J 1994; 13(8):704–708.
3. Denny FW Jr: A 45-year perspective on the streptococcus and rheumatic fever: The Edward H. Kass Lecture

4. Roberts WC, Perloff JK: Mitral valvular disease: A clinicopathologic survey of the conditions causing the mitral valve to function abnormally. Ann Intern Med 1972; 77:939–975.
5. Edwards JE: Pathology of left ventricular outflow tract obstruction. Circulation 1965; 31:586–599.
6. Roberts WC: Anatomically isolated aortic valvular disease: The case against its being a rheumatic etiology. Am J Med 1970; 49:151–159.
7. Roberts WC: The congenitally bicuspid aortic valve: A study of 85 autopsy cases. Am J Cardiol 1970; 26:72–83.
8. Roberts WC: The structure of the aortic valve in clinically isolated aortic stenosis: An autopsy study of 162 patients over 15 years of age. Circulation 1970; 42:91.
9. Roberts WC, Perloff JK, Costantino T: Severe valvular aortic stenosis in patients over 65 years of age: A clinicopathologic study. Am J Cardiol 1971; 27:497.
10. Edwards JE: Pathology of acquired valvular disease of the heart. Semin Roentgenol 1979; 14:96.
11. Edwards JE: Pathology of aortic incompetence. In Silver MD (ed): Cardiovascular Pathology, Vol. 1. New York, Churchill Livingstone, 1983, pp 619–631.
12. Oeconomos NS, Camiliaris DH, Petritis J, et al: Congenital tricuspid valvular stenosis. J Cardiovasc Surg 1975; 16:100–103.
13. Dennis JL, Hansen AE, Corpening TN: Endocardial fibroelastosis. Pediatrics 1953; 12:130–139.
14. Millman S: Tricuspid stenosis and pulmonary stenosis complicating carcinoid of the intestine with metastasis to the liver. Am Heart J 1943; 25:391–398.
15. Gibson R, Wood P: The diagnosis of tricuspid stenosis. Br Heart J 1955; 17:552–562.
16. Silverman NA, Levitsky S, Spigos DG, et al: Massive hemoptysis and recurrent tricuspid infective endocarditis in a heroin addict. Chest 1982; 82:195–196.
17. Lee ME, Chaux A: Unusual complications of endocardial pacing. J Thorac Cardiovasc Surg 1980; 80:934–940.
18. Cintron GB, Snow JA, Fletcher RD, et al: Pericarditis mimicking tricuspid valvular disease. Chest 1977; 71:772–774.
19. Lyons HA, Kelly JJ Jr, Nusbaum N, et al: Right atrial myxoma: A clinical study of a patient in whom diagnosis was made by angiocardiography during life (surgically removed). Am J Med 1958; 25:321–326.
20. Thomas JH, Panoussopoulos DG, Jewell WR, et al: Tricuspid stenosis secondary to metastatic melanoma. Cancer 1977; 39:1732–1737.
21. DeCock KM, Gikonyo DK, Lucas SB, et al: Metastatic tumor of right atrium mimicking constrictive pericarditis and tricuspid stenosis. Br Med J 1982; 285:1314.
22. Rippe JM, Angoff G, Sloss LJ, et al: Multiple floppy valves: An echocardiographic syndrome. Am J Med 1979; 66:817–824.
23. Gorlin G, Gorlin SG: Hydraulic formula for calculation of the area of the stenotic mitral valve, other cardiac valves, and central circulatory shunts. Am Heart J 1951; 41:1–29.
24. Gorlin R: Calculations of cardiac valve stenosis: Restoring an old concept for advanced applications. J Am Coll Cardiol 1987; 10:920–922.
25. Dumesnil JG, Yoganathan AP: Theoretical and practical differences between the Gorlin formula and the continuity equation for calculating aortic and mitral valve areas. Am J Cardiol 1991; 67:1268–1272.
26. Cohen MV, Gorlin R: Modified orifice equation for the calculation of mitral valve area. Am Heart J 1972; 84:839–840.
27. Thomas JD, Weyman AE: Doppler mitral pressure half-

time: A clinical tool in search of theoretical justification. J Am Coll Cardiol 1987; 10:923–929.

28. Anderson FL, Tsagaris TJ, Tikoff G, et al: Hemodynamic effects of exercise in patients with aortic stenosis. Am J Med 1969; 46:872–885.

29. Bache RJ, Wang Y, Jorgensen ER: Hemodynamic effects of exercise in isolated valvular aortic stenosis. Circulation 1971; 44:1003–1013.

30. Ubago JL, Figueroa A, Colman T, et al: Hemodynamic factors that affect calculated orifice area in the mitral Hancock xenograft valve. Circulation 1980; 61:388–394.

31. Cannon SR, Richards KL, Crawford M: Hydraulic estimation of stenotic orifice area: A correction of the Gorlin formula. Circulation 1985; 71:1170–1178.

32. Segal J, Lerner DJ, Miller DC, et al: When should Doppler-determined valve area be better than the Gorlin formula? Variation in hydraulic constants in low-flow states. J Am Coll Cardiol 1987:1294–1305.

33. Casale PN, Palacios IF, Abascal VM, et al: Effects of dobutamine on Gorlin and continuity equation valve areas and valve resistance in valvular aortic stenosis. Am J Cardiol 1992; 70:1175–1179.

34. Martin TW, Moody JM, Bird JJ, et al: Effect of exercise on indices of valvular aortic stenosis. Cathet Cardiovasc Diagn 1992; 25:265–271.

35. Clark C: The fluid mechanics of aortic stenosis: I. Theory and steady-flow experiments. J Biomech 1976; 9:521–528.

36. Clark C: The fluid mechanics of aortic stenosis: II. Unsteady flow experiments. J Biomech 1976; 9:567–573.

37. Rivas MA, Shapiro AH: On the theory of discharge coefficients for rounded entrance flowmeters and Venturis. Trans Am Soc Mech Eng 1956; 54(a98):489–497.

38. Dow JW, Levine HD, Elkin M, et al: Studies of congenital heart disease: IV. Uncomplicated pulmonic stenosis. Circulation 1950; 1:267–282.

39. Silver EN, Prec O, Grossman N, Katz LN: Dynamics of isolated pulmonary stenosis. Am J Med 1951; 10:21–26.

40. Ford LE, Feldman T, Chiu YC, Carroll JD: Hemodynamic resistance as a measure of functional impairment in aortic valvular stenosis. Circ Res 1990; 66:1–7.

41. Ford LE, Feldman T, Carroll JD: Valve resistance. Circulation 1994; 89:893–895.

42. Hillis LD, Firth BG, Winniford MD: Analysis of factors affecting the variability of Fick versus indicator dilution measurements of cardiac output. Am J Cardiol 1985; 56:764–768.

43. Peterson KL: Volume overload. In Greenberg BH, Murphy E (eds): Valvular Heart Disease. Littleton, MA, PSG, 1987.

44. Guidry LD, Wood EH, Burchell HB: Application of a method for detecting and estimating severity of aortic regurgitation alone or in association with mitral regurgitation. Mayo Clin Proc 1958; 33:596–599.

45. Conn HL Jr: Use of indicator-dilution curves in the evaluation of acquired heart disease. Progr Cardiovasc Dis 1959; 2:166.

46. Frank MJ, Casanegra P, Nadimi M, et al: Measurement of aortic regurgitation by upstream sampling with continuous infusion of indicator. Circulation 1966; 33:545–557.

47. Frank MJ, Nadimi M, Hilmi KI, et al: Measurement of mitral regurgitation in man by the upstream sampling method using continuous indicator infusion. Circulation 1967; 35:100.

48. Nichols WW, Pepine CJ, Conti CR, et al: Quantitation of aortic insufficiency using a catheter-tip velocity transducer. Circulation 1981; 64:375–380.

49. McLoughlin MJ, Morch JE: Cineangiography in mitral regurgitation: A comparison of cineangiography with other methods of assessment, particularly constant infusion of ^{133}Xe. Invest Radiol 1971; 6:416–425.

50. Sandler H, Dodge HT, Hay RE, et al: Quantitation of valvular insufficiency in man by angiocardiography. Am Heart J 1963; 65:501–513.

51. Miller GAH, Kirklin JW, Swan HJC: Myocardial function and left ventricular volumes in acquired valvular insufficiency. Circulation 1965; 31:374–384.

52. Taubman JO, Goodman DJ, Steiner RE: The value of contrast studies in the investigation of aortic valve disease. Clin Radiol 1966; 17:23–31.

53. Baron MG: Angiocardiographic evaluation of valvular insufficiency. Circulation 1971; 43:599–605.

54. Mennel RG, Joyner CR Jr, Thompson PD, et al: The preoperative and operative assessment of aortic regurgitation: Cineaortography versus electromagnetic flowmeter. Am J Cardiol 1972; 29:360–366.

55. Hunt D, Baxley WA, Kennedy JW, et al: Quantitative evaluation of cineaortography in the assessment of aortic regurgitation. Am J Cardiol 1973; 31:696–700.

56. Rackley CE, Hood WP Jr: Quantitative angiographic evaluation and pathophysiologic mechanisms in valvular heart disease. Prog Cardiovasc Dis 1973; 15:427–447.

57. Croft CH, Lipscomb K, Mathis K, et al: Limitations of qualitative angiographic grading in aortic or mitral regurgitation. Am J Cardiol 1984; 53:1593–1598.

58. St John-Sutton MG, St John-Sutton M, Oldershaw P, et al: Valve replacement without preoperative cardiac catheterization. N Engl J Med 1981; 305:1233–1238.

59. Brandenberg RO: No more routine catheterization for valvular heart disease? N Engl J Med 1981; 305:1277–1278.

60. Roberts WC: Reasons for cardiac catheterization before cardiac valve replacement. N Engl J Med 1982; 306:1291–1293.

61. Rahimtoola SH: The need for cardiac catheterization and angiography in valvular heart disease is not disproven. Ann Intern Med 1982; 97:433–439.

62. Lange RA, Moore DM, Cigarroa RG, Hillis LD: Use of pulmonary capillary wedge pressure to assess severity of mitral stenosis: Is true left atrial pressure needed in this condition? J Am Coll Cardiol 1989; 13:825–829.

63. Minnear FL, Barie PS, Malik AB: Effects of large transient increases in pulmonary vascular pressure on lung fluid balance. J Appl Physiol 1983; 55:983.

64. Cross CE, Shaver JA, Wilson RJ, Robin ED: Mitral stenosis and pulmonary fibrosis: Special reference to pulmonary edema and lung lymphatic function. Arch Intern Med 1970; 125:248.

65. Coalson JJ, Jacques WE, Campbell GS, Thompson WM: Ultrastructure of the alveolar capillary membrane in congenital and acquired heart disease. Arch Pathol 1967; 83:377.

66. Kay JM, Edwards FR: Ultrastructure of the alveolar capillary wall in mitral stenosis. J Pathol 1973; 111:239.

67. Braunwald E, Braunwald NS, Ross J Jr, Morrow AG: Effects of mitral valve replacement on the pulmonary vascular dynamics of patients with pulmonary hypertension. N Engl J Med 1965; 273:509.

68. Ward C, Hancock BW: Extreme pulmonary hypertension caused by mitral valve disease: Natural history and results of surgery. Br Heart J 1975; 37:74.

69. Dalen JE, Matloff JM, Evans GL, et al: Early reduction of pulmonary vascular resistance after mitral valve replacement. N Engl J Med 1967; 277:387.

70. Jordan SC, Hicken P, Watson DA, et al: Pathology of the lungs in mitral stenosis in relation to respiratory function and pulmonary hemodynamics. Br Heart J 1966; 23:101.

71. Kasalicky J, Hurych J, Widimsky J, et al: Left heart hemodynamics at rest and during exercise in patients with mitral stenosis. Br Heart J 1968; 30:188–195.

72. Gorlin R, Sawyer CG, Haynes FW, et al: Effects of exercise on circulatory dynamics in mitral stenosis. Am Heart J 1951; 41:192–203.

73. Blackmon JR, Rowell LB, Kennedy JW, et al: Physiological significance of maximal oxygen intake in "pure" mitral stenosis. Circulation 1967; 36:497–510.

74. Ross J Jr, Gault JH, Mason DT, et al: Left ventricular performance during muscular exercise in patients with and without cardiac dysfunction. Circulation 1966; 34:597–608.

75. Saxton GA, Rabinowitz M, Dexter L, Haynes F: The relationship of pulmonary compliance to pulmonary vascular pressures in patients with heart disease. J Clin Invest 1956; 35:611–618.

76. White HC, Butler J, Donald KIW: Lung compliance in patients with mitral stenosis. Clin Sci 1958; 17:667–679.

77. Cohen-Solal A, Aupetit JF, Dahan M, et al: Peak oxygen uptake during exercise in mitral stenosis with sinus rhythm or atrial fibrillation: Lack of correlation with valve area. Eur Heart J 1994; 15:37–44.

78. Horwitz LD, Mullins CB, Payne RM, Curry GC: Left ventricular function in mitral stenosis. Chest 1973; 64:609–614.

79. Gash AK, Carabello BA, Cepin D, Spann JF: Left ventricular ejection performance and systolic muscle function in patients with mitral stenosis. Circulation 1983; 67:148–154.

80. Heller SJ, Carleton RA: Abnormal left ventricular contraction in patients with mitral stenosis. Circulation 1970; 42:1099.

81. Curry GC, Elliot LP, Ramsey HW: Quantitative left ventricular angiocardiographic findings in mitral stenosis. Am J Cardiol 1971; 29:621–627.

82. Holzer JA, Karliner JS, O'Rourke RA, Peterson KL: Quantitative angiographic analysis of the left ventricle in patients with isolated rheumatic stenosis. Br Heart J 1973; 35:497.

83. Silverstein DM, Hansen DP, Ojiambo HP, Griswold HE: Left ventricular function in severe mitral stenosis as seen at the Kenyatta National Hospital. Am Heart J 1980; 99:727–733.

84. Gash AK, Carabello BA, Cepin D, Spann JF: Left ventricular ejection performance and systolic muscle function in patients with mitral stenosis. Circulation 1983; 67:148–154.

85. Mohan JC, Khalilullah M, Arora R: Left ventricular intrinsic contractility in pure rheumatic mitral stenosis. Am J Cardiol 1989; 64:240–242.

86. Bolen JL, Lopez MG, Harrison DC, Alderman EL: Analysis of left ventricular function in response to afterload changes in patients with mitral stenosis. Circulation 1975; 52:894.

87. Johnston DL, Kostuk WJ: Left and right ventricular function during symptom-limited exercise in patients with isolated mitral stenosis. Chest 1986; 89:186–191.

88. Urschel CW, Covell JW, Sonnenblick EH, et al: Myocardial mechanics in aortic and mitral valvular regurgitation: The concept of instantaneous impedance as a determinant of the performance of the intact heart. J Clin Invest 1968; 47:867–883.

89. Urschel CW, Covell JW, Graham TP, et al: Effects of acute valvular regurgitation on the oxygen consumption of the canine heart. Circ Res 1968; 23:33.

90. Corin WJ, Murakami T, Monrad ES, et al: Left ventricular passive diastolic properties in chronic mitral regurgitation. Circulation 1991; 83:797.

91. Kihara Y, Sasayama S, Miyazaki S, et al: Role of the left atrium in the adaptation of the heart to chronic mitral regurgitation in conscious dogs. Circ Res 1988; 62:543.

92. Braunwald E, Awe WC: The syndrome of severe mitral regurgitation with normal left atrial pressure. Circulation 1963; 27:29.

93. Levinson GE, Frank MJ, Schwartz CG: The effect of rest and physical effort on the left ventricular burden in mitral and aortic regurgitation. Am Heart J 1970; 80:791–801.

94. Chatterjee K: Vasodilator therapy for mitral regurgitation. In Duran C, Angell WW, Johnson AD, Oury JH (eds): Recent Progress in Mitral Valve Disease. London, Butterworths, 1984, pp 138–148.

95. Rapaport E: Natural history of aortic and mitral valve disease. Am J Cardiol 1975; 35:221.

96. Crawford MH, Souchek J, Oprian CA, et al: Determinants of survival and ventricular performance after mitral valve replacement. Circulation 1990; 81:1173–1181.

97. Carabello BA, Barry WH, Grossman W: Changes in arterial pressure during left heart pullback in patients with aortic stenosis: A sign of severe aortic stenosis. Am J Cardiol 1979; 44:424.

98. Folland ED, Parisi AF, Carbone C: Is peripheral arterial pressure a satisfactory substitute for ascending aortic pressure when measuring aortic valve gradients? J Am Coll Cardiol 1984; 4:1207.

99. Gorlin R, McMillan IKR, Medd WE, et al: Dynamics of the circulation in aortic valvular disease. Am J Med 1955; 18:855–870.

100. Anderson FL, Tsagaris TJ, Tikoff G, et al: Hemodynamic effects of exercise in patients with aortic stenosis. Am J Med 1964; 46:872–885.

101. Lee SJK, Johnson B, Bevegard S, et al: Hemodynamic changes at rest and during exercise in patients with aortic stenosis of varying severity. Am Heart J 1970; 79:318–331.

102. Richardson JW, Anderson FL, Tsagaris TJ: Rest and exercise hemodynamic studies in patients with isolated aortic stenosis. Cardiology 1979; 64:1–11.

103. Sasayama S, Ross J Jr, Franklin D, et al: Adaptations of the left ventricle to chronic pressure overload. Circ Res 1976; 38:172–178.

104. Grossman W, Jones D, McLaurin LP: Wall stress and patterns of hypertrophy in the human left ventricle. J Clin Invest 1975; 56:56.

105. Peterson KL, Tsuji J, Johnson A, et al: Diastolic left ventricular pressure-volume and stress-strain relations in patients with valvular aortic stenosis and left ventricular hypertrophy. Circulation 1978; 58:77–89.

106. Peterson KL, Ricci D, Tsuji J, Sasayama S, Ross J Jr: Evaluation of chamber and myocardial compliance in pressure overload hypertrophy. Eur J Cardiol 1978; 7(Suppl):195–211.

107. Hess OM, Ritter M, Schneider J, et al: Diastolic stiffness and myocardial structure in aortic valve disease before and after valve replacement. Circulation 1984; 69:855–865.

108. Peterson KL: Instantaneous force-velocity-length relations of the left ventricle: Methods, limitations, and applications in humans. In Fishman AP (ed): Heart Failure. Washington, Hemisphere, 1978, pp 121–132.

109. Gunther S, Grossman W: Determinants of ventricular function in pressure-overload hypertrophy in man. Circulation 1979; 59:679–688.

110. Carabello BA, Green LH, Grossman W, et al: Hemodynamic determinants of prognosis of aortic valve replacement in critical aortic stenosis and advanced congestive heart failure. Circulation 1980; 62:42–48.

111. Glancy DL, Freed TA, O'Brien KP, et al: Calcium in the aortic valve: Roentgenologic and hemodynamic

correlations in 148 patients. Ann Intern Med 1969; 71:245–250.

112. Morganroth J, Perloff JK, Zeldis SM, et al: Acute severe aortic regurgitation: Pathophysiology, clinical recognition, and management. Ann Intern Med 1977; 87:225.

113. Perloff JK: Acute severe aortic regurgitation: Recognition and management. J Cardiovasc Med 1983; 8:209.

114. Downes TR, Nomeir A-M, Hackshaw BT, et al: Diastolic mitral regurgitation in acute but not chronic aortic regurgitation: Implications regarding the mechanism of mitral closure. Am Heart J 1989; 117:1106.

115. Levinson GE, Grank MJ, Schwartz CJ: The effect of rest and physical effort on the left ventricular burden in mitral and aortic regurgitation. Am Heart J 1970; 80:791–801.

116. Lewis RP, Bristow JD, Griswald HE: Exercise hemodynamics in aortic regurgitation. Am Heart J 1970; 80:171–176.

117. Nusrat A, Massie BM: The role of exercise measure-ments in the evaluation of valvular heart disease. *In* Greenberg BH, Murphy E (eds): Valvular Heart Disease, Littleton, MA, PSG, 1987.

118. Massie BM, Kramer BL, Loge D, et al: Ejection fraction response to supine exercise in asymptomatic aortic regurgitation: Relation to simultaneous hemodynamic measurements. J Am Coll Cardiol 1985; 5:847–855.

119. Greves J, DeMots H, Murphy E, et al: Transthoracic left ventricular puncture and angiography in patients with double valve disease. Circulation 1979; 60-II:99.

120. Baxley WA, Soto B: Hemodynamic evaluation of patients with combined aortic and mitral prostheses. Am J Cardiol 1980; 45:42–47.

121. Gash AK, Carabello BA, Kent RL, et al: Left ventricular performance in patients with coexistent mitral stenosis and aortic insufficiency. J Am Coll Cardiol 1984; 3:703–711.

122. Braunwald E: Valvular heart disease. *In* Braunwald E (ed): Heart Disease, 4th ed. Philadelphia, W. B. Saunders, 1992.

Chapter 19

Catheterization and Angiography in Coronary Heart Disease

KIRK L. PETERSON
VALMIK BHARGAVA
PASCAL NICOD

Despite a recent decline over the last 3 decades, coronary artery disease remains a major cause of morbidity and mortality worldwide. In 1988, 511,050 people in the United States died of coronary artery disease. In a 20-year follow-up analysis of 5209 men or women aged 30 to 62 years from the Framingham study, the most common manifestation of the disease was myocardial infarction (45%), whereas in women it was angina pectoris (56%).[1]

In either the symptomatic or asymptomatic patient, evaluation of the risk profile, combined with noninvasive stress testing (electrocardiography, alone or with radionuclide or sonographic cardiac imaging), generally allows detection of significant coronary artery obstruction. Once the diagnosis is established, global left ventricular function and the extent of regional myocardium at risk become major determinants of prognosis. Thus, in many patients further diagnostic studies in the cardiac catheterization laboratory are used to evaluate comprehensively the severity and extent of disease and specific choices for medical, interventional, or surgical therapy.

Selective coronary angiography remains the primary diagnostic method for the study of coronary artery disease in the cardiac catheterization suite. Other than its use to define the extent and severity of disease and to determine the feasibility and efficacy of coronary angioplasty, bypass surgery, and thrombolysis, coronary angiography is also being used to assess coronary vasomotion and regression of atherosclerotic lesions after various medical or dietary interventions. Specific indications for coronary angiography have been formulated by an American College of Cardiology–American Heart As-

sociation joint task force[2]; the recommendations of this committee are also reviewed in Chapter 9. Those conditions for which coronary angiography is considered are grouped into the following three classes:

Class 1—represents conditions for which there is general agreement that coronary angiography is justified

Class 2—represents conditions for which coronary angiography is frequently performed, but there is a divergence of opinions with respect to its justification in terms of value and appropriateness

Class 3—represents conditions for which there is general agreement that coronary angiography is not justified

The task force has evaluated indications for coronary angiography in the following groups:

I. Patients with known or suspected coronary heart disease that is (A) asymptomatic and (B) symptomatic

II. Patients with atypical chest pain of uncertain origin

III. Patients after myocardial infarction that is (A) evolving; (B) completed; and (C) convalescent

A summary of the task force criteria is presented in Table 19–1.

INTERPRETATION OF CORONARY ANGIOGRAPHY: RELATION TO PROGNOSIS

Subjective interpretation of a coronary arteriogram is confounded by significant intraob-

Table 19–1. American College of Cardiology–American Heart Association Task Force Criteria for Coronary Angiography

I.A. Asymptomatic Patients with Known or Suspected Coronary Artery Disease

This group includes patients with previous (>8-week-old) myocardial infarction, coronary artery bypass surgery, or angioplasty (known coronary artery disease) and those with rest- or exercise-induced ECG abnormalities suggesting silent myocardial ischemia, often associated with other risk factors (suspected coronary artery disease).

Class 1
1. Evidence of high-risk status on noninvasive testing
   a. Exercise ECG testing
      (1) Horizontal or downsloping ST depression
         - Onset at heart rate <120 beats/min, off β-adrenergic blocking agents, or ≤6.5 METS*
         - Magnitude ≥2 mm of ST segment depression
         - Postexercise duration of ST segment depression ≥6 min
         - ST segment depression in multiple leads
      (2) Abnormal systolic blood pressure response during exercise
         - Sustained decrease of >10 mm Hg or flat blood pressure response (≤130 mm Hg), associated with ECG evidence of ischemia
      (3) Other determinants
         - Exercise-induced ST segment *elevation* in leads other than aVR (in the absence of previous Q wave infarction)
         - Exercise-induced ventricular tachycardia
   b. Thallium scintigraphy
      - Abnormal rest or exercise thallium distribution in more than one myocardial region
      - Increase in lung uptake in absence of severely depressed left ventricular function at rest
   c. Radionuclide ventriculography
      - ≥10% fall in left ventricular ejection fraction during exercise
      - Rest or exercise left ventricular ejection fraction ≤50%, when suspected to be due to coronary artery disease
2. Occupations involving the safety of others (such as drivers and pilots) or requiring sudden vigorous activity (such as firefighters and athletes)
3. Survival after resuscitation from cardiac arrest, with no obvious cause but a suspicion of coronary artery disease

Class 2
1. Presence of ≥1 but ≤2 mm of ST depression during exercise, confirmed as ischemia by an independent noninvasive stress test (radionuclide or echocardiographic study), without high-risk criteria listed above
2. Presence of two or more risk factors (smoking, hypertension, hypercholesterolemia, positive family history, diabetes) and a positive exercise test in men (without known coronary artery disease)
3. Presence of prior myocardial infarction at rest and evidence of ischemia by noninvasive testing (without high-risk criteria)
4. After revascularization procedures (angioplasty or coronary artery bypass surgery) in the presence of ischemia by noninvasive testing
5. Before high-risk noncardiac surgery in patients who have evidence of ischemia by noninvasive testing
6. Post-cardiac transplantation periodic evaluation

Class 3
1. Screening for coronary artery disease, without prior use of noninvasive testing
2. Follow-up after revascularization, without evidence of ischemia on noninvasive testing
3. Presence of abnormal ECG exercise test alone, excluding patients defined in classes 1 and 2

I.B. Symptomatic Patients with Known or Suspected Coronary Artery Disease

Class 1
1. Symptoms that responded inadequately to medical, interventional, or surgical treatment, or a combination of them, that significantly interfere with daily life
2. Unstable angina pectoris
3. Prinzmetal's variant angina pectoris
4. Angina pectoris in association with any of the following:
   a. Evidence of high risk as defined for asymptomatic patients. Other high-risk criteria include failure to complete stage II of the Bruce protocol or an equivalent work load, and an exercise heart rate ≤120 beats/min at the onset of symptoms
   b. Coexistence of a history of previous myocardial infarction or hypertension and ST segment depression on baseline ECG
   c. Intolerance to medical therapy
   d. Occupation or lifestyle involving unusual risk, or "need to know" for insurance or job-related purposes
   e. Recurrent episodes of pulmonary edema or left ventricular failure of unknown origin
5. Preoperative evaluation for major vascular surgery, in the presence of angina or objective evidence of ischemia
6. After resuscitation for cardiac arrest or sustained ventricular tachycardia in the absence of acute myocardial infarction

Class 2
1. Angina pectoris
   a. In women <40 years of age (with objective, noninvasive evidence of ischemia)
   b. In men <40 years of age
   c. In patients <40 years of age with previous myocardial infarction
   d. In patients requiring major nonvascular surgery, if there is evidence of ischemia on noninvasive testing
   e. In patients with progressively more abnormal noninvasive stress test on serial evaluations

2. Severe angina pectoris (Canadian class III or IV) that changes to mild angina on medical therapy, in the absence of high-risk criteria (see above)
3. Patients who cannot be evaluated by noninvasive testing

Class 3
1. Mild, clinically stable angina pectoris, in the absence of impaired left ventricular function, high-risk exercise studies, or criteria listed in classes 1 and 2
2. Well-controlled angina pectoris in patients with limited life expectancy because of age or the presence of other illness

II. Patients with Atypical Chest Pain

Class 1
1. Presence of high-risk criteria as defined above
2. Suspicion of coronary spasm
3. Associated symptoms or signs of left ventricular dysfunction

Class 2
1. Noninvasive testing equivocal or impossible to perform
2. Severe recurrent symptoms, even in the absence of noninvasive evidence of ischemia

Class 3
1. Previous normal coronary angiogram and normal noninvasive testing

III. A. Patients Following an Evolving Myocardial Infarction (initial hours)

Class 1
None
Class 2
1. Patients for whom revascularization is considered (angioplasty, bypass surgery, or thrombolysis), if angiography can be performed within 6 hours of onset of clinical syndrome (see Chapter 27)
2. When angioplasty or coronary bypass surgery is considered immediately after thrombolysis (see Chapter 27)
Class 3
None

III. B. Patients Following a Completed Myocardial Infarction (after the intial 6 hours but not including the predischarge evaluation)

Class 1
1. Recurrent ischemic chest pain
2. Suspected mitral regurgitation or interventricular septal rupture causing left ventricular failure or shock
3. Suspected postinfarction pseudoaneurysm

Class 2
1. After thrombolysis, particularly in the presence of signs of reperfusion
2. Congestive heart failure, hypotension, or both, despite medical therapy
3. Recurrent malignant ventricular arrhythmia despite medical therapy
4. Cardiogenic shock
5. When infarction is suspected to be the consequence of coronary embolization

Class 3
1. Myocardial infarction after which no acute mechanical or surgical intervention is contemplated

III. C. Patients Convalescing After Myocardial Infarction (predischarge up to 8 weeks)

Class 1
1. Angina pectoris occurring at rest or with minimal physical activity
2. In selected patients with heart failure during the evolving phase, or left ventricular ejection fraction <0.45%, primarily when associated with evidence of recurrent myocardial ischemia or with significant ventricular arrhythmias
3. Evidence of myocardial ischemia on noninvasive testing
4. Non-Q wave myocardial infarction

Class 2
1. Mild angina pectoris
2. Age <50 years, despite absence of symptoms
3. Need to return to unusually active and vigorous physical employment
4. Past history of myocardial infarction or stable angina, or both, present for >6 months before current infarction
5. Thrombolytic therapy during the evolving phase, particularly with evidence of reperfusion

Class 3
1. Advanced physiologic age
2. Coexisting illnesses limiting life expectancy
3. Severe left ventricular dysfunction (ejection fraction <0.2%) in the absence of angina or noninvasive evidence of ischemia, with the exception of patients considered for aneurysmectomy and cardiac transplantation
4. Ventricular arrhythmias, in the absence of symptoms or signs of ischemia, and no evidence of aneurysm formation, with the exception of refractory ventricular tachycardia

---

*Energy expenditure at rest, equivalent to an oxygen uptake of approximately 3.5 mL O_2/kg body weight.
ECG, electrocardiograph.

server and interobserver variability.[3, 4] Nevertheless, studies dating back to the 1960s that categorize the extent, severity, and location of disease have provided valuable insights into patient prognosis.

Chronic Stable Angina

Shortly after the use of coronary angiography became widespread, reports from the Cleveland Clinic[5, 6] and Duke University[7] showed a relation between the number of diseased coronary vessels and prognosis. Lim and associates[5] showed a 5-year mortality of 51% in patients with 50% or greater left main coronary artery stenosis. Harris and colleagues[7] reported in the Duke data bank an annual mortality rate of 1.6%, 3%, 7.2%, and 12.6% for patients with one-vessel, two-vessel, three-vessel, and left main coronary artery disease, respectively. In the subset with reduced left ventricular function, 5-year survival was 38% compared with 89% in those with normal ventricular function. In the 1970s, several large studies of medical versus surgical treatment for coronary artery disease largely confirmed these early observations. In the Coronary Artery Surgery Study (CASS) registry,[8] patients with proximal narrowing of one, two, and three vessels, had a 6-year survival of 77%, 58%, and

40%, respectively, compared with 88%, 74%, and 56% for those with nonproximal stenoses. Left ventricular ejection fraction (LVEF) had a significant impact on survival: 58% of patients with an LVEF lower than 35% survived at 4 years versus 92% for those with LVEF higher than 50%. Zack and coworkers[9] have identified a subgroup of patients with left main equivalent (proximal stenosis of the left anterior descending and the circumflex arteries) with an overall 8-year survival of 43% only, a statistic again markedly influenced by LVEF.

In the European Coronary Surgery Study,[10] annual mortality in the medically treated group was 2.4%, 3.6%, and 6.4% for two-vessel, three-vessel, and left main coronary artery disease, respectively. Proximal involvement of the left anterior descending artery decreased 12-year survival to 65% compared with 83% for nonproximal stenoses (Fig. 19–1).[11] In the Veterans Administration Study,[12] annual mortality for one-vessel, two-vessel, and three-vessel disease was 3.2%, 2.8%, and 4.5%, respectively. A major influence of LVEF on survival was also found. Thus, these studies have reiterated the important influence of left main disease, the severity and upstream location of coronary stenosis (particularly when in the left anterior descending), and LVEF on prognosis.

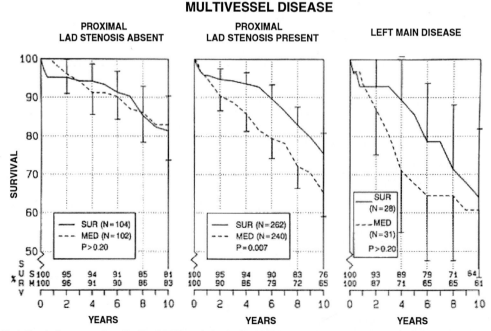

Figure 19–1. Survival curves of medically (MED) and surgically (SUR) treated patient cohorts, segregated by left main coronary artery disease and the presence or absence of a proximal left anterior descending (LAD) stenosis. Note the adverse influence on survival of both left main disease and the presence of a proximal lesion in the LAD group. (Modified from Varnauskas E, European Coronary Surgery Study Group: Twelve-year follow-up of survival in the randomized European Coronary Surgery Group. N Engl J Med 1988; 319:332–337.)

Findings from cardiac catheterization must be evaluated with other clinical features to better assess prognosis. The presence of severe angina, abnormal exercise testing, and previous myocardial infarction significantly worsen prognosis.[13-15] These clinical parameters may explain differences in survival between studies. For instance, in the European study, only patients with mild to moderate angina and normal LVEF were included, explaining a favorable overall 5-year survival.

Evidence of progression of coronary artery disease from one angiogram to another may be another factor portending a poor prognosis. Waters and associates[16] showed a relative risk of cardiac death of 7.3 in a group of patients with evidence of progression compared with a non-progressor group. This emphasizes the need to find medical strategies that prevent progression or even induce regression of coronary artery disease.

Unstable Angina

In unstable angina, the extent of coronary artery disease varies between studies, depending on the criteria used for patient inclusion. In an early study, Alison and colleagues[17] reported an 11% incidence of normal coronary arteries and an 11% incidence of left main coronary artery disease. Most complications (overall 4.5% fatal and 3% nonfatal infarctions in the first 2 weeks) occurred in patients with left main or three-vessel coronary artery disease, particularly when associated with left ventricular dysfunction. In the National Cooperative Study Group,[18, 19] pa-

tients with left main coronary artery disease, those with an LVEF less than 30%, and those with severe distal coronary occlusions were excluded. All patients had ischemic ST segment or T wave changes, and 90% of them had pain at rest. In this study, 76% of patients had multivessel coronary artery disease. In the medically treated group, the in-hospital mortality and nonfatal myocardial infarction rates were 7% and 11%, respectively, and were particularly increased in those with spontaneous episodes of ST segment elevation. In the randomized Veterans Administration Cooperative Study,[20, 21] 35% of the patients had two-vessel and 46% had three-vessel coronary artery disease. Prognosis was markedly influenced by LVEF.

In the CASS registry of patients who received bypass surgery for unstable angina, 50% had three-vessel and 14% had left main coronary artery disease.[22] However, in a subset of patients with new-onset unstable angina and no history of chronic stable angina or previous infarction, the incidence of single-vessel artery disease has been reported to be significantly higher.[23]

CLASSIFICATION OF LESION TYPES

Unstable angina and myocardial infarction both may be triggered by plaque rupture or ulceration (Fig. 19-2), platelet aggregation, thrombosis, and vasoconstriction.[24] Postmortem studies have shown a correlation between the presence of irregular (or complex) lesions on angiography and the presence of plaque rup-

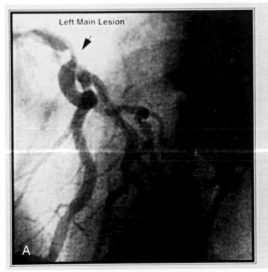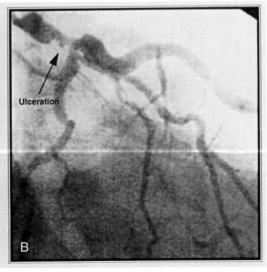

Figure 19-2. Left *(A)* and right *(B)* anterior oblique coronary angiograms of a patient with unstable angina, a high-grade left main lesion, and an ulceration within the obstructive plaque.

CONCENTRIC LESIONS

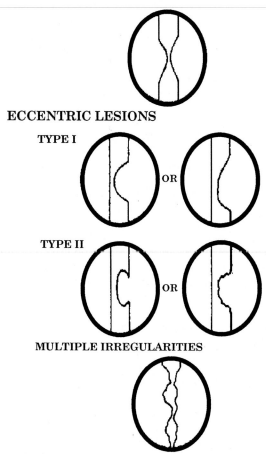

ECCENTRIC LESIONS

TYPE I

OR

TYPE II

OR

MULTIPLE IRREGULARITIES

Figure 19–3. Classification of lesion types based on their appearance on coronary angiography. (Reprinted with permission from the American College of Cardiology [Journal of the American College of Cardiology, 1985; 5:609–616].)

ture, subintimal hemorrhage within the plaque, and fresh or recanalized thrombi on histologic examination.[25] In 1985, Ambrose and coworkers[26] proposed the following angiographic classification of coronary stenoses (Fig. 19–3):

1. Concentric stenosis—symmetric narrowing of a coronary artery; the borders of the lesion are smooth or only slightly irregular
2. Eccentric stenosis—asymmetric narrowing of a coronary artery. Two subgroups were defined
   a. Type 1—those with smooth borders and a broad neck
   b. Type 2—those with a convex intraluminal obstruction with a narrow base or neck due to one or more overhanging edges or borders, which may be irregular or scalloped
3. Multiple irregularities—the presence of three

or more serial, severe (≥70%), closely spaced obstructions; this also includes coronary arteries with severe diffuse irregularities or arteries in which a segment between two severe obstructions contains diffuse irregularities

Using this classification, Ambrose and coworkers[26] showed that 12 (48%) of 25 patients with stable angina had concentric lesions and 8 (32%) of 25 had eccentric, type 1 lesions. Only 4 (16%) of 25 and 1 (4%) of 25 had eccentric, type 2 lesions or multiple irregularities, respectively. Patients with unstable angina more often had eccentric, type 2 lesions (6 [14.6%] of 41) or multiple irregularities (29 [70.7%] of 41). Few had concentric lesions (6 [14.6%] of 41). These observations have been largely confirmed by others. Angiographic evidence of intracoronary thrombus is seen mostly in patients with unstable angina, but its incidence varies between studies because of difficulties with interpretation of angiograms and wide variations in the interval from onset of symptoms to the angiogram. In Holmes's[27] and Zack's[28] group studies, the low incidence (<12%) of intracoronary thrombi may be explained by a delayed angiogram (within 30 days from symptoms). Others have found incidence of thrombus as high as 58%, particularly when angiograms were performed within 24 hours from the last symptoms.[29, 30] On the other hand, angiographic evidence of intracoronary thrombi is rare in patients with stable angina.

The prognostic value of the interpretation of coronary lesions in acute coronary syndromes is not well known. This is in part because of the high incidence of interventions performed in unstable patients, particularly in the subgroup who undergo a diagnostic angiogram. According to Haft and Al-Zarka,[31] severe irregular lesions (90%) tended to progress to complete occlusion in 46% of the patients undergoing a second angiogram an average of 2.6 years later. Less severe, irregular lesions usually remained stable but irregular over time. On the other hand, most new irregular coronary lesions originated from less severe smooth stenoses.

In another study, Davies and associates[32] suggested that the presence of lesion irregularities had a negative prognostic value in a subset of patients with an acute coronary syndrome. In an analysis from the CASS registry, Ellis and colleagues[33] found a fourfold increase in the risk of myocardial infarction in medically treated patients with irregular left anterior descending coronary artery stenoses compared with those with smooth stenoses. All these studies, however, were influenced by patient selection, timing of angiography from onset of symptoms, and variations in the severity of underlying stenoses.[34]

LIMITATIONS OF CORONARY ANGIOGRAPHY

The severity of atherosclerotic lesions seen on coronary angiography does not correlate well with functional impairment of coronary flow, as shown by White and coworkers.[35] Furthermore, wall thickness and composition of the atherosclerotic plaque cannot be evaluated with coronary angiography, which only assesses the lumen of the vessel. Atherosclerosis may thicken the arterial wall despite only a small reduction of the lumen seen on angiography, because of compensatory outward expansion of the vessel wall.[36]

Recent techniques using Doppler flow-wires (see Chapter 6), quantitative myocardial perfusion parametric imaging (see digital coronary angiography, Chapter 10), inducible wall motion disturbances (see later discussion), or coronary translesional pressure measurements[37–39] may be better predictors of coronary flow reserve and give a superior evaluation of the functional severity of a given lesion. Improvement in intravascular sonographic techniques may, in the future, allow assessment of both vessel thickness and composition. Both panel reading (multiple observers with a combined consensus) and automated analysis of digitally processed angiograms also help reduce the variability in the ultimate interpretation.

Although the qualitative and quantitative interpretations of coronary lesions may have some prognostic value, as stated earlier, the clinical evolution of coronary artery disease is often unpredictable. Several angiographic studies have shown that myocardial infarction may occur in sites of the coronary tree where only minor stenoses were present on previous angiograms.[40, 41] Thus, coronary angiograms must be evaluated together with other clinical parameters such as age, symptoms, efficacy of medical treatment, and results of noninvasive testing, when the need for revascularization is being assessed. Any coronary lesion, even of lesser importance, may be the cause of myocardial infarction, which emphasizes the need for medical therapy and reduction of risk factors. In addition, subsets of patients for whom revascularization procedures have been shown to be superior to medical therapy should be identified on the basis of clinical and angiographic parameters.

CORONARY ARTERIAL TONE

Both physiologic and pharmacologic interventions in the catheterization laboratory have been shown to affect coronary arterial tone. This has led to a better understanding of the role of vasomotion and the endothelium in the pathogenesis of ischemia.

Physiologic Stimuli

Many stimuli, including exercise,[42, 43] pacing,[44] cold pressor testing,[45] and mental stress,[46] have a coronary vasodilatory effect in normal humans. The mechanism of vasodilation may differ for each stimulus. However, in most patients, increase in shear stress due to increased coronary blood flow and driving pressure is likely to produce an endothelial-dependent relaxing factor (EDRF)-mediated vasodilation. There is evidence that this factor is nitric oxide itself or a byproduct.[47, 48] Sympathetic stimulation may have opposing effects on vascular tone, including an α_1-adrenergic receptor–mediated vasoconstrictive effect on large epicardial coronary arteries[49]; a minor β_1-adrenergic receptor–mediated vasodilatory effect; and an α_2-adrenergic receptor–mediated release of EDRF, if endothelial function is intact.[50]

Several studies have shown that during such stimuli, a paradoxical coronary vasoconstriction may be seen in patients with various stages of atherosclerosis as a result of an alteration in the vasodilatory properties of the endothelium.[42–46] In their study, for instance, Yeung and associates[46] have elegantly shown that mental stress, a common occurrence in daily life, has a vasoconstrictive effect only in parts of the coronary tree with irregularities or stenoses. Zeiher and colleagues[51] have shown a progressive impairment of endothelial function during various stages of early atherosclerosis, using three different endothelial-mediated stimuli: (1) cold pressor testing, (2) intracoronary acetylcholine infusion, and (3) papaverine infusion. They have observed that early changes in patients with hypercholesterolemia and smooth arteries consisted in an abnormal response to acetylcholine, whereas flow-dependent vasodilation was preserved. On the other hand, later stages of atherosclerosis were associated with abnormal responses to all stimuli. They suggest that early atherosclerosis impairs first receptor-mediated, before flow-mediated, release of EDRF. Seiler and coworkers[52] have demonstrated a progressive impairment of exercise-induced coronary vasodilation correlated with increasing levels of plasma cholesterol. They also suggest that the effect of hypercholesterolemia or early athero-sclerosis affects endothelial-mediated vasodilation.

Pharmacologic Stimuli

Various pharmacologic agents have been used in the cardiac catheterization laboratory to influence coronary arterial tone. Some are endothelial dependent (such as acetylcholine, serotonin, histamine, and substance P), whereas others are endothelial independent (such as nitroglycerin and ergonovine).

The best-studied agent is acetylcholine. The technique used for acetylcholine infusion in our laboratory is the following[53]:

All antianginal drugs are discontinued at least 24 hours before the catheterization and angiographic procedure. After completion of diagnostic catheterization, a 3-French infusion catheter is placed subselectively into the proximal segment of the coronary artery to be studied through a standard 8-French guiding catheter, and pacing at 80 beats/min is secured from the right atrium. Biplane angiography is performed in the control state and after serial 3-minute infusions by a Harvard pump of acetylcholine at concentrations of 10^{-6} M, 10^{-5} M, and 10^{-4} M; assuming a coronary artery flow of 80 mL/min, intracoronary acetylcholine concentrations are 10^{-8}, 10^{-7}, and 10^{-6} M, respectively. Coronary arteriography is performed by electrocardiographic-gated power injection of 9 mL of nonionic contrast agent (Omnipaque, 350 mg/mL) at 6 mL/sec using a Medrad Mark IV injector (Medrad, Inc., Pittsburgh, PA).

All images are acquired maintaining identical x-ray gantry, table height, and source-to-image intensifier distance; that is, the magnifications and projections are maintained constant throughout the imaging sequences. Projections are selected to (1) optimally display the maximum length of the vessel parallel to the image plane to minimize foreshortening; (2) minimize superimposition of branches and other arteries; and (3) minimize overlap of the artery with the diaphragm, spine, and lung field. To assess comprehensively changes in vasomotor tone, we have developed quantitative coronary angiography software that allows detection of coronary artery dimensions over multiple segments of a given coronary artery (Fig. 19–4).[53] This computer routine also interpolates the pharmacologically stressed, whole-artery diameter function against the control injection so as to ensure that fiducial points (branch takeoffs) are corresponding (Fig. 19–5). It has also been demonstrated in multiple, sequential control injections (without pharmacologic stress) that the limit of reproducibility for the average diameter over an

approximately 5-mm segment has an SD of 0.153 mm.[53] Thus, in our laboratory a change in average diameter of at least 0.31 mm (2 SDs) over a segment of this size would be required to have a 95% confidence level that a detected change in vasomotion was not the result of the inherent error of measurement by quantitative angiography.

Ludmer and associates[54] first reported paradoxical vasoconstriction to acetylcholine in patients with coronary artery disease. Subsequently, several groups have confirmed and extended these findings by demonstrating a similar phenomenon in patients with elevated cholesterol levels, a family history of coronary artery disease, hypertension, male sex, advanced age, and smoking.[55–62] In some patients, paradoxical vasoconstriction seems to be present even before alterations in endothelial morphology are found. This paradoxical response to acetylcholine is interpreted as a dysfunction of endothelial-mediated vasodilation, with liberation of the direct muscarinic vasoconstrictive effect of acetylcholine on smooth muscle. Such dysfunction of receptor-mediated, endothelial-dependent vasodilation seems to occur before dysfunction of flow-mediated, endothelial-dependent vasodilation, in a hierarchical fashion, as described earlier.[51]

This paradoxical vasoconstriction may be highly heterogenous along the coronary tree. In our research, significant vasodilation and vasoconstriction are found in the same coronary artery in almost half the patients studied.[53] This suggests that inclusion of the entire analyzable region of a coronary artery is mandatory, particularly if sequential angiograms are to be compared over time. Reversal of paradoxical vasoconstriction after cholesterol level reduction has been shown to occur in localized segments.[63–65]

In patients with variant angina and coronary spasm, a good correlation between acetylcholine and ergonovine-induced spasm has been reported.[66]

Other agents, such as serotonin and substance P, have been used to assess endothelial function. Golino and colleagues[67] have reported a significant paradoxical vasoconstriction after graded serotonin infusion (at doses of 0.1, 1, and 10 μg/kg of body weight) in patients with coronary artery disease that was reversed by administration of ketanserin (which blocks 5-hydroxytryptamine$_2$ [5HT$_2$] receptors). Again, such a phenomenon may be explained by a dysfunction of endothelial-mediated vasodilation, with liberation of the direct vasoconstrictive effect of serotonin. Blockade of the paradoxical vasoconstriction by ketanserin suggests

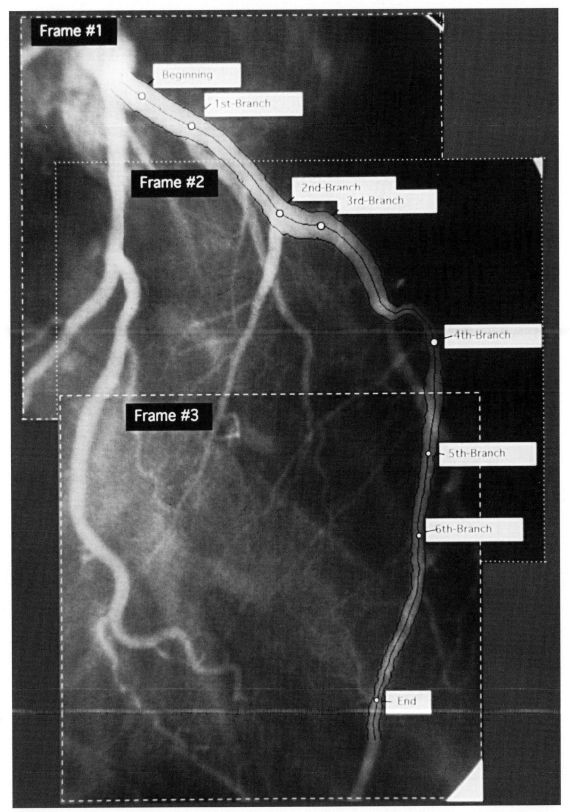

Figure 19–4. Digitally spliced image of a left anterior descending coronary artery (three separate end-diastolic frames) with superimposed vessel edges determined by edge recognition algorithm, annotated fiducial (branch) points, and beginning and end points of diameter function. (Reprinted with permission from the American College of Cardiology [Journal of the American College of Cardiology, 1995; 25:1046–1055].)

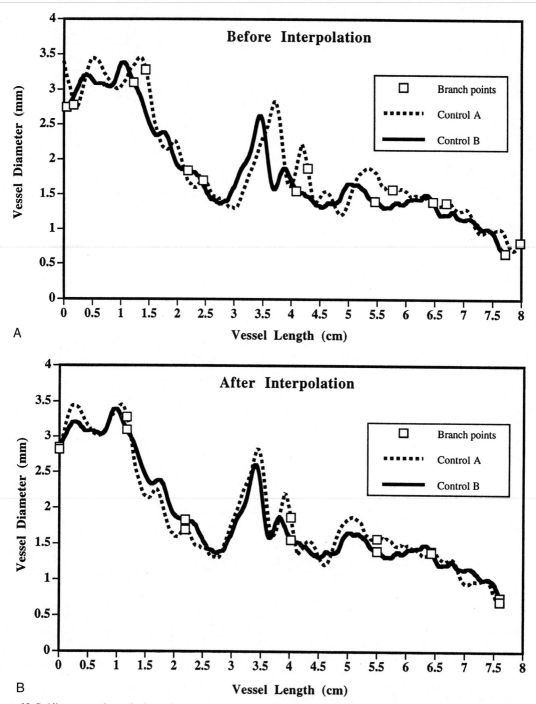

Figure 19–5. Alignment of vessels through interpolation. *A,* Vessel diameter (millimeter) versus length (centimeter) functions for two successive coronary angiograms. Note the slight change in overall length and lack of registration of branch points. *B,* Same curves as in *A.* The injection A diameter function has now been interpolated to that of injection B to effect anatomic registration of the beginning point, end point, and definable branch points.

a prominent role for $5HT_2$ receptors. After coronary angioplasty, a marked vasoconstrictive effect is seen at the site of angioplasty compared with nondilated segments.[68] This also suggests a role of the endothelium in serotonin-mediated vasomotion, although another explanation could be that smooth muscle cells may become hypersensitive to serotonin after angioplasty.

In patients with variant angina,[69] coronary spasm may be triggered by serotonin, which cannot be prevented by ketanserin, suggesting a role of $5HT_1$ receptors in this condition. The intracoronary infusion of serotonin may be less safe than acetylcholine because it may also activate platelet aggregation. A few cases of temporary coronary occlusion have occurred as a result of spasm and possible coronary thrombosis.[70]

Substance P has also been used to test endothelial-dependent vasodilation. This agent is particularly interesting because it lacks the direct vasoconstrictive effect on smooth muscle that acetylcholine and serotonin have. In patients with variant angina, it produces vasodilation even at sites of known spasms when given intracoronary at doses of 13.5, 40, and 135 ng over 1 minute.[71, 72] These studies suggest that coronary spasm in patients with variant angina results from vascular hyperreactivity rather than endothelial dysfunction.

Ergonovine, a coronary vasoconstrictor acting on both α-adrenergic and serotonergic receptors, can be used to induce focal spasm and test for variant anginal syndrome during coronary angiography. Its use should be restricted to patients with only mild coronary stenosis or normal arteries. The drug (0.05 to 0.4 mg) is given intravenously in 0.05-mg increments (at 3- to 5-minute intervals) and under clinical, electrocardiographic, and angiographic monitoring[73, 74]; nitroglycerin is kept available for immediate intracoronary administration in the event that ergonovine causes sustained spasm, ischemia, and ventricular arrhythmias. If intracoronary nitroglycerin is unsuccessful in relieving refractory spasm, repeated low doses of verapamil, 0.1 mg intracoronary, may be used, but the patient should be watched carefully for bradycardia or worsening hypotension, or both. Falsely negative responses to ergonovine may be noted if the patient is not withdrawn from calcium channel blockers and long-acting nitrates for at least 24 hours before the procedure.

The sensitivity of the ergonovine challenge for induction of focal spasm is highly dependent on the population of patients chosen for study.[75] Those with known variant angina prove frequently to have a positive response. Conversely, the response is positive in fewer than 5% of those patients whose symptoms do not suggest Prinzmetal's variant anginal syndrome. Diffuse coronary arterial narrowing in response to ergonovine, as opposed to focal segmental spasm, is usually noted in normal subjects and should not be misinterpreted as indicative of variant anginal syndrome.[76]

FUNCTIONAL ASSESSMENT OF THE SEVERITY OF CORONARY ARTERY OBSTRUCTION

Because assessment of the severity of coronary artery obstruction by coronary angiography is plagued by observer variability[3, 4] and relatively poor correlation with the actual pathology of a given lesion,[77-79] considerable attention has been focused on measuring physiologic or metabolic parameters that reflect sufficient compromise of vessel lumen cross-sectional area to cause myocardial ischemia. These parameters include (1) reduction in coronary flow reserve; (2) rest and maximal vasodilatory coronary translesional pressure gradient; (3) electrocardiographic changes of ischemia during a physiologic stress; (4) metabolic byproducts of ischemia at rest or during a physiologic stress; (5) left ventricular function abnormalities during a physiologic stress; and (6) inducible left ventricular wall motion disturbances. Of these, the electrocardiographic and left ventricular function abnormalities have been most readily assessed; however, considerable progress has been made in the direct assessment of coronary flow reserve (see Chapter 6) by Doppler velocity catheters or digital angiography (see Chapter 10), proximal and distal coronary artery pressure measurements, and improved display and quantitation of regional dyssynergy.

DETECTION OF MYOCARDIAL ISCHEMIA BY CARDIAC PACING

In patients with one or several relatively fixed coronary obstructions, regional coronary perfusion generally remains adequate to meet basal myocardial oxygen requirements. Pathophysiologic manifestations of ischemia are apparent, therefore, only during periods of heightened myocardial oxygen demand or reduced coronary perfusion (oxygen supply) brought about by superimposed coronary artery spasm or thrombosis. It follows that comprehensive detection of myocardial ischemia is best accomplished by provocative techniques that tran-

Table 19–2. **Pathophysiologic Findings Provoked During Myocardial Ischemia by Cardiac Pacing**

Electrocardiographic Changes

ST segment depression >1 mm
Rate-dependent left bundle branch block
Ventricular extrasystoles

Myocardial Metabolism

Decreased lactate extraction or lactate production
Increased potassium release
Changes in amino acid uptake and release
Prostaglandin release

Left Ventricular Function

Elevation of left ventricular end-diastolic pressure
Increase in fiber stretch in ischemic area; with variable
effect on end-diastolic volume
Delayed pressure decline during isovolumic relaxation
Increase in myocardial stiffness
Regional asynergy and synchrony of ventricular wall
Variable effect on chamber ejection fraction, depending
on the size or area of ischemia

Coronary Blood Flow

Increase in coronary flow in normal areas, with decrease
in perfusion in those areas served by a
hemodynamically significant coronary artery
obstruction
Redistribution of flow away from the endocardium and
toward the subepicardium

siently and safely enhance myocardial oxygen demand or reduce oxygen supply. In the cardiac catheterization laboratory, induction of tachycardia by atrial and ventricular pacing has been the physiologic stress most commonly used to elicit a number of pathophysiologic and metabolic abnormalities associated with myocardial ischemia (Table 19–2). Other interventions that have been used include isometric exercise with hand-gripping, isotonic and isometric exercise using a bicycle ergometer, infusion of a β_1-adrenergic agent (such as isoproterenol and dobutamine), or combining pacing tachycardia with a sympathomimetic agent.

Cardiac pacing influences myocardial oxygen consumption primarily through its potential for augmenting heart rate and, indirectly, its effect on myocardial contractility (force-frequency relation) and wall stress development per minute. In an experimental preparation where the heart was forced to contract isovolumetrically and where peak systolic wall stress was held constant, a twofold increase in heart rate caused a doubling of the myocardial oxygen consumption per beat.[80] By analyzing beats immediately after pacing tachycardia, one can also study the heart during periods of residual increased contractility yet while wall stress per beat is enhanced compared with individual beats during pacing. This latter approach has

been found particularly useful for the study of left ventricular dimensions and wall motion during ischemia as compared with the basal state.

Electrocardiographic Responses to Pacing-induced Ischemia

Although others initially found electrocardiographic responses to pacing-induced ischemia to be relatively nonspecific and poorly sensitive, Heller and colleagues[81] later reported improved sensitivity (94%) and specificity (83%) provided a 12-lead electrocardiographic system was used, a change of 1 mm or more in horizontal or downsloping ST depression was used as the criterion for positivity, and a heart rate of 85% or greater of maximal age-predicted heart rate was achieved. Occasionally, atropine, 0.6 mg, needs to be given to inhibit atrioventricular block with pacing and to achieve a relatively rapid heart rate. Endocardial electrocardiograms, recorded locally in areas of suspected ischemia using a 0.064-inch unipolar electrode wire, also have been reported to improve the sensitivity for detection of pacing-induced ischemia.[82]

Metabolic Responses to Pacing-induced Ischemia

Because of its ability to augment myocardial oxygen demand while at the same time maintaining a relative steady state, cardiac pacing has been used to assess metabolic derangements associated with myocardial ischemia. Most commonly, the difference in lactate concentration between a systemic artery and the coronary sinus has been measured[83]; under normal circumstances, the myocardium does not produce a net amount of lactate, and the concentration in the venous effluent is significantly less than that in the coronary arteries. During myocardial ischemia oxidative phosphorylation is blocked and pyruvate accumulates and is reduced to lactate, which, in turn, is released. In addition, within myocardial cells lactic acid accumulates rapidly and serves to either directly or indirectly inhibit the activity of several important enzymes in the glycolytic pathway, including phosphofructokinase, phosphorylase kinase, hexokinase, and glyceraldehyde-3-phosphate dehydrogenase. Moreover, fatty acids, the other major fuel source of the heart, are inhibited from entering into the citric acid (Krebs) cycle because of a reduction in the activity of carnitine palmitoylcoenzyme A, a mitochondrial enzyme important in the oxidation of fatty acids. Ultimately, this sequence leads to a significant drop in oxidative phosphorylation with depressed production of

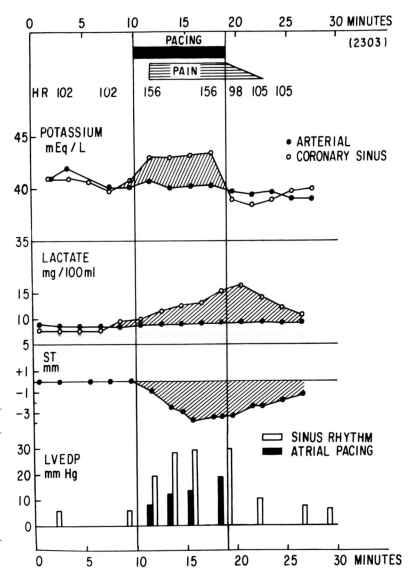

Figure 19–6. Alterations in potassium and lactate concentrations in coronary sinus blood during anginal pain provoked by pacing-induced tachycardia in a patient with coronary artery disease. Note that the concentration rise of these metabolic indices of ischemia correlated with depression of the ST segment on electrocardiogram and the rise of the left ventricular end-diastolic pressure (LVEDP). (From Parker JO, Chiong MA, West RO, Case RB: The effect of ischemia and alterations of heart rate on myocardial potassium balance in man. Circulation 1970; 42:205. Reproduced with permission of Circulation. Copyright 1970 American Heart Association.)

high-energy phosphate compounds, most importantly adenosine triphosphate. Demonstration of excess lactate production thus provides specific evidence of deranged glycolytic and oxidative metabolism in the presence of myocardial ischemia (Fig. 19–6).

Other metabolic indicators of ischemia that have been measured in the coronary sinus blood of humans during pacing-induced ischemia include serum potassium, amino acids, and prostaglandins. Parker and coworkers[84] demonstrated that potassium ion concentration in the coronary sinus increases in response to heart rate augmentation (see Fig. 19–6), a finding that had previously been described in the experimental animal. In 18 of 30 patients who ostensibly developed myocardial ischemia dur-

ing pacing (increase in lactate production and ST segment depression), potassium release into the coronary sinus was significantly greater than in patients without manifestations of ischemia. They found that approximately 1 mEq of potassium was lost for each 2 mmol of lactate produced.

As with skeletal muscle, there is evidence to suggest that alanine and glutamic acid play a central metabolic function in oxygen-deprived myocardial tissue. Mudge and associates[85] studied 19 patients (8 normal subjects and 11 with proven coronary artery disease) at rest and during pacing-induced tachycardia in order to test the hypothesis that cardiac amino acid metabolism, as defined by the arteriovenous difference, might be altered in chronic ischemic heart disease. They found that (1) alanine release from the normal myocardium occurred only during pacing stress and not at rest, whereas the diseased heart released alanine during both states; and (2) at rest, significant uptake of glutamate occurred in both normal and diseased hearts but was statistically greater in the coronary group; during pacing the arteriovenous difference in the normal group decreased to zero, whereas in the coronary group glutamate uptake persisted. Calculation of net amino acid fluxes ([arteriovenous difference] $\times$ [coronary sinus blood flow $\times$ hematocrit]) yielded similar conclusions to the arteriovenous differences alone. It was hypothesized from these results that during chronic ischemia a metabolic adaptation occurs whereby lactate accumulation causes a retardation (mass action effect) of pyruvate conversion to lactate with subsequent augmentation of glutamate-pyruvate transamination. During pacing the enhanced uptake of glutamate and release of alanine in the patients with coronary artery disease suggested that altered myocardial amino acid metabolism could then be used as a chemical marker of myocardial ischemia.

Berger and coworkers[86] reported that prostaglandin F, a substance that may serve a homeostatic function if it is inhibiting cardiac lysosomal enzyme release during coronary occlusion, was found in significantly higher quantities in blood withdrawn from the coronary sinus during anginal pain induced by atrial pacing. No such release could be shown by a similar radioimmunoassay for prostaglandins E and A.

Although these metabolic markers cited in the studies just mentioned are quite specific to myocardial ischemia, their use has been significantly compromised by the time and effort necessary to selectively catheterize the coronary sinus. They are primarily used in cardiac catheterization laboratories devoted to clinical research protocols.

Left Ventricular Responses to Pacing-induced Ischemia

Myocardial ischemia has significant effects on systolic and diastolic functions of the left ventricle. Important parameters to measure include the left ventricular end-diastolic pressure, the left ventricular end-diastolic volume, the maximum rate of systolic pressure change (peak [+]dP/dt), the maximum rate of isovolumetric pressure decay (peak [−]dP/dt), and the time constant of isovolumetric left ventricular pressure decay (Tau [T]). The simplest of these indices to quantitate is the left ventricular end-

diastolic pressure; it can be measured with reasonable accuracy using a fluid-filled catheter placed retrograde through the aortic valve into the left ventricle. Evaluation of other pressure parameters (peak [+]dP/dt, dP/dt at a given developed pressure, peak [−]dP/dt, or T), requires the use of a high-fidelity tip manometer pressure transducer (see Chapters 3, 4, 11, and 12).

Pacing-induced ischemia is associated with characteristic abnormalities of left ventricular end-diastolic pressure. Observations have been made both during and immediately after the cessation of pacing. Patients with induced ischemia show a modest elevation of the left ventricular end-diastolic pressure during pacing, and then on the cessation of pacing, during prolonged periods of diastolic filling, the end-diastolic pressure can reach levels between 20 and 40 mm Hg (Fig. 19–7). Dwyer[87] and Pasternac and colleagues[88] have reported that during pacing-induced ischemia, left ventricular end-diastolic volume either remained stable or declined in most subjects. In their observations, however, it is likely that left ventricular dimensions were influenced by the restriction of diastolic filling time during rapid pacing. Others have found that with immediate postpacing ischemia there was an increase in beginning- as well as end-diastolic volume, although the most notable effect was an upward shift in the diastolic pressure-volume relationship.[89, 90] These observations in humans, along with supportive experimental data, indicate that ischemia causes an increase in end-diastolic fiber length and in muscle stiffness, which together cause an upward and rightward shift of the end-diastolic pressure-volume relationship. Other factors that may contribute to this shift include (1) a constraining influence of the pericardium; (2) coronary hyperemia with consequential increase in myocardial turgor; (3) altered viscoelastic (velocity-dependent) properties of muscle during ischemia; and (4) delayed relaxation during early diastole, extending into the rapid filling phase (see later discussion).

In the presence of myocardial ischemia, either during pacing-induced tachycardia or in the immediate postpacing period, both peak (+)dP/dt and peak (−)dP/dt decrease, presumably in response, respectively, to a reduced force and extent of systolic contraction and a delay in relaxation in ischemic zones of the left ventricle. There is also evidence that during ischemia, regional asynchrony or temporal dispersion of contraction also may play an important role in the decrease of these indices (Fig. 19–8).

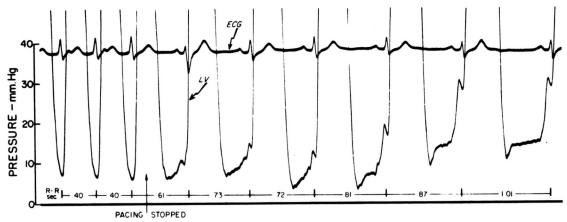

Figure 19–7. Left ventricular (LV) pressure at high gain and immediately after cessation of pacing. Note the increase in end-diastolic pressure in the six beats following the end of pacing, reflecting the persistence of ischemia. See text for discussion of possible mechanisms. (From O'Brien KP, Higgs LM, Glancy DL, et al: Hemodynamic accompaniments induced by exercise and by atrial pacing. Circulation 1969; 39:735–742. Reproduced with permission of Circulation. Copyright 1969 American Heart Association.)

Delayed relaxation, or pressure decline, during the isovolumetric phase after aortic valve closure is also noted with ischemia. Because the left ventricular pressure during the isovolu-metric relaxation phase decays near monoexponentially, the delay in relaxation can be quantitated by calculating a rate constant for this decay[91] (see Chapter 12). T, the negative inverse

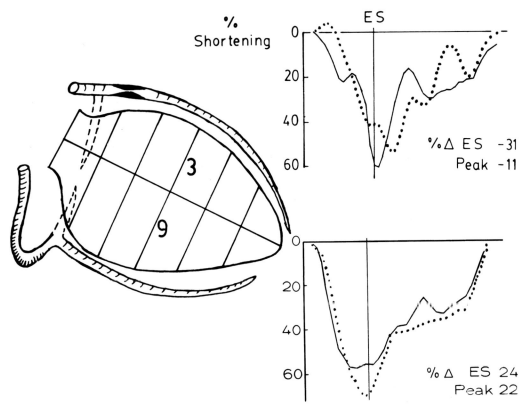

Figure 19–8. Chordal analysis of regional shortening of the left ventricular wall in control state *(solid line)* and during myocardial ischemia *(dotted line).* Chord 3 is shown in the upper panel, and chord 9 is shown in the lower panel. On the chord 3 plot, note the time delay of peak shortening during postpacing ischemia when compared with end-systole (ES) on the control ventriculogram.

of the rate constant, may be estimated by the slope of a straight line fitted to the natural log of pressure versus time, from peak negative pressure to a pressure just before the opening of the mitral valve. This mathematic model for the exponential decay assumes a zero asymptote. Alternatively, a three-constant, monoexponential model can be fitted to the pressure versus time data, over the same time span, according to the following equation (Fig. 19–9):

$$P = a + be^{-ct}$$

where P is pressure, a is the pressure asymptote as t approaches infinity, and c is the rate con-

stant. In this model, T is defined as $-1/c$. Figure 19–9 also demonstrates the shift in T in an experimental model of heart failure induced by long-term rapid pacing where subendocardial ischemia is believed to play a significant role in depression of myocardial shortening and delay of relaxation.

CORONARY PRESSURE AND VELOCITY MEASUREMENTS

Coronary atherosclerotic obstruction causes a significant pressure decrease across the lesion, particularly when the percent area obstruction

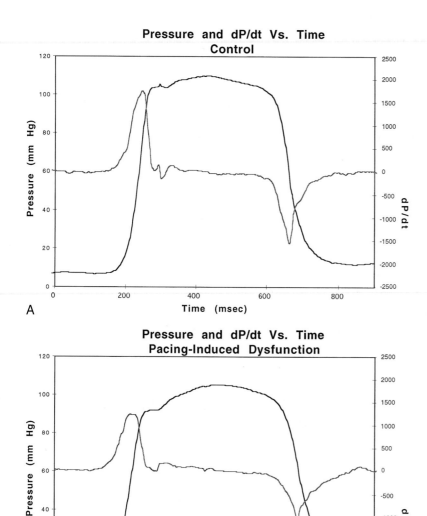

A

B

Figure 19–9. A, Left ventricular pressure and the first derivative (dP/dt) of pressure in the control state. B, Left ventricular pressure and first derivative (dP/dt) of pressure during pacing-induced dysfunction of the left ventricle.

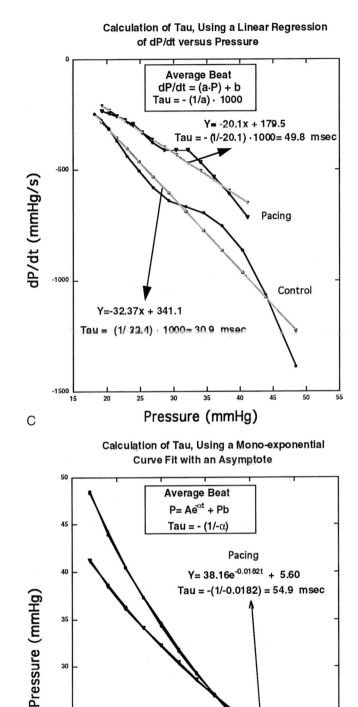

Figure 19–9 *Continued C,* Calculation of Tau (T) (rate constant of pressure decline during isovolumetric relaxation) based on a linear regression of dP/dt versus pressure relationship. See text for details of calculation. *D,* Calculation of Tau (rate constant of pressure decline during isovolumetric relaxation) based on a three-constant monoexponential mathematic model. See text for details of calculation.

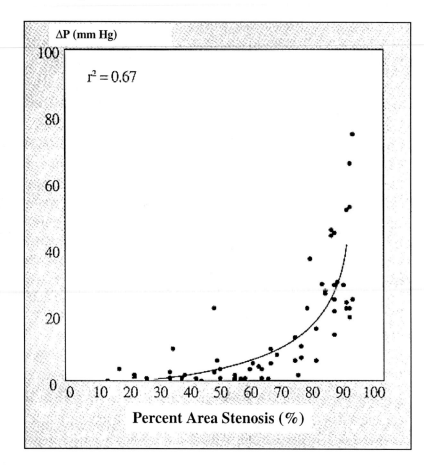

Figure 19–10. Relationship between the basal translesional pressure gradient (vertical axis) and the percent area stenosis by quantitative coronary angiography (horizontal axis) in patients with coronary artery disease. (From De Bruyne B, Pijls NHJ: Coronary pressure measurements. Primary Cardiol 1995; 21[5]:29.)

is 70% or greater (Fig. 19–10). The actual pressure gradient can be predicted by the following fluid dynamic equation:

$$\Delta P = \frac{8\pi\mu L}{A_s^2} \cdot Q + \frac{\rho}{2} \cdot \left(\frac{1}{A_s} - \frac{1}{A_n}\right)^2 \cdot Q^2$$

where ΔP is the pressure gradient, π is 3.1416, μ is the blood viscosity constant, L is stenosis length, Q is blood flow, ρ is blood density constant, A_s is stenotic area, and A_n is the normal area.

The first term in this equation relates to energy losses associated with viscous friction, as estimated by Poiseuille's law. The second term relates to the convective acceleration of blood, where the resultant pressure drop is estimated by the law of Bernoulli. From this equation it is apparent that the translesional pressure gradient is dependent on transstenotic flow. This dependency has been confirmed by direct translesional pressure measurements in humans, as shown in Figure 19–11.

Thus, to assess the functional importance

of a given coronary lesion under basal conditions, both flow (Q) and the pressure gradient (ΔP) must be measured. Doppler guide wire velocity measurements are now available (see Chapter 6) but are confounded by a dependence on measurement of cross-sectional area to convert velocity to flow. Moreover, basal flow measurements are influenced by regional myocardial oxygen demand and the distribution area of the artery in which it is being measured. Consequently, Pijls and associates[92] have proposed that the pressure gradient, measured during a period of maximal microcirculation vasodilation, should be used as an index of flow reserve. Maximum flow through a stenotic artery is compared with what maximum flow would be in that same artery in the absence of a stenosis. This ratio is termed the *fractional flow reserve* (FFR). If the coronary resistance is minimized (and thereby flow maximized) by pharmacologic dilation (e.g., papaverine or adenosine) of the microcirculation, then the translesional pressure gradient is measured under the condition of maximally achievable flow. Using these concepts, myocardial FFR (FFR_{myo}),

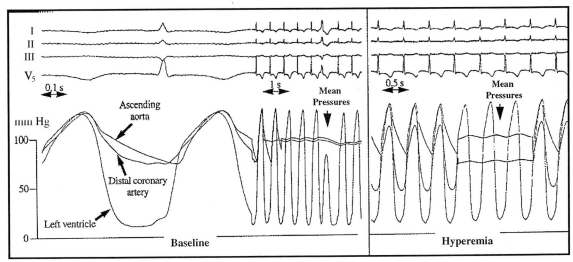

Figure 19–11. Pressure tracings (ascending aorta, left ventricle and distal coronary artery) showing the dependency of a translesional pressure gradient on flow in a patient with a mild obstructive lesion in the proximal part of the coronary vessel. The *left panel* shows a minimal gradient during diastole during basal flow conditions. In the *right panel,* under hyperemic conditions, the pressure gradient increases markedly and is present during systole and diastole. (From De Bruyne B, et al: Intracoronary pressure measurements with a 0.015-inch fluid-filled angioplasty guide wire. *In* Serruys PW, Foley DP, de Feyter PJ [eds]: Quantitative Coronary Angiography in Clinical Practice. Norwell, MA, Kluwer Academic, 1994; pp 147–165. Reprinted by permission of Kluwer Academic Publishers.)

coronary FFR (FFR$_{cor}$), and collateral FFR (FFR$_{coll}$) have been calculated as[38, 39, 92]

$$FFR_{myo} = 1 - (P_{ao} - P_c)/(P_{ao} - P_v)$$
$$= 1 - \Delta P/(P_{ao} - P_v)$$
$$FFR_{cor} = 1 - (P_{ao} - P_c)/(P_{ao} - P_w)$$
$$FFR_{myo} = 1 - \Delta P/(P_{ao} - P_w)$$
$$FFR_{coll} = FFR_{myo} - FFR_{cor}$$

where P_{ao} is the mean aortic pressure, P_c is the distal coronary pressure, P_v is the mean right atrial pressure, and P_w is the mean coronary wedge pressure or distal coronary pressure during balloon inflation. A more extensive theoretical background for the validity of these equations has been presented recently.[92] Subsequently, De Bruyne and coworkers[93] compared FFR in human measurements to information derived from quantitative coronary angiography and relative flow reserve (RFR)—the ratio of hyperemic flow in the stenotic region to hyperemic flow in the contralateral normal region—as assessed by positron emission tomography (PET).[88] They found a close correlation between RFR obtained by PET and both FFR$_{myo}$ ($r = .87$) and FFR$_{cor}$ obtained by pressure recordings ($r = .86$). The correlations between RFR by PET and stenosis measurements from quantitative angiography were significantly weaker (minimal obstruction area, $r = .66$; percent area stenosis, $r = -.70$; and stenosis flow reserve, $r = 0.68$).

Mancini and associates[94, 95] have proposed the instantaneous hyperemic flow versus pressure slope index as a more sensitive index than coronary flow reserve for detection of significant coronary stenoses.[89, 90] Ideally, routine determination of this index in humans would require the incorporation of both a Doppler velocity probe and a high-fidelity pressure transducer on the same small guide wire. However, in one initial human study, Di Mario and colleagues[96] found that simultaneous registration of an ascending aortic, fluid-filled guiding catheter pressure and an intracoronary Doppler flow wire recording of velocity allowed construction of a full pressure-flow velocity relationship throughout the cardiac cycle (Fig. 19–12). The slope of the instantaneous hyperemic diastolic pressure-velocity relationship (IHDPVS), between peak maximal diastolic velocity and the beginning of the phase of rapid decrease of flow velocity induced by ventricular contraction, distinguished between arteries with and without coronary stenoses and showed a significant inverse correlation with the severity of stenosis. The IHDPVS index also manifested similar sensitivity with Doppler velocity coronary flow reserve in differentiating lesions with a cross-sectional area smaller than 1.5 mm^2.[96]

Application of the Doppler guide wire alone has also been found promising for validation of lesion severity. In 84 patients with lesions ranging from 28% to 98% diameter narrowing,

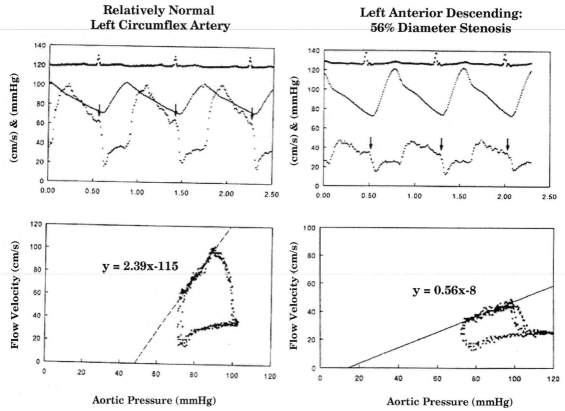

Figure 19–12. Upper, Electrocardiogram, ascending aortic pressure, and flow-velocity waveforms acquired during maximal hyperemia in a circumflex coronary artery with minimal irregularities *(left)* and in a left anterior descending coronary artery distal to a significant, 56% diameter, stenosis *(right)*. The maximal velocity and the rapid decrease in velocity due to the beginning of myocardial contraction *(arrows)* signify the start and end point for the diastolic hyperemic pressure-velocity relation plotted below. *Lower,* Pressure-velocity loops, throughout the cardiac cycle, of the same beats shown in the *upper panels.* A linear regression line has been calculated from the mid-data points of the diastolic interval indicated in the *upper panel.* Note the steeper slope of the pressure-velocity linear regression line in the normal coronary artery. (From Di Mario C, Krams R, Gil R, Serruys PW: Slope of the instantaneous hyperemic diastolic coronary flow velocity–pressure relation: A new index for assessment of the physiological significance of coronary stenosis in humans. Circulation 1994; 90:1215–1224. Reproduced with permission of Circulation. Copyright 1994 American Heart Association.)

a strong correlation (r = .8, $P<0.001$) was noted between basal translesional pressure gradients and the ratios of the proximal to distal total flow velocity integrals.[97]

It is unclear which of a number of velocity- and pressure-derived indices will prove to be the most reliable for assessment of lesion severity.

REGIONAL WALL MOTION ANALYSIS IN CORONARY HEART DISEASE

In the 1960s it was recognized that regional, as opposed to global, abnormalities of left ventricular contraction accompanied myocardial ischemia or infarction, or both. Since then a number of approaches have been undertaken to quantify regional dysfunction or dyssynergy. The more commonly used constructs (orthogonal axes, radial axes, and centerline methods) are discussed in Chapter 11. In general, four categories of dysfunction may be noted: (1) hypokinesis, where the myocardium exhibits reduced extent of shortening and wall thickening; (2) akinesis, where the myocardium manifests absence of shortening or thickening; (3) dyskinesis, where the myocardium exhibits paradoxical movement, or expansion while the remainder of the myocardium is in systolic contraction; and (4) dyssynchrony, where the region is contracting out of phase with the remainder of the left ventricle. The latter temporal disturbance is seen frequently in concert with an abnormality of the extent of shortening (see Fig. 19–8).

Regional dysfunction may be irreversible and secondary to an area of myocardial infarction; alternatively, the myocardium may be reversibly dysfunctional, or "stunned."[98] Such behavior not only has been observed experimentally after temporary coronary occlusion but also in humans after thrombolytic reperfusion for an evolving myocardial infarction,[99, 100] after ischemia induced by partial coronary stenosis and increased oxygen demand (e.g., with exercise in the presence of partial coronary occlusion or with left ventricular hypertrophy), after cardiopulmonary bypass,[101] and after prolonged balloon angioplasty occlusion of a coronary artery.[102] In the circumstance of stunning, it may take days to a week after restoration of normal myocardial perfusion for a wall motion disturbance to return to normal. A persistent wall motion disturbance, ultimately reversible after coronary revascularization, may be seen with chronic ischemia; in this instance the myocardium has been considered to be "hibernating."[103] It is hypothesized that the contractile function of hibernating myocardium is depressed to reduce myocardial oxygen demand (i.e., protect the heart) in the face of reduced oxygen supply.

Demonstration of worsening of regional wall motion by left ventriculography (and now by two-dimensional echocardiography or radionuclide angiography) during periods of physiologic or pharmacologic stress has become a common mode for detecting heart muscle that is ischemic but still viable and its topographic location. In our catheterization laboratories, we have found digitally processed intravenous left ventriculography, at control and immediately after pacing, to be particularly useful for recognition, quantitation, and display of inducible wall motion disturbances.[104–106]

NEW APPROACHES TO REGIONAL WALL MOTION ANALYSIS

An important development in cardiac angiography in the last decade has been the use of digital processing for quantitation and display of cardiac images. By segmenting the gray scale left ventricular angiographic image into a matrix of small pixels, each of which can be manipulated mathematically, powerful options are available for detecting and quantitating regional dyssynergy. Four new approaches have been taken: (1) use of shape information in conjunction with artificial intelligence (curvature method[107–110] and normalized curvature difference function[111]); (2) regional videodensitometric methods[105]; (3) temporal Fourier analysis with use of the phase and amplitude of the first harmonic[112–116]; or (4) intensity-based (slope) methods.[106, 117–119] Both videointensity and videodensitometric methods use the third-

dimension information (depth) embedded in the shades of gray, all of which require significant data processing. For these last two methods to perform well it is essential that sequential ventricular images be stored in a video or digital format and acquired with a constant x-ray potential throughout the imaging run. Moreover, motion artifacts need to be avoided during image acquisition.

Curvature Method

The curvature method has been developed to use information that reflects normal and abnormal changes in shape of the left ventricle throughout the cardiac cycle.[107–110] This approach requires edge detection and permits evaluation of only a limited portion of the endocardium (that part responsible for casting the edge shadow). The endocardial silhouette is traced from the anterior aspect of the aortic valve to the junction of aortic and mitral valve. At 100 equispaced points along the silhouette in a clockwise direction, the left ventricular silhouette is fitted with circular arcs. Curvature is defined as the inverse of the radius of the arc and is normalized by multiplying by the perimeter length to yield a dimensionless quantity. Right-handed curves are assigned positive curvature and left-handed, negative values. Point-by-point curvature values are smoothed and plotted to yield a unique quantitative measure of the shape of the ventricle.

Analysis is performed on end-diastolic and end-systolic frames. Data from normal subjects are used to determine the limits for the curvature in each region along the ventricular silhouette. When the curvature for a given subject deviates outside this limit, then it is considered to be abnormal.

Mancini and coworkers[107–110] showed that there is minimal information in change in curvature from end-diastole to end-systole, that is, difference in the two curvatures. Marcus and colleagues[111] have shown, on the other hand, that the normalized curvature difference function is diagnostically useful. They define, slightly differently, the shape based on a transform of the silhouette and estimate the normalized curvature difference function as the point-by-point difference between end-diastole and end-systole.

One advantage of the curvature method, like the centerline method (see Chapter 11), is that it is independent of a reference and coordinate system. But like most other methods it depends on edge detection. Furthermore, this technique analyzes the curvature of the endocardial surface and not its motion. It is the only method, nevertheless, capable of analyzing an isolated single frame to assess the normality in shape of a left ventricular silhouette.

Videodensitometry and Videointensity Methods

Automated edge detection is difficult mainly because of suboptimal opacification of the cavity and the inherent trabeculation along the edges. Image enhancement improves edge detection and visually assists the clinician but results in loss of densitometric information. Visualized edges represent only a small part of the endocardial surface, whereas methods that use videodensitometry or videointensity are capable of evaluating a larger volume of the ventricular wall.[105, 106, 112–119] Computer processing of image data is essential here because changes in videodensity at each pixel location are evaluated throughout the cardiac cycle (frame by frame), requiring a large amount of data analysis and storage. On the other hand, videointensity or videodensitometry methods analyze the image sequence from the entire cardiac cycle either as one event (phase and amplitude) to derive two parametric images or as slope images for each small increment of time as in the slope method.[117, 118]

Pixel-by-pixel temporal Fourier analysis of one cardiac cycle is performed as shown in Figure 19–13A (see also the color section). For each pixel in the ventricular region of interest, a time-intensity or time-density curve is calculated and fitted to a sine wave. The amplitude and phase of the sine wave are then mapped as a number between 0 and 255, representing a shade of gray, to derive two parametric images. The amplitude-parametric image portrays peak-to-peak excursion in the brightness of the image over a cardiac cycle. The phase-parametric image displays the phase angle of the sine wave, reflecting the relative synchrony of these changes. Regions that are ischemic or infarcted display a delayed phase and decreased amplitude (Fig. 19–13B; see also the color section). In the presence of a paradoxically moving aneurysm (dyskinesis), the amplitude may be maintained but its phase is approximately 180 degrees out of synchrony. Thus, in phase-amplitude analysis it is helpful that the two parametric images be visualized and evaluated simultaneously. Also, for the phase-amplitude method to be applied to two sequential ventriculograms, it is important to assess function at comparable heart rates. At slow heart rates the systolic portion of the curve encompasses about one third of the RR interval, and at higher heart rates

systolic and diastolic intervals become equal. In other words, the sine wave is a good approximation to the shape of the time-intensity curve at higher heart rates and deviates from this assumption at slower heart rates. The extent to which the heart rate variations affect the phase when the morphology deviates from a sine wave is unclear. Therefore, to evaluate the effect of interventions, ventriculographic data should be acquired at similar paced heart rates.

A number of studies[112–116] have reported identification of an ischemic region by analyzing the phase and amplitude of the fundamental harmonic of the temporal Fourier transform. The mean and SD of the amplitude and phase for a normal population are calculated in the anterior and inferior regions. Assuming a gaussian distribution, if either the mean value of regional amplitude or the mean phase angle falls outside 2 SDs (derived from normal subjects) for that region, then the region is considered abnormal. Alternatively, the mean ± 2 SDs of the global left ventricular region of interest can be used to normalize the comparable image filmed during an intervention to induce ischemia. This serves to identify changes in intensity brought about by reduced contraction in an area of ischemia (see Fig. 19–13B). Because phase and amplitude data are sensitive to heart rate, or RR interval, a comparison of these images when RR intervals are not matched is problematic.

Regional ejection fraction, another method developed in our laboratory, can also be calculated from videodensitometric data.[105] In this method a region of interest is manually drawn over the left ventricular silhouette encompassing the ventricular region of interest at both end-diastole and end-systole. The center of gravity of this region is calculated. Radial lines are drawn from the anterior aspect of the aortic valve, the apex, and the inferior aspect of the mitral valve to the center of gravity. These regions are further subdivided into three segments, each to yield six regions of interest. Time-density curves are generated for the six regions of interest. A horseshoe-shaped background region of interest is drawn just outside the end-systolic silhouette. The average videodensity in the background region of interest is calculated. From these values the regional ejection fraction is calculated as background-corrected end-diastolic density minus end-systolic density divided by the end-diastolic density. For each of the six segments, the lower limit of regional ejection fraction is defined as the mean minus 2 SDs of a normal population both at

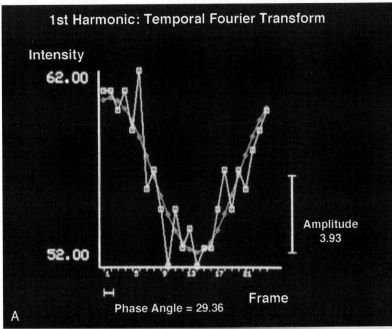

Figure 19–13. A, Plot of gray scale (intensity) versus time (cine-frame) throughout the cardiac cycle for a single pixel. The first harmonic of a temporal Fourier transform is shown, in red, superimposed. Amplitude and phase angle for the first harmonic are displayed. *B,* Parametric image display of the amplitudes calculated, pixel by pixel over the left ventricular region of interest. Pseudocolor coding below shows low amplitudes as purple, whereas high amplitudes are shown as shades of red. The ventricle was filmed in the right anterior oblique projection. Note the reduced pixel amplitudes on the control injection along the high inferior wall in the area of an old inferoposterior myocardial infarction. During the immediate postpacing ischemia, the area of reduced amplitudes along the inferior wall enlarges, indicating reduced wall motion in this region. (See color section.)

rest and after pacing. This method has been shown to be sensitive in discriminating regions perfused by normal vessels with those perfused by stenotic vessels in patients. The regional ejection fraction sensitivity increased from 50% at control to 83% after pacing in detecting low regional ejection fractions in patients with known coronary artery disease. Chappuis and associates[105] also showed the sensitivity of this method to be superior, both at rest and after pacing, to the geometric area and radial methods.

A further new technique developed in our laboratory is the so-called slope method (Figs. 19–14 to 19–16).[117] In this method the average videointensity over the left ventricular region of interest is calculated over a cardiac cycle. A given pixel's videointensity over a short interval (100 or 50 ms) is linearly regressed with the average intensity. If the changes in shades of gray at this location change by more than the average over the whole ventricular region of interest, then the slope of the linear regression will be greater than or equal to one and is defined as normal. If the changes in shades of gray are less than that for the whole ventricle,

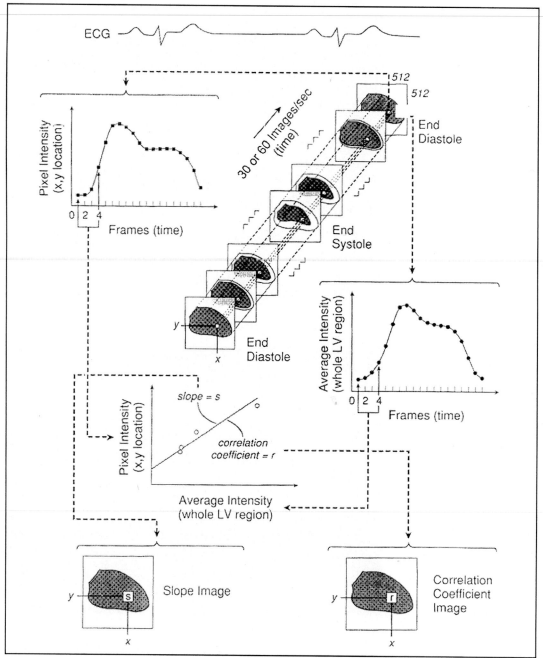

Figure 19–14. Schematic summary of the so-called slope method for detection of regional wall motion disturbance. Time sequence of cardiac images, comprising an array of 512 × 512 pixels × 8 bits, is shown. Two curves are extracted from the image sequence: an average time intensity of the region over the left ventricle (LV) and a time-intensity curve of a single pixel. For sequential 100-msec intervals, the intensity of a given pixel is correlated with that of the average global region of interest, and the slope and correlation coefficient values of linear regression are computed. These values are scaled between 0 and 255 and then mapped into output parametric images as shades of gray. This analysis is repeated for all pixels in the assigned region of interest for the left ventricle. The next 100 msec, overlapping the previous interval by 67 msec, is then analyzed until the whole cardiac cycle has been analyzed and displayed. (From Bhargava V, Sunnerhagen KS, Rashwan M, et al: Detection and quantitation of ischemic left ventricular dysfunction using a new video intensity technique for regional wall motion evaluation. Am Heart J 1990; 120:1058–1072.)

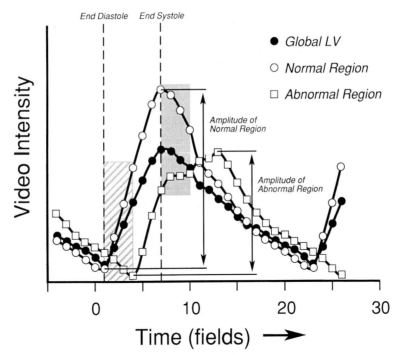

Figure 19–15. Time-intensity curves of the global left ventricle (LV) and normal and ischemic regions from end diastole to end-diastole are shown. Vertical lines indicate end-systole. Discordance between global and ischemic (abnormal) curve is seen, particularly in early diastole. Note also the discrepancy in amplitude of the normal, as opposed to abnormal, regions. (From Bhargava V, Sunnerhagen KS, Rashwan M, et al: Detection and quantitation of ischemic left ventricular dysfunction using a new video intensity technique for regional wall motion evaluation. Am Heart J 1990; 120:1058–1072.)

Patient With Left Anterior Descending Lesion: 62% Diameter Stenosis

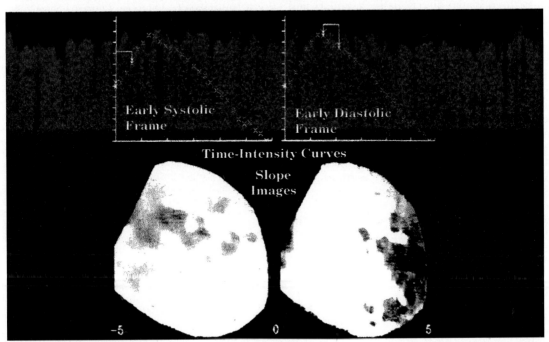

Figure 19–16. Upper, Average time-intensity curves for whole ventricle. Arrows on the time-intensity curves indicate the time interval of the data analyzed. Left panel, For early diastole; right panel, during early diastole. Lower, Slope parametric images. Early diastolic apical abnormality is seen as the dark region mapped in the lower right panel, in distribution of the left anterior descending coronary artery (62% diameter stenosis). (From Bhargava V, Sunnerhagen KS, Rashwan M, et al: Detection and quantitation of ischemic left ventricular dysfunction using a new video intensity technique for regional wall motion evaluation. Am Heart J 1990; 120:1058–1072.)

the slope of the linear regression is less than one and is considered hypokinetic. Finally, if the changes are opposite in direction to that of the whole ventricle, then the slope will be negative and the wall motion is considered to be paradoxical. Correlation coefficient values are also calculated and used to confirm the goodness of fit of the linear regression. This analysis is repeated for each pixel within the left ventricular region of interest. Both slope and correlation coefficient values are mapped as values between 0 and 255 shades of gray to create parametric images (and displayed in pseudocolor). This analysis is repeated for an interval overlapping the previous data by dropping the first data point (image) and adding one new data point from the next video image. The whole cardiac cycle is analyzed sequentially by dropping one image and adding a successive one.

The advantages of the slope method are that (1) it does not require a normal population to define abnormal regional function; (2) it analyzes the whole cardiac cycle on a pixel-by-pixel as well as frame-by-frame basis (i.e., both systole and diastole); (3) it can define the duration of both systolic and diastolic abnormalities; (4) it can quantitate the size of an abnormality relative to the end-diastolic ventricular silhouette size; (5) it assesses function in four dimensions (three spatial directions [x, y, and z] and time); and (6) it does not require edge detection.

The method has been evaluated in 80 patients with coronary artery disease. The sensitivity of the method at rest (against a 50% measured diameter stenosis) was found to be 79%.[118] In another study from our laboratory in 42 patients with coronary artery disease (30 without and 12 with prior myocardial infarction), the slope method showed a higher sensitivity (81%) than either the radial or centerline method.[119] In this same study the centerline method had a sensitivity of 44%, and the radial method had one of 38%. In a limited comparison of 15 patients, studied before and after pacing, the phase-amplitude and slope methods showed a similar sensitivity before pacing for detection of a presumed ischemic region. The phase-amplitude method showed some improvement in sensitivity after pacing. More extensive studies are needed to comprehensively determine the relative value of these new approaches to detection of regional dyssynergy.

REFERENCES

1. Dawler TR: The Framingham Study: The epidemiology of atherosclerotic disease. Cambridge, MA, Harvard University Press, 1980.

2. Subcommittee on Coronary Angiography: Guidelines for Coronary Angiography: A report of the American College of Cardiology/American Heart Association Task Force on Assessment of Diagnostic and Therapeutic Cardiovascular Procedures. J Am Coll Cardiol 1987; 10:935–950.

3. Zir LM, Miller SW, Dinsmore RE, et al: Interobserver variability in coronary angiography. Circulation 1976; 52:979–986.

4. DeRouen TA, Murray JA, Owen W: Variability in the analysis of coronary arteriograms. Circulation 1977; 55:324–328.

5. Lim JS, Proudfit WL, Sones FM Jr: Left main coronary arterial obstruction: Long-term follow-up of 141 nonsurgical cases. Am J Cardiol 1975; 36:131–135.

6. Webster JS, Moberg C, Rincon G: Natural history of severe proximal coronary artery disease as documented by coronary cineangiography. Am J Cardiol 1974; 33:195–200.

7. Harris PJ, Harrel FE, Lee KL, et al: Survival in medically treated coronary artery disease. Circulation 1979; 60:1259–1269.

8. Ringquist I, Fisher LD, Mock M, et al: Prognostic value of angiographic indices of coronary artery disease from the Coronary Artery Surgery Study (CASS). J Clin Invest 1983; 71:1854–1866.

9. Zack PM, Chaitman BR, Davis KB, et al: Survival pattern in clinical and angiographic subsets of medically treated patients with combined proximal left anterior descending and proximal left circumflex coronary artery disease (CASS). Am Heart J 1989; 118:220–227.

10. European Coronary Surgery Study Group: Long-term results of prospective, randomized study of coronary artery bypass surgery in stable angina pectoris. Lancet 1982; 2:1173–1180.

11. Varnauskas E, European Coronary Surgery Study Group: Twelve-year follow-up of survival in the randomized European Coronary Surgery Group. N Engl J Med 1988; 319:332–337.

12. Veterans Administration Coronary Artery Bypass Surgery Cooperative Study Group: Eleven-year survival in the Veterans Administration randomized trial of coronary bypass surgery for stable angina. N Engl J Med 1984; 311:1333, 1339.

13. Bonow KO, Bacharach SL, Green MV, et al: Prognostic implications of symptomatic versus asymptomatic (silent) myocardial ischemia induced by exercise in mildly symptomatic and in asymptomatic patients with angiographically documented coronary artery disease. Am J Cardiol 1987; 60:778–783.

14. Cohn P, Harris P, Barry WH, et al: Prognostic importance of anginal symptoms in angiographically defined coronary artery disease. Am J Cardiol 1981; 47:233–237.

15. Kaiser GC, Davis KB, Fisher LD, et al: Survival following coronary bypass grafting in patients with severe angina pectoris (CASS). J Thorac Cardiovasc Surg 1985; 89:512–524.

16. Waters D, Craven TE, Lesperance J: Prognostic significance of progression of coronary atherosclerosis. Circulation 1993; 87:1067–1075.

17. Alison HW, Russell RO Jr, Mantle JA, et al: Coronary anatomy and arteriography in patients with unstable angina pectoris. Am J Cardiol 1978; 41:204–209.

18. Russell RO Jr, Moraski RE, Kouchoukos N, et al: Unstable angina pectoris: National cooperative study group to compare surgical and medical therapy. Am J Cardiol 1978; 42:839–848.

19. Russell RO Jr, Moraski RE, Kouchoukos N, et al: Unstable angina pectoris: National cooperative study group

to compare medical and surgical therapy. Am J Cardiol 1981; 48:517–524.

20. Luchi RJ, Scott SM, Deupree RH, Principal investigators and their associates of Veterans Administration Cooperative Study: Comparison of medical and surgical treatment for unstable angina pectoris. N Engl J Med 1987; 316:977–984.

21. Scott SM, Luchi RJ, Deupree RH, and Veterans Administration Unstable Angina Cooperative Study Group: Veterans Administration Cooperative Study for treatment of patients with unstable angina. Circulation 1988; 78:I-113–I-121.

22. McCormick JR, Schick EC Jr, McCabe CH, et al: Determinants of operative mortality and long-term survival in patients with unstable angina: The CASS experience. J Thorac Surg 1985; 89:683–688.

23. Roberts KB, Califf RM, Harrell FE Jr, et al: The prognosis for patients with new-onset angina who have undergone cardiac catheterization. Circulation 1983; 68:970–978.

24. Willerson JT, Campbell WB, Winniford MD, et al: Conversion from chronic to acute coronary artery disease: Speculation regarding mechanisms. Am J Cardiol 1984; 54:1349.

25. Levin DC, Fallon JT: Significance of the angiographic morphology of localized coronary stenoses: Histopathologic correlation. Circulation. 1982; 66:316.

26. Ambrose JA, Winters SL, Stern A, et al: Angiographic morphology and the pathogenesis of unstable angina pectoris. J Am Coll Cardiol 1985; 5:609–616.

27. Holmes DR, Hartzler GO, Smith HC, Fuster V: Coronary artery thrombosis in patients with unstable angina. Br Heart J 1981; 45:411–416.

28. Zack PM, Ischinger T, Aker VT, et al: The occurrence of angiographically detected intracoronary thrombus in patients with unstable angina pectoris. Am Heart J 1984; 108:1408–1411.

29. Kusuaka H, Mishima M, Inoue M, Kamada T: The role of intracoronary thrombus in unstable angina: Angiographic assessment and thrombolytic therapy during ongoing anginal attacks. Circulation 1988; 77:526–534.

30. Cowley MJ, Disciascio G, Rehr RB, Vetrovec GW: Angiographic observations and clinical relevance of coronary thrombus in unstable angina pectoris. Am J Cardiol 1989; 63:E-108–E-113.

31. Haft JI, Al-Zarka AM: Comparison of the natural history of irregular and smooth coronary lesions: Insights into the pathogenesis, progression, and prognosis of coronary atherosclerosis. Am Heart J 1993; 126:551–561.

32. Davies SW, Marchant B, Lyons JP, et al: Irregular coronary lesion morphology after thrombolysis predicts early clinical instability. J Am Coll Cardiol 1991; 18:669–674.

33. Ellis S, Alderman EL, Cain K, et al: Morphology of left anterior descending coronary territory lesions as a predictor of anterior myocardial infarction: A CASS registry study. J Am Coll Cardiol 1989; 13:1481–1491.

34. Ambrose JA: Prognostic implications of lesion irregularity on coronary angiography. J Am Coll Cardiol 1991; 18:675–676.

35. White CW, Wright CB, Doty DB, et al: Does visual interpretation of the coronary arteriogram predict the physiologic importance of a coronary stenosis? N Engl J Med 1984; 310:819.

36. Glagov SE, Weisenberg E, Zarins CK, et al: Compensatory enlargement of human atherosclerotic coronary arteries. N Engl J Med 1987; 316:1371–1375.

37. Emanuelsson H, Dohnal M, Lamm C, Tenerz L: Initial experiences with a miniaturized pressure transducer during coronary angioplasty. Cathet Cardiovasc Diagn 1991; 24:137–143.

38. De Bruyne B, Pijls NHJ, Paulus WJ, et al: Transstenotic coronary pressure gradient measurement in humans: In vitro and in vivo evaluation of a new pressure monitoring angioplasty guide wire. J Am Coll Cardiol 1993; 22:119–126.

39. De Bruyne B, Baudhuin T, Melin JA, et al: Coronary flow reserve calculated from pressure measurements in humans: Validation with positron emission tomography. Circulation 1994; 89:1013–1022.

40. Ambrose JA, Tannenbaum MA, Alexopoulos D, et al: Angiographic progression of coronary artery disease and the development of myocardial infarction. J Am Coll Cardiol 12:56–62.

41. Little WC, Constantinescu M, Applegate RJ, et al: Can coronary angiography predict the site of a subsequent myocardial infarction in patients with mild-to-moderate coronary artery disease? Circulation 1988; 78:1157–1166.

42. Gage JE, Hess OM, Murakami T, et al: Vasoconstriction of stenotic coronary arteries during dynamic exercise in patients with classic angina pectoris: Reversibility by nitroglycerin. Circulation 1986; 73:865–876.

43. Gordon JB, Ganz P, Nabel EG, et al: Atherosclerosis influences the vasomotor response of epicardial coronary arteries to exercise. J Clin Invest 1989; 83:1940–1952.

44. Nabel EG, Selwyn AP, Ganz P: Paradoxical narrowing of atherosclerotic arteries induced by increases in heart rate. Circulation 1990; 81:850–859.

45. Nabel EG, Ganz P, Gordon JB, et al: Dilation of normal and constriction of atherosclerotic coronary arteries caused by the cold pressor test. Circulation 1988; 77:43–52.

46. Yeung AC, Vershtein VI, Krantz DS, et al: The effect of atherosclerosis on the vasomotor response of coronary arteries to mental stress. N Engl J Med 1991; 325:1551–1556.

47. Palmer RM, Ferrige AG, Moncada S: Nitric oxide release accounts for the biological activity of endothelium-derived relaxing factor. Nature 1987; 327:524–526.

48. Myers PR, Minor RL, Guerra R, et al: Vasorelaxant properties of the endothelium-derived relaxing factor more closely resembles s-nitrocysteine than nitric oxide. Nature 1990; 345:161–163.

49. Cohen RA, Shepherd JT, Vanhoutte PM: Effects of the adrenergic transmitter on epicardial coronary arteries. Fed Proc 1984; 43:2862–2866.

50. Cohen RA, Weisbrod RM: Endothelium inhibits norepinephrine release from adrenergic nerves of rabbit carotid artery. Am J Physiol 1988; 254:H-871–H-878.

51. Zeiher AM, Drexler H, Wollschlager H, Just H: Modulation of coronary vasomotor tone in humans: Progressive endothelial dysfunction with different early stages of coronary atherosclerosis. Circulation 1991; 83:391–401.

52. Seiler C, Hess OM, Buechi M, et al: Influence of serum and cholesterol and other coronary risk factors on vasomotion of angiographically normal coronary arteries. Circulation 1993; 88:2139–2148.

53. Penny WF, Rockman H, Long J, et al: Heterogeneity of vasomotor response to acetylcholine along the human coronary artery. J Am Coll Cardiol 1995; 25:1046–1055.

54. Ludmer PL, Selwyn AP, Shook TI, et al: Paradoxical vasoconstriction induced by acetylcholine in atherosclerotic coronary arteries. N Engl J Med 1986; 315:1046–1051.

55. Horio Y, Yasue H, Rokutanda M, et al: Effects of intra-

coronary injection of acetylcholine on coronary arterial diameter. Am J Cardiol 1986; 57:984–989.

56. Werns SW, Walton JA, Hsia HH, et al: Evidence of endothelial dysfunction in angiographically normal coronary arteries of patients with coronary artery disease. Circulation 1989; 79:287–291.

57. Hodgson JMB, Marshall JJ: Direct vasoconstriction and endothelium-dependent vasodilation: Mechanisms of acetylcholine effects on coronary flow and arterial diameter in patients with nonstenotic coronary arteries. Circulation 1989; 79:1043–1051.

58. Vita JA, Treasure CB, Nabel EG, et al: Coronary vasomotor response to acetylcholine relates to risk factors for coronary artery disease. Circulation 1990; 81:491–497.

59. Yasue H, Maysuyama K, Okumara K, et al: Responses of angiographically normal human coronary arteries to intracoronary injection of acetylcholine by age and segment: Possible role of early coronary atherosclerosis. Circulation 1990; 81:482–490.

60. Brush JE Jr, Faxon DP, Salmon S, et al: Abnormal endothelium-dependent vasomotion in hypertensive patients. J Am Coll Cardiol 1992; 19:809–815.

61. Nitenberg A, Antony I, Foult JM: Acetylcholine-induced coronary vasoconstriction in young, heavy smokers with normal coronary arteriographic findings. Am J Med 1993; 95:71–77.

62. Reddy KG, Nair RN, Sheehan HM, Modgson JM: Evidence that selective endothelial dysfunction may occur in the absence of angiographic or ultrasound atherosclerosis in patients with risk factors for atherosclerosis. J Am Coll Cardiol 1984; 23:833–843.

63. Leung WH, Lau CP, Wong CK: Beneficial effect of cholesterol-lowering therapy on coronary endothelium-dependent relaxation in hypercholesterolemic patients. Lancet 1993; 341:1496–1500.

64. Treasure CB, Klein JL, Weintraub WS, et al: Beneficial effects of cholesterol-lowering therapy on the coronary endothelium in patients with coronary artery disease. N Engl J Med 1995; 332:481–487.

65. Anderson TJ, Meredith IT, Yeung AC, et al: The effect of cholesterol-lowering and antioxidant therapy on endothelium-dependent coronary vasomotion. N Engl J Med 1995; 332:488–493.

66. Suzuki Y, Tokunaga S, Ikeguchi S, et al: Induction of coronary artery spasm by intracoronary acetylcholine: Comparison with intracoronary ergonovine. Am Heart J 1992; 124:39–47.

67. Golino P, Piscione F, Willerson JT, et al: Divergent effects of serotonin on coronary artery dimensions and blood flow in patients with coronary atherosclerosis and control patients. N Engl J Med 1991; 324:641–648.

68. McFadden EP, Bauters C, Lablanche JM, et al: Response of human coronary arteries to serotonin after injury by coronary angioplasty. Circulation 1993; 88:I-2076–I-2085.

69. McFadden EP, Bauters C, Lablanche JM, et al: Effect of ketanserin on proximal and distal coronary constrictor responses to intra-coronary infusion of serotonin in patients with stable angina, patients with variant angina, and control patients. Circulation 1992; 86:187–195.

70. Vrints CJM, Bult H, Bosmans J, et al: Paradoxical vasoconstriction as result of acetylcholine and serotonin in diseased human coronary arteries. Eur Heart J 1992; 13:824–831.

71. Egashira K, Inoue T, Yamada A, et al: Preserved endothelium-dependent vasodilation at the vasospastic site in patients with variant angina. J Clin Invest 1992; 89:1047–1052.

72. Okumura K, Yasue H, Ishizaka H, et al: Endothelium-dependent dilator response to substance P in patients with coronary spastic angina. J Am Coll Cardiol 1992; 20:838–844.

73. Schroeder JS, Bolen JL, Quint RA, et al: Provocation of coronary spasm with ergonovine maleate: New test with results in 57 patients undergoing coronary arteriography. Am J Cardiol 1977; 40:487.

74. Heupler FA Jr, Proudfit WL, Razavi M, et al: Ergonovine maleate provocative test for coronary arterial spasm. Am J Cardiol 1978; 41:631.

75. Bertrand ME, Lablanche JM, Tilmant PY, et al: Frequency of provoked coronary arterial spasm in 1089 consecutive patients undergoing coronary arteriography. Circulation 1982; 65:1299–1306.

76. Cipriano PR, Guthaner DF, Orlick AE, et al: The effects of ergonovine maleate on coronary arterial size. Circulation 1979; 59:82.

77. Vlodaver Z, Frech R, Van Tassel RA, Edwards JE: Correlation of the antemortem coronary angiogram and the postmortem specimen. Circulation 1973; 47:162–169.

78. Grondin CM, Dyrda I, Pasternac A, et al: Discrepancies between cineangiographic and post mortem findings in patients with coronary artery disease and recent myocardial revascularization. Circulation 1974; 49:703–708.

79. Arnett E, Isner J, Redwood D, et al: Coronary artery narrowing in coronary heart disease: Comparison of cineangiographic and necropsy findings. Ann Intern Med 1979; 91:350–356.

80. Boerth RC, Covell JW, Pool PE, Ross J Jr: Increased myocardial oxygen consumption and contractile state associated with increased heart rate in dogs. Circ Res 1969; 24:725.

81. Heller GV, Aroesty JM, McKay RG, et al: The pacing stress test: A reexamination of the relation between coronary artery disease and pacing induced electrocardiographic changes. Am J Cardiol 1984; 54:50.

82. Nabel EG, Shook TL, Meyerovitz M, et al: Detection of pacing-induced myocardial ischemia by endocardial electrograms recorded during cardiac catheterization. J Am Coll Cardiol 1988; 11:983.

83. Krasnow N, Gorlin R: Myocardial lactate metabolism in coronary insufficiency. Ann Intern Med 1965; 59:781.

84. Parker JO, Chiong MA, West RO, Case RB: The effect of ischemia and alterations of heart rate on myocardial potassium balance in man. Circulation 1970; 42:205.

85. Mudge GH, Mills RM Jr, Taegtmeyer H, et al: Alterations of myocardial amino acid metabolism in chronic ischemic heart disease. J Clin Invest 1976; 58:1185.

86. Berger HJ, Zaret BL, Specoff L, et al: Cardiac prostaglandin release during myocardial ischemia induced by atrial pacing in patients with coronary artery disease. Am J Cardiol 1977; 39:481.

87. Dwyer EM Jr: Left ventricular pressure-volume alterations and regional disorders of contraction during myocardial ischemia induced by atrial pacing. Circulation 1970; 42:1111.

88. Pasternac A, Gorlin R, Sonnenblick EH, et al: Abnormalities of ventricular motion induced by atrial pacing in coronary disease. Circulation 1972; 45:1195

89. Mann T, Brodie BR, Grossman W, McLaurin LP: Effect of angina on the left ventricular diastolic pressure-volume relationship. Circulation 1976; 55:761.

90. Mann T, Goldberg S, Mudge GH Jr, Grossman W: Factors contributing to altered left ventricular diastolic properties during angina pectoris. Circulation 1979; 59:14.

91. Weiss JL, Frederiksen JW, Weisfeldt ML: Hemodynamic determinants of the time-course of fall in canine left ventricular pressure. J Clin Invest 1976; 58:751.

92. Pijls NHJ, van Son JA, Kirkeeide RL, et al: Experimental basis of determining maximum coronary, myocardial, and collateral blood flow by pressure measurements for assessing functional stenosis severity before and after percutaneous transluminal coronary angioplasty. Circulation 1993; 86:1354–1367.

93. De Bruyne B, Baudhuin T, Melin JA, et al: Coronary flow reserve calculated from pressure measurements in humans: Validation with positron emission tomography. Circulation 1994; 89:1013–1022.

94. Mancini GBJ, McGillem MJ, DeBoe SF, Gallagher KP: The diastolic hyperemic flow versus pressure relation: A new index of coronary stenosis severity and flow reserve. Circulation 1989; 80:941–950.

95. Mancini GBJ, Cleary RM, DeBoe SF, et al: Instantaneous hyperemic flow-versus-pressure slope index: Microsphere validation of an alternative to measures of coronary reserve. Circulation 1991; 84:862–870.

96. Di Mario C, Krams R, Gil R, Serruys PW: Slope of the instantaneous hyperemic diastolic coronary flow velocity-pressure relation: A new index for assessment of the physiological significance of coronary stenosis in humans. Circulation 1994; 90:1215–1224.

97. Donohue TJ, Kern MJ, Aguirre FV, et al: Assessing the hemodynamic significance of coronary artery stenoses: Analysis of translesional pressure-flow relations in patients. J Am Coll Cardiol 1993; 22:449–458.

98. Braunwald E, Kloner RA: The stunned myocardium: Prolonged, post-ischemic ventricular dysfunction. Circulation 1982; 55:1146–1149.

99. Touchstone DA, Beller GA, Hygaard TW, et al: Effects of successful intravenous reperfusion therapy on regional myocardial function and geometry in humans: A tomographic assessment using two-dimensional echocardiography. J Am Coll Cardiol 1989; 13:1506–1513.

100. Sheehan FH, Doerr R, Schmidt WG, et al: Early recovery of left ventricular function after thrombolytic therapy for acute myocardial infarction: An important determinant of survival. J Am Coll Cardiol 1988; 12:289–300.

101. Ballantyne CM, Verani MS, Short HD, et al: Delayed recovery of severely "stunned" myocardium with the support of a left ventricular assist device after coronary artery bypass graft surgery. J Am Coll Cardiol 1987; 10:710–712.

102. Wijns W, Serruys PW, Slager CJ, et al: Effect of coronary occlusion during percutaneous transluminal angioplasty in humans on left ventricular chamber stiffness and regional diastolic pressure-radius relations. J Am Coll Cardiol 1986; 7:455–463.

103. Rahimtoola SH: The hibernating myocardium. Am Heart J 1989; 117:211–221.

104. Mancini GBJ, Peterson KL, Gregoratos G, Higgins CB: Effect of atrial pacing on global and regional left ventricular function in coronary heart disease assessed by digital intravenous ventriculography. Am J Cardiol 1984; 53:456–461.

105. Chappuis FP, Widmann TF, Niood P, Peterson KL: Densitometric regional ejection fraction: A new three-dimensional index of regional left ventricular function—comparison with geometric methods. J Am Coll Cardiol 1988; 11:72–82.

106. Bhargava V, Sunnerhagen KS, Rashwan M, et al: Effect of atrial pacing on left ventricular regional wall motion using a new video-intensity technique. Coron Artery Dis 1990; 1:65–74.

107. Mancini GBJ, LeFree MT, Vogel RA: Curvature analysis of normal ventriculograms: Fundamental framework for the assessment of shape changes in man. IEEE Comput Cardiol 1985; 141–144.

108. Mancini GBJ, DeBoe SF, Anselmo E, et al: Quantitative regional curvature analysis: An application of shape determination for the assessment of segmental function in man. Am Heart J 1987; 113:326–334.

109. Mancini GBJ, DeBoe SF, Anselmo E, LeFree MT: A comparison of traditional wall motion assessment and quantitative shape analysis: A new method for characterizing ventricular function in man. Am Heart J 1987; 114:1183–1191.

110. Mancini GBJ, DeBoe SF, McGillem MJ, Bates ER: Quantitative regional curvature analysis: A prospective evaluation of ventricular shape and wall motion measurements. Am Heart J 1988; 116:1616–1621.

111. Marcus E, Barta E, Beyar R, et al: Characterization of regional left ventricular contraction by curvature difference analysis. Basic Res Cardiol 1988; 83:486–500.

112. Katayama K, Guth B, Widmann T, et al: Temporal Fourier transformation of digital angiograms for left ventricular regional wall motion analysis. Jpn Circulation J 1988; 52:607–616.

113. Widmann TF, Tubau JF, Ashburn WL, et al: Evaluation of regional wall motion by phase and amplitude analysis of intravenous contrast ventricular fluoroangiography: Technical aspects and computation. In Sigwart U, Heintzen PH (eds): Ventricular Wall Motion, International Symposium Lausanne. New York, Georg Thieme Verlag, 1982, pp 24–33.

114. Botvinick EH, Frais MA, Shosa DW, et al: An accurate means of detecting and characterizing abnormal patterns of ventricular activation by phase image analysis. Am J Cardiol 1982; 50:289–298.

115. Ratib O, Righetti A, Brandon G, Rasoamanambelo L: Usefulness of phase analysis for the evaluation of regional wall motion asynchrony from digitized contrast ventriculography. In Heintzen PH, Brennecke R (eds): Digital Imaging in Cardiovascular Radiology. New York, Georg Thieme Verlag, 1983, pp 299–304.

116. Lyons J, Norell M, Gardener J, et al: Phase and amplitude analysis of exercise digital left ventriculograms in patients with coronary disease. Br Heart J 1989; 62:102–111.

117. Bhargava V: A new videointensity-based wall motion analysis technique. Comput Med Imaging Graph 1990; 14:107–118.

118. Bhargava V, Sunnerhagen KS, Rashwan M, et al: Detection and quantitation of ischemic left ventricular dysfunction using a new videointensity technique for regional wall motion evaluation. Am Heart J 1990; 120:1058–1072.

119. Sunnerhagen K, Smith SC, Joshi DE, Bhargava V: Ischemic heart disease and regional left ventricular wall motion: A study comparing radial, centerline, and a videointensity based slope technique. Int J Card Imaging 1991; 6:85–96.

Chapter 20

Cardiac Catheterization and Angiography in Dilated Cardiomyopathy and Heart Failure

RALPH SHABETAI
VALMIK BHARGAVA
PASCAL NICOD

Circulatory failure can result from a variety of cardiovascular disorders. In this chapter, we focus on heart failure caused by either primary or secondary myocardial pathology sufficiently severe to cause ventricular dysfunction. Systolic dysfunction is emphasized because it is more common and more easily treated, but diastolic dysfunction is included here, as well as in Chapters 12 and 22.

The major causes of ventricular dysfunction include idiopathic dilated cardiomyopathy, ischemic cardiomyopathy, and extensive myocardial damage from other cardiac diseases and malformations, such as valvular heart disease. In this chapter, we concentrate on dilated cardiomyopathy because it provides the best model of heart failure.

The aims of cardiac catheterization vary among cases. An important goal is to establish the etiology. In this connection, it is important to determine whether dilated cardiomyopathy is idiopathic or secondary to severe coronary atherosclerosis. A second aim is to assess the severity of heart failure and the extent of myocardial reserve, and to distinguish true myocardial damage from the effects of adverse loading conditions. These aims are met by the following procedures:

1. Measurement of resting and exercise hemodynamics.
2. Measurement of hemodynamics during other interventions such as pharmacologic interventions or pacing.
3. Assessment of left and right ventricular function by contrast ventriculography.

4. Assessment of coronary anatomy using coronary arteriography.
5. Endomyocardial biopsy.

In this chapter, we review the practice and the use of cardiac catheterization in dilated cardiomyopathy. Myocardial biopsy will not be reviewed, because it is well described in Chapter 16.

GENERAL PROCEDURES

In patients with dilated cardiomyopathy, particular attention should be given to close monitoring of electrical and hemodynamic parameters during the entire procedure. Cardiac arrhythmias are frequent in patients with dilated cardiomyopathy and may be worsened by the passage of catheters and the injection of dye. Repositioning or removal of catheters may be required during the procedure. In patients with left bundle branch block, a common conduction abnormality in dilated cardiomyopathy, prophylactic placement of a temporary pacemaker may be advisable prior to right-sided heart catheterization. The use of balloon flotation catheters does not entirely abolish the risk of complete heart block in patients with left bundle branch block. Worsening of heart failure can occur during cardiac catheterization owing to the negative inotropic effect of dye given for intracoronary injections or ventriculography, although the severity of this problem is reduced when a nonionic contrast agent is used. The increase in volume and preload may also exacerbate heart failure. Therefore, frequent measurements of pulmonary capillary wedge pressure during cardiac catheterization may be a useful precaution in patients with severe heart failure. If heart failure worsens, the procedures should be temporarily stopped and the patient should be treated appropriately, using diuretics, morphine sulfate, vasodilators, or catecholamines, as needed. Patients should never be sent back to their room until the hemodynamics are stable. There is no better place to intervene promptly, if necessary, than a cardiac catheterization laboratory. In patients with severe heart failure, the risk of worsening heart failure is minimized by the use of nonionic contrast agents and by limiting the volume of dye and saline given. In many instances, left ventriculography can be replaced by echocardiography.

Following cardiac catheterization, a Swan-Ganz catheter should be left in place in unstable patients to monitor hemodynamic parameters for the next 24 to 48 hours. Whereas preload may be increased during the procedure, osmotic diuresis may follow cardiac catheterization and lead to hypotension and renal failure.

PLANNING THE STUDY

Cardiac catheterization for evaluation of dilated cardiomyopathy or congestive heart failure provides a good example of the general principle that cardiac catheterization is a generic procedure. Different patients require different diagnostic procedures, and the priority assigned to the components of the study must be tailored to the individual. When the study is performed to assess severity, therapeutic response, and prognosis, highest priority should be assigned to hemodynamics at rest, the responses to exercise, and to ventricular function. Access by the internal jugular vein and an upper limb artery facilitates the procedure. In some cases, etiology is the critical question, so coronary angiography and endomyocardial biopsy should be accomplished early in the procedure. When biopsy is needed, the operator has two choices, the first being to undertake the biopsy before administering a systemic dose of heparin. If coronary arteriography and ventriculography are subsequently required, heparin can be administered once it is established that the procedure was uncomplicated. In circumstances in which the likelihood of coronary artery disease is substantial and biopsy would not be undertaken were this confirmed, angiography can be performed before biopsy, after which the heparin effect

is reversed with protamine and the biopsy is performed.

A full exercise study, endomyocardial biopsy, and diagnostic left-sided and right-sided heart catheterization is a large undertaking for a single sitting, particularly for a patient with advanced heart failure. Under those circumstances, it is sometimes preferable to perform the right-sided heart catheterization, endomyocardial biopsy, and an exercise study at a time other than when angiography is performed. A proportion of patients with advanced dilated heart failure, in addition, require electrophysiologic studies, especially when the use of an implantable defibrillator is contemplated.

When a patient is being studied with a view to cardiac transplantation, assessment of pulmonary hypertension and pulmonary vascular reactivity must receive high priority. When a patient has been on the transplant waiting list for more than a few months and is known to have significant pulmonary hypertension, these studies may have to be repeated when it is judged that a donor heart may soon become available.

HEMODYNAMIC PARAMETERS

Resting left-sided and right-sided pressures are recorded at baseline, before any dye is injected. Nearly simultaneous measurement of cardiac output and vascular pressures allows calculation of systemic and pulmonary resistances. Resting hemodynamic parameters correlate poorly with symptoms or functional capacity in a given patient[1, 2] and do not predict the long-term response to treatment well.[3] However, they give useful information on resting cardiac function and prognosis. Patients with elevated left ventricular filling pressure, increased systemic vascular resistance, and decreased cardiac index have a poor prognosis,[4–8] although few studies have failed to show a correlation between resting hemodynamic parameters and survival.[9–10] Differences between studies may be due to characteristics of the populations studied and to the influence of factors other than heart failure, such as ischemia or arrhythmias, on survival. An association between elevated right atrial pressure and mortality has been reported.[6, 8, 11] This increase in right atrial pressure can be a secondary effect of increased pulmonary arterial pressure, but alternatively, it may be due to intrinsic right ventricular failure.[12] A strong association between pulmonary arterial pressure and morbidity and mortality has been reported,[13–15] which is mainly attributed to impairment of left ventricular function and postcapillary pulmonary hypertension but could be secondary to coexisting lung disease in some cases. A difference between pulmonary arterial diastolic pressure and pulmonary wedge pressure exceeding 10 mm Hg suggests that pulmonary vascular resistance is increased and is compatible with lung disease or increased pulmonary arteriolar tone.

Measurement of cardiac output when it is low may be best performed using the Fick method[16] (see Chapter 5). However, indicator dilution techniques may be also acceptable. Associated mitral regurgitation further impairs the indocyanine green dye method, just as tricuspid regurgitation impairs the thermodilution technique[17] (see Chapter 5).

Elevated pulmonary vascular resistance in patients with dilated cardiomyopathy should be carefully elevated, particularly if cardiac transplantation is being considered. Fixed elevation of pulmonary resistance suggests occlusive pulmonary arteriolar disease. Transplantation of a normal heart in the presence of fixed increased pulmonary vascular resistance may cause the transplanted right ventricle to fail. Until recently, assessment of pulmonary vascular resistance for the purpose of evaluating cardiac transplantation was performed by cautious intravenous infusion of nitroprusside. This agent causes a sharp drop in pulmonary vascular resistance when the increase in resistance reflects increased tone rather than occlusion of pulmonary arteries or arterioles. However, nitroprusside may not be the agent of choice, because it dilates the systemic as well as the pulmonary vascular bed, thereby considerably complicating the interpretation of the data. Furthermore, it must be recognized that when pulmonary vascular resistance drops but, as a result, cardiac output increases substantially, no decrease in pulmonary arterial pressure may occur. Therefore, it is preferable to employ agents that act on the pulmonary arterial vasculature but not on the systemic vasculature. In previous years, pulmonary vascular reactivity was assessed by infusing acetylcholine directly into the pulmonary artery, because this substance is completely deactivated in the lung by cholinesterase and thus does not reach the systemic circulation. However, doses of acetylcholine used for this intervention, as compared with those used for assessment of reactivity of the coronary vascular bed, are large and consequently not easily available. Inhaled oxygen is useful in this context only when hypoxemia exists. It is possible that inhaled nitric oxide at a concentration of 80 ppm may become the agent of choice in the future. Inhaled nitric oxide is deactivated when it combines with hemoglobin, and therefore, this agent also is a selective pulmonary arteriolar vasodilator without direct effects on the systemic circulation.[18]

HEMODYNAMICS DURING EXERCISE

Many patients sent for evaluation of heart failure are asymptomatic at rest; therefore, hemodynamic data obtained while the patient is exercising often are needed. Furthermore, the New York Heart Association classification does not correlate well with measured indices of exercise tolerance.[19] The techniques we use were developed recognizing that patients with heart failure receiving good medical treatment often have normal or nearly normal hemodynamics when studied supine at rest, and because of the need to distinguish between dyspnea of pulmonary and cardiac origin and to assess the severity of pulmonary hypertension and the reactivity of the pulmonary vascular bed. We apply the technique described in the following section to patients being considered for cardiac transplantation and to many patients in whom the cause of symptoms or response to treatment needs to be clarified.

We prefer upright exercise over supine exercise because it is more physiologic and more closely related to the symptoms complained of by patients with heart failure. Furthermore, most patients can achieve a higher workload walking on a treadmill or sitting on a stationary bicycle than when they attempt cycle ergometry in a supine position. Data obtained with supine exercise are not interchangeable with upright exercise.[20]

A catheter is placed via the right internal jugular vein and positioned so that pulmonary wedge or pulmonary arterial pressure can be obtained quickly and at will by inflation of the balloon. Arterial pressure is measured via a small thin-walled catheter placed in either the radial or brachial artery, usually the former. Pressures are measured simultaneously from the right atrium, the systemic artery, and the pulmonary artery alternating with the pulmonary wedge position. Cardiac output is estimated by thermal dilution and by the direct method of Fick. Oxygen consumption is measured as described in Chapter 5, and arterial and venous blood samples are removed in duplicate to determine blood gas content. Obtaining duplicate samples is important because an error in the mixed venous oxygen saturation can lead to profound misinterpretation of the pathophysiology.

Initially, the patient is studied supine and

at rest. The catheters are disconnected from the transducers and capped, and the puncture sites are covered with a sterile dressing. The patient then gets off the table and sits on a stool so that the location of the proximal port of the catheter, through which a small amount of contrast is injected, can be seen through a fluoroscope. Its height is marked on the chest wall. The patient then sits on a bicycle ergometer. The electrocardiogram (ECG) electrodes and transducers are reconnected, and the transducers are leveled to the mark on the skin indicating the height of the tip of the Swan-Ganz catheter.

A second collection of expired air for determination of oxygen consumption is begun once the patient is comfortably seated on the bicycle and is continued until the heart rate, the respiratory rate, oxygen consumption, blood pressure, and the gas exchange ratio indicate that the patient is in steady state. Pulmonary arterial and pulmonary wedge pressures are measured again. Determining the height of the right atrium with patients sitting erect and releveling the transducers ensures that changes from the pressures measured with the patient supine are physiologic and related to the change of posture and are not an artifact related to the height of the right atrial pressure transducer. Blood samples are obtained again from the pulmonary and systemic arteries for oxygen content.

The patient is instructed to pedal at 60 revolutions per minute, which is monitored by an analog revolution counter. The exercise protocol comprises 3-minute stages beginning at 25 watts (150 kilopound meters) and is increased by 25-watt steps until the patient's exercise capacity is exhausted.

Mean pressures from the three sites are recorded continuously at 10 mm/sec. Periodically, short bursts of phasic pressure are recorded to ensure that damping has not taken place. At 90 seconds into each stage, the balloon at the tip of the Swan-Ganz catheter is inflated and pulmonary wedge pressure is recorded until it is constant, after which the balloon is deflated. At 150 seconds into each stage, blood samples are withdrawn for measurement of oxygen content. At the end of each exercise stage, the patient is asked to indicate the level of perceived exertion on a large chart showing the Borg scale held in the visual field. Heart rate is measured off-line from the last 30 seconds of data during each stage of exercise.

Examples are shown in the tables and figures. Table 20–1 shows the data recorded from a 43-year-old man referred for cardiac transplantation because of severe left ventricular systolic dysfunction and moderate diastolic dysfunction. The radionuclide ejection fraction was 25%, the echocardiographic left ventricular end-diastolic dimension was 6.0 cm, and the shortening fraction was 15%. The patient exercised into the seventh stage, that is, 175 watts (1150 kilo pound meters), illustrating nicely the well-known lack of correlation between left ventricular systolic function and exercise capacity.[2, 3] He was able to achieve a maximum oxygen consumption of 18.9 mL/kg/min, which would

Table 20–1. Hemodynamic Data During Exercise in a 43-Year-Old Man Referred for Cardiac Transplantation*

Parameters	Rest-Bike	25 Watts	50 Watts	75 Watts	100 Watts	125 Watts	150 Watts	175 Watts
VO_2 (mL/min)	492	899	1104	1410	1622	1825	2017	2084
VO_2 (mL/min/kg)	4.5	8.2	10.0	12.8	14.7	16.6	18.3	18.9
VCO_2 (mL/min)	387	719	916	1218	1528	1763	2172	2388
RQ	0.79	0.80	0.83	0.86	0.94	0.97	1.08	1.15
Borg Scale		10	10	12	13	14	16	20
RAP (mm Hg)	3	4	5	5	5	6	9	11
PAP (mm Hg)	23	29	31	33	35	39	47	52
PWP (mm Hg)	8	11	13	14	17	18	27	33
BAP (mm Hg)	103	117	124	126	132	135	142	142
BA SAT %	97.1	97.2	96.9	97.1	97.1	97.1	97.5	97.4
PA SAT %	66.0	55.4	50.2	43.7	39.4	34.6	27.0	19.1
BA Hemoglobin	14.2	14.7	14.7	14.5	14.7	15	15.1	15.4
PA Hemoglobin	14.4	14.7	13.9	14.2	14.4	14.8	15.2	15.3
AV-O_2 Diff	5.8	8.4	9.9	10.7	11.7	12.8	14.4	16.4
CO (L/min)	8.4	10.8	11.2	13.2	13.9	14.2	14.0	12.7
CI (L/min/M²)	3.1	4.0	4.1	4.8	5.1	5.2	5.1	4.7
HR (beats/min)	102	110	115	129	140	155	160	170
SV (mL)	83	98	97	102	99	92	87	75
SVR (Woods Units)	11.8	10.5	10.7	9.2	9.2	9.1	9.5	10.3
PVR (Woods Units)	1.8	1.7	1.6	1.4	1.3	1.5	1.4	1.5
Ex-factor		568	202	652	331	168	−126	−1909

*SK: date, 8/21/91; weight, 110 kg; BSA, 2.72 M².

correspond with only mild exercise intolerance in spite of a devastated ventricle. This response was in part due to an excellent chronotropic response, the maximum heart rate being 170 bpm. The systemic vascular resistance fell in an appropriate manner. Patients with uncomplicated heart failure do not show systemic arterial oxygen desaturation during exercise,[21] a feature that is documented in the table for this patient. Oxygen extraction was avid so that he dropped his mixed venous oxygen saturation from 66% to 19.1% as exercise progressed. Correspondingly, the arteriovenous oxygen difference increased progressively from 5.8 vol% down to a low of 16.4 vol% when he was performing 175 watts of work. Pulmonary vascular resistance fell slightly. Mean pulmonary wedge pressure rose from 8 to 33 mm Hg and pulmonary arterial pressure climbed from 23 to 52 mm Hg. Right atrial pressure increased from 3 to 11 mm Hg, indicating concurrent right ventricular failure unmasked by exercise. These data are characteristic of severe heart failure in which, for any submaximal workload, oxygen consumption and heart rate are normal, whereas the arteriovenous oxygen difference is increased so that cardiac output is less than normal. The peak workload of which the patient is capable is reduced.

Based on these data, the patient therefore was considered to have severe left ventricular dysfunction with greatly abnormal increases in filling pressures during exercise but only moderate heart failure. He mounted an excellent chronotropic response and was able to achieve a relatively high maximum oxygen consumption. On the basis of these data, it was decided that he would probably be a candidate for cardiac transplantation in the future but, in the meantime, should not be placed on the active waiting list.

Subsequently, this patient underwent percutaneous cholecystectomy without cardiac complication. During the investigation for gallbladder disease, a renal cell carcinoma was discovered and this, too, was surgically removed without cardiovascular complications. In the 18 months since this study was performed, the patient has shown slight clinical deterioration. His current maximum oxygen consumption is 21.7 mL/kg/min.

Special attention is paid to the rate of rise of pulmonary wedge and pulmonary arterial pressure. At the end of each stage of exercise, the oxygen consumption, the respiratory gas exchange ratio, the perceived severity of exertion, the mixed venous oxygen saturation, and the cardiac output and stroke volume are noted.

The exercise factor, that is, the amount that the cardiac output increases with each 100 mL/min of total oxygen consumption, is also derived.

In Table 20–2, we show the data obtained from a patient whose complaint was extreme shortness of breath. Walking a very short distance, for instance, across a room on the level, produced severe dyspnea. The patient had aortic stenosis, but on several echocardiographic evaluations, the aortic valve area was found to be approximately 1.5 cm². At cardiac catheterization, a value of 1.3 cm² was obtained. A moderate degree of aortic regurgitation was demonstrated by contrast injection into the aortic root.

The study was performed to elucidate the major discrepancy between moderate aortic valve disease and extreme exertional dyspnea. When the patient was supine, right atrial pulmonary arterial and pulmonary wedge pressures were normal, but the end-diastolic pressure in the left ventricle was increased to 18 mm Hg. Mixed venous oxygen saturation was normal, yielding a cardiac output based on predicted oxygen consumption of 3.2 L/m²/min. The left ventricular ejection fraction was 67%, and pulmonary function studies at rest were also normal.

This patient was able to complete only three stages of exercise (50 watts, 300 kg/pound meter) and was able to increase his oxygen consumption only from 4.7 to 11.9 mL/min/kg, confirming the severe exercise incapacity of which he complained. The gas exchange ratio

Table 20–2. **Data from a Young Man with Mild Aortic Valve Disease But Late Stage 3 New York Heart Association Classification for Dyspnea***

Parameters	Rest-Bike	25 Watts	50 Watts
VO₂ (mL/min)	356	700	895
VO₂ (mL/min/kg)	4.7	9.3	11.9
VCO₂ (mL/min)	278	826	1047
RQ	0.78	1.18	1.17
RAP (mm Hg)	−4	−2	−4
PAP (mm Hg)	9	13	13
PWP (mm Hg)	0.5	3	6
BAP (mm Hg)	80	105	105
BA SAT %	97.4	98.8	99.2
PA SAT %	68.0	63.3	57.9
BA Hemoglobin	14.6	14.1	14.4
PA Hemoglobin	14.5	14.4	14.5
AV-O₂ Diff	5.9	6.5	8.0
CO (L/min)	6.0	10.7	11.2
CI (L/min/M²)	3.5	6.2	6.5
HR (beats/min)	80	96	114
SV (mL)	75	111	98
SVR (Woods Units)	14.0	10.0	9.8
PVR (Woods Units)	1.4	0.9	0.6
Ex-factor		1362	249

*DE: weight, 75 kg; BSA, 1.72 M².

Table 20–3. **Data from a Patient with Severe**
Left Ventricular Dysfunction and Severe Obstructive Airways Disease*

Parameters	Rest-Bike	25 Watts	75 Watts	100 Watts
VO_2 (mL/min)	412	674	1032	1454
VO_2 (mL/min/kg)	4.2	6.9	10.5	14.8
VCO_2 (mL/min)	313	613	1021	1600
RQ	0.76	0.91	0.99	1.10
PAP (mm Hg)	25	40	42	42
PWP (mm Hg)	10	12	10	10
BAP (mm Hg)	100	103	105	105
BA SAT %	95.4	95.3	95.2	96.4
PA SAT %	60.2	41.6	28.8	28.7
BA Hemoglobin	15.8	16.3	15.1	17.3
PA Hemoglobin	16	15.5	15.1	16.9
AV-O_2 Diff	7.4	12.4	13.6	16.1
CO (L/min)	5.6	5.5	7.6	9.0
Cl (L/min/M^2)	2.6	2.5	3.5	4.2
HR (beats/min)	105	108	112	128
SV (mL)	53	51	68	71
SVR (Woods Units)	18.0	18.9	13.9	11.6
PVR (Woods Units)	2.7	5.1	4.2	3.5
Ex-factor		− 43	590	349

*HWH: weight, 98.2 kg; BSA, 2.17 M^2.

was normal at rest but indicated anaerobic metabolism when he was performing a mere 25 watts of exercise. The increase in pulmonary arterial and pulmonary wedge pressures during exercise was negligible. Investigation of the biochemical function of his lower extremity musculature did not reveal any defect in tissue metabolism. Thus far, the severity of dyspnea is unexplained but has not been attributed to aortic valve disease. The study was helpful because it provided objective data that confirmed a most unusual clinical circumstance, although unfortunately it did not explain the cause of such severe exercise limitation.

Table 20–3 shows the results of a study performed in a patient with severe left ventricular dysfunction who also had significant obstructive airways disease. The main complaint was dyspnea on exertion. In this patient, the rise in pulmonary arterial pressure was considerable, but there was little increase in pulmonary wedge pressure. These data indicated that dyspnea was largely secondary to lung disease and that treatment should be directed mainly toward improving respiratory function.

Table 20–4 shows the data obtained when studying a patient with idiopathic dilated cardiomyopathy. He was able to increase the heart rate to almost 200 bpm. Oxygen consumption rose to 19.5 mL/kg/min, a respectable value for a patient with class 3 heart failure, but the corresponding increase in cardiac output was meager, rising only from 6.1 to 10.7 L/min. The mixed venous oxygen content was low to start with but fell to 25.9 vol%, indicating the

importance of increased tissue extraction of oxygen for this patient. Figures 20–1 and 20–2 show the limited response of cardiac output compared with oxygen consumption.

As would be anticipated from the literature on heart failure, a broad spectrum of responses may be observed when oxygen consumption and hemodynamics are measured simultaneously in patients with heart failure. Some patients who have extremely severe left ventricular dysfunction, with or without accompanying right ventricular dysfunction, can achieve a remarkably good maximum level of oxygen consumption around 20 mL/kg/min. In most such patients, the chronotropic response is excellent. Because our protocol calls for maximum exercise, all patients achieve the anaerobic threshold as estimated by gas exchange and this event usually occurs toward 75% of peak exercise. All patients reach 16 and most reach 19 or more on the Borg scale. As expected,[21] we have not seen hypoxemia develop during exercise, nor have we observed any patient in whom systemic vascular resistance did not decline appropriately. Pulmonary vascular resistance, on the other hand, often fails to decrease during exercise and sometimes increases slightly. Stroke volume is usually reduced at rest, increases in the early stages of exercise, and then reaches a steady value during progressive exercise. The exercise factor, that is, the increase in cardiac output per 100 mL increase in oxygen consumption during exercise, is greatly reduced but is not always linear, as it is in normal subjects. The increase in cardiac output and oxygen con-

Table 20–4. **Severe Idiopathic Dilated Cardiomyopathy*†**

Parameters	Rest-Bike	25 Watts	50 Watts	75 Watts	100 Watts	125 Watts
VO$_2$ (mL/min)	519	711	1035	1206	1494	1641
VO$_2$ (mL/min/kg)	6.2	8.5	12.3	14.4	17.8	19.5
VCO$_2$ (mL/min)	393	601	893	1044	1517	1775
RQ	0.76	0.85	0.86	0.87	1.02	1.08
Borg Scale	0	9	12	13	15	17
RAP (mm Hg)	5	1	7	7	9	11
PAP (mm Hg)	25	22	37	36	40	42
PWP (mm Hg)	11	20	26	30	28	30
BAP (mm Hg)	70	70	75	74	70	70
BA SAT %	97.2	97.2	97.4	97.2	97.5	97.5
PA SAT %	55.3	44.0	38.2	33.7	29.9	25.9
BA Hemoglobin	15.5	15.2	15.7	15.8	15.7	15.9
PA Hemoglobin	16	16	15.8	15.9	15.9	16.3
AV-O$_2$ Diff	8.5	10.5	12.6	13.6	14.4	15.3
CO (L/min)	6.1	6.8	8.2	8.9	10.4	10.7
CI (L/min/M^2)	2.9	3.2	3.9	4.2	5.0	5.1
HR (beats/min)	110	165	180	180	180	198
SV (mL)	56	41	46	49	58	54
SVR (Woods Units)	10.6	10.2	8.3	7.6	5.9	5.5
PVR (Woods Units)	2.3	0.3	1.3	0.7	1.2	1.1
Ex factor		324	451	378	535	195

*RDS: date, 3/3/92; weight, 84 kg; BSA, 2.1 M^2.

†In this patient, oxygen consumption during exercise was close to normal but was the result of greatly increased extraction by the peripheral tissues. Cardiac output response was greatly depressed.

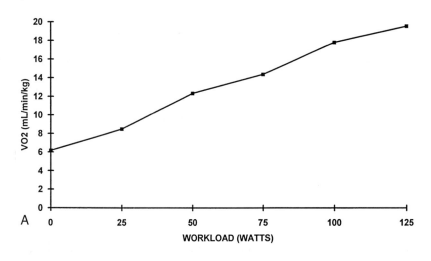

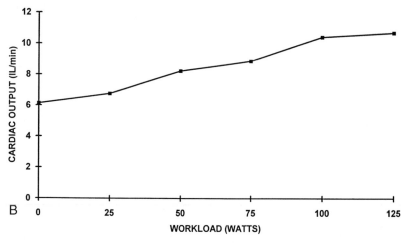

Figure 20–1. *A,* Plot of oxygen consumption during exercise against workload. Maximum oxygen consumption is relatively well preserved. *B,* Cardiac output plotted against workload in the patient whose data appear in *A.* In spite of the relative preservation of oxygen consumption during exercise, the cardiac output response to exercise is severely blunted.

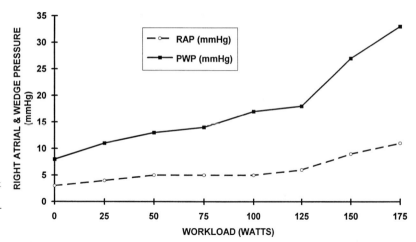

Figure 20–2. Plot of right atrial and pulmonary wedge pressure during upright bicycle exercise showing a steeper rise in wedge pressure compared with right atrial pressure. These data do not support the hypothesis of cardiac enlargement during exercise causing the heart to engage the pericardium.

sumption at the submaximal workloads observed during the studies are relatively normal, but anaerobic threshold, maximal oxygen consumption, and cardiac output occur at a much lower than normal workload.

Reduced maximal oxygen uptake during exercise has been associated with decreased survival[23–26] in some but not all studies.[12] Differences between studies may be due to characteristics of the populations studied. Studies in which patients with severe heart failure and significant functional limitations are included together with less symptomatic subjects are more likely to show in association between survival and functional capacity, compared with studies including only patients with moderate failure.[12]

It has been reported[22] that, in patients with heart failure, when the already enlarged heart increases in volume during performance of exercise, it engages the pericardium, thereby limiting performance. This development is characterized by an equal slope of increasing right atrial and pulmonary wedge pressure and an invariant stroke volume. Before the heart engages the pericardium, or when it fails to do so, the rate of rise of pulmonary wedge pressure exceeds that of right atrial pressure. We have not observed this phenomenon. Most patients increase pulmonary wedge pressure during exercise on a considerably steeper slope than that of right atrial pressure increase (see Fig. 20–2).

ETIOLOGY OF DYSPNEA

A significant number of patients with severe heart failure have lung disease. Sometimes, this takes the form of unrelated obstructive airways disease, but in addition, there is often a component of restrictive lung disease secondary to

heart failure. In such patients, it is essential to determine as clearly as possible whether dyspnea is principally of cardiac or pulmonary origin. Pulmonary function studies are of course helpful in this assessment, but it is important to recognize that heart failure itself depresses pulmonary function and that maximal oxygen consumption in these patients is correlated with pulmonary function at rest.[27] Finally, many of the patients have moderate to severe pulmonary hypertension, and here again, it is often important to determine whether the increased pulmonary arterial pressure is primarily the result of heart failure or of lung disease. When the rate of rise of pulmonary wedge pressure is modest in relation to that of pulmonary artery pressure, one should suspect that lung disease plays a major role. Likewise, a difference between pulmonary arterial diastolic pressure and pulmonary wedge pressure exceeding 10 mm Hg suggests that pulmonary vascular resistance is increased and is compatible with lung disease. Patients with a significantly elevated pulmonary wedge pressure at rest that rises appreciably during exercise but in whom the increase in pulmonary arterial pressure is disproportionate probably have both severe heart and lung disease. Pulmonary disease makes an important contribution to dyspnea when the ratios of maximal tidal volume to functional vital capacity, maximal ventilation during exercise to maximal voluntary ventilation, and maximal exercise flow rate to peak flow rate rise above their normal levels of around 50% to as high as 70%.[28] The importance of exercise testing is apparent when one considers the lack of correlation between the New York Heart Association classification and measured exercise capacity or oxygen consumption or changes[29] in oxygen delivery to exercising muscle. Changes in lower extremity oxygen consumption are of great importance to symptoms of heart failure[30] but are not considered in this chapter.

VENTRICULAR FUNCTION

Many patients undergoing hemodynamic investigation for heart failure have had exhaustive noninvasive studies of left ventricular function. Thus, it is not always necessary to perform a contrast left ventriculogram at the time of cardiac catheterization, especially when there is concern about the status of renal function. In some cases, the clinician may require better quantification of mitral regurgitation than was obtained by echo Doppler, necessitating a left ventriculogram from which global and segmental ventricular function can be assessed, along with the severity of mitral regurgitation. Even in the absence of significant epicardial coronary arterial narrowing and the presence of severe global hypokinesis, regional abnormalities are frequent.[31] Hypokinesis is often most extreme near the cardiac apex, and in many cases, ventricular wall motion is best preserved in the basal portion of the ventricle (Fig. 20–3).

On average, one expects better preservation of right ventricular function in patients with ischemic heart disease than in those with idiopathic dilated cardiomyopathy, but right ventriculography need not be performed unless it is necessary to assess tricuspid regurgitation. For this purpose, contrast media should be injected slowly through a low-resistance catheter directed toward the cardiac apex.

When assessing pulmonary hypertension and right ventricular dysfunction, the clinician should pay special attention to the left ventricular diastolic pressure. In many cases in which exercise intolerance is ascribed to intrinsic right ventricular failure, right ventricular dysfunction is, in large part, secondary to the increase in pressure and volume of the left ventricle, with subsequent deformation of the right ventricle and pulmonary hypertension.

Left Ventriculography

Left ventricular volumes and ejection fraction should be calculated according to the method described in Chapter 8. The accuracy of these calculations may be limited by the global and segmental distortions of left ventricular geome-

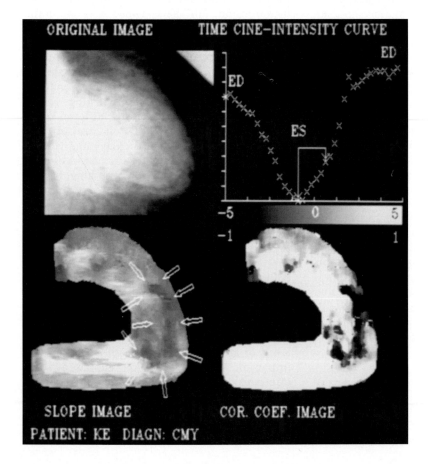

Figure 20–3. Upper left, End-systolic angiographic image in a patient with dilated cardiomyopathy. Upper right, time-intensity curve for the cardiac cycle analyzed. Arrows on the curve indicate a 100-msec segment of the data analyzed to derive the parametric images in the lower panels. Lookup table shown below the time-intensity table shows the mapping of shades of gray to slope values (−5 to 5) and correlation coefficient values (−1 to 1). Lower left and right, Slope and correlation coefficient parametric images derived in early diastole. Slope values >1 are considered normal. Arrows point to the abnormal area that appears darker (slope values <−1), compared with the rest of the shell in white (slopes >2) representing normal functioning ventricle.[31] ED, end-diastole, ES, end-systole.

try seen in patients with dilated cardiomyopathy, because calculations of left ventricular volumes are based on the assumption that the left ventricle has an elliptic shape. By definition, left ventricular ejection fraction is always decreased in patients with dilated cardiomyopathy. Correlation between left ventricular ejection fraction and symptoms or functional capacity is not strong.[1, 2, 19] Furthermore, a correlation between left ventricular ejection fraction and survival has been found in a few studies[6, 24] but not in others.[8, 9]

The extent of ventricular dilation varies widely between patients. It used to be claimed that lesser degrees of ventricular dilation were seen in milder forms of cardiomyopathy and were associated with better survival.[5, 32, 33] Recent studies,[6, 34, 35] however, have not found larger left ventricular volumes in nonsurvivors with dilated cardiomyopathy. Furthermore, a group of patients with mildly dilated congestive cardiomyopathy has been reported.[36, 37] These patients often had a family history of heart failure (56%) and a poor prognosis, except for those who improved their ejection fraction during follow-up. In one study, prognosis was more related to the shape than to the size of the left ventricle.[38] Those patients who displayed a more spherical left ventricular cavity had decreased survival compared with those with an ellipsoidal ventricle. This finding was associated with a more uniform distribution of wall stress and an increased meridional stress in patients with a spherical left ventricle.

Regional wall motion abnormalities are seen in both idiopathic and ischemic dilated cardiomyopathy.[31, 39–43] However, segmental abnormalities are generally more prominent in ischemic cardiomyopathy and often involve two or more adjacent segments.[43] These regional abnormalities may be due to regional variations in both contractility and in loading conditions. The inhomogeneous distribution of fibrosis and cardiomyopathic lesions may contribute to segmental asynergy.[39, 44] However, regional wall stress may be increased in homogeneously in the various left ventricular segments, resulting in regional afterload mismatch and asynergy.[42] At that anatomic location, abnormalities are often seen around the apex and in the anteroapical region, where wall stress is mostly increased in the presence of spherical ventricles, whereas basal wall motion is often better preserved[31] (see Fig. 20–3).

Diastolic relaxation abnormalities occur in dilated cardiomyopathy[45, 46] and may be due to regional asynchrony or the cardiomyopathic process itself. Regional asynchrony may, in turn,

be load dependent, because it is more prominent in segments displaying increased wall stress and usually improves following afterload reduction.[45]

CORONARY ARTERIOGRAPHY

Many of the patients require coronary arteriography in addition to studies of hemodynamics and ventricular function. When it is readily apparent that no major stenosis is present in a large epicardial vessel, the number of injections should be strictly limited to save contrast for uses more critical and relevant to heart failure. When severe epicardial coronary artery disease is demonstrated, even in the presence of severe left ventricular dysfunction, the patient should be carefully evaluated by appropriate studies of myocardial function and viability.

Detection of significant coronary artery disease may be important both for prognosis and for treatment. Recent studies have shown that surgical revascularization in subsets of patients with dilated cardiomyopathy due to coronary disease may benefit even when ventricular systolic function is severely depressed.[47, 48]

When severe coronary artery disease is found, areas of viable hibernating myocardium should be differentiated from scar tissue, because only viable myocardium may recover function following revascularization. A number of methods have been described for this purpose, some of which assess regional left ventricular functional reserve, whereas others assess perfusion, membrane integrity, and metabolism.[49] Assessment of myocardial viability is, however, rarely performed in the catheterization laboratory because of time constraints and the necessity of limiting contrast load. Many noninvasive methods are being tested, such as positron emission tomography and dobutamine echocardiography, but their description lies beyond the scope of this chapter.

REFERENCES

1. Franciosa JA: Functional capacity of patients with chronic left ventricular failure: Relationship of bicycle exercise performance to clinical and hemodynamic characterization. Am J Med 1979; 67:460–466.
2. Engler R, Ray R, Higgins CB, et al: Clinical assessment and follow-up of functional capacity in patients with chronic congestive cardiomyopathy. Am J Cardiol 1982; 49:1832–1837.
3. Massie BM, Kramer BL, Topic N: Lack of relationship between the short-term hemodynamic effects of captopril and subsequent clinical responses. Circulation 1984; 69:1135–1141.

4. Franciosa JA, Wilen M, Ziesche S, Cohn JN: Survival in men with severe chronic left ventricular failure due to either coronary heart disease or idiopathic dilated cardiomyopathy. Am J Cardiol 1983; 51:831–836.

5. Fuster V, Gersh ER, Tajik AJ, et al: The natural history of idiopathic dilated cardiomyopathy. Am J Cardiol 1981; 47:525–531.

6. Unverferth DV, Magorien DR, Moeschberger ML, et al: Factors influencing the one year mortality of dilated cardiomyopathy. Am J Cardiol 1984; 54:147–152.

7. Massie B, Ports T, Chatterjee K, et al: Long-term vasodilator therapy for heart failure: Clinical response and its relationship to hemodynamic measurements. Circulation 1981; 63:269–278.

8. Creager MA, Faxon DP, Halperin JL, et al: Determinants of clinical response and survival in patients with congestive heart failure treated with captopril. Am Heart J 1982; 104:1147–1154.

9. Wilson JR, Schwartz JS, St. John Sutton M, et al: Prognosis in severe heart failure: Relation to hemodynamic measurements and ventricular ectopic activity. J Am Coll Cardiol 1983; 2:403–410.

10. Lee WH, Packer M: Prognostic importance of serum sodium concentration and its modification by converting-enzyme inhibition in patients with severe chronic heart failure. Circulation 1986; 73:257–267.

11. Lee WH, Packer M: Importance of right ventricular function as the primary determinant of clinical response and long-term survival in patients with severe heart failure treated with converting-enzyme inhibitors [abstract]. J Am Coll Cardiol 1985; 5:461.

12. Franciosa JF: Why patients with heart failure die: Hemodynamic and functional determinants of survival. Circulation 1987; 75(Suppl IV):20–27.

13. Romeo F, Pelliccia F, Cianfrocca C, et al: Determinants of end-stage idiopathic dilated cardiomyopathy: A multivariate analysis of 104 patients. Clin Cardiol 1989; 12:387–392.

14. Ikram H, Williamson HG, Won M, et al: The course of idiopathic dilated cardiomyopathy in New Zealand. Br Heart J 1987; 57:521–527.

15. Abramson SV, Burke JF, Kelly JJ Jr, et al: Pulmonary hypertension predicts mortality and morbidity in patients with dilated cardiomyopathy. Ann Intern Med 1992; 116:888–895.

16. Grossman W: Blood flow measurement: The cardiac output. In Grossman W (ed): Cardiac Catheterization and Angiography. Philadelphia, Lea & Febiger, 1980, p 101.

17. Hillis LD, Firth BG, Winniford MD: Analysis of factors affecting the variability of Fick versus indicator dilution measurements of cardiac output. Am J Cardiol 1985; 56:764–768.

18. Roberts JD Jr, Lang P, Bigatello LM, et al: Inhaled nitric oxide in congenital heart disease. Circulation 1993; 87:447–453.

19. Higginbotham MB, Morris KG, Conn EH, et al: Determinants of variable exercise performance among patients with severe left ventricular dysfunction. Am J Cardiol 1983; 51:52–60.

20. Bonzheim SC, Franklin BA, DeWitt C, et al: Physiologic responses to recumbent versus upright cycle ergometry, and implications for exercise prescription in patients with coronary artery disease. Am J Cardiol 1992; 69:40–44.

21. Franciosa JA, Leddy CL, Wilen M, Schwartz DE: Relation between hemodynamic and ventilatory responses in determining exercise capacity in severe congestive heart failure. Am J Cardiol 1984; 53:127–134.

22. Janicki JS: Influence of the pericardium and ventricular interdependence on left ventricular diastolic and systolic function in patients with heart failure. Circulation 1990; 81(Suppl 2):115–120.

23. Griffin BP, Shah PK, Ferguson J, Rubin SA: Incremental prognostic value of exercise hemodynamic variables in chronic congestive heart failure secondary to coronary artery disease or to dilated cardiomyopathy. Am J Cardiol 1991; 67:848–853.

24. Likoff MJ, Chandler SL, Kay HR: Clinical determinants of mortality in chronic congestive heart failure secondary to idiopathic dilated or to ischemic cardiomyopathy. Am J Cardiol 1987; 59:634–638.

25. Szlachcic J, Massie BM, Kramer BL, et al: Correlates and prognostic implication of exercise capacity in chronic congestive heart failure. Am J Cardiol 1985; 55:1037–1042.

26. Cohn JN, Johnson GR, Shabetai R, et al: Ejection fraction, peak exercise oxygen consumption, cardiothoracic ratio, ventricular arrhythmias, and plasma norepinephrine as determinants of prognosis in heart failure. Circulation 1993; 87(Suppl VI):VI5–VI16.

27. Kraemer MD, Kubo SH, Rector TS, et al: Pulmonary and peripheral vascular factors are important determinants of peak exercise oxygen uptake in patients with heart failure. J Am Coll Cardiol 1993; 21:641–648.

28. Weber KT, Janicki JS: Cardiopulmonary exercise testing for evaluation of chronic cardiac failure. Am J Cardiol 1985; 55:22A–31A.

29. Franciosa JA, Ziesche S, Wilen M: Functional capacity of patients with chronic left ventricular failure—relationship of bicycle exercise performance to clinical and hemodynamic characterization. Am J Med 1979; 67:460–466.

30. Wilson JR, Ferraro N: Exercise intolerance in patients with chronic left failure: Relation to oxygen transport and ventilatory abnormalities. Am J Cardiol 1983; 51:1358–1363.

31. Sunnerhagen KS, Bhargava V, Shabetai R: Regional left ventricular wall motion abnormalities in idiopathic dilated cardiomyopathy. Am J Cardiol 1990; 65:364–370.

32. Goodwin JF: Prospects and predictions for the cardiomyopathies. Circulation 1974; 50:210–219.

33. Oackley C: Diagnosis and natural history of congested (dilated) cardiomyopathies. Postgrad Med J 1978; 54:440–447.

34. Gavazzi A, DeMaria R, Giuliano R, et al: The spectrum of left ventricular size in dilated cardiomyopathy: Clinical correlates and prognostic implications. Am Heart J 1993; 125:410–422.

35. Baker BJ, Leddy CL, Galie N, et al: Predictive value of M-mode echocardiography in patients with congestive heart failure. Am Heart J 1986; 111:697–702.

36. Keren A, Billingham ME, Weintraub D, et al: Mildly dilated congestive cardiomyopathy. Circulation 1985; 72:302–309.

37. Keren A, Gottlieb S, Tzivoni D, et al: Mildly dilated congestive cardiomyopathy: Use of prospective diagnostic criteria and description of the clinical course without heart transplantation. Circulation 1990; 81:506–517.

38. Douglas PS, Morrow R, Ioli A, Reichek N: Left ventricular shape, afterload and survival in idiopathic dilated cardiomyopathy. J Am Coll Cardiol 1989; 13:311–315.

39. Ritchie JL, Clarke LJ, Reichenbach D: Congestive cardiomyopathy with segmental wall motion abnormalities and a non-uniform pattern of fibrosis. Cathet Cardiovasc Diagn 1979; 5:283–287.

40. Kreulen TH, Gorlin R, Herman VH: Ventriculographic patterns and hemodynamics in primary myocardial disease. Circulation 1973; 47:299–308.

41. Wallis DE, O'Connell JB, Henkin RE, et al: Segmental wall motion abnormalities in dilated cardiomyopathy: A

common finding and good prognostic sign. J Am Coll Cardiol 1984; 4:674–679.

42. Hayashida W, Kumada T, Nohara R, et al: Left ventricular regional wall stress in dilated cardiomyopathy. Circulation 1990; 82:2075–2083.

43. Hare JM, Walford GD, Hruban RH, et al: Ischemic cardiomyopathy: Endomyocardial biopsy and ventriculographic evaluation of patients with congestive heart failure, dilated cardiomyopathy and coronary artery disease. J Am Coll Cardiol 1992; 20:1318–1325.

44. Roberts WC, Ferrans VJ: Pathological aspects of certain cardiomyopathies. Circ Res 1974; 34(Suppl II):128–144.

45. Hayashida W, Kumada T, Kohno F, et al: Left ventricular relaxation in dilated cardiomyopathy: Relation to loading conditions and regional nonuniformity. J Am Coll Cardiol 1992; 20:1082–1091.

46. Grossman W, McLaurin LP, Rolett EL: Alteration in left ventricular relaxation and diastolic compliance in congestive cardiomyopathy. Cardiovasc Res 1979; 13:514–522.

47. Kron IL, Flanagan TL, Blackbourne LH, et al: Coronary revascularization rather than cardiac transplantation for chronic ischemic cardiomyopathy. Ann Surg 1989; 210:348–354.

48. Louie HW, Laks H, Milgalter E, et al: Ischemic cardiomyopathy: Criteria for coronary revascularization and cardiac transplantation. Circulation 1991; 84(Suppl III):290–295.

49. Dilsizian V, Bonow RO: Current diagnostic techniques of assessing myocardial viability in patients with hibernating and stunned myocardium. Circulation 1993; 87:120.

Chapter 21

Catheterization and Angiography in Hypertrophic Cardiomyopathies

PETER VOLLENWEIDER
URS SCHERRER
RALF POLIKAR
PASCAL NICOD

Hypertrophic cardiomyopathy is a primary myocardial disease in which gross myocardial hypertrophy develops in the absence of increased wall stress. The hypertrophy, which may be homogeneous or, more often, heterogeneous, is not accompanied by dilation of the left ventricle.

The condition was first described on pathologic examination by Teare.[1] Soon thereafter, several clinical studies published simultaneously recognized the dynamic nature of the left ventricular outflow tract obstruction.[2-4] A variety of terms were used to describe this new entity. In Europe, *hypertrophic obstructive cardiomyopathy* was usually used, whereas *idiopathic hypertrophic subaortic stenosis* was preferred in the United States. It would seem that *hypertrophic cardiomyopathy* is the most appropriate term, because it refers to a primary disease of the cardiac muscle that includes obstructive and nonobstructive, asymmetric and symmetric forms.[5]

The incidence and prevalence of the disease vary widely depending on the study design and the diagnostic criteria used. A population-based study using routine clinical evaluation found an incidence of 2.5:100,000 and a prevalence of 19.7:100,000.[6] Studies using echocardiographic screening of selected populations[7, 8] found prevalence rates of 830:100,000 and 170:100,000, respectively. Thus, until reliable genetic markers of the disease are found, its diagnosis will rely on descriptive clinical and noninvasive criteria, and estimations of its incidence and prevalence will depend on the study design used.

In most patients the disease appears to be inherited in a pattern suggestive of an autosomal dominant trait.[9, 10] In some families, the disease seems to be linked to a missense mutation of the β-cardiac myosin heavy-chain gene.[11, 12] However, using echocardiographic screening of families with index cases, Maron and associates[13] identified other cases of the disease in only 55% of the families, whereas in 45% no other cases were found. The latter finding suggests either sporadic occurrence or other modes of inheritance such as autosomal recessive transmission with reduced penetrance.

CLASSIFICATION

The classification of the various forms of hypertrophic cardiomyopathy relies on morphologic and clinical criteria and therefore is not uniform in the medical literature. It is likely that a better understanding of the underlying genetic defects will lead to a more precise classification of the different subtypes of hypertrophic cardiomyopathy. For the time being, four forms have been described, as discussed in the following sections.

ASYMMETRIC SEPTAL HYPERTROPHY. This condition is the most commonly encountered form. Wall thickening is heterogeneous and involves parts of the interventricular septum and of the anterior, lateral, or posterior free wall. Various patterns have been described by Maron and colleagues.[14, 15] Subaortic obstruction is often found in patients with a thickened basal septum, whereas in the nonobstructive form the thickening usually involves more distal parts of the septum.

APICAL HYPERTROPHIC CARDIOMYOPATHY. This condition was first described in Japan[16]; it is characterized by a spadelike appearance of the end-diastolic left ventricular contour and the presence of giant T waves on the precordial leads of the electrocardiogram. Subsequently, this entity has also been described in Western countries but often has somewhat different features.[17, 18] Apical hypertrophy is usually not as pronounced; thus, the spadelike left ventricular deformity is often lacking. There is no outflow obstruction because the basal septum is not hypertrophied. However, mid-ventricular systolic obstruction has occasionally been documented.[17]

SYMMETRIC HYPERTROPHIC CARDIOMYOPATHY. Depending on the studies, 2% to 20% of the patients with hypertrophic cardiomyopathy have no asymmetric septal hypertrophy.[19-21] This form may not represent a separate entity, because it has been found in relatives of the asymmetric variety. An obstructive and a nonobstructive form have been described.

HYPERTROPHIC CARDIOMYOPATHY IN THE ELDERLY. Recently, this form has been described as a distinct entity.[22, 23] Although many hemodynamic features, including the degree of obstruction, are similar in old and young patients with hypertrophic cardiomyopathy, differences exist in the shape of the left ventricle. In young patients, marked thickening and a reversed curvature of the interventricular septum lead to a crescent-shaped left ventricle, whereas in the elderly, the left ventricle usually retains its normal ovoid shape and septal curvature. The only clinical feature that seems more common in the elderly is mild hypertension. In the future, a better understanding of the underlying genetic defects will probably clarify whether this form represents a distinct entity or a different manifestation of the same disease as in the young.

PATHOLOGY

Several other features, in addition to myocardial hypertrophy, are characteristic of hypertrophic cardiomyopathy. Gross cellular disorganization is present at the level of the interventricular septum and often involves the left ventricular free wall.[24, 25] The marked angulation of myocytes probably contributes to diastolic left ventricular dysfunction and may represent the substrate for the frequently encountered arrhythmias. The small intramural coronary arteries are often thickened and their lumina are narrowed.[26] This may offer a possible explanation for the frequent occurrence of myocardial ischemia and patchy myocardial scarring in these patients. Large myocardial scars may also be found in the absence of macroscopic coronary artery disease.[27]

PATHOPHYSIOLOGY

Left Ventricular Pressure Gradient and Anatomic Correlates

The presence of a dynamic systolic gradient between the left ventricular body and the outflow tract is the hallmark of obstructive hypertrophic cardiomyopathy[2-4, 28] (Fig. 21–1). At rest, the gradient is present in only 25% of the patients.[29, 30] However, during physiologic or pharmacologic maneuvers designed to provoke obstruction, it can be demonstrated in about 70% of the patients.

Because in such patients, more than 75% of the left ventricular stroke volume is ejected during the first third of systole,[31-34] questions have arisen as to whether this systolic gradient is due to true outflow tract obstruction or to cavity obliteration resulting in catheter entrapment. However, careful angiographic, hemodynamic, and echocardiographic studies have provided conclusive evidence that the systolic pressure gradient is coincident with outflow tract narrowing.[35-38] Ross and coworkers[31] measured elevated left ventricular systolic inflow tract pressures while demonstrating a free, not-entrapped catheter tip in the left ventricular cavity. These authors also located the obstruction in the outflow tract of the left ventricle. Indeed, they could find no location within the left ventricle, proximal to the obstruction, that showed low pressure, such as would have been expected if distal cavity obliteration was the cause of the systolic gradient. Finally, in patients undergoing surgery, the authors demonstrated that 70% of the left ventricular ejection occurred while there was already evidence of outflow tract obstruction (Fig. 21–2).

Echocardiographic studies have largely confirmed these angiographic observations.[35, 37, 38] The systolic outflow tract gradient occurs at the time of systolic approach and apposition (systolic anterior motion) of the mitral valve to the basal interventricular septum (Fig. 21–3). Furthermore, the degree of obstruction correlates with the degree and the time length of the systolic mitral valve apposition to the septum.[35] An early-systolic traction of the anterior leaflet toward the septum is conceived logically to result from a Venturi effect.[39] The latter phenomenon is caused presumably by the high blood flow velocity in the outflow tract, favored by its

OBSTRUCTIVE HYPERTROPHIC CARDIOMYOPATHY

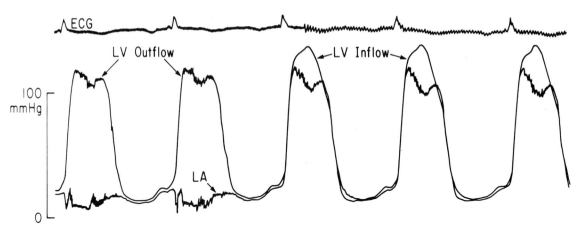

Figure 21–1. Micromanometric aortic, left atrial (LA), and left ventricular (LV) pressure recordings in a patient with obstructive hypertrophic cardiomyopathy. One catheter is advanced from the femoral artery to the central aorta. The second catheter is advanced using a transseptal approach from the LA to the inflow tract of the LV, under fluoroscopic guidance and manual injections of contrast agents. Note the presence of a systolic pressure gradient. (From Peterson KL, Karliner JS, Ross JR Jr: Profiles in congestive and hypertrophic cardiomyopathies. *In* Grossman W [ed]: Cardiac Catheterization and Angiography, 2nd ed. Philadelphia, Lea & Febiger, 1980, p 350.)

narrowing due to basal septal hypertrophy. Later in mid-systole and late-systole, forward aortic flow and velocity continue during the period of obstruction, even though they decrease markedly, and the aortic valve closes partially at the time of mitral-septal apposition.[40]

Systolic anterior motion is not specific for hypertrophic cardiomyopathy and occurs occasionally in other congenital or acquired cardiac diseases. However, in such patients it generally does not cause significant outflow obstruction.

Left Ventricular Pressure Gradient and Hydrodynamic Correlates

The dynamic and polymorphic systolic gradient of hypertrophic cardiomyopathy causes a partic-

ular aortic wave form, sometimes referred to as the "spike and dome" configuration. The early spike is associated with a high early-systolic ejection velocity, whereas the late dome is coincident with the deceleration when obstruction intervenes (Fig. 21–4).

In recent years ejection dynamics also have been usefully described according to the unsteady Bernoulli equation, where

$$\Delta P = \alpha \cdot \rho \cdot \frac{dv_r}{dt} + \beta \cdot \frac{\rho}{2} \cdot v_r^2 \qquad (1)$$

$$\Delta P = A \cdot \frac{dQ_r}{dt} + B \cdot Q_r^2 \qquad (2)$$

In these equations, ΔP = total instantaneous

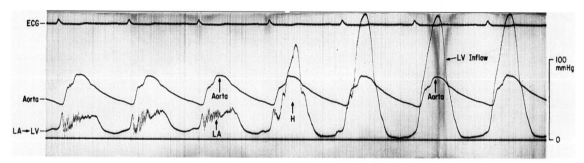

Figure 21–2. Micromanometric left atrial (LA), left ventricular (LV) inflow, and ascending aortic (aorta) pressure recordings using the technique described in Figure 21–1. A hybrid (H) pressure is recorded just as the catheter is crossing the mitral valve. Note the marked systolic gradient at rest between the LV inflow and aorta in this patient with hypertrophic cardiomyopathy. No gradient was demonstrated on pullback across the aortic valve. Note the high-frequency oscillations on the left atrial pressure pulse; the patient also had significant mitral valve regurgitation.

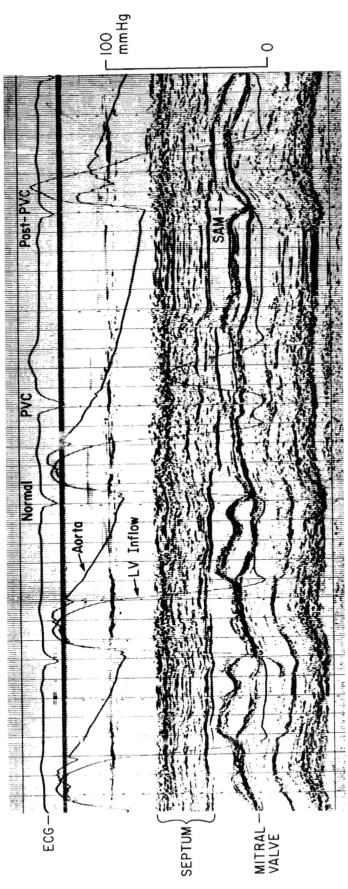

Figure 21–3. Simultaneous electrocardiographic (ECG), micromanometric left ventricular (LV) inflow and aortic pressure, and M-mode echocardiographic recordings in a patient with obstructive hypertrophic cardiomyopathy. After a premature ventricular contraction (PVC on the ECG tracing), there is an increase in the LV pressure gradient that correlates well with a close septal apposition of the anterior leaflet of the mitral valve. Note the decrease in pulse pressure (Brockenbrough sign) and the spike-and-dome configuration of the aortic pressure waveform in the post-PVC beat. SAM, systolic anterior motion. (From Peterson KL, Karliner JS, Ross JR Jr: Profiles in congestive and hypertrophic cardiomyopathies. *In* Grossman W [ed]: Cardiac Catheterization and Angiography, 2nd ed. Philadelphia, Lea & Febiger, 1980, p 354.)

POSTEXTRASYSTOLIC POTENTIATION

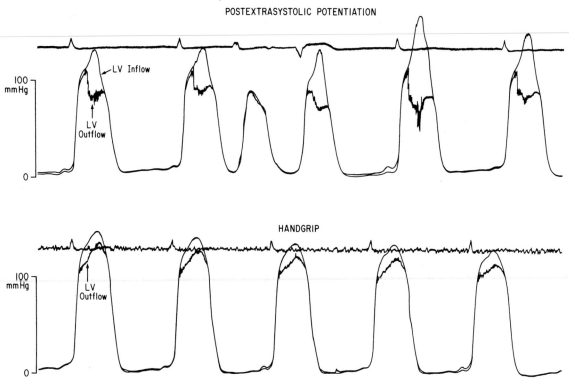

Figure 21–4. Simultaneous micromanometric left ventricular (LV) inflow and outflow tract pressure recordings using the technique described in Figure 21–2. The upper recording shows an increased intraventricular systolic gradient and a slightly decreased aortic pressure, following two premature ventricular beats. On the lower recording, a hand-grip maneuver results in a marked decrease of the intraventricular systolic gradient and a change in profile during systole of both inflow and outflow pressure recordings.

pressure drop, ρ = mass per unit volume, $\left(\alpha \cdot \rho \cdot \dfrac{dv_r}{dt}\right)$ and $\left(A \cdot \dfrac{dQ_r}{dt}\right)$ are local acceleration components, and $\left(\beta \cdot \dfrac{\rho}{2} \cdot v_r^2\right)$ and $\left(\beta \cdot Q_r^2\right)$ are convective acceleration components; the subscript r signifies a reference position; for example, the aortic ring for measurement of velocity v_r or flow rate Q_r and their derivatives, $\alpha\beta$, are geometric coefficients, and A and B depend on the instantaneous geometry and the density of blood.[41] By this model, in obstructive hypertrophic cardiomyopathy it is the interaction of outflow tract narrowing with increased early-systolic velocities and accelerations (convective effects) that underlies the augmentation of the outflow tract gradient during early ejection. However, in mid-systole and late-systole, a substantive gradient is generated, even after aortic flow has returned to zero or is negative, suggesting that local viscous hydrodynamic shear forces and local acceleration components are also playing an important role in the overall pressure gradient measured.[41]

Factors that Influence the Magnitude of the Pressure Gradient

Several factors may contribute to a closer apposition of the mitral valve on the interventricular septum and, in turn, to greater narrowing of the outflow tract. These include the following: (1) increased myocardial contractility; (2) decreased left ventricular preload; and (3) a fall in left ventricular afterload resulting in a decreased size of the left ventricle (Table 21–1).

An increase in left ventricular contractility occurs typically following an extrasystole. Normally, such postextrasystolic potentiation of myocardial contractility results in an increase in stroke volume and pulse pressure. Conversely, as described by Brockenbrough and associates,[42] in hypertrophic cardiomyopathy increased postextrasystolic contractility may worsen the outflow tract pressure gradient (see Fig. 21–4, *upper*) and blunt the increase or frankly decrease the ascending aortic pulse pressure (see Fig. 21–3). Exercise or positive inotropic agents such as isoproterenol may have similar effects. Decreased preload or afterload, such as seen dur-

Table 21–1. **Factors Modifying the Left Ventricular Systolic Outflow Tract Gradient in Hypertrophic Cardiomyopathy**

Maneuvers Increasing the Left Ventricular Outflow Gradient
   Agents or interventions that increase contractile force
      Post-ventricular premature contraction
      Increased sympathetic drive during exercise
      Digitalis
      Isoproterenol
   Agents or interventions that decrease preload
      Valsalva maneuver
      Hemorrhage
      Nitroglycerin
   Agents or interventions that decrease afterload
      Nitroglycerin
      Amyl nitrite
      Hemorrhage
Maneuvers Decreasing the Left Ventricular Outflow Gradient
   Agents or interventions that decrease contractile force
      β-adrenergic blockade
      Verapamil
   Agents or interventions that increase preload
      Increase in venous preload
      Blood volume expansion
   Agents or interventions that increase afterload
      Phenylephrine
      Angiotensin
      Squatting
      Hand-grip exercise

ing a Valsalva maneuver and administration of vasodilators, may also worsen significantly the left ventricular outflow tract pressure gradient. On the other hand, decreasing left ventricular contractility with β-blockers or increasing preload or afterload by squatting, hand-grip exercise, or infusion of phenylephrine lessen the left ventricular pressure gradient (see Fig. 21–4, *lower*).

Left Ventricular Diastolic Function

Anomalies in both left ventricular compliance and relaxation have been well documented in patients with hypertrophic cardiomyopathy.[43, 44]

That decreased compliance is common is suggested by the frequent finding of a high end-diastolic pressure in the presence of a small left ventricular end-diastolic volume, demonstrating a leftward and upward shift of the diastolic pressure-volume relationship. Several mechanisms, such as increased muscle stiffness secondary to fibrosis,[45] cellular disarray,[46] and left ventricular hypertrophy,[47, 48] may contribute to decreased compliance.

Impaired left ventricular relaxation has been documented by a prolonged isovolumetric relaxation time[47, 49] and a slow decline in early-diastolic left atrial[50] and ventricular pressure. This impaired relaxation may be due to different factors such as impaired calcium sequestra-

tion in the sarcoplasmic reticulum,[51] myocardial ischemia,[51] and load-dependent mechanisms.[52, 53]

These diastolic function abnormalities result in a decreased early-diastolic filling and an increased atrial contribution to diastolic filling. Initially, these filling dysfunctions were documented using left ventricular pressure-volume curves, M-mode echocardiography, or radionuclide ventriculography. The recent development of Doppler echocardiography has allowed noninvasive evaluation of the left ventricular filling pattern, demonstrating a delayed, low-amplitude early filling (E wave) and a prominent atrial filling (A wave).[54, 55] However, the validity of such noninvasive measurements of left ventricular filling is limited by the fact that they may be altered by changes in preload or afterload.

Myocardial Ischemia

In patients with hypertrophic cardiomyopathy, clinical presentation and results of noninvasive evaluation are often consistent with the diagnosis of myocardial ischemia. However, both chest pain and exercise-induced electrocardiographic or myocardial scintigraphic perfusion abnormalities occur frequently in the absence of coronary artery disease.[56] In such patients, pacing performed during cardiac catheterization often induces myocardial ischemia accompanied by chest pain, increased transcardiac production of lactate, and abnormalities in left ventricular diastolic function.

The causes for impaired coronary reserve and myocardial ischemia are multiple. In patients with significant left ventricular outflow tract obstruction, myocardial oxygen demand is augmented because of left ventricular hypertrophy and increased left ventricular systolic pressure. Various mechanisms may contribute to impaired oxygen delivery, including (1) systolic compression of coronary arteries in the absence of coronary artery disease; (2) abnormal intramyocardial coronary arteries; (3) inadequate myocardial capillary density; and (4) decreased coronary vasodilator reserve.[57]

PROGNOSIS

The event most feared in patients with hypertrophic cardiomyopathy is sudden premature death, which is associated with an annual mortality rate of 2% to 3%.[58] Few clinical or hemodynamic features may predict the occurrence of such an event. Only the occurrence of ventricular tachycardia on electrocardiographic monitoring and a positive family history have been consistently associated with an increased risk of sudden death.[58, 59] Therefore, it is likely that ventricular tachycardia and fibrillation[60] are the cause for sudden death in a substantial number of such patients, even though other mechanisms such as left ventricular obstruction and supraventricular arrhythmias[61] may also occasionally contribute to such events. Ventricular arrhythmias may be triggered by myocardial cellular disarray, ischemia, or scarring.[27] Hypertrophic cardiomyopathy of the elderly[22] and apical hypertrophic cardiomyopathy[18] seem to have a more favorable prognosis than asymmetric septal hypertrophy.

INDICATIONS FOR CARDIAC CATHETERIZATION

The indications for cardiac catheterization in patients with hypertrophic cardiomyopathy are not well established in the medical literature. This may be related to the following factors: (1) there are no hemodynamic features predictive of sudden death, the most feared complication of hypertrophic cardiomyopathy; (2) recent technologic developments allow a reliable noninvasive assessment of left ventricular systolic and diastolic function and the degree of obstruction; and (3) the effects of medical treatment can be adequately followed by noninvasive means.

However, cardiac catheterization may be indicated in the following selected subsets of patients:

1. Those with symptoms refractory to medical treatment—in such patients, invasive hemodynamic measurements and left ventricular angiography contribute to determining the feasibility of surgery. In addition, coronary angiography may be useful to establish the presence or absence of epicardial coronary artery disease.

2. Those who present with chest pain—in such patients, cardiac catheterization with coronary angiography is the only reliable technique to establish the presence or absence of epicardial coronary artery disease. Indeed, exercise testing may reveal electrocardiographic and scintigraphic myocardial perfusion abnormalities even in the absence of epicardial coronary artery disease.

3. Those in whom, after complete noninvasive evaluation, the diagnosis of hypertrophic cardiomyopathy is still in doubt—in such rare patients, cardiac catheterization together with hemodynamic measurements during maneuvers designed to provoke obstruction may help definitively establish or rule out the diagnosis. In patients suspected of having coexisting cardiac malformations such as valvular, subvalvular, and supravalvular membranous obstructions, cardiac catheterization may help quantitate the hemodynamic contribution of each pathoanatomic problem.

TECHNIQUES OF CARDIAC CATHETERIZATION

Left-sided cardiac catheterization may be difficult because of catheter entrapment and instability resulting from a hypercontractile left ventricle and cavity obliteration.

An end-hole catheter is used for pressure measurement. To ensure its position in the inflow tract of the left ventricle, fluoroscopy and small injections of contrast agents are used. Aspiration of blood through the catheter during a complete cardiac cycle helps rule out catheter entrapment. If the position of the catheter is unstable or if there is any doubt that the increased systolic left ventricular pressure is caused by entrapment, a transseptal approach may allow a better and more stable positioning of the catheter in the inflow tract of the left ventricle. Simultaneous pressure recordings in the inflow tract of the left ventricle and in the aorta or in the outflow tract of the left ventricle accurately identify the presence or absence of subvalvular obstruction. Catheter pullback is another way for documenting obstruction.

Standard techniques and catheters are used for ventriculography and coronary angiography.

HEMODYNAMIC FINDINGS

Cardiac Output

Cardiac output is usually normal or even increased in patients with hypertrophic cardiomyopathy.[62] A decreased cardiac output may be seen either as a result of decreased preload (secondary to the use of diuretics or vasodilators) or in a subset of patients who develop a dilated type of cardiomyopathy in the final stages of their disease.[63–65]

Right-sided Pressures

In patients with hypertrophic cardiomyopathy, right atrial and ventricular pressures are usually within the normal range. However, in the following rare circumstances they may be elevated:

(1) a right-sided outflow tract gradient, secondary to right ventricular involvement by hypertrophic cardiomyopathy, may rarely occur and cause an increase in right ventricular systolic pressure; (2) elevated pulmonary capillary pressure, particularly in patients with mitral regurgitation, may cause retrograde elevation of pulmonary artery and right ventricular pressures; and (3) right ventricular hypertrophy secondary to long-standing elevation of systolic right ventricular pressure may result in elevated end-diastolic right ventricular and right atrial pressure.[28, 62]

Left-sided Pressures

As already mentioned in the section on pathophysiology, a left ventricular systolic pressure gradient is a hallmark of hypertrophic cardiomyopathy. In the resting state, the gradient may be (1) latent, that is, seen only during provocative maneuvers (see Table 21–1); (2) persistent; or (3) labile, that is, appearing and disappearing during cardiac catheterization. A labile pressure gradient, appearing and disappearing beat by beat, is only rarely seen and is probably caused by fluctuating changes in preload and afterload (due to inspiration and altered blood pressure), or contractility (Fig. 21–5).

In a study of 126 patients with hypertrophic cardiomyopathy, Frank and Braunwald[62] measured pressure gradients as high as 175 mm Hg, with an average value of 54 mm Hg. The magnitude of the pressure gradient was generally not correlated with the patient's symptoms or functional class.

In a given patient, however, the left ventricular systolic gradient may vary with time. An increase in pressure gradient is one of the causes for worsening symptoms.[66] In occasional patients, the pressure gradient may disappear secondary to myocardial infarction or to the occurrence of dilated cardiomyopathy, which has a poor prognosis.

CONTRAST VENTRICULOGRAPHY

Contrast ventriculography typically reveals a small left ventricular cavity with marked hypertrophy and vigorous systolic contraction resulting in near cavity obliteration. Systolic anterior motion of the mitral valve can be assessed using an anteroposterior or left anterior oblique view, with or without cranial angulation, or a left lateral view (Fig. 21–6). In patients considered for surgical myotomy-myomectomy, it may be helpful to perform a simultaneous right ventricular injection in a cranial angulation that allows optimal visualization of the interventricular septum. In the right oblique projection, the left ventricle often has a banana shape due to thickened papillary muscles. In apical hypertrophic cardiomyopathy, particularly the Japanese variety, the end-diastolic left ventricular contours show a spade shape (Fig. 21–7). In the variety seen in Western countries, a marked mid-ventricular obstruction occasionally causes a "shelflike" appearance of the interventricular septum (Fig. 21–8).

In patients displaying systolic anterior motion of the mitral valve,[67] mitral regurgitation is often found. It is usually mild but occasionally may be hemodynamically significant. Its severity appears to be related to the extent of the systolic anterior motion of the mitral valve.

CORONARY ANGIOGRAPHY

Coronary arteries may be enlarged and tortuous in hypertrophic cardiomyopathy, similarly to what is seen in other hypertrophic states such as aortic valvular stenosis. Systolic compression may be seen, particularly at the level of the left anterior descending artery and its septal branches. Such compression may occasionally cause systolic coronary lumen obliteration or result in a characteristic "sawfish" appearance of the vessel[68] (Fig. 21–9). Systolic compression may lead to myocardial ischemia or even myo-

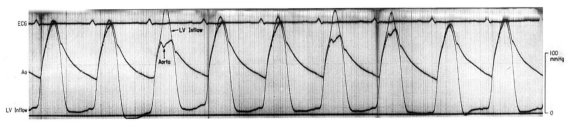

Figure 21–5. Simultaneous micromanometric left ventricular (LV) inflow and ascending aortic (Ao) pressure recordings at rest and during spontaneous respiration. Note the labile, beat-to-beat pressure gradient with the associated changes in the profile of the ascending aortic pressure pulse.

SYSTOLE   DIASTOLE

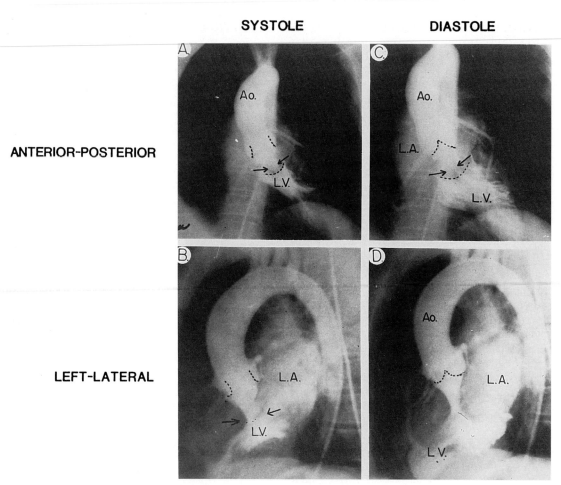

ANTERIOR-POSTERIOR

LEFT-LATERAL

Figure 21–6. Biplane contrast left ventriculography in a patient with hypertrophic cardiomyopathy. By end-systole *(A and B)*, there is near cavity obliteration. In the outflow tract of the left ventricle (shown by *arrows* in the anteroposterior view), apposition of the mitral valve to the interventricular septum causes an area of decreased contrast. In the left lateral view, at end-systole, the apposition of the anterior leaflet of the mitral valve against the interventricular septum is clearly shown *(arrow).* Mitral regurgitation is present. *(A and B* Reproduced and modified with permission from Ross J Jr, Braunwald E, Gault JH, et al: The mechanism of the intraventricular pressure gradient in idiopathic hypertrophic subaortic stenosis. Circulation 1966; 34:558. Copyright 1966 American Heart Association.)

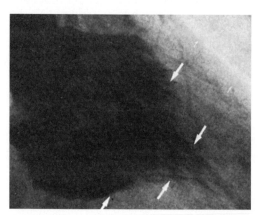

Figure 21–7. Contrast left ventriculography in a patient with apical hypertrophic cardiomyopathy at end-diastole (right oblique anterior projection). Note the spadelike ventricular configuration and the marked increase in free wall thickness toward the apex *(arrows).* (From Hada Y, Sakamoto T, Amano K, et al: Prevalence of hypertrophic cardiomyopathy in a population of adult Japanese workers as detected by echocardiographic screening. Am J Cardiol 1987; 59:183–184.)

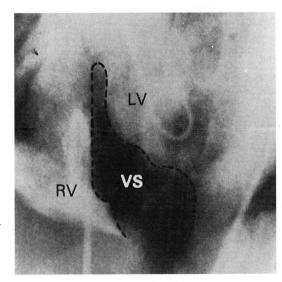

Figure 21–8. Biventricular contrast angiography in the left anterior oblique projection during diastole in a patient with apical hypertrophic cardiomyopathy. Contrast material fills the left ventricular (LV) and right ventricular (RV) cavities simultaneously, delineating the ventricular septum (VS), which is outlined by the broken line. The cephalad portion of the septum is of normal thickness and the left and right endocardial surfaces are parallel. Toward the apex the septum increases abruptly in thickness, resulting in a "shelflike" appearance. (From Maron BJ, Bonow RO, Seshagiri TNR, et al: Hypertrophic cardiomyopathy with ventricular septal hypertrophy localized to the apical region of the left ventricle [apical hypertrophic cardiomyopathy]. Am J Cardiol 1982; 49:1838–1848. Reprinted with permission from American Journal of Cardiology.)

cardial infarction in patients with hypertrophic cardiomyopathy and normal coronary arteries.

CONCLUSION

Indications for cardiac catheterization in hypertrophic cardiomyopathy are limited. In patients with refractory symptoms, it may help to determine the main underlying mechanism, which may include (1) dynamic systolic left ventricular outflow tract obstruction, (2) abnormal diastolic function, and (3) myocardial ischemia. Thereby, it may lead to the identification of patients with marked obstruction who may benefit either from surgical myotomy-myomectomy or new pacing modalities that, in some instances, may alleviate the obstruction.[69, 70] Furthermore, it helps establish whether associated coronary artery disease is contributing to symptoms, particularly in older patients who may benefit from specific treatment. Finally, it may help identify the most appropriate medical treatment for patients depending on whether left ventricular systolic obstruction, left ventricular diastolic dysfunction, or myocardial ischemia is the predom-

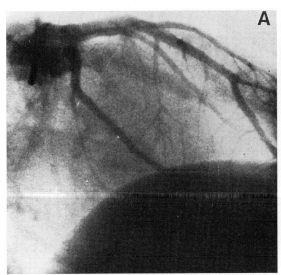

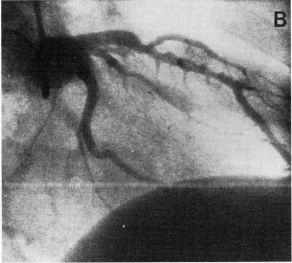

Figure 21–9. Left coronary angiograms in the right anterior oblique projection with caudocranial angulation. Diastolic (A) and systolic (B) frames are shown. "Sawfish" appearance of the left anterior descending coronary artery is the result of systolic compression. Note the associated systolic compression of the septal, second diagonal, and intermediate branches. (From Brugada P, Bär FW, De Zwann C, et al: "Sawfish" systolic narrowing of the left anterior descending coronary artery: An angiographic sign of hypertrophic cardiomyopathy. Circulation 1982; 66:800–803.)

inant pathophysiologic abnormality leading to symptoms.

REFERENCES

1. Teare D: Asymmetrical hypertrophy of the heart in young adults. Br Heart J 1958; 20:1–8.
2. Goodwin JF, Hollman A, Cleland WP, Teare D: Obstructive cardiomyopathy simulating aortic stenosis. Br Heart J 1960; 22:403–414.
3. Morrow AG, Braunwald E: Functional aortic stenosis: A malformation characterized by resistance to left ventricular outflow without anatomic obstruction. Circulation 1959; 20:181–189.
4. Wigle ED, Heimbecker RO, Gunton RW: Idiopathic ventricular septal hypertrophy causing muscular subaortic stenosis. Circulation 1962; 26:325–340.
5. Maron BJ, Epstein SE: Hypertrophic cardiomyopathy: A discussion of nomenclature. Am J Cardiol 1979; 43:1242–1244.
6. Codd MB, Sugrue DD, Gersh BJ, Melton LJ III: Epidemiology of idiopathic dilated and hypertrophic cardiomyopathy: A population-based study in Olmsted County, Minnesota, 1975–1984. Circulation 1989; 80:564–572.
7. Hada Y, Sakamoto T, Amano K, et al: Prevalence of hypertrophic cardiomyopathy in a population of adult Japanese workers as detected by echocardiographic screening. Am J Cardiol 1987; 59:183–184.
8. Savage DD, Castelli WP, Abbott RD, et al: Hypertrophic cardiomyopathy and its markers in the general population: The great masquerader revisited: The Framingham study. J Cardiovasc Ultrasonogr 1983; 2:41–47.
9. Maron BJ, Mulvihill JJ: The genetics of hypertrophic cardiomyopathy. Ann Intern Med 1986; 105:610–613.
10. Clark CE, Henry WL, Epstein SE: Familial prevalence and genetic transmission of idiopathic hypertrophic subaortic stenosis. N Engl J Med 1978; 289:709–714.
11. Geisterfer-Lowrance AAT, Kass S, Tanigawa G, et al: A molecular basis for familial hypertrophic cardiomyopathy: A β cardiac myosin heavy chain gene missense mutation. Cell 1990; 62:999–1006.
12. Watkins H, Rosenzweig A, Hwang DS, et al: Characteristics and prognostic implications of myosin missense mutations in familial hypertrophic cardiomyopathy. N Engl J Med 1992; 326:1108–1114.
13. Maron BJ, Nichols PF, Pickle LW, et al: Patterns of inheritance in hypertrophic cardiomyopathy: Assessment by M-mode and two-dimensional echocardiography. Am J Cardiol 1984; 53:1087–1094.
14. Maron BJ, Bonow RO, Cannon RO, et al: Hypertrophic cardiomyopathy: Interrelations of clinical manifestations, pathophysiology, and therapy. N Engl J Med 1987; 316:780–789.
15. Maron BJ, Bonow RO, Cannon RO, et al: Hypertrophic cardiomyopathy: Interrelations of clinical manifestations, pathophysiology, and therapy. N Engl J Med 1987; 316:844–852.
16. Yamaguchi H, Ishimura T, Nishiyama S, et al: Hypertrophic nonobstructive cardiomyopathy with giant negative T waves (apical hypertrophy): Ventriculographic and echocardiographic features in 30 patients. Am J Cardiol 1979; 44:401–412.
17. Maron BJ, Bonow RO, Seshagiri TNR, et al: Hypertrophic cardiomyopathy with ventricular septal hypertrophy localized to the apical region of the left ventricle (apical hypertrophic cardiomyopathy). Am J Cardiol 1982; 49:1838–1848.
18. Webb JG, Sasson Z, Rakowski H, et al: Apical hypertrophic cardiomyopathy: Clinical follow-up and diagnostic correlates. J Am Coll Cardiol 1990; 15:83–90.
19. Maron BJ, Gottdiener JS, Roberts WC, et al: Left ventricular outflow tract obstruction due to systolic anterior motion of the anterior mitral leaflet in patients with concentric left ventricular hypertrophy. Circulation 1978; 57:527–533.
20. Come PC, Bulkly BH, Goodman ZD, et al: Hypercontractile cardiac states stimulating hypertrophic cardiomyopathy. Circulation 1977; 55:901–908.
21. Shapiro LM, McKenna WJ: Distribution of left ventricular hypertrophy in hypertrophic cardiomyopathy: A two-dimensional echocardiographic study. J Am Coll Cardiol 1983; 2:437–444.
22. Topol EJ, Traill TA, Fortuin NJ: Hypertensive hypertrophic cardiomyopathy of the elderly. N Engl J Med 1985; 312:277–283.
23. Lever HM, Karam RF, Currie PJ, Healy BP: Hypertrophic cardiomyopathy in the elderly: Distinctions from the young based on cardiac shape. Circulation 1989; 79:580–589.
24. Ferrans VJ, Morrow AG, Roberts WC: Myocardial ultrastructure in idiopathic hypertrophic subaortic stenosis: A study of operatively excised left ventricular outflow tract muscle in 14 patients. Circulation 1972; 45:769–792.
25. Bulkley BH, Weisfeldt ML, Hutchins GM: Isometric cardiac contraction: A possible cause of the disorganized myocardial pattern of idiopathic hypertrophic subaortic stenosis. N Engl J Med 1977; 296:135–139.
26. Maron BJ, Wolfson JK, Epstein SE, Roberts WC: Intramural ("small vessel") coronary artery disease in hypertrophic cardiomyopathy. J Am Coll Cardiol 1986; 8:545–557.
27. Maron BJ, Epstein SE, Roberts WC: Hypertrophic cardiomyopathy and transmural myocardial infarction without significant atherosclerosis of the extramural coronary arteries. Am J Cardiol 1979; 43:1086–1102.
28. Braunwald E, Lambrew CT, Rockoff SD, et al: Idiopathic hypertrophic subaortic stenosis. Part I: A description of the disease based upon an analysis of 64 patients. Circulation 1964; 30(Suppl 4):IV-3–IV-119.
29. Ciro E, Nichols PF III, Maron BJ: Heterogeneous morphologic expression of genetically transmitted hypertrophic cardiomyopathy: Two-dimensional echocardiographic analysis. Circulation 1983; 67:1227–1233.
30. Spirito P, Maron BJ: Absence of progression of left ventricular hypertrophy in adult patients with hypertrophic cardiomyopathy. J Am Coll Cardiol 1987; 9:1013–1017.
31. Ross J Jr, Braunwald E, Gault JH, et al: The mechanism of the intraventricular pressure gradient in idiopathic hypertrophic subaortic stenosis. Circulation 1966; 34:558–578.
32. Siegel RJ, Criley JM: Comparison of ventricular emptying with and without a pressure gradient in patients with hypertrophic cardiomyopathy. Br Heart J 1985; 53:283–291.
33. Sugrue DD, McKenna WJ, Dickie S, et al: Relation between left ventricular gradient and relative stroke volume ejected in early and late systole in hypertrophic cardiomyopathy: Assessment with radionuclide cineangiography. Br Heart J 1984; 52:602–609.
34. Maron BJ, Gottdiener JS, Arce J, et al: Dynamic subaortic obstruction in hypertrophic cardiomyopathy: Analysis by pulsed Doppler echocardiography. J Am Coll Cardiol 1985; 6:1–8.
35. Pollick C, Rakowski H, Wigle ED: Muscular subaortic stenosis: The quantitative relationship between systolic

anterior motion and the pressure gradient. Circulation 1984; 69:43–49.

36. Murgo JP, Alter BR, Dorethy JF, et al: Dynamics of left ventricular ejection in obstructive and nonobstructive hypertrophic cardiomyopathy. J Clin Invest 1980; 66:1369–1382.

37. Shah PM, Gramak R, Kramer DH: Ultrasound location of left ventricular outflow obstruction in hypertrophic obstructive cardiomyopathy. Circulation 1969; 40:3–11.

38. Henry WL, Clark CE, Glaney DL, Epstein SE: Echocardiographic measurement of the left ventricular outflow gradient in idiopathic hypertrophic subaortic stenosis. N Engl J Med 1973; 288:989–993.

39. Wigle ED, Adelman AG, Silver MD: Pathophysiological considerations in muscular subaortic stenosis. *In* Wolstenholme GEW, O'Connor M (eds): Hypertrophic Obstructive Cardiomyopathy [Ciba Foundation Study Group, No. 47]. London, Churchill, 1971, pp 63–75.

40. Yock PG, Hatle L, Popp RL: Patterns and timing of Doppler-detected intracavitary and aortic flow in hypertrophic cardiomyopathy. J Am Coll Cardiol 1986; 8:1047–1058.

41. Pasipoularides A: Clinical assessment of ventricular ejection dynamics with and without outflow obstruction. J Am Coll Cardiol 1990; 15:859–882

42. Brockenbrough EC, Braunwald E, Morrow AG: A hemodynamic technic for the detection of hypertrophic subaortic stenosis. Circulation 1961; 23:189–194.

43. Goodwin JF: Congestive and hypertrophic cardiomyopathies: A decade of study. Lancet 1970; 1:731–739.

44. Wigle ED, Sasson Z, Henderson MA, et al: Hypertrophic cardiomyopathy—the importance of the site and the extent of hypertrophy: A review. Prog Cardiovasc Dis 1985; 28:1–83.

45. Tanaka M, Fujiwara H, Onodera T, et al: Quantitative analysis of myocardial fibrosis in normals, hypertensive hearts, and hypertrophic cardiomyopathy. Br Heart J 1986; 55:575–581.

46. St John Sutton MG, Lie JT, Anderson KR, et al: Histopathological specificity of hypertrophic obstructive cardiomyopathy: Myocardial fibre disarray and myocardial fibrosis. Br Heart J 1980; 44:433–443.

47. Gaasch WH, Levine HJ, Quinones MA, Alexander JK: Left ventricular compliance: Mechanisms and clinical implications. Am J Cardiol 1976; 38:645–653.

48. Grossman W, McLaurin LP: Diastolic properties of the left ventricle. Ann Intern Med 1976; 84:316–326.

49. St John Sutton MG, Tajik AJ, Gibson DG, et al: Echocardiographic assessment of left ventricular filling and septal and posterior wall dynamics in idiopathic hypertrophic subaortic stenosis. Circulation 1978; 57:512–520.

50. Stewart S, Mason DT, Braunwald E: Impaired rate of left ventricular filling in idiopathic hypertrophic subaortic stenosis and valvular aortic stenosis. Circulation 1968; 37:8–14.

51. Nayler WC, Williams A: Relaxation in heart muscle: Some morphological and biochemical considerations. Eur J Cardiol 1978, 7(Suppl):35–50.

52. Hess OM, Grimm J, Krayenbühl HP: Diastolic function in hypertrophic cardiomyopathy: Effects of propanolol and verapamil on diastolic stiffness. Eur Heart J 1983; 4(Suppl):F47–F56.

53. Brutsaert DL, Rademakers FE, Sys SU: Triple control of relaxation: Implications in cardiac disease. Circulation 1984; 69:190–196.

54. Yellin EL, Nikolic S, Frater RWM: Left ventricular filling dynamics and diastolic function. Prog Cardiovasc Dis 1990; 32:247–271.

55. Mirsky I, Pasipoularides A: Clinical assessment of diastolic function. Prog Cardiovasc Dis 1990; 32:291–318.

56. Pitcher D, Wainwright R, Marsey M, et al: Assessment of chest pain in hypertrophic cardiomyopathy using exercise thallium 201 myocardial scintigraphy. Br Heart J 1980; 44:650–656.

57. Cannon RO III, Rosing DR, Maron BJ, et al: Myocardial ischemia in patients with hypertrophic cardiomyopathy: Contribution of inadequate vasodilator reserve and elevated left ventricular filling pressures. Circulation 1985; 71:234–243.

58. Maron BJ, Savage DD, Wolfson JK, Epstein SE: Prognostic significance of 24-hour ambulatory electrocardiographic monitoring in patients with hypertrophic cardiomyopathy: A prospective study. Am J Cardiol 1981; 48:252–257.

59. McKenna WJ, England D, Doi YL, et al: Arrhythmia in hypertrophic cardiomyopathy. Part I: Influence on prognosis. Br Heart J 1981; 46:168–172.

60. Nicod P, Polikar R, Peterson KL: Hypertrophic cardiomyopathy and sudden death. N Engl J Med 1988; 318:1255–1257.

61. Krikler DM, Davies MJ, Rowland E, et al: Sudden death in hypertrophic cardiomyopathy: Associated accessory atrioventricular pathways. Br Heart J 1980; 43:245–251.

62. Frank S, Braunwald E: Idiopathic hypertrophic subaortic stenosis: Clinical analysis of 126 patients with emphasis on the natural history. Circulation 1968; 37:759–788.

63. Spirito P, Maron BJ, Bonow RO: Occurrence and significance of progressive left ventricular wall thinning and relative cavity dilatation in patients with hypertrophic cardiomyopathy. Am J Cardiol 1987; 59:123–129.

64. Spirito P, Maron BJ, Bonow RO, Epstein SE: Severe functional limitation in patients with hypertrophic cardiomyopathy and only mild localized left ventricular hypertrophy. J Am Coll Cardiol 1986; 8:537–544.

65. ten Cate FJ, Roelandt J: Progression to left ventricular dilatation in patients with hypertrophic obstructive cardiomyopathy. Am Heart J 1979; 97:762–765.

66. Agatston AS, Polakoff R, Hippogoankar R, et al: The significance of increased left ventricular outflow tract velocities in the elderly measured by continuous wave Doppler. Am Heart J 1989; 117:1320–1326.

67. Kinoshita N, Nimura Y, Okamoto M, et al: Mitral regurgitation in hypertrophic cardiomyopathy: Noninvasive study by two-dimensional Doppler echocardiography. Br Heart J 1983; 49:574–583.

68. Brugada P, Bär FWHM, De Zwann C, et al: "Sawfish" systolic narrowing of the left anterior descending coronary artery: An angiographic sign of hypertrophic cardiomyopathy. Circulation 1982; 66:800–803.

69. Jeanrenaud X, Kappenberger L, Goy JJ: Hemodynamic and therapeutic effects of dual-chamber pacing in patients with hypertrophic obstructive cardiomyopathy. Lancet 1992; 339:1318–1323.

70. Fananapazir L, Canon RO III, Tripodi D, Panza JA: Impact of dual-chamber permanent pacing in patients with obstructive hypertrophic cardiomyopathy with symptoms refractory to verapamil and beta-adrenergic blocker therapy. Circulation 1992: 85:2149–2161.

Catheterization and Angiography in Restrictive and Constrictive Disorders of the Heart

RALF POLIKAR
PASCAL NICOD
RALPH SHABETAI

Three categories of patients with pericardial disease are likely to be referred for cardiac catheterization: those with a large pericardial effusion, those with cardiac tamponade, and those suspected of constrictive pericarditis in whom the differential diagnosis of restrictive cardiomyopathy may also need to be considered.

CARDIAC TAMPONADE

Role of Cardiac Catheterization in Establishing the Diagnosis: Atypical Tamponade

In some patients, cardiac catheterization is requested or required for the purpose of establishing definitively whether or not cardiac tamponade is present. This indication for cardiac catheterization is becoming uncommon, because in most patients, the diagnosis of cardiac tamponade and an assessment of its severity are established based on clinical and echocardiographic findings. Cardiac catheterization carried out primarily to establish the diagnosis is therefore almost confined to atypical cases. For example, right ventricular diastolic collapse[1] and right atrial compression[2] may have been identified on an echocardiogram of a patient in whom the clinical features of cardiac tamponade are absent. Pulsus paradoxus is not found in cardiac tamponade when a large proportion of the filling of one or both ventricles is independent of the phase of respiration, as in aortic regurgitation[3] or atrial septal defect.[4] A more common cause of absent pulsus paradoxus in cardiac tamponade is preexisting heart disease in which the diastolic pressure of one of the ventricles is significantly higher than that of the other.[5] For example, in patients with severe left ventricular diastolic dysfunction, the left ventricular end-diastolic pressure may be elevated to a level higher than those of the right ventricle and intrapericardial space. A left ventricular diastolic pressure higher than that of the right ventricle and pericardium prevents the development of pulsus paradoxus in cardiac tamponade. Likewise, severe right ventricular diastolic dysfunction, for example, secondary to severe right ventricular hypertrophy, would result in a tamponade complex in which the pericardial pressure rises to equal the left ventricular diastolic pressure but remains lower than right ventricular diastolic pressure. Again, under these circumstances, pulsus paradoxus is not found. In some cases, notoriously those secondary to recent cardiac surgery, pericardial effusion is localized and perhaps complicated by the presence of clot.[6, 7] These patients frequently lack the classic clinical findings; furthermore, the echocardiographic findings may be atypical or absent.

In some patients a clinical diagnosis of cardiac tamponade appears straightforward, but echocardiographic findings such as right ventricular diastolic collapse are absent. This phenomenon may be observed in patients with severe right ventricular hypertrophy. The hypertrophied right ventricle is less susceptible to compression by an increase in intrapericardial pressure. Likewise, severe heart failure with increased jugular venous pressure may prevent the occurrence of right atrial compression.

Classically, in cardiac tamponade, the jugular venous pressure is elevated and has a characteristic waveform, but there are cases of so-called low-pressure cardiac tamponade,[8] mainly associated with severe hypovolemia. In a few cases, the jugular venous pressure simply cannot be evaluated at the bedside, necessitating direct measurement of central venous pressure.

In these patients with discrepancy between the echocardiographic and clinical findings or with other atypical features, cardiac catheterization may be requested to resolve the discrepancy, explain atypical features, and make a definitive decision regarding the presence or absence of cardiac tamponade and assess its severity if present.

Cardiac Catheterization in Patients with Clinically Established Cardiac Tamponade

Much more commonly, cardiac catheterization is requested in patients in whom the diagnosis of cardiac tamponade has already been firmly established. In many such patients, cardiac catheterization becomes less a diagnostic procedure and more an adjunct to pericardiocentesis.

The major objectives are to obtain accurate measurements of intracardiac pressure simultaneously with intrapericardial pressure, to measure the cardiac output, to assess left ventricular function if it has not been accomplished satisfactorily by the preceding noninvasive studies, and to assess the hemodynamic changes induced by pericardiocentesis.

Several categories of patients with or suspected of having cardiac tamponade may be brought to the laboratory for cardiac catheterization. These include patients who recently have sustained a catastrophic event such as rupture of the heart or aorta, or a penetrating wound of the heart. These patients are usually brought either from the emergency department or from a coronary or medical intensive care unit. Another group of patients is that with pericardial effusion secondary to medical diseases such as carcinoma of the breast or lung, lymphoma, acquired immunodeficiency syndrome (AIDS), viral or idiopathic pericarditis, collagen vascular disorders, and renal failure. Cardiac tamponade in these patients is usually less acute[9]; consequently, their noninvasive studies tend to be more comprehensive. Patients coming from the surgical intensive care unit, sometimes hours or days after cardiac surgery, often have atypical clinical and echocardiographic findings as mentioned earlier. In these instances, cardiac catheterization is sometimes indicated several days, and sometimes even weeks, after discharge from intensive care.[10]

These patients also often have atypical cardiac tamponade.

PROCEDURE

Diastolic equilibration of pressures is the hallmark of cardiac tamponade. Therefore, accurate measurement of pressures in the various right-sided and left-sided chambers is mandatory. Two pressure transducers—or if pericardiocentesis is to be carried out, three transducers—are calibrated simultaneously against a standard mercury manometer or electrically and are leveled to the same height, that is, that corresponding to the level of the right atrium. Strictly speaking, to measure the difference between pressures most accurately, each transducer should be leveled to the height of the corresponding catheter tip as determined fluoroscopically. However, in most laboratories, this refinement is omitted. The pressure tracings should be recorded simultaneously via identical catheters at high gain and fast paper speed along with systemic arterial pressure, the respiratory cycle, and the electrocardiogram.[11] Ideally, both right-sided and left-sided cardiac catheterization should be carried out to demonstrate accurately diastolic equalization of pressures. However, if pulmonary capillary wedge pressure is of good quality and if clinical, noninvasive, and hemodynamic features are consistent with cardiac tamponade, left-sided heart catheterization may be omitted. At times, pulmonary capillary wedge pressure is difficult to obtain or is elevated compared with right-sided diastolic pressures because of mitral regurgitation with a large V wave. In such patients, left-sided cardiac catheterization is useful. Left-sided heart catheterization should not be omitted in patients when associated left-sided cardiac or coronary artery disease is suspected or reasonably likely.

If pericardiocentesis is to be performed, heparin should not be administered until the pericardium has been safely cannulated. Before heparinization, the time during which the catheter is placed above the aortic arch should be kept as short as possible to avoid embolic complications.

With the availability of echocardiography, angiographic studies are rarely necessary in pericardial tamponade. The distance of the catheter positioned in the right atrium from the border of the cardiac silhouette on fluoroscopy provides a good estimate of the size of the pericardial effusion.[12] If angiography is performed, 50 to 75 mL of contrast material should be injected at 25 mL/sec through an 8-French NIH

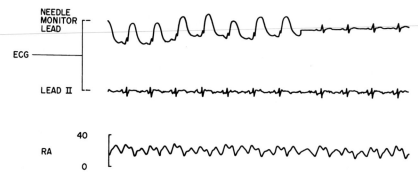

Figure 22–1. Monitoring the electrocardiogram (ECG) directly from a pericardiocentesis needle. *Upper tracing,* ECG is recorded from the needle; *middle tracing,* lead II; *lower tracing,* right atrial (RA) pressure (mm Hg). For the first eight complexes, the needle is in contact with the epicardium, during which time the tracing monitored from the needle shows a virtually monophasic ECG that returns to normal when the needle is withdrawn 1 to 2 mm. The ST segment shift in lead II is barely perceptible. RA pressure is elevated to 20 mm Hg.

or Eppendorfer catheter at the superior vena caval–right atrial junction. Images should be recorded at 30 frames/sec in a slight right anterior oblique projection.

Pericardiocentesis

Pericardiocentesis should be carried out or at least be closely supervised only by an experienced physician.[13–16] Unless the situation is so urgent that the necessary delay could prove fatal, an echocardiographic evaluation should be obtained before or during the pericardial tap. Guidance of the procedure by echocardiography may minimize the risk.[17] When the study shows that the pericardial effusion is small, especially when the pericardiocentesis is aimed more at making an etiologic diagnosis than relieving tamponade, the procedure can be abandoned in favor of a surgical approach.

The subxyphoid route is usually preferred because it reduces the risk of pneumothorax.[15–17] Rarely, when pericardial effusion is very large, the anteroposterior route can be chosen, where the pericardial space is entered via the third or fourth left intercostal space, about 1 cm laterally from the sternum, to avoid puncture of the internal mammary artery when too medial, or the pleura when too lateral. Puncture near the cardiac apex is an acceptable alteration.

The patient's chest should be propped up to an angle of about 45 degrees to redistribute the pericardial effusion anteriorly and inferiorly, making the pericardial puncture easier. The skin should be anesthetized 1 cm below the xyphoid process, slightly to the left. The tissue is incised, and a small tunnel is created using a mosquito clamp.

An 18-gauge trocar and cannula or an 18-gauge short-beveled needle connected to a syringe may be used. The needle is connected to the V_1 lead of an electrocardiograph through a sterile alligator clamp. The resulting electrocardiogram is recorded along with a standard limb lead throughout the procedure (Fig. 22–1), watching for the appearance of ventricular or, more rarely, atrial arrhythmias and of ST segment elevation when the needle touches the myocardium. The electrocardiograph must be properly grounded to avoid electric stimulation of the heart by a current leak, which can cause ventricular fibrillation. The needle is inserted in the subcutaneous tissue in an anteroposterior direction with a cephalad tilt, until it touches the inferior aspect of the rib cage. If pain occurs, 2% lidocaine should be administered slowly through the needle. The needle should then be slipped under the rib cage and directed more cephalad, with a posterior angulation of about 10 of 30 degrees. The needle is advanced gently under careful hemodynamic and electrocardiographic monitoring. Entry into the pericardial space may be suspected when less resistance is felt; sometimes it is accompanied by a distinct popping sensation. Aspiration should reveal pericardial fluid. If the aspirate is bloody, immediate steps should be taken to ascertain whether the needle tip is free in the pericardial space or has penetrated the heart. Aspiration that is difficult or intermittent in nature may be the first clue to improper placement. Next, the nature of the fluid must be ascertained, bearing in mind that the composition of the fluid depends on the etiology. Thus, pericardial effusion may be blood stained or even look like blood but has a lower hematocrit than peripheral blood. Its dilute nature can be rapidly recognized by placing a few milliliters on a sponge. The resulting appearance is quite different from a pure blood stain. If this simple maneuver does not answer the question with certainty, hematocrit results can be compared between the aspirate and blood from a catheter. Pericardial fluid contains lytic agents and therefore does not clot. On the other hand, fresh hemorrhage into the pericardium most certainly does clot. The other way to determine where the needle tip is immediately after puncture is to record the pressure. A ventricular pressure speaks for itself, but a venous-appearing tracing could come from either the pericardial cavity or an atrium, usually the right. A small volume of contrast material injected under fluoroscopy will immediately settle the issue. When injected into the atrium, the contrast material will be seen to "puff away" in the circulation. If it is the pericardium that has been injected, the contrast material soon pools in the most dependent portion of the pericardium. When aspiration is difficult, a tiny amount of contrast material can be injected to search for myocardial staining.

Once it has been established for certain that the needle tip is free in the pericardial space, a soft-tipped guide wire should be introduced under fluoroscopic guidance. A 6- to 7-French dilator is advanced carefully over the wire before a 6- to 7-French high-flow pigtail catheter with multiple side holes is placed in the pericardium.[18, 19] Before any fluid is withdrawn for analysis, the catheter is connected to a pressure transducer for simultaneous measurement of right atrial, pulmonary wedge, and intrapericardial pressures. If the catheter does not pass easily, the passage should be further dilated using large-bore introducers. Pericardial fluid is aspirated by syringe, usually one with a 50-mL capacity. The first samples should be put into containers suitable for cytologic and chemical assay because later samples may become more bloody. Samples for culture can be taken at any time. Periodically, the pressures should be remeasured to monitor the hemodynamic effects of removing intrapericardial fluid. Air or, preferably, carbon dioxide can be injected to image the pericardium (Fig. 22–2); however, because pericardiocentesis has usually been preceded by noninvasive imaging, this step is often unnecessary. Pericardial drainage can be continued through a tubing attached to a closed-suction system. For this purpose the catheter may be left in place for a few days, although care must be taken to avoid superinfection. Rinsing may be required if the fluid is thick but should not be performed unless necessary.

Hemodynamic Findings

The hemodynamic findings on which a diagnosis of cardiac tamponade can reliably be made depend on two principal factors: the severity of the cardiac tamponade and the presence or absence of preexisting underlying cardiac disease. It has been shown that even a small pericardial effusion with minimal increase in intrapericardial pressure exerts detectable hemodynamic effects, principally by increasing respiratory variation in arterial blood pressure and ventricular function.[20] However, from the point of view of the clinician performing cardiac catheterization to evaluate cardiac tamponade, it is more appropriate to consider that cardiac tamponade begins when intrapericardial pressure has increased to equal right atrial pressure. The hemodynamics of cardiac tamponade can best be appreciated by considering the total volume of the intrapericardial contents, that is, the volume of pericardial fluid plus the volume of the cardiac chambers and those portions of the great vessels contained in the pericardial sac. When intrapericardial pressure increases as a result of effusion or bleeding, the venous pressure rises, thereby maintaining intracardiac volume. In early cardiac tamponade without preexisting heart disease, the intrapericardial and right atrial pressures are equal but only slightly elevated. Hemodynamic compromise is absent; furthermore, pulmonary wedge or left atrial pressure remains higher than right atrial and intrapericardial pressures. This constellation of finding constitutes a very early stage of cardiac tamponade and therefore is seldom encountered in the cardiac catheterization laboratory. Indeed, cardiac tamponade of this small magnitude seldom, if ever, justifies cardiac catheterization and certainly pericardiocentesis.

When cardiac tamponade becomes more severe, the right atrial and intrapericardial pressures remain equal and rise progressively according to the severity of the cardiac tamponade. The point at which these pressures come to equal the left atrial and pulmonary wedge pressures defines classic cardiac tamponade as understood clinically and hemodynamically.[5, 21]

Scrupulous technique is an invaluable aide to establishing the correct diagnosis of cardiac tamponade. Right atrial and pulmonary wedge pressures should be recorded simultaneously rather than sequentially for adequate recognition that two pressures are indeed equal.[11] There must be no error in the calibration of

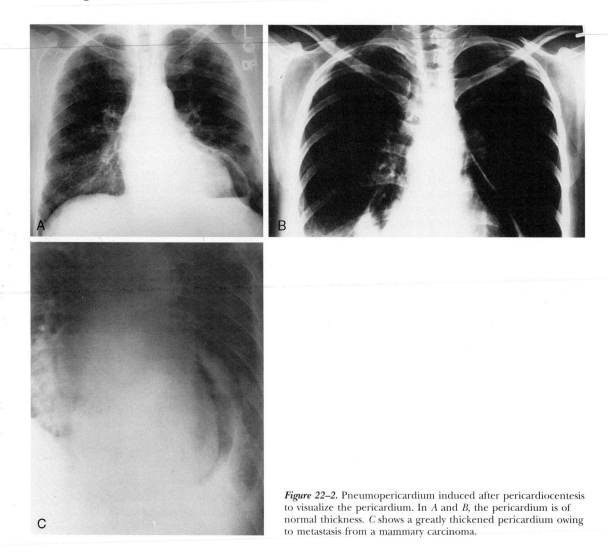

Figure 22-2. Pneumopericardium induced after pericardiocentesis to visualize the pericardium. In *A* and *B*, the pericardium is of normal thickness. *C* shows a greatly thickened pericardium owing to metastasis from a mammary carcinoma.

leveling of the two transducers. Where an unsuspected difference between right atrial and pulmonary wedge pressures is found, it is advisable to reverse the connections between the two transducers and the catheters to rule out the possibility of a technical artifact. Equilibration of venous pressures on the two sides of the heart is much closer in cardiac tamponade than in constrictive pericarditis, because in cardiac tamponade, respiratory variation of right atrial pressure is preserved and therefore pulmonary wedge and right atrial pressures track each other well throughout the respiratory cycle (Fig. 22–3A). In constrictive pericarditis, however, respiratory variation of right atrial pressure is significantly diminished, whereas pulmonary wedge pressure declines normally during inspiration. Therefore, in constrictive pericarditis as opposed to cardiac tamponade, tracking between the two pressures is inconsistent throughout the respiratory cycle (Fig. 22–3B).

The height to which the venous pressures is elevated depends on the severity of cardiac tamponade. In milder cases, these pressures range from about 7 to 10 mm Hg. In moderate cases, the pressures are 10 to 15 mm Hg and are often accompanied by reduction in cardiac output and arterial blood pressure. Severe cardiac tamponade is characterized by pressures in the range of 15 to 30 mm Hg usually accompanied by profound decrease in cardiac output and arterial blood pressure, which at that stage demonstrates pulsus paradoxus.

In establishing the diagnosis of cardiac tamponade in the cardiac catheterization laboratory, special attention must be paid to the waveform of right atrial, and to a lesser extent, pulmonary wedge pressures. Of paramount importance, inspiratory decrease in right atrial pressure should be observed (Fig. 22–4). If right atrial pressure fails to decrease during inspiration, the physician should suspect complicating

CARDIAC TAMPONADE

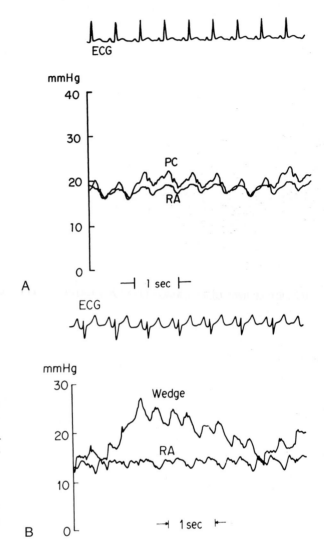

Figure 22–3. *A*, Pulmonary capillary (PC) wedge and right atrial (RA) pressures simultaneously recorded in a patient with moderate to severe cardiac tamponade. Note the tight tracking of the two pressures throughout the respiratory cycle, with only mild deviation during expiration. *B*, Pulmonary wedge and RA pressures recorded from a patient with moderately severe constrictive pericarditis. Because of marked respiratory variation in the pulmonary wedge pressure but absence of such variation in RA pressure, the two pressures equilibrate only during the inspiratory phase of respiration. (From Shabetai R: The Pericardium. New York, Grune & Stratton, 1981.)

constrictive pericarditis, that is, effusive-constrictive pericarditis or underlying heart disease. Cardiac tamponade exerts its abnormal pressure on heart chambers throughout the cardiac cycle. However, ventricular ejection is faster than venous return, causing cardiac volume to decrease. With this event, there is a slight decline in intrapericardial pressure because of the decrease in total intrapericardial content. For this reason, venous return is confined to the period of ventricular systole that translates to prominence of the *x* descent and absence of the *y* descent of venous pressure (Fig. 22–5).[22] Thus, in typical cardiac tamponade, right atrial pressure is elevated equal to pulmonary wedge pressure and shows an inspiratory drop and absence of the *y* descent.

It is necessary to distinguish between cardiac filling, that is, venous return, and ventricular filling. Blood is transferred from the atria to the ventricles; consequently, cardiac volume is constant except during rapid ejection. The atria fill the ventricles slowly throughout diastole and therefore the ventricular diastolic pressure fails to show the dip-and-plateau phenomenon characteristic of constrictive pericarditis (Fig. 22–6) and restrictive cardiomyopathy. Rather, ventricular diastole in cardiac tamponade is characterized by elevation of the diastolic pressure that slopes in a linear fashion from early diastole to the onset of systole (Fig. 22–7). In typical cardiac tamponade, in the absence of underlying heart disease, the diastolic pressures of the ventricles are exactly equal to one another. If, as

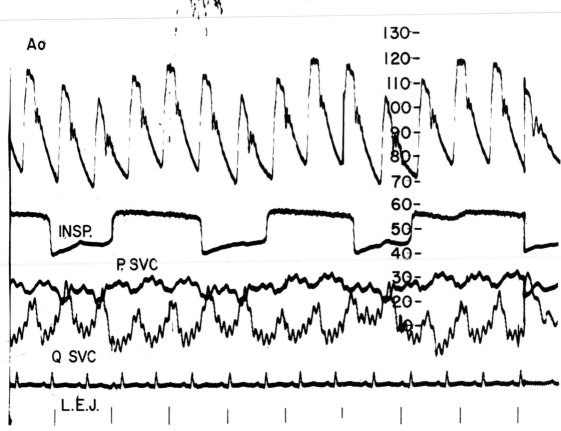

Ao

INSP.

P. SVC

Q SVC

L.E.J.

Figure 22–4. Simultaneous recordings of aortic pressure (Ao), the respiratory cycle (INSP, inspiration), superior vena caval pressure (P SVC), and flow (Q SVC) measured by an electromagnetic velocity probe catheter in a patient with severe cardiac tamponade. During inspiration, systemic venous return is increased and Ao is decreased (pulsus paradoxus). Note that P SVC decreases during inspiration. (From Shabetai R: The Pericardium. New York, Grune & Stratton, 1981.)

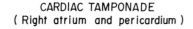

CARDIAC TAMPONADE
(Right atrium and pericardium)

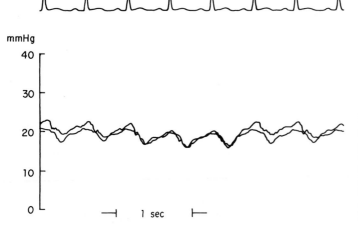

ECG

mmHg

40

30

20

10

0

1 sec

Figure 22–5. Simultaneously recorded right atrial and intrapericardial pressures in the same patient illustrated in Figure 22–3A. Note the extremely tight coupling between the two pressures, the prominence of the *x* descent with absence of the *y* descent, and the presence of normal respiratory variation. (From Shabetai R: The Pericardium. New York, Grune & Stratton, 1981.)

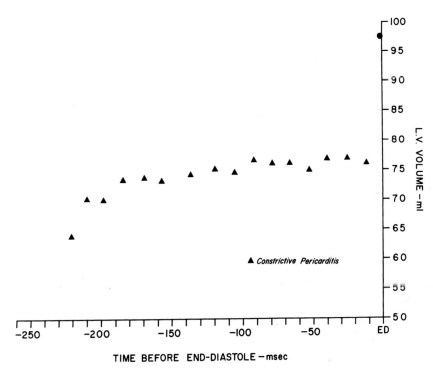

Figure 22–6. Left ventricular (LV) volume changes during diastole in a patient with severe constrictive pericarditis. Note that all ventricular filling occurs in early diastole. The LV end-diastolic volume is significantly reduced.

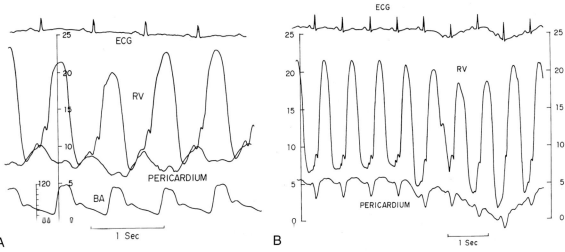

Figure 22–7. Mild cardiac tamponade. *A,* Right ventricular (RV) diastolic pressure is moderately elevated. There is no dip-and-plateau configuration of ventricular diastolic pressure. Pericardial and RV diastolic pressures are equal, indicating the presence of tamponade. Blood pressure is normal, and pulsus paradoxes are absent. BA, brachial artery. *B,* The same patient after pericardiocentesis. No significant change has occurred in arterial blood pressure or RV systolic pressure. However, pericardial pressure is now lower than RV diastolic pressure throughout the respiratory and cardiac cycles, indicating that mild cardiac tamponade has been abolished by the procedure. (From Shabetai R: The Pericardium. New York, Grune & Stratton, 1981.)

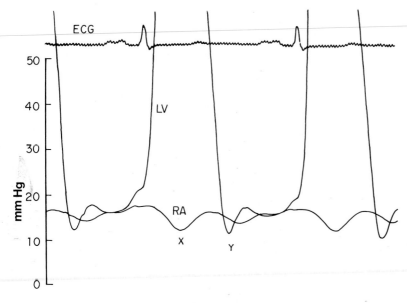

Figure 22–8. Right atrial (RA) and high-gain left ventricular (LV) pressures recorded during the study of a patient with moderately severe cardiac tamponade. This combination of pressures is helpful when it is difficult to obtain a good-quality record of RV pressure. The y descent is attenuated, and the ventricular pressure is underdamped.

sometimes occurs, artifact is present in the right ventricular pressure tracing, this equalization of diastolic pressures on two sides of the heart can be established by a simultaneous recording of left ventricular and right atrial pressures (Fig. 22–8).

Systemic arterial pressure remains normal in magnitude and waveform characteristics when cardiac tamponade is mild. When cardiac tamponade becomes more severe, pulsus paradoxus appears apparent. *Pulsus paradoxus* is defined as an abnormally large inspiratory decrease in systemic arterial systolic pressure and pulse pressure. During inspiration, systemic arterial systolic pressure falls to an abnormal degree with little change in diastolic pressure (Fig. 22–9). The decreased pulse pressure represents diminished systemic stroke volume during inspiration. We lack a truly satisfactory quantitative definition of pulsus paradoxus. The literature commonly states that the normal inspiratory decrease in systemic arterial pressure ought not to exceed 10 mm Hg.[23] However, in patients with respiratory distress, respiratory variation exceeding this magnitude is often documented in the cardiac catheterization laboratory. Furthermore, it has been suggested that pulsus paradoxus should be defined not by an absolute number but rather as a percentage of systolic pressure. A decrease exceeding 10% of peak systolic pressure from expiration to inspiration has been suggested as an alternative definition. In many severe cases, pulsus paradoxus is pronounced and may range from 20 to 40 mm Hg, obviating the need for a precise quantitative definition. With mild or moderate cardiac tam-

ponade, systemic arterial blood pressure is maintained reasonably close to normal, but hypotension develops when cardiac tamponade becomes more severe. In some instances, although not commonly, the excessive excretion of catecholamines in response to cardiac tamponade generates hypertension rather than the expected hypotension.[24]

In mild cardiac tamponade the cardiac output remains normal.[25] With increasing severity of cardiac tamponade, cardiac output progressively diminishes in response to decreased venous return and severe compression of ventricular end-diastolic volume. Decreased systolic function of the ventricles is an end-stage phenomenon in cardiac tamponade. Diminished stroke volume is a consequence solely of diminished left ventricular end-diastolic volume. End-systolic volume is also reduced with, if anything, hypercontractility of the ventricles. Tachycardia and increased ventricular contractility serve partially to compensate for the reduction in end-diastolic volume and stroke volume.

The Influence of Preexisting Heart Disease

The hemodynamics described in the previous paragraphs apply to patients with no underlying heart disease and are particularly characteristic of traumatic cardiac tamponade and tamponade resulting from rupture of the aorta. This clinical picture is also characteristic of young patients with cardiac tamponade secondary to idiopathic or viral pericarditis.

In a number of patients, however, cardiac

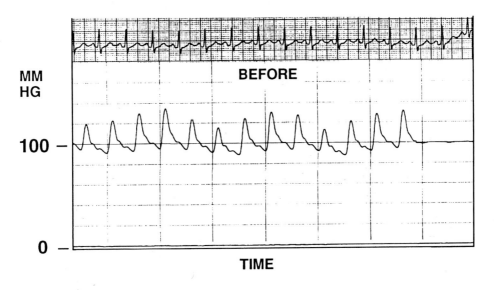

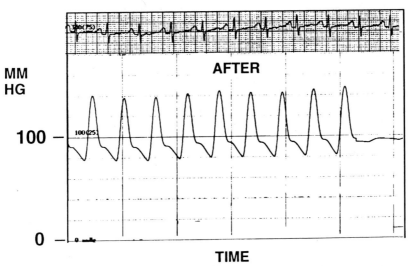

Figure 22–9. Aortic pressure tracing in a patient with cardiac tamponade before *(upper)* and after *(lower)* pericardiocentesis. Note the presence of pulsus paradoxus, which disappears after pericardiocentesis.

tamponade develops against a background of preexisting heart disease and, under this circumstance, the hemodynamic findings are significantly modified. The most common cardiac factor modifying the hemodynamics of cardiac tamponade is left ventricular dysfunction with elevation of left ventricular diastolic pressures. Take, for example, an elderly patient with hypertensive or ischemic heart disease who has developed cardiac tamponade secondary to a malignant pericardial effusion. In such a patient, the pericardial and right atrial pressures may be elevated, for example, to 10 mm Hg,

but because of heart disease, the left ventricular diastolic pressure may be 25 mm Hg. This preexisting left ventricular diastolic hypertension must mean that in spite of cardiac tamponade defined by equalization of right atrial and pericardial pressures, equalization of right atrial and pulmonary wedge pressures does not occur. Were the right atrial and intrapericardial pressures to increase further to 20 mm Hg, cardiac tamponade would be severe and yet equalization of left and right atrial pressures would still be absent. Classic cardiac tamponade would not be present until right atrial and pericardial pressures had climbed to 25 mm Hg. In addition, the clinician should not anticipate pulsus paradoxus in the presence of preexisting elevation of left ventricular diastolic pressure. In classic uncomplicated cardiac tamponade, the principal mechanism responsible for pulsus paradoxus is the fixed intrapericardial volume contained within a pericardium that cannot stretch in response to the inspiratory increase in systemic venous return. The common diastolic pressure shared by both ventricles causes their effective diastolic compliance to be exactly equal. Increased diastolic volume of the right-sided heart chambers therefore decreases the diastolic volumes of the left-sided chambers so that pulsus paradoxus becomes apparent. When cardiac tamponade supervenes in the presence of preexisting elevation of left ventricular diastolic pressure, pulsus paradoxus and equalization of right and left venous pressures remain absent until such time as the intrapericardial pressure has risen to the level of the elevated left ventricular diastolic pressure.

The obvious way out of the dilemma that may be caused by preexisting left ventricular disease is to measure right atrial and pericardial pressures simultaneously. Cardiac tamponade is characterized by a remarkably precise equilibration between right atrial and intrapericardial pressures (see Fig. 22–3).

A less common, perhaps more difficult, cardiac cause of atypical cardiac tamponade is preexisting right-sided heart disease. In patients with right-sided heart disease, for example, secondary to chronic lung disease, right ventricular diastolic pressure may be elevated above the level of the pulmonary wedge pressure. In instances of this sort, intrapericardial pressure becomes equal to pulmonary wedge pressure before it has risen to the level of right atrial pressure. Therefore, cardiac tamponade may be present in the absence of equilibration of left and right atrial pressures or pulsus paradoxus. Here, the hemodynamic diagnosis is made by simultaneous measurement of pulmonary wedge and intrapericardial pressures.

Low-pressure Cardiac Tamponade

Uncommonly, severe hemodynamic compromise secondary to cardiac tamponade may develop in the absence of the expected great elevation of systemic venous pressure (Fig. 22–10).[8] The most common cause for this phenomenon is severe hypovolemia. The hypovolemia in traumatic cases is often due to significant hemorrhage elsewhere in the body. In other cases, hypovolemia may be the result of ill-judged forceful diuretic treatment, usually administered in the belief that the patient has cardiac rather than pericardial disease.

The Influence of Valvular Disease of the Heart

From the earlier discussion, it comes as no surprise that preexisting valvular disease modifies the hemodynamics of cardiac tamponade. Severe aortic valve disease is apt to reduce ventricular diastolic compliance and increase diastolic pressure of the left ventricle; therefore, equalization of left-sided and right-sided heart filling pressures and pulsus paradoxus is often absent in such patients. Another situation when pulsus

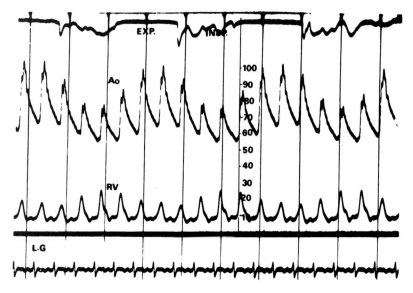

Figure 22–10. Marked pulsus paradoxus in a patient with low-pressure cardiac tamponade. Note the following features: right ventricular (RV) diastolic pressure of 10 mm Hg, absence of dip and plateau, minimum RV pressure not corresponding with maximal aortic (Ao) pressure, and inspiratory decrease in pulse pressure and hypotension. EXP, expiration; INSP, inspiration. (From Shabetai R, Fowler NO, Fenton JC, Masangkay M: Pulsus paradoxus. Reproduced from The Journal of Clinical Investigation, 1965; 44:1882–1898 by copyright permission of The American Society for Clinical Investigation.)

paradoxus may be absent in severe cardiac tamponade is when filling of a cardiac ventricle occurs independently of the respiratory cycle, such as in patients with atrial septal defect.[4] By a variety of mechanisms, mitral valve disease may also modify the hemodynamics. This is the reason why it is advisable to obtain good simultaneous measurements of pulmonary wedge and left ventricular pressures during the evaluation of cardiac tamponade. In many instances, a thorough evaluation of ventricular function and structural or functional abnormalities of the cardiac valves will have been obtained noninvasively before the patient is subjected to cardiac catheterization, but it is a relatively simple task to reassess valvular function hemodynamically after pericardiocentesis has been completed.

Tricuspid valve disease, almost always tricuspid regurgitation, is another factor that may obfuscate the diagnosis of cardiac tamponade. In this instance, instead of a right atrial pressure pulse characteristic of cardiac tamponade, a giant systolic wave may be recorded. We have encountered a patient with cardiac tamponade secondary to an automobile accident. The patient was admitted directly from the emergency department to the cardiac catheterization laboratory with a diagnosis of traumatic cardiac tamponade. The pericardial pressure was greatly elevated and promptly returned to normal after pericardiocentesis. However, right atrial pressure failed to decline and was characterized by a large abnormal systolic wave. A right ventriculogram was then performed showing that the trauma had resulted not only in cardiac tamponade but also in rupture of the tricuspid valve apparatus. The patient therefore went from the cardiac catheterization laboratory to the operating room for repair of the tricuspid valve. This case illustrates the need for full cardiac evaluation in any situation when there is a reasonable likelihood of underlying cardiac disease.

Cardiac Tamponade as a Complication of Cardiac Surgery

The cardiologist is seldom asked to perform cardiac catheterization to rule in or out the diagnosis of cardiac tamponade in the patient who has recently undergone cardiac surgery. Cardiac tamponade in these patients may be delayed and frequently is atypical because of loculation or complicating clot in the pericardial effusion. Most often, the diagnosis is established by the combination of clinical and echocardiographic evaluations; often, when the condition is suspected, the surgeon will explore the chest without asking for prior cardiac catheterization. In the few cases that do come to cardiac catheterization, careful integration of the hemodynamic and noninvasive findings is essential because of the potential modification of the classic findings related to factors such as a poorly functioning prosthetic or repaired valve and ventricular dysfunction.

Cardiac Tamponade as a Complication of Cardiac Catheterization

Acute cardiac tamponade can complicate any intracardiac procedure. Occasionally, the coronary sinus is ruptured when an operator mistakenly believes that the catheter is being advanced through the right ventricle to the pulmonary artery. Cardiac tamponade may result when endomyocardial biopsy is directed to the free wall of the right ventricle instead of the interventricular septum. Cardiac tamponade may also occur if the aorta is inadvertently punctured during transseptal cardiac catheterization of the left ventricle or if the operator mistakes the atrial appendage for the mitral orifice and attempts to advance the transseptal catheter into the left ventricle. Pacemaker insertion may also be associated with cardiac tamponade.

The patient usually complains of pain, often pleuritic in nature. Blood pressure and the clinical status deteriorate. Pulsus paradoxus develops early. A critically important finding is disappearance of cardiac pulsations as observed under the fluoroscope. Prompt pericardiocentesis is essential and, if not immediately successful, should be followed by substernal pericardiostomy.

Evaluating the Hemodynamic Results of Pericardiocentesis

During pericardiocentesis, intrapericardial, right and left atrial and left ventricular diastolic pressures decline progressively. During this time, hypotension is gradually corrected, pulsus paradoxus diminishes and finally disappears, and cardiac output increases. During the progressive decline in intrapericardial pressure, right atrial and intrapericardial pressures fall below the pulmonary wedge or left ventricular diastolic pressure but remain equal to each other. Thereafter, further aspiration of pericardial fluid causes the intrapericardial pressure to fall below right atrial pressure throughout the respiratory and cardiac cycles. From this point onward, further aspiration of pericardial fluid does not result in any measurable hemodynamic improvement (Fig. 22–11).

In uncomplicated cardiac tamponade, once pericardial pressure has been reduced to zero or to its subatmospheric level, right atrial and pulmonary wedge pressures should be normal, the pulmonary wedge pressure should be higher than right atrial pressure, and the right atrial pressure waveform should be normal. When the pulmonary wedge or left ventricular diastolic pressure remains elevated after pericardiocentesis, the operator should consider preexisting heart muscle disease or valvular disease.

When right atrial pressure fails to normalize, effusive-constrictive disease of the pericardium must be considered. This entity is described in the section dealing with constrictive pericarditis.

Angiocardiography

Adequate echocardiographic evaluation preceding cardiac catheterization usually obviates the

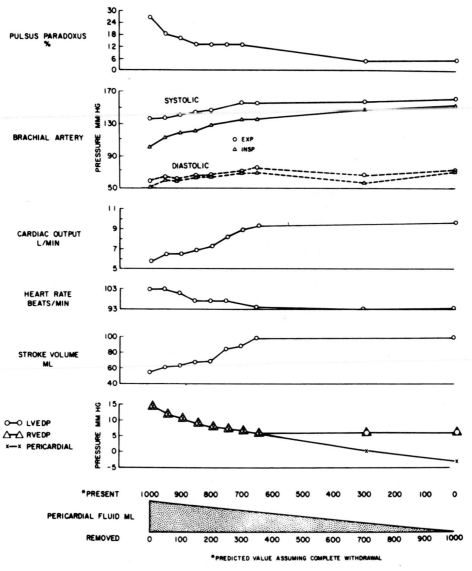

A

Figure 22–11. Hemodynamic effects of pericardiocentesis for cardiac tamponade. *A,* Theoretical construct. The bottom shaded area represents pericardiocentesis of a 1-L pericardial effusion. With pericardiocentesis, cardiac tamponade becomes progressively less severe as right (RVEDP) and left ventricular (LVEDP) diastolic and pericardial pressures decline from 15 to 5 mm Hg. Thereafter, the ventricular diastolic pressures stabilize, but pericardial pressure drops to a subatmospheric value. During the time that cardiac tamponade is becoming less severe, stroke volume increases, heart rate declines, cardiac output and blood pressure increase, and pulsus paradoxus decreases. Aspiration of pericardial fluid after pericardial pressure separates from ventricular diastolic pressure, no further hemodynamic benefit can be documented.
(*A* from Reddy PS, Curtiss EI, O'Toole JD, Shaver JA: Cardiac tamponade: Hemodynamic observations in man. Circulation 1978; 58:265–272.)

need for angiocardiographic studies. However, in acute cases in which it has not been possible to obtain an echocardiogram of good quality and when the hemodynamic findings following pericardiocentesis suggest underlying heart disease, opaque contrast medium injection is justified. An example of the necessity for a right ventriculogram in a patient with combined cardiac tamponade and tricuspid valve avulsion has already been cited. Certainly, elevation of left ventricular diastolic pressure after pericardiocentesis unexplained by prior echocardiography may necessitate the need for a left ventriculogram. In selected patients, coronary arteriography may also need to be carried out after pericardiocentesis.

Before the era of high-quality echocardiography, it was common practice to inject contrast medium at the superior vena caval–right atrial junction. This injection visualized the small hy-peractive ventricles contracting within a large cardiac silhouette. These studies also demonstrated the slow continuous filling at the ventricles during diastole. Currently, there is seldom justification for carrying out this injection just to evaluate cardiac tamponade.

Percutaneous Balloon Pericardiotomy

Percutaneous balloon pericardiotomy is advocated in appropriate patients in place of the surgical creation of a pericardial window. Most patients treated have had malignant pericardial effusion, although lesser numbers with AIDS or idiopathic pericarditis and pericardial effusion of other causes have been treated in this manner. In the first series to be reported,[26] balloon pericardiotomy was done as a secondary procedure for patients with a malignant pericardial effusion treated by pericardiocentesis and place-

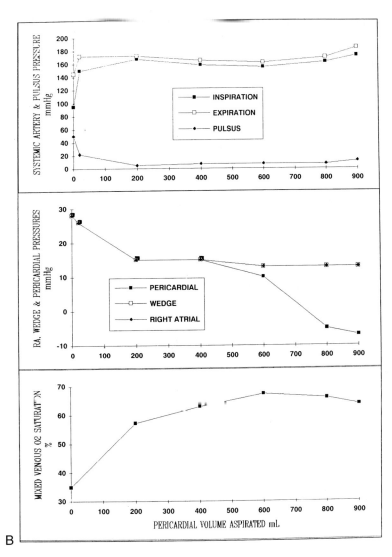

Figure 22–11 Continued B, Hemodynamic data from a patient with severe cardiac tamponade. Before pericardiocentesis, pericardial, right atrial, and pulmonary wedge pressures are 28 mm Hg *(middle)* and pulsus paradoxus is 50 mm Hg. The patient demonstrates systolic hypertension in spite of severe cardiac tamponade. With pericardiocentesis, right atrial, pulmonary wedge, and pericardial pressures drop to 14 mm Hg. Thereafter, pericardial pressure progressively falls to a substantially subatmospheric pressure, whereas the right atrial and pulmonary wedge pressures remain elevated because of a component of constrictive pericarditis. The bottom panel illustrates an increase in the mixed venous oxygen saturation, indicating increased cardiac output that plateaus near the point at which pericardial pressure separates from the atrial pressures.

Illustration continued on following page **B**

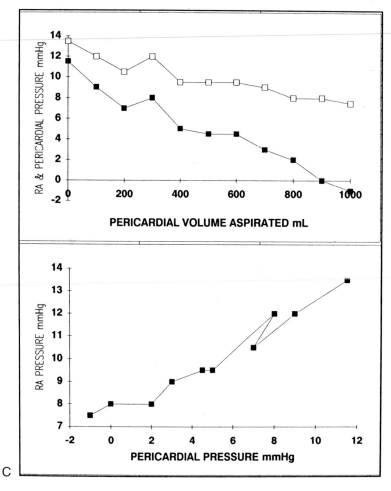

Figure 22–11 Continued C, Hemodynamic changes following aspiration of a very large pericardial effusion causing mild cardiac tamponade. The upper panel illustrates the progressive fall of right atrial and pericardial pressures, and the bottom panel further illustrates the interdependence of right atrial and pericardial pressures.

ment of a catheter for subsequent pericardial drainage. The patients selected were those in whom pericardial drainage through the indwelling catheter exceeded 100 mL per day. Not surprisingly, this attractive technique is now performed in many cardiac catheterization laboratories. With further experience recorded in a multicenter registry,[27] percutaneous balloon pericardiotomy is now often performed at the time of the initial pericardiocentesis. However, when pericardiocentesis is performed in an emergency setting, it is preferable to leave in a catheter for pericardial drainage and perform percutaneous balloon pericardiotomy, if indicated later, in a controlled environment. Most candidates will have malignant pericardial effusion, and the procedure is usually indicated either because of cardiac tamponade or because of the large size of the pericardial effusion.

Technique

A 0.034- to 0.038-inch stiff J-tipped guide wire is advanced into the pericardial space following standard subxyphoid pericardial puncture. As in standard pericardiocentesis, the guide wire should loop in the pericardial space—this maneuver protects from inadvertent passage of the guide wire into the myocardium or through the right-sided heart chambers to the pulmonary artery. With the guide wire satisfactorily positioned, the tract through the skin of subcutaneous tissue is progressively dilated with at least an 8-French dilator. An 8-French pigtail or straight catheter with side holes is then advanced into the pericardial space. Pericardial pressure is then measured and fluid is withdrawn for appropriate studies. Because a second pericardial puncture may be needed, 200 to 300 mL of fluid should be left in the pericardial space. About 20 mL of 50% radiographic contrast material is injected into the pericardial space. A 0.038-inch extra-stiff J-tipped guide wire is then advanced into the pericardial space. The catheter is then removed. Different authors have recommended different balloons, but in the registry study,[27] a 20-mm wide, 3-cm long dilating balloon (Mansfield) containing 30% radiographic contrast medium was used. The balloon catheter is advanced to straddle the pericardial border and is then gently inflated to locate the margin of the pericardium. If the proximal portion of balloon fails to dilate, it can be assumed that the pericardium is apposed to the chest wall. Under those circumstances, the catheter is gently advanced while the skin is pulled in the opposite direction; thereafter, the balloon is manually inflated to create the window.

After dilation, the balloon is removed and the pericardial catheter is put back. To verify successful creation of a window, contrast medium is injected through the catheter while it is slowly withdrawn until the side holes are just within the pericardial space. At that time, 10 to 15 mL of dilute contrast material can be injected rapidly to document flow through the window to the pleural space or into the peritoneal cavity. However, the procedure can be successful even when this free flow cannot be documented in the laboratory.

Of course the Mansfield catheter is not the only device suitable for percutaneous balloon pericardiostomy. Some investigators[28] prefer the Inoue self-positioning catheter. Here, the distal portion of the balloon catheter can be inflated first and the catheter can then be pulled back gently until resistance is felt as the distal balloon anchors itself at the parietal pericardium. The balloon catheter can then be rapidly inflated manually to its full extent. Whether or not this more expensive device is really necessary for balloon pericardiostomy is debatable, but in any event, the particular device used and the details of the technique vary among laboratories and interventional cardiologists.

Pericardioscopy

The poor yield of exfoliative cytology for the definitive diagnosis of malignant pericardial effusion, combined with the desire to avoid open surgery, was the stimulus to develop a pericardioscopic technique[29–31] so that the pericardium and epicardium can be directly inspected and lesions targeted for biopsy. Both rigid and flexible instruments have been used. The instrument is advanced into the pericardial space through a sheath, that is, 0.5 cm shorter than the pericardioscope. The procedure is preceded by evacuation of the pericardial fluid followed by the extensive rinsing of the pericardial space with normal saline to make the sac clear and thus permit adequate pericardioscopy. Biopsy specimens are taken from areas identified as abnormal at the preceding pericardioscopy. Pericardioscopy is still an investigational technique,

and as of this writing has not found wide application in standard cardiac catheterization laboratories.

CONSTRICTIVE PERICARDITIS

Constrictive pericarditis and cardiac tamponade have in common a number of important hemodynamic characteristics, but each has its distinctive hemodynamics; therefore, the two conditions ought not to be confused with each other in the cardiac catheterization laboratory. Common to both conditions is restriction to diastolic filling with consequent elevation of systemic and pulmonary venous pressures but preservation in most patients of normal systolic ventricular function.[32] Except in atypical cases both constrictive pericarditis and cardiac tamponade involve all four cardiac chambers with resulting equalization of their diastolic pressures. In both, when compression is severe, ventricular end-diastolic volume and stroke volume are reduced and reduced stroked volume may be partially compensated by tachycardia.

In spite of the overall similarity of these two compressive disorders of the heart, important hemodynamic differences distinguish them. Common to both conditions is elevation of jugular venous pressure. However, in constrictive pericarditis, respiratory variation of the jugular venous pressure is greatly attenuated with inspiration. The y descent becomes deeper, steeper, and more prominent, but there is usually no perceptible change in mean jugular venous or right atrial pressure during quiet breathing (Fig. 22–12). This characteristic is the opposite of preservation of the normal and respiratory decline in right atrial pressure seen in cardiac tamponade, however severe (see Figs. 22–3A and 22–4). In constrictive pericarditis, respiratory variation of the pulmonary wedge pressure is not diminished; therefore, although equilibration of right atrial and pulmonary wedge pressures is a diagnostic criterion for constrictive pericarditis, the equilibration cannot be expected to be tight throughout the respiratory cycle as it is in cardiac tamponade (Fig. 22–13). Another important difference between constrictive pericarditis and cardiac tamponade is the morphology of the jugular venous and right atrial pulse. In the description of the venous pressure pulse in cardiac tamponade, we explained why the y descent is attenuated or abolished. In constrictive pericarditis, however, there is little or no impediment to cardiac filling at end-systole, therefore both the x descent associated with ventricular ejection and the y de-

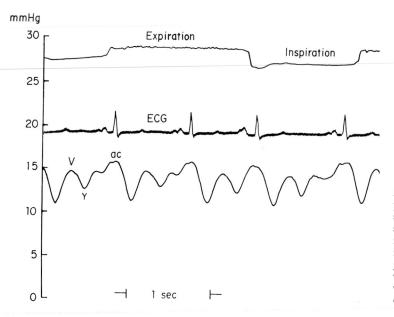

Figure 22–12. Right atrial pressure in a patient with moderately severe constrictive pericarditis. In this case, as sometimes occurs, the *x* descent is more prominent than the *y*. However, in contradistinction to tamponade, the *y* descent is well preserved. Respiratory variation of right atrial pressure is severely attenuated. V, V wave; ac, a and c waves.

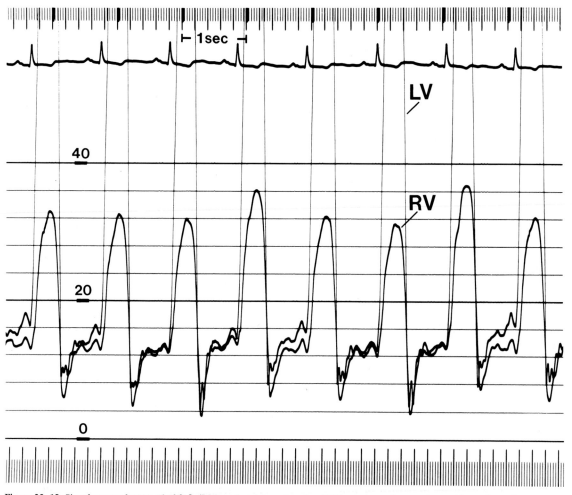

Figure 22–13. Simultaneously recorded left (LV) and right ventricular (RV) pressures in a patient with moderately severe constrictive pericarditis. Note the dip-and-plateau configuration of the diastolic pressure of both ventricles. The plateaus equilibrate, but the degree of equilibration varies somewhat with the respiratory cycle. Systolic pulmonary hypertension is not severe, a characteristic of constrictive pericarditis.

scent associated with early rapid filling of the ventricle are present (see Figs. 22–12 and 22–13). Indeed, these two descents, especially the *y* descent, are apt to be considerably more prominent than their normal counterparts. The ventricles in constrictive pericarditis tend to be small and therefore have exaggerated recoil in early diastole. Frame-by-frame analysis of left ventriculogram in patients with constrictive pericarditis has shown that filling of the left ventricle during the first third of diastole is considerably more rapid than normal.[33] The ventricles abruptly cease to fill at the end of the early rapid filling period, after which further diastolic expansion of cardiac volume is prevented by the constricting pericardium. From this point on, further filling of the ventricle is greatly attenuated or completely absent. This abnormality of the filling pattern of the left ventricle is reflected in its diastolic pressure pulse. Early diastole is characterized by a deep rapidly inscribed drop in pressure which then rapidly rises to an abnormally high value, where it remains for the remainder of diastole. This configuration of the diastolic pressure of the ventricles has been labeled the dip-and-plateau phenomenon, or alternatively, the square root sign, first described in 1951. The authors speculated that the early diastolic dip represented extremely fast early ventricular filling and that the plateau of pressure represented prolonged diastasis. This speculation was duly confirmed

following the advent of quantitative analysis of cine left ventriculograms.

The same degree of care regarding the hydrostatic leveling and calibration of the transducers required for evaluation of cardiac tamponade is also a necessity for the hemodynamic evaluation of constrictive pericarditis. When left and right ventricular diastolic pressures are recorded simultaneously, the plateaus of pressure from mid-diastolic to end-diastolic are equal in the two ventricles (see Fig. 22–13).[11] Also, during this portion of the cardiac cycle the atrial pressures also plateau at a level close to that of the ventricular diastolic pressure plateaus (Fig. 22–14).

Two exceptions must be emphasized: in some patients with constrictive pericarditis, the typical dip-and-plateau pattern is not present; in addition, a dip-and-plateau configuration may be seen in patients without constrictive pericarditis or restrictive cardiomyopathy. In patients with considerable tachycardia, diastole is shortened at the expense of the diastolic plateau, which is of no hemodynamic benefit because no ventricular or atrial filling takes place. Thus, the early diastolic dip of pressure is followed by the next systolic rise without separation by a diastolic plateau. When this situation arises in patients with sinus tachycardia, the clinician should induce a ventricular extrasystole because the diastolic plateau of pressure becomes quite evident in the postextrasystolic

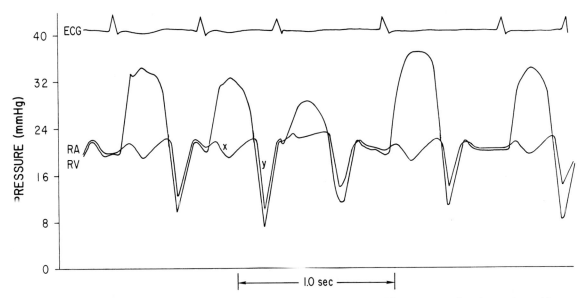

Figure 22–14. Simultaneous recording of right atrial (RA) and right ventricular (RV) pressure tracings in a patient with constrictive pericarditis. Note the prominent early diastolic dip of ventricular diastolic pressure and the corresponding sharp *y* descent of right atrial (RA) pressure that characterize the typical square root sign. This patient has atrial fibrillation; therefore, the diastolic plateau is evident only in beats with a long R-R interval. The RA and RV plateau pressures are increased to a value more than one third of RV systolic pressure, a common finding in constrictive pericarditis.

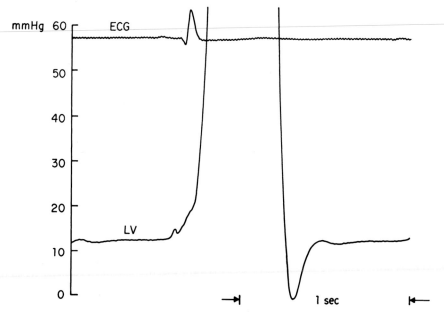

Figure 22–15. Left ventricular (LV) pressure tracing obtained during routine diagnostic cardiac catheterization in a patient without pericardial disease or restrictive cardiomyopathy. The tracings illustrate a false dip-and-plateau phenomenon. (From Shabetai R: The role of the pericardium in the pathophysiology of heart failure in congestive heart failure. *In* Hosenpud JD, Greenberg BH [eds]: Congestive Heart Failure: Pathophysiology, Diagnosis, and Comprehensive Approach to Management. New York, Springer-Verlag, 1993.)

beat. In patients with atrial fibrillation, a common late sequel of chronic constrictive pericarditis, spontaneous variation in the R-R interval may allow recognition of the mid-diastolic and late-diastolic plateau without the need for inducing extrasystoles. There is a variant of constrictive pericarditis that has been called *elastic constrictive pericarditis.*[34] In patients with this condition, many of the classic findings of constrictive pericarditis are present, but the pericardium is slightly more compliant than the essentially inelastic pericardium of typical constrictive pericarditis. Therefore, in these patients, a prominent a wave with a corresponding increase in ventricular diastolic volume can occur with atrial systole.

A false-positive dip-and-plateau sign owing to underdamped pressure recordings is a fairly common artifact in the cardiac catheterization laboratory (Fig. 22–15). Unless there is clinical suspicion of constrictive pericarditis or restrictive cardiomyopathy, most clinicians ignore this finding, but they agonize over it when some question of possible restriction or constriction has arisen. Left ventricular pressure is frequently measured through a large-bore thin-walled pigtail catheter designed specifically for ease and rapidity of contrast medium injection. These characteristics of the catheter that favor angiography tend to result in significant underdamping of the pressure tracing. The suggestion has even been made that the dip-and-plateau phenomenon of diastolic ventricular pressure is an artifact even in patients with constrictive pericarditis. However, studies employing catheter-tipped transducers that have a frequency response an order of magnitude higher than that required for a true high-fidelity pressure tracing have shown that the dip-and-plateau phenomenon is in fact a real feature of constrictive pericarditis. However, when this technique is employed, the tip does not reach zero, still less subatmospheric levels. Thus, the dip and plateau in constrictive pericarditis recorded by conventional fluid-filled catheter transducer systems is a real phenomenon exaggerated by underdamping (Fig. 22–16).

Another difference between constrictive pericarditis and cardiac tamponade is that pulsus paradoxus is common in cardiac tamponade and highly unusual in constrictive pericarditis. Absence of pulsus paradoxus in constrictive pericarditis is perhaps surprising in view of echo-Doppler studies that show abnormal respiratory variation in mitral and tricuspid inflow and in aortic and pulmonary outflow velocities.[35, 36] Based on these observations, it has been stated that respiratory variation of pulmonary arterial and aortic pressures in constrictive pericarditis ought to be 180 degrees out of phase. In actuality, however, peak systolic pressure in these two great vessels in constrictive pericardi-

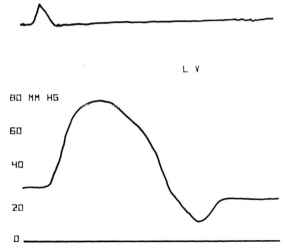

Figure 22–16. Computer printout of the left ventricular (LV) pressure tracing in a patient with severe constrictive pericarditis. The record was obtained with a high-fidelity catheter-tip transducer. The computer printed out the average of 100 beats. The early diastolic dip is less prominent than when conventional catheter transducer systems are employed. (From Shabetai R: The pathophysiology of cardiac tamponade and constriction in pericardial diseases. Cardiovasc Clin 1976; 7:67–89.)

tis is neither in phase, nor 180 degrees out of phase, but somewhere in between, as would be anticipated considering the complex variables that determine the respiratory variation of systemic and pulmonary arterial pressures (Fig. 22–17).

In the typical severe case of constrictive pericarditis, left and right ventricular diastolic pressures plateau around 20 mm Hg (see Fig. 22–13). Lower pressures may be due either to less severe constriction or to the effect of diuretics or vasodilators. When preparing a patient with severe chronic constrictive pericarditis for cardiac catheterization, the use of diuretics should be restrained and vasodilators should be avoided. Patients with severe chronic constrictive pericarditis coming to the cardiac catheterization laboratory free from edema and ascites and with normal or nearly normal jugular venous pressure have certainly been overtreated, usually to their detriment. The better course is to avoid vasodilators and use diuretics sparingly to reduce edema and ascites to the point where they no longer cause discomfort and dyspnea. Whereas characteristically in constrictive pericarditis the diastolic pressures in the four chambers are the same in at least one phase of the respiratory cycle, unusual cases of localized constriction can occur. Localized constriction can produce reasonably faithful imitations of mitral stenosis, tricuspid stenosis (Fig. 22–18), and pul-

monary stenosis. These valves are indeed narrowed, but by extrinsic local pericardial constriction, not by intrinsic valvular disease.

Occult Constrictive Pericarditis

In patients in whom the clinician suspects constrictive pericarditis but cannot elicit the characteristic hemodynamic findings at cardiac catheterization, many physicians rapidly administer a large intravenous volume load, for example, a liter of saline in 10 minutes, in an attempt to bring out the hemodynamic features of constrictive pericarditis. This (in our opinion too commonly applied) test is based on the concept of occult constrictive pericarditis described in 1977.[37] This report described patients with chest pain, many of whom had a remote history of acute pericarditis. The venous and ventricular diastolic pressures at baseline were not particularly suggestive of constrictive pericarditis, but following rapid volume expansion, right atrial pressure lost its respiratory variation, developed the typical deep x and y descents of constrictive pericarditis and was equal to the pulmonary wedge pressure. The patients who responded in this manner underwent pericardiectomy. The surgical findings confirmed constrictive pericarditis and the associated pericardial biopsy showed fibrosis and thickening of the pericardia. Most patients challenged with fluid infusion to bring out constrictive pericarditis do not fit the clinical description of the original series. Furthermore, in the original series there were, understandably, no control subjects. What is known is that in animals, rapid infusion of a large volume of fluid raises right atrial pressure considerably, but it also raises intrapericardial pressure so that there is only a small change in transmural right atrial pressure. Furthermore, the right atrial pressure under these circumstances has a waveform similar to that of constrictive pericarditis. It is thus distinctly possible that normal human subjects respond in an equivalent manner to rapid fluid infusion. The other problem is that in patients with underlying heart disease, rapid fluid infusion could raise pulmonary venous pressure to the level at which pulmonary edema would occur or become imminent, thus endangering the patient besides invalidating the data. In original series, the patients' complaint was chest pain, whereas most patients challenged in this way do not complain of chest pain. Finally, once it is recognized that constrictive pericarditis is so mild as to be inapparent until the patient had been abnormally volume loaded, pericardiectomy cannot be justified on the basis of this test.

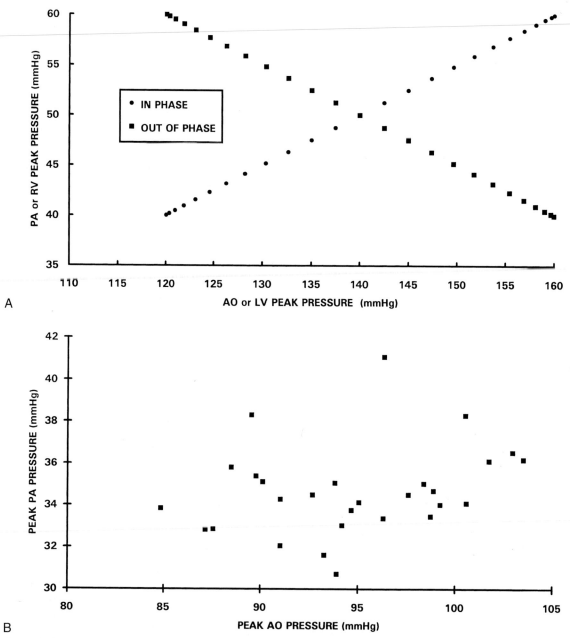

Figure 22–17. Peak left ventricular (LV) and right ventricular (RV) systolic pressures were plotted throughout several respiratory cycles in patients with severe constrictive pericarditis. Data from one of the patients are shown to determine the phase 1 relationship during normal quiet breathing. These pressures are neither in-phase nor 180 degrees out of phase. *A* shows how the plot would appear were the pressures completely in-phase or 180 degrees out of phase. *B* shows typical data from a patient with constrictive pericarditis. Ao, aortic; PA, pulmonary artery.

Angiocardiography or left ventriculography, when carried out, shows the increased thickness of the pericardium (Fig. 22–19) and confirms normal systolic function of the ventricles, which often are small and somewhat distorted in shape. An element of mitral or tricuspid regurgitation is not uncommon.

In severe constriction, however, left ventricular end-diastolic and stroke volumes are low, but cardiac output is partially maintained by compensatory tachycardia. The systolic indices of left ventricular contractility are normal or increased.[32, 38] In particular, myocardial failure, the so-called myocardial factor, cannot be documented in the cardiac catheterization laboratory.

The coronary arteriogram may show charac-

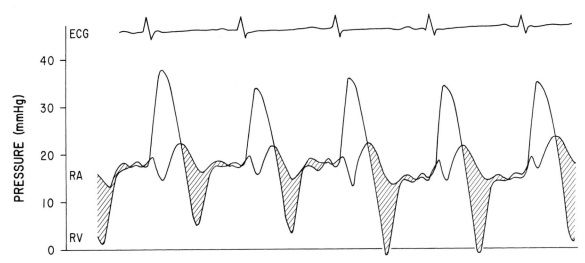

Figure 22–18. Simultaneous right atrial (RA) and right ventricular (RV) pressure tracings in a patient with extrinsic tricuspid stenosis secondary to localized constrictive pericarditis. Note the prominent *y* descent of the ventricular tracing and the atrioventricular pressure gradient present mostly in early diastole. The gradient increases during inspiration because RV pressure decreases with inspiration, whereas RA pressure is constant throughout the respiratory cycle.

teristic abnormalities in patients with constrictive pericarditis. Coronary arteriography can hardly be justified simply to demonstrate this appearance but is frequently indicated in all the patients in whom subsequent pericardiectomy is contemplated. The coronary arteries often show markedly reduced motion because of the epicardial scarring.[39] In contrast, the septal ar-

teries show increased motion.[40] Extension of the cardiac shadow beyond the epicardium as defined by the opacified coronary arteries may be a clue to increase pericardial thickness.

Effusive Constrictive Pericarditis

Effusive constrictive pericarditis[34] is an entity in which there is a pericardial effusion together

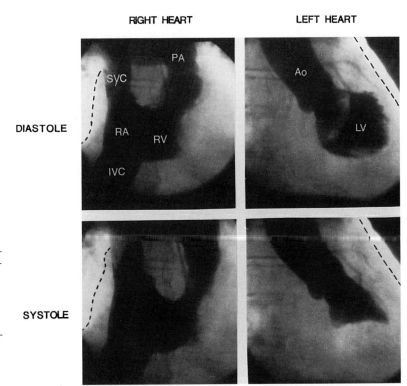

Figure 22–19. Right and left ventriculograms in a patient with constrictive pericarditis. Note the opacity of the cardiopericardial silhouette beyond the right atrial (RA) edge. When the left ventricle (LV) is opacified, the cardiac shadow extends beyond the epicardium as defined by the coronary arteries. Ao, aortic; PA, pulmonary artery; SVC, superior vena cava; IVC, inferior vena cava.

with thickening and decreased compliance of the pericardium. Common causes are tuberculous pericarditis and prior precordial radiation. Typically, the patient presents with evidence of cardiac compression, that is, with raised venous pressure, edema, and dyspnea. Detailed examination usually favors cardiac tamponade over constrictive pericarditis. Pulsus paradoxus is frequently present, and the jugular venous pressure lacks a prominent *y* descent. An echocardiogram to document the presence of pericardial effusion should be done in these cases, as in others, before invasive studies are undertaken. After the catheters have been placed in the right atrium, pulmonary wedge position, and pericardium, the characteristic findings of cardiac tamponade are usually found. Pericardiocentesis lowers the intrapericardial pressure in the expected manner, but right atrial pressure, although it may decrease somewhat, remains elevated and frequently develops characteristic sharp *x* and *y* descent and the absence of respiratory variation. Thus, when the patients first present, it is usually with the picture of cardiac tamponade, but after pericardiocentesis, the picture is that of constrictive pericarditis (Fig. 22–20).

RESTRICTIVE CARDIOMYOPATHY

In some patients sent to the laboratory for evaluation of constrictive pericarditis, the clinical and noninvasive laboratory diagnosis has been well established beforehand. In other instances, however, patients are sent to the laboratory in an attempt to establish the differential diagnosis between constrictive pericarditis and restrictive cardiomyopathy. For the purposes of this discussion, *restrictive cardiomyopathy* can be defined as a primary or secondary myocardial disorder without ventricular dilation and without significant ventricular hypertrophy in which a compliance abnormality of the myocardium produces diastolic heart dysfunction that closely mimics constrictive pericarditis. Typically, the patient presents the classic constrictive or restrictive pattern with dyspnea, raised jugular venous pressure with prominent *x* and *y* descents, and edema but no indication as to whether the fault lies in the myocardium or pericardium. Thus, the electrocardiogram shows only repolarization abnormalities, calcification of the pericardium is absent, and imaging fails to show a convincingly thick and abnormal pericardium. The right atrial pressure is indistinguishable from that of constrictive pericarditis, and the ventricular pressures show the typical dip-and-plateau configuration (Fig. 22–21). This observation has been reported by the majority of investigators, although it has been challenged by Hirota and associates,[41] who believe that the dip-and-plateau configuration of ventricular diastolic pressure is not found in restrictive cardiomyopathy.

When during cardiac catheterization, a

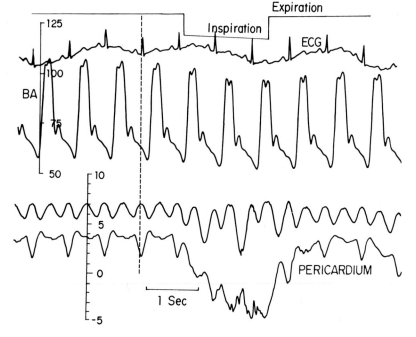

AFTER TAP

Figure 22–20. Effusive constrictive pericarditis. Tracings from top down: phase of respiration, electrocardiogram (ECG), brachial arterial (BA) pressure, right atrial pressure (unlabeled), and pericardial pressure. The right atrial pressure remains elevated to 7 mm Hg and displays prominent *x* and *y* descents, with respiratory variation limited to the *y* descent. (From Shabetai R: The Pericardium. New York, Grune & Stratton, 1981.)

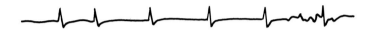

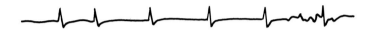

Figure 22–21. Right atrial (RA) and ventricular pressure recordings from a patient with restrictive cardiomyopathy secondary to hemochromatosis. More commonly, hemochromatosis causes reversible dilated cardiomyopathy.

large difference is found between left ventricular and right ventricular diastolic pressures, the diagnosis is much more likely to be restrictive cardiomyopathy than constrictive pericarditis. However, and in contradistinction to earlier teaching,[42] equal diastolic pressures in the two ventricles is equally consistent with constrictive pericarditis or restrictive cardiomyopathy; the finding simply is not helpful. Tyberg and colleagues[33] reported that patients with constrictive pericarditis achieved on average 85% of left ventricular filling in the first half of diastole compared with 45% in patients with restrictive cardiomyopathy. We[43] and others[44] have often found no difference in the early ventricular filling rate between patients with constrictive pericarditis and those with restrictive cardiomyopathy. Thus, although slow filling favors myocardial disease, rapid filling fails to distinguish between restrictive cardiomyopathy and constrictive pericarditis. If at the conclusion of a complete hemodynamic study the differential diagnosis has not become apparent, endomyocardial biopsy should be carried out.[44] In most patients with restrictive cardiomyopathy, the biopsy shows fibrosis, infiltrate, or radiation injury. A normal endomyocardial biopsy is highly persuasive evidence that the patient has constrictive pericarditis not restrictive cardiomyopathy. Therefore, when the hemodynamic study fails to uncover the diagnosis and endomyocardial biopsy reveals no abnormality, surgical exploration is fully justified.

Some patients have mixed constrictive pericarditis and restrictive cardiomyopathy. This constellation is commonly the result of radiation, which may injure both the myocardium and pericardium. It is difficult to sort out on hemodynamic grounds the relative contribu-

tions of pericardial and myocardial disease in many of these patients, so that the decision regarding exploration is often based on the severity of the pathology as disclosed by endomyocardial biopsy.

REFERENCES

1. Leimgruber PP, Klopfenstein HS, Wann LS, Brooks HL: The hemodynamic derangement associated with right ventricular diastolic collapse in cardiac tamponade: An experimental echocardiographic study. Circulation 1983; 68:612–620.
2. Gillam LD, Guyer DE, Gibson TC, et al: Hydrodynamic compression of the right atrium: A new echocardiographic sign of cardiac tamponade. Circulation 1983; 68:294–301.
3. Shabetai R, Fowler NO, Fenton JC, Masangkay M: Pulsus paradoxus. J Clin Invest 1965; 44:1882–1898.
4. Winer HE, Kronzon I: Absence of paradoxical pulse in patients with cardiac tamponade and atrial septal defects. Am J Cardiol 1979; 44:378–380.
5. Reddy PS, Curtiss EI, O'Toole JD, Shaver JA: Cardiac tamponade: Hemodynamic observations in man. Circulation 1978; 58:265–272.
6. Nottestad SY, Mascette AM: Loculated pericardial effusion and cardiac tamponade late after cardiac surgery. Chest 1992; 101:852.
7. Russo AM, O'Connor WH, Waxman HL: Atypical presentations and echocardiographic findings in patients with cardiac tamponade occurring early and late after cardiac surgery. Chest 1993; 104:71–78.
8. Antman EM, Cargill V, Grossman W: Low-pressure cardiac tamponade. Ann Intern Med 1979; 91:403–406.
9. Guberman BA, Fowler NO, Engel PJ, et al: Cardiac tamponade in medical patients. Circulation 1981; 64:633–640.
10. Hardesty RL: Delayed postoperative cardiac tamponade: Diagnosis and management. In Reddy PS, Leon DF, Shaver JA (eds): Pericardial Disease. New York, Raven Press, 1982, pp 341–348.
11. Shabetai R, Fowler NO, Guntheroth WG: The hemodynamics of cardiac tamponade and constrictive pericarditis. Am J Cardiol 26:480–489, 1970.

12. Spitz HB, Holmes JC: Right atrial contour in cardiac tamponade. Radiology 1972; 103:69–75.

13. Krikorian JG, Hancock EW: Pericardiocentesis. Am J Med 1978; 65:808–814.

14. Wong B, Murphy J, Chang CJ, et al: The risk of pericardiocentesis. Am J Cardiol 1979; 44:1110–1114.

15. Kilpatrick ZM, Chapman CB: On pericardiocentesis. Am J Cardiol 1965; 16:722–728.

16. Wolfe MW, Edelman ER: Transient systolic dysfunction after relief of cardiac tamponade. Ann Intern Med 1993; 119:42–44.

17. Martin RP, Rakowski H, French J, Popp RL: Localization of pericardial effusion with wide-angle phased-array echocardiography. Am J Cardiol 1978; 42:904–912.

18. Lock JE, Bass JL, Kulik TJ, Fuhrman BP: Chronic percutaneous pericardial drainage with modified pigtail catheters in children. Am J Cardiol 1984; 53:1179–1182.

19. Stewart JR, Gott VL: The use of a Seldinger wire technique for pericardiocentesis following cardiac surgery. Ann Thorac Surg 1983; 35:467–468.

20. Wayne VS, Bishop RL, Spodick DH: Dynamic effects of pericardial effusion without tamponade: Respiratory responses in the absence of pulsus paradoxus. Br Heart J 1984; 51:202–204.

21. Reddy PS, Curtiss EI: Cardiac tamponade. Cardiol Clin 1990; 8:627–637.

22. DeCristofaro D, Liu CK: The haemodynamics of cardiac tamponade and blood volume overload in dogs. Cardiovasc Res 1969; 3:292–298.

23. Shabetai R, Fowler NO, Braunstein JR, Gueron M: Transmural ventricular pressures and pulsus paradoxus in experimental cardiac tamponade. Dis Chest 1961; 39:557–568.

24. Brown J, MacKinnon D, King A, Vanderbush E: Elevated arterial blood pressure in cardiac tamponade. N Engl J Med 1992; 327:463–466.

25. Klopfenstein HS, Schuchard GH, Wann LS, et al: The relative merits of pulsus paradoxus and right ventricular diastolic collapse in the early detection of cardiac tamponade: An experimental echocardiographic study. Circulation 1985; 71:829–833.

26. Palacios IF, Tuzcu EM, Ziskind AA, et al: Percutaneous balloon pericardial window for patients with malignant pericardial effusion and tamponade. Cathet Cardiovasc Diagn 1991; 22:244–249.

27. Ziskind AA, Pearce AC, Lemmon CC, et al: Percutaneous balloon pericardiotomy for the treatment of cardiac tamponade and large pericardial effusions: Description of technique and report of the first 50 cases. J Am Coll Cardiol 1993; 21:1–5.

28. Chow W-H, Chow T-C, Cheung K-L: Nonsurgical creation of a pericardial window using the Inoue balloon catheter. Am Heart J 1992; 124:1100–1102.

29. Kondos GT, Rich S, Levitsky S: Flexible fiberoptic pericardioscopy for the diagnosis of pericardial disease. J Am Coll Cardiol 1986; 7:432–434.

30. Maisch B, Drude L: Pericardioscopy—a new diagnostic tool in inflammatory diseases of the pericardium. Eur Heart J 1991; 12(Suppl D):2–6.

31. Little AG, Ferguson MK: Pericardioscopy as adjunct to pericardial window. Chest 1986; 89:53–55.

32. Gaasch WH, Peterson KL, Shabetai R: Left ventricular function in chronic constrictive pericarditis. Am J Cardiol 1974; 34:107–110.

33. Tyberg TI, Goodyer AVN, Hurst VW, et al: Left ventricular filling in differentiating restrictive amyloid cardiomyopathy and constrictive pericarditis. Am J Cardiol 1981; 47:791–796.

34. Hancock EW: Subacute effusive-constrictive pericarditis. Circulation 1971; 43:183–192.

35. Hatle LK, Appleton CP, Popp RL: Differentiation of constrictive pericarditis and restrictive cardiomyopathy by Doppler echocardiography. Circulation 1989; 79:357–370.

36. Oh JK, Hatle LK, Seward JB, et al: Diagnostic role of Doppler echocardiography in constrictive pericarditis. J Am Coll Cardiol 1994; 23:154–162.

37. Bush CA, Stang JM, Wooley CF, Kilman JW: Occult constrictive pericardial disease: Diagnosis by rapid volume expansion and correction by pericardiectomy. Circulation 1977; 56:924–930.

38. Lewis BS, Gotsman MS: Left ventricular function in systole and diastole in constrictive pericarditis. Am Heart J 1973; 86:23–41.

39. Alexander J, Kelley MJ, Cohen LS, Langou RA: The angiographic appearance of the coronary arteries in constrictive pericarditis. Radiology 1979; 131:609–617.

40. Soto B, Shin MS, Arciniegas J, Ceballos R: The septal arteries in the differential diagnosis of constrictive pericarditis. Am Heart J 108:332–336, 1984.

41. Hirota Y, Kohriyama T, Hayashi T, et al: Idiopathic restrictive cardiomyopathy: Differences of left ventricular relaxation and diastolic wave forms from constrictive pericarditis. Am J Cardiol 1983; 52:421–423.

42. Wood P: Chronic constrictive pericarditis. Am J Cardiol 1961; 7:48–61.

43. Meaney E, Shabetai R, Bhargava V, et al: Cardiac amyloidosis, constrictive pericarditis, and restrictive cardiomyopathy. Am J Cardiol 1976; 38:547–556.

44. Schoenfeld MH, Supple EW, Dec GW, et al: Restrictive cardiomyopathy versus constrictive pericarditis: Role of endomyocardial biopsy in avoiding unnecessary thoracotomy. Circulation 1987; 75:1012–1017.

Chapter 23

Catheterization and Angiography in Pulmonary Hypertension

WILLIAM AUGER
KENNETH MOSER
KIRK L. PETERSON

Pulmonary angiography in patients with known pulmonary hypertension often elicits trepidation on the part of the angiographer. This concern is fueled by the belief that pulmonary angiography in this patient population is frequently accompanied by life-threatening complications, such as acute right ventricular failure and arrhythmias, or may even result in the patient's death. Based primarily on anecdotal and old reports, these concerns can potentially delay or inhibit the complete evaluation of a given patient's pulmonary hypertensive disease.

This chapter examines the issue of pulmonary angiography in the setting of pulmonary hypertension, with two areas of emphasis. First, the belief that this radiographic procedure is "dangerous" in a pulmonary hypertensive patient is addressed. This belief has been challenged by several series dealing with patients with significant pulmonary hypertension[1-4]; these papers have affirmed both the safety and diagnostic importance of this procedure. Second, potentially lifesaving surgical techniques have emerged for patients with severe pulmonary hypertension, for example, pulmonary thromboendarterectomy for chronic, major-vessel thromboembolic disease[5, 6] and lung transplantation for severe small-vessel pulmonary hypertensive disorders.[7] Such new therapies increase the need for accurate preoperative determination of etiology. Therefore, the angiographer plays an essential role in defining the pulmonary vascular anatomy in those patients undergoing an evaluation of their pulmonary hypertensive disease.

SAFETY AND TECHNICAL CONSIDERATIONS

Concerns about pulmonary angiography in the patient with pulmonary hypertension originate in several early case reports of fatalities related to this procedure.[8-12] Not only was patient mortality associated with angiography in the setting of pulmonary hypertension but right-sided heart catheterization alone was reported as potentially hazardous.[13] These reports were followed by series dealing with pulmonary angiography in larger groups of patients, primarily in the diagnosis of acute pulmonary embolic disease. Complications such as the induction of transient arrhythmias, myocardial perforation, endocardial injections, contrast agent reactions, and cardiopulmonary arrest were described but not specifically attributed to the presence of pulmonary hypertensive disease. However, deaths resulting from this diagnostic procedure seemed to occur most commonly in the patient with "severe pulmonary hypertension," albeit at a low incidence relative to the total population reviewed. In 1971, Dalen and associates[14] reported one death in 367 angiographic studies of the pulmonary vessels. This death occurred in a patient with "terminal" primary pulmonary hypertension after the injection of 40 mL of contrast agent. Marsh and colleagues[15] described a similar event in a patient with a pulmonary artery systolic pressure of 70 mm Hg (mean pulmonary artery pressure of 33 mm Hg and a right atrial pressure of 27 mm Hg) after a subselective hand injection of 10 mL of contrast medium; the total number of patients in this series was 106. Moses and coworkers,[16] in 1974, reviewed 298 patients undergoing pulmonary angiography and reported two deaths in patients with severe pulmonary vascular obstruction. In a large study in 1980 with 1350 pulmonary angiographic procedures, Mills and associates[17] described three deaths (an incidence of 0.2%). All three patients had severe pulmonary hypertension and elevated right ventricular end-diastolic pressure (RVEDP) (20 mm Hg or higher). Although the mortality in Marsh and colleagues' series[15] was associated with an elevation in right atrial pressure, Mills and associates' study[17] was unique in its implication that right ventricular dysfunction in the patient with pulmonary hypertension may represent a subcategory of patients particularly susceptible to complications of pulmonary angiography.

Although the articles just referenced clearly identify the patients with pulmonary hypertension as prevalent in the group dying from pulmonary angiography, the mortality incidence of the total number of patients with pulmonary hypertension undergoing this procedure was not clearly defined. In one report,[15] the presence of significant pulmonary hypertension represented an exclusion criterion for performance of pulmonary angiography.

Attention has been directed to substantiation of these concerns. Perlmutt and associates[4] reviewed pulmonary angiography between 1967 and 1985 in 1434 patients, 313 patients with moderate pulmonary hypertension (pulmonary artery systolic pressure 40 to 70 mm Hg) and 75 patients with severe (pulmonary artery systolic pressure >70 mm Hg) elevation of pulmonary arterial pressures. In the pulmonary hypertensive group, two patients, both with severe pulmonary hypertension, died (0.5%) after a main pulmonary artery injection. Consistent with the experience of Mills and associates,[17] both patients had an RVEDP of 20 mm Hg or higher. No deaths occurred in the nonhypertensive patients, although the percentage of nonfatal complications was comparable in the two groups.

Additionally, two large series of patients with severe pulmonary hypertensive disease undergoing diagnostic pulmonary angiography have been reported. Nicod and coworkers[1] described 67 patients with chronic thromboembolic pulmonary hypertension. Mean pulmonary arterial pressure in this group of patients was 47 ± 13 mm Hg, with an RVEDP of 13 ± 6 mm Hg and a cardiac index of 2.2 ± 0.7 L/min. There were no deaths attributed to pulmonary angiography. This series has expanded (1987 to 1991) to include more than 300 patients, without a death.[2] Complications related

to pulmonary angiography in this group included the occurrence of a seizure in a patient with a known seizure disorder, a few cases of transient systemic hypotension (none requiring vasoactive medications), and three cases of reversible, contrast agent–related renal dysfunction (none requiring dialysis). The National Heart Lung and Blood Institute registry for primary pulmonary hypertension completed in 1987 included 50 patients who underwent diagnostic pulmonary angiography without a death.[3] Transient hypotension occurred in only one of these patients. Ten of the 187 patients who had cardiac catheterization experienced an adverse reaction from this procedure: five instances of transient hypotension, one episode of post-catheterization hemoptysis (these six events probably related to the presence of pulmonary hypertension), inadvertent arterial puncture, oversedation, and pneumothorax (unrelated to the presence of pulmonary hypertension). The 187 patients in this series had severe pulmonary hypertension (pulmonary artery mean pressure of 60.7 ± 19.7 mm Hg in males and 60.3 ± 26.5 mm Hg in females) with significant compromise of their cardiac function (cardiac index of 2.35 ± 1.0 L/min/m^2 in males and 2.21 ± 0.9 L/min/m^2 in females).

This review indicates that although precautions are warranted in the setting of pulmonary hypertension, pulmonary angiography can be performed with acceptable risk by experienced operators in this patient population. The difference between earlier reports of hazard associated with angiography and more recent reports is probably heavily influenced by technical advances that have occurred over time in both right-sided heart catheterization and pulmonary angiography.

One such advance has been in the contrast media used. The injection of *ionic* or high-osmolality contrast agents into the right cardiac chambers or the pulmonary vessels has been noted to cause significant hemodynamic changes. In both animal[18–20] and human[21–23] studies, reflex systemic hypotension, abrupt increases in pulmonary arterial pressure, and acute depression of myocardial contractility have been described after injection of this type of contrast medium. Additionally, in pulmonary hypertensive patients in whom arterial oxygenation is partially dependent on mixed venous Po_2, an abrupt decline in cardiac output may adversely affect gas exchange.[24] Consequently, *ionic* contrast agent injection in such patients may have contributed to the negative outcomes observed in earlier series. The advent of *nonionic* and low-osmolality contrast agents has resulted in a reduction of adverse patient reactions[25, 26] and hemodynamic perturbations[2, 22, 23] (see Chapter 7).

Second, advances in both cardiac catheter design, promoting precise catheter placement, and carefully programmed pressure injectors have enhanced safety. Catheter placement directly into the pulmonary arteries (rather than in the right atrium or ventricle) reduces the likelihood of cardiac perforation and of contrast agent injection at locations likely to induce arrhythmias. Furthermore, such placement allows use of smaller amounts of contrast agent.

Third, diagnostic advances such as two-dimensional echocardiography, noninvasive leg venous studies, and radionuclide lung ventilation-perfusion scanning prior to cardiac catheterization and pulmonary angiography have contributed to patient safety. Echocardiography with Doppler estimation of pulmonary arterial pressures allows a precatheterization assessment of the patient's severity of illness. In addition, detection of thrombi or tumor in either the right atrium or right ventricle appropriately warns the angiographer so that inadvertent dislodgment of thrombi into the pulmonary vascular bed can be avoided.

Noninvasive assessment of the patency of the femoral-iliac–inferior vena caval system also can define the presence of thrombi there so that catheterization via the neck or arm, rather than the leg, can similarly prevent potential dislodgment of venous thrombi. Perfusion lung scanning further allows a precatheterization assessment as to the location and severity of pulmonary vascular obstruction. Such assessments are particularly useful when dealing with vascular obstruction to an entire lobe or lung.

Finally, continuous measurement of oxygen saturation allows provision of adequate oxygen therapy. Monitoring of systemic and pulmonary arterial blood pressures and heart rate and rhythm during right-sided heart catheterization and pulmonary angiography allows immediate detection, and hence, prompt administration of antiarrhythmic or inotropic medications in the event of significant cardiopulmonary compromise.

Although methodology may differ from institution to institution and from patient to patient, some general principles relating to minimizing risk have been established. At the University of California, San Diego, Medical Center (UCSD), more than 500 patients with severe pulmonary hypertension secondary to chronic thromboembolic disease or primary pulmonary hypertension have undergone right-sided heart catheterization and pulmonary angiography between 1970 and 1993. Several aspects

of the procedure routinely performed in the cardiac catheterization laboratory can be summarized as follows:

1. Heart rhythm, oxygen saturation, and systemic and pulmonary arterial blood pressures are monitored continuously during the procedure; supplemental oxygen is provided to maintain an oxygen saturation level higher than 90%.

2. Scout films are first obtained to ensure patient positioning that optimizes visualization of the main, lobar, and segmental pulmonary vessels.

3. Access to the pulmonary arteries is preferentially via the neck or arm to avoid potential dislodgment of unsuspected venous thrombi involving the femoral vein, iliac vein, or inferior vena cava. Because most of the pulmonary hypertensive patient population at UCSD has chronic thromboembolic disease, this approach can be justified. In the case of small-vessel pulmonary vascular disease, neck or arm access may not be as critical.

4. Relatively stiff, side-hole catheters (7-French or 8-French NIH or Berman angiography catheters) are most commonly used. Because the catheter is preshaped with a curve at the tip, torque control and hence manipulation through a frequently enlarged right ventricle are improved; catheter retraction and "whip" during injection are also minimized.

5. Unilateral, sequential injection of contrast agent into each main pulmonary artery is preferred. The catheter is positioned near the origin of the lower lobe vessels, and the contrast agent is allowed to fill retrograde the upper lobes.

6. The amount of contrast agent required for definition of the pulmonary vascular anatomy is gauged by noting the patient's thermodilution cardiac output and the speed of run-off during a small hand injection. A slow run-off or low cardiac output indicates the need for lesser amounts of contrast agent. In this series, the total amount of contrast medium ranged from 40 to 60 mL, injected at a rate of 20 mL/sec. Cut-film angiograms are obtained at a speed of 2 images/sec for 4 seconds, then 1 image/sec for 4 seconds. The adequacy of the study is confirmed on review of the films before injection of the contralateral pulmonary artery.

7. Nonionic contrast medium is used; this has resulted in less adverse patient reactions (such as coughing and "flushing") and minimal hemodynamic compromise.

Although pulmonary angiography is an invasive procedure with attendant risk, appropriate precautions and an experienced angiographer allow this diagnostic procedure to be available to all patients who require definition of their pulmonary vascular anatomy, even if this is in the setting of significant pulmonary hypertension.

PULMONARY ANGIOGRAPHY: INTERPRETATION IN THE PATIENT WITH PULMONARY HYPERTENSION

In most instances, pulmonary angiography represents the final diagnostic step in the evaluation of a patient with elevated pulmonary artery pressures. Delineation of precapillary causes of pulmonary hypertension is the primary goal of this diagnostic procedure. "Postcapillary" causes, such as long-standing pulmonary venous hypertension (e.g., left-sided heart failure and mitral valve disease), or other pulmonary vascular disorders, such as those associated with venous occlusion, generally present clinical and laboratory features that provide the diagnosis. However, left-sided heart catheterization, coronary angiography, regional pulmonary capillary wedge determinations, and retrograde pulmonary venography may be required to confirm or exclude these diagnoses. Consequently, the usual goal of pulmonary angiography in the pulmonary hypertensive patient is to define the prearteriolar anatomy to distinguish between major-vessel (main, lobar, and segmental) and small-vessel disease.

Proper interpretation of the pulmonary angiogram requires a knowledge of the usual anatomy of the pulmonary arterial vasculature. The reader is encouraged to study carefully the idealized model of the lung vascular trees depicted in Figures 23–1 (right lung) and 23–2 (left lung). The distribution and arborization of both pulmonary arteries are best appreciated when interpreted from biplane angiographic films.

On the anteroposterior view of the right lung, there is usually good separation of the apical, posterior, and anterior branches of the

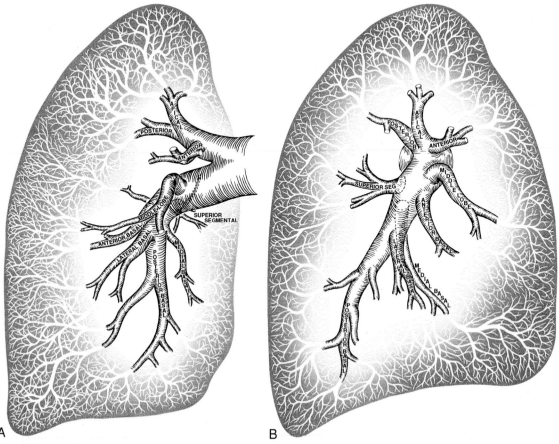

A   B

Figure 23–1. *A,* Three-dimensional perspective shown in a schematic drawing of the anterorposterior view of the right pulmonary artery and its major branches. *B,* The lateral view of the same artery shown in *A.* Note the ready separation of the middle lobe artery from the branches to the segments of the right lower lobe.

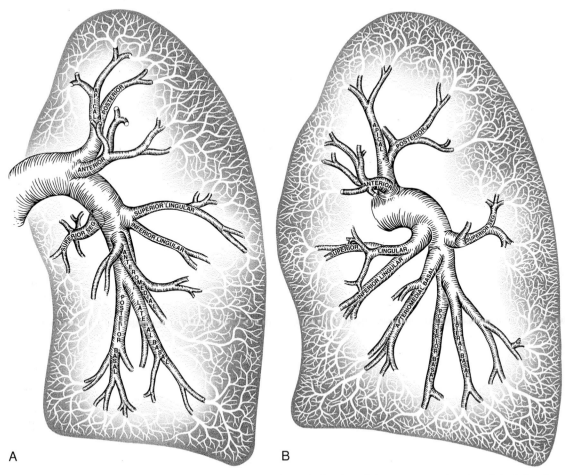

A   B

Figure 23–2. *A,* Three-dimensional perspective shown in a schematic drawing of the anteroposterior view of the left pulmonary artery and its major branches. *B,* The lateral view of the same artery shown in *A.* Note the ready separation of the segmental branches to the left lower lobe.

major branch to the right upper lobe; however, there is generally significant overlap of the branch to the right middle lobe with the superior, anterobasal, mediobasal, and laterobasal segmental tributaries to the right lower lobe. The lateral projection assists greatly in separating out these branches. Occasionally, the mediobasal and laterobasal branches overlap partially the posterobasal branch in the anteroposterior projection; again, the lateral projection helps to separate these structures.

The most problematic overlap of the left pulmonary arterial tree is that of the anteromedial, laterobasal, and posterobasal branches to the left lower lobe. The lateral projection helps significantly in separating these structures. Also, the superior and inferior branches to the lingula, the branch to the superior segment of the left lower lobe, and the anterior, apical, and posterior branches to the left upper lobe are well separated on the lateral projection, al-

though these same structures are also well examined on the anteroposterior view.

Accurate interpretation of pulmonary angiograms in a patient with pulmonary hypertension requires also an understanding of certain physiologic principles and recognition of interpretive pitfalls. As an example, the presence of significantly elevated pulmonary arterial pressures necessarily implies extensive *bilateral* involvement of the pulmonary vascular bed. Consequently, unilateral and regional subselective pulmonary angiography have limited usefulness. However, after bilateral pulmonary angiography is performed, a subselective, low-volume contrast study may be required to better define pertinent regions of the pulmonary vascular bed. A pitfall to be avoided is heavy reliance on the lung perfusion scan to dictate selective regional angiography. In the case of chronic thromboembolic pulmonary hypertension, the lung perfusion scan can significantly underestimate the degree of obstructive vascular disease,[27] with regions of lung parenchyma that appear gray by macroaggregated albumin (MAA) scan, but not devoid of flow. This discrepancy is related to partially occlusive but significantly obstructing vascular lesions, allowing radiolabeled MAA to pass into the distal pulmonary vascular bed. Because absence of flow requires a narrowing of 80% or more of the arterial lumen, failure to attempt visualization at angiography of such gray zones results in an inadequate evaluation.

Another pitfall is the quite striking difference in angiographic appearance between "fresh" and chronic pulmonary emboli. The sharply defined intraluminal filling defects diagnostic of fresh thrombi[28] are distinct from the unusual angiographic patterns seen in chronic thromboembolic disease (Fig. 23–3). Further, small acute emboli cannot be implicated as the sole cause of significantly elevated pulmonary artery pressures. Sutton and colleagues[29] and others[30, 31] have demonstrated that marked pulmonary hypertension from acute thromboem-

bolic disease does not typically occur; that is, a mean pulmonary artery pressure higher than 35 mm Hg is distinctly unusual. Consequently, the presence of an intraluminal filling defect on angiography in the markedly pulmonary hypertensive patient suggests acute thrombus superimposed on chronic thromboembolic disease (Figs. 23–4), complications of another vascular process, or other disorders such as pulmonary vascular tumors[32, 33] (Fig. 23–5).

The need for interpretive caution is particularly important in patients with suspected chronic major-vessel thromboembolic disease. Recognition of this diagnosis, as opposed to the vascular "pruning" pattern of small-vessel pulmonary vascular hypertension (Fig. 23–6), makes a substantial difference in therapeutic approach. The patient with surgically accessible chronic thromboembolic disease becomes a potential candidate for pulmonary thromboendarterectomy.[5, 6] The patient with small-vessel disease, for example, primary pulmonary hypertension, is a candidate for a vasodilator drug trial[34] or possible lung transplantation.[7] Thus, angio-

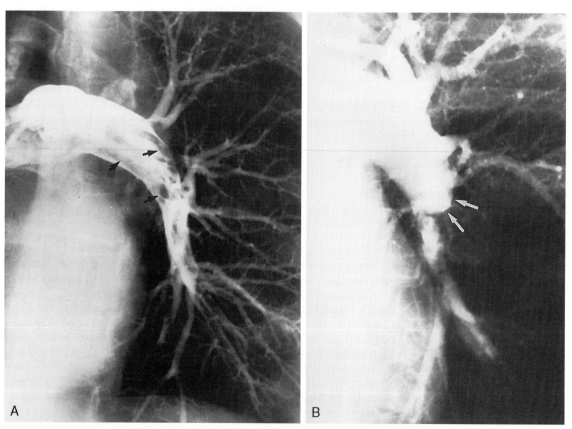

A

B

Figure 23–3. *A*, Numerous filling defects involving the left descending pulmonary artery (PA), consistent with acute thromboemboli *(arrows)*. *B*, In contrast with *A*, this left pulmonary angiogram shows central PA enlargement; the "pouching" abnormality *(arrows)* in the left descending PA and several obstructed left lower lobe vessels are abnormalities seen in chronic thromboembolic disease.

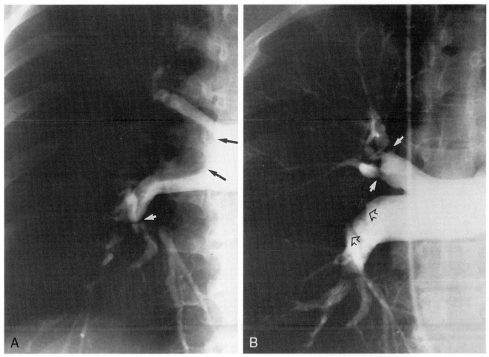

Figure 23–4. *A,* Pulmonary angiogram performed in a patient with acute dyspnea. A saddle embolus involves the proximal right upper lobe and descending pulmonary arteries (PAs) *(black arrows).* PA pressure is 100 mm Hg systolic; PA mean pressure is 70 mm Hg. Proximal right lower lobe "webs" *(white arrow)* suggest the presence of chronic thromboembolic disease. *B,* Repeat angiogram 3 months later, after an initial course of streptokinase and subsequent anticoagulation. The fresh thrombus is gone with angiographic evidence of chronic thromboembolic disease involving the right upper lobe ("webs," *white arrows*) and right descending PA (absent middle lobe vessels and intimal irregularities, *open arrows*).

graphic interpretation leads to major branches in therapeutic decision making.

Several angiographic patterns have come to be recognized as indicating the presence of chronic thromboembolic material.[2] These patterns include "pouching" abnormalities; vascular "webs" or bandlike constrictions; intimal irregularities; abrupt narrowing of major pulmonary vessels; and obstruction of major pulmonary vessels, frequently at points of origin (Figs. 23–7 through 23–11). These unusual angiographic findings represent recanalized and organized thromboemboli. It is speculated that in a small number of pulmonary embolic survivors the process of clot organization is either incomplete or "hyperaggressive," leading to partial recanalization, vessel obstruction, and vessel retraction. As previously mentioned, these angiographic patterns are distinct from the well-defined, intraluminal filling defects of acute emboli and the peripheral vascular pruning of such diseases as primary (idiopathic) pulmonary hypertension. The classic findings in primary pulmonary hypertension include normal (or dilated) central elastic arteries with pruning of the small, nonelastic arteries. The normal arteriolar-capillary "blush" as dye transverses the

small, distal vessels is absent. One must be cautious, however, in interpreting pruning limited to certain portions of the lung as indicative of primary pulmonary hypertension. In primary pulmonary hypertension, the pruning is global. However, in thromboembolic pulmonary hypertension, apparent regional pruning may simply reflect obstruction of the more proximal elastic artery by thrombus.

There are, however, competing diagnoses when several of the angiographic findings characteristic of chronic, major-vessel thromboembolism are present. Pulmonary arterial webs were originally described as evidence of chronic thromboemboli.[35] Nonetheless, these bandlike narrowings traversing the width of major pulmonary vessels can also be seen with congenital stenotic lesions of the pulmonary arteries[36, 37] and with nonspecific arteritis of large pulmonary vessels (Takayasu's arteritis).[38–40] In the case of congenital pulmonary arterial stenosis, coexisting cardiac anomalies are typically present, with patients usually presenting at an early age. Takayasu's arteritis of the pulmonary vessels is observed in 50% of patients with systemic manifestations, and in addition to weblike narrowings, vessel occlusion, luminal irregularities,

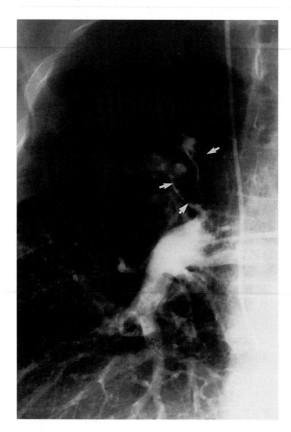

Figure 23–5. Right pulmonary angiogram in a 73-year-old male with exertional dyspnea and pulmonary hypertension (pulmonary artery pressure, 80/30 mm Hg). Right upper lobe intraluminal filling defects *(arrows)* were discovered at surgery to be secondary to a primary pulmonary vascular tumor.

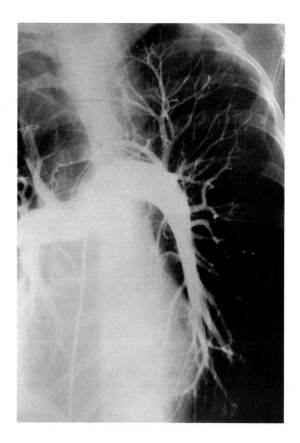

Figure 23–6. Classic angiographic pattern of primary pulmonary hypertension. All segmental vessels are present, with a reduction of vascular density or ''pruning'' toward the lung periphery.

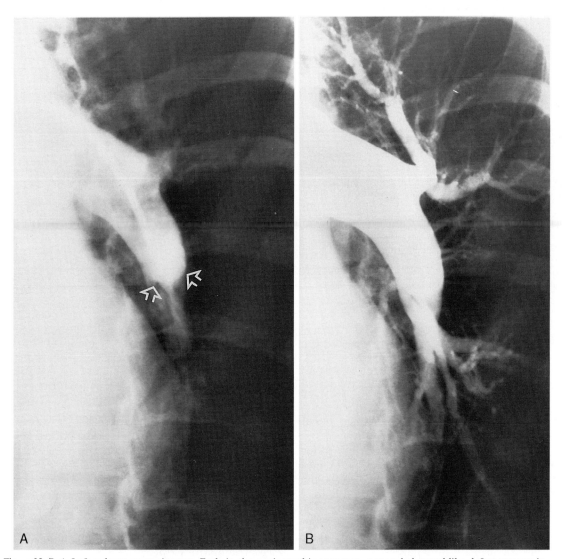

Figure 23–7. *A,* Left pulmonary angiogram. Early in the angiographic sequence, a rounded, pouchlike defect appears in the mid-left descending pulmonary artery *(open arrows).* Distal left lower lobe segmental vessels eventually opacify. *B,* Pulmonary angiogram. A chronic thrombus was removed from this vessel at the time of surgery.

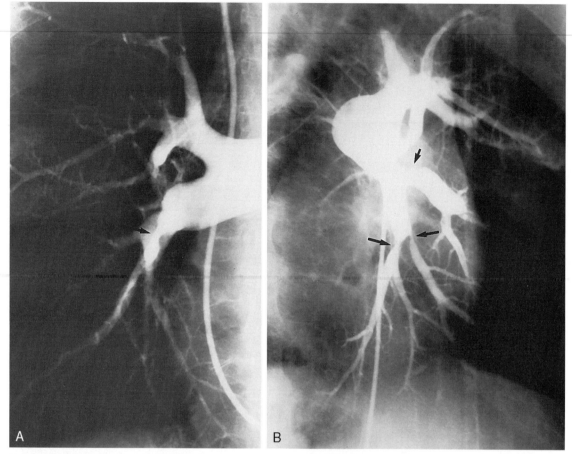

Figure 23–8. Posteroanterior *(A)* and lateral *(B)* views of a right pulmonary angiogram. Discrete bandlike narrowings or "webs" involve several right lower lobe branches *(long arrows)*. Proximal intimal irregularities *(short arrows)* with distal obstruction are seen in a middle lobe vessel.

and pulmonary arterial aneurysms can be observed at angiography.

In addition, total obstruction or abrupt narrowing of major pulmonary arteries, particularly at the level of the main and lobar vessels, may complicate a number of other disease entities. Examples include extrinsic compression from extensive mediastinal or hilar lymphadenopathy,[41] fibrosing mediastinitis,[42, 43] and pulmonary vascular or primary lung carcinoma.[41, 44, 45] The extent of vascular involvement may be enough to cause pulmonary hypertension; the distinction from chronic thromboembolic disease is frequently dependent on additional historical information and other diagnostic studies such as computed tomography and magnetic resonance imaging.

Particular attention should be given to the occurrence of a unilaterally absent main pulmonary vessel. Although frequently attributed to pulmonary artery agenesis, this appearance can be secondary to chronic thromboembolic disease.[46] Especially in the setting of a pulmonary hypertensive patient, careful review of contralateral vascular anatomy and prior radiographic and perfusion lung scan information may clarify the differential diagnosis.

The angiographic patterns suggestive of chronic thromboembolic disease do not occur in isolation. Several vascular abnormalities typically occur in the same patient, in both lung fields. It is also commonplace that subtle vascular irregularities can mark the presence of significant amounts of chronic thrombi (see Fig. 23–9). Experience in interpretation, therefore, becomes an important component not only in establishing the correct diagnosis but in patient selection for surgical intervention.

PULMONARY ANGIOSCOPY AND INTRAVASCULAR ULTRASONOGRAPHY

The varied angiographic appearances associated with chronic major-vessel thromboembolic pul-

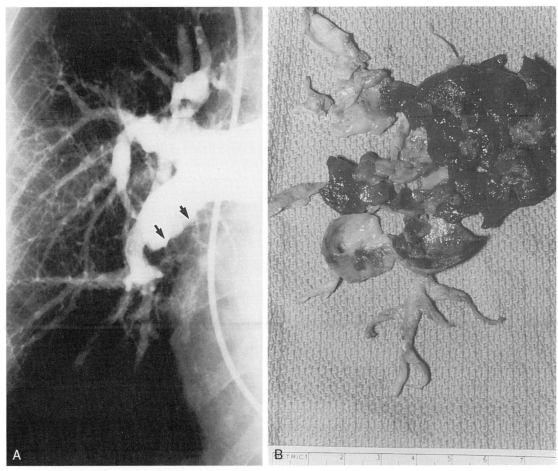

Figure 23–9. *A,* Intimal irregularities *(arrows)* involving the proximal right descending pulmonary artery. Vascular irregularities also involve the right upper lobe vessels, with diminished flow to the right lower lobe. *B,* Large amount of organized thrombus removed at surgery. Intimal irregularities on the angiogram corresponded to an organizing thrombus adherent to the vessel wall.

monary hypertension are, with experience, sufficiently characteristic to allow the diagnosis to be established. However, another question arises when this diagnosis is established: Are the chronic thrombi accessible to surgical removal? To qualify for removal, the thrombi must begin in the lobar arteries or at the origins of the segmental arteries. If this is not the case, successful endarterectomy currently is impossible. In many patients, although diagnostic abnormalities are present by angiogram, their proximal extent is unclear. Often, an obstructing lesion (e.g., a web) apparently isolated to a segmental or subsegmental artery is just the distal extension of much more proximal thrombus. Attempted endarterectomy in a severely hypertensive patient whose thrombi prove too distal to allow removal is associated with a high mortality risk or, with survival, unabated pulmonary hypertension.

To resolve this issue, fiberoptic angioscopy has been developed to allow direct visualization of the interior of the central pulmonary arteries.[47] The angioscope is a 120-cm fiberoptic device, 3 mm in diameter, which is inserted via the same sheath used for angiography. The distal portion of the device can be flexed and extended by proximal controls. A balloon is fastened over its distal end; it can be inflated, when desired, by a small channel. Carbon dioxide is used as the inflating gas. After manipulation into the pulmonary artery tree, balloon inflation allows excellent visualization of the pulmonary arterial walls. The normal arterial walls are white and glistening; in pulmonary hypertensive patients, there are occasional small, yellowish atherosclerotic plaques. Chronic thrombi present as irregularities in the arterial wall; transluminal bands or webs; and puckered, irregular vessel ostia. Combined with fluoroscopy to establish position of the angioscope, angioscopy can define the point at which these

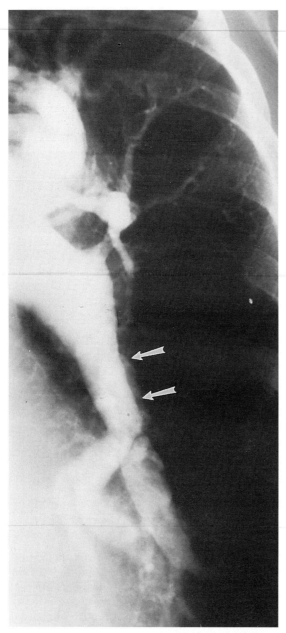

Figure 23–10. Recanalized thrombus abruptly narrowing the left descending pulmonary artery. Both lingular branches are occluded. Intimal irregularity is indicated by the arrows.

plane, with a thrombus of sufficient thickness so that it will not tear or fracture as dissection proceeds distally. To answer this question, efforts are underway to use intravascular ultrasonographic imaging of areas at issue.[48] Preliminary results have been encouraging, and investigations of this approach continue.

Thus, in summary, the diagnostic evaluation of the patient with pulmonary hypertension of uncertain etiology presents special challenges. These challenges must be met because errors in

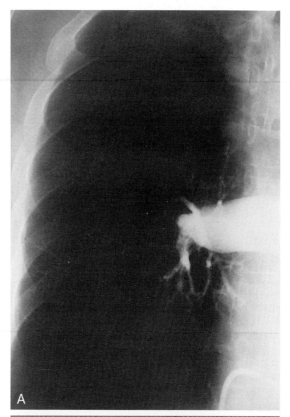

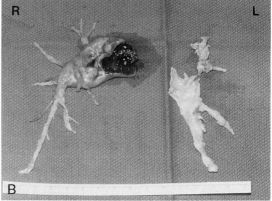

Figure 23–11. A, Near-complete obstruction of a right main pulmonary artery. *B,* Chronic thrombus removed at the time of pulmonary thromboendarterectomy.

chronic thrombi begin and establish whether they are within surgical reach. The procedure has not been associated with significant morbidity. With experience, "mapping" of the major vessels can be accomplished in 15 to 20 minutes.

Even angioscopy, however, may leave one residual question of importance in chronic thromboembolic pulmonary disease; namely, how thick are these proximal thrombi? Surgical removal requires establishment of a dissection differential diagnosis can place these patients on incorrect therapeutic pathways. With modern cardiac catheterization techniques and the availability of pulmonary angiography, pulmonary angioscopy, and other emerging modalities, the correct differential diagnosis is now within reach in most of these patients so that appropriate therapy can be selected.

REFERENCES

1. Nicod P, Peterson KL, Levine M, et al: Pulmonary angiography in severe chronic pulmonary hypertension. Ann Intern Med 1987; 107:565–568.
2. Auger WR, Fedullo PF, Moser KM, et al: Chronic major-vessel thromboembolic pulmonary artery obstruction: Appearance at angiography. Radiology 1992; 182:393–398.
3. Rich S, Dantzker DR, Ayres SM, et al: Primary pulmonary hypertension: A national prospective study. Ann Intern Med 1987; 107:216–223.
4. Perlmutt LM, Braun SD, Newman GE, et al: Pulmonary arteriography in the high-risk patient. Radiology 1987; 162:187–189.
5. Moser KM, Auger WR, Fedullo PF: Chronic major-vessel thromboembolic pulmonary hypertension. Circulation 1990; 81:1735–1743.
6. Rich S, Levitsky S, Brundage BH: Pulmonary hypertension from chronic pulmonary thromboembolism. Ann Intern Med 1988; 108:425–434.
7. Trulock EP, Cooper JD, Kaiser LR, et al: The Washington University–Barnes Hospital experience with lung transplantations. JAMA 1991; 266:1943–1946.
8. Dotter CT, Jackson FS: Death following angiocardiography. Radiology 1950; 54:527–533.
9. Diamond EG, Gonlubol F: Death following angiocardiography: Report of two cases after administration of Diodrast and Neo-iopax, respectively. N Engl J Med 1953; 249:1029–1031.
10. Rowe GG, Huston JH, Tuchman H, et al: The physiologic effect of contrast media used for angiocardiography. Circulation 1956; 13:896–904.
11. Alexander JK, Gonzales DA, Fred HL: Angiographic studies in cardiorespiratory diseases: Special reference to thromboembolism. JAMA 1966; 198:575–578.
12. Snider GL, Ferris E, Gaensler EA, et al: Primary pulmonary hypertension: A fatality during pulmonary angiography. Chest 1973; 64:628–635.
13. Caldini P, Gensini GG, Hoffman MS: Primary pulmonary hypertension with death during right heart catheterization. Am J Cardiol 1959; 519–527.
14. Dalen JE, Brooks HL, Johnson LW, et al: Pulmonary angiography in acute pulmonary embolism: Indications, techniques, and results in 367 patients. Am Heart J 1971; 81:175–185.
15. Marsh JD, Glynn M, Torman HA: Pulmonary angiography: Application in a new spectrum of patients. Am J Med 1983; 75:763–770.
16. Moses DC, Silver TM, Bookstein JJ: The complementary roles of chest radiography, lung scanning, and selective pulmonary angiography in the diagnosis of pulmonary embolism. Circulation 1974; 49:179–188.
17. Mills SR, Jackson DC, Older RA, et al: The incidence, etiologies, and avoidance of complications of pulmonary angiography in a large series. Radiology 1980; 136:295–299.
18. Almen T, Aspelin P, Levin B: Effect of ionic and non-ionic contrast medium on aortic and pulmonary arterial pressure: An angiocardiographic study in rabbits. Invest Radiol 1975; 10:519–525.
19. Ingleby TV, Raizner AE, Hanley HG, Skinner S Jr: Cardiovascular reflexes induced by selectively altering pulmonary osmolarity. Am J Physiol 1972; 222:302–307.
20. Agarwal JB, Baile EM, Palmer WH: Reflex systemic hypotension due to hypertonic solutions in pulmonary circulation. Am J Physiol 1969; 27:251–255.
21. Watson H: Severe pulmonary hypertension episodes following angiocardiography with sodium metrizoate. Lancet 1964; 2:732–733.
22. Tajima H, Kumazaki N, Tajima N, Ebata K: Effect of iohexol and diatrizoate on pulmonary arterial pressure following pulmonary angiography: A clinical comparison in man. Acta Radiol 1988; 29:487–490.
23. Kumazaki T: Ioxaglate versus diatrizoate in selective pulmonary angiography. Part II: Cardiovascular responses. Acta Radiol 1985; 26:635.
24. Kapitan KS, Buchbinder M, Wagner PD, Moser KM: Mechanisms of hypoxia in chronic thromboembolic pulmonary hypertension. Am Rev Respir Dis 1989; 139:1149–1154.
25. Saeed M, Braun SD, Cohan RH, et al: Pulmonary angiography with iopamidol: Patient comfort, image quality, and hemodynamics. Radiology 1987; 165:345–349.
26. Smith DC, Lois JF, Gomes AS, et al: Pulmonary angiography: Comparison of cough stimulation effects of diatrizoate and ioxaglate. Radiology 1987; 162:617–618.
27. Ryan KL, Fedullo PF, Davis GB, et al: Perfusion scan findings understate the severity of angiographic and hemodynamic compromise in chronic thromboembolic pulmonary hypertension. Chest 1988; 93:1180–1185.
28. Greenspan RH: Angiography in pulmonary embolism. *In* Abrams HL (ed): Angiography: Vascular and Interventional Radiology, 3rd ed. Boston, Little, Brown, 1983, pp 803–876.
29. Sutton GC, Hall RJC, Kerr IH: Clinical course and late prognosis of treated subacute massive, acute minor, and chronic pulmonary thromboembolism. Br Heart J 1977; 39:1135–1142.
30. McDonald IG, Hirsh J, Hale GS: Early rate of resolution of major pulmonary embolism. Br Heart J 1971; 33:432–437.
31. Dalen JE, Banas JS Jr, Brooks HL, et al: Resolution rate of acute pulmonary embolism in man. N Engl J Med 1969; 1194–1199.
32. Olsson HE, Spitzer RM, Erston WF: Primary and secondary artery neoplasia mimicking acute pulmonary embolism. Radiology 1976; 118:49–53.
33. Misra DP, Sunderrajan EV, Rosenholtz MJ, Hurst DJ: Malignant fibrous histiocytoma in the lung masquerading as recurrent pulmonary thromboembolism. Cancer 1983; 51:538–541.
34. Rich S, Brundage BH: High-dose calcium channel–blocking therapy for primary pulmonary hypertension: Evidence for long-term reduction in pulmonary arterial pressure and regression of right ventricular hypertrophy. Circulation 1987; 76:135–141.
35. Peterson Kirk L, Fred HL, Alexander JK: Pulmonary arterial webs: A new angiographic sign of previous thromboembolism. N Engl J Med 1967; 277:33.
36. D'Cruz IA, Agustsson MH, Bicoff JP, et al: Stenotic lesions of the pulmonary arteries: Clinical and hemodynamic findings in 84 cases. Am J Cardiol 1964; 13:441–450.
37. Delaney TB, Nadas AS: Peripheral pulmonic stenosis. Am J Cardiol 1964; 13:451–461.
38. Lupi E, Sanchez GT, Horwitz S, Gutierrez EF: Pulmonary artery involvement in Takayasu's arteritis. Chest 1975; 67:69–74.

39. Haas A, Stiehm R: Takayasu's arteritis presenting as pulmonary hypertension. Am J Dis Child 1986; 140:372–374.

40. Yamato M, Lecky JW, Hiramatsu K, Kohda E: Takayasu's arteritis: Radiographic and angiographic findings in 59 patients. Radiology 1986; 161:329–334.

41. Cho S-R, Tisnado J, Cockrell CH, et al: Angiographic evaluation of patients with unilateral massive perfusion defects in the lung scan. Radiographics 1987; 7:729–745.

42. Berry DF, Buccigrossi D, Peabody J, et al: Pulmonary vascular occlusion and fibrosing mediastinitis. Chest 1986; 89:296–301.

43. Arnett EN, Bacos JM, Macher AM, et al: Fibrosing mediastinitis causing pulmonary arterial hypertension without pulmonary venous hypertension. Am J Med 1977; 63:634–643.

44. Carlin BW, Moser KM: Pulmonary artery obstruction due to malignant fibrous histiocytoma. Chest 1987; 92:173–175.

45. Schermoly M, Overman J, Pingleton SK: Pulmonary artery sarcoma—unusual pulmonary angiographic findings–a case report. Angiology 1987; 617–621.

46. Moser KM, Olson LK, Schlusselberg M, et al: Chronic thromboembolic occlusion in the adult can mimic pulmonary agenesis. Chest 1989; 95:503–508.

47. Shure D, Gregoratos G, Moser KM: Fiberoptic angioscopy: Role in the diagnosis of chronic pulmonary arterial obstruction. Ann Intern Med 1985; 103:844–850.

48. Ricou F, Nicod PH, Moser KM, Peterson KL: Catheter-based intravascular ultrasound imaging of chronic thromboembolic pulmonary disease. Am J Cardiol 1991; 67:749–752.

Chapter 24

Catheterization and Angiography in Chronic Obstructive Pulmonary Disease

JAMES K. ALEXANDER

This chapter is designed to provide some background regarding experience with cardiac catheterization in patients with obstructive lung disease, summarizing anatomic and physiologic factors of importance in the analysis of catheterization data obtained under various conditions and indicating potential uses of the procedure. Technical aspects, discussed elsewhere in this text, are alluded to only in special settings. A reasonably comprehensive coverage of cardiovascular aspects of the disease is attempted, but without exhaustive review.

ANATOMY OF THE PULMONARY VASCULAR BED

Although the incidence in patients with obstructive lung disease is not well defined, muscularization of the precapillary arterioles is found on histologic examination postmortem in a significant number. This involves hyperplasia of smooth muscle cells distally in the media of small pulmonary arterioles to encompass the entire circumference of precapillary vessels that normally have little or no smooth muscle component.[1-3] These changes are also found in other settings of chronic alveolar hypoxia such as juvenile adenoid hyperplasia and residence at high altitudes, occurring in conjunction with hypoxic pulmonary vasoconstriction at this anatomic level.[3] The same histologic pattern can be induced in rats subjected to alveolar hypoxia for several weeks or longer, with reversal of the lesion on alleviation of hypoxia.[4-7] Electron microscopic studies show extrusion of the cytoplasm of smooth muscle cells through deficiencies in the outer elastic lamina into the adventi-

tia.[3] In addition, there may be increased medial thickness of the muscular pulmonary arteries, often associated with right ventricular hypertrophy, but the degree of thickening does not correlate with right ventricular weight.[8, 9]

HEMODYNAMIC CONSIDERATIONS

Pulmonary Vascular Resistance

Under normal conditions, pulmonary blood flow may be increased several-fold with little or no change in pulmonary artery pressure. The two predominant mechanisms accounting for this phenomenon appear to be recruitment of additional blood vessels previously unperfused and significantly increased distensibility of the pulmonary vascular bed as compared with the systemic. The relation between pressure and flow may be characterized in terms of the pulmonary vascular resistance. This is defined as the ratio of the pressure gradient across the pulmonary vascular bed, and the pulmonary blood flow

$$PVR = (PA_m - LA_m) \div CO$$

where PVR is pulmonary vascular resistance, PA_m is mean pulmonary artery pressure (mm Hg), LA_m is mean left atrial pressure (mm Hg), and CO is cardiac output (L/min).

The reproducibility of this calculation is of the order of $\pm 10\%$ using thermodilution or Fick methodology to assess flow and a fluid-filled catheter for pressure measurement. Results may be expressed as Wood units or millimeters of mercury per liter or converted to the unit dyne $\cdot$ sec^{-1} $\cdot$ cm^{-5}, multiplying by the conversion factor 80. In virtually all studies in patients with obstructive lung disease, pulmonary venous pressure, as reflected by pulmonary wedge or balloon occlusion pressure, has been substituted for left atrial pressure. This may condition interpretation of the result to some extent (see later). A pulmonary vascular resistance index may be derived by substituting cardiac index for cardiac output in the calculation. The usefulness of pulmonary vascular resistance is significantly limited by a number of factors that play a role in its determination. These include pulmonary blood volume, distensibility of the pulmonary vascular bed, pulmonary blood flow, lung inflation, left atrial pressure, alveolar Po_2, and arterial blood pH. Thus, the interpretation of this calculated parameter must be approached cautiously. Probably its usefulness relative to obstructive lung disease is greatest in assessing the hemodynamic effect of an acute intervention.

Pulmonary Artery Pressure

Determinants of pulmonary artery pressure in patients with obstructive lung disease include the size of the pulmonary vascular bed and its compliance, the degree of pulmonary vasomotor activity, pulmonary blood volume and flow, pulmonary venous pressure, blood viscosity, and intrathoracic pressure.[10, 11] Alveolar septation and the loss of pulmonary capillaries accompanying the development of obstructive lung disease with emphysema result in a decrement of pulmonary blood volume and reduced distensibility of the vascular bed with leg raising or exercise.[12] Diminished compliance of the pulmonary vascular tree also makes for an increase in pulse pressure at comparable stroke volume. Thus, in patients with obstructive lung disease and quasi-normal or elevated mean pulmonary artery pressures at rest, substantial increments may take place with exercise, associated with little change in arterial blood gas levels and pulmonary vascular resistance.[13–15] These observations support the conclusion that a decrement in the size of the pulmonary vascular bed secondary to a decreased number of vessels or structural alterations (thickened walls and reduced luminal size) in them may lead to an elevated pulmonary vascular resistance and flow-related pulmonary hypertension in some patients with obstructive lung disease.

In addition, pulmonary vasomotor activity related to alveolar oxygen tension and pulmonary blood pH may play an important role in the pathogenesis of pulmonary hypertension with obstructive lung disease. The importance of hypoxemia in the genesis of pulmonary hy-

pertension in patients with obstructive lung disease is emphasized by the strong negative correlation between arterial Po_2 and pulmonary artery pressure in the natural history of the disease,[16–18] an increase in pulmonary artery pressure with induced hypoxemia,[19, 20] and a decrease in pressure with oxygen administration.[14, 18, 21, 22] Another mechanism of pulmonary hypertension with some supportive data is the presence of increased alveolar and intrapleural pressure secondary to airway obstruction.[18, 23] The pulmonary capillary blood volume is decreased in emphysema.[24] The level of pulmonary artery pressure and increments in it correlate positively with central blood volume, total blood volume, and increments in them. However, blood viscosity has little effect in a range of hematocrits as high as 60% to 65%.[25]

Mechanisms of Hypoxic Vasoconstriction and Oxygen Therapy

Hypoxic pulmonary vasoconstriction is an important mechanism in the matching of perfusion to ventilation and therefore the maintenance of arterial oxygen tension. Thus, poorly ventilated lung segments receive lesser perfusion. Both alveolar oxygen tension and pulmonary arterial blood oxygen tension contribute to the hypoxic response, although the alveolar component is predominant.[26] Vasoconstriction in a hypoventilated lung segment is accompanied by a decrement in lung volume[27] and diversion of blood flow from the hypoxic site.[28] Most investigators appear to agree that the site of vasoconstriction is at the location of the precapillary pulmonary arteries.

The mechanism of hypoxic vasoconstriction in terms of a sensor-mediator-effector cycle has not been defined. Indeed, whether the response is mediated or results from the direct effect of reduced oxygen tension on the blood vessel is unknown. Calcium dependency of response appears to be established on the basis of enhancement in the setting of increased calcium influx and diminution with blockage of calcium entry into some lung cells.[29] In vitro studies of pulmonary artery rings from patients with hypoxic cor pulmonale, obtained at the time of heart-lung transplantation, have indicated impairment of relaxation mediated by endothelium-derived relaxing factor.[30] Several investigations of intracellular mechanisms include hypoxia-induced depolarization of smooth muscle cells of the pulmonary artery, increased sensitivity to hypoxia with inhibition of oxidative phosphorylation, inhibition of the pressor re-

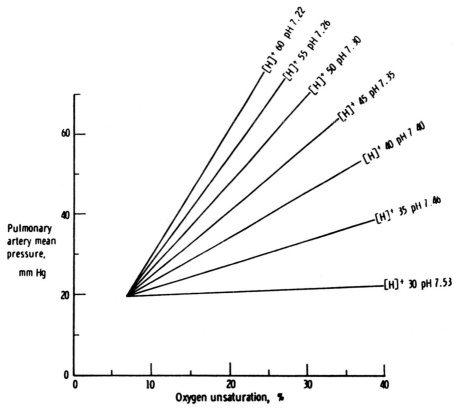

Figure 24–1. Relationship among pulmonary artery mean pressure, arterial blood oxyhemoglobin unsaturation, and hydrogen ion concentration. (From Enson Y, Giuntini C, Lewis ML, et al: The influence of hydrogen in concentration and hypoxia on the pulmonary circulation. Reproduced from The Journal of Clinical Investigation, 1964; 43:1146–1162 by copyright permission of The American Society for Clinical Investigation.)

sponse by hydrogen peroxide, and increased pulmonary leukotriene synthesis with hypoxia.[29]

Acidosis potentiates hypoxic vasoconstriction,[31] and, by infusion of alkalizing agents with and without hypoxic effects, it has been shown that the hypoxic pulmonary pressor response in patients with obstructive lung disease is a function of blood pH[32] (Fig. 24–1). Thus, hypercapnia, either acute or chronic, has important hemodynamic implications in these patients.

Hypoventilation and transient arterial oxygen desaturation during rapid-eye-movement sleep frequently occur in patients with obstructive lung disease, precipitating recurrent nocturnal pulmonary hypertension,[33, 34] possibly accelerating the development of structural changes in the pulmonary vessels,[35] and contributing to the progressive rise in pulmonary artery pressure with declining arterial PO_2 over the long term.[16, 36] Transient elevation of pulmonary artery pressure, cardiac output, and right ventricular filling pressure may accompany the superimposition of an acute respiratory infection in patients with preexisting obstructive lung disease,[37, 38] subsiding with treatment.

Response to both acute and chronic oxygen administration is quite variable in obstructive lung disease. In the acute setting, it has been found that most patients experience an increase in ventilatory dead space during oxygen administration. This suggests that, in the group of patients with hypoxic vasoconstriction, this is lessened by oxygen administration, with diversion of blood flow to poorly ventilated areas and consequent augmentation of dead space. Thus, the hypoxemic vasoconstrictive response favors matching of ventilation and perfusion at the expense of higher pulmonary artery pressure, whereas absence of the vasoconstrictive response favors a lesser degree of pulmonary hypertension at the expense of increased hypoxemia and hypercapnia. This latter response appears to be associated with better prognosis in some studies[39] but not in others.[13]

Acute oxygen administration to patients with pulmonary hypertension and obstructive lung disease usually results in modest decrements in pulmonary artery pressure or vascular resistance, and pressure virtually never normalizes.[13, 21, 22] This has been interpreted as indicating a diminished distensibility of the pulmonary vascular bed, making for a component of pulmonary hypertension independent of vasomotor effects. However, the degree of right ventricular hypertrophy does not correlate with the degree of emphysematous change.[40, 41] In the setting of acute respiratory failure precipitated by lung infection, oxygen administration usually effects little change in pulmonary artery pressure, but, despite a fall in cardiac output, enhanced oxygen delivery may be possible in patients with severe hypoxemia.[42]

Studies of long-term oxygen administration in patients with obstructive lung disease have demonstrated modest reduction in pulmonary artery pressure or failure of pulmonary hypertension to progress.[17, 43–46] The favorable effect on mortality in these studies does not appear to be well correlated with the improvement in pulmonary hemodynamic patterns. The response to acute administration of oxygen may be predictive of the long-term effect on pulmonary artery pressure[47] but not on survival.[48]

Interaction of the structural and vasomotor factors, in part related to the airway obstructive defect, appears to be the predominant mechanism for the genesis of pulmonary hypertension at rest, but more particularly during exercise.[49, 50]

Cardiac Output

A variety of factors may affect cardiac output in patients with obstructive lung disease, including the size of the pulmonary vascular bed, arterial blood oxygen pressure or saturation, pulmonary artery pressure, pulmonary vascular resistance, blood volume, blood viscosity, right and left ventricular loading conditions, and respiratory work. Although it has been possible to assign relative degrees of importance to some of these factors, a unifying hypothesis to account for regulation of cardiac output has proved elusive.

In most patients, cardiac index at rest tends to fall in a normal range, and the increment with exercise is normal relative to the increment in oxygen consumption.[25, 51, 52] Markedly elevated pulmonary vascular resistance and right ventricular afterload, with or without depressed myocardial contractility, is the generally accepted basis for reduced cardiac output at rest and during exercise in the setting of frank cor pulmonale with systemic venous congestion and edema. However, cardiac output is often at normal levels in these patients, associated with low systemic arterial pressure; reduced renal plasma flow; and elevated levels of plasma norepinephrine, renin, vasopressin, atrial natriuretic peptide, and growth hormone.[53] The development of edema in such patients appears to be more related to the renal and neurohumoral effects of hypercapnia and vasodilation than to the levels of pulmonary artery pressure and cardiac output.[53, 54]

The basis for significant limitation of cardiac output during exercise, associated with concomitant limitation of maximal oxygen uptake and exercise tolerance in many other patients, has not been clearly defined. In obstructive lung disease, the adequacy of oxygen delivery relative to demand is reflected by the mixed venous blood oxygen tension or saturation.[55] The importance of cardiac output is emphasized by studies showing that the level of mixed venous oxygen tension can be maintained with or without arterial hypoxemia if systemic blood flow is adequately sustained,[56] even though polycythemia may play a partially compensatory role in the setting of severe arterial hypoxemia.[57] Exercise tolerance, oxygen uptake, and cardiac output appear to be limited by ventilatory mechanics and respiratory work in some patients. In one study of patients with comparable and moderately elevated pulmonary artery pressure at rest and during exercise, the subjects could be divided into two groups of low and high cardiac output response to exercise.[58] Although pulmonary vascular resistance was higher and arterial PO_2 slightly lower in the low-output group, the chief differentiating factors were lower exercise ventilation and first second forced expiratory volume, and a higher ratio of functional residual capacity to total lung volume. Finally, in two clinical types of chronic lung disease, cardiac output tends to be significantly different: In the patients having a predominantly bronchitic component to the disease with severe hypoxemia, hypoventilation, polycythemia, and pulmonary hypertension ("blue bloaters"), cardiac index is usually normal or elevated, whereas in those with predominant emphysema, hyperventilation, and lesser degrees of hypoxemia ("pink puffers"), cardiac index tends to be reduced.[59–61]

Pulmonary Wedge Pressure

The pulmonary wedge pressure may be assessed either by mechanical wedging of an open-ended catheter, such as a Cournand catheter, into a distal pulmonary artery or by measurement of pressure in a pulmonary artery distal to balloon occlusion. The wedge pressure provides a measurement of left atrial pressure based on the assumption that flow beyond the occlusion is stopped with the distal vasculature functioning as inert tubing, transmitting pressure changes in the left atrium. Whichever technique is used, the pressure contour should reflect that characteristic of the left atrium with a and v waves in the absence of valvular or pericardial disease, and the pulmonary artery pressure waveform should appear promptly on withdrawal of the catheter from the wedge position or on deflation of the balloon. Another criterion for adequacy of the wedge pressure as a reflection of left atrial pressure is the aspiration of pulmonary capillary blood with an oxygen saturation higher than that of systemic arterial blood.[62] Integration of pressure curves for three or more respiratory cycles to obtain mean wedge pressure usually yields levels 2 or 3 mm Hg less than those at end-expiration in patients with obstructive lung disease.

Interpretation of wedge pressure levels in patients with obstructive lung disease may be difficult, especially if the levels are elevated. Levels may be different at various wedging sites in the same lung, more so with distal wedging than balloon occlusion, and aspiration of an appropriately wedged catheter may yield blood oxygen saturation levels as much as 3% below systemic in areas of abnormal perfusion as indicated by absence of capillary blush on wedge angiogram.[63] There is generally good agreement between values obtained by distal wedging and balloon occlusion, but the difference may be as much as 13 mm Hg higher with distal wedging.[63] These higher distal pressures may reflect local perfusion inhomogeneity secondary to venous constriction or collapse rather than left atrial pressure.[64, 65] Balloon occlusion appears to be associated with less pressure variability at different sites than is catheter wedging in obstructive lung disease. Abnormal elevation of wedge pressure during exercise may sometimes be observed secondary to marked increase in intrapleural pressure.[66] When absolute (relative to atmosphere) and effective (atmosphere minus intrapleural) wedge pressures are compared, agreement is often within 3 mm Hg, but with respiratory intrathoracic pressure variations that exceed 20 mm Hg, mean absolute pressures may be 6 to 17 mm Hg higher.[67] Comparison of wedge and left ventricular end-diastolic pressures at rest in patients with obstructive lung disease usually yields good agreement, but wedge pressure is higher in some patients for the reasons noted earlier.[68] Reasonable procedures would be measurement of wedge pressure at more than one site if elevated and use of a single site for serial measurements assessing the effect of an intervention.[63]

In patients with obstructive lung disease, mean wedge pressure at rest is usually in a normal range (3 to 12 mm Hg), but with frank cor pulmonale and systemic venous congestion, it is often elevated.[66, 69–72] A rise to abnormal levels (>12 to 15 mm Hg) during exercise frequently occurs, particularly if there is a concomitant rise in right atrial pressure.[69, 73, 74] The correlation between right and left atrial pressure increases during hyperventilation as well as exercise has led to the suggestion that tachypnea with consequent gas trapping may result in lower lobe distention, increased pressure around the heart (juxtacardiac pressure), and cardiac compression, that is, a tamponade effect.[75, 76] Wedge pressure does faithfully reflect left ventricular end-diastolic pressure to a large extent during exercise,[77] and esophageal (intrathoracic) pressures often do not rise.[75, 77]

THE RIGHT VENTRICLE

In those patients with hepatomegaly, edema, or other evidence of systemic venous congestion, right ventricular dilation and hypertrophy can usually be demonstrated on echocardiographic or postmortem examination,[78, 79] but correlation with the extent of anatomic pulmonary involvement is often poor.[80, 81] The functional significance of right ventricular hypertrophy in such patients remains somewhat controversial. Assessment of function has largely involved measurement of right ventricular ejection fraction by radionuclide methods. Right ventricular ejection fraction is normal in most patients and depressed in others, generally those with a diagnosis of cor pulmonale.[82–84] A negative correlation between ejection fraction at rest and pulmonary artery pressure has been found in some studies[85, 86] but not in others.[78, 87] Failure of right ventricular ejection fraction to rise normally with exercise is frequently observed[83, 87–89] Severe hypoxemia during exercise may be associated with a decrement in right ventricular ejection fraction, little modified by acute oxygen administration or long-term therapy, which result in modest reduction in pulmonary artery pressure and little effect on ejection fraction.[87]

Because ejection fraction is sensitive to ventricular afterload, reduction in ejection fraction or its failure to increase normally may be secondary either to augmented afterload or to compromised ventricular contractility. Under acute conditions, it has been shown in the animal laboratory that the slope of the end-systolic pressure volume relationship in the left ventricle is linear, independent of preload and end-systolic pressure, as well as indicative of the ventricular inotropic state.[90] Other laboratory studies have demonstrated a similar relationship for the right ventricle.[91] Although studies of this relationship in humans have established some usefulness in relation to left ventricular function,[92, 93] there is little information regarding its usage for appraisal of right ventricular performance. Such appraisal in patients with obstructive lung disease is complicated by (1) chronic change in ventricular configuration or hypertrophy necessitating the use of end-systolic stress-volume relationship for definition of a linear result[94]; (2) right ventricular dilation and hypertrophy occurring concomitantly in virtually all patients with chronic lung disease[95]; and (3) questionable accuracy of right ventricular wall stress estimates due to cavity configuration. In one study of seven patients using sodium nitroprusside infusion to define two points on the right ventricular end-systolic pressure-volume slope, assuming a linear relation, there was poor correlation between the slope and the ejection fraction.[88] In addition, the resting end-systolic pressure-volume ratio correlated poorly with the slope. The authors concluded that the ejection fraction and resting pressure-volume ratio were unreliable indices of right ventricular contractile state in obstructive lung disease. Ventricular wall stress data were not available for this analysis.

In another study, the pressure-volume ratio was examined during leg raising and exercise as compared with the resting value.[96] In patients with significantly elevated pulmonary vascular resistance and no significant increase in ejection fraction during exercise, there was an abnormal response, that is, a fall in the ratio during leg raising. However, there was some modest increment during exercise, leading the authors to conclude that even in those patients with depressed contractile function, enhancement could occur during exercise.

Right ventricular end-systolic pressure-volume and stress-volume index ratios in patients with chronic obstructive lung disease at rest and during exercise were defined in another study, examining the relation between these findings and the ejection fraction, as well as the presence or absence of ventricular hypertrophy.[78] Two groups of patients were identified: those with an increase in pressure-volume ratio during exercise and those without. In those with significant hypertrophy, ratios tended to increase during exercise, despite variable changes in ejection fraction, suggesting preserved contractile performance in the setting of increased afterload. In those without an increased ratio during exercise, an inappropriate systolic wall stress developed, and ejection fractions fell significantly more. Thus, it appears that assessment

of the right ventricular contractile state remains elusive in the clinical setting, but significant depression of ejection fraction (5% to 15%) on exercise implies a deficit.

Little information is available regarding right ventricular diastolic function in obstructive lung disease. Elevated right ventricular diastolic pressure at rest or during exercise is commonly present in this setting, secondary to several factors. These include diminished right ventricular compliance associated with the hypertrophy itself, increased ventricular afterload, elevated intrathoracic pressure, and augmented blood volume.[15]

The right atrial emptying rate during early ventricular diastole is slowed in the presence of pulmonary hypertension compatible with the altered ventricular filling dynamics of hypertrophy.[97]

THE LEFT VENTRICLE

The question of structural and functional alterations in the left heart consequent to chronic obstructive lung disease has attracted some interest, with a number of investigations addressing it. A major obstacle to the definition of such effects is the frequency of concomitant entities such as systemic hypertensive, coronary, valvular, or myopathic disease. Thus, cardiac catheterization to include coronary arteriography and myocardial biopsy would presumably be necessary to rule out accompanying disease with confidence and isolate the effects of lung disease, per se. Rigorous studies of this order are almost nonexistent, yet postmortem observations, laboratory experiments, and clinical studies do provide some insight.

In postmortem studies excluding other cardiac disease and using left ventricular weight as the criterion for diagnosis of hypertrophy in obstructive lung disease, the incidence appears to be low.[98–100] If left ventricular thickness is taken as the criterion,[101] the incidence is reported to be 25%. A partial explanation for the finding of left ventricular hypertrophy in the presence of right ventricular hypertrophy may relate to the fact that the middle layer of the ventricular septum is composed of fibers that are continuous with those of the left ventricular free wall.[102]

A single report of recurrent left ventricular failure, elevated left ventricular diastolic pressures, Kerley's B lines on chest radiography, and biventricular dilation and hypertrophy on postmortem examination in eight patients with obstructive lung disease appeared in 1968.[103]

These patients were virtually free of coronary disease at autopsy and gave no history of alcoholism. The authors concluded that cor pulmonale in these patients might be regarded as a generalized cardiomyopathy, with severe left ventricular failure occasionally presenting as the dominant clinical feature. No further reports of this kind have appeared. The salient feature distinguishing these patients from others reported is the finding of marked left ventricular dilation. An equally or perhaps more plausible view would be that these patients represent a group with idiopathic dilated cardiomyopathy with some element of concomitant obstructive lung disease.[104]

Laboratory studies have provided evidence for ventricular interdependence, both anatomically and biochemically. Pulmonary artery banding in dogs results in greater myocardial cell length and intercalated disk width, with longer sarcomere length in both ventricles.[105] In cats with right ventricular pressure load hypertrophy, myocardial collagen as indicated by hydroxyproline concentration increases in both ventricles.[106] In the setting of right ventricular failure secondary to pressure overload, left ventricular myofibrillar adenosine triphosphatase activity and creatinine phosphate levels are depressed.[107, 108] Norepinephrine stores in both ventricles are depressed in dogs with heart failure secondary to pulmonary artery constriction and tricuspid insufficiency.[109]

Insight into the hemodynamic and mechanical effects of ventricular interaction in the setting of acute and chronic pulmonary hypertension has resulted from experimental observations. In the closed-chest dog, for example, acute elevation of pulmonary artery mean pressure to 60 mm Hg is associated with right ventricular dilation and a tripling of end-diastolic pressure, accompanied by a 20% to 30% decrease in left ventricular end-diastolic volume and a fall in end-diastolic pressure, stroke volume, and ejection fraction.[110] Septal bulging brings about a shortening of the mid-ventricular diameter in diastole and systole. However, very high pulmonary artery pressures are required for these changes, there being little effect on these left ventricular parameters with pulmonary artery mean pressures as high as 30 mm Hg. In dogs with severe chronic pulmonary hypertension, there is a decrease in left ventricular chamber compliance, together with a reduction in peak left ventricular maximum rate of tension development and peak contractile element velocity.[111] It is unclear whether these changes in systolic performance represent an impairment in contractility or a mechanical effect secondary to altered geometry.

Another animal study of left ventricular performance with right ventricular dilation and hypertrophy relates to brisket disease in cattle secondary to hypoxic pulmonary hypertension at high altitude.[112] Using the relationship of left ventricular stroke work to filling pressure as an index of function, improvement in function curves was demonstrated when the animals were taken to a lower altitude, pulmonary artery pressures decreased, and manifestations of the disease regressed.

In patients with obstructive lung disease, studies of standard left ventricular function curves relating filling pressure to stroke volume or stroke work under conditions of increasing afterload have demonstrated little deviation from normal.[113-116] However, abnormal responses to exercise in left ventricular ejection fraction have been found in patients with and without cor pulmonale.[117] Failure to increase stroke volume or ejection fraction, or both, has been ascribed to elevated pulmonary vascular resistance and diminished left ventricular inflow.[116-119] Abnormal left ventricular ejection fractions at rest and during exercise in patients with obstructive lung disease and free of other cardiac disease are poorly correlated with hypoxemia, hypercarbia, and acidosis.[120] In one study, elevated left ventricular end-diastolic pressures and function curves were found after angiotensin infusion,[121] but left ventricular volumes and pulmonary and systemic artery pressures were not recorded after infusion, and angiotensin may have caused ventricular dysfunction.[122]

Little information is available regarding diastolic left ventricular function in obstructive lung disease. One study was carried out in such patients, excluding those with hypertension or coronary disease and characterizing response according to subgroups without congestive failure, history of failure, or current frank manifestations of failure.[123] Left ventricular end-diastolic pressures were in a normal range in all patients at rest, as were indices of systolic function on exercise. However, during exercise and after angiotensin infusion, both right and left ventricular diastolic pressures rose to abnormal levels (Fig. 24–2). Elevated left ventricular diastolic pressures have also been found in patients with obstructive lung disease, normal coronary arteriograms, and decreased mitral E-F slope on echocardiogram.[124] Abnormal left ventricular end-diastolic pressure-volume relationships suggestive of diminished chamber compliance have been reported in a single study.[125]

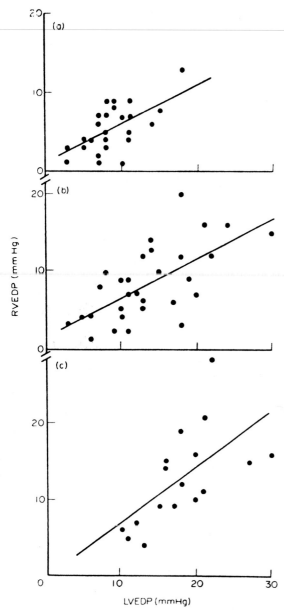

Figure 24–2. Relationship between left and right end-diastolic pressures at rest (a), during exercise (b), and during angiotensin infusion (c). (From Jezek V, Schrijen F: Left ventricular function in chronic obstructive pulmonary disease with and without cardiac failure. Clin Sci Mol Med 1973; 45:267–279.)

PHARMACOLOGIC INTERVENTIONS

Recent pharmacologic interventions in obstructive lung disease have largely involved trials of agents designed to produce pulmonary vasodilation. Most of these trials have monitored acute or short-term effects, with few relating to long-term administration. A pulmonary vasodilator effect has not always been achieved, and some-

times systemic circulatory effects have predominated. Side effects have been frequent, and, in many patients, hypoxemia has been worsened because of increased perfusion of poorly ventilated regions. There appears to be no selective pulmonary vasodilator agent. Symptomatic benefit has been variable, with no evidence that survival is prolonged. Arrest or reversal of bronchial or pulmonary vascular disease has not been demonstrated.[126, 127]

Parameters examined at cardiac catheterization usually include pulmonary artery and wedge pressures, pulmonary blood flow, and right ventricular filling pressure. Concomitant effects on systemic and pulmonary blood oxygen tension or saturation and systemic arterial pressure are also monitored. In all such studies attempting to assess the effects of an intervention, the degree of spontaneous variation in measured parameters is of critical importance. Although the average changes in patients with obstructive lung disease studied at rest over a 30-minute period for mean pulmonary artery and wedge pressures approximate 3 to 4 mm Hg, the range for pulmonary artery pressure is up to 5 mm Hg and, for wedge pressure, up to 7 mm Hg.[128] Standard deviations for the differences in mean pulmonary artery pressure may be 14%; for pulmonary vascular resistance, 20%; and for pulmonary blood flow, 14%.[129, 130] In acute studies involving repeat exercise, pulmonary artery and wedge pressures may be lower without any intervention,[131] and, if repeat studies are done at 10-minute intervals during exercise, the coefficients of variation may be 13% for mean pulmonary artery pressure, 11% for pulmonary blood flow, and 34% for pulmonary vascular resistance.[132] Observations of this type serve to emphasize that demonstration of statistical significance for differences in data points with an intervention may or may not carry physiologic impact, and the data must be examined in relation to spontaneous variation and repeatability.

No attempt is made here to critically review the results of various pharmacologic interventions carried out in the setting of obstructive lung disease, but those agents receiving the most attention are mentioned, together with some notation of their effects.

Acute hemodynamic studies of the frequently used bronchodilator agents theophylline and terbutaline have demonstrated reduction in pulmonary vascular resistance.[133, 134] Improved right ventricular ejection fraction has been observed with both agents, although cardiac index tends to increase only with terbutaline.[135] Sustained improvement in right ventricular ejection fraction with oral theophylline therapy over a 4-month period has been observed.[136]

Of the direct-acting vasodilator agents, hydralazine has probably received the greatest attention. In some studies, hydralazine has been reported to improve cardiac output and mixed venous blood oxygen saturation, sometimes with reduction in pulmonary artery pressure and resistance[137] and sometimes not.[138, 139] Neither acute nor longer-term hydralazine therapy increases maximal oxygen consumption during exercise, but it does produce an increase in ventilation,[140, 141] often with increased dyspnea.[140]

Of the calcium channel blocking agents, nifedipine has been investigated most frequently and appears to be somewhat more effective than diltiazem and verapamil in reducing pulmonary vascular resistance in patients with obstructive lung disease.[142] At rest and during upright cycle exercise, increased pulmonary blood flow is accompanied by a decrement in mean pulmonary artery pressure after acute administration of oral or sublingual nifedipine but with no increase in exercise tolerance.[143, 144] Although nifedipine attenuates the pulmonary vasoconstrictive effect of acutely induced hypoxia,[145] its effect on arterial oxygen tension may[146] or may not[143, 144] be deleterious. With long-term administration, the increase in pulmonary vascular resistance is attenuated or virtually disappears, and the response to oxygen administration is blocked.[146, 147] Neither verapamil[148] nor diltiazem[149] appears to produce consistent salutary effects on pulmonary hemodynamics in obstructive lung disease, and long-term clinical benefit of nifedipine therapy has not been demonstrated.[150, 151]

Studies on the effects of angiotensin-converting enzyme inhibitors in patients with obstructive lung disease are virtually all acute, limited to the use of captopril, and often associated with predominantly systemic circulatory changes. Captopril appears to block the development of hypoxic pulmonary vasoconstriction in rats[152] but not in cats,[153] with variable effect in humans. Acute studies in patients with obstructive lung disease have demonstrated little change in arterial blood gases, a fall in systemic arterial blood pressure, and, in some patients, salutary effects on pulmonary hemodynamics.[154–156] Decrements in mean pulmonary artery pressure and pulmonary vascular resistance have been observed with an increase in cardiac output. However, in other studies, these changes have not been found,[157–160] and it is unclear what factors may account for these diverse results.

Two prostaglandins, prostaglandin E_1 (PGE$_1$)

and prostacyclin, possessing both systemic and pulmonary vascular dilating effects, have received limited trials in patients with obstructive lung disease. During intravenous infusion of PGE$_1$, decrements in pulmonary artery pressure and vascular resistance, in conjunction with increased cardiac output and oxygen transport, have been demonstrated,[161, 162] as well as after administration of an oral analog over 8 hours.[163] Similar results have been obtained during infusion of prostacyclin,[164, 165] but decrements in arterial blood oxygen tension and oxygen transport occur in some patients. PGE$_1$ does not inhibit hypoxic pulmonary vasoconstriction in normal subjects,[161, 166] and side effects of headache, malaise, hypotension, facial flushing, and diarrhea have proved to be vexing problems associated with both agents.

Almitrine, an orally administered peripheral chemoreceptor agonist, tends to improve arterial blood oxygen tension and saturation in patients with hypoxic obstructive lung disease, usually to a greater extent than can be accounted for on the basis of the increase in ventilation alone. Although not apparent in one study,[167] in others this effect was accompanied by an increment in pulmonary artery pressure both acutely and over the long term at rest and during exercise, as well as incapacitating dyspnea in some patients.[168, 169] Neither the mechanisms for the improvement in oxygenation nor the pulmonary hypertension appear to be well understood, although the latter may be conditioned by decreased distensibility of the pulmonary arteries,[170] and stimulation of the chemoreceptors does increase pulmonary artery pressure in the dog.[171]

Although noninvasive modalities such as echocardiography and radionuclide studies may provide useful information in the evaluation of pharmacologic-agent effects in patients with obstructive lung disease, right-sided heart catheterization remains the accepted standard.

PULMONARY ANGIOGRAPHY

In patients with predominant emphysema (pink puffers), the pulmonary angiogram usually demonstrates enlargement of both left and right proximal pulmonary arteries, which diminish rapidly in diameter, giving rise to a less than normal number of relatively small pulmonary arteries.[172] The distal arterial tree divides in a divaricate wide-angled manner with few branches, ending in small, fine, straight terminal twigs. The upper lobe arteries fill with contrast agent more rapidly and completely than do the lower lobe arteries. Injected lung specimens at postmortem demonstrate marked reduction in the number of side branches from the axial pathway, but still more pulmonary artery branches than airway branches.[173]

In patients with predominantly bronchitic disease (blue bloaters), the proximal pulmonary arteries also tend to be enlarged, but there is no abnormal diminution in size distally, and the terminal vascularization has a fastigatum type of branching. However, some of the smaller branches may be occluded. There is no regional variation in vascular opacification.[172]

Pulmonary artery wedge arteriography involving hand injection of a small amount of contrast material through the end hole of the wedged catheter may be useful in characterizing the distal pulmonary vasculature. Normally, multiple arborizing vessels are opacified from the central artery with a capillary background "blush" and early filling of paralobular veins (Fig. 24–3). With obstructive lung disease, changes of varying severity may take place.[174–176] These include less arborization, later progression to small vessel dilation and irregular filling defects, and poor capillary blush. In the advanced stage, there is terminal truncation of the arterial tree, absent capillary blush, and diminished venous filling (Fig. 24–4).

Some correlation may exist between the severity of pulmonary wedge angiographic changes and the transpulmonic vascular driving pressure (pulmonary artery mean pressure minus wedge pressure),[176] but these changes are not predictive, and, in other studies, correlation of wedge angiographic findings with hemodynamic parameters has been relatively poor.[174, 175]

The dichotomy between pulmonary vascular anatomy and blood flow in obstructive lung disease is emphasized by the frequently observed discrepancy between the findings on arteriography and radionuclide scintillation scanning.[177] From a practical standpoint, it appears that pulmonary angiography in obstructive lung disease can be performed relatively safely and is most useful in the setting of suspected pulmonary embolism.

INDICATIONS FOR CARDIAC CATHETERIZATION IN PATIENTS WITH CHRONIC OBSTRUCTIVE LUNG DISEASE

Indications for cardiac catheterization in patients with chronic obstructive lung disease include the following:

1. Right-sided heart catheterization to include measurement of cardiac output and pulmonary wedge, pulmonary artery, and right ventricular diastolic or right atrial pressures, together with blood gas analyses, should be carried out in conjunction with interventions such as vasodilator or almitrine therapy in an acute setting or serially over the long term. These data are useful not only in assessing the qualitative effect of these interventions but also in providing guidance relative to dosage.

2. Routine right-sided heart catheterization

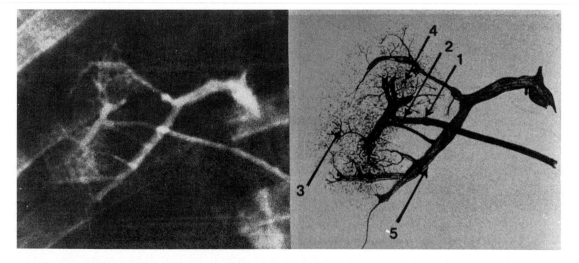

Figure 24–3. Peripheral wedge angiogram in healthy lung *(left)*. The diagrammatic sketch *(right)* shows (**1**) a wedged catheter; (**2**) a normal central lobular artery; (**3**) divided into two branches, normal arborizing vessels; (**4**) normal capillary background blush; and (**5**) paralobular veins. (From Bracchi G, Barbaccia P, Vezzoli F, et al: Peripheral pulmonary wedge angiography in chronic obstructive pulmonary disease: Relationship to pulmonary function, chest x-ray film, and hemodynamic data. CHEST 1977; 7:718–724.)

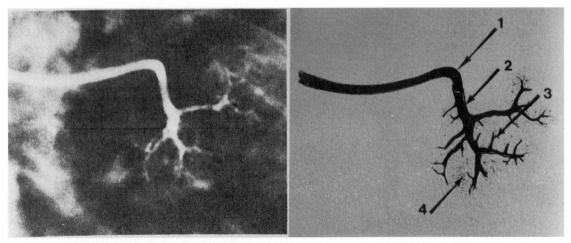

Figure 24–4. Peripheral wedge angiogram, arterial phase, in a patient with severe pulmonary emphysema *(left)*. The diagrammatic sketch *(right)* shows (1) a wedged catheter; (2) a normal lobular artery; (3) a marked decrease in the number of arborizing vessels; and (4) loss of capillary background blush. (From Bracchi G, Barbaccia P, Vezzoli F, et al: Peripheral pulmonary wedge angiography in chronic obstructive pulmonary disease: Relationship to pulmonary function, chest x-ray film, and hemodynamic data. CHEST 1977; 7:718–724.)

prior to initiation of long-term oxygen therapy is controversial.[178, 179] Although the presence of pulmonary hypertension is not an essential criterion and may not directly reflect results, knowledge of pulmonary and right-sided heart hemodynamics may provide an additional impetus one way or the other for decision making in some instances.

3. In patients with documented or suspected sleep apnea, nocturnal studies to include right-sided heart catheterization may provide information useful in determining the mode of therapy and, with serial observations, its effectiveness.

4. In the setting of acute and life-threatening illness, particularly in the differentiation of cardiogenic and noncardiogenic pulmonary edema, appraisal of pulmonary hemodynamics to include cautious interpretation of pulmonary wedge pressure may provide information critical to appropriate therapy.

5. The indications for left-sided heart catheterization in conjunction with coronary, myocardial, or valvular heart disease are, in most patients, not greatly different from those in patients without lung disease, but concomitant right-sided heart catheterization will provide information useful in diagnosis and therapy.

REFERENCES

1. Hicken P, Heath D, Brewer B, Whitaker W: The small pulmonary arteries in emphysema. J Pathol Bacteriol 1965; 90:107–114.
2. Hasleton PS, Heath D, Brewer DB: Hypertensive pulmonary vascular disease in states of chronic hypoxia. J Pathol Bacteriol 1968; 95:431–440.
3. Heath D, Smith P: Electron microscopy of hypertensive pulmonary vascular disease. Br J Dis Chest 1983; 77:1–13.
4. Heath D: Reversibility of cardiopulmonary changes in rats induced by simulated high altitude. Prog Respir Res 1975; 9:118–120.
5. Leach E, Howard P, Barer GR: Resolution of hypoxic changes in the heart pulmonary arterioles of rats during intermittent correction of hypoxia. Clin Sci Mol Med 1976; 52:153–162.
6. Kay JM: Effect of intermittent normoxia on chronic hypoxic pulmonary hypertension, right ventricular hypertrophy, and polycythemia in rats. Am Rev Respir Dis 1980; 121:993–1001.
7. Kay JM, Sutma KL, Keave PM: Effect of intermittent normoxia on muscularization of pulmonary arterioles induced by chronic hypoxia in rats. Am Rev Respir Dis 1981; 123:484–488.
8. Wagenvoort CA, Wagenvoort N: Hypoxic pulmonary vascular lesions in man at high altitude and in patients with chronic respiratory disease. Pathol et Microbiol 1973; 39:276–282.
9. Siemmens M, Reid L: Pulmonary arterial muscularity and right ventricular hypertrophy in chronic bronchitis and emphysema. Br J Dis Chest 1974; 68:253–263.
10. McFadden ER Jr, Braunwald E: Cor pulmonale and pulmonary thromboembolism. In Braunwald E (ed): Heart Disease: A Textbook of Cardiovascular Medicine. Philadelphia, WB Saunders, 1987, pp 1572–1598.
11. Agarwal JB, Tattoo R, Palmer WH: Relative viscosity of blood at varying hematocrits in pulmonary circulation. J Appl Physiol 1970; 29:866–871.
12. Schrijen F, Urtiaga B: Pulmonary blood volume in chronic lung disease changes with legs raised and during exercise. Chest 1982; 81:544–549.
13. Ashutosh K, Mead G, Dunsky M: Early effects of oxygen administration and prognosis in chronic pulmonary disease and cor pulmonale. Am Rev Respir Dis 1983; 127:399–404.
14. Finlay M, Middleton MC, Peake MD, Howard P: Cardiac output, pulmonary hypertension, hypoxaemia,

and survival in patients with chronic obstructive airways disease. Eur J Respir Dis 1983; 64:252–263.

15. Jezek V, Schrijen F, Sadoul P: Right ventricular function and pulmonary hemodynamics during exercise in patients with chronic obstructive bronchopulmonary disease. Cardiology 1973; 58:20–31.

16. Weitzenblum E, Loiseau A, Hirth C, et al: Course of pulmonary hemodynamics in patients with chronic obstructive pulmonary disease. Chest 1979; 75:656–662.

17. Report of the Medical Research Council Working Party: Long-term domiciliary oxygen therapy in chronic hypoxic cor pulmonale complicating chronic bronchitis and emphysema. Lancet 1981; 1:680–685.

18. Wright JL, Lawson L, Pare PD, et al: The structure and function of the pulmonary vasculature in mild chronic obstructive pulmonary disease. Am Rev Respir Dis 1983; 128:702–707.

19. Fishman AP, McClement J, Himmelstein A, Cournand A: Effects of acute anoxia on the circulation and respiration in patients with chronic pulmonary disease studied during the "steady state." J Clin Invest 1952; 31:770–781.

20. Abraham HS, Hedworth Whitty RB, Bishop JM: Effects of acute hypoxia and hypervolemia singly and together upon the pulmonary circulation in patients with chronic bronchitis. Clin Sci 1967; 33:371–380.

21. Hunt JM, Copland J, McDonald CF, et al: Cardiopulmonary response to oxygen therapy in hypoxaemic chronic airflow obstruction. Thorax 1989; 44:930–936.

22. Saadjian A, Philip JF, Levy S, Arnaud A: Vascular and cardiac reactivity in pulmonary hypertension due to chronic obstructive lung disease: Assessment with various oxygen concentrations. Eur Respir J 1992; 5:525–530.

23. Harris P, Segel M, Green I, Housley E: The influence of airways resistance and alveolar pressure on the pulmonary vascular resistance in chronic bronchitis. Cardiovasc Res 1968; 2:84–92.

24. Morrison NJ, Abboud RT, Muller NL, et al: Pulmonary capillary blood volume in emphysema. Am Rev Respir Dis 1990; 141:53–61.

25. Segel N, Bishop JM: The circulation in patients with chronic bronchitis and emphysema at rest and during exercise, with special reference to the influence of changes in blood viscosity and blood volume on the pulmonary circulation. J Clin Invest 1966; 45:1555–1568.

26. Bergofsky EH, Haas F, Porcelli R: Determination of the sensitive sites from which hypoxia and hypercapnia elicit rises in pulmonary arterial pressure. Fed Proc 1968; 27:1420–1425.

27. Dawson CA, Grimm DJ, Livehan JH: Influence of hypoxia on the longitudinal distribution of pulmonary vascular resistance. J Appl Physiol 1978; 44:493–498.

28. Marshall BE, Marshall C, Benumoff J, Saidman W: Hypoxic pulmonary vasoconstriction in dogs: Effects of lung segment size and oxygen tension. J Appl Physiol 1981; 51:1543–1551.

29. Voelkel NF: Mechanisms of hypoxic pulmonary vasoconstriction. Am Rev Respir Dis 1986; 133:1186–1195.

30. Dinh-Xuan AT, Higenbottam TW, Wallwork J: Relationship between chronic hypoxia and in vitro pulmonary relaxation mediated by endothelium-derived relaxing factors in human chronic obstructive lung disease. Angiology 1992; 43:350–356.

31. Marshall C, Lindgren L, Marshall BE: Metabolic and respiratory hydrogen ion effects on hypoxic pulmonary vasoconstriction. J Appl Physiol 1984; 57:545–550.

32. Enson Y, Giuntini C, Lewis ML, et al: The influence of hydrogen in concentration and hypoxia on the pulmonary circulation. J Clin Invest 1964; 43:1146–1162.

33. Boysen PG: Nocturnal oxygen therapy and hemodynamic changes in COPD. Chest 1984; 85:2–3.

34. Fletcher EC, Levin DC: Cardiopulmonary hemodynamics during sleep in subjects with chronic obstructive pulmonary disease. Chest 1984; 85:6–14.

35. Block AJ, Boysen PG, Wynne JW: The origins of cor pulmonale: A hypothesis. Chest 1979; 75:109–110.

36. Levi-Valensi P, Weitzenblum E, Rida Z, et al: Sleep-related oxygen desaturation and daytime pulmonary haemodynamics in COPD patients. Eur Respir J 1992; 5:301–307.

37. Ferrer MI: Cor pulmonale (pulmonary heart disease): Present-day status. Am Heart J 1975; 89:657–664.

38. Weitzenblum E, Hirth C, Parini JP, et al: Clinical, functional, and pulmonary hemodynamic course of patients with chronic obstructive pulmonary disease followed up over three years. Respiration 1978; 36:1–9.

39. Lindsay DA, Read J: Pulmonary vascular responsiveness in the prognosis of chronic obstructive lung disease. Am Rev Respir Dis 1972; 105:242–250.

40. Cromie JB: Correlation of anatomic pulmonary emphysema and right ventricular hypertrophy. Am Rev Respir Dis 1961; 84:657–662.

41. Hicken P, Heath D, Brewer D: The relation between the weight of the right ventricle and the percentage of abnormal air space in the lung in emphysema. J Pathol Bacteriol 1966; 92:519–546.

42. Degante UP, Domenighetti G, Naeije R, et al: Oxygen delivery in acute exacerbation of chronic obstructive pulmonary disease. Am Rev Respir Dis 1981; 124:26–30.

43. Gluskowski J, Jedrezejewska-Makowska M, Hawrylkiewicz I, et al: Effects of prolonged oxygen therapy on pulmonary hypertension and blood viscosity in patients with advanced cor pulmonale. Respiration 1983; 44:177–183.

44. Nocturnal Oxygen Therapy Trial Group: Continuous or nocturnal oxygen therapy in hypoxemic chronic obstructive lung disease. Ann Intern Med 1980; 93:391–398.

45. Weitzenblum E, Sautegeau A, Ehrhart M, et al: Long-term oxygen therapy can reverse the progression of pulmonary hypertension in patients with chronic obstructive lung disease. Am Rev Respir Dis 1985; 131:493–498.

46. Weitzenblum E, Oswald M, Mirhom R, et al: Evolution of pulmonary haemodynamics in COLD patients under long-term oxygen therapy. Eur Respir J Suppl 1989; 7:669s–673s.

47. Klein G, Matthys H: Acute and long-term effects of chronic obstructive lung diseases. Pneumologie 1990; 44:188–190.

48. Sliwinski P, Hawrylkiewicz I, Gorecka D, Zielinski J: Acute effect of oxygen on pulmonary arterial pressure does not predict survival on long-term oxygen therapy in patients with chronic obstructive pulmonary disease. Am Rev Respir Dis 1992; 146:665–669.

49. Siebold H, Wieshammer S, Kress P: Relation of pressure and flow of pulmonary circulation in patients with chronic obstructive pulmonary disease. Clin Physiol Biochem 1988; 6:29–35.

50. Siebold H, Bunjes D, Kohler J, Schmidt A: Relation of noninvasive parameters and pulmonary artery mean pressure in patients with chronic obstructive lung disease. Clin Physiol Biochem 1988; 6:106–116.

51. Wade OL, Bishop JM: Cardiac Output and Regional Blood Flow. Oxford, Blackwell, 1962, p 149.

52. Findley M, Middleton HC, Peake MD, Howard P: Cardiac output, pulmonary hypertension, hypoxaemia,

and survival in patients with chronic obstructive airways disease. Eur J Respir Dis 1983; 64:252–263.

53. Anand IS, Chandrashekhar Y, Ferrari R, et al: Pathogenesis of congestive state in chronic obstructive pulmonary disease: Studies of body water and sodium, renal function, hemodynamics, and plasma hormones during edema and after recovery. Circulation 1992; 86:12–21.

54. Harris P: Are pulmonary haemodynamics of importance to survival in chronic obstructive lung disease? Eur Respir J Suppl 1989; 7:674s–677s.

55. Tenney SM, Mithoeffer JC: The relationship of mixed venous oxygenation to oxygen transport with special reference to adaptation to high altitude and pulmonary disease. Am Rev Respir Dis 1982; 125:474–479.

56. Mithoeffer JC, Ramirez C, Cook W: The effect of mixed venous oxygenation on arterial blood in chronic obstructive pulmonary disease. Am Rev Respir Dis 1978; 117:259–264.

57. Vanderelst AMC, Vanderwerf T: Some circulatory aspects of the oxygen transport in patients with emphysema. Respiration 1985; 48:310–320.

58. Stewart RI, Lewis CM: Cardiac output during exercise in patients with COPD. Chest 1986; 89:199–205.

59. Filley GF, Beckwitt HJ, Reeves JT, Mitchell RS: Chronic obstructive bronchopulmonary disease, Part II: Oxygen transport in two clinical types. Am J Med 1968; 44:26–37.

60. Bishop JM: Cardiovascular complications of chronic bronchitis and emphysema. Med Clin North Am 1973; 57:771–780.

61. Matthay RA, Berger HJ: Cardiovascular performance in chronic obstructive pulmonary disease. Med Clin North Am 1981; 65:489–524.

62. Morris AH, Chapman RH: Wedge pressure confirmation by aspiration of pulmonary capillary blood. Crit Care Med 1985; 13:756–759.

63. Henriquez AH, Schrijen FV, Redondo J, Delorme N: Local variations of pulmonary arterial wedge pressure and wedge angiograms in patients with chronic lung disease. Chest 1988; 94:491–495.

64. Rabinowitz M, Niden AH, Pickard SD, et al: Evidence for pulmonary venous obstruction in pulmonary emphysema. J Lab Clin Med 1962; 60:1006–1007.

65. Shelton D, Keal E, Reid L: The pulmonary circulation in chronic bronchitis and emphysema. Chest 1977; 71:303–306.

66. Charms BL, Brofman BL, Adicoff A: Factors affecting the pulmonary "capillary" pressure. Am J Cardiol 1960; 5:328–332.

67. Rice DL, Awe RJ, Gaasch WH, et al: Wedge pressure measurements in obstructive pulmonary disease. Chest 1974; 66:628–632.

68. Lockhart A, Tsareva M, Schrijen F, Sadoul P: Etudes hemodynamiques des decompensations respiratoires aigues des bronchopneumopathies chroniques. Bull Physiopathol Respir 1967; 3:645–667.

69. Albert RK, Muramoto A, Caldwell J, et al: Increases in intrathoracic pressure do not explain the rise in left ventricular end-diastolic pressure that occurs during exercise in patients with chronic obstructive pulmonary disease. Am Rev Respir Dis 1985; 132:623–627.

70. Burrows B, Kettel LJ, Niden AH, et al: Patterns of cardiovascular dysfunction in chronic obstructive lung disease. N Engl J Med 1972; 286:912–918.

71. Noseda A, Verbeet T, Verhas M, et al: Left ventricular function in obstructive chronic bronchopneumopathy. Presse Med 1989; 18:967–971.

72. Herles F, Jezek V, Daum S: Site of resistance in cor pulmonale in chronic bronchitis. Br Heart J 1968; 30:654–660.

73. Kitchin AH, Lowther CP, Matthews MV: The effects of exercise and of breathing oxygen-enriched air on the pulmonary circulation in emphysema. Clin Sci 1961; 21:93–106.

74. Horsfield K, Segel N, Bishop JM: The pulmonary circulation in chronic bronchitis at rest and during exercise breathing air and 80% oxygen. Clin Sci 1968; 34:473–483.

75. Butler J, Schrijen F, Henriquez A, et al: Cause of the raised wedge pressure on exercise in chronic obstructive pulmonary disease. Am Rev Respir Dis 1988; 138:350–354.

76. Butler J, Schrijen F, Henriquez A, et al: Cause of increased right and left atrial pressures in patients with obstructed airflow disease. Chest 1988; 93(Suppl 3):171s–172s.

77. Lockhart A, Tzareva M, Nader F, et al: Elevated pulmonary artery wedge pressure at rest and during exercise in chronic bronchitis: Fact or fancy? Clin Sci 1969; 37:503–517.

78. Seibold H, Grossman G, Weishammer S, et al: Effect of right ventricular hypertrophy on cardiac performance and the relation between right ventricular systolic peak pressure and end-systolic volume. Clin Physiol Biochem 1987; 5:27–37.

79. Murphy ML, Hutcheson F: The electrocardiographic diagnosis of right ventricular hypertrophy in chronic obstructive pulmonary disease. Chest 1974; 65:622–627.

80. Hasleton PS: Right ventricular hypertrophy in emphysema. J Pathol 1973; 110:27–36.

81. Mitchell RS, Stanford RE, Silvers GW, Dart G: The right ventricle in chronic airway obstruction: A clinico-pathologic study. Am Rev Respir Dis 1976; 114:147–154.

82. Marshall RC, Gottschalk A, Zaret BL: Assessment of cardiac performance with quantitative radionuclide angiocardiography: Right ventricular ejection fraction with reference to findings in chronic obstructive pulmonary disease. Am J Cardiol 1978; 41:897–905.

83. Olvey SK, Reduto LA, Stevens PM, et al: First-pass radionuclide assessment of right and left ventricular ejection fraction in chronic pulmonary disease. Chest 1980; 78:4–9.

84. MacNee W: Right ventricular function in cor pulmonale. Cardiology 1988; 75(Suppl 1):30–40.

85. Brent BN, Berger HJ, Matthay RA, et al: Physiologic correlates of right ventricular ejection fraction in chronic obstructive pulmonary disease: A combined radionuclide and hemodynamic study. Am J Cardiol 1982; 50:255–262.

86. Morrison D, Goldman S, Wright AL, et al: The effect of pulmonary hypertension on systolic function of the right ventricle. Chest 1983; 84:250–257.

87. MacNee W, Morgan AD, Wathen CG, et al: Right ventricular performance during exercise in chronic obstructive pulmonary disease. Respiration 1985; 48:206–215.

88. Mahler DA, Brent BN, Loke J, et al: Right ventricular performances and central circulatory hemodynamics during upright exercise in patients with chronic obstructive pulmonary disease. Am Rev Respir Dis 1984; 130:722–729.

89. Oliver RM, Fleming JS, Waller DG: Right ventricular function at rest and during exercise in chronic obstructive pulmonary disease: Comparison of two radionuclide techniques. Chest 1993; 103:74–80.

90. Sagawa R: The ventricular pressure-volume diagram revisited. Circ Res 1978; 43:677–683.

91. Maughan WL, Skoukas AA, Sagawa K, Weisfeld ML: Intravenous pressure-volume relationship of the canine right ventricle. Circ Res 1979; 44:309–315.

92. Grossman W, Braunwald E, Mann T, et al: Contractile state of the left ventricle in man as evaluated from end-systolic pressure-volume relations. Circulation 1977; 56:845–852.

93. Mehmel HC, Stockins B, Luffmann K, et al: The linearity of the end-systolic pressure-volume relationship in man and its sensitivity for assessment of left ventricular function. Circulation 1981; 63:1216–1222.

94. Sasayama S, Franklin D, Ross J Jr: Hyperfunction with normal inotropic state of the hypertrophied left ventricle. Am J Physiol 1977; 232:H418–H425.

95. Horan LG, Flowers NC, Haveeda CJ: Relation between right ventricular mass and cavity size: An analysis of 1500 human hearts. Circulation 1981; 64:132–138.

96. Schrijen F, Redondo J, Henriquez A, Polu JM: Right ventricular pressure-volume relationship at rest and during exercise in patients with chronic lung disease. Chest 1990; 97(Suppl 3):87s–88s.

97. Dittrich HC, Chow LC, Nicod PH: Early improvement in left ventricular diastolic function after relief of chronic right ventricular pressure overload. Circulation 1989; 80:823–830.

98. Murphy ML, Adamson J, Hutcheson F: Left ventricular hypertrophy in patients with chronic bronchitis and emphysema. Ann Intern Med 1974; 81:307–313.

99. Rahlf G, Komori R: Der Linke Ventrikel bei chronischem Cor Pulmonale. Virchows Arch A Pathol Anat Histopathol 1975; 336:237–247.

100. Ishikawa S, Fattal GA, Popiewicz J, Wyatt JP: Functional morphometry of myocardial fibers in cor pulmonale. Am Rev Respir Dis 1972; 105:358–367.

101. Fluck DC, Chandrasekar RG, Gardner FV: Left ventricular hypertrophy in chronic bronchitis. Br Heart J 1966; 28:92–97.

102. Strester DD Jr: Gross morphology and fiber geometry of the heart. In Berne RM, Sperdakis N (eds): Handbook of Physiology. Baltimore, Williams & Wilkins, 1979, pp 61–112.

103. Rao BS, Cohn KE, Eldridge FL, Hancock EW: Left ventricular failure secondary to chronic pulmonary disease. Am J Med 1968; 45:229–241.

104. Herer B, Le-Gros V, Lascault G, Thomas D: Left ventricular insufficiency in chronic obstructive bronchopneumopathies: A cause to look for dilated cardiomyopathy. Presse Med 1987; 16:2051–2054.

105. Laks MM, Morady F, Swan HJC: Canine right and left ventricular cell sarcomere lengths after banding the pulmonary artery. Circ Res 1969; 24:705–710.

106. Buccino RA, Harris E, Spann JF: Response of myocardial connective tissue to development of experimental hypertrophy. Am J Physiol 1969; 216:425–428.

107. Chandler BM, Sonnenblick EH, Spann JF, Pool PE: Association of depressed myofibrillar adenosine triphosphate and reduced contractility in experimental heart failure. Circ Res 1967; 21:717–725.

108. Pool PE, Spann JF, Buccino RA, et al: Myocardial high-energy phosphate stores in cardiac hypertrophy and heart failure. Circ Res 1967; 21:3365–3373.

109. Chidsey CA, Kaizer GA, Sonaenblick EA, et al: Cardiac norepinephrine stores in experimental heart failure in the dog. J Clin Invest 1964; 43:2386–2393.

110. Stool EW, Mullins CB, Leshin SJ, Mitchell JH: Dimensional changes of the left ventricle during acute pulmonary arterial hypertension in dogs. Am J Cardiol 1974; 33:866–875.

111. Kelly DT, Spotnitz HM, Reiser GD, et al: Effects of chronic right ventricular volume and pressure loading on left ventricular performance. Circulation 1971; 44:403–412.

112. Hecht HH, Kinda H, Tsagaris J: Brisket disease. Part IV: Impairment of left ventricular function in a form of cor pulmonale. Trans Assoc Am Physicians 1962; 75:263–276.

113. Williams JF, Childress RH, Boyd DL, et al: Left ventricular function in patients with chronic obstructive pulmonary disease. J Clin Invest 1968; 47:1143–1153.

114. Davies H, Overy HR: Left ventricular function in cor pulmonale. Chest 1970; 58:8–14.

115. Matthay RA, Ellis JH Jr, Steele PP: Methoxamine-induced increase in afterload: Effect on left ventricular performance in chronic obstructive pulmonary disease. Am Rev Respir Dis 1978; 117:871–877.

116. Khaja F, Parker JO: Right and left ventricular performance in chronic obstructive pulmonary disease. Am Heart J 1971; 82:319–327.

117. Slutsky R, Hooper W, Ackerman W, et al: Evaluation of left ventricular function in chronic pulmonary disease by exercise-gated equilibrium radionuclide angiography. Am Heart J 1981; 101:414–420.

118. Frank MJ, Weisse AB, Moschos CB, Leviason GE: Left ventricular function, metabolism and blood flow in chronic cor pulmonale. Circulation 1973; 47:798–806.

119. Unger K, Shaw D, Karliner JS, et al: Evaluation of left ventricular performance in acutely ill patients with chronic obstructive lung disease. Chest 1975; 68:135–142.

120. Steele P, Ellis JH Jr, Van Dyke D, et al: Left ventricular ejection fraction in severe chronic obstructive airways disease. Am J Med 1975; 59:21–28.

121. Baum GL, Schwartz A, Llamas R, Castillo C: Left ventricular function in chronic obstructive lung disease. N Engl J Med 1971; 285:361–365.

122. Frank MJ, Nadimi M, Casanegra P, et al: Effect of angiotensin on myocardial function. Am J Physiol 1970 218:1267–1272.

123. Jezek V, Schrijen F: Left ventricular function in chronic obstructive pulmonary disease with and without cardiac failure. Clin Sci Mol Med 1973; 45:267–279.

124. Song GJ, Oldershaw PJ: Left ventricular dysfunction in obstructive lung disease: An echocardiographic and angiographic study of cor pulmonale patients with decreased mitral E-F slope. Int J Cardiol 1989; 25:47–54.

125. Gabinski C, Courty G, Besse P, Castaing R: La fonction ventriculaire gauche au cours des bronchopneumopathies chroniques obstructives. Bull Eur Physiopathol Respir 1979; 15:755–772.

126. Denolin H: Clinical trials with long-term treatment of pulmonary hypertension due to lung disease. Eur Heart J 1988; 9(Suppl J):29–32.

127. Howard P: Vasodilator drugs in chronic obstructive airways disease. Eur Respir J Suppl 1989; 7:678s–681s.

128. Nemens EF, Woods SL: Normal fluctuations in pulmonary artery and pulmonary capillary wedge pressures in acutely ill patients. Heart Drug 1982; 11:393–398.

129. Mammosser M, Schrijen F, Henriquez A: Stabilite hemodynamique et gasometrique au cours du catheterisme cardiaque droit dans les bronchopneumopathies chroniques. Bull Eur Physiopathol Respir 1986; 22:133–136.

130. Schrijen F, Jezkova J: Natural variability of pulmonary hemodynamics. Eur Heart J 1988; 9(Suppl J):19–22.

131. Schrijen F, Jezek V: Hemodynamic variables during repeated exercise in chronic lung disease. Clin Sci Mol Med 1978; 55:485–590.

132. Schrijen F, Jezek V: Constitution et maintien d'un etat stable hemodynamique et ventilatoire au cours d'an exercice de 40 watts chez des pulmonaires chroniques. Bull Eur Physiopathol Respir 1970; 6:819–832.

133. Parker JO, Ashekian PB, DiHiorgi S, West RO: Hemodynamic effects of aminophylline in chronic obstructive pulmonary disease. Circulation 1967; 35:365–372.

134. Matthay RA, Berger HJ, Lake J, et al: Effects of amino-

phylline upon right and left ventricular performance in chronic obstructive pulmonary disease: Noninvasive assessment by radionuclide angiocardiography. Am J Med 1978; 65:903–910.

135. Brent BN, Mahler D, Verger HJ, et al: Augmentation of right ventricular performance in chronic obstructive pulmonary disease by terbutaline: A combined radionuclide and hemodynamic study. Am J Cardiol 1982; 50:313–319.

136. Matthay RA, Berger HJ, Davies R, et al: Improvement in cardiac performance by oral long-acting theophylline in chronic obstructive pulmonary disease. Am Heart J 1982; 104:1022–1026.

137. Rubin W, Peter RH: Hemodynamics at rest and during exercise after oral hydralazine in patients with cor pulmonale. Am J Cardiol 1981; 47:116–122.

138. Lupi-Henera E, Seoare M, Verdejo J: Hemodynamic effect of hydralazine in advanced stable chronic obstructive lung disease with cor pulmonale. Chest 1984; 85:156–163.

139. Dal Nogare AR, Rubin LJ: The effects of hydralazine on exercise capacity in pulmonary hypertension secondary to chronic obstructive pulmonary disease. Am Rev Respir Dis 1986; 133:385–389.

140. Tuxen DV, Powles ACP, Mathur PN, et al: Detrimental effects of hydralazine in patients with chronic air-flow obstruction and pulmonary hypertension. Am Rev Respir Dis 1984; 129:388–395.

141. Gassner A, Fridrich L, Magometschnigg D, et al: Vasodilator therapy in pulmonary hypertension and chronic obstructive lung disease (COPD). Herz 1986; 11:207–216.

142. Gassner A, Sommer G, Fridrich L, et al: Differential therapy with calcium antagonists in pulmonary hypertension secondary to COPD: Hemodynamic effects of nifedipine, diltiazem, and verapamil. Chest 1990; 98:829–834.

143. Muramoto A, Caldwell J, Albert RK, et al: Nifedipine dilates the pulmonary vasculature without producing symptomatic systemic hypotension in upright resting and exercising patients with pulmonary hypertension secondary to chronic obstructive pulmonary disease. Am Rev Respir Dis 1985; 132:963–966.

144. Singh H, Ebejer MJ, Higgins DA, et al: Acute hemodynamic effects of nifedipine at rest and during maximal exercise in patients with chronic cor pulmonale. Thorax 1985; 40:910–914.

145. Barghuber OC: Nifedipine attenuates acute hypoxic pulmonary vasoconstriction in patients with chronic obstructive pulmonary disease. Respiration 1983; 52:86–93.

146. Melot C, Hallemans R, Naeije R, et al: Deleterious effect of nifedipine on pulmonary gas exchange in chronic obstructive pulmonary disease. Am Rev Respir Dis 1984; 130:612–616.

147. Agostari P, Doria E, Galli C, et al: Nifedipine reduces pulmonary pressure and vascular time during short- but not long-term treatment of pulmonary hypertension in patients with chronic obstructive pulmonary disease. Am Rev Respir Dis 1989; 139:120–125.

148. Brown SE, Linden GS, King RR, et al: Effects of verapamil on pulmonary hemodynamics during hypoxaemia, at rest, and during exercise in patients with chronic obstructive pulmonary disease. Thorax 1983; 38:840–844.

149. Clozel JP, Delorme N, Battistella P, et al: Haemodynamic effects of intravenous diltiazem in hypoxic pulmonary hypertension. Chest 1987; 91:171–175.

150. Domenighetti GM, Saglini VG: Short- and long-term hemodynamic effects of oral nifedipine in patients with pulmonary hypertension secondary to COPD and lung fibrosis: Deleterious effects in patients with restrictive disease. Chest 1992; 102:708–741.

151. Vestri R, Philip-Joet F, Surpas P, et al: One-year clinical study on nifedipine in the treatment of pulmonary hypertension in chronic obstructive lung disease. Respiration 1988; 54:139–144.

152. Kentera D, Susie D, Evetkovic A, Djordjevic G: Effects of SQ 14,225, an orally active inhibitor of angiotensin-converting enzyme, on hypoxic pulmonary hypertension and right ventricular hypertrophy in rats. Basic Res Cardiol 1981; 76:344–351.

153. Previtt EL, Leffler CW: Feline hypoxic pulmonary vasoconstriction is not blocked by the angiotensin I converting enzyme inhibitor, captopril. J Cardiovasc Pharmacol 1981; 3:293–298.

154. Burke CM, Herte M, Duncan J, et al: Captopril and domiciliary oxygen in chronic airflow obstruction. Br Med J 1985; 290:1251.

155. Bertolli L, Fusco M, Loucero S, et al: Influence of ACE inhibition on pulmonary haemodynamics and function in patients in whom beta-blockers are contraindicated. Postgrad Med J 1986; 62(Suppl 1):47–51.

156. Takada K, Hayashi M, Takahashi K, Yasui S: Acute effects of oral captopril on hemodynamics in patients with cor pulmonale. Jpn Circ J 1986; 50:1055–1061.

157. Richard C, Ricome JL, Rimailho A, et al: Effects of captopril on pulmonary haemodynamics. Eur J Clin Pharmacol 1984; 27:35–39.

158. Baschetti E, Tautucei C, Cocchieri M, et al: Acute effects of captopril in hypoxic pulmonary hypertension. Respiration 1985; 48:296–302.

159. Zielinski J, Hawrylkiewicz I, Gorecka D, et al: Captopril effects on pulmonary and systemic hemodynamics in chronic cor pulmonale. Chest 1986; 90:562–565.

160. Patakas D, Georgopoulos D, Rodini H, Christaki P: Effects of captopril in patients with chronic obstructive pulmonary disease and secondary pulmonary hypertension. Postgrad Med J 1988; 64:193–195.

161. Naeije R, Melot C, Mols P, Hallemans R: Reduction in pulmonary hypertension by prostaglandin E, in decompensated chronic obstructive pulmonary disease. Am Rev Respir Dis 1982; 125:1–5.

162. Long WA, Rubin LJ: Prostacyclin and PGE₁ treatment of pulmonary hypertension. Am Rev Respir Dis 1987; 136:773–776.

163. Ishizaki T, Nuyabo S, Mifune J, et al: OP-1206, a prostaglandin E₁ derivative: Effects of oral administration to patients with chronic lung disease. Chest 1984; 85:382–386.

164. Rubin LJ, Mendoza J, Leng W: Rest and exercise hemodynamic effects of intravenous prostaglandin I₂ in chronic cor pulmonale. Am Rev Respir Dis 1987; 135:A301.

165. Jones K, Higenbotham T, Wallwork J: Pulmonary vasodilation with prostacyclin in primary and secondary pulmonary hypertension. Chest 1989; 96:784–789.

166. Mols P, Nasiye R, Melot C, Hallemans R: Failure of prostaglandin E to inhibit hypoxic pulmonary vasoconstriction in man. Acta Ther 1980; 6:45.

167. Peng W, Duan SF: Hemodynamic and hemorrheologic effect of ligustrazini in chronic obstructive pulmonary disease with cor pulmonale. Chin Med J (Engl) 1987; 100:965–970.

168. Powles ACP, Tuxen DV, Mahood CB, et al: The effect of intravenously administered almitrine, a peripheral chemoceptor agonist, on patients with chronic air-flow obstruction. Am Rev Respir Dis 1983; 127:284–289.

169. MacNee W, Connaughton JJ, Rhind GB, et al: A comparison of the effects of almitrine or oxygen breathing on pulmonary artery pressure and right ventricular

ejection fraction in hypoxic chronic bronchitis and emphysema. Am Rev Respir Dis 1986; 134:559–565.

170. Herve PH, Musset D, Simonneau G, et al: Almitrine decreases the distensibility of the pulmonary artery in man. Chest 1989; 96:572–577.

171. Deburgh JH, Daly M, Ungar A: Comparison of the reflex responses elicited of separately perfused carotid and aortic body chemoreceptors in the dog. J Physiol (Lond) 1966; 182:379–403.

172. Scarrow GD: The pulmonary angiogram in chronic bronchitis and emphysema. Clin Radiol 1966; 17:54 67.

173. Reid L: The angiogram and pulmonary artery structure and branching (in the normal and with reference to disease). Proc R Soc Med 1965; 58:681–684.

174. Schrijen F, Jezek V: Haemodynamics and pulmonary wedge angiography findings in chronic bronchopulmonary disease. Scand J Respir Dis 1977; 58:151–158.

175. Bracchi G, Barbaccia P, Vezzoli F, et al: Peripheral pulmonary wedge angiography in chronic obstructive pulmonary disease: Relationship to pulmonary function, chest x-ray film, and hemodynamic data. Chest 1977; 7:718–724.

176. Khattri HN, Jindal SK, Singh HJ, Sodhi JS: Peripheral pulmonary angiography in chronic bronchitis and emphysema. Indian Heart J 1979; 31:255–258.

177. Bryant LR, Cohn JE, O'Neill RP, et al: Pulmonary blood flow distribution in chronic obstructive airway disease. Am Rev Respir Dis 1968; 97:832–842.

178. MacNee W: Should patients have cardiac catheterization prior to long-term oxygen treatment? Lung 1990; 168(Suppl):800–808.

179. Weitzenblum E, Apprill M, Ehrhart M, Oswald M: Should patients have right heart catheterization prior to long-term oxygen treatment? Lung 1990; 168 (Suppl):794–799.

Chapter 25

Catheterization and Angiography in Congenital Heart Disease of the Adult

KIRK L. PETERSON
GABRIEL GREGORATOS

Over the last half-century notable progress has been made in the diagnosis and treatment of congenital lesions of the heart.[1] Cardiac catheterization and angiography have been integral to these achievements by providing accurate characterization of the pathophysiologic and patho-anatomic features of acyanotic and cyanotic lesions. In the 1990s, noninvasive techniques, particularly two-dimensional echocardiography, Doppler ultrasonography, and magnetic resonance imaging, provide a high degree of diagnostic accuracy and ready detection of congenital lesions at an early age.[2] Nevertheless, in the presence of a suspected congenital defect, catheterization and angiography continue to provide important confirmatory information before lesion palliation or correction. Catheter techniques are also being used therapeutically to alter the degree of valvular or vascular obstruction, to close off abnormal pathways of shunting, or to palliate inadequate pulmonary blood flow by opening up or enlarging pathways to the lung.

The adult cardiologist confronts congenital heart disease primarily in patients who, for whatever reason, have not received close medical scrutiny in childhood and adolescence, or where the clinical characteristics of their lesion or lesions have been subtle and have evaded detection. A second class of patients, now seen ever more frequently, is those who have undergone previous corrective or palliative surgery in childhood and who need ongoing surveillance for late complications of their disease or operative intervention.

In this chapter the general principles of cardiac catheterization and angiography in congenital heart disease are considered. The salient pathophysiologic and pathoanatomic features of the common acyanotic and cyanotic lesions

of the adult are also reviewed. No effort is made to comprehensively cover all potential lesions; others have admirably provided more exhaustive reference sources.[3, 4]

GENERAL PRINCIPLES

Because in congenital lesions of the heart the cardiac chambers and great vessels frequently are situated in an anomalous position, the operator should be familiar with the full spectrum of pathologic abnormalities and alert to possible misinterpretation of exact catheter tip location by fluoroscopy. Thus, training, under the close supervision of an experienced tutor, should be undertaken before the clinician independently performs heart catheterization and angiography in congenital heart disease; this admonition applies particularly for those conditions that involve anatomic malpositions and right-to-left shunting (cyanotic lesions).

Catheter Selection and Passage

When congenital heart disease is suspected, the operator must bear in mind the potential for air, thrombus, or foreign bodies reaching the left side of the circulation by way of an abnormal anatomic connection or patent shunt. Thus, in our laboratory we are cautious about using balloon flotation catheters for the right-sided heart examination unless there is difficulty in entering the pulmonary artery. In this instance, a balloon flotation catheter can be employed, but with carbon dioxide rather than air used for balloon inflation. To direct the tip of a catheter into an atrial septal defect, anomalous pulmonary venous connection, displaced tricuspid valve, abnormally placed right-sided ventricle, and so forth, it is advantageous to use a relatively stiff catheter with a 15- to 30-degree angle at the terminal 3 to 4 cm of the tip. For ready withdrawal of blood samples, it is useful to insert a catheter with both an end-hole as well as side-holes near the tip. In our laboratories the Goodale-Lubin catheter is often used because it shares these characteristics. In contrast, a multilumen, balloon flotation, thermodilution catheter is often too flexible to torque, and it does not allow quick withdrawal of blood samples. For angiographic studies it is desirable to insert a catheter that not only allows rapid delivery of large amounts of contrast but one that is readily manipulated into anomalously placed anatomic structures. Although relatively stiff, the curved NIH catheter, with side-holes and no end-hole, exhibits excellent torque response and is useful for this purpose (see Chapter 2). As an alternative, a Berman angiographic catheter can be used, particularly if flotation with a CO_2-filled balloon is desirable. The most diagnostically accurate and revealing cineangiograms in congenital heart disease are those where adequate contrast medium has been given to identify subtle pathoanatomic features and to overcome the dilutional effects of relatively large intracardiac shunts.

Detection of Shunts

Shunting of blood can occur either as an inappropriate left-to-right admixture of arterial blood with the venous return into the right heart, an inappropriate right-to-left admixture of systemic venous blood into the left heart, or a combination of both (bidirectional shunting). Shunts are common pathophysiologic abnormalities in many forms of congenital heart disease and should be searched for diligently at the time of cardiac catheterization and angiography. Today, because of findings on two-dimensional and Doppler ultrasonographic imaging, the presence of shunting usually is known or suspected before the catheterization procedure. Alternatively, there may be a strong suspicion based on a careful analysis of other clinical findings, including physical signs at the bedside; the electrocardiogram; or the appearance of the cardiac silhouette, great vessels, and pulmonary vasculature on the chest roentgenogram. Occasionally, the operator is alerted to the presence of the shunt only at the time of the catheterization procedure. Clues to the presence of an unexpected intracardiac shunt include (1) an abnormal catheter passage (e.g., entrance into an anomalous pulmonary venous connection into the superior vena cava, right

atrium, or inferior vena cava); (2) a relatively low systemic arterial oxygen saturation or tension in the absence of significant lung disease, reflecting systemic venous admixture of arterial blood; and (3) a relatively high oxygen saturation or tension in the pulmonary artery, reflecting arterial admixture with the normal systemic venous blood return.

Because of the potential discovery of unexpected shunts, we routinely measure both pulmonary arterial and systemic arterial oxygen saturation and the arteriovenous oxygen content difference in all patients undergoing cardiac catheterization, including those patients referred only for coronary angiography and left ventriculography. Any patient with a pulmonary artery oxygen saturation higher than 80% has a full oxygen saturation run performed throughout the right side of the heart; in the patient with a systemic arterial desaturation less than 88%, a careful probing is made of the area of the foramen ovale (looking for a source of right-to-left shunting), and if the left atrium is easily entered, oxygen saturation samples are taken through the left side of the heart.

PERFORMANCE OF OXYGEN SATURATION RUN. An oxygen saturation run consists of blood specimens, taken in duplicate and in rapid sequence, for analysis of an inordinate change in oxygen saturation. In the right-sided heart circulation, the first specimen is collected in either the right or left pulmonary artery branches, with the catheter positioned not much beyond the mediastinal shadow to avoid inadvertent sampling from pulmonary capillary wedge or near wedge positions. A specimen is obtained from the contralateral branch followed by a third from the main pulmonary artery. The catheter is then withdrawn across the pulmonic valve, and a specimen is obtained high in the right ventricular outflow tract just beneath the valve. The catheter is subsequently withdrawn further to the junction of inflow and outflow tracts (mid-right ventricle) and a sample taken from this location. A third right ventricular sample also is obtained just beneath the tricuspid valve. At least three samples are obtained in the right atrium. With the catheter tip rotated toward the lateral wall of the right atrium, samples are aspirated from "high" (just below the junction of the right atrium with the superior vena cava), "mid," and "low" (lower one-third) positions. The superior vena cava specimen is obtained at least 2 to 3 cm above the upper margin of the right atrium. Inferior vena cava sampling can be problematic. Care must be exercised to maintain the catheter tip in the center of the

Figure 25–1. Effects of intracardiac shunts on an indicator-dilution curve (e.g., indocyanine green) into the right atrium with sampling in a systemic artery downstream to the site of shunting. A right-to-left (R to L) shunt is detected as an early appearance of the indicator; a left-to-right (L to R) shunt is detected as a delay in disappearance (recirculation) of the indicator on the downslope. Note also that the peak concentration of indicator, as compared with a normal curve, is diminished in the presence of the shunts.

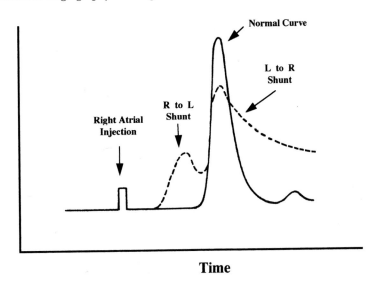

vessel and to avoid selective sampling of a hepatic vein. If an arterial catheter has been previously introduced, an aortic sample is also now obtained. Thus, a right heart oxygen saturation run, used to detect a left-to-right shunt, consists of 12 specimens obtained within 10 minutes. This is modified appropriately for specific malformations, especially when shunt volume is believed to be low. Specimens from a common origin are averaged and the means are compared (Table 25–1).

If there is ready access to the left atrium via an atrial septal defect or probe-patent foramen ovale, oxygen saturation specimens from the left heart chambers also are used to assess intrapulmonary and right-to-left intracardiac shunts. The initial specimen is usually taken from the mid-left atrium, just above the mitral valve and then across the mitral valve in the inflow position of the left ventricle. If the left atrial saturation is less than 98%, specimens should also be obtained from as many of the four pulmonary veins as can be readily and safely entered. A retrograde catheter, positioned in the ascending aorta, is generally used to assess the systemic arterial saturation. Other aortic saturations may be taken further downstream if there is evidence of right-to-left shunting into the transverse or descending thoracic aorta (e.g., reversed shunting through a patent ductus arteriosus).

Left-to-Right Shunts

Proof of inappropriate arterial admixture of the venous return to the right heart involves detection of one or more of the following:

1. An inappropriately high concentration of an indicator, such as oxygen, at some locale in the right heart

2. Either recirculation of an indicator, such as indocyanine green, delivered as a bolus into the right or left side of the heart, proximal to the shunt, with sampling downstream to the shunt (Fig. 25–1), or early appearance of inhaled hydrogen gas (Fig. 25–2) or injected ascorbic acid (Fig. 25–3) at a platinum-tipped electrode catheter positioned at or distal to the site of shunt in the right heart

3. Direct angiographic visualization of immediate passage of iodinated contrast medium from a left heart chamber into a right heart chamber

In the 1990s, quantification of the degree of left-to-right shunting is performed most commonly using the sequential determinations of oxygen saturation from various anatomic loci in the right and left heart as well as connecting vessels.

The first use of oxygen content (measured by the Van Slyke method) as an indicator of systemic arterial admixture of right heart blood was reported by Dexter and associates in their classic study published in 1947.[5] Subsequently, other methods for assessing relative oxygen content, including reflectance oximetry for saturation and an electrochemical fuel-cell method (Lex-O_2-Con) for content,[6] have been developed and are now used in most catheterization laboratories. Irrespective of the method for measurement of oxygen content, from the time of Dexter and associates' original investigation the question has arisen as to what constitutes a sufficient "step-up" in oxygen concentration in the right heart so as to document the presence of a left-to-right shunt.

Table 25–1. Minimal Step-ups for Detection of Intracardiac Left-to-Right Shunts by Oximetry

References*	O_2 Measurement Technique	Comparison of Samples	Site of Shunt in Right Heart			
			Atrium	Ventricle	Great Vessel	Any Level (SVC to great vessel)
Dexter et al[5]	Van Slyke	Difference of maximum value in two chambers	2.0 O_2 vol%	1.0 O_2 vol%	0.5 O_2 vol%	
Barratt-Boyes and Wood[7]	Cuvette oximeter	Difference of means of 2 paired samples	8 units O_2 %sat	3 units O_2 %sat	2 units O_2 vol%	
Rudolph and Caylor[8]	Cuvette oximeter	1 pair of samples 2 pairs of samples 3 pairs of samples	10 units O_2 %sat 7 units O_2 %sat 5 units O_2 %sat	7 units O_2 %sat 5 units O_2 %sat 3 units O_2 %sat	5 units O_2 %sat 3 units O_2 %sat 3 units O_2 %sat	
Freed et al[9]	Reflectance oximeter or transmission spectrophotometer	Difference of means of all samples obtained in each chamber	8 units O_2 %sat	6 units O_2 %sat	5 units O_2 %sat	
Antman et al[10]	Whole blood O_2 fuel cell analyzer	Difference of means of all samples obtained in each chamber	7 units O_2 %sat or 1.3 O_2 vol%	5 units O_2 %sat or 1.0 O_2 vol%	5 units O_2 %sat or 1.0 O_2 vol%	7 units O_2 %sat or 1.3 O_2 vol%
		Difference of maximum value in two chambers	11 units O_2 %sat or 2.0 O_2 vol%	10 units O_2 %sat or 1.7 O_2 vol%	5 units O_2 %sat or 1.0 O_2 vol%	8 units O_2 %sat or 1.5 O_2 vol%

*Chronologic order of publication.
O_2 vol% = 1 mL O_2/100 mL of blood; O_2 units %sat = percent saturation of O_2; SVC, superior vena cava.

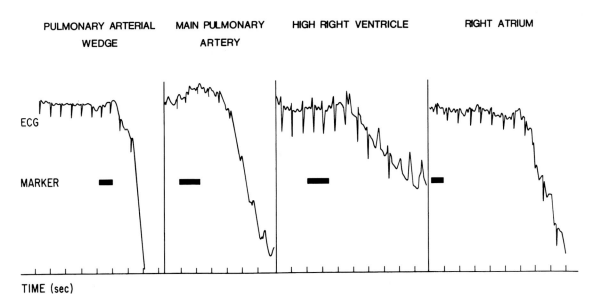

PULMONARY ARTERIAL WEDGE   MAIN PULMONARY ARTERY   HIGH RIGHT VENTRICLE   RIGHT ATRIUM

ECG

MARKER

TIME (sec)

Figure 25–2. Hydrogen curves in membranous ventricular septal defects: detection and localization of a left-to-right shunt by use of inhaled hydrogen gas and an electrocardiographic (ECG) platinum-tipped electrode catheter, positioned at various loci within the right heart and pulmonary vasculature. The time of administration of the gas is annotated by the black mark. Contact with inhaled hydrogen causes an immediate change in the voltage on the recording of the intracardiac electrogram. In this instance, an early appearance time is picked up in the high right ventricle and the main pulmonary artery, indicating a shunt in the membranous portion of the ventricular septum. The immediate appearance in the pulmonary arterial wedge position is used to test the integrity of the detection system.

Dexter and colleagues, using the Van Slyke method for measurement of oxygen content, found that samples from the right atrium, right ventricle, and pulmonary artery in normal subjects could vary by as much as 2, 1, and 0.5 vol%, respectively, at each of these sites of blood withdrawal (see Table 25–1).[5] This significant variability in oxygen content, particularly in the right atrium, in subjects without a left-to-right shunt can be explained by the diverse origins of systemic venous return with widely varying oxygen content (superior and inferior vena cavae, coronary sinus) as well as by streaming or laminar flow patterns.

Others later used cuvette oximetry for determination of oxygen saturation and found that a minimum step-up of 5 to 10 percentage saturation units was necessary to detect reliably a shunt at the atrial level, 3 to 7 units at the right ventricular level, and 2 to 5 units at the great vessel (usually pulmonary artery) level.[7–9] Rudolph and Caylor demonstrated that this minimum step-up requirement could be narrowed by taking multiple samples (see Table 25–1).[8] Antman and associates[10] reappraised prospectively the variation in both blood oxygen content and calculated saturation in all relevant loci of the right heart in a series of patients with diverse cardiac diagnoses, including valvular, coronary, and cardiomyopathic heart disease as well as pulmonary thromboembolism (see Table

25–1). They found that proof of a left-to-right shunt at the atrial level, in a subject with a normal serum hemoglobin concentration of 14 gm%, requires that the mean chamber samples between the systemic veins and right atrium differ by at least 7 oxygen saturation percentage points or 1.33 vol% oxygen content; at the ventricular level, the step-up between the mean values in the right atrium and right ventricle must be equal to or exceed 5 oxygen saturation percentage points or 1.0 vol%; and, finally, at the pulmonary artery level, the mean right ventricular and pulmonary artery samples had to be equal to or differ by more than 5 oxygen saturation percentage points or 1.0 vol%. Assuming that the systemic blood flow index is approximately 3 L/min/M[2], this degree of variability limits the detection of left-to-right shunts at the atrial level to an approximate ratio of total pulmonary blood flow (Qp) to total systemic blood flow (Qs) of 1.5, and at the ventricular or pulmonary artery level to a Qp/Qs of 1.3.[10]

These same authors have emphasized the influence of the absolute level of systemic blood flow, and, in particular, its inverse effect on arteriovenous oxygen content difference and the mixed venous oxygen saturation.[10] The higher the systemic output and systemic venous return, the narrower the arteriovenous oxygen difference and the less the variability in the right atrial oxygen saturations from the multiple

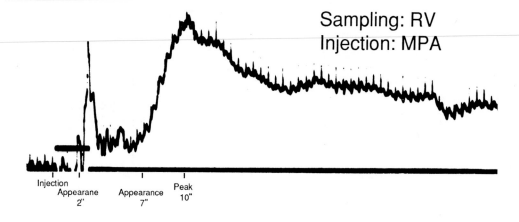

Sampling: RV
Injection: MPA

Injection   Appearane   Appearance   Peak
2"   7"   10"

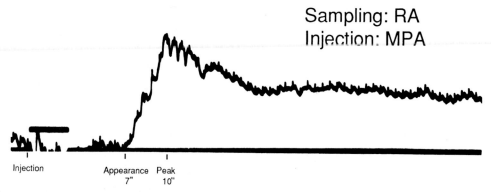

Sampling: RA
Injection: MPA

Injection   Appearance   Peak
7"   10"

Figure 25–3. Detection and localization of left-to-right shunt by ascorbic acid indicator-dilution technique in a patient with a small ventricular septal defect. *Upper,* Ascorbic acid injected in the main pulmonary artery is detected within 2 seconds (early appearance) by the platinum electrode in the right ventricle. The main bolus of the indicator is detected by the electrode at 7 seconds after completing the systemic circuit. *Lower,* The platinum electrode has been withdrawn into the right atrium. There is no early appearance of the indicator, confirming the presence of the left-to-right shunt at the ventricular level only (presuming a competent tricuspid valve). RV, right ventricle; RA, right atrium; MPA, main pulmonary artery.

contributing sources of venous return. Thus, in the setting of a high systemic output, smaller degrees of oxygen step-up could indicate a significant left-to-right shunt.

It is also logical that any given oxygen saturation percentage step-up translates into a variable oxygen content step-up, depending on the hemoglobin concentration. Oxygen content can be calculated as (see equation at bottom of page). Thus, as shown in Figure 25–4, the slope of the relation between blood oxygen content and hemoglobin oxygen saturation becomes steeper with increasing levels of hemoglobin concentration in the blood. Stated alternatively, the higher the hemoglobin concentration, a step-up in any given amount of oxygen saturation translates into an even larger step-up in oxygen content.

One final consideration in the use of oxygen to calculate intracardiac shunts concerns the most accurate algorithm for determining the *average* oxygen saturation or content of the diverse sources of the systemic various return. Obviously, as discussed earlier, the more downstream from the point of admixture of venous sources, the greater is going to be the efficiency of mixing and the more likely that a given sample will reflect the *average* oxygen content for mixed venous blood. This issue is particularly germane in shunts that occur in close anatomic proximity to the right atrium where venous tributaries first manifest confluence of the blood that they carry. In patients without a shunt, the oxygen concentration of the pulmonary arterial blood may be closely approximated by a three-times weighting of the superior vena caval as

$$O_2 \text{ content} = O_2\text{-carrying capacity } (1.36 \text{ mL } O_2/\text{gm}) \cdot \text{Hg (gm/100 mL)} \cdot O_2 \text{ saturation } (\%)$$

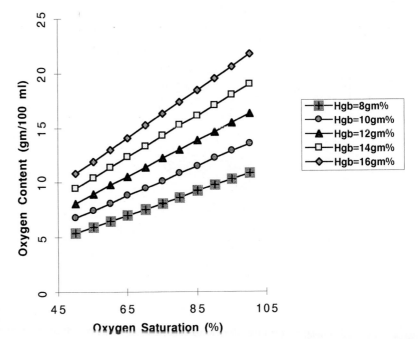

Figure 25–4. Relation between oxygen content in vol% (vertical axis) and oxygen saturation (percent) (horizontal axis) at various levels of hemoglobin concentration (isopleths). As hemoglobin concentration increases, the slope of relation between oxygen content and oxygen saturation becomes steeper. See text for discussion.

compared to the inferior caval caval blood samples.[11] Thus, by the "Flamm equation,"

$$C_{MVO_2} = \frac{3C_{SVCO_2} + C_{IVCO_2}}{4}$$

where C is concentration, MVO_2 is mixed venous oxygen, $SVCO_2$ is superior vena caval oxygen, and $IVCO_2$ is inferior vena caval oxygen. This weighting is most useful in an atrial septal defect where inadequate mixing of the three sources of blood return (superior vena cava, inferior vena cava, and coronary sinus) complicates the use of right atrial blood samples alone to evaluate the oxygen content of systemic venous blood.

The indocyanine green method, with injection of indicator into the left side of the heart, allows resolution of the site of shunting by comparison of the appearance time at sampling sites in the right side of the heart (right atrium, right ventricle, or pulmonary artery); the absolute degree of shunting is not determined by this method. Inhaled hydrogen gas is particularly useful as an indicator for detection of arterial admixture of systemic venous blood but does not allow quantification of absolute flow; moreover, because the gas is explosive, local fire regulations in recent years have interdicted the application of this sensitive technique. Cineangiographic demonstration of shunting is at best semiquantitative and dependent on the subjective interpretation of the angiogram. Nevertheless, when filmed in a biplane mode, cineangiography provides clear demonstration of the anatomic site of shunting and often uncovers associated lesions, such as a cleft mitral valve associated with a primum atrial septal defect and infundibular stenosis associated with the ventricular septal defect and aortic override of the ventricular septum in tetralogy of Fallot.

Right-to-Left Shunts

Proof of systemic venous admixture with already oxygenated blood is performed using one of the following:

1. Analysis of oxygen saturation or concentration from blood samples taken from various loci of the right and left sides of the heart
2. An early appearance of an indicator injected into the right side of the circulation with sampling from a systemic arterial source, such as indocyanine green (see Fig. 25–1)
3. Cineangiographic visualization of inappropriate early passage of iodinated contrast medium into the left heart when injected into the right side of the heart

Other indicators, including ascorbic acid, saccharin, ether, and Evans blue, have been used in the past but are not applied in modern catheterization laboratories. As with left-to-right shunts, the oxygen method alone is used for quantification of the magnitude of shunting, whereas the cineangiographic method is sensitive but, at best, semiquantitative.

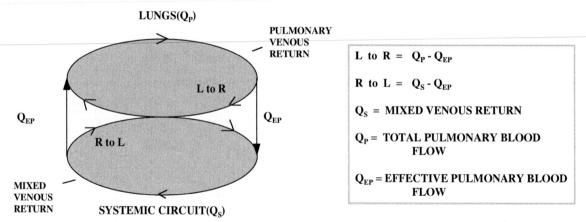

Figure 25–5. Schematic diagram of the components of flow and their calculation by the Fick principle in the circulation in the presence of left-to-right and right-to-left shunts. Q_{EP} is the hypothetical amount of blood flow, having been oxygenated in the lungs, that would be required to be delivered to the systemic circuit to account for total $\dot{V}O_2$. Q_S, total blood flow through systemic circuit; Q_P, total blood flow through lungs.

Quantification of Absolute Values of Intracardiac Shunting

Quantification of absolute values of intracardiac shunting, using oxygen as the indicator, is performed using equations derived from the Fick principle. Absolute pulmonary blood flow, Q_P, is calculated by measuring the oxygen uptake in the lungs, $\dot{V}O_2$, and dividing by the measured difference between the oxygen concentrations in samples of blood taken from the pulmonary veins (C_{PVO_2}) and pulmonary artery (C_{PAO_2}). Absolute systemic blood flow (Q_S) is calculated by assuming that oxygen uptake in the lungs is equivalent to total oxygen extraction in the systemic circuit.

Again, $\dot{V}O_2$ is divided by the arteriovenous oxygen concentration difference across this circuit, or, the difference between the concentration of oxygen in a major systemic artery, usually the ascending aorta (C_{AOO_2}), and the average concentration of oxygen in a mixed systemic venous return sample (C_{MVO_2}). The formulas for calculation of absolute amounts of left-to-right and right-to-left shunting also derive from the basic equations for Q_P and Q_S, as follows:

$$Q_{L\rightarrow R} = Q_P \cdot \frac{(C_{MVO_2} - C_{PAO_2})}{(C_{MVO_2} - C_{PVO_2})}$$

$$Q_{R\rightarrow L} = Q_P \cdot \frac{(C_{PVO_2} - C_{SAO_2})(C_{PAO_2} - C_{PVO_2})}{(C_{SAO_2} - C_{MVO_2})(C_{MVO_2} - C_{PVO_2})}$$

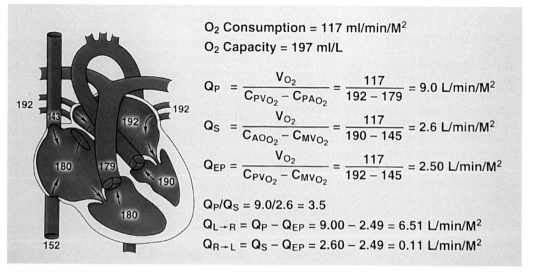

Figure 25–6. Schematic diagram of blood oxygenation in the heart in the presence of a relatively large interatrial septal defect with left-to-right shunting of oxygenated blood and normal pulmonary vascular resistance. A step-up in oxygen content is noted in the right atrium. Note the equations used for calculation of pulmonary blood flow (Q_P), systemic blood flow (Q_S), and effective pulmonary blood flow (Q_{EP}). (See also color section.)

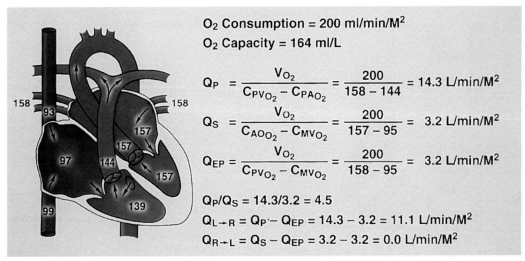

$$O_2 \text{ Consumption} = 200 \text{ ml/min/M}^2$$
$$O_2 \text{ Capacity} = 164 \text{ ml/L}$$

$$Q_P = \frac{V_{O_2}}{C_{PVO_2} - C_{PAO_2}} = \frac{200}{158 - 144} = 14.3 \text{ L/min/M}^2$$

$$Q_S = \frac{V_{O_2}}{C_{AOO_2} - C_{MVO_2}} = \frac{200}{157 - 95} = 3.2 \text{ L/min/M}^2$$

$$Q_{EP} = \frac{V_{O_2}}{C_{PVO_2} - C_{MVO_2}} = \frac{200}{158 - 95} = 3.2 \text{ L/min/M}^2$$

$$Q_P/Q_S = 14.3/3.2 = 4.5$$

$$Q_{L \to R} = Q_P - Q_{EP} = 14.3 - 3.2 = 11.1 \text{ L/min/M}^2$$

$$Q_{R \to L} = Q_S - Q_{EP} = 3.2 - 3.2 = 0.0 \text{ L/min/M}^2$$

Figure 25–7. Schematic diagram of blood oxygenation in the heart in the presence of a relatively large left-to-right shunt at the ventricular level and normal pulmonary vascular resistance. Sometimes, in the presence of tricuspid regurgitation, the step-up is detectable at the low right atrial level. Alternatively, with a high membranous ventricular septal defect, the step-up may be detectable in the pulmonary artery. (See also color section.)

Using simpler equations, it is also possible to estimate the absolute magnitude of intracardiac shunting by calculating the amount of effective pulmonary blood flow (Q_{EP}), which is the theoretic amount of blood flow, having been oxygenated in the lungs, that would be required to be delivered to the systemic circuit to account for total $\dot{V}_{O_2}$ (Fig. 25–5). This component of flow is calculated as $\dot{V}_{O_2}$ divided by the difference between the concentration of oxygen in the pulmonary veins (C_{PVO_2}) and the average concentration of oxygen in a mixed venous systemic return sample (C_{MVO_2}). In the presence of a right-to-left shunt ($Q_{R \to L}$), Q_S is approximated by the sum of Q_{EP} and $Q_{R \to L}$. In like fashion, in the presence of a left-to-right shunt ($Q_{L \to R}$), Q_P is approximated by the sum of Q_{EP} and $Q_{L \to R}$. These approximate calculations are used in most catheterization laboratories and are given in detail in specific congenital lesions in Figures 25–6 through 25–11 (see also the color section). Note that in the case of transposition of the great vessels (see Figs. 25–10 and 25–11), where the pulmonary and systemic circuits function in parallel rather than in series, and where there must be an open intracardiac shunt for systemic venous blood to reach the pulmonary circuit for oxygenation, the Q_{EP}, $Q_{R \to L}$, and $Q_{L \to R}$ are all equal.

Quantification of Relative Values of Intracardiac Shunting

In many instances, $\dot{V}_{O_2}$ is either not measured or inaccurate; thus, calculation of absolute blood flow through the pulmonary and systemic circuits cannot be made. Moreover, the absolute quantification of both $Q_{R \to L}$ and $Q_{L \to R}$ cannot be accomplished without knowing $\dot{V}_{O_2}$. However, because $\dot{V}_{O_2}$ drops out of the equation, the ratio of Q_P to Q_S can yet be calculated based on the measurement of oxygen percentage saturation alone in the systemic artery (aorta), pulmonary artery, pulmonary vein, and the systemic veins (inferior and superior vena cavae). Moreover, because oxygen-carrying capacity and blood hemoglobin concentration are presumably constant in all parts of the circulation, a simple measure of oxygen saturation on repeated blood samples allows estimation of the relative flows in the pulmonary and systemic circuits. Thus, (see equation at bottom of page). When combined with mean pressure ($\bar{P}$) measurements, the ratio of resistances in the pulmonary and systemic circuits (R_P/R_S) can also be calculated, without knowing the $\dot{V}_{O_2}$, as

$$R_P/R_S = \frac{(\bar{P}_{PA} - \bar{P}_{PV})(C_{PVO_2} - C_{PAO_2})}{(\bar{P}_{AO} - \bar{P}_{RA})(C_{AO\,O_2} - C_{MVO_2})}$$

$$Q_P/Q_S = \frac{\text{Systemic arterial } O_2 \text{ saturation (\%)} - \text{mixed venous } O_2 \text{ saturation (\%)}}{\text{Pulmonary arterial } O_2 \text{ saturation (\%)} - \text{pulmonary venous } O_2 \text{ saturation (\%)}}$$

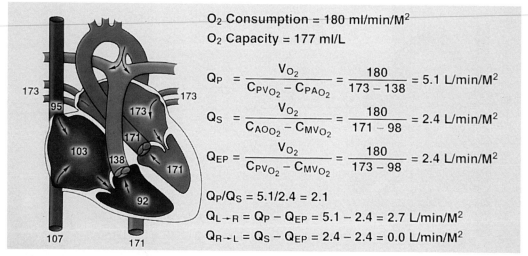

Figure 25–8. Schematic diagram of blood oxygenation in the heart in the presence of a patent ductus arteriosus and normal pulmonary vascular resistance. The arterial admixture of venous blood is best detected near the site of the shunt but may also be notable above the pulmonic valve and into the right pulmonary artery. (See also color section.)

In normal subjects, this ratio of the vascular resistances in the pulmonary and systemic circuits is less than 0.25. It serves as an important predictor in the patient with congenital heart disease of mortality risk during or shortly after operative correction. Broadly stated, in a patient with bidirectional shunting and elevated pulmonary resistance, the operative risk will be exceedingly high, or the clinical outcome poor, if the net shunt is right-to-left and the R_P/R_S is close to 1.0. Conversely, if the net shunt is left-to-right and the R_P/R_S is less than 0.50, the operative risk is relatively small and the clinical outcome more assured. Of course, many other factors impact on these decisions for surgical correction and affect the ultimate outcome.

COMMON ACYANOTIC CONGENITAL LESIONS OF THE HEART

Atrial Septal Defects

Excluding congenital valvular lesions (bicuspid aortic valve, mitral valve prolapse), an atrial septal defect is the most common lesion encountered by the cardiologist performing heart cath-

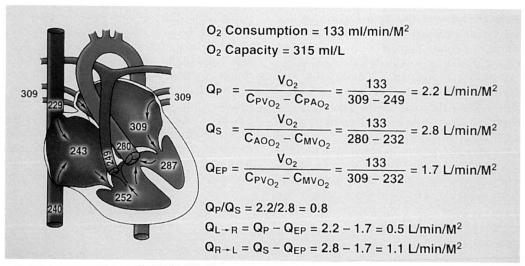

Figure 25–9. Schematic diagram of blood oxygenation in a heart with tetralogy of Fallot and bidirectional shunting at the high ventricular septal level. Left-to-right shunting is relatively small owing to obstruction to the pulmonary vascular bed by pulmonary stenosis. Right-to-left shunting is facilitated by aortic override of the ventricular septum. (See also color section.)

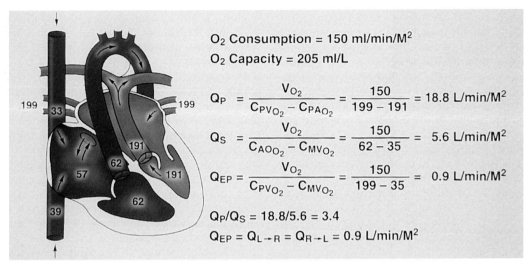

$$O_2 \text{ Consumption} = 150 \text{ ml/min/M}^2$$

$$O_2 \text{ Capacity} = 205 \text{ ml/L}$$

$$Q_P = \frac{V_{O_2}}{C_{PVO_2} - C_{PAO_2}} = \frac{150}{199 - 191} = 18.8 \text{ L/min/M}^2$$

$$Q_S = \frac{V_{O_2}}{C_{AOO_2} - C_{MVO_2}} = \frac{150}{62 - 35} = 5.6 \text{ L/min/M}^2$$

$$Q_{EP} = \frac{V_{O_2}}{C_{PVO_2} - C_{MVO_2}} = \frac{150}{199 - 35} = 0.9 \text{ L/min/M}^2$$

$$Q_P/Q_S = 18.8/5.6 = 3.4$$

$$Q_{EP} = Q_{L \to R} = Q_{R \to L} = 0.9 \text{ L/min/M}^2$$

Figure 25–10. Schematic diagram of blood oxygenation in a heart with D-transposition of the great vessels and an atrial septal defect. Note that the pulmonary and systemic circuits function in parallel; effective pulmonary blood flow (Q_{EP}) is dependent on the intracardiac shunt. In the absence of left ventricular outflow obstruction, pulmonary blood flow is increased. (See also color section.)

eterization and angiography in adults. Even in the 1990s, this class of lesion may escape detection because it uncommonly produces symptoms in childhood, and the physical findings may be readily overlooked or confused with functional flow murmurs.

The patent connection between the right and left atria allows bidirectional shunting to occur, although owing to the relatively greater compliance of the right versus the left ventricle, most shunting is left to right. Laminar flow, nevertheless, out of the inferior vena cava directly toward the secundum defect, allows some right-to-left shunting in all patients, particularly when the intrathoracic pressure is increased, such as by a Valsalva maneuver, and then as right-sided filling increases during the post-Valsalva phase. As long as there is a predominant left-to-right shunt, a volume overload exists on the right side of the circulation that may, in time, lead to an increase in the pulmonary vascular resistance (Eisenmenger reaction) and failure of the right ventricular myocardium. In contrast, with aging, acquired heart diseases that decrease left ventricular compliance, such as systemic hypertension and ischemic heart dis-

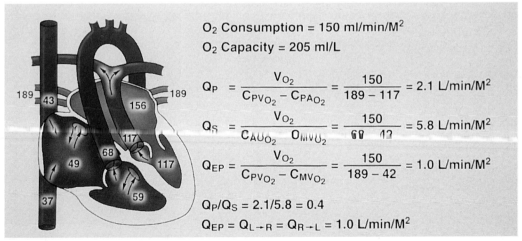

$$O_2 \text{ Consumption} = 150 \text{ ml/min/M}^2$$

$$O_2 \text{ Capacity} = 205 \text{ ml/L}$$

$$Q_P = \frac{V_{O_2}}{C_{PVO_2} - C_{PAO_2}} = \frac{150}{189 - 117} = 2.1 \text{ L/min/M}^2$$

$$Q_S = \frac{V_{O_2}}{C_{AOO_2} - C_{MVO_2}} = \frac{150}{68 - 42} = 5.8 \text{ L/min/M}^2$$

$$Q_{EP} = \frac{V_{O_2}}{C_{PVO_2} - C_{MVO_2}} = \frac{150}{189 - 42} = 1.0 \text{ L/min/M}^2$$

$$Q_P/Q_S = 2.1/5.8 = 0.4$$

$$Q_{EP} = Q_{L \to R} = Q_{R \to L} = 1.0 \text{ L/min/M}^2$$

Figure 25–11. Schematic diagram of blood oxygenation in a heart with D-transposition of the great vessels, an atrial septal defect, a ventricular septal defect, and subpulmonic stenosis. In this case, Q_{EP} contributes approximately the same proportion of Q_S. Because of the subpulmonic stenosis, pulmonary blood flow is reduced and Q_P/Q_S is diminished. (See also color section.)

ease, may contribute to ever greater left-to-right shunting. Late in the clinical course of an atrial septal defect, however, the degree of left-to-right shunting may decrease owing to a gradual increase in pulmonary vascular resistance, attendant pressure overload on the right ventricle, and failure and decreased compliance of the right ventricular myocardium. Such patients present with signs of right ventricular failure, atrial arrhythmias (atrial fibrillation), and increasing degrees of arterial hypoxemia owing to an increase in right-to-left shunting.

Defects in the interatrial septum occur most commonly at the site of the fossa ovalis (a secundum defect) but also are encountered high in the septum (sinus venosus defect) or directly above the atrioventricular valves (primum defect) (Fig. 25–12). The secundum defect in most patients is associated with a right ventricular conduction delay (rSr' pattern in precordial lead V_1) on the scalar electrocardiogram. The primum atrial septal defect is associated with a leftward mean QRS axis and a counterclockwise loop in the frontal plane leads; it may also be associated with clefts of the atrioventricular valves. The sinus venosus defect is frequently accompanied by partial anomalous pulmonary venous connections (Fig. 25–13) and is often suspected before catheterization by a leftward shift in the mean P axis (an ectopic atrial rhythm).

Technique of Catheter Passage

The preferred approach to catheterization of the right heart is via the right or left femoral vein. Once the catheter tip is in the right atrium, a 30- to 60-degree posteromedial rotation of the catheter allows ready probing of the septal defect and entrance into the left atrium. Engagement of the right atrial appendage can be recognized by the characteristic movement of the catheter tip with each atrial contraction as well as by the anteromedial position of the catheter tip in the upper one third of the right atrium. The type of atrial septal defect can often by suspected by whether the catheter crosses the septum just above the atrioventricular valves (a primum defect), high and posterior in the right atrium (a sinus venosus defect), or midway up the septum between the tricuspid valve and the superior vena cava (a secundum defect). If catheter passage via the femoral vein is not feasible, the septum can be traversed via the superior vena cava, but usually a full looping of the catheter in the right atrium is required and even then may be unsuccessful in entering the left atrium and ventricle. Because of its inferior location in the atrial septum, a primum defect is easier to cross from the superior vena cava than are either the secundum or sinus venosus types of defects. Mere passage of a catheter across the interatrial septum does not confirm an atrial septal defect but rather may prove only the existence of a probe-patent flap across the fossa ovalis.

Once the left atrium has been successfully entered, the catheter can often be introduced into the four pulmonary veins (Fig. 25–14) by applying external torque to the curved tip of the catheter and carefully advancing the catheter while watching on fluoroscopy for its passage beyond the geometric limits of the cardiac silhouette. Particular care should be taken to

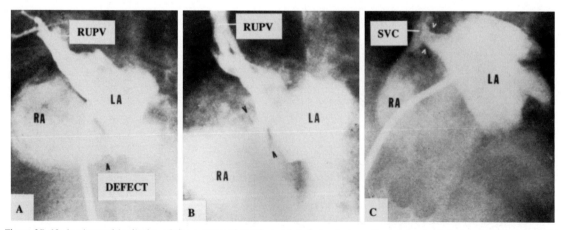

Figure 25–12. Angiographic display of three types of atrial septal defects. *A,* An ostium primum defect is demonstrated at the lower portion of the interatrial septum. *B,* An ostium secundum defect is shown. *C,* A sinus venosus defect high in the interatrial septum is demonstrated. RA, right atrium; LA, left atrium; SVC, superior vena cava; RUPV, right upper lobe pulmonary vein. (*A* to *C* from Elliott LP, Bargeron LM, Bream PR, et al: Axial cineangiography in congenital heart disease. II: Specific lesions. Circulation 1977; 56:1084–1093.)

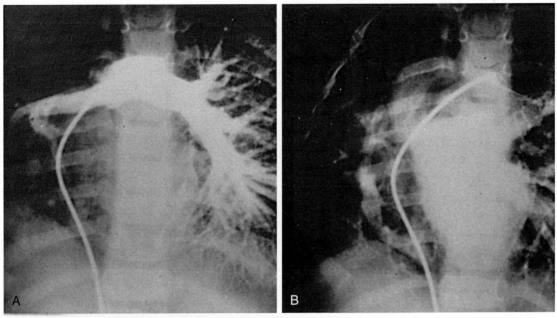

Figure 25–13. Angiographic display (arterial *[left]* and venous *[right]*) of partial anomalous pulmonary venous drainage, a lesion often associated with a sinus venosus atrial septal defect. The venous phase *(right)* of pulmonary angiography demonstrates an anomalous pulmonary vein connecting into the inferior vena cava. The curved, swordlike shadow of this vein can oftentimes be seen on the standard chest roentgenogram, giving rise to the so-called scimitar syndrome.

avoid entering the left atrial appendage, where injudicious application of pressure by the operator can lead to a perforation of the heart. Finally, counterclockwise and anterior rotation of the catheter is often successful in allowing traversal of the mitral valve and entrance into the left ventricle. This latter maneuver is best visualized while viewing the heart in the right anterior oblique projection with the left atrium and left

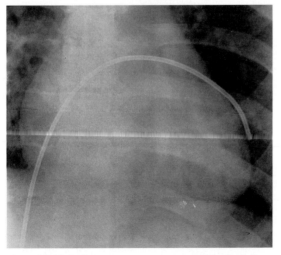

Figure 25–14. Catheter passage across an atrial septal defect into the left lower lobe pulmonary vein (anteroposterior projection).

ventricle separated, in profile, by the atrioventricular groove. Whenever the operator is uncertain as to the exact anatomic location of the catheter tip, a small injection of iodinated contrast medium serves to define its true position.

Intracardiac Pressures

When the size of the interatrial communication is not restrictive, the mean pressures in the right and left atria equalize, and no gradient can be detected on pull-back of the catheter from the left to the right atrium. Moreover, the phasic pressure pulse is similar in the two chambers, with the right atrial v wave manifesting usually a dominance over the a wave, in like fashion to what is observed normally in the left atrium. Late in the course of the lesion, as the right and left ventricles hypertrophy and the atria dilate, the a wave may become dominant, reflecting the increased operational stiffness of the ventricles during atrial contraction. Generally, the mean atrial pressures are not elevated unless there is considerable ventricular hypertrophy and dilation as might be seen late in the course of the lesion.

If the interatrial communication is small and restrictive, then a measurable pressure gradient can be demonstrated on pull-back across the septum. The presence of this gradient is also suggestive that the communication may, in fact, be a probe-patent foramen ovale.

Oximetric Data

As noted earlier, a left-to-right shunt at the atrial level is characterized by a step-up in oxygen saturation or content at the atrial level (see Fig. 25–6). Because of streaming effects and inadequate mixing, however, the magnitude of oxygen concentration increase required to prove the existence of a shunt is greater than shunts occurring further downstream in the right heart. As shown in Table 25–1, a step-up of 7 to 8 percent saturation units, or 1.3 to 2.0 vol% units, is necessary to reliably differentiate the effects of inadequate mixing from those of a true shunt. To best approximate an average mixed venous oxygen sample, considering all the sources of venous return, most laboratories use the weighted average of the Flamm equation (see earlier).

Detection of a step-up in oxygen concentration or saturation at the right atrial level is not specific for an atrial septal defect. Other relatively common causes of arterial admixture of venous blood at this level include (1) a ventricular septal defect, associated with some degree of tricuspid regurgitation; (2) a coronary arteriovenous fistula, draining into the coronary sinus; (3) a separate anomalous venous connection into the right atrium, with an associated atrial septal defect; and (4) a ruptured sinus of Valsalva aneurysm into the right atrium.

Angiography

Selective injection of contrast medium into the left atrium, or preferably the right upper lobe pulmonary vein, can be useful for subjectively quantitating the degree of left-to-right shunting across the atrial septum and for identifying the type of defect. This contrast angiogram is optimally performed in the left anterior oblique, approximately 45-degree cranial angulated, position. This four-chamber projection serves to place the atrial and ventricular septa in profile and allows ready identification of contrast agent streaming along and across the interatrial septum as well as the mitral valve (see Fig. 25–12). This view also allows identification of a coexistent ventricular septal defect, occurring as part of an endocardial cushion defect. In the adult, obtaining a true hepatoclavicular projection is at times difficult. A steep left anterior oblique projection (50 to 60 degrees) with 30-degree cranial angulation can be substituted successfully.

Selective contrast left ventriculography can also be useful for identifying the mitral valve abnormalities seen in some patients with an atrial septal defect. Mitral valve prolapse, usually with associated mild mitral regurgitation, can be seen with a secundum atrial septal defect. Also, patients with a primum atrial septal defect frequently exhibit a cleft of the anterior leaflet of the mitral valve and a mild to severe mitral regurgitation and manifest the classic "gooseneck" deformity of the left ventricular outflow tract (Fig. 25–15). The appearance of a gooseneck is caused by elongation of the left ventricular outflow tract owing to the mitral valve abnormality.

Ventricular Septal Defects

A ventricular septal defect may occur anywhere in the ventricular septum but occurs most commonly in the anterior region of the membranous, as opposed to the muscular, septum. Occasionally, when the defect is immediately beneath the aortic valve, its right coronary or noncoronary cusp will prolapse into the mouth of the membranous defect and cause associated

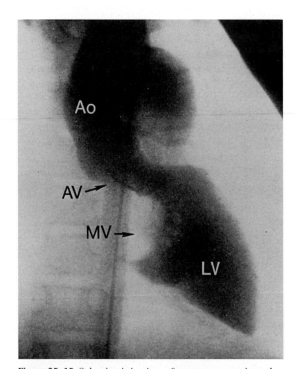

Figure 25–15. Selective injection of contrast agent into the left ventricle that displays a partial endocardial cushion defect with the typical "gooseneck" deformity created by the defective (cleft) mitral valve and the left ventricular outflow tract in patients with an ostium primum atrial septal defect. LV, left ventricle; Ao, aorta; AV, aortic valve *(upper arrow)*; MV, mitral valve *(lower arrow)*.

mild to moderate aortic regurgitation. The most anterior of the membranous defects are those that are subpulmonary, situated in the cone between the aorta and pulmonary arteries. Alternatively, the defect may be part of an endocardial cushion defect and occur predominantly in the posterior portion of the membranous septum. These defects may communicate directly with the right atrium (the so-called Gerbode defect) or show seeming direct regurgitation from the left ventricle into the right atrium via a ventricular septal defect and the tricuspid valve.

Defects in the muscular ventricular septum can also occur at any site between the apex and the high anterior or posterior muscular wall. Most commonly they occur in the mid-septal area immediately beneath the moderator band of the right ventricle. Multiple small defects can coexist, giving rise to a so-called sieve ventricular septal defect.

Because of the usually higher systolic pressures in the left than in the right ventricle, most shunting across a ventricular septal defect is left to right and during systole. However, right-to-left shunting can be present in coexisting conditions where the right ventricular systolic pressure is either high or progressively rises, for example, severe pulmonic stenosis or an Eisenmenger reaction in the lung, respectively. The degree of shunting is also influenced importantly by the afterload conditions on the two ventricles. To wit, a severe coarctation of the aorta, associated with a high systolic pressure in the proximal aorta, causes a relatively high proportion of the left ventricular stroke volume to unload across the ventricular septal defect into the pulmonary artery. Conversely, a potent systemic arteriolar vasodilator reduces aortic impedance and favors unloading into the aorta as opposed to the path across the ventricular septal defect.

The natural history of a patient with a ventricular septal defect is determined by the size of the defect and the response of the pulmonary vascular bed. If a patient has signs of pulmonary plethora (significant volume overload of the lungs), catheterization and angiography are recommended with a view toward early closure of the defect to avoid an Eisenmenger reaction. This latter reaction, an acquired disease of the resistance vessels of the lung, leading to irreversible pulmonary hypertension, occurs in approximately 5% to 10% of patients with large nonrestrictive ventricular septal defects. Many smaller ventricular septal defects spontaneously close by age 5 years. Thus, medical management is advised in those patients who are asymptomatic and have signs of a restrictive defect.

Technique of Catheter Passage

Most procedures for a suspected ventricular septal defect are accomplished by percutaneous insertion of catheters into the right femoral vein and artery. An arm approach can just as readily be used, however. Generally, with advancement of the right heart catheter into the right ventricle, it passes preferentially into the pulmonary artery. An exception to this circumstance is when the aorta straddles partially the plane of the ventricular septum (an "overriding aorta," as in tetralogy of Fallot), promoting direct entry into the aorta via a membranous septal defect (Fig. 25–16). To record the systolic pressure difference across the ventricular septal defect, both left and right ventricular pressures are recorded simultaneously.

Pressure Data

In the presence of a ventricular septal defect, a systolic pressure gradient (between the left and right ventricles) across the ventricular septal defect signifies a restrictive defect of relatively small size. On the other hand, the absence of a pressure gradient does not indicate necessarily a large, nonrestrictive defect. Either an elevated pulmonary vascular resistance, secondary to an Eisenmenger reaction, or an elevated right ventricular systolic pressure secondary to coexistent obstruction of the right ventricular outflow, pulmonic valve, or supravalvular pulmonary artery can cause equalization of systolic left and right ventricular pressures even in the face of a small ventricular septal defect.

Oximetric Data

Serial sampling of blood throughout the right heart, ascending aorta, and left ventricle allows calculation of the left-to-right and right-to-left shunting across a ventricular septal defect (see Fig. 25–7). In some patients presumably because of streaming or a defect situated immediately beneath the pulmonic valve, the step-up of oxygen saturation or content appears to be at the level of the main pulmonary artery. Also, in the presence of a large left-to-right shunt and tricuspid regurgitation, the step-up may be detected first at the level of the right atrium. Thus, the level of oxygen step-up cannot be depended on reliably for localization of the defect. Even in the face of a step-up in the right ventricle, it

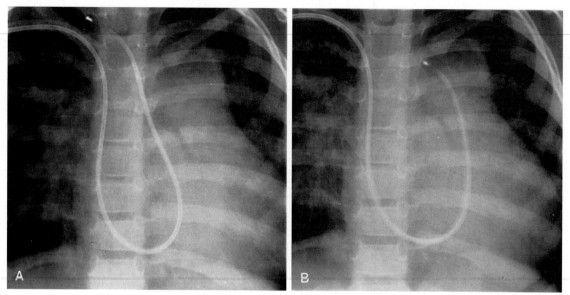

Figure 25–16. Catheter passage across a large ventricular septal defect into the ascending aorta *(A)*. Anteroposterior projection. Note the location of the catheter medially when compared in the same patient with the catheter location in the dilated main pulmonary artery *(B)*.

may be related to more than one ventricular septal defect.

Angiography

Modern biplane cineradiographic installations, with near-universal angulating capabilities for biplane x-ray gantries (see Chapter 7), have allowed precise localization by angiography of ventricular septal defects. Bargeron and Elliott and colleagues first described explicitly the views most optimal for demonstration of the location of various types of defects.[12, 13]

One particularly useful set of radiographic projections is as follows: (1) the patient is kept supine on the table, (2) the vertical x-ray system is positioned *left anterior oblique* (45-degree) and also angulated *cranially* (approximately 45-degree), and (3) the lateral system is positioned *posterior oblique* (45-degree) and also angulated *cranially* (15 to 20 degrees). Alternatively, while the patient is rotated rightward, the left shoulder brought up 45 degrees, and the feet brought to the right at 15 to 20 degrees to the long axis of the x-ray table, the vertical x-ray gantry is kept in an upright, anteroposterior orientation, and the lateral gantry is kept horizontal and directly orthogonal to the x-ray table. Either of these set-ups provides a so-called *hepatoclavicular* or *four-chamber* view in the vertical plane; the lateral plane provides complementary information. Using these views, the posterior portion of the ventricular septum is first seen while the sinus and the attachment of the

posterior leaflet of the mitral valve are visualized en face. The junction of the posterior mitral valve and the anterior mitral valve commissure with the posterior and free wall of the ventricular septum is well seen at the left margin of the mitral valve. Both mitral regurgitation and a left ventricular-to-right atrial shunt are particularly well seen in the vertical plane view. Moreover, with these projections, the anterior leaflet of the mitral valve can be visualized to be either normal or cleft. The full length of the ventricular septum can be seen in profile, and the location of a defect to the membranous or muscular portion can be readily determined (Fig. 25–17).

The *long axial oblique* view differs from the hepatoclavicular view in that (1) the vertical gantry is positioned at a *right anterior oblique* projection (15 to 20 degrees) while angulated *caudally* (20 to 30 degrees), (2) the lateral x-ray gantry is positioned in a steep *left anterior oblique* (approximately 60 to 70 degrees) and angulated *cranially* (approximately 20 to 30 degrees). It is the lateral system in this set-up that provides a particularly good view of the anterior ventricular septum; defects of the membranous septum or the conal area are particularly well seen.

Patent Ductus Arteriosus

A patent ductus arteriosus is a persistent conduit from fetal life between the underside of the aortic arch, usually immediately distal to the take-off of the left subclavian, that terminates in the left pulmonary artery. Rarely, the patent

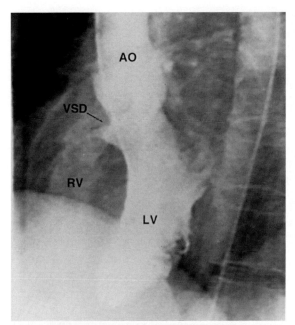

Figure 25–17. Selective left ventriculogram, filmed in the left anterior oblique projection, caudally angulated (four-chamber) view that displays a membranous ventricular septal defect. AO, aorta; VSD, ventricular septal defect; RV, right ventricle; LV, left ventricle.

ductus arteriosus arises from an anomalous left subclavian artery associated with a right-sided aortic arch. Prostaglandin E production during fetal life promotes patency of the conduit, and after birth premature infants are particularly prone to exhibit this lesion. A persistently patent ductus arteriosus occurs more frequently in females than in males (70:30 ratio) and accounts for about 5% to 10% of all forms of congenital heart disease confronted in the adult patient. The size and length of the ductus arteriosus vary widely, and may in later life become either calcified or aneurysmal.

In the adult, the physiologic impact of the open ductus arteriosus depends primarily on its size. If small, there is minimal hemodynamic derangement and the major risk of the lesion is that of a predisposition to infective endocarditis. If moderate to large, however, there is then a substantial left-to-right shunt that creates a volume overload on the left atrium and ventricle and predisposes the patient long-term to an Eisenmenger reaction of the pulmonary vascular bed. If this reaction occurs, the patient ultimately exhibits mitigation or loss of the left-to-right shunt and may exhibit right-to-left shunting with consequential differential cyanosis and clubbing of the toes as opposed to the right hand.

Technique of Catheter Passage

In general, the patient with a suspected patent ductus arteriosus, associated with a substantive shunt, requires only a right heart catheterization. Passage of the right heart catheter from the leg, arm, or neck into the left pulmonary artery allows ready access to the distal end of the ductus. If the ductus cross-sectional area is sufficiently large, gentle probing with a catheter allows advancement across the ductus into the descending thoracic aorta (Fig. 25–18). Visualization of the catheter in the left anterior oblique projection often facilitates this passage. If a catheter cannot be advanced successfully across the ductus, then display of its presence requires a retrograde arterial catheterization for performance of contrast angiography.

Pressure Data

If there is normal pulmonary vascular resistance and a moderate- to large-sized ductal conduit, then the conditions exist for diastolic "run-off" of systemic arterial blood into the pulmonary circuit. This creates a widened arterial pulse pressure, exaggeration of the systolic arterial pressure, and a lowering of the diastolic pressure. However, most ductal conduits are not large enough to create these conditions, and the arterial pressure pulse remains normal.

As the pulmonary vascular resistance begins to rise in response to a substantive left-to-right shunt, then the pulmonary artery systolic, diastolic, and mean pressures all increase concomitantly. The pulmonary arterial wedge pressure should remain relatively normal, although in some patients a high-quality wedge tracing may be difficult to obtain. Any apparent increase in the mean or phasic wedge tracing should be confirmed by repeating the measurement in other loci of the pulmonary vasculature. If an ambiguous wedge tracing is obtained in multiple sites, then an effort should be made to measure the left atrial pressure directly by crossing a probe-patent foramen ovale.

In an occasional adult patient with persistent left-to-right shunt and elevated pulmonary vascular resistance, the question arises as to whether the elevated pulmonary vascular resistance and pulmonary hypertension are reversible. In this circumstance, exposure of the patient to either inhaled 100% oxygen, or the administration of a vasodilator such as tolazoline, and careful observation for a decrease in the pulmonary artery pressure as flow remains constant or increases allows differentiation of reactive versus a fixed increase in the pulmonary vascular resistance.

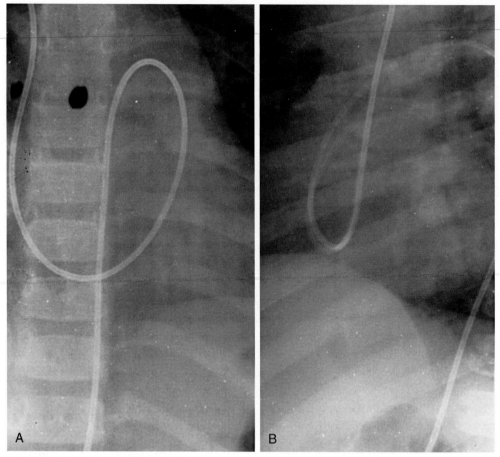

Figure 25–18. Typical catheter passage across a patent ductus arteriosus into the descending aorta. Projections are antero-posterior *(A)* and lateral *(B)*.

Oximetric Data

Sampling for pulmonary artery blood oxygen level in the setting of a patent ductus arteriosus is complicated by incomplete mixing both proximal and distal to the level of the shunt. With a left-to-right shunt, a sample drawn downstream to the shunt in the left pulmonary artery exhibits the highest oxygen saturation or content; however, there can be significant retrograde arterial admixture of mixed venous blood entering the main pulmonary artery, and to a lesser extent, that in the right pulmonary artery (see Fig. 25–8). Thus, calculation of a "mixed" pulmonary artery saturation or concentration is, at best, an estimate. In the presence of a right-to-left shunt, there is considerable discrepancy, without reliable downstream mixing, of samples taken from the descending and ascending portions of the aorta. Again, it is difficult to calculate accurately a mixed systemic arterial oxygen content. Consequently, the size of a shunt across a patent ductus arteriosus, calculated

from standard equations, must be correlated with other clinical and hemodynamic findings.

Angiography

When demonstration of a patent ductus arteriosus is deemed necessary, angiography is optimally performed in the left lateral projection (with the ascending, transverse, and descending thoracic aortic segments roughly parallel to the plane of view). Usually, this projection separates the ductal conduit from both the aorta and left pulmonary artery. Contrast medium needs to be injected in relatively high volume and near the take-off of the ductus from the aorta.

COMMON CONGENITAL OBSTRUCTIVE LESIONS OF THE HEART AND GREAT VESSELS

Pulmonic Valvular Stenosis

A congenital obstruction of the pulmonic valve generally allows survival into adulthood without surgical intervention. Moreover, mild obstruction of this valve has been noted to remain relatively stable throughout life and manifest little evidence of progression in severity. Late in life, the valve may exhibit calcification, although not to the degree seen in congenital malformations of the aortic valve. The stenosis is most commonly caused by fusion of the commissures, associated with thickening, increased rigidity, and doming during systole. In some patients there is dysplasia of the valve leaflets with only a small central orifice.

Moderate to severe obstruction of the pulmonic valve places a pressure overload on the right ventricle that, in turn, leads to significant right ventricular hypertrophy. Pressure measurements on right-sided heart catheterization confirm the diagnosis; usually, a slow "pull-back" tracing is recorded with an end-hole catheter under constant fluoroscopy, starting in the left or right pulmonary artery, and the operator looks for a sudden increase in systolic pressure (Fig. 25–19). Visual correlations are then made between catheter position and the point at which the pressure gradient appears. In some patients, both valvular pulmonic stenosis and right ventricular infundibular stenosis coexist; this can be detected by recording pressure gradients at two successive levels on slow pull-back of an end-hole catheter from the main pulmonary artery into the body of the right ventricle.

Selective right ventriculography is useful for demonstrating not only the site of right ventricular outflow tract obstruction but also the typical features of pulmonary valvular stenosis, including doming and thickening of the leaflets

and a central jet. Visualization of the right ventricular outflow tract is usually optimal in the lateral projection (Fig. 25–20). Coexistent infundibular stenosis can also be documented from the same injection. Alternatively, a straight anteroposterior projection with 25- to 35-degree cranial angulation also allows good visualization of the right ventricular outflow tract and pulmonic valve (Fig. 25–21). These two views are frequently obtained simultaneously in a biplane cineangiogram.

Infundibular Pulmonary Stenosis

Obstruction of the right ventricular outflow tract, between the crista supraventricularis and the pulmonic valve, is referred to as *infundibular stenosis*. An obstruction in this area can be the result of either a discrete or a relatively diffuse subvalvular muscle bundle. The lesion may be part of a constellation of lesions, as in tetralogy of Fallot, or it may be isolated. It may also coexist with valvular pulmonic stenosis.

Proof of the lesion by catheterization is dependent on a careful pull-back tracing, preferably using an end-hole catheter, from the main pulmonary artery into the immediate subvalvular area and thence into the body of the right ventricle. The systolic pressure gradient should be noted between the infundibular chamber, immediately beneath the pulmonic valve, and the body of the right ventricle (Fig. 25–22).

Selective cine-right ventriculography, positioned as shown in Figure 25–20, is usually diagnostic.

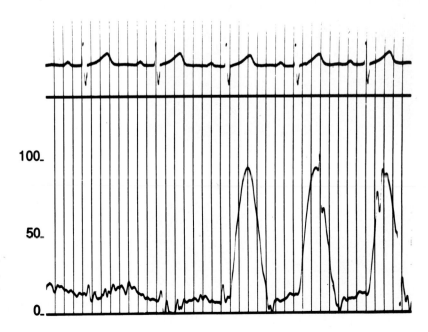

Figure 25–19. Pressure tracing of a "pull-back" in a case of severe valvular pulmonic stenosis (pressure scale in millimeters of mercury).

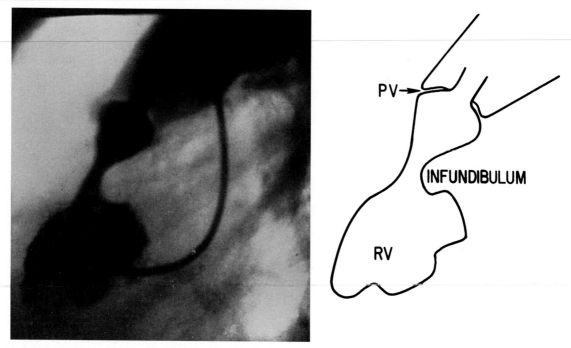

Figure 25–20. Selective right ventriculogram, filmed in the lateral projection, demonstrating narrowing of the right ventricular (RV) outflow tract at the infundibulum and the typical angiographic findings of pulmonic valvular stenosis (central jet, thickened and domed leaflets, and poststenotic dilation of pulmonary artery). PV, pulmonic valve.

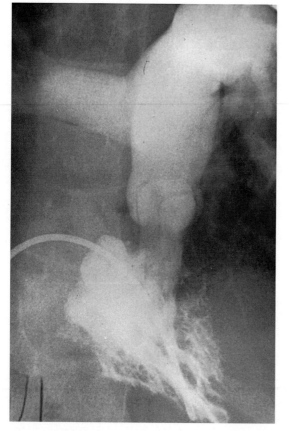

Figure 25–21. Cineangiogram of the right ventricle, right ventricular outflow tract, and proximal pulmonary arteries of an adolescent with pure valvular pulmonic stenosis (anteroposterior projection with 20-degree cranial angulation). In this systolic frame the cusps of the pulmonic valve are easily seen in a "domed" position. The infundibulum is widely patent with no evidence of subvalvular stenosis.

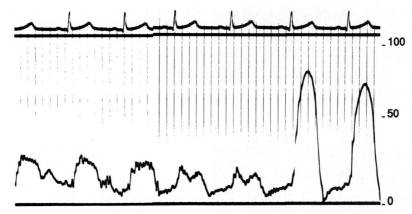

Figure 25–22. Pressure tracing of a "pull-back" from the main pulmonary artery to the infundibulum and thence to the body of the right ventricle in a patient with tetralogy of Fallot and infundibular pulmonic stenosis. Note the systolic pressure gradient between the infundibulum and the body of the right ventricle and the absence of a pressure gradient across the pulmonic valve. Note also that in diastole the infundibular chamber pressure is that of the body of the right ventricle and differs significantly from the diastolic pressure in the pulmonary artery. This finding helps confirm the location of the catheter tip proximal to (below) the pulmonic valve.

Aortic Stenosis

Congenital malformation of the aortic valve, leading to stenosis, constitutes approximately 5% of the total population of patients with congenital heart disease. The spectrum of pathoanatomy in this lesion spans from a unicuspid to a bicuspid valve with commissural fusion and an eccentric orifice between the left coronary and noncoronary cusps to a tricuspid valve with fused commissures and a solitary central orifice.

The severity of valve obstruction is based on calculation of a valve orifice size (Gorlin and Gorlin equation, see Chapter 18) and measurement of the transvalvular pressure gradient during systole. The hemodynamic burden is considered to be severe when the valve orifice area is 0.5 cm²/m² (indexed to body surface area) or the gradient is 80 mm Hg or more. Assessment of the valve orifice area is critically dependent on an accurate measurement of cardiac output and systolic flows across the valve. Ideally, the pressure gradient should be measured with one catheter inserted transseptally into the left ventricle and a second positioned just above the aortic valve. More commonly, however, the pressure gradient is assessed by a pull-back tracing taken with a catheter positioned retrograde into the left ventricle. In this circumstance, the catheter itself contributes to the severity of the measured pressure gradient (see Chapter 18).

Both a cine-left ventriculogram and an ascending aortogram serve to demonstrate the pathologic characteristics of congenital valvular aortic stenosis. The valve leaflets are thickened, manifest increased rigidity, and can be seen to dome during systole. Often a jet of contrast

agent helps to subjectively estimate the severity of narrowing of the valve orifice.

It is important to differentiate the various forms of subvalvular from valvular aortic stenosis, including (1) asymmetric hypertrophy associated with an obstructive hypertrophic cardiomyopathy (see Chapter 21); (2) a fixed subvalvular membrane that is often situated immediately beneath the aortic valve; (3) a fibromuscular tunnel obstruction; (4) anomalous muscle bundles of the left ventricular outflow tract; and (5) obstructive tumors in the outflow tract.

Supravalvular aortic stenosis is also part of the differential diagnosis of the various types of left ventricular outflow tract obstruction. Usually, the obstruction above the aortic valve is caused by an hourglass deformity caused by significant thickening of the media just above the sinuses of Valsalva. This lesion has been associated with a nonfamilial form, characterized by elfin facies, mental retardation, stenosis of systemic arterial as well as pulmonary arterial branches, strabismus, poor dentition, and an inguinal hernia (Williams syndrome). There also appears to be a familial form, carried as an autosomal dominant gene and associated with arterial stenoses of larger arteries. A further type of supravalvular stenosis is that associated with hypoplasia of the ascending aorta (Fig. 25–23).

Coarctation of the Aorta

A coarctation of the aorta is a congenital vascular obstruction secondary to a shelflike membrane, of variable thickness, across the lumen of the thoracic aorta (see Fig. 25–23). It coexists with a bicuspid aortic valve in approximately

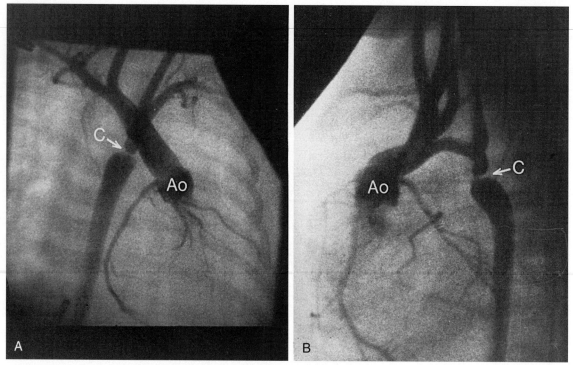

Figure 25-23. A biplane aortic root (Ao) injection, right anterior oblique *(A)* and left anterior oblique *(B)* with display of the ascending, hypoplastic transverse, and descending thoracic aorta and major tributaries, in a patient with coexistent coarctation of the aorta *(C)* associated with L-transposition of the great vessels.

85% of patients. Most commonly it is situated in close proximity to the ligamentum arteriosum (remnant of the ductus arteriosus), just distal to the take-off of the left subclavian artery from the thoracic aorta. Isolated cases have a coarctation that is proximal to the origin of the left subclavian. If the obstruction is sufficiently severe, the vascular tree above the coarctation exhibits significant hypertension while the abdominal aorta and its tributaries exhibit a relatively low systemic arterial pressure. The effect of the obstruction can be mitigated, however, by the presence of collateral vessels. In the adult with severe aortic coarctation the number and size of collateral vessels can be prodigious (Fig. 25-24).

Despite the accuracy of physical findings and noninvasive imaging in establishing the site and severity of the obstruction, cardiac catheterization and angiography are performed commonly in the patient with aortic coarctation. Their frequent application relates to the use of percutaneous balloon angioplasty at the same sitting for relief of the obstruction.

COMMON CYANOTIC CONGENITAL LESIONS OF THE HEART

Tetralogy of Fallot

In the adult patient, tetralogy of Fallot represents the most common congenital heart condi-

tion associated with systemic arterial desaturation or cyanosis. The four requisite lesions consist of (1) pulmonary stenosis, usually infundibular but possibly supravalvular or valvular; (2) a ventricular septal defect, usually infracristal, occasionally intracristal, rarely multiple; (3) right ventricular hypertrophy; and (4) an aortic root that overrides the ventricular septum.

In some patients there may also be an associated anomaly of the left anterior descending coronary artery arising from the right. This latter abnormality is particularly important to recognize before an attempt at surgical correction of the constellation of lesions. Also, in approximately 5% to 10% of patients there are aortopulmonary artery connections that mitigate the effects of obstructed access to the lungs out of the right ventricle.

Usually in this disease the ventricular septal defect is large enough to equalize the ventricular pressures between the right and left ventricles. Because access to the lungs is obstructed, right ventricular blood is ejected preferentially into the aorta, creating a significant right-to-left shunt and a deficiency of pulmonary blood flow. The severity of the right-to-left shunt is determined primarily by the degree of obstruction at the right ventricular outflow tract. Over a period of years, a patient with tetralogy of

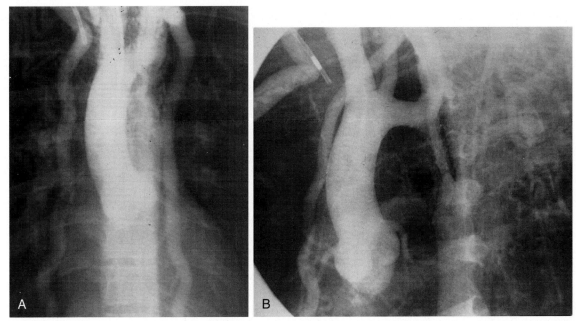

Figure 25–24. Biplane aortogram, shown in anteroposterior *(A)* and lateral *(B)* projections, in a patient with severe coarctation of the aorta. Note the large and numerous collateral vessels, including the huge internal mammary arteries.

Fallot usually develops ever-increasing worsening of obstruction across the right ventricular infundibulum.

Technique of Catheter Passage

Study of the patient with tetralogy of Fallot is best accomplished via the right femoral vein. The catheter can then be passed readily via the right ventricle, across the ventricular septal defect and into the aorta; also, unless the pulmonary valve is completely atretic, the catheter, with careful manipulation, can also be directed across the right ventricular outflow direct into the pulmonary artery. Risks of this passage include transient induction of complete heart block or a hypercyanotic spell (as pulmonary blood flow is further reduced). In many patients, the foramen ovale is probe patent, and clockwise rotation (posterior–left lateral orientation) of a curve-tipped catheter along the interatrial septum allows access to the left atrium and then subsequently the pulmonary veins and left ventricle. Generally, these maneuvers are readily accomplished with a relatively stiff NIH angiographic catheter that is curved at the tip by approximately 30 degrees. In any cyanotic patient, air-filled balloon flotation catheters are to be avoided unless carbon dioxide is used for balloon distension.

Pressure Data

Pressure recordings in tetralogy of Fallot usually reveal normal right and left atrial pressures,

normal diastolic pressures in both ventricles, and equalization of the systolic pressures across the unrestrictive ventricular septal defect. The magnitude of the pressure gradient between the bodies of the right and left ventricles and the pulmonary arteries depends, obviously, on the severity of the obstruction and the status of the intravascular volume. Pulmonary artery pressures are usually reduced, and the pressure gradient can be as high as 100 mm Hg. There may also be a pressure gradient at multiple levels across the right ventricular outflow tract, that is, both infundibulum and valvular.

Oximetric Data

As shown in Figure 25–9, the step-down in oxygen content in the left heart occurs at the level of the ventricular septal defect, although because of streaming, it may not be detected until the ascending aorta. Because of inadequate pulmonary blood flow, and a modest to absent left-to-right shunt, the Q_{EP} is significantly reduced. Systemic blood flow at rest, accounted for by Q_{EP} and the right-to-left shunt, is usually normal, although the mixed venous saturation in the right atrium is reduced.

Angiography

Axial biplane cineangiography is essential for diagnostic evaluation of the pathoanatomic features of patients with tetralogy of Fallot. The

454   Diagnosis

aims of the angiographic study are to assess (1) the site and number of ventricular septal defects; (2) the position of the aorta with respect to the ventricular septum; (3) the anatomy of the right ventricular outflow tract and the level of obstruction; and (4) the anatomy of the pulmonary artery from the supravalvular area up to and past its bifurcation into the right and left pulmonary arteries. The vertical hepatoclavicular (four-chamber) view is particularly useful for display of the ventricular septal defect and the pulmonary artery. The orthogonal lateral view is then particularly useful for displaying in profile right ventricular outflow tract and the infundibulum (Fig. 25–25).

Transposition of the Great Vessels

It is relatively unusual today for a patient with any form of transposition of the great vessels to present de novo to the cardiologist who primarily treats adults. By contrast, many such patients have either palliative or corrective surgery early in life and are now living into adulthood. The most common form of this anomaly is D-transposition, where the aorta is anterior and rightward to the pulmonary artery and arises from the anatomic right ventricle while the pulmonary artery is posterior and leftward to the aorta and comes off the left ventricle. A number of variants of these malpositions also exist; a full discussion of them is beyond the scope of this chapter.

With uncorrected D-transposition of the great vessels, the systemic and pulmonary circuits function in parallel, rather than in series. Therefore, for unoxygenated blood returning to the heart to access the lungs, there must be a communication between the right and left sides of the heart or a persistently patent ductus arteriosus. In most patients, an open interatrial communication (atrial septal defect, patent foramen ovale) exists that provides access to the lungs for the systemic venous return. Also, in 40% of patients with D-transposition, there is an associated ventricular septal defect (see Figs. 25–10 and 25–11).

In a steady state the degree of right-to-left and left-to-right shunting must be equivalent or blood would accumulate in one circuit at the expense of the other. By definition, $Q_{L \to R}$, $Q_{R \to L}$, and Q_{EP} must all be equal. Obviously, in the setting of transposition of the great vessels, the effectiveness of the heart in delivering oxygen to the periphery is highly dependent on the magnitude of Q_{EP}.

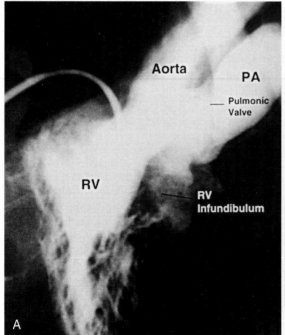 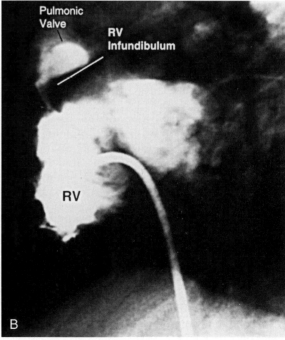

Figure 25–25. Biplane angiogram of tetralogy of Fallot, filmed in the anteroposterior (AP), with cranial angulation *(A)*, and lateral projections *(B)*. Contrast is injected selectively into the right ventricle (RV). The AP projection demonstrates the near-simultaneous opacification of the ascending aorta and pulmonary artery (PA). A narrow, slitlike opening of subvalvular infundibulum obstruction is demonstrated in both planes. Because the ventricular septum is not shown in profile, the overriding of the aorta is not demonstrated. (Courtesy of Abraham Rothman, MD.)

Technique of Catheter Passage

The best approach to the heart in the presence of transposition of the great vessels is via the right femoral vein. Either an atrial septal defect or a probe-patent foramen ovale most often allows access to the left atrium followed by the left ventricle. With skillful manipulation, or by use of a balloon flotation catheter or tip deflector, the pulmonary artery coming off the left ventricle can then be accessed.[14] In the absence of an interatrial communication, the operator can alternatively access the left ventricle via a ventricular septal defect. However, manipulation of a catheter into the pulmonary artery requires considerably more skill and persistence.

Pressure Data

Because the anatomic right ventricle is the systemic ventricle in simple D-transposition of the great vessels, the peak systolic pressure in this chamber is equivalent to that in the aorta. The right atrial pressure reflects the degree of elevation of the right ventricular diastolic pressure. In adult life, the right ventricle can fail or become significantly stiffer, and the right atrial pressure is then significantly elevated. The anatomic left ventricular pressure depends on the presence or absence of a ventricular septal defect, its size, and the resistance in the pulmonary vasculature. Also, in some patients with transposition of the great arteries, there is associated subpulmonic obstruction of the outflow tract of the left ventricle. Thus, the peak systolic pressure in the left ventricle may be significantly higher than that measured in the pulmonary artery. The pulmonary artery pressure, and also that in the left ventricle, can also be influenced by the presence or absence of a patent ductus arteriosus.

Oximetric Data

In most patients with transposition of the great vessels, the ductus arteriosus closes soon after birth. Thereafter, the degree of systemic arterial desaturation is determined solely by the size of the intracardiac shunt. As shown in a sample case depicted in Figure 25–10, Q_{EP}, $Q_{L \rightarrow R}$, and $Q_{R \rightarrow L}$ are all quite low at the same time that there is a relatively high flow through the lungs owing to a normal pulmonary vascular resistance. An atrial septal defect represents the only connection between the two parallel circuits. In this instance, therefore, there is an extremely low systemic arterial saturation, and the patient is in dire need of a procedure to promote access of mixed venous blood to the pulmonary circuit.

In other instances when there is obstruction to left ventricular outflow by pulmonic stenosis, the pulmonary blood flow is relatively low (see Fig. 25–11). At the same time, the degree of systemic arterial desaturation is dependent on the degree of shunting provided by either an atrial or ventricular septal defect. If perfect mixing were present, the saturations in the pulmonary artery and the systemic arteries would equalize. Generally, if the difference in saturation between the pulmonary and systemic arteries is greater than 10%, then a palliative procedure to increase intracardiac shunting (balloon or blade septostomy) is indicated.

Angiography

Both right and left ventriculography help delineate the abnormal relationship between the great vessels and the two ventricles and other associated anomalies in transposition of the great vessels. The right ventriculogram reveals the systolic function of the right ventricle, the presence or absence of tricuspid regurgitation, the presence or absence of a patent ductus arteriosus, and, in some instances, the coronary artery anatomic structure. The left ventriculogram demonstrates the anatomy of the outflow tract and the presence or absence of a ventricular septal defect. Occasionally, a left atrial injection is performed to visualize the size of an atrial defect.

Single Ventricle

The term *single* or *common ventricle* refers to a spectrum of congenital lesions, all of which are characterized by at least one ventricular chamber that receives blood through both the tricuspid and mitral valves or a common atrioventricular valve. Detailed classifications of this entity revolve around the presence or absence of varying contributions of muscle mass from the left and right ventricles. Also, the great vessels are frequently transposed, some in the D-configuration and others in the L-configuration; a few patients have great vessels that are normally related.

Other lesions are frequently encountered with single ventricle, most notably pulmonic stenosis, and play an important role in pathophysiology and prognosis. Other factors impacting on natural history are ventricular function, insufficiency of the atrioventricular valve or valves, and the presence or absence of subaortic stenosis. Pulmonic stenosis protects the lung against excessive pulmonary blood flow and ultimate congestive heart failure. On the other hand, if pulmonic stenosis is too severe, pulmonary blood flow is inadequate, and systemic arterial desaturation is excessive. Relatively few patients with single ventricle, without palliation, survive into adulthood.

Pressure and Oximetric Data

The pressure and oximetric findings in the various types of single ventricle depend greatly on the specific type and any associated abnormalities. Every effort should be made to enter both the aorta and the pulmonary artery to delineate outlet obstruction beneath either of these vessels. In addition, to calculate systemic and pulmonary resistances, it is important to measure both the pressure and the oxygen saturation in each great vessel. The common ventricle serves as a mixing chamber for both pulmonary and systemic venous return, but streaming effects can lead to a significant disparity in oxygen saturation or content between the aorta and the main pulmonary artery.

Angiography

The most important angiographic examination in single ventricle is a biplane ventriculogram. This study, usually performed in straight anteroposterior and lateral projections, identifies the anatomy and competency of the atrioventricular valves, the integrity of ventricular myocardial function, the presence or absence of outlet obstruction, the presence or absence of transposed great vessels, and the relative contributions of the morphologic right and left ventricles to the single ventricle.

REFERENCES

1. McNamara DG: The adult with congenital heart disease. Curr Prob Cardiol 1989; 14:57–114.
2. Higgins CB, Silverman NH, Kersting-Sommerhoff BA, Schmidt K (eds): Congenital Heart Disease: Echocardiography and Magnetic Resonance Imaging. New York, Raven, 1990.
3. Nadas AS, Fyler DC (eds): Pediatric Cardiology. Philadelphia, WB Saunders, 1972.
4. Rudolph AM (ed): Congenital Disease of the Heart: Clinical-Physiologic Considerations in Diagnosis and Management. Chicago, Year Book, 1974.
5. Dexter L, Haynes FW, Burwell CS, et al: Studies of congenital heart disease. II: The pressure and oxygen content of blood in the right auricle, right ventricle, and pulmonary artery in control patients, with observations on the oxygen saturation and source of pulmonary "capillary" blood. J Clin Invest 1947; 26:554.
6. Kusumi F, Butts WC, Ruff WL: Superior analytical performance of electrolytic cell analysis of blood oxygen content. J Appl Physiol 1973; 35:299–300.
7. Barratt-Boyes BF, Wood EH: The oxygen saturation of blood in the venae cavae, right heart chambers, and pulmonary vessels of healthy subjects. J Lab Clin Med 1957; 50:93–106.
8. Rudolph Am, Caylor GC: Cardiac catheterization in infants and children. Pediatr Clin North Am 1958; 5:907–943.
9. Freed MD, Miettinen OS, Nadas AS: Oximetric detection of intracardiac left-to-right shunts. Br Heart J 1979; 42:690–694.
10. Antman EM, Marsh JD, Green LH, Grossman W: Blood oxygen measurements in the assessment of intracardiac left-to-right shunts: A critical appraisal of methodology. Am J Cardiol 1980; 46:265.
11. Flamm MD, Cohn KE, Hancock EW: Measurement of systemic cardiac output at rest and exercise in patients with atrial septal defect. Am J Cardiol 1969; 23:258–265.
12. Bargeron LM, Elliott LP, Soto B, et al: Axial cineangiography in congenital heart disease. Section I: Concept, Technical, and Anatomic Considerations. Circulation 1977; 56:1075–1083.
13. Elliott LP, Bargeron LM, Bream PR, et al: Axial cineangiography in congenital heart disease. Section II: Specific lesions. Circulation 1977; 56:1084–1093.
14. Kelly DT, Krovetz LJ, Rowe RD: Double-lumen flotation catheter for use in complex congenital cardiac anomalies. Circulation 1971; 44:910–913.

Chapter 26

Catheterization in Disorders of Cardiac Rhythm

PENG-SHENG CHEN
GREGORY K. FELD

Electrophysiologic studies are commonly performed in the catheterization laboratory for the diagnosis and treatment of cardiac rhythm disorders. No single person can claim the sole credit for the development of clinical electrophysiology as a subspecialty, and several landmark events have allowed significant advances to current electrophysiologic practices. These events include the development of pacemakers,[1] programmed stimulation,[2] the electrophysiologically guided surgical treatment of Wolff-Parkinson-White syndrome[3, 4] and ventricular tachycardia,[5, 6] the automatic implantable defibrillator,[7, 8] and the techniques of catheter ablation-modification of the atrioventricular (AV) node and the accessory pathways using direct current[9, 10] or radiofrequency energy.[11, 12] With the availability of these diagnostic and therapeutic methods, electrophysiologic studies have greatly contributed to patient care.

EVALUATION OF BRADYCARDIA

Inappropriate sinus bradycardia or AV block can result in serious symptoms or sudden cardiac death; in general, if symptomatic bradycardia is documented by electrocardiographic (ECG) recordings in the absence of reversible causes, such as the use of bradycardic medications, patients should have a permanent pacemaker implanted and an electrophysiologic study would be inappropriate.[13] However, in certain patients in whom symptomatic bradycardia is suspected but cannot be documented because of its rare occurrence, electrophysiologic study can provide evidence supporting this diagnosis and thus justify the use of a permanent pacemaker.

The most commonly used test parameter for the evaluation of the sinus node is the sinus node recovery time. It is well known that pacemaker cells can be suppressed by overdrive pacing.[14] In patients with sick sinus syndrome, however, the recovery time of the sinus or AV node to resume normal activity after a period of rapid atrial pacing is often prolonged.[14-17] The techniques used in measuring the sinus node recovery time are illustrated in Figure 26–1. The patient presented is a 62-year-old man who underwent two previous coronary artery bypass procedures. He was experiencing fatigue, weakness, and frequent episodes of slow, incessant, atrial flutter with a 2:1 AV conduction and a ventricular rate of 105 to 120 beats/min. Atrial pacing was performed from the high right atrium, and a rhythm strip was recorded to determine baseline spontaneous sinus rate. Atrial pacing at a cycle length slightly shorter than that of the spontaneous sinus cycle length was performed for 30 seconds. The pacing was then abruptly terminated, and the time from the last pacing spike to the first spontaneous P wave was designated as the sinus node recovery time. If the first beat after pacing had not been preceded by a P wave, the time from the last pacing spike to the onset of the first QRS complex would have been used as the sinus node recovery time. The corrected sinus node recovery time is calculated as the difference between the sinus node recovery time and the average of three baseline sinus cycle lengths. An abnormal response is defined as a corrected sinus node recovery time of 550 msec or longer.[18] During the study of this patient (see Fig. 26–1), the corrected sinus node recovery time was found to be prolonged to 1150 msec, and a dual-chamber pacemaker was implanted. Subsequently, the patient noticed a marked improvement in exercise capacity. His atrial flutter was

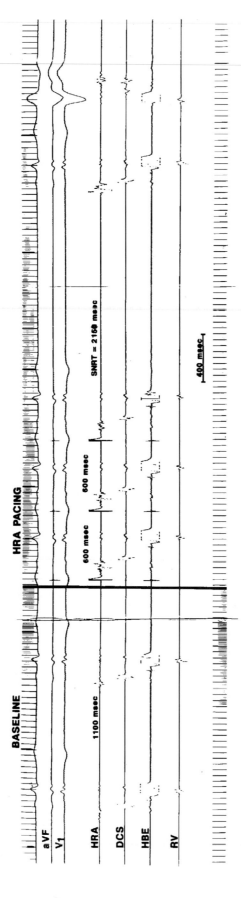

Figure 26–1. Sinus node recovery time testing. The patient is a 62-year-old man who had a history of coronary artery disease and recurrent atrial flutter since coronary artery bypass grafting surgery. The electrocardiographic leads I, aVF, and V_1 and intracardiac leads from high right atrium (HRA), distal coronary sinus (DCS), His bundle (HBE), and right ventricle (RV) are shown. The baseline cycle length was 1100 msec. The ventricles were then paced at a 600-msec cycle length for 30 seconds. When pacing was terminated, the sinus rhythm recovered in 2150 msec. The corrected sinus node recovery time is the difference between 2150 msec and 1100 msec, or 1050 msec.

well controlled, and his antiarrhythmic medications were discontinued.

AV nodal conduction can be evaluated by recording the His electrogram[19, 20] (Fig. 26–2). The normal values of the AH interval range from 45 to 140 msec and those of the HV interval from 25 to 55 msec.[18] In the presence of complete AV block, the site of the block can be

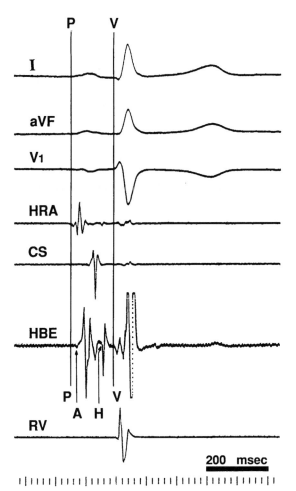

200 msec

Figure 26–2. His bundle electrogram recording. Electrocardiographic (ECG) leads I, aVF, V$_1$, and intracardiac electrogram recorded at high right atrium (HRA), coronary sinus (CS), His bundle (HBE), and right ventricle (RV) are shown. The HBE was recorded by a quadripolar electrode catheter with 1-cm spacing between the electrodes. The high-pass filter was set at 30 Hz and the low-pass filter at 500 Hz. The notch filter was off. The HBE was identified by a sharp deflection registered between the A and the V waves. The AH interval was measured from the onset of the local A wave to the onset of the local H wave, and the HV interval was measured from the onset of the H wave to the onset of the surface ECG QRS complex. To determine accurately the onset of surface QRS complexes, more than one ECG channel should be recorded. In this example, if aVF was the only ECG recorded, the onset of QRS complex could be miscalculated by more than 20 msec because the initial part of QRS complex on aVF was isoelectric.

either supra-Hisian (where an A wave is not followed by a His bundle deflection) or infra-Hisian (where an A wave is followed by a His deflection but not by ventricular activation). Despite the earlier reports about the increased risks of sudden death in patients with prolonged HV intervals,[21] subsequent studies have demonstrated that the clinical course in asymptomatic patients is usually benign.[22, 23] Thus, there is no indication to perform His bundle recording in this group. In symptomatic patients (patients with syncope or near syncope), for whom His-Purkinje block is suspected but not proved, electrophysiologic evaluation is indicated.[13] It is our experience that His bundle electrogram recordings are rarely the only factor that determines whether or not a patient should have a permanent pacemaker implanted.

The upright-tilt test[24] has been reported to be useful in evaluating patients with unexplained syncope; it may be performed at the end of electrophysiologic study. There are at least two common methods used to perform this test: the first is to position the patient upright at an angle of 80 degrees for 10 minutes,[24] and the second is to position the patient at 60 degrees until symptoms occur.[25] Using the latter method, the mean time to syncope after tilt is 25 minutes, according to Raviele and associates.[25] We have used the 60-degree, long duration–tilt method[25] in our laboratory. The blood pressure and the heart rate are closely monitored. If syncope develops, the test is positive. The patient is then rapidly lowered to a supine position. If syncope is not induced, an infusion of isoproterenol is started at a dose of 1 µg/min and increased gradually to 5 µg/min. If the isoproterenol infusion results in syncope, the test is positive. The test is negative in absence of syncope at the maximal dose of isoproterenol or if the heart rate reaches 150 beats/min.[24]

There is no consensus about how to treat patients with a positive tilt test. However, both α-adrenergic and β-adrenergic antagonists (blockers) have been used in a small number of patients, with good results being observed during a short term follow up period.[25]

ELECTROPHYSIOLOGIC STUDY FOR SUPRAVENTRICULAR TACHYCARDIA

The recent development of radiofrequency catheter ablation techniques[11, 12] has drastically changed electrophysiologic approaches to supraventricular tachycardia. Calkins and colleagues[12] reported a 90% cure rate by catheter ablation techniques in a group of 106 patients referred for electrophysiologic studies at their institution, with virtually no complications. We have had the same experience at our institution. Because of the high degree of success and the low morbidity and mortality associated with ablation procedures, electrophysiologic study of patients with drug-resistant supraventricular tachycardia should be used not only for diagnosis but also for treatment. Ideally, both diagnosis and treatment should be performed during the same procedure to avoid a second electrophysiologic study at additional cost and risk.

Ectopic Atrial Tachycardia

Ectopic atrial tachycardia is an uncommon cause of supraventricular tachycardia.[12] The mechanisms of this arrhythmia are unknown and pharmacologic treatment is often unsatisfactory. Persistent atrial tachycardia can eventually lead to cardiomyopathy and heart failure. Before the availability of catheter ablation techniques, surgical treatment of the arrhythmia could lead to reversibility of the cardiomyopathy.[26] However, with the availability of catheter ablation techniques, some of these patients can be cured without surgery.[27]

During electrophysiologic study, a coronary sinus catheter should be inserted to determine the sequence of activation on the left atrial side of the AV groove. A His bundle catheter should be placed to determine the time of atrial activation at the AV junction and the time of the His bundle electrogram. A right ventricular electrode is needed for right ventricular pacing and recordings. A modified Brockenbrough[28] catheter is then positioned in the high right atrium. The times of activation throughout the right atrial endocardial surface will be determined by moving the catheter in an up-and-down fashion, starting from the high lateral right atrium and then moving either clockwise or counterclockwise inside the atrium. When the earliest activation site is found in the right atrium, catheter ablation can be attempted at that site.

Figures 26–3 through 26–5 illustrate a patient who has been mapped and cured. The patient is a 33-year-old man who developed incessant atrial tachycardia at a rate as high as 240 beats/min 10 years ago. He was treated with various antiarrhythmic agents, but none resulted in suppression of the arrhythmia. He was then placed on a combination of propranolol and flecainide, which decreased the heart rate to approximately 100 beats/min. Because of in-

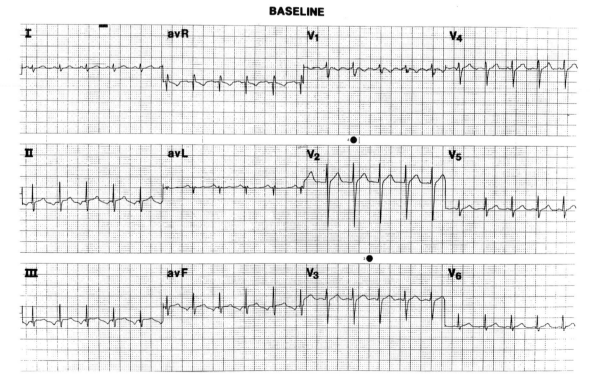

BASELINE

Figure 26–3. Ectopic atrial tachycardia. This electrocardiogram was taken from a 33-year-old man with incessant tachycardia. There were inverted P waves in leads II, III, and aVF and a positive P wave in leads I and aVL, indicating that the origin of the tachycardia is probably located in the low lateral right atrium.

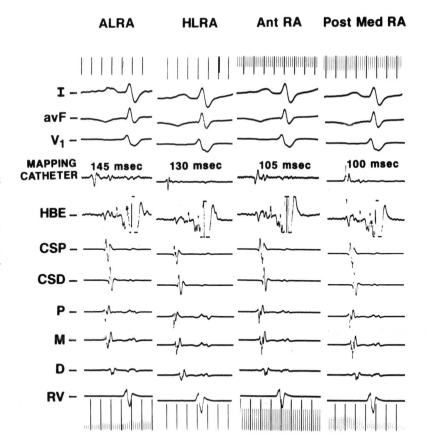

Figure 26–4. Endocardial mapping of ectopic atrial tachycardia. The mapping catheter was moved systemically inside the right atrium. The earliest activation occurred in the anterolateral right atrium (ALRA), with local A wave occurring 145 msec prior to the onset of QRS complex. When the catheter was moved to other locations, the timing of local electrogram was progressively later. HLRA, high lateral right atrium; Ant RA, anterior right atrium; Post Med RA, posteromedial right atrium; HBE, His bundle electrogram; CSP, bipolar coronary sinus proximal electrogram; CSD, bipolar coronary sinus distal electrogram; P, M, D, proximal, mid, and distal unipolar coronary sinus electrogram, respectively; RV, right ventricular electrogram.

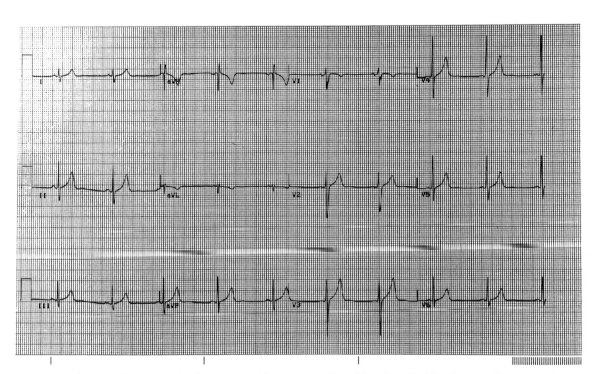

Figure 26–5. Electrocardiogram after radiofrequency ablation of ectopic atrial tachycardia. The electrocardiogram was taken 6 months after ablation and showed normal sinus rhythm.

tolerable side effects to these medications, the patient was admitted for electrophysiologic study. The baseline ECG (see Fig. 26–3) showed ectopic atrial tachycardia with a negative P wave in leads II, III, and aVF and a positive P wave in lead I, indicating a possible low right atrial focus. Endocardial mapping (see Fig. 26–4) showed that the earliest activation site was located in the anterolateral right atrium. Radiofrequency energy was then applied to this area multiple times and successfully converted the patient to sinus rhythm (see Fig. 26–5). The patient remained in sinus rhythm during the 1-year follow-up period.

Supraventricular Tachycardia due to Atrioventricular Nodal Reentry

The clinical presentation of supraventricular tachycardia due to AV nodal reentry includes frequent, intermittent palpitations and an ECG manifesting a narrow QRS complex. The tachycardia can be terminated either by vagal maneuver or by an intravenous injection of verapamil[29] or adenosine.[30] After termination, there is no evidence of preexcitation on the ECG. The differentiation by ECG between AV nodal reentrant tachycardia and AV reentrant tachycardia due to an accessory pathway can be difficult. The presence or absence of preexcitation during normal rhythm cannot be used as a definitive diagnostic test. Patients with concealed accessory pathways can have a normal surface ECG. On the other hand, patients with preexcitation are not immune to AV nodal reentrant tachycardia.[31] The presence of a retrograde P wave during tachycardia is a helpful clue in diagnosing AV reentry due to an accessory pathway, because the ventriculoatrial (VA) interval is usually prolonged when the tachycardia uses the ventricle as a part of the reentrant circuit.[32] However, because the P wave is of low amplitude, the determination of the presence or absence of the P wave may be difficult.

The techniques for studying AV nodal reentrant tachycardia and other supraventricular tachycardia of unknown mechanisms include the insertion of catheters in the coronary sinus, the right ventricle, the His bundle area, and the right atrium. Programmed stimulation can then be performed by giving a single premature stimulus to the atrium and the ventricle and by rapid atrial and ventricular pacing. During atrial premature stimulation, the A_2H_2 intervals are measured for each S_1S_2 (or A_1A_2) interval. The presence of dual AV nodal pathways[33] is defined as an increase in the A_2H_2 interval by more than 55 msec when the A_1A_2 interval is decreased by

10 to 20 msec.[18] This sudden increase in the A_2H_2 interval indicates a conduction block in the fast pathway, leaving the slow pathway to conduct alone. Dual AV nodal pathways can also be determined by ventricular programmed stimulation when a sudden increase in the VA conduction interval is noted.

Figure 26–6 shows an example of AV nodal reentrant tachycardia. Figure 26–6A shows that with an S_1S_2 interval of 560 msec, the A_2H_2 interval was 140 msec. Figure 26–6B shows that when the S_1S_2 interval was shortened by 20 msec, the A_2H_2 interval increased dramatically, to 360 msec, suggesting the presence of a dual AV nodal pathway. During tachycardia (Fig. 26–6C), the anterograde conduction was through the slow pathway, resulting in a long AH interval. The retrograde conduction was through the fast pathway, resulting in a very short HA interval. As a result, the A and V waves were superimposed. This latter finding is classic for AV nodal reentrant tachycardia. According to one report,[32] the differentiation between AV nodal reentrant tachycardia and AV reentrant tachycardia using an accessory pathway can be made by measuring the VA intervals. During reciprocating tachycardia, an interval between V and the earliest recorded retrograde A wave of 61 msec or less and an interval between the V and the high right atrium A wave of 95 msec or less exclude the presence of an accessory pathway.[32]

The anatomic location of the slow and fast pathways may be quite separate. The fast pathway usually is located near the AV node, whereas the slow pathway is more posterior, near the coronary sinus orifice.[34] Because of the anatomic distance between these two pathways, the selective ablation of one of the two pathways by surgery[35, 36] or by catheter techniques[12] can result in the cure of AV nodal reentrant tachycardia while avoiding complete heart block.

McGuire and coworkers[37] reported that the reentrant circuit of AV nodal reentrant tachycardia is not confined to the AV node and that perinodal atrium is an essential part of the circuit. These authors suggested that the traditional scheme of the AV nodal reentrant circuit (Fig. 26–7A) is incorrect, because it implies that the whole circuit is intranodal. These authors, instead, proposed several alternative models that may explain their findings (Fig. 26–7B through D). Among these models, the one shown in Figure 26–7D incorporates perinodal tissue as a part of the reentrant circuit and is most compatible with current electrophysiologic findings and surgical results.[37] Based on the experience of radiofrequency catheter ablation, in which successful results can be achieved by

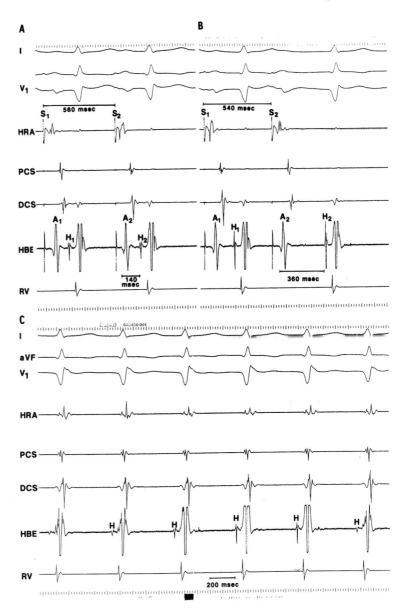

Figure 26–6. Atrioventricular nodal reentrant tachycardia. See text for details.

ablating tissue outside of the AV node, we agree with these authors that the extranodal tissue is probably an essential part of the reentrant circuit.

Supraventricular Tachycardia due to Atrioventricular Reentry

Wolff-Parkinson-White syndrome is characterized by the presence of an accessory AV pathway. The degree of preexcitation is determined by the location and the anterograde conduction properties of the accessory pathway. Because the sinus node is in the right atrium, an accessory pathway located in the right atrium or the septal area tends to be associated with more

apparent preexcitation because of the proximity of the accessory pathway to the sinus node. However, when the accessory pathway is located in the left lateral AV groove, the impulse originating from the sinus node travels a long distance before reaching the accessory pathway. Thus, the ventricles are excited more by way of the AV node and the His-Purkinje system and less by way of the accessory pathway. In this instance, the preexcitation can be minimal or absent on the surface ECG. Furthermore, the accessory pathway may not conduct bidirectionally. If the accessory pathway conducts only in the retrograde direction, there will be no preexcitation regardless of the pathway location. Such a concealed accessory pathway can nevertheless

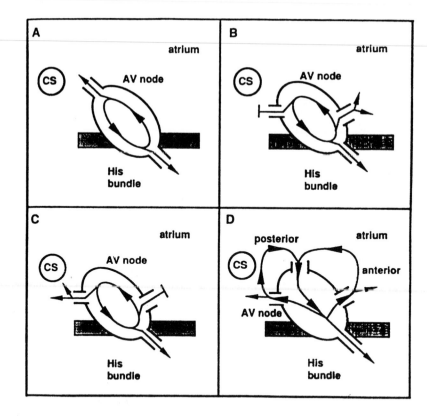

Figure 26–7. Possible mechanisms of atrioventricular (AV) nodal reentrant tachycardia. *A,* Schematic of commonly accepted mechanism, that is, intranodal reentry with common pathway of nodal tissue above and below the reentrant circuit. *B* through *D,* Alternative mechanisms of AV nodal reentrant tachycardia. Among them, *D* shows reentry using perinodal atrium as part of the circuit. CS, coronary sinus. (From McGuire MA, Lau K-C, Johnson DC, et al: Patients with two types of atrioventricular [AV] nodal reentrant tachycardia. Circulation 1991; 83:1245.)

be associated with narrow QRS complex supraventricular tachycardia. Concealed accessory pathways are not rare. For example, at Duke University Medical Center,[38] a total of 342 patients were operated on for symptomatic tachycardia related to Wolff-Parkinson-White syndrome between 1968 and 1986. Of these patients, 40 (12%) had a single concealed accessory pathway. Thus, the absence of preexcitation does not rule out Wolff-Parkinson-White syndrome.

Patients with Wolff-Parkinson-White syndrome present classically with AV reentrant tachycardia that uses the accessory pathway as an essential part of the tachycardia circuit. In more than 90% of these patients, anterograde conduction occurs by way of the AV node and retrograde conduction by way of the accessory pathway (the orthodromic reciprocating tachycardia). In 10% of patients, however, the accessory pathway is used as the anterograde limb and the retrograde activation occurs by way of either the AV node or another accessory pathway.[39] Because the accessory pathway is an essential part of the reentry circuit in either kind of tachycardia, ablation of the accessory pathway by surgery[3] or by catheter ablation techniques[11, 12, 40, 41] can result a cure. In our laboratory, both the diagnostic and the therapeutic

procedures are usually performed during the same electrophysiologic study.

Electrophysiologic studies should be performed after all antiarrhythmic medications have been discontinued for at least five half-lives. To position the coronary sinus catheter, we prefer to use the left basilic vein as the catheter entry site. In patients whose basilic veins are too small to be cannulated, the right internal jugular vein is used. A 5-French or 6-French electrode catheter is then inserted. Once the coronary sinus catheter is positioned, the left femoral vein is cannulated for the insertion of the right ventricular and the His bundle catheters; 6-French catheters are usually used in these locations. The right femoral vein is then cannulated and a 7-French sheath is used. If the surface ECG shows evidence of preexcitation compatible with conduction by way of a right free wall or septal pathway, a modified Brockenbrough[28] catheter is inserted to map the AV groove during reciprocating tachycardia. In patients with a left free wall accessory pathway, a 6-French quadripolar catheter is inserted instead, because tricuspid ring mapping is unnecessary for these patients in our opinion. Ventricular premature stimulation and rapid pacing is then performed to determine the retrograde atrial activation sequence and to induce reciprocating tachycardia. If the accessory pathway is located in the left free wall, the coronary sinus catheter will be pulled back 1 cm at a time to determine the changes of activation sequences (Fig. 26–8). The location of the accessory pathway is determined by the electrode that registered the shortest VA interval. At this time, we usually pull the catheter back from the high right atrium into the inferior vena cava to serve as the ground and then connect each of the four poles on the coronary sinus catheter to the ground. This usually results in satisfactory unipolar recordings. The coronary sinus pull-back techniques are then repeated to determine if we can "bracket" the activation sequence by registering the earliest retrograde A wave on the no. 2 or 3 electrodes of the quadripolar catheter. These techniques usually result in the accurate localization of the accessory pathway.

If the accessory pathway is located in the right free wall or the septum, a modified Brockenbrough catheter is used to map the AV groove and to determine the site of the earliest retrograde A wave during reciprocating tachycardia. Coronary sinus pull-back techniques are then used to exclude the presence of a left-sided pathway. Once the location of the accessory pathway is determined, a radiofrequency ablation catheter can be inserted to ablate the accessory pathway. For most pathways, the ablation catheters can be inserted by way of the right femoral vein access in exchange with the recording electrode catheter. In other patients, however, the catheter may need to be inserted by way of the right internal jugular vein to ablate the pathway.

In the use of ablation techniques, it is important to identify the accessory pathway potential.[42] These potentials are seen usually as sharp deflections between the A and the V waves occurring at the onset of the δ wave in the surface ECG or slightly earlier (Fig. 26–9). Discrete accessory pathway potentials can also be identified during reciprocating tachycardia (Fig. 26–10). Although successful ablation does not always require the identification of a discrete accessory

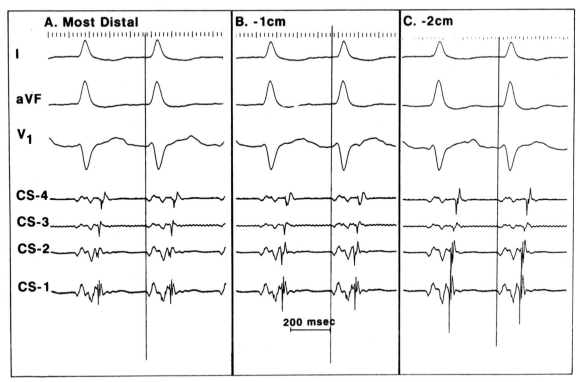

Figure 26–8. Coronary sinus pullback. This figure shows reciprocating atrioventricular reentrant tachycardia using a left posterior free wall accessory pathway as the retrograde limb of the reentrant circuit. CS-1, CS-2, CS-3, and CS-4 represent the four electrodes on the coronary sinus catheter, CS-1 being the most distal and CS-4 the most proximal electrode. *A,* When the coronary sinus catheter was in the most distal position, the CS-2 electrogram was earlier than the CS-1 and CS-3 electrograms. This "bracketing" phenomenon indicates that the accessory pathway was located near the CS-2 electrode. *B* and *C,* The electrograms when the catheter was pulled back by 1 and 2 cm, respectively, are shown. When the catheter was pulled back, the more distal electrode came closer to the accessory pathway. *C,* The retrograde activation sequence has changed, with the electrogram registered by CS-1 electrode being the earliest.

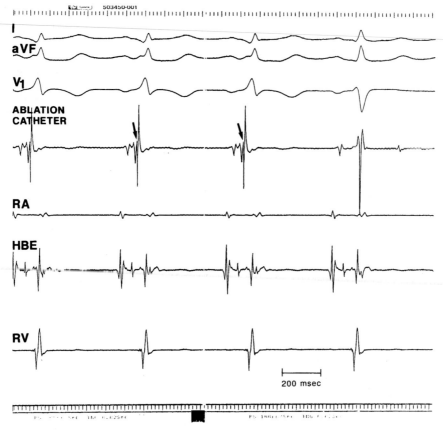

503450-001

I

aVF

V1

ABLATION
CATHETER

RA

HBE

RV

200 msec

Figure 26–9. Accessory pathway potential. These electrograms were recorded from a patient with left lateral free wall accessory pathway. The ablation catheter was positioned under the mitral apparatus near the atrioventricular groove, where both atrial and ventricular electrograms were recorded during sinus rhythm. A sharp deflection was registered at that location *(arrows)* in beats 1 to 3. The timing of this sharp deflection was earlier than the onset of the surface QRS complex and represents the accessory pathway potential. Beat 4 was a normally conducted beat without evidence of preexcitation. The accessory pathway potential was not seen on this beat.

pathway potential in the ablation catheter, the presence of such a potential is a strong predictor of success.

Although the procedure may fail and catheter ablation of the accessory pathway is often successful, some patients may still require surgery. A more complete electrophysiologic investigation is usually necessary before the surgical procedure to rule out the presence of multiple accessory pathways. For instance, induction of atrial fibrillation should always be part of a preoperative evaluation. Different δ wave morphology may be observed during atrial fibrillation and suggest the presence of a second accessory pathway.[43] In some pathways, the conduction occurs only during the supernormal period[44] and is therefore undetectable during sinus rhythm or programmed stimulation.

The following example demonstrates how induction of atrial fibrillation uncovered the presence of a second pathway. The patient is a 31-year-old woman who had a history of near

syncope and recurrent tachycardia. Baseline ECG showed only minimal preexcitation. During electrophysiologic study, two different preexcited morphologies were observed (Fig. 26–11). The second morphology was seen only after atrial premature stimulations. When atrial fibrillation was induced (Fig. 26–12), two different preexcited QRS morphologies were observed. This finding confirmed the presence of a second accessory pathway, which could conduct with short RR intervals. Furthermore, the location of a second pathway could be suspected based on the morphology of maximally preexcited QRS complexes observed during atrial fibrillation. In this patient, it was apparent that one pathway was located in the left lateral free wall and the other in the posteroseptal space. Both pathways were documented by intraoperative mapping studies and were successfully ablated.[45] With the availability of catheter ablation techniques, the induction of atrial fibrillation is usually unnecessary, because the second acces-

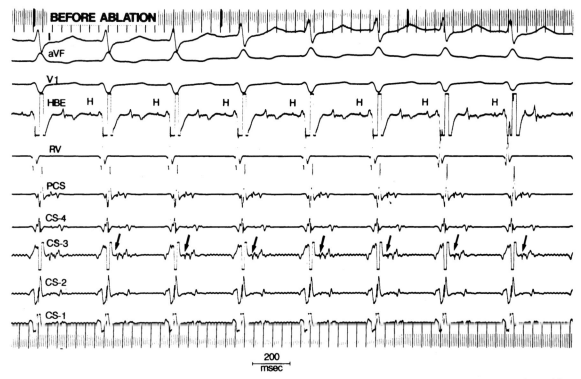

Figure 26–10. Accessory pathway potential registered during reciprocating tachycardia. This figure was from a patient with retrograde-only accessory pathway that recurred after an apparently successful ablative surgery. During repeat electrophysiologic study, accessory pathway potential was clearly demonstrated *(arrows)*. Radiofrequency catheter ablation at this site successfully ablated the accessory pathway. (From Chen P-S, Feld GK, Dembitsky WP, et al: Successful radiofrequency catheter ablation of accessory pathways that recurred after surgery. Am J Cardiol 1991; 68:825–827.)

sory pathway will become evident when the first pathway is ablated.

ELECTROPHYSIOLOGIC STUDY FOR VENTRICULAR TACHYCARDIA

To study ventricular tachycardia, at least two catheters are needed: One is positioned on the His bundle and the other in the right ventricular apex. Some electrophysiologists insert a third catheter in the right ventricular outflow tract to avoid moving the catheter during the study. After the catheters are positioned, programmed stimulation can be performed to induce tachycardia. The ventricular pacing threshold is first determined. Ventricular pacing is then performed at one and one-half or two times the pacing threshold. It is important not to use higher currents because single, strong premature stimuli can result in ventricular fibrillation even in normal hearts.[46] The higher the current, the more likely that the ventricular fibrillation threshold will be reached. There is no consensus as to what constitutes the standard protocol for programmed stimulation. We use eight baseline (S_1) stimulations followed by an S_2 stimulation given at the right ventricular apex to determine the effective refractory period. Three S_1 cycle lengths (600, 500, and 400 msec) are used. This step is followed by the delivery of double premature stimulation at the same site. If sustained monomorphic ventricular tachycardia is not induced, the catheter will be repositioned to the right ventricular outflow tract, where single, double, and triple premature stimuli will be given to induce ventricular tachycardia. If the results are still negative, the catheter is then repositioned to the right ventricular apex where triple premature stimuli are given to complete the protocol. A positive study is one that is associated with the induction of at least one episode of sustained monomorphic ventricular tachycardia. If the results are positive, 10 to 15 mg/kg of procainamide will be given, followed by a 2 mg/min infusion. The programmed stimulation will then be repeated. The suppression of inducibility by procainamide usually indicates that the patient has a better prognosis[47]; however, not every electrophysiologist regards the procainamide infusion test as a necessary part of the

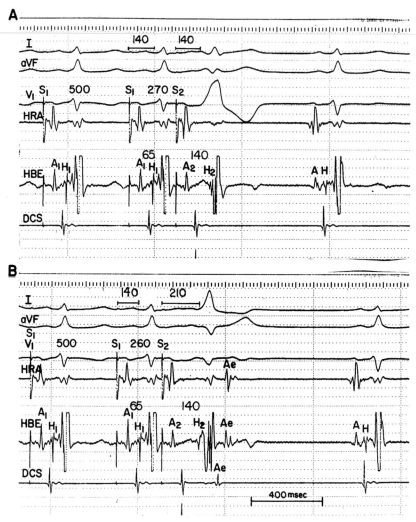

Figure 26–11. Two different preexcited QRS morphologies during electrophysiologic study. In *A*, with S_1S_2 of 500 msec and S_1S_2 of 270 msec, the QRS morphology after S_2 showed a positive δ wave in lead V_1 compatible with conduction over a left-sided accessory pathway. In *B*, with S_1S_2 shortened to 260 msec, the QRS morphology after S_2 stimulation changed to a second morphology, with near-isoelectric δ wave and predominantly negative QRS complex in lead V_1. One atrial echo beat (Ae) was observed. This second accessory pathway was not seen during sinus rhythm but could be easily identified during atrial fibrillation (see Fig. 26–12). (From Chen P-S, Dembitsky WP, Fleck RP, et al: Demonstration of accessory pathway interaction by computerized mapping in preexcitation syndrome. PACE Pacing Clin Electrophysiol 1990; 13:839–844.)

procedure. Regardless of the results of the procainamide infusion test, the patient will be given an antiarrhythmic agent and the electrophysiologic study will be repeated to determine whether or not the tachycardia is still inducible. Great controversy, however, still exists as to whether a negative study necessarily indicates that the antiarrhythmic drug protects a patient from recurrent episodes of life-threatening ventricular tachycardia or sudden death,[48] especially in patients with poor ventricular function. With the improvement of implantable cardioverter-defibrillators, it is likely that many of the high-risk patients will be treated with these devises rather than by pharmacologic agents alone.

Macroreentrant Ventricular Tachycardia

Macroreentrant ventricular tachycardia attributed to bundle branch reentry is an unusual form of tachycardia that accounts for 6% of patients with ventricular tachycardia.[49, 50] Although most patients with this form of tachycardia exhibit idiopathic dilated cardiomyopathy, patients with coronary artery disease are not immune to this arrhythmia.[49–51] Because the reentrant pathway of this tachycardia uses the

ATRIAL FIBRILLATION

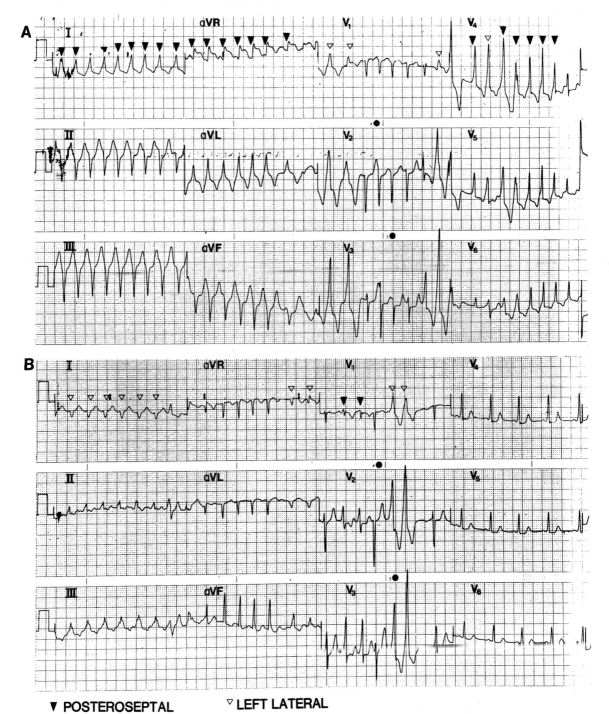

▼ POSTEROSEPTAL   ▽ LEFT LATERAL

Figure 26–12. Identification of two different QRS morphologies during atrial fibrillation. *A* and *B* are two 12-lead electrocardiographic recordings during atrial fibrillation. The unfilled triangles are QRS morphologies that are compatible with left lateral accessory pathway conduction; the filled triangles are QRS morphologies that are compatible with conduction over the posteroseptal accessory pathway. The spontaneous conversion of atrial fibrillation to sinus rhythm was noted in *B*.

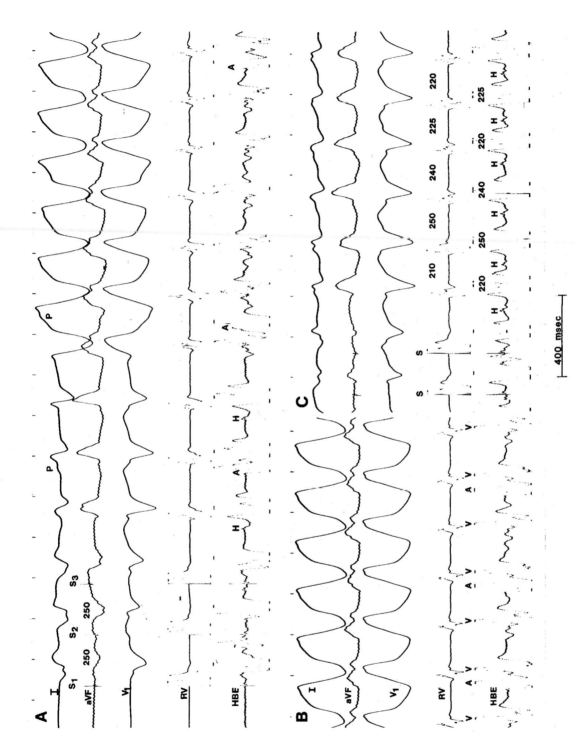

Figure 26–13 See legend on opposite page

left and right bundle branches, catheter ablation of the right bundle branch can result in the cure of this arrhythmia.[49, 51] The electrophysiologic study techniques used for this condition are the same as those described earlier. The criteria for the diagnosis of macroreentrant tachycardia[49] include (1) that each QRS complex be preceded by a His bundle or right bundle branch electrogram; (2) the presence of a constant HV interval; (3) the absence of a His or right bundle branch electrogram during ventricular pacing at the cycle length of the tachycardia; (4) that the surface ECG during ventricular tachycardia resembles left bundle branch block; and (5) that spontaneous variations in the VV interval are preceded, rather than followed, by similar changes in the HH intervals. Once the diagnosis is made, catheter ablation of the right bundle branch either with direct-current or radiofrequency energy can result in the cure of the arrhythmia.[49, 51] We have reported an unusual case of macroreentrant tachycardia.[51] The patient was a 62-year-old man with both coronary artery disease and cerebrotendinous xanthomatosis. He was resuscitated from sudden cardiac death. During electrophysiologic study, he displayed two different kinds of ventricular tachycardia. Figure 26–13A shows the induction of the ventricular tachycardia. At the onset of the ventricular tachycardia, a His bundle electrogram was registered, which preceded the QRS complex. The QRS morphology exhibited during the tachycardia was compatible with left bundle branch block. The tachycardia then spontaneously converted to a different tachycardia with right bundle branch block morphology and the His bundle deflection was no longer seen (Fig. 26–13B). After rapid ventricular pacing, the tachycardia was converted back to the first morphology (Fig. 26–13C). Each QRS complex was again preceded by a His bundle deflection. Furthermore, the alterations of the HH interval preceded, rather than followed, the alteration of the cycle length of the tachycardia. Thus, the tachycardia with the left bundle branch block pattern was the macroreentrant tachycardia, which was no longer inducible after direct-current catheter ablation of the right bundle branch. However, the ventricular tachycardia with the right bundle branch block pattern was still inducible. Treatment with quinidine suppressed the inducibility of this second tachycardia. This case was reported because it shows that two different mechanisms of ventricular tachycardia can occur in the same patient.

Recognition of the presence of macroreentrant ventricular tachycardia can result in the relatively easy cure of the tachycardia and the prevention of sudden cardiac death. Thus, the His bundle electrogram should always be recorded during the first electrophysiologic study.

VENTRICULAR TACHYCARDIA MAPPING AND ABLATION

In a highly select group of patients, ventricular tachycardia can be cured by electrophysiology-guided subendocardial resection.[5, 6] These patients usually have a discrete ventricular aneurysm with relatively well-preserved left ventricular function in the area outside the aneurysm. During the preoperative electrophysiologic study, the site of origin of the ventricular tachycardia should be determined for each inducible ventricular tachycardia morphology. This step is important because in some patients sustained ventricular tachycardia may not be inducible once the patient is anesthetized, or it may turn out that the induced morphology is different than the clinical ventricular tachycardia. There is more than one way to map ventricular tachycardia. We prefer to insert a steerable mapping catheter into the left ventricular cavity during the sinus rhythm. The left ventricle is then paced at a rate similar the ventricular tachycardia rate, from different sites on the endocardium. Figures 26–14 and 26–15 show a patient who had experienced recurrent ventricular tachycardia that was refractory to pharmacologic treatment. The patient had experienced a previous anterior wall infarction complicated by

Figure 26–13. Induction of macroreentrant ventricular tachycardia. Surface electrocardiographic leads I, aVF, V$_1$, and intracardiac right ventricular (RV) apical and His bundle electrograms (HBE) were recorded simultaneously. *A*, Induction of ventricular tachycardia with S$_1$ cycle length of 600 msec, S$_1$S$_2$ of 250 msec, and S$_2$S$_3$ of 250 msec is shown. The first three beats of the ventricular tachycardia had left bundle branch block morphology; His bundle activation was seen in the first and third beat. The tachycardia then spontaneously converted to right bundle branch block morphology after the fourth beat and the His bundle potential was no longer observed. *B*, 2:1 ventriculoatrial conduction during ventricular tachycardia with right bundle branch block morphology is shown. *C*, Conversion to left bundle branch block ventricular tachycardia by ventricular pacing is shown. There was His bundle potential before each beat. (From Chen P-S, Fleck RP, Calisi CM, et al: Macroreentrant ventricular tachycardia and coronary artery disease in cerebrotendinous xanthomatosis. Am J Cardiol 1989; 64:680–682.)

A   **Ventricular Tachycardia**

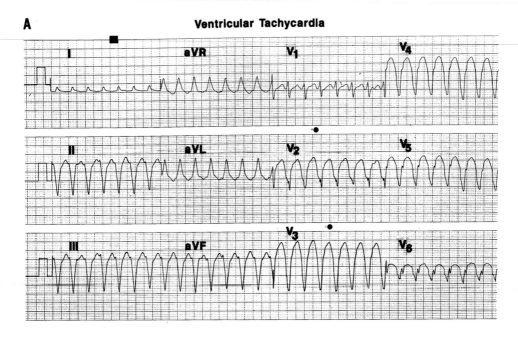

B   **Pacemap**

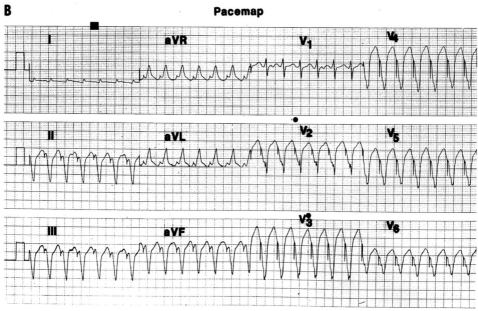

Figure 26–14. Pacemap of sustained monomorphic ventricular tachycardia. *A,* The baseline morphology of sustained monomorphic ventricular tachycardia that was easily induced in the laboratory is shown. *B,* The result of pacemap producing exactly the same QRS morphology as in the ventricular tachycardia is shown, indicating that the site of pacing is close to the origin of ventricular tachycardia.

the formation of a large anteroapical aneurysm. Left ventricular pacing at the anterior and apical part of the septum resulted in a QRS morphology almost identical to that recorded during induced and spontaneous ventricular tachycardia (see Fig. 26–14). Ventricular tachycardia was then induced and the earliest activa-

tion was recorded at the same site (see Fig. 26–15A). Furthermore, the activation at this site during ventricular tachycardia preceded the QRS complex on the surface ECG, confirming that the site was at or near the origin of the ventricular tachycardia. By first performing pacemapping, and then endocardial mapping

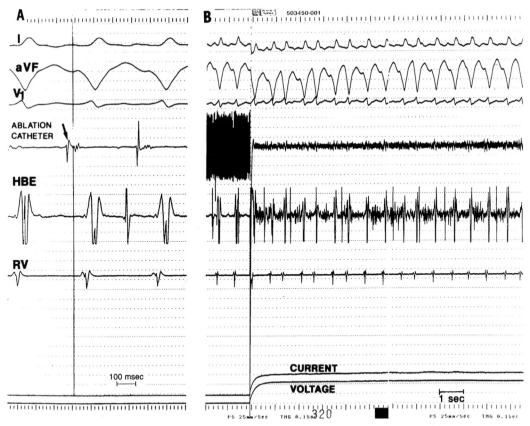

Figure 26–15. Mid-diastolic potential during ventricular tachycardia. *A,* The intracardiac recording during ventricular tachycardia is shown. The ablation catheter registered intracardiac activation during diastole, before the onset of the surface QRS complex (indicated by the *vertical line*). *B,* The radiofrequency energy applied at the same site failed to terminate tachycardia.

during ventricular tachycardia, the duration and the number of episodes of ventricular tachycardia triggered during electrophysiologic study could be minimized. The patient underwent successful surgical ablation of the tachycardia foci. Intraoperative computerized mapping demonstrated that the tachycardia originated from the same area as predicted by the preoperative electrophysiologic study. The efficacy of catheter ablation of the tachycardia foci varies greatly, depending on patient selection and the presence of a number of other factors.[52, 53] One of the most useful predictors of successful direct-current ablation appears to be the presence of a mid-diastolic potential[52]; this observation, however, was made on a small patient population. Other investigators have reported much lower success rates using direct-current shocks.[53] The efficacy of radiofrequency ablation of ventricular tachycardia has been even less well documented. In the previous patient, we attempted multiple subendocardial radiofrequency ablation at the site where the mid-diastolic potential

was recorded and were not able to terminate the tachycardia (see Fig. 26–15).

SUMMARY

With the advancement of pacemaker technology, implantable defibrillators, intraoperative computerized mapping, catheter mapping, and ablation techniques, cardiac catheterization in disorders of cardiac rhythm has become an important diagnostic and therapeutic procedure. With an appropriately staffed and equipped laboratory, many forms of supraventricular tachycardia can be diagnosed and cured during a single electrophysiologic study.[12] The same cure rate can be applied to macroreentrant ventricular tachycardia.[49] Thus, despite the fact that electrophysiologic study often takes a long time to perform—especially in the case of catheter ablation—the results are often highly satisfactory, both for the patients and for their physicians.

REFERENCES

1. Lagergren H: How it happened: My recollection of early pacing. PACE Pacing Clin Electrophysiol 1978; 1:140–143.
2. Durrer D, Schoo L, Schuilenburg RM, Wellens HJJ: The role of premature beats in the initiation and termination of supraventricular tachycardia in the Wolff-Parkinson-White syndrome. Circulation 1967; 36:622–644.
3. Cobb FR, Blumenschein SD, Sealy WC, et al: Successful surgical interruption of the bundle of Kent in a patient with Wolff-Parkinson-White syndrome. Circulation 1968; 38:1018–1029.
4. Gallagher JJ, Pritchett ELC, Sealy WC, et al: The preexcitation syndromes. Prog Cardiovasc Dis 1978; 20:285–327.
5. Guiraudon G, Fontaine G, Frank R, et al: Encircling endocardial ventriculotomy: A new surgical treatment for life-threatening ventricular tachycardias resistant to medical treatment following myocardial infarction. Ann Thorac Surg 1978; 26:438–444.
6. Josephson ME, Harken AH, Horowitz LN: Endocardial excision: A new surgical technique for the treatment of recurrent ventricular tachycardia. Circulation 1979; 60:1430–1439.
7. Schuder JC, Stoeckle H, Gold JH, et al: Experimental ventricular defibrillation with an automatic and completely implanted system. Trans Am Soc Artif Intern Organs 1970; 16:207–212.
8. Mirowski M, Reid PR, Mower MM, et al: Termination of malignant ventricular arrhythmias with an implanted automatic defibrillator in human beings. N Engl J Med 1980; 303:322–324.
9. Gallagher JJ, Svenson RH, Kasell JH, et al: Catheter technique for closed-chest ablation of the atrioventricular conduction system: A therapeutic alternative for the treatment of refractory supraventricular tachycardia. N Engl J Med 1982; 306:194–200.
10. Scheinman MM, Morady F, Hess DS, Gonzalez R: Catheter-induced ablation of the atrioventricular junction to control refractory supraventricular arrhythmia. JAMA 1982; 248:851–855.
11. Jackman WM, Wang X, Friday KJ, et al: Catheter ablation of accessory atrioventricular pathways (Wolff-Parkinson-White syndrome) by radiofrequency current. N Engl J Med 1991; 324:1605–1611.
12. Calkins H, Sousa J, El-Atassi R, et al: Diagnosis and cure of the Wolff-Parkinson-White syndrome or paroxysmal supraventricular tachycardias during single electrophysiologic test. N Engl J Med 1991; 324:1612–1618.
13. Zipes DP, Akhtar M, Denes P, et al: Guidelines for clinical intracardiac electrophysiologic studies: A report of the American College of Cardiology/American Heart Association Task Force on Assessment of Diagnostic and Therapeutic Cardiovascular Procedures (Subcommittee to Assess Clinical Intracardiac Electrophysiologic Studies). Circulation 1989; 80:1925–1939.
14. Lange G: Actions of driving stimuli from intrinsic and extrinsic sources on in situ cardiac pacemaker tissues. Circ Res 1965; 17:449–459.
15. Mandel WJ, Hayakawa H, Danzig R, Marcus HS: Evaluation of sinoatrial node function in man by overdrive suppression. Circulation 1971; 44:59–66.
16. Narula OS, Samet P, Javier RP: Significance of the sinus node recovery time. Circulation 1972; 45:140–158.
17. Strauss HC, Bigger JT, Sardoff AC, Giardina EG: Electrophysiologic evaluation of sinus node function in patients with sinus node dysfunction. Circulation 1976; 53:763–776.
18. Josephson ME, Seides SF: Clinical Cardiac Electrophysiology: Techniques and Interpretations. Philadelphia, Lea & Febiger, 1979.
19. Scherlag BJ, Lau SH, Helfant RH, et al: Catheter technique for recording his bundle activity in man. Circulation 1969; 39:13–18.
20. Wit AL, Weiss MB, Berkowitz WD, et al: Patterns of atrioventricular conduction in the human heart. Circ Res 1970; 27:345–359.
21. Scheinman MM, Peters RW, Modin G, et al: Prognostic value of infranodal conduction time in patients with chronic bundle branch block. Circulation 1977; 56:240–244.
22. Dhingra R, Denes P, Wu D, et al: Prospective observations in patients with chronic bundle branch block and marked HV prolongation. Circulation 1976; 53:600–604.
23. McAnulty JH, Murphy E, Rahimtoola SH: Prospective evaluation of intrahisian conduction delay. Circulation 1979; 59:1035–1039.
24. Almquist A, Goldenberg IF, Milstein S, et al: Provocation of bradycardia and hypotension by isoproterenol and upright posture in patients with unexplained syncope. N Engl J Med 1989; 320:346–351.
25. Raviele A, Gasparini G, DiPede F, et al: Usefulness of head-up tilt test in evaluating patients with syncope of unknown origin and negative electrophysiologic study. Am J Cardiol 1990; 65:1322–1327.
26. Packer DL, Bardy GH, Worley SJ, et al: Tachycardia-induced cardiomyopathy: A reversible form of left ventricular dysfunction. Am J Cardiol 1986; 57:563–570.
27. Davis J, Scheinman MM, Ruder MA, et al: Ablation of cardiac tissues by an electrode catheter technique for treatment of ectopic supraventricular tachycardia in adults. Circulation 1986; 74:1044–1053.
28. Gallagher JJ, Pritchett ELC, Benditt DG, et al: New catheter techniques for analysis of the sequence of retrograde atrial activation in man. Eur J Cardiol 1977; 6:1–14.
29. Wit AL, Cranefield PF: Effect of verapamil on the sino-atrial and atrioventricular nodes of the rabbit and the mechanism by which it arrests reentrant atrioventricular nodal tachycardia. Circ Res 1974; 35:413–425.
30. Lerman BB, Belardinelli L: Cardiac electrophysiology of adenosine: Basic and clinical concepts. Circulation 1991; 83:1499–1509.
31. Zardini M, Leitch JW, Guiraudon GM, et al: Atrioventricular nodal reentry and dual atrioventricular node physiology in patients undergoing accessory pathway ablation. Am J Cardiol 1990; 66:1388–1389.
32. Benditt DG, Pritchett ELC, Smith WM, Gallagher JJ: Ventriculoatrial intervals: Diagnostic use in paroxysmal supraventricular tachycardia. Ann Intern Med 1979; 91:161–166.
33. Moe GK, Preston JB, Burlington H: Physiologic evidence for a dual AV transmission system. Circ Res 1956; 4:357–375.
34. Sung RJ, Waxman HL, Saksena S, Juma Z: Sequence of retrograde atrial activation in patients with dual atrioventricular nodal pathways. Circulation 1981; 64:1059–1067.
35. Ross DL, Johnson DC, Denniss AR, et al: Curative surgery for atrioventricular junctional ("AV nodal") reentrant tachycardia. J Am Coll Cardiol 1985; 6:1383–1392.
36. Cox JL, Holman WL, Cain ME: Cryosurgical treatment of atrioventricular node reentrant tachycardia. Circulation 1987; 6:1329–1336.
37. McGuire MA, Lau K-C, Johnson DC, et al: Patients with two types of atrioventricular junctional (AV nodal) reentrant tachycardia: Evidence that a common pathway of nodal tissue is not present above the reentrant circuit. Circulation 1991; 83:1232–1246.

38. Chen P-S, Pressley JC, Tang ASL, et al: New observations on atrial fibrillation before and after surgery in patients with Wolff-Parkinson-White syndrome. J Am Coll Cardiol 1992; 19:974–981

39. Bardy GH, Packer DL, German LD, Gallagher JJ: Preexcited reciprocating tachycardia in patients with Wolff-Parkinson-White syndrome: Incidence and mechanisms. Circulation 1984; 70:377–391.

40. Warin J-F, Haissaguerre M, Lemetayer P, et al: Catheter ablation of accessory pathways with a direct approach: Results in 35 patients. Circulation 1988; 78:800–815.

41. Chen P-S, Feld GK, Dembitsky WP, et al: Successful radiofrequency catheter ablation of accessory pathways that recurred after surgery. Am J Cardiol 1991; 68:825–827.

42. Jackman WM, Friday KJ, Scherlag BJ, et al: Direct endocardial recording from an accessory atrioventricular pathway: Localization of the site of block, effect of antiarrhythmic drugs, and attempt at nonsurgical ablation. Circulation 1983; 5:906–916.

43. Fananapazier L, German LD, Gallagher JJ, et al: Importance of preexcited QRS morphology during induced atrial fibrillation to the diagnosis and localization of multiple accessory pathways. Circulation 1990; 81:578–585.

44. Chen P-S, Prystowsky EN: Role of concealed and supernormal conduction during atrial fibrillation in the preexcitation syndrome. Am J Cardiol 1991; 68:1329–1334.

45. Chen P-S, Dembitsky WP, Fleck RP, et al: Demonstration of accessory pathway interaction by computerized mapping in preexcitation syndrome. PACE Pacing Clin Electrophysiol 1990; 13:839–844.

46. Wiggers CJ, Wegria R: Ventricular fibrillation due to single, localized induction and condenser shocks applied during the vulnerable phase of ventricular systole. Am J Physiol 1940; 128:500–505.

47. Waxman HL, Buxton AE, Sadowski LM, Josephson ME: The response to procainamide during electrophysiologic study for sustained ventricular tachyarrhythmias predicts the response to other medications. Circulation 1983; 67:30–37.

48. Poole JE, Mathisen TL, Kudenchuk PJ, et al: Long-term outcome in patients who survive out-of-hospital ventricular fibrillation and undergo electrophysiologic studies: Evaluation by electrophysiologic subgroups. J Am Coll Cardiol 1990; 16:657–665.

49. Tchou PT, Jazayeri M, Denker S, et al: Transcatheter electrical ablation of right bundle branch: A method of treating macroreentrant ventricular tachycardia attributed to bundle branch reentry. Circulation 1988; 78:246–257.

50. Caceres J, Jazayeri M, McKinnie J, et al: Sustained bundle branch reentry as a mechanism of clinical tachycardia. Circulation 1989; 79:256–270.

51. Chen P-S, Fleck RP, Calisi CM, et al: Macroreentrant ventricular tachycardia and coronary artery disease in cerebrotendinous xanthomatosis. Am J Cardiol 1989; 64:680–682.

52. Fitzgerald DM, Friday KJ, Wah, JA, et al: Electrogram patterns predicting successful catheter ablation of ventricular tachycardia. Circulation 1988; 77:806–814.

53. Garan H, Kuchar D, Freeman C, et al: Early assessment of the effect of map-guided transcatheter intracardiac electric shock on sustained ventricular tachycardia secondary to coronary artery disease. Am J Cardiol 1988; 61:1018–1023.

THERAPY

Thrombolysis, Coronary Angiography, and Coronary Angioplasty in Acute Coronary Syndromes

KIRK L. PETERSON

Beginning in the early 1970s, thrombolytic agents emerged as a major innovation in the pharmacologic treatment of intracoronary thrombi and acute coronary syndromes.[1-3] Use of thrombolytic therapy intensified with reports that total or partial coronary artery occlusion by thrombus often was noted in patients with acute myocardial infarction[4, 5] (Fig. 27–1). These agents have been administered intravenously and directly by catheter into the coronary artery and have become both complementary and competitive to the use of coronary angioplasty in those coronary syndromes associated with acute myocardial ischemia and infarction. Moreover, because successful reperfusion in acute myocardial infarction often leaves salvaged muscle at future risk, large clinical trials have been organized to define the indications for angiography and percutaneous transluminal coronary angioplasty (PTCA) after the use of thrombolytic agents.

This chapter considers the types, modes of action, contemporary indications, and clinical outcomes after use of thrombolytic agents. Those clinical trials that address the issues of coronary angiography and PTCA after thrombolysis and those that compare primary balloon angioplasty with intravenous thrombolysis in the treatment of acute coronary syndromes also are reviewed.

MAJOR THROMBOLYTIC AGENTS

General Characteristics

Thrombolytic agents augment the intrinsic fibrinolytic system by accelerating the conversion of plasminogen to plasmin, which, in turn, through its proteolytic enzyme activity degrades fibrin, fibrinogen, prothrombin, and clotting factors V and VIII. Normally, a_2-antiplasmin, a plasmin inhibitor, serves to neutralize plasmin; however, the increased amount of plasmin generated by thrombolysis exhausts the supply of this inhibitor, and the resultant decrease in clotting factors eventuates in defective hemostasis.

Types

Historically, non–clot-specific thrombolytic agents were discovered first and include streptokinase (SK), urokinase (UK), and anisoylated plasminogen-streptokinase activator complex (APSAC) (Table 27–1). Modern recombinant technology has allowed mass production of clot-specific agents, including tissue-type plasminogen activator (t-PA), prourokinase, and fibrin-specific monoclonal antibodies, all of which activate plasminogen directly at the site of the clot.

THROMBOLYSIS IN ACUTE MYOCARDIAL INFARCTION

Mortality

The ultimate goal of coronary reperfusion is reduction in the significant mortality rate associated with acute myocardial infarction. A number of randomized, as well as observational, trials have confirmed that survival can be significantly improved by use of these agents in the early hours of a coronary thrombotic occlusion; most studies reveal that the earlier the myocardium is reperfused, the greater the improvement in the survival rate.

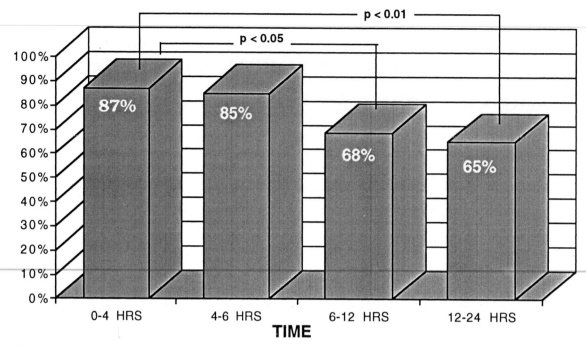

Figure 27–1. Percentage of patients with total thrombotic coronary artery occlusion during the early hours of acute myocardial infarction. The reduction in occlusion with time is believed to be secondary to spontaneous thrombolysis. (Data from DeWood MA, Spores J, Notske R, et al: Prevalence of total coronary occlusion during the early hours of transmural myocardial infarction. N Engl J Med 1980; 303:897–902.)

The Gruppo Italiano per lo Studio della Streptochinasi nell'Infarto Miocardico (GISSI-1) and the Second International Study of Infarct Survival (ISIS-2) were the first large, placebo-controlled trials to report a survival benefit of intravenous SK.[6, 7] The GISSI-1 protocol enrolled patients of any age who were encountered within 12 hours of the onset of their pain and who manifested an ST segment shift of more than 1 mm in any limb lead or more than 2 mm in one or more precordial leads, or both. The treated group of 5860 patients received 1.5 million units of SK over 60 minutes; no specific adjunctive antiplatelet or anticoagulant regimen was required. The overall mortality in the SK group was 10.7% as compared with 13% in the placebo group, providing a risk reduction of 18%. In those patients treated within 1 and 3 hours of the onset of their infarct syndrome, the risk reduction was 47% and 23%, respectively.

Table 27–1. **Major Thrombolytic Agents**

Characteristic	Streptokinase	APSAC	Urokinase	rt-PA
Origin	Bacterial culture	Anisoylated SK-plasminogen complex	Renal cell culture	Recombinant DNA
Clot specific	No	No	No	Yes
Antigen	Yes	Yes	No	No
Plasminogen activation	Indirect	Indirect	Direct	Direct
Systemic lysis	Severe	Severe	Moderate	Mild
Half-life (min)	23	90	16	5
Patency rates (%)				
90 min	55–64	70–72	66	69–79
24–72 hr	88	72	73	71–85
1–3 wk	75	77	71	76–83
Persistent favorable effect on long-term survival	Yes	Yes	Unproved	Yes

rt-PA, recombinant tissue plasminogen activator; DNA, deoxyribonucleic acid; APSAC, anisoylated plasminogen-streptokinase activator complex.

The ISIS-2 trial confirmed in a large cohort of 17,187 patients the results of GISSI-1; there were no electrocardiographic criteria and no upper age limit for enrollment. Adjunctive treatment was not prescribed. Patients were randomized into four groups (placebo, aspirin alone [ASA], SK alone, and ASA with SK); the dose of SK administered was 1.5 million units over 1 hour. SK alone or ASA alone was associated with a 25% and 23% reduction in 5-week follow-up mortality, respectively, but the greatest reduction of 43% was noted in the combination SK/ASA group. Some differences were noted in comparison with the GISSI-1 results: (1) mortality was reduced in those patients treated between 6 and 24 hours after the onset of symptoms; and (2) the survival benefit applied to patients older than 65 years of age and in those with an inferior wall myocardial infarction.

The APSAC Intervention Mortality Study (AIMS) was the largest noncomparative investigation of the therapeutic efficacy of APSAC.[8] This study enrolled 1258 patients who were within 6 hours of the onset of their infarct syndrome, younger than 70 years of age, and exhibited at least 0.1 mV of ST segment elevation in two or more standard limb leads or at least 0.2 mV in one or more of the precordial leads of the electrocardiogram, or both. Thirty units of APSAC were administered over a 5-minute period, and heparin was then started 6 hours later. No other specific adjunctive therapy was prescribed. Those patients treated with APSAC showed a mortality of 6% as compared with 12% in the placebo group (a mortality reduction of 50%). Patients treated with APSAC in less than 4 hours showed no survival benefit compared with those treated within 4 to 6 hours of the onset of the infarct syndrome.

The German Activator Urokinase Study (GAUS) constitutes the most prominent multicenter investigation of UK as a primary thrombolytic agent in acute myocardial infarction.[9] In this comparative study, 246 patients were randomized to treatment with either intravenous UK (1.5 million-unit initial bolus and a total of 3 million units over a 90-minute period) or t-PA (10 mg initial bolus and a total of 70 mg over a 90-minute period). A placebo group was not enrolled in this comparative study. The death occurrence in the UK group was 5 in 117 patients (4.3%).

The Anglo-Scandinavian Study of Early Thrombolysis (ASSET) analyzed in a randomized, double-blinded protocol the effect on mortality rate of t-PA with heparin versus heparin alone in 5013 patients younger than 75 years of age.[10] ASA and other antiplatelet or anticoagulant agents were excluded as adjunctive agents. There were no specific electrocardiographic criteria for entry, and all patients were treated within 5 hours of the onset of symptoms. Recombinant t-PA (rt-PA) was administered as a 10-mg bolus followed by an infusion of 50 mg in 1 hour then 20 mg in each of the next 2 hours; all patients received in addition an initial intravenous bolus of 5000 units of heparin followed by a heparin infusion at 1000 units/hr for 21 hours. At 1 month the overall mortality rates were 7.2% and 9.8% in the t-PA and placebo groups, respectively, a relative reduction of 26%. Similar to AIMS, there was no difference in the mortality benefit between those treated within the first 3 hours and at 3 to 5 hours. There was a greater mortality benefit with t-PA treatment with increasing age as compared with placebo. Finally, at 6 months follow-up, the initial mortality benefit appeared to be sustained with a risk reduction of 26%.

Subsequent trials have made comparative randomized analyses of the mortality benefit of SK and t-PA when used with variable regimens of adjunctive antiplatelet and anticoagulant agents.[11, 12] In the GISSI-2 and the rt-PA/SK International Mortality Trial (IMT) patients received intravenous, single-chain t-PA (alteplase), 100 mg over 3 hours, or intravenous SK, 1.5 million units over 1 hour, with or without heparin, 12,500 units subcutaneously twice daily, started 12 hours after thrombolytic therapy. ASA and intravenous β-blockers were used if there were no contraindications. In these analyses no statistical difference was observed between patient groups treated with t-PA and SK, with or without heparin. Subgroup analysis also failed to show any differences between the two thrombolytic agents.

The ISIS-3 trial analyzed in a randomized protocol a very large population (41,299 patients) in which the effects of double-chain rt-PA (duteplase), SK, and APSAC on mortality were compared at 35 days and at 6 months after myocardial infarction.[13] ASA, 162 mg, was given immediately to all patients; half of these patients were allocated to subcutaneous calcium heparin (12,500 units starting at 4 hours and given twice daily for 7 days or until discharge) and the other half was scheduled to receive ASA. No statistically significant difference in mortality was observed between the three thrombolytic agents, with all individual cohorts showing mortality rates between 0 and 35 days of approximately 10.5%. Moreover, the use of subcutaneous heparin with ASA, as compared with ASA alone, conferred no benefit on either early or late mortality rates.

Whether an optimal t-PA dosage schedule and maintenance of patency by adequate anticoagulation were achieved in the GISSI-2, the rt-PA/SK IMT, and the ISIS-3 has been questioned. For example, Turpie and associates[14] reported that the administration of subcutaneous heparin, 12,500 units every 12 hours for 10 days, results in a mid-dose, average partial thromboplastin time of 47.8 ± 12.3 seconds; at 24 to 36 hours after the beginning of heparin administration this same mid-dose, average partial thromboplastin time was only 35 seconds. Front-loaded t-PA (an initial bolus of 15 mg followed by an infusion of 50 mg over 30 minutes and 35 mg over 60 minutes) had been noted in the rt-PA–APSAC Patency Study (TAPS) to provide a patency rate by coronary angiography of 84.4% at 90 minutes as compared with 70.3% for APSAC.[15] In addition, double-chain rt-PA is a variant of human t-PA in that a methionine is substituted for a valine at position 245 in the Kringle 2 region of the amino acid sequence. Other analyses with double-chain t-PA suggest that its early patency rate at 90 minutes (Thrombolysis in Myocardial Infarction [TIMI]) grade 2 or 3 flow of the infarct-related artery at angiography[16] (Table 27–2) is between 67% and 71%,[17–19] questionably lower than the 69% to 79%[9, 20] patency rate reported with single-chain t-PA (see Table 27–1).

Because of concerns, particularly in the medical community of the United States, that prompt thrombolytic treatment in conjunction with immediate anticoagulation had not yet reached its full potential, the Global Utilization of Streptokinase and t-PA for Occluded Coronary Arteries (GUSTO) trial was organized; its salient results have now been published.[21, 22] Patients admitted to GUSTO were first given ASA, 160 mg, then thereafter 160 to 325 mg daily. The patients then were randomized to one of the following four regimens:

1. SK (intravenous at 1.5 million unit/60 min) and subcutaneous heparin (12,500 units beginning 4 hours after the start of SK, followed by 12,500 units subcutaneously every 12 hours for 7 days)
2. SK (intravenous at 1.5 million unit/60 min) and heparin (a 5000-unit bolus given immediately, followed by a 1000 unit/hr drip adjusted to keep the partial thromboplastin time between 60 and 85 seconds)
3. t-PA, front loaded, weight adjusted (<100 mg) over a 90-minute period and heparin (a 5000-unit bolus given immediately followed by

Table 27–2. Definitions of Perfusion in the TIMI-1 Trial[15]

Grade	Definition
0	No antegrade flow beyond the point of occlusion
1	Penetration without perfusion, i.e., the contrast material passes beyond the area of obstruction but "hangs up" and fails to opacify the entire coronary bed distal to the obstruction for the duration of the cineangiographic filming sequence
2	Partial perfusion, i.e., the contrast material passes across the obstruction and opacifies the coronary bed distal to the obstruction. However, the rate of entry of contrast material into the vessel distal to the obstruction or its rate of clearance from the distal bed (or both) are perceptibly slower than its entry into or clearance from comparable areas not perfused by the previously occluded vessel, e.g., the opposite coronary artery or the coronary bed proximal to the obstruction
3	Complete perfusion, i.e., antegrade flow into the bed distal to the obstruction occurs as promptly as antegrade flow into the bed proximal to the obstruction, and clearance of contrast material from the involved bed as rapid as clearance from an uninvolved bed in the same vessel or the opposite artery

TIMI-1, Thrombolysis in Myocardial Infarction trial, phase 1.

a 1000 unit/hr drip adjusted to keep the partial thromboplastin time between 60 and 85 seconds)
4. t-PA (intravenous at <90 mg/60 min) plus SK (intravenous at 1 million unit/60 min) and heparin (a 5000-unit bolus given immediately, followed by a 1000 unit/hr drip adjusted to keep the partial thromboplastin time between 60 and 85 seconds)

The hypothesis underlying GUSTO is that an artery that is opened and reperfused early and sustained as an open artery in follow-up will have a favorable influence on both immediate and long-term survival and subsequent coronary events.

Analysis of the various drug treatments tested in GUSTO has revealed that an accelerated t-PA regimen, in combination with immediate and sustained anticoagulation with heparin, was associated with an early 30-day mortality rate of 6.3% as compared with a 7.2% mortality rate with SK and subcutaneous heparin and 7.4% with SK and intravenous heparin; thus, a statistically significant mortality risk reduction of 14% was uncovered (Fig. 27–2). Early 24-hour mortality was found to be 2.3% in the t-PA cohort and 2.8% in both the t-PA plus SK and SK (pooled) groups. Of importance, the

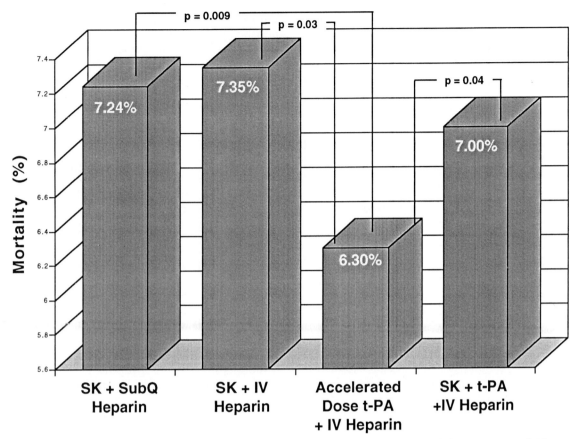

Figure 27–2. Mortality at 30 days after thrombolytic therapy (four separate randomized groups) for acute myocardial infarction in the Global Utilization of Streptokinase and t-PA for Occluded Coronary Arteries (GUSTO) trial. Note the statistically significant reduction of mortality with an accelerated dosage schedule for t-PA with intravenous heparin. See text for details. (Data from Neuhas KL, von Essen R, Tebbe U, et al: Improved thrombolysis in acute myocardial infarction with front-loaded administration of alteplase: Results of the rt-PA–APSAC Patency Study [TAPS]. J Am Coll Cardiol 1992; 19:885–891.)

overall mortality odds ratio for accelerated t-PA versus SK was 0.86 (95% confidence interval = 0.78 to 0.94), whereas in ISIS-3 and GISSI-2 International (where a standard t-PA dosage schedule was used) these odds ratios were 0.97 (0.90 to 1.05) and 1.04 (0.95 to 1.15), respectively (Fig. 27–3). The longer-term follow-up data on patients entered into the GUSTO protocol will be forthcoming.

The design of the GUSTO trial and the interpretation of its results have been criticized on the following grounds[23–25]: (1) it was an "open label" investigation and therefore potentially subject to physician bias; (2) the accelerated t-PA cohort ultimately had a higher incidence of coronary artery bypass graft surgery, possibly influencing ultimate mortality in this "intention-to-treat" analysis; (3) the mortality benefit of t-PA was restricted to patients treated within the United States; (4) the superiority of the t-PA to the SK regimens was not consistent for all subgroups of the cohorts; and (5) the

magnitude of the treatment differences and the cost disparity between t-PA and SK arms made the number of patients needed to treat to avoid one clinical event relatively high and expensive, respectively. In fact, with a mortality rate difference of 1%, 100 patients would need to get t-PA rather than SK to save one life.[26]

Nevertheless, in the GUSTO trial the association of reduced mortality with early arterial patency supports the important paradigm that, in sequence, early reperfusion of an occluded infarct-related artery leads to myocardial salvage, preservation of regional wall thickening, preservation of global left ventricular function, and improved patient survival.[27]

Global and Regional Left Ventricular Function

Thrombolytic therapy is aimed at reperfusing residual ischemic myocardium in a territory un-

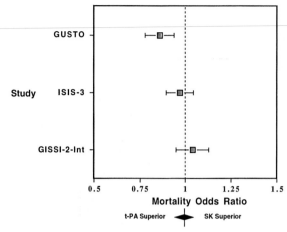

Figure 27–3. Mortality odds ratios (with 95% confidence intervals) for tissue plasminogen activator (t-PA) versus streptokinase (SK) in three large, randomized trials. Note the statistically significant superiority of t-PA in the Global Utilization of Streptokinase and t-PA for Occluded Coronary Arteries (GUSTO) study as compared with the Third International Study of Infarct Survival Trial (ISIS-3) and the Second Gruppo Italiano per lo Studio della Streptochinasi nell'Infarto Miocardico (GISSI-2-Internaltional) trial.

dergoing infarction; to the extent that ischemia is relieved, concomitant improvement of regional myocardial shortening theoretically should be observed. Assessment of the effects of thrombolysis on left ventricular function is complicated by several well-recognized pathophysiologic processes: (1) hyperkinesis of myocardial shortening in the noninfarct zone, in response to the reduced, absent, or paradoxical systolic shortening in the infarct zone, serves to maintain a normal global left ventricular ejection fraction despite significant regional dysfunction in the infarct territory; and (2) even in the presence of adequate reperfusion, regional myocardial shortening and lengthening in the infarct territory may not recover for days to weeks because of so-called stunning. Thus, to assess the end effect of reperfusion on left ventricular function, an analysis must await full recovery from myocardial stunning and maximal restoration of aerobic myocardial energetics. Use of left ventricular ejection fraction as an end-point also has been complicated by missing values as a result of patients who die, failure to obtain an accurate measure of the index, or technical inadequacy of the imaging modality.[28]

Nevertheless, some clinical studies have shown that thrombolytic therapy is associated with a reduction in left ventricular dysfunction[29] and support the notion that salvage of reversibly ischemic myocardium is integral to the clinical benefit brought about by reperfusion.[30-35] However, in a host of placebo-controlled trials of

intravenous thrombolytic agents, a clear relationship between mortality reduction and improvement in ejection fraction has not been demonstrated.[32-37] In fact, those trials that have shown the most improvement in ejection fraction have tended to demonstrate the least mortality reduction.[28] It is also accepted, based on several comparative trials, that there is no significant difference between APSAC with t-PA and t-PA with SK in their effect on left ventricular function.[38, 39]

Sheehan and the TIMI-1 study group coinvestigators[39] found from paired left ventriculograms (pretreatment and predischarge) that global ejection fraction increased after thrombolysis only in those patients who achieved reperfusion by 90 minutes after the onset of therapy or who initially had subtotal occlusions. Recovery of regional dysfunction was greater in those patients who achieved reperfusion earlier versus later than 4 hours after symptom onset and in patients with some collateral circulation to the infarct-related territory. Longer-term follow-up at 6 weeks by TIMI investigators and at 6 months by Thrombolysis and Angioplasty in Myocardial Infarction (TAMI) investigators have revealed only minimal further improvement in left ventricular ejection fraction.[40, 41]

In the GUSTO trial[22] analysis of a random subgroup at 90 minutes after treatment with an accelerated t-PA regimen as compared with SK with intravenous heparin was associated with a smaller area of regional dyssynergy in the infarct zone and a higher percentage of the group with preserved regional wall motion. However, these favorable comparisons did not hold on the left ventriculograms performed at 5 to 7 days after treatment. And, in fact, at 5 to 7 days the global ejection fraction was equivalent at 57% to 59% in all treatment arms.

If thrombolytic therapy does not benefit appreciably the ejection fraction, what other characteristics, if any, of ventricular function, geometry, and remodeling are affected favorably by successful use of these reperfusion agents? A number of investigations have revealed that pathophysiologic changes occurring in the later phase, that is, weeks or months after a myocardial infarction, have significant influence on patient survival, clinical status, and left ventricular function and geometry. These events include expansion of the myocardium in the area of the infarct, dilation of the left ventricular chamber at end-diastole, increase in left ventricular chamber volume at end-systole, and development of eccentric hypertrophy in the noninfarct zone.[42-46] Mitigation of these adverse pathophysiologic changes by vasodilators, including nitrates and angiotensin-converting enzyme inhibitors, has also been shown experimentally and in clinical trials.[47–52] It is unclear to what extent these favorable influences of vasodilators also might be dependent on preservation of perfusion into the region of the myocardial infarct. One analysis in patients who received thrombolytic therapy for an anterior wall myocardial infarction (left anterior descending territory) suggests that the degree of residual stenosis of the infarct-related artery before hospital discharge has a significant influence on left ventricular end-diastolic and end-systolic volumes, as well as ejection fraction, at 6 months and 1 year after infarction (Fig. 27–4).[53]

Infarct-related Artery Patency

In view of the confirmation that acute coronary syndromes are related, at least in part, to the formation of an intracoronary thrombus, the patency of the affected artery after thrombolysis becomes an important end-point of therapy. There is accumulating evidence that a persistently open artery after myocardial infarction has important implications to both short-term and long-term prognosis.[26–29, 54–57] In the Western Washington trial of intracoronary streptokinase, the 12-month mortality was 15% in those patients with an occluded artery as opposed to 2% in those with a patent artery[57] (Fig. 27–5).

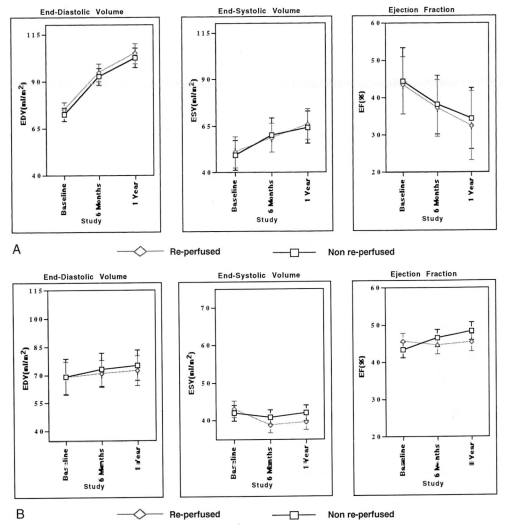

Figure 27–4. A, Effect of total occlusion of the left anterior descending coronary artery on the natural history of left ventricular end-diastolic volume, end-systolic volume, and ejection fraction. Clinical signs of reperfusion appeared to have no effect on eventual parameters at 6 months and 1 year. B, Effect of residual infarct-artery patency (left anterior descending) of greater than 1.5 mm minimal luminal diameter on serial changes in left ventricular end-diastolic volume, end-systolic volume, and ejection fraction. (A and B data from Leung W-H, Lau C-P: Effect of severity of the residual stenosis of the infarct-related coronary artery on left ventricular dilation and function after acute myocardial infarction. J Am Coll Cardiol 1992; 20:307–313.)

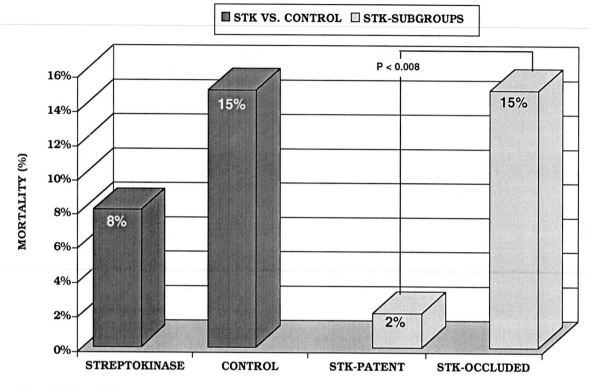

Figure 27–5. Beneficial effect of a patent infarct artery on 12-month mortality in the Western Washington randomized trial of intracoronary streptokinase (STK) versus placebo in acute myocardial infarction. (Data from Kennedy JW, Ritchie JL, Davis KB, et al: The Western Washington randomized trial of intracoronary streptokinase in acute myocardial infarction: A 12-month follow-up report. N Engl J Med 1985; 312:1073–1080.)

The TAMI study group[56] found in-hospital mortality of 4% and 12.8% for those patient groups with a patent and an occluded infarct-related artery, respectively. Also, a patent artery has been observed to favorably influence the incidence of inducible ventricular tachycardia and the frequency of late potentials by signal-averaged electrocardiography.[58, 59] Finally, an open artery provides a potential source of collateral flow to other ischemic territories in the patient with multivessel coronary heart disease.

To assess vessel patency, coronary angiography customarily has been performed at 90 minutes after administration of the thrombolytic agent. For example, in the data of the GUSTO trial released in 1993,[22] patency of the infarct-related artery (TIMI grades 2 or 3 flow) at 90 minutes after treatment was confirmed by coronary angiography in 55.6% of the SK (subcutaneous heparin), 61.0% of the SK (intravenous heparin), 80.8% of the t-PA (intravenous heparin), and 73.1% of the rt-PA plus SK (intravenous heparin) groups, confirming the efficacy of t-PA with immediate heparinization for achieving an early open artery (Fig. 27–6). These early patency differences, however, were not found to be significant if the patency rate was assessed at 180 minutes after treatment. In the GUSTO trial,[22] a TIMI grade 2 or 3 flow at 90 minutes after treatment conferred a mortality reduction of 35.6% (9.0% in TIMI grade 0 or 1, 5.8% in TIMI grade 2 or 3, P<.05). Currently, t-PA has been associated with the highest rate of vessel patency[9, 20] (see Table 27–1). However, if patency is then assessed at 1 to 3 days and at 3 weeks after thrombolytic treatment, the rates of patency for t-PA, SK, and APSAC become essentially equivalent.[22, 38, 60–67] The limited angiographic follow-up data on vessel patency after administration of UK indicated longer-term patency rates of the same magnitude as for other thrombolytic agents.[9]

Complications

Cerebrovascular events are important complications of the use of thrombolytic agents and must be considered in any decision to administer the drug. In older, placebo-controlled trials of SK, a stroke rate in the treated group of 0.6% to 1.1% (average of 0.84%) has been observed, whereas in the placebo group the rate observed

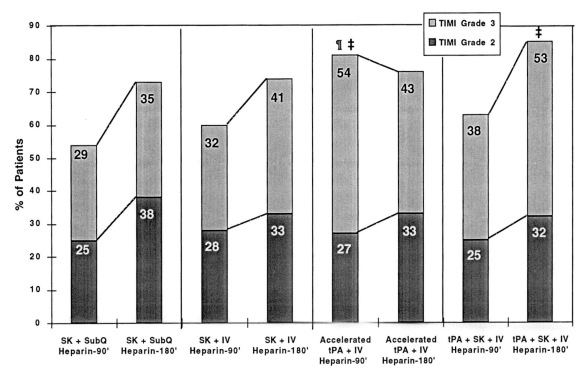

Figure 27–6. Patency of the infarct-related artery at 90 and 180 minutes after thrombolytic therapy in the Global Utilization of Streptokinase and t-PA for Occluded Coronary Arteries (GUSTO) trial, by treatment group. Note that an accelerated tissue plasminogen activator (t-PA) regimen with intravenous heparin provides a statistically significant improvement in 90-minute patency; however, this superiority no longer holds at 180 minutes. See text for discussion.

has been 0.0 to 0.9 (average of 0.79%).[6, 7, 36, 68, 69] Of all stroke events, intracranial hemorrhage constituted 22% and ischemic cerebral infarction accounted for 26%; 52% could not be classified. By comparison, in two separate placebo-controlled trials of t-PA, the rate of cerebrovascular events was observed to be 2% in the treated group and 0.5% and 1.4% (average of 1.26%) in the control group.[10, 37, 70] Intracranial hemorrhage constituted 36%, ischemic cerebral infarction 38%, unclassifiable events 24%, and subdural hematoma 2% of the total stroke events in these two studies. A placebo-controlled trial of APSAC revealed a stroke rate of 1.3% and 0.63% in the treated and control cohorts, respectively.[8, 71]

Considering the results of some large comparative trials, there appears to be a small but significant increased risk of stroke with use of t-PA as opposed to SK. In ISIS-3, strokes of all types occurred in 1.1% of SK-treated and 1.4% of t-PA–treated patients (*P*<.01).[13] Cerebral hemorrhage was more common in the t-PA–treated than in the SK-treated group. Similarly, in ISIS-3 APSAC was associated with a small but significant increase in the incidence of stroke of any type as well as of cerebral hemorrhage. Other studies, however, performed with single-chain, rather than double-chain, t-PA have not confirmed intracranial hemorrhage rates of this magnitude. For example, the TIMI-2 trial[72] of 3016 patients reported an intracranial bleeding rate of 0.4% for single-chain t-PA as opposed to 0.7% for double-chain t-PA in 12,841 patients enrolled in ISIS-3.[13] Overall stroke rates in ISIS-3 did not appear to be influenced by the use, or nonuse, of heparin. In the GUSTO trial[21] the investigators reported a 1.31% and 1.55% incidence of stroke in the SK and rt-PA groups, respectively (*P* = .091).

Bleeding complications in placebo-controlled trials of thrombolytic agents range from 0% to 6.3%, depending on the categorization of the bleeding manifestation as major or minor. Generally, minor bleeds require no transfusions and are characterized by small volumes of blood loss in the sputum and urine or at puncture sites. Major bleeding episodes have been characterized by the need for blood transfusion, usually 2 units or more.

In ISIS-3 there were no significant differences between SK, APSAC, and double-chain t-PA, blood transfusion being required in each treatment group with an incidence of 0.9% to 1%.[13] Generally, immediate use of intravenous, as opposed to subcutaneous, heparin has not been associated with a statistically significant increase in the incidence of major bleeding.

Allergic reactions can be seen not uncommonly in patients receiving SK or APSAC and are rarely seen with t-PA. For example, in the ISIS-3 trial,[13] allergic reactions were reported in 3.6%, 5.1%, and 0.8% of those patients treated with SK, APSAC, and t-PA, respectively. Frank anaphylactic shock, however, is relatively uncommon, having been noted in only 0.1% of patients treated in GISSI-1.[6] Prior administration of SK or APSAC, therefore, constitutes a relatively strong contraindication to their use.

Hypotensive responses may or may not be manifestations of an immune response to a thrombolytic agent. They occur commonly toward the end of the administration of the drug and usually respond to administration of intravenous fluids to augment circulating blood volume. Atropine or dopamine administration may also be necessary in some patients. In ISIS-2 the incidence of hypotension was found to be fivefold greater in the SK group than in the control group,[7] and in the Intravenous Streptokinase in Acute Myocardial Infarction (ISAM) study group, the incidence of hypotension with SK was approximately twofold greater (9.7% in the SK group and 5.1% in the control group).[36] In AIMS the incidence of hypotension was 24.7% with APSAC treatment, whereas it was 18.1% in a control group.[8]

Arrhythmias may or may not be related to the effects of thrombolysis. Both atrial and ventricular tachyarrhythmias are relatively common in acute myocardial infarction, and most studies have shown no significant ability of thrombolytic agents to reduce their incidence. Also, there appears to be no significant difference in the incidence of arrhythmias in comparative studies of various thrombolytic regimens, with and without heparin. The International Study Group showed no statistically significant difference in the incidence of ventricular fibrillation between the groups treated with SK alone, SK and heparin, t-PA alone, and t-PA with heparin.[12] Similarly, APSAC in AIMS had no significant effect on ventricular fibrillation when compared with a placebo arm of the trial.[8] By contrast, in this same trial the incidence of ventricular tachycardia was higher in the APSAC-treated cohort (15.7%) than in a control group (10.5%, P = .006). Sustained ventricular tachycardia occurred with equivalent frequency in GISSI-2 (3.7% in SK, 3.8% in rt-PA).[11] Likewise in the GUSTO trial,[21] sustained ventricular tachycardia occurred in 5.6%, 6.6%, and 6.1% in the t-PA, pooled SK and t-PA, and SK groups, respectively; these values were not statistically different. Bradyarrhythmias, on the other hand, particularly asystole and sinus bradycardia, have

been found to occur more frequently in some studies. In GISSI-1 asystole was higher in the treated group than in the placebo group (2.2% vs. 1.6%, respectively).[6] APSAC treatment in AIMS[8] was associated with a 17.2% incidence of sinus bradycardia as opposed to 9.9% in the control group (P<.001).

Reinfarction rate is a further important endpoint to evaluate in the patient treated with thrombolytic agents. An overview or meta-analysis of 33 randomized, controlled trials prior to 1985 of both intravenous and intracoronary fibrinolytic therapy concluded that the in-hospital reinfarction rate averaged 3.3% in an SK group and 2.4% in the control group (P<.001). More recently published trials have also confirmed that patients treated with thrombolytic agents are more likely to experience reinfarction.[6, 7, 36, 39, 62] In addition, the reinfarction rate appears relatively equal irrespective of the agent used for thrombolytic treatment.[11–13] In the GUSTO trial, the reinfarction rate was observed to be 4% in the t-PA and the combination t-PA/SK groups and 3.7% in the SK pooled group; these differences were not significant.[21] In ISIS-2, ASA alone or in combination with SK reduced the reinfarction rate significantly as compared with the rate in those patients who received neither of these agents.[7]

Recurrent ischemia after thrombolysis occurs in 18% to 32% of patients treated for acute myocardial infarction.[73] Recently, the GUSTO trial[21] found similarly that approximately 18% to 19% of patients exhibited recurrent ischemia after thrombolysis, irrespective of their treatment regimen. Early reports suggested that the presence of a high-grade residual stenosis predicted recurrent ischemia.[74–78] Several of these studies also suggested that a high degree of residual stenosis was associated with a higher reocclusion rate.[74, 76, 77] However, the TAMI investigators were not able to demonstrate a relationship between the degree of residual stenosis after intravenous t-PA and recurrent ischemic events and reocclusion in 192 patients studied by quantitative coronary angiography.[73] Recurrent ischemia also was not predicted by the specific infarct-related artery, TIMI grade flow at 90 minutes after treatment, percentage of diameter stenosis, absolute diameter stenosis, angiographically defined thrombus, diffuse disease or ectasia in the infarct-related artery, or specific morphology of the lesion. Moreover, in 733 consecutive patients, 42% of whom were treated with coronary balloon angioplasty, these same investigators observed a similar degree of residual stenosis in the infarct-related artery acutely in patients who sustained either patency or reocclusion.[56]

THROMBOLYSIS AND PTCA

After a myocardial infarction has been treated with thrombolysis, PTCA has been used to (1) open further a residual high-grade stenosis of a successfully reperfused infarct artery and (2) restore antegrade coronary flow in the patient in whom thrombolytic therapy is unsuccessful ("rescue" PTCA).

PTCA After Successful Thrombolysis

The relatively high incidence of recurrent ischemia and reocclusion after thrombolysis has engendered a number of clinical trials to assess the effects of PTCA (including its timing, i.e., immediate versus deferred) on patient survival and clinical status. Three large, comparative trials of immediate PTCA versus a conservative intervention strategy after t-PA thrombolysis have been reported[79-82] (Table 27–3). Despite some differences in trial design and the actual time of randomization of patients, the conclusions of the three studies were mutually supportive: (1) each concluded that immediate PTCA did not improve either global or regional myocardial shortening during the early convalescent period; and (2) immediate intervention was associated with a greater incidence of procedural complications, including the need for emergency surgical intervention and blood transfusions, a trend toward higher in-hospital mortality rates, and no reduction in the frequency of reocclusion and reinfarction.

A lack of significant difference in both short-term and long-term clinical outcomes also was noted by Erbel and coworkers[83] in a study in which both intravenous and intracoronary thrombolysis were initially given followed by either immediate PTCA or mechanical recanalization using a flexible guide wire.

Although a number of reasons can be cited for the lack of therapeutic benefit of immediate PTCA after thrombolysis, the overriding factor appears to be that balloon dilation itself is deleterious and associated with intramural hemorrhage at the site of dilation, resulting in subtotal occlusion of the dilated vessel.[84-86]

PTCA After Unsuccessful Thrombolysis

In approximately 10% to 25% of patients with an acute myocardial infarction, thrombolytic therapy is unsuccessful in restoring antegrade coronary blood flow. PTCA can be used to open the vessel immediately or during the subsequent hours or days after the onset of the coronary event. The aims of the recanalization are to salvage remaining viable (usually ischemic) myocardium and to improve long-term survival by providing sustained arterial patency.

The strategy of salvage PTCA is hampered, however, by a lack of reliable and timely criteria for identifying clinically the failure of thrombolytic therapy to re-establish antegrade coronary blood flow. Simple clinical criteria, such as relief of chest pain, reversion of ST segment elevation, and reperfusion arrhythmias, fail to pre-

Table 27–3. **Randomized Trials of Immediate and Deferred Interventional Strategies After Intravenous Tissue Plasminogen Activator**

Clinical Characteristic	TAMI (n = 386)	TIMI-2A (n = 367)	ECSG (n = 389)
Point of randomization	After determination of suitability for PTCA	Before diagnostic coronary angiography	Before diagnostic coronary angiography
Immediate group undergoing PTCA (%)	100	72	92
Reocclusion (%)			
Immediate	11	NA	13
Deferred	13	NA	11
Emergency CABG (%)			
Immediate	7	3	3
Deferred	2	0	0
Left ventricular ejection fraction (%)			
Immediate	53	50	51
Deferred	56	49	51
In-hospital mortality (%)			
Immediate	4	8	8
Deferred	1	5	5

TAMI, Thrombolysis and Angioplasty in Myocardial Infarction trial[79]; TIMI-2A, Thrombolysis in Myocardial Infarction trial, phase 2A[80, 81]; NA, not assessed; ECSG, European Cooperative Study Group[82]; CABG, coronary artery bypass graft; PTCA, percutaneous transluminal coronary angioplasty.

dict accurately perfusion status after intravenous thrombolysis.[87] Routine coronary angiography, therefore, is the only recourse for accurate diagnosis but itself is complicated by bleeding at the site of arterial entrance and by excessive cost.

PTCA in the postthrombolytic patient who exhibits a persistently occluded infarct-related artery has been investigated, although not in a randomized study. The TAMI investigators[88] performed a retrospective analysis of 607 patients with successful thrombolysis as compared with 169 patients with successful rescue PTCA after failed thrombolytic treatment. The in-hospital mortality rates in these two groups were not different (4.6% and 5.9%, respectively), but the incidence of reocclusion was significantly higher in the rescue PTCA cohort than that after successful thrombolysis (21% vs. 11%, $P<.001$, respectively). In addition, the rescue PTCA group showed less improvement in regional wall motion in the area of the infarction. However, reocclusion after rescue PTCA was much higher in patients treated with t-PA than with either UK or a combination of t-PA and UK. Others have also reported lower reocclusion rates when using thrombolytic agents with significant systemic fibrinolytic potential.[89–91] The TAMI investigators also organized a prospective study (TAMI-5) that compared an aggressive interventional strategy with a more conservative one.[92] The hypotheses tested were as follows: (1) by using a combination of t-PA and UK for thrombolytic therapy, vessel patency, left ventricular function, and clinical outcomes could be improved; and (2) if thrombolytic therapy fails to open the infarct-related artery, or if there is ongoing ischemia after thrombolysis, then rescue PTCA could improve left ventricular function and clinical outcomes. In this analysis, the patients treated with the combination therapy had a lesser adverse clinical event rate based on a composite end-point (death, stroke, reinfarction, reocclusion, heart failure, or recurrent ischemia). Global ejection fraction was no different between the two strategies, but regional wall shortening in the infarct zone was better in the aggressive than in the deferred catheterization group.

Based on these somewhat divergent data, the role of rescue PTCA is yet to be fully defined. The Randomized Evaluation of Salvage Angioplasty with Combined Utilization of Endpoints (RESCUE) trial, an international multicenter study of patients with left anterior descending coronary artery occlusion, is now providing greater insight into the ultimate value of rescue angioplasty. When applied to a patient with a first anterior infarction, rescue angioplasty appears useful in prevention of death or severe heart failure, with improvement in exercise, but not resting, ejection fraction.[93]

Noninvasive Postthrombolytic Strategy

In light of the nonbeneficial, and possibly deleterious, effect of immediate PTCA after thrombolysis on clinical outcomes, a conservative strategy based on noninvasive testing for residual ischemia was formulated and tested against a deferred PTCA strategy in several randomized studies[65, 94] (Table 27–4). Both of these trials compared PTCA for patients with spontaneous or exercise-induced ischemia after infarction versus an invasive strategy of routine catheterization and PTCA at 18 to 48 hours. At follow-up the number of deaths, the incidence of repeat infarctions, and the resting ejection fraction were not statistically different between the conservative and routine catheterization groups. In TIMI-2, however, there was evidence that patients with a prior myocardial infarction were preferably managed with an aggressive or invasive strategy before discharge.[95]

Although the issue of when to implement PTCA after thrombolysis is reasonably well established, based on the aforementioned randomized trials in the United States and Europe, there remains controversy as to the indications for diagnostic coronary angiography after thrombolysis. There are no definitive studies that would support either selective or routine cardiac catheterization and coronary angiography. The best alternative to angiography for risk stratification would be a noninvasive test with high predictive accuracy for identification of residual ischemia and territory at risk. However, essentially all studies addressing the accuracy of noninvasive tests after myocardial infarction have been conducted in patients who did not receive thrombolysis.[96] Of those studies published on noninvasive functional testing after intravenous thrombolysis, all have raised the issue of the value of these examinations in detecting residual ischemia and prognosticating natural history in a patient who has reperfused.[97–99] In addition, it has been reported that the most common explanation for a fixed or peri-infarct redistribution defect on thallium scintigraphy after thrombolytic treatment for acute myocardial infarction is a completed or nearly complete infarct, not a total coronary occlusion of the infarct-related artery.[100] Moreover, prognosis after thrombolysis may be related not to a physiologically significant narrowing of the reperfused coronary artery but rather to the underlying pathoanatomy of the

Table 27–4. **Randomized Trials of a Deferred, Elective Interventional Strategy Versus a Conservative, Noninvasive Strategy After Thrombolysis**

Clinical Characteristic	TIMI-2B: t-PA (n = 3262)	SWIFT: APSAC (n = 800)
Point of randomization	After drug administration	After 24 hr of clinical stability
Period of follow-up	6 wk	1 yr
Invasive group undergoing PTCA or CABG (%)	56.7	57
Conservative group undergoing PTCA or CABG (%)	13.2	14.7
Mortality (%)		
Invasive	5.2	5.8
Noninvasive	4.7	5.0
Reinfarction (%)		
Invasive	6.4	15.1
Noninvasive	5.8	12.9
Resting left ventricular ejection fraction (%)		
Invasive	50.5	50.7
Noninvasive	49.9	51.7
Incidence of exercise-induced myocardial ischemia (%)		
Invasive	12.8	
Noninvasive	17.7*	
Blood transfusion (%)		
Invasive	5.5	19.9
Noninvasive	4.3	16.1

*$P < .001$

TIMI-2B, Thrombolysis in Myocardial Infarction;[95] SWIFT, Should We Intervene Following Thrombolysis? trial[94]; see Tables 27–1 and 27–3 for other abbreviations.

arterial wall and its predisposition to fissure and incite thrombosis. Direct visualization of the arterial lesion, either by intravascular ultrasonography or angioscopy, may be proved in time to be the best method for identifying the patient at highest risk after thrombolysis.[96] Only further clinical follow-up studies, coupled perhaps with a refinement of existing or development of new diagnostic techniques, will settle the uncertainty over the indications for coronary angiography after thrombolysis.

PRIMARY PTCA

Although thrombolysis has been proven in multiple, large randomized trials to significantly improve survival after myocardial infarction, this form of therapy continues to have significant limitations. These include the following:

1. The therapy is applied currently in only one third of patients proved to have an acute myocardial infarction
2. Many patients have contraindications to the use of thrombolytic agents
3. The average time to thrombolytic therapy for acute myocardial infarction has been 2.5 to 5 hours after symptom onset, even though the maximum benefit is attained if the therapy begins within 60 to 90 minutes
4. Usually full clot lysis does not occur for

approximately 45 minutes after initiation of therapy
5. In 20% to 25% of patients there is a failure to achieve patency of the infarct-related artery
6. Serious bleeding complications can eventuate even in the well-screened patient
7. There is an increased risk of myocardial ischemia after thrombolytic treatment

A number of interventional cardiologists therefore have advocated direct balloon angioplasty to mechanically lyse and relieve the underlying obstruction in a patient with an acute myocardial infarction. A number of observational, nonrandomized studies have indicated that immediate angioplasty, early in the course of an acute myocardial infarction, can achieve a high rate of reperfusion, an increase in ejection fraction, and a low in-hospital mortality rate.[101–103]

Only recently have further randomized prospective trials of primary, direct PTCA versus intravenous thrombolysis been completed and reported[104–106] (Table 27–5). It can be concluded from these investigations that immediate PTCA was more effective than thrombolysis in restoring vessel patency and preventing reocclusion of the infarct-related artery. Moreover, patients undergoing primary PTCA had a shorter hospital stay, similar in-hospital but reduced follow-up costs, and fewer readmissions than those treated with thrombolytic therapy. Finally, the three studies indicate that although PTCA is no

Table 27–5. **Randomized Trials of Primary, Immediate Coronary Balloon Angioplasty Versus Intravenous Thrombolytic Therapy**

Clinical Characteristic	PAMI	ZWOLLE (Netherlands)	MAYO Clinic
Thrombolytic agent	rt-PA	Streptokinase	rt-PA
Number of patients	395	142	108
Point of randomization	Within 12 hr of MI; after heparin and aspirin	Within 6 hr of MI; after heparin and aspirin	Within 12 hr of MI; after heparin and aspirin
Period of follow-up	Through 6 mo	Through hospital discharge	Through hospital discharge
In-hospital death rate (%)			
PTCA	2.6	0	2.1
Thrombolysis only	6.5	6	0
In-hospital reinfarction (%)			
PTCA	2.6	0	0
Thrombolysis only	6.5	13	3.6
6-mo death or reinfarction rate (%)			
PTCA	8.5*		
Thrombolysis only	16.8		
In-hospital stroke rate (%)			
PTCA	0	0	
Thrombolysis only	3.5	3	
Ejection fraction at rest (%)			
PTCA	53	NA	53
Thrombolysis only	53	NA	50
Myocardial salvage (as percentage of left ventricle) by myocardial scintigraphy			
PTCA			15 ± 19
Thrombolysis only			13 ± 19

*P = .02 versus thrombolysis only.

rt-PA, recombinant tissue plasminogen activator; MI, myocardial infarction; PAMI, Primary Angioplasty in Myocardial Infarction study[105]; ZWOLLE, randomized study performed in Zwolle, The Netherlands[106]; MAYO Clinic, randomized study performed at the Mayo Clinic[104]; NA, not assessed.

more effective than thrombolysis in salvaging myocardium, the interventional procedure led to a lower incidence of recurrent ischemia, reinfarction, and death. Direct PTCA was particularly efficacious in those patients at high risk, for example, those older than 75 years of age, exhibiting an anterior infarction, or experiencing persistent tachycardia. Based on these conclusions, direct PTCA is recommended in the patient with acute myocardial infarction who is first evaluated in close proximity to a catheterization laboratory that is staffed by personnel capable of executing expertly and promptly coronary angiography and balloon angioplasty.

THROMBOLYSIS IN UNSTABLE ANGINA

As with acute myocardial infarction, recent studies have confirmed the importance of coronary thrombi in unstable angina.[107–109] Not surprisingly, therefore, ASA and heparin, both individually and together, have been shown to reduce the relative risk of both fatal and nonfatal myocardial infarction in patients with unstable ischemic syndromes.[110–113] However, the efficacy of thrombolytic agents has not been conclusive and remains controversial.

The largest study published, the TIMI-3A trial, analyzed 308 patients with coronary angiography within the first 24 hours after an episode of chest pain.[114] If a culprit coronary artery lesion was identified (excluding a left main artery), patients were randomized to t-PA (dose of 0.8 mg/kg, one third given as bolus and the remainder infused over 90 minutes, to a maximal dose of 80 mg) or to placebo.[114] A second coronary angiogram was performed within 18 to 48 hours; the culprit lesion at baseline was quantitated as an 84% ± 9% (SD) stenosis (0.45 ± 0.28 mm minimal diameter) and improved by 6.2% (0.17 ± 0.29 mm) with t-PA and by 4.6% (0.14 ± 0.2 mm) with placebo (difference not significant). Other placebo-controlled studies of thrombolytic therapy also have failed to confirm any significant improvement in subtotal luminal obstruction in unstable anginal syndromes.[115–118] For example, in the Unstable Angina Study Using Sminase (UNASEM) trial, excluding those patients with a complete occlusion of the coronary artery, there was a 5% and 3% (difference not significant) improvement in luminal diameter for the thrombolytic and placebo groups, respectively.[115]

If the end-point of therapy is angiographic improvement of coronary flow, and patients with total thrombotic occlusion are included, some salutary effect of thrombolysis can be identified. In the TIMI-3A trial,[114] t-PA was successful in increasing coronary perfusion by two TIMI grades or in the percentage of stenosis by 20% in 15% of patients and in only 5% of those given placebo. In the UNASEM investigation, 12 of 17 patients with a totally occluded artery showed restoration of blood flow after rt-PA, whereas all 11 patients in the placebo group remained totally occluded.[115]

If, however, the end-points of therapy are clinical events, then addition of thrombolytic therapy to conventional medical treatment in unstable angina does not provide a clinical benefit to patients with unstable angina.[115–119] In the UNASEM trial, recurrent angina and severe bleeding were both more commonly noted after treatment in the thrombolytic group as compared with the placebo cohort.[115] Death, myocardial infarction, and urgent surgery were not statistically affected by thrombolytic therapy in the study reported by Freeman and colleagues.[117] In the TIMI-3B investigation (a randomized, 2 × 2 factorial design), patients with either unstable angina or non–Q wave myocardial infarction who received thrombolysis did not differ for unfavorable outcome when compared with those receiving standard medical therapy with placebo. Moreover, an early invasive strategy (cardiac catheterization, left ventriculography, and coronary angiography) did not affect patient outcome favorably.[119]

REFERENCES

1. Chazov EL, Mateera LS, Masaev AV, et al: Intracoronary administration of fibrinolysis in acute myocardial infarction. Ter Arkh 1976; 48:8–19.
2. Rentrop KP, Blanke H, Karsch KR, Kreuzer H: Initial experience with transluminal recanalization of the recently occluded infarct-related coronary in acute myocardial infarction: Comparison with conventionally treated patients. Clin Cardiol 1979; 1:92.
3. Kennedy JW, Ritchie JL, Davis KB, Fritz JK: Western Washington randomized trial of intracoronary streptokinase in acute myocardial infarction. N Engl J Med 1983; 309:1477–1482.
4. DeWood MA, Spores J, Notske R, et al: Prevalence of total coronary occlusion during the early hours of transmural myocardial infarction. N Engl J Med 1980; 303:897–902.
5. Falk E: Plaque rupture with severe pre-existing stenosis precipitating coronary thrombosis: Characteristics of coronary atherosclerotic plaques underlying fatal occlusive thrombi. Br Heart J 1983; 50:127–134.
6. Gruppo Italiano per lo Studio della Streptochinase Nell'Infarto Miocardico (GISSI): Effectiveness of intravenous thrombolytic treatment in acute myocardial infarction. Lancet 1986; 1:397–402.
7. ISIS (International Study of Infarct Survival) Collaborative Group: Randomized trial of intravenous streptokinase, oral aspirin, both, or neither among 17,187 cases of suspected acute myocardial infarction: ISIS-2. Lancet 1988; 2:349–360.
8. AIMS Trial Study Group: Effect of intravenous APSAC on mortality after acute myocardial infarction: Preliminary report of a placebo-controlled clinical trial. Lancet 1988; 1:545–549.
9. Neuhas KL, Tebbe U, Gottwik M, for the GAUS group: Intravenous recombinant tissue plasminogen activator (rt-PA) and urokinase in acute myocardial infarction: Results of the German Activator Urokinase Study (GAUS). J Am Coll Cardiol 1988; 12:581–587.
10. Wilcox RG, Olsson CG, Skene AM, et al: Trial of tissue plasminogen activator for mortality reduction in acute myocardial infarction: Anglo-Scandinavian Study of Early Thrombolysis (ASSET). Lancet 1988; 2:525–530.
11. GISSI-2: A factorial randomized trial of alteplase versus streptokinase and heparin versus no heparin among 12,490 patients with acute myocardial infarction. Lancet 1990; 336:65–71.
12. International Study Group: In-hospital mortality and clinical course of 20,891 patients with suspected acute myocardial infarction randomized between alteplase and streptokinase with or without heparin. Lancet 1990; 336:71–75.
13. ISIS-3 (Third International Study of Infarct Survival) Collaborative Group: ISIS-3: A randomized comparison of streptokinase vs. tissue plasminogen activator vs. anistreplase and of aspirin plus heparin vs. aspirin alone among 41,299 cases of suspected acute myocardial infarction. Lancet 1992; 339:753–770.
14. Turpie AGG, Robinson JG, Doyle DJ, et al: Comparison of high-dose with low-dose subcutaneous heparin to prevent left ventricular mural thrombus in patients with acute transmural anterior myocardial infarction. N Engl J Med 1989; 320:352–357.
15. Neuhas KL, von Essen R, Tebbe U, et al: Improved thrombolysis in acute myocardial infarction with front-loaded administration of alteplase: Results of the rt-PA–APSAC Patency Study (TAPS). J Am Coll Cardiol 1992; 19:885–891.
16. Chesebro JH, Knatterud G, Roberts R, et al: Thrombolysis in Myocardial Infarction (TIMI) Trial, Phase I: A comparison between intravenous tissue plasminogen activator and intravenous streptokinase. Clinical findings through hospital discharge. Circulation 1987; 76:142–154.
17. Malcolm A, on behalf of ESPRIT Study Group: European Study of the Prevention of Reocclusion after Initial Thrombolysis (ESPRIT) with duteplase in acute myocardial infarction. 1992. Unpublished, but cited in reference 13.
18. Grines CL, Karlsberg R, Stadius M, for The Burroughs Wellcome Study Group: Infarct vessel patency and bleeding complications after weight-adjusted dosing of a double-chain tissue plasminogen activator [final report]. J Am Coll Cardiol 1990; 15:2A.
19. Kalbfleish J, Kumik P, Thadani U, et al, for The Burroughs Wellcome Study Group: Infarct-artery patency

and reocclusion rates after treatment with duteplase at the dose used in ISIS-3. 1992. Unpubished, but cited in reference 13.

20. Topol EJ, George BS, Kereiakes DJ, et al: A randomized, controlled trial of intravenous tissue plasminogen activator and early intravenous heparin in acute myocardial infarction. Circulation 1989; 79:281–286.

21. The GUSTO Investigators: An international randomized trial comparing four thrombolytic strategies for acute myocardial infarction. N Engl J Med 1993; 329:673–682.

22. GUSTO Investigators: The effects of tissue plasminogen activator, streptokinase, or both on coronary artery patency, ventricular function, and survival after acute myocardial infarction. N Engl J Med 1993; 329:1615–1622.

23. Ridker PM, O'Donnell C, Marder VJ, Hennekens CH: Large-scale trials of thrombolytic therapy for acute myocardial infarction: GISSI-2, ISIS-3, and GUSTO-1 [editorial]. Ann Intern Med 1993; 119:530–532.

24. Rapaport E: GUSTO: Assessment of the preliminary results. J Myocard Ischemia 1993; 5:15–24.

25. Conti RC: Myocardial infarction, thrombolytic therapy, and economics [editorial]. Clin Cardiol 1993; 16:635.

26. Farkouh ME, Larig JD, Sackett DL: Thrombolytic agents: The science of the art of choosing the better treatment. Ann Intern Med 1994; 120:886–888.

27. Kim CB, Braunwald E: Potential benefits of late reperfusion of infarcted myocardium: The open artery hypothesis. Circulation 1993; 88:2426–2436.

28. Califf RM, Harrelson-Woodlief L, Topol EJ: Left ventricular ejection fraction may not be useful as an endpoint of thrombolytic therapy comparative trials. Circulation 1990; 82:1847–1853.

29. Braunwald E: Myocardial reperfusion, limitation of infarct size, reduction of left ventricular dysfunction, and improved survival: Should the paradigm be expanded? Circulation 1989; 79:441–444.

30. Sheehan FH, Doerr R, Schmidt WG, et al: Early recovery of left ventricular function after thrombolytic therapy for acute myocardial infarction: An important determinant of survival. J Am Coll Cardiol 1988; 12:289–300.

31. Mathey DG, Schoffer J, Sheehan FH, et al: Improved survival up to four years after early coronary thrombolysis. Am J Cardiol 1988; 61:524–529.

32. O'Rourke M, Baron D, Keogh A, et al: Limitation of myocardial infarction by early infusion of recombinant–type plasminogen activator. Circulation 1988; 77:1131–1135.

33. White HD, Norris RM, Brown MA, et al: Effect of intravenous streptokinase on left ventricular function and early survival after acute myocardial infarction. N Engl J Med 1987; 317:850–855.

34. Guerci AD, Gerstenbith G, Brinker JA, et al: A randomized trial of intravenous tissue plasminogen activator for acute myocardial infarction with subsequent randomization to elective coronary angioplasty. N Engl J Med 1987; 317:1613–1618.

35. National Heart Foundation of Australia Coronary Thrombolysis Group: Coronary thrombolysis and myocardial salvage by tissue plasminogen activator given up to four hours after onset of myocardial infarction. Lancet 1988; 1:203–207.

36. ISAM Study Group: A prospective trial of intravenous streptokinase in acute myocardial infarction (ISAM). N Engl J Med 1986; 314:1465–1471.

37. Van de Werf F, Arnold AER, for the European Cooperative Study Group: Intravenous tissue plasminogen activator and size of infarct, left ventricular function, and survival in acute myocardial infarction. Br Med J 1988; 297:1371–1379.

38. Bassand JP, Machecourt J, Cassagnes J, et al, for the APSIM Study Investigators: Multicenter trial of intravenous anisoylated plasminogen streptokinase activator complex (APSAC) in acute myocardial infarction: Effects on infarct size and left ventricular function. J Am Coll Cardiol 1989; 13:988–997.

39. Sheehan FH, Braunwald E, Canner P, TIMI-I Group: The effect of intravenous thrombolytic therapy on left ventricular function: A report on tissue-type plasminogen activator and streptokinase from the thrombolysis in myocardial infarction (TIMI phase I) trial. Circulation 1987; 75:817–829.

40. Henzlova MJ, Bourge RC, Tauxe L, Rogers WJ: Is preservation of left ventricular function after thrombolytic therapy sustained [abstract]? Circulation 1989; 80(Suppl II):II-312.

41. Harrison JK, Skelton TN, Davidson CJ, et al: Regional and global left ventricular function evaluated acutely at 7 days, and at 6 months following thrombolytic therapy [abstract]. Circulation 1989; 80(Suppl II):II-313.

42. Hutchins GM, Bulkley BH: Infarct expansion versus extension: Two different complications of acute myocardial infarction. Am J Cardiol 1978; 41:1127.

43. Weisman HF, Healy B: Myocardial infarct expansion, infarct extension, and reinfarction: Pathophysiologic concepts. Prog Cardiovasc Dis 1987; 30:73–110.

44. Pfeffer MA, Braunwald E: Ventricular remodeling after myocardial infarction: Experimental observations and clinical implications. Circulation 1990; 81:1161–1172.

45. McKay RG, Pfeffer MA, Pasternak RC, et al: Left ventricular remodeling after myocardial infarction: A corollary to infarct expansion. Circulation 1986; 74:693–702.

46. White HD, Norris RM, Brown MA, et al: Left ventricular end-systolic volume as the major determinant of survival after recovery from myocardial infarction. Circulation 1987; 76:44–51.

47. Pfeffer JM, Pfeffer MA, Braunwald E: Influence of chronic captopril therapy on the infarcted left ventricle of the rat. Circ Res 1985; 57:84–95.

48. Pfeffer MA, Lamas GA, Vaughan DE, et al: Effect of captopril on progressive ventricular dilatation after anterior myocardial infarction. N Engl J Med 1988; 319:80–86.

49. Sweet CS, Kemment SE, Stabilito II, Ribeiro LGT: Increased survival in rats with congestive heart failure treated with enalapril. J Cardiovasc Pharmacol 1987; 10:636–642.

50. Pfeffer MA, Pfeffer JM, Steinberg C, Finn P: Survival after an experimental myocardial infarction: Beneficial effects of long-term therapy with captopril. Circulation 1985; 72:406–412.

51. Jugdutt BI, Schwarz-Michorowski Bl, Khan MI: Effect of long-term captopril therapy on left ventricular remodeling and function during healing of canine myocardial infarction. J Am Coll Cardiol 1992; 19:713–721.

52. Jugdutt BI, Warnica JW: Intravenous nitroglycerin therapy to limit myocardial infarct size, expansion, and complications: Effect of timing, dosage, and infarct location. Circulation 1988; 78:906–919.

53. Leung W-H, Lau C-P: Effect of severity of the residual stenosis of the infarct-related coronary artery on left ventricular dilation and function after acute myocardial infarction. J Am Coll Cardiol 1992; 20:307–313.

54. Cigarroa RG, Lange RA, Hillis LD: Prognosis after acute myocardial infarction in patients with and without residual anterograde coronary blood flow. Am J Cardiol 1989; 64:155–160.

55. Lange RA, Cigarroa RG, Hillis LD: Influence of residual antegrade coronary blood flow on survival after

myocardial infarction in patients with multivessel coronary artery disease. Coronary Artery Dis 1990; 1:59–63.

56. Ohman EF, Califf RM, Topol EJ, et al: Consequences of reocclusion after successful reperfusion therapy in acute myocardial infarction. Circulation 1990; 82:781–791.

57. Kennedy JW, Ritchie JL, Davis KB, et al: The Western Washington randomized trial of intracoronary streptokinase in acute myocardial infarction: A 12-month follow-up report. N Engl J Med 1985; 312:1073–1080.

58. Kersschot IE, Brugada P, Ramentol M, et al: Effects of early reperfusion in acute myocardial infarction on arrhythmias induced by programmed stimulation: A prospective, randomized study. J Am Coll Cardiol 1986: 7:1234–1242.

59. Lange RA, Cigarroa RG, Wells PJ, et al: Influence of anterograde flow in the infarct artery on the incidence of late potentials after acute myocardial infarction. Am J Cardiol 1990; 65:554–558.

60. Verstraete M, Bory M, Collen D, for the ECSG group: Randomized trial of intravenous recombinant tissue–type plasminogen activator versus intravenous streptokinase in acute myocardial infarction: Report from ECSG for tissue-type plasminogen activator. Lancet 1985; 1:842–847.

61. PRIMI Trial Study Group: Randomized double-blind trial of recombinant pro-urokinase against streptokinase in acute myocardial infarction. Lancet 1989; 1:863–867.

62. White HD, Rivers JT, Maslowski AH, et al: Effect of intravenous streptokinase as compared with that of tissue plasminogen activator on left ventricular function after first myocardial infarction. N Engl J Med 1989; 320:817–821.

63. Bleich SD, Nichols T, Shumacher RR, et al: Effect of heparin on coronary arterial patency after thrombolysis with tissue plasminogen activator in acute myocardial infarction. Am J Cardiol 1990; 66:1412–1417.

64. Bassand JP, Cassagnes J, Machecourt J, et al: Comparative effects of APSAC and rt-PA on infarct size and left ventricular function in acute myocardial infarction: A multicenter, randomized study. Circulation 1991; 84:1107–1117.

65. TIMI Study Group: Comparison of invasive and conservative strategies after treatment with intravenous tissue plasminogen activator in acute myocardial infarction: Results of the Thrombolysis in Myocardial Infarction (TIMI) Phase II Trial. N Engl J Med 1989; 320:618–627.

66. Van de Werf F, for the ECSG for rt-PA Trial: Lessons from the European cooperative recombinant tissue–type plasminogen activator. J Am Coll Cardiol 1988; 12:14A–19A.

67. Anderson JL, Sorensen SG, Moreno FL, et al: Multicenter patency trial of intravenous anistreplase compared with streptokinase in acute myocardial infarction. Circulation 1991; 83:126–140.

68. Rovelli F, Devita C, Feruglio MG, et al: GISSI trial: Early results and late follow-up. J Am Coll Cardiol 1987; 10(Suppl):33B–39B.

69. Schroder R, Neuhas KL, Leizorovicz A, et al, for the ISAM Study Group: A prospective placebo-controlled double-blind multicenter trial of intravenous streptokinase (ISAM): Long-term mortality and morbidity in acute myocardial infarction. J Am Coll Cardiol 1987; 9:197–203.

70. Wilcox RG, von der Lippe G, Olsson CG, et al: Effects of alteplase on acute myocardial infarction: Six-month results from the ASSET Study. Lancet 1990; 335:1175–1178.

71. AIMS Trial Study Group: Long-term effects of intravenous anistreplase in acute myocardial infarction: Final report of the AIMS study. Lancet 1990; 335:427–431.

72. Gore JM, Sloan M, Price TR, et al: Intracerebral hemorrhage, cerebral infarction, and subdural hematoma after acute myocardial infarction and thrombolytic therapy in the thrombolysis in myocardial infarction study: Thrombolysis in Myocardial Infarction, Phase II, Pilot and Clinical Trial. Circulation 1991; 83:448–459.

73. Ellis SG, Topol EJ, George BS, et al: Recurrent ischemia without warning: Analysis of risk factors for in-hospital ischemic events following successful thrombolysis with intravenous tissue plasminogen activator. Circulation 1989; 80:1159–1165.

74. Gold HK, Leinbach RC, Palacios IF, et al: Coronary reocclusion after selective administration of streptokinase. Circulation 1983; 68(Suppl IV):IV-50–IV-54.

75. Serruys PW, Wijns W, Van den Brand M, et al: Is transluminal coronary angioplasty mandatory after successful thrombolysis? Quantitative coronary angiographic study. Br Heart J 1983; 50:257–265.

76. Harrison DG, Furguson DW, Collins SM, et al: Rethrombosis after reperfusion with streptokinase: Importance of geometry of residual lesions. Circulation 1984; 69:991–999.

77. Gash AK, Spann JF, Sherry S, et al: Factors influencing reocclusion after coronary thrombolysis for acute myocardial infarction. Am J Cardiol 1986; 57:175–177.

78. Badger RS, Brown BG, Kennedy JW, et al: Usefulness of recanalization to luminal diameter of 0.6 mm or more with intracoronary streptokinase during acute myocardial infarction in predicting "normal" perfusion status, continued arterial patency, and survival at one year. Am J Cardiol 1987; 59:519–522.

79. Topol EJ, Califf RM, George BS, et al: A randomized trial of immediate versus delayed elective angioplasty after intravenous tissue plasminogen activator in acute myocardial infarction. N Engl J Med 1987; 317:581–588.

80. The TIMI Research Group: Immediate versus delayed catheterization and angioplasty following thrombolytic therapy for acute myocardial infarction: TIMI-IIA results. JAMA 1988; 260:2849–2858.

81. Rogers WJ, Baim DS, Gore JM, et al: Comparison of immediate invasive, delayed invasive, and conservative strategies after tissue-type plasminogen activator: Results of the Thrombolysis in Myocardial Infarction (TIMI) Phase II-A Trial. Circulation 1990; 81:1457–1476.

82. Simoons ML, Arnold AER, Betriu A, et al: Thrombolysis with tissue plasminogen activator in acute myocardial infarction: No additional benefit from immediate percutaneous coronary angioplasty. Lancet 1988; 1:197–202.

83. Erbel R, Pop T, Diefenbach C, Meyer J: Long-term results of thrombolytic therapy with and without percutaneous transluminal coronary angioplasty. J Am Coll Cardiol 1989; 14:276–285.

84. Muller DWM, Topol EJ: Thombolytic therapy: Adjuvant mechanical intervention for acute myocardial infarction. Am J Cardiol 1992; 69:60A–70A.

85. Duber C, Jungbluth A, Rumpelt H-J, et al: Morphology of the coronary arteries after combined thrombolysis and percutaneous coronary angioplasty for acute myocardial infarction. Am J Cardiol 1986; 58:698–703.

86. Waller BF, Rothbaum DA, Pinkerton CA, et al: Status of the myocardium and infarct-related coronary artery in 19 necropsy patients with acute recanalization using pharmacologic (streptokinase, r-tissue plasminogen activator), mechanical (percutaneous transluminal coronary angioplasty) or combined types of reperfusion therapy. J Am Coll Cardiol 1987; 9:785–801.

87. Califf RM, O'Neill WW, Stack RS, et al: Failure of simple clinical measurements to predict perfusion sta-

tus after intravenous thrombolysis. Ann Intern Med 1988; 108:658–662.

88. Abbotsmith CW, Topol EJ, George BS, et al: Fate of patients with acute myocardial infarction with patency of the infarct-related vessel achieved with successful thrombolysis versus rescue angioplasty. J Am Coll Cardiol 1990; 16:770–778.

89. Grines CL, Nissen SE, Booth DC, et al: A new thrombolytic regimen for acute myocardial infarction using combination half-dose tissue-type plasminogen activator with full-dose streptokinase: A pilot study. J Am Coll Cardiol 1989; 14:573–580.

90. Holmes DR, Gersch BJ, Bailey KR, et al: Emergency "rescue" percutaneous transluminal coronary angioplasty after failed thrombolysis with streptokinase: Early and late results. Circulation 1990; 81(Suppl IV):IV-51–IV-56.

91. Whitlow PL, CRAFT Study Group: Catheterization/Rescue Angioplasty Following Thrombolysis (CRAFT) Study: Results of rescue angioplasty [abstract]. Circulation 1990; 82:III-308.

92. Califf RM, Topol EJ, Stack RS, et al: Evaluation of combination thrombolytic therapy and timing of cardiac catheterization in acute myocardial infarction: Results of thrombolysis and angioplasty in myocardial infarction—phase 5 randomized trial. Circulation 1991; 83:1543–1556.

93. Ellis SG, da Silva ER, Heyndrickx G, et al: Randomized comparison of rescue angioplasty with conservative management of patients with early failure of thrombolysis for acute anterior myocardial infarction. Circulation 1994; 90:2280–2284.

94. SWIFT (Should We Intervene Following Thrombolysis?) Trial Study Group: SWIFT trial of delayed elective intervention versus conservative treatment after thrombolysis with anistreplase in acute myocardial infarction. Br Med J 1991; 302:555–560.

95. Mueller HS, Cohen LS, Braunwald E, et al: Predictors of early morbidity and mortality after thrombolytic therapy of acute myocardial infarction: Analyses of patient subgroups in the Thrombolysis in Myocardial Infarction (TIMI) Trial, Phase II. Circulation 1992; 85:1254–1264.

96. Topol EJ, Holmes DR, Rogers WJ: Coronary angiography after thrombolytic therapy for acute myocardial infarction. Ann Intern Med 1991; 114:877–885.

97. Touchstone DA, Beller GA, Nygaard TW, et al: Functional significance of predischarge exercise thallium 201 findings following intravenous streptokinase therapy during acute myocardial infarction. Am Heart J 1988; 116:1500–1507.

98. Weiss AT, Maddahi J, Shah PK: Exercise-induced ischemia in the streptokinase-reperfused myocardium: Relationship to extent of salvaged myocardium and degree of residual coronary stenosis. Am Heart J 1989; 118:9–16.

99. Simoons ML, Vos J, Tijssen JG, et al: Long-term benefit of early thrombolytic therapy in patients with acute myocardial infarction: Five-year follow-up of a trial conducted by the Interuniversity Cardiology Institute in the Netherlands. J Am Coll Cardiol 1989; 14:1609–1615.

100. Sutton JM, Topol EJ: Significance of a negative exercise thallium test in the presence of a critical residual stenosis after thrombolysis for acute myocardial infarction. Circulation 1991; 83:1278–1286.

101. O'Keefe JH Jr, Rutherford BD, McConahay DR, et al: Early and late results of coronary angioplasty without antecedent thrombolytic therapy for acute myocardial infarction. Am J Cardiol 1989; 64:1221–1230.

102. Ellis SG, O'Neill WW, Bates ER, et al: Coronary angioplasty as primary therapy for acute myocardial infarction 6 to 48 hours after symptom onset: Report of an initial experience. J Am Coll Cardiol 1989; 13:1122–1126.

103. Rothbaum DA, Linnemeier TJ, Landin RJ, et al: Emergency percutaneous transluminal coronary angioplasty in acute myocardial infarction: A three-year experience. J Am Coll Cardiol 1987; 10:264–272.

104. Gibbons RJ, Holmes DR, Reeder GS, et al: Immediate angioplasty compared with the administration of a thrombolytic agent followed by conservative treatment for myocardial infarction. N Engl J Med 1993; 328:685–691.

105. Grines CL, Browne KIF, Marco J, et al: A comparison of immediate angioplasty with thrombolytic therapy for acute myocardial infarction. N Engl J Med 1993; 328:673–679.

106. Zijlstra F, de Boer MJ, Hoorntje JCA, et al: A comparison of immediate coronary angioplasty with intravenous streptokinase in acute myocardial infarction. N Engl J Med 1993; 328:680–684.

107. Falk E: Unstable angina with fatal outcome: Dynamic coronary thrombosis leading to infarction and/or sudden death: Autopsy evidence of recurrent mural thrombosis with peripheral embolization culminating in total vascular occlusion. Circulation 1985; 71:699–708.

108. Davies MJ, Thomas AC: Thrombosis and acute coronary artery lesions in sudden ischemic death. N Engl J Med 1984; 310:1137–1140.

109. Sherman CT, Litvack F, Grundfest W, et al: Coronary angioscopy in patients with unstable angina pectoris. N Engl J Med 1986; 315:913–919.

110. Theroux P, Ouimet H, McCans J, et al: Aspirin, heparin, or both to treat acute unstable angina. N Engl J Med 1988; 319:1105–1111.

111. Lewis HD, Davis JW, Archibald DG, et al: Protective effects of aspirin against myocardial infarction and death in men with unstable angina. N Engl J Med 1983; 309:396–403.

112. Cairns JA, Gent M, Singer J, et al: Aspirin, sulfinpyrazone, or both in unstable angina. N Engl J Med 1985; 313:1369–1375.

113. The RISC Group: Risk of myocardial infarction and death during treatment with low-dose aspirin and intravenous heparin in men with unstable coronary disease. Lancet 1990; 336:827–830.

114. TIMI-3A Investigators: Early effects of tissue plasminogen activator, added to conventional therapy, on the culprit coronary lesion in patients presenting with unstable angina. J Am Coll Cardiol 1985; 5:609–616.

115. Bar FW, Verheugt FW, Col J, et al: Thrombolysis in patients with unstable angina improves the angiographic but not the outcome: Results of UNASEM, a multicenter, randomized, placebo-controlled clinical trial with anistreplase. Circulation 1992; 86:131–137.

116. Williams DO, Topol EJ, Califf RM, et al: Intravenous recombinant tissue–type plasminogen activator in patients with unstable angina pectoris: Results of a placebo-controlled, randomized trial. Circulation 1990; 82:376–383.

117. Freeman MR, Langer A, Wilson RF, et al: Thrombolysis in unstable angina: Randomized double-blind trial of t-PA and placebo. Circulation 1992; 85:150–157.

118. Ardissino D, Barberis P, De Servi S, et al: Recombinant tissue–type plasminogen activator followed by heparin compared with heparin alone for refractory unstable angina pectoris. Am J Cardiol 1990; 66:910–914.

119. The TIMI III-B Investigators: Effects of tissue plasminogen activator and a comparison of early invasive and conservative strategies in unstable angina and non–Q wave myocardial infarction. Circulation 1994; 89:1545–1556.

Chapter 28

Coronary Balloon Angioplasty
Methods and Results

CHRISTOPHE BAUTERS
JEAN-MARC LaBLANCHE
MICHEL E. BERTRAND

Percutaneous transluminal coronary angioplasty (PTCA) was first introduced by Andreas Gruentzig and associates[1] in 1977 as an alternative form of myocardial revascularization for patients with coronary artery disease. During the early years of its application, PTCA was limited to patients with single proximal coronary artery disease, well-preserved left ventricular function, and stable angina refractory to medical treatment. Since then, PTCA has become a well-established technique for myocardial revascularization of patients with unstable angina,[2] patients with an evolving myocardial infarction,[3] patients with multivessel disease,[4] and patients with depressed left ventricular function.[5] An estimated 300,000 angioplasty procedures were performed in the United States in 1990, a more than 10-fold increase over the past decade.[6] Rapid improvement in technology and growing operator experience are responsible for the high rate of procedural success obtained in most institutions despite the increase in complexity of the dilated lesions. In this chapter, we review the current knowledge concerning the practice and the results of PTCA. The technology of PTCA, however, is constantly evolving, and its results and indications must be constantly updated.

CURRENT TECHNIQUE OF BALLOON ANGIOPLASTY

Elective PTCA is usually performed during a brief hospitalization; patients are admitted to the hospital the day before or the morning of the procedure and are discharged after 24 to 48 hours in the event of an uncomplicated procedure.

The only mandatory pretreatment for a PTCA procedure is antiplatelet therapy. Fracture of the stenotic lesion, medial disruption, and stretching of the external vessel diameter are necessary for a successful angioplasty[2]; endothelial denudation, platelet deposition, and mural thrombus formation occur immediately after injury and may lead to acute occlusion.[7] Antiplatelet therapy has been shown to reduce the incidence of acute thrombotic occlusion and periprocedural Q wave myocardial infarction in patients receiving full anticoagulation with heparin. Schwartz and associates[8] randomized patients to a pretreatment with aspirin, 330 mg/day, plus dipyridamole, 225 mg/day, versus placebo; patients receiving antiplatelet therapy had a significantly lower incidence of Q wave myocardial infarction than the patients in the placebo group (1.6% and 6.9%, respectively). A similar beneficial effect has been reported for ticlopidine.[9]

At the time of PTCA a guiding catheter is positioned at the ostium of the involved coronary artery, and systemic anticoagulation is achieved using 10,000 units of intravenous heparin. The activated clotting time can be monitored during the procedure and should be longer than 300 seconds to avoid thrombus formation. Baseline angiography of the target vessel is then performed in multiple projections after intracoronary injection of nitroglycerin; these pre-PTCA angiograms should provide a good visualization not only of the target lesion but also of the segments proximal and distal to the stenosis (Fig. 28–1A).

A guide wire is then passed across the steno-

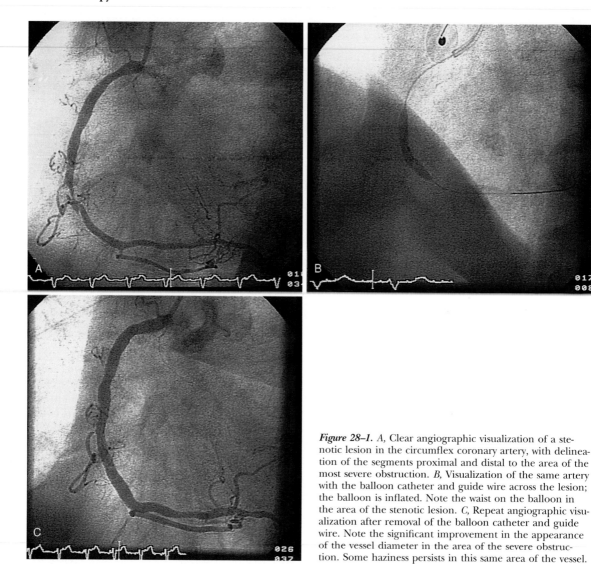

Figure 28–1. *A,* Clear angiographic visualization of a stenotic lesion in the circumflex coronary artery, with delineation of the segments proximal and distal to the area of the most severe obstruction. *B,* Visualization of the same artery with the balloon catheter and guide wire across the lesion; the balloon is inflated. Note the waist on the balloon in the area of the stenotic lesion. *C,* Repeat angiographic visualization after removal of the balloon catheter and guide wire. Note the significant improvement in the appearance of the vessel diameter in the area of the severe obstruction. Some haziness persists in this same area of the vessel.

sis and positioned in the distal segment of the vessel. Currently, available guide wires vary from 0.10 to 0.18 inches in diameter. Good torque control, radiographic visibility, and soft atraumatic tips allow these devices to be easily manipulated. The position of the guide wire in the coronary tree can be revealed by contrast medium injection through the guiding catheter. The deflated dilation catheter can then be advanced over the guide wire to the stenotic site. Improvements in technology have allowed the development of very-low-profile deflated dilation catheters that can be used to cross severe stenoses in tortuous and distal vessels. The size of the inflated balloon (between 2 and 4 mm) is chosen to approximate the normal "reference" segment adjacent to the stenosis. Oversizing the balloon may be responsible for a higher risk of vessel dissection that may lead to acute closure;

in a randomized trial involving 336 patients Roubin and colleagues[10] showed that oversizing the balloon by 13% relative to the adjacent reference segment led to 2.5 times the incidence of acute complications with the use of a balloon 7% undersized. The dilation balloon catheter is then inflated at the stenotic site (Fig. 28–1*B*); usual inflation pressures vary between 4 and 10 atm, but recent devices have the ability to tolerate pressures as high as 20 atm and can thus be used to dilate rigid stenoses. Adequate dilation is then confirmed using repeat angiography after intracoronary injection of nitroglycerin and in the same projections as before PTCA (Fig. 28–1*C*). Translesional gradient and measurements of flow velocity can also be useful in some circumstances to assess the functional result of the procedure (see later).

Immediately after PTCA, attention is directed to monitoring for evidence of recurrent ischemia and to ensuring appropriate hemostasis at the site of catheter insertion. Intravascular sheaths can be removed 3 to 6 hours after an uncomplicated procedure. Most patients can be safely discharged from the hospital within 24 to 48 hours after an uncomplicated PTCA. In low-risk patients, a prolonged (18 to 24-hour) intravenous infusion of heparin is not associated with a reduction in the risk of ischemic complication compared with control patients treated by placebo[11]; however, in high-risk patients such as patients with large dissection or intraluminal thrombus, a continuous infusion of heparin is often resumed for 24 to 48 hours.

After discharge, patients can typically return to work within 1 week. Despite a satisfactory primary result, the high risk of restenosis (30% to 60%) implies that the patients should be followed at least 6 months for evidence of recurrent ischemia.

HOW TO DEFINE A SUCCESSFUL PROCEDURE

Deciding that the result of the procedure is adequate and that, consequently, no further arterial damage should be risked in an attempt to improve the result is not always an easy task for the physician performing PTCA. Assessment of the result of a PTCA procedure is most often made using coronary angiography. A successful angioplasty procedure is defined as a 20% change in luminal diameter, with the final-diameter stenosis of less than 50% and without the occurrence of death or acute myocardial infarction or the need for emergency bypass operation during hospitalization.[6] An optimal angiographic result is also defined by the absence of angiographically visible intimal tear or dissection that is associated with a higher risk of subsequent acute closure.[12] Angiography should always be performed in multiple projections to obtain an adequate visualization of the dilated lesion(s).

The method used to determine the severity of a residual stenosis after PTCA is also an important determinant of the rate of angiographic success. Visual estimates of lesion severity are highly subjective; they tend to overestimate the preangioplastic stenosis and to underestimate the residual stenosis after angioplasty. In a study, we compared visual estimates of lesion severity performed by experienced interventional cardiologists versus computerized quantitative angiographic measurements of lesion severity in 305 patients before and after PTCA.[13]

Before PTCA the visual estimate of the mean percentage of stenosis severity, 81%, was significantly ($P<.001$) higher than the equivalent value, 73%, obtained with use of quantitative angiography; immediately after PTCA the visual estimate of the mean residual stenosis, 19%, was significantly ($P<.0001$) lower than the equivalent quantitative estimate, 37%; additionally, the residual stenosis was more frequently (18% vs. 3%) classified as significant (>50%) by quantitative angiography. Consequently, the primary success rate defined as a residual stenosis of less than 50% was significantly overestimated with visual assessment in comparison with quantitative angiography.

Similar findings have been observed in the Coronary Angioplasty Versus Excisional Atherectomy Trial (CAVEAT).[14] As visually estimated by site investigators, the success rate (the rate at which a reduction in stenosis to 50% or less was achieved) was 96.4% in both groups. By quantitative angiography, however, the primary success rate was only 89% in the patients treated by atherectomy and 80% in the patients who underwent balloon angioplasty. Similarly, the mean residual stenosis assessed visually by site was 15% after atherectomy and 20% after balloon angioplasty, but 29% and 36%, respectively, when assessed quantitatively by angiographic laboratory. It appears that the rate of primary success after balloon angioplasty is dependent not only on the definition of a successful procedure but also on the method used to analyze the angiographic result. Most of the recent studies analyzing the immediate or midterm angiographic outcome after PTCA used quantitative angiographic estimates of lesion severity.[14] In clinical practice, however, although on-line quantitative angiographic systems that allow immediate measurements of lesion severity are available, the estimation of the immediate outcome after PTCA is performed mostly by visual analysis and may consequently lead to a significant overestimation of the true success rate.

In addition to angiography, techniques that analyze the physiologic impact of the PTCA procedure may be useful in some circumstances. Before the advent of low-profile balloon catheters and large-lumen guiding catheters, adequate angiographic assessment of a PTCA result was sometimes difficult. Because of this limitation operators often assess their results using the translesional gradient. Fluid dynamic models suggest that the translesional gradients should be inversely proportionate to the diameter of stenosis and directly proportionate to the blood flow through the dilated lesion.[15] Although these measurements had some imperfections (such as artifacts because of high balloon:artery ratio), high translesional gradient has been associated with a higher risk of acute closure[12] or even restenosis[16] after PTCA.

Other functional measures of the PTCA results have also been explored. Investigations using Doppler coronary artery catheters to assess blood flow velocity and vasodilator reserve in proximal coronary arteries have provided inconsistent results, with some patients demonstrating an immediate return to normal hyperemic/baseline flow:reserve ratio and others showing little improvement or even a decrease in flow:reserve ratio.[17, 18] Recently, a 0.018-inch Doppler coronary artery flow guide wire has been validated in vitro and in vivo[19, 20] (see Chapter 6). The major advantage of this system in comparison with the older Doppler coronary catheter is that its small size allows a precise measurement of blood flow velocity variables distal to a significant coronary artery stenosis without depressing the peak velocity of blood flow in the sample volume.[19] Segal and coworkers[21] measured blood flow velocity, flow reserve, and diastolic:systolic velocity ratio both proximal and distal to the stenosis in patients undergoing PTCA. They demonstrated that proximal measurements were of limited usefulness to assess the results of PTCA; by contrast, the measurements performed distal to the stenosis showed a significant increase in mean time of average peak velocity after angioplasty and a normalization in the mean diastolic:systolic velocity ratio. These preliminary data suggest that distal measurements of flow velocity parameters may be of usefulness to assess the functional results of a PTCA procedure.

Finally, defining a successful procedure as a low-residual stenosis immediately after PTCA may be an oversimplification of the problem. PTCA induces a certain degree of injury of the vascular wall that in turn is responsible for a restenotic process leading to progressive renarrowing of the dilated site. This phenomenon, which occurs principally during the first few months after PTCA,[22, 23] leads to a significant (>50%) stenosis in 30% to 60% of the patients. The appreciation of the final result of a PTCA procedure should therefore be delayed for a few months; at this time, if there is no clinical or angiographic evidence of restenosis, the procedure can be considered to have been successful. It has been suggested that an important "acute gain" during PTCA (leading to a good immediate angiographic result) may be associated with an important amount of "late loss" during the follow-up period[24]; consequently, such patients may have restenosis despite an excellent initial result.

MAJOR COMPLICATIONS

The major complications of PTCA (need for emergency bypass surgery, myocardial infarction, and death) are mainly a consequence of acute coronary artery closure. In 1979, The National Heart, Lung, and Blood Institute established a PTCA registry to evaluate the safety and the results of the technique. The results of this first registry, including 3079 patients, were published in 1982: The primary success rate was 61%; 4.9% of the patients had a nonfatal myocardial infarction; 5.8% had emergency coronary artery bypass surgery; and the mortality rate was 1.2%.[25] In 1985, because of the technical advances and changes in indications, a new registry was opened. The results published in 1988 showed a significant increase in the procedural success rate (78%) and a decrease in the rates of myocardial infarction (4.3%) and emergency bypass surgery (3.4%). The mortality rate (1%) was unchanged.[26]

Predicting the Risk of Acute Closure

Abrupt vessel closure during PTCA occurs in 3% to 8% of procedures.[6] Although acute closure is occasionally caused by thrombus or spasm, its usual cause is coronary dissection.[27]

Coronary angiography provides the best procedural assessment of the risk of acute closure during or immediately after PTCA and allows for the identification of high-risk patients before the procedure. We have analyzed 3679 successive coronary angioplasty procedures performed in native coronary vessels in our institution between 1988 and 1991. Total occlusions before angioplasty were excluded. All the angiograms before and after angioplasty were analyzed using quantitative angiography by an independent observer. A qualitative assessment of the lesion was performed before angioplasty by the interventional cardiologist who performed the angioplasty. An analysis of the data showed that an acute closure occurred in 201 of the 3679 dilated sites (5.5%). Three factors were associated by multivariate analysis with the occurrence of an acute closure: (1) a severe stenosis by quantitative angiography ($P<.0001$); (2) the location in a bend that is 45 degrees or more ($P<.003$); and (3) the location in the left coronary artery ($P<.05$). Because in experimental preparations dissections have been found most often in areas containing thick, multiple atherosclerotic plaques,[28] it is not surprising that acute closure may be related to lesion severity that appears to correlate with the amount of atherosclerotic material at the site of balloon inflation. As previously suggested by Ellis and associates[29] and Savage and colleagues,[30] eccentric lesions were associated with the same rate of acute closure as concentric lesions. Other anatomic factors such as long lesions[31] or the presence of an angiographically visible thrombus before the procedure[12, 29] have also been associated with a high risk of acute closure. Thus, a careful analysis of the preangioplasty angiogram may allow for an estimation of the risk of a PTCA procedure. A cumulative effect of each risk factor has been demonstrated[32]; the risk of the procedure is increasing from less than 2% in the absence of risk factor to as high as 15% for four or more risk factors.

Predicting the Hemodynamic Risk

Distinct from predicting the risk of acute closure by analyzing the angiographic characteristics of the target lesion is the prediction of the risk of cardiovascular collapse and death if abrupt closure complicates PTCA. The hemodynamic risk of coronary angioplasty has been extensively studied.[33, 34] Certain variables have been shown to be useful in prospectively identifying patients at risk of hemodynamic complications if acute closure occurs during PTCA. An important determinant of the risk of PTCA is left ventricular function before the procedure. Park and associates[35] found that a preangioplasty ejection fraction was the most powerful predictor of death in 5413 patients undergoing PTCA. However, the hemodynamic risk of a procedure is not only determined by the level of ventricular dysfunction before the procedure but also by the amount of myocardium at risk during the procedure. A myocardial jeopardy score has been described in an attempt to quantify the amount of potentially ischemic myocardium during angioplasty.[34, 36] This score divides the coronary tree into six segments and takes into account not only the areas that are akinetic or hypokinetic at baseline but also those likely to become akinetic in the event of an abrupt closure. Ellis and colleagues,[36] using this scoring system, demonstrated that patients with a score of more than 2.5/6 had a 10% mortality rate in the event of an acute closure, whereas those with a score of less than 2.5/6 had a 2% mortality. Other clinical variables have been shown to influence the mortality in the event of an abrupt closure. They include advanced age[35] and female gender.[35, 36]

Management of an Acute Closure

In the event of acute closure, after a rapid evaluation of its hemodynamic consequence, the first step is to determine its cause. The most common causes of acute closure during a PTCA procedure are coronary dissection and formation of an intracoronary thrombus. When the angiographic appearance is conclusive for the cause of the occlusion (i.e., an evident dissection or intraluminal filling defect indicating a thrombus), a specific treatment can be discussed immediately. Frequently, the angiographic diagnosis of the cause is more problematic. Coronary dissection is much more common than thrombus formation except in patients with severe unstable angina (angina at rest with ischemic electrocardiographic changes during the episodes), where intracoronary thrombus is a common cause of acute occlusion.

When dissection appears to be the cause of abrupt vessel closure, recrossing the occluded segment and repeating balloon inflation can frequently re-establish coronary artery patency and relieve ischemia.[37] The management of abrupt closure has been improved with the advent of perfusion catheters,[38] which can be placed across the occluded segment to permit perfusion of the distal bed and redilation of the stenotic site simultaneously; these catheters allow long inflations (15 to 30 minutes) to be performed that may lead to angiographic success. In some circumstances, directional atherectomy may also be useful to treat an occlusive coronary dissection.[39] Preliminary results have shown that coronary stenting may be useful in the management of coronary dissection after PTCA.[40–42] Hearn and coworkers[42] demonstrated that 74% of the patients treated for acute closure by coronary stenting had a clinical success defined as a final diameter stenosis less than 50% without death, Q wave myocardial infarction, or bypass surgery.

After stent implantation the management of the patients requires a careful balance between adequate anticoagulation to prevent thrombosis and avoidance of bleeding complication. The incidence of angiographic restenosis within the stent appears higher in implantation for acute closure[42] than in elective implantation.[43] When thrombus appears to be the cause of abrupt closure, low doses of intracoronary urokinase (100,000 to 250,000 units) in combination with redilation of the occluded site may reopen the vessel.[44]

If early indication of successful reperfusion is not seen and more than a minor myocardial infarction is believed likely to ensue, the patient should undergo immediate surgery. Emergency coronary artery bypass grafting under these circumstances can be done effectively but with an operative mortality higher than that encountered in comparable patients managed with primary elective surgery.[45, 46]

MINOR COMPLICATIONS

Peripheral vascular complications (false aneurysms or bleeding) may occur but are less frequent with PTCA than with other techniques of endoluminal revascularization that imply either the use of a larger catheter (directional atherectomy) or the periprocedural use of heparin (coronary stenting). Other risk factors for peripheral complications include prolonged procedures, advanced age, and use of fibrinolytic agents.[47] Intracoronary embolization of atherosclerotic or thrombotic material is a rare event during coronary angioplasty, except when dilation is performed in the presence of a thrombus or when the site of angioplasty is a stenosis located in a diffusely diseased saphenous vein graft.[48] Guide wire embolization is very uncommon; when it occurs, the retained fragment can be removed using a bioptome or a snare loop technique.[49, 50] Rupture of a coronary artery during PTCA is also exceedingly rare; it has been related to guide wire perforation, inflation of the balloon in a subintimal location, or overexpansion of the coronary artery.[51, 52]

RESTENOSIS AFTER BALLOON ANGIOPLASTY

Restenosis that occurs in 30% to 60% of patients despite a successful procedure remains the major limitation of PTCA. Assuming that 300,000 PTCA procedures are performed each year in the United States,[6] more than 100,000 patients experience restenosis every year. Although some restenoses may be silent, most of these patients present stable or unstable symptoms, and a significant proportion need a new revascularization procedure. Decreasing the rate of restenosis would sharply lower the long-term cost of PTCA; in the United States, a reduction of the rate of restenosis from a hypothetical 33% to 25% might save as much as $300 million annually.[53]

Mechanisms

The exact mechanism responsible for the occurrence of restenosis after a successful balloon angioplasty is still unclear. It probably involves the combination of different factors: (1) elastic recoil[54] and remodeling of the vessel; (2) thrombus formation and incorporation into the vascular wall[55]; and (3) a response of the smooth muscle cells leading to intimal thickening.[56]

In experimental models, balloon denudation of a normal artery induces a series of events that ultimately lead to the formation of a neointima.[56] The platelets play a major initial role; they adhere and aggregate in large numbers and release vasoconstrictive factors (such as serotonin and thromboxane A_2) and growth factors (such as platelet-derived growth factors). After angioplasty and as a result of the activation by growth factors, vasoactive hormones, and mechanical stretch, a significant proportion of the smooth muscle cells of the media shift from a contractile to a synthetic phenotype.[57] Between 1 day and 2 weeks after the initial injury, the smooth muscle cells proliferate and migrate from the media to the intima. From 2 weeks to 3 months after injury the neointimal thickening increases further, mainly as a consequence of the synthesis of extracellular matrix components by the synthetic smooth muscle cells.

The response of the arterial wall after PTCA in humans has been studied by several investigators.[55, 58] These studies have shown that the restenotic lesion is characterized by synthetic smooth muscle cells in a loose extracellular matrix. Serruys and coworkers[22] and Nobuyoshi and associates[23] have shown that the restenotic process after coronary angioplasty in humans is occurring within the first 6 months after the procedure.

Definitions

Many different definitions of restenosis have been used, and there is still no consensus among interventional cardiologists about the best definition. As shown by Rensing and colleagues,[59] the restenotic process can be quantified as a continuous variable because the distribution of the loss in minimal luminal diameter from immediately after angioplasty to follow-up follows a near-gaussian distribution. Continuous measurements of the degree of luminal obstruction such as percentage of luminal diameter stenosis and minimal luminal diameter are therefore preferable for studies analyzing the impact of different interventions on the restenosis rate. The use of a continuous variable to measure restenosis has the advantage of reflecting the processes of interest whether or not an arbitrarily defined threshold of obstruction is reached and offers greater statistical power for detecting treatment effects in randomized clinical trials. However, in clinical practice, a binary definition of restenosis (yes/no) provides more relevant information to the interventional cardiologist. Various binary definitions of restenosis have been used in the literature; these different definitions may identify different patients as having or not having restenosis.[53] The most common binary definition of restenosis is the presence of a stenosis 50% or greater in diameter at follow-up angiography. This definition does not take into account the changes in luminal diameter from the postangioplasty angiogram to the follow-up angiogram; consequently, stenoses dilated with an "acceptable" immediate result (e.g., 45% residual stenosis) are more likely to be classified as restenosed at follow-up than stenoses dilated with an "excellent" immediate result (e.g., 20% residual stenosis).

The technique used for measuring the severity of the stenosis at follow-up is as important as the definition of restenosis. As indicated earlier, visual estimation may lead to a significant underestimation of residual stenosis after PTCA. The problem is the same for the assessment of the severity of the stenosis on the follow-up angiogram. Quantitative angiography systems enable more precise continuous measurements to be made. Most modern angioplasty laboratories now have on line quantitative angiography systems that allow the investigators to obtain the objective measurements of any stenosis during the procedure and may thus be useful for the decision-making process in conjunction with the clinical status of the patient and the results of functional tests.

Predictive Factors

Various factors have been associated with an increased likelihood of restenosis. However, although the combination of some of these factors may actually increase or decrease the probability of recurrence, the occurrence of a restenosis remains mainly an unpredictable event.

Diabetes mellitus appears to be an important risk factor for restenosis[60]; the increase in risk is particularly marked for diabetic patients receiving insulin.[61] Califf and coworkers,[53] in an analysis of the available information between 1984 and 1989, suggest a doubling of relative risk in diabetic patients compared with nondiabetic patients. Variable results have been reported concerning a possible relationship between serum cholesterol levels and restenosis. Some studies have suggested that a high serum

level of Lp(a) lipoprotein may increase the risk of restenosis.[62]

The clinical setting in which the angioplasty is performed may also affect the probability of restenosis. Patients with unstable angina (chest pain at rest with ischemic electrocardiographic changes within the episodes) have a much higher risk of restenosis than do stable patients. In patients with unstable angina undergoing multivessel angioplasty, the high propensity for restenosis appears to be confined to the culprit lesion, suggesting a role for local factors rather than for patient-related factors.[63] Similarly, patients with variant angina have a marked increase in the restenosis rate.[64]

Multiple lesion- and procedure-related factors have been implicated in the pathogenesis of restenosis. They include saphenous vein graft angioplasty, total occlusions before PTCA, bend location, presence of collateral vessels before angioplasty, stenosis length, ostial lesions, higher post-PTCA residual stenosis, inflation time and pressure, and a low balloon:artery ratio.

Detection of Restenosis

The "gold standard" for the detection of restenosis after PTCA remains coronary angiography. The classic primary end-point for clinical trials on restenosis is an angiographic end-point (minimal luminal diameter at follow-up, percentage of diameter stenosis at follow-up, and late loss in minimal luminal diameter from postangioplasty to follow-up). When angiography is performed to detect restenosis, the optimal time is 6 months after angioplasty, because it has been shown that the changes in luminal diameter are occurring mainly in the first few months after angioplasty.[22, 23]

In clinical practice noninvasive methods for detection of restenosis are widely used to select patients who should undergo angiographic follow-up. The ability of an exercise treadmill test to detect restenosis, however, may be limited by a low predictive value because of incomplete revascularization.[53] Exercise redistribution thallium 201 scintigraphy and tomographic thallium imaging have better positive and negative predictive values and may allow for the detection of the ischemic territory.[65]

Treatment of Restenosis

Symptomatic patients with restenosis need a repeat revascularization procedure. Although in some instances bypass surgery may be indicated, most of the patients undergo a second angioplasty procedure. The primary success rate of a repeat PTCA is higher than that of a first PTCA. This undoubtedly reflects in part the biased nature of the population in that such patients have already had a successful procedure at the target site but may also be the result of differences in the physical properties of restenotic compared with primary lesions. The rate of recurrent restenosis after a repeat PTCA appears similar to that observed after a first PTCA.[66, 67]

REFERENCES

1. Gruentzig A, Senning A, Siegenthaler WE: Nonoperative dilatation of coronary artery stenosis: Percutaneous transluminal coronary angioplasty. N Engl J Med 1979; 301:61.
2. de Feyter PJ, Serruys PW, Wijns W, van den Brand M: Emergency PTCA in unstable angina pectoris refractory to optimal medical treatment. N Engl J Med 1985; 313:342–346.
3. Grines CL, Browne KF, Marco J, et al: Comparison of immediate angioplasty with thrombolytic therapy for acute myocardial infarction. N Engl J Med 1993; 328:673–679.
4. Cowley MJ, Vetrovec GW, DiSciascio G, et al: Coronary angioplasty of multiple vessels: Short-term outcome and long-term results. Circulation 1985; 72:1314–1320.
5. Vogel RA: Elective supported angioplasty registry: Benefit of prophylactic cardiopulmonary bypass support in low ejection fraction [abstract]. Circulation 1992; 86(Suppl II):I-787.
6. Ryan TJ, Bauman WB, Kennedy JW, et al: Guidelines for percutaneous transluminal coronary angioplasty: A report of the American Heart Association/American College of Cardiology task force on assessment of diagnostic and therapeutic cardiovascular procedures (Committe on Percutaneous Transluminal Coronary Angioplasty). Circulation 1993; 88:2987–3007.
7. Steele PM, Chesebro JH, Stanson AW, et al: Ballon angioplasty: Natural history of the pathophysiological response to injury in a pig model. Circ Res 1985; 57:105–112.
8. Schwartz L, Bourassa MG, Lesperance J, et al: Aspirin and dipyridamole in the prevention of restenosis after percutaneous transluminal coronary angioplasty. N Engl J Med 1988; 318:1714–1719.
9. White CW, Chaitman B, Lassar TA, and the Ticlopidine Study Group: Antiplatelet agents are effective in reducing the immediate complications of PTCA: Results from the ticlopidine multicenter trial [abstract]. Circulation 1987; 76(Suppl IV):IV-400.
10. Roubin GS, Douglas JS, King SB, et al: Influence of balloon size on initial success, acute complications, and restenosis after percutaneous transluminal coronary angioplasty. Circulation 1988; 78:557–565.
11. Ellis SG, Roubin GS, Wilentz J, et al: Effect of 18 to 24 hours' heparin administration for prevention of restenosis after uncomplicated coronary angioplasty. Am Heart J 1989; 117:777–782.
12. Ellis SG, Roubin GS, King SB, et al: Angiographic and clinical predictors of acute closure after native vessel coronary angioplasty. Circulation 1988; 77:372–379.
13. Bertrand ME, Lablanche JM, Bauters C, et al: Discordant results of visual and quantitative estimates of stenosis severity before and after coronary angioplasty. Cathet Cardiovasc Diagn 1993; 28:1–6.
14. Topol EJ, Leya F, Pinkerton CA, et al: A comparison of

15. Klocke FJ: Measurements of coronary blood flow and degree of stenosis: Current clinical implications and continuing uncertainties. J Am Coll Cardiol 1983; 1:31–41.
16. Leimgruber PP, Roubin GS, Hollman J, et al: Restenosis after successful coronary angioplasty in patients with single-vessel disease. Circulation 1986; 73:710–717.
17. Serruys PW, Juilliere Y, Zijlstra F, et al: Coronary blood flow velocity during percutaneous transluminal coronary angioplasty as a guide for assessment of the functional result. Am J Cardiol 1988; 61:253–259.
18. Wilson RF, Johnson MR, Marcus ML, et al: The effect of coronary angioplasty on coronary flow reserve. Circulation 1988; 77:873–885.
19. Doucette JW, Corl PD, Payne HM, et al: Validation of a Doppler wire for intravascular measurements of coronary artery flow velocity. Circulation 1992; 85:1899–1911.
20. Vanyi J, Bowers T, Jarvis G, White CW: Can an intracoronary Doppler wire accurately measure changes in coronary blood flow velocity? Cathet Cardiovasc Diagn 1993; 29:240–246.
21. Segal J, Kern MJ, Scott NA, et al: Alterations of phasic coronary artery flow velocity in humans during percutaneous coronary angioplasty. J Am Coll Cardiol 1992; 20:276–286.
22. Serruys PW, Luijten HE, Beatt KJ, et al: Incidence of restenosis after successful coronary angioplasty—a time-related phenomenon: A quantitative angiographic study in 342 consecutive patients at 1, 2, 3, and 4 months. Circulation 1988; 77:361–371.
23. Nobuyoshi M, Kimura T, Nosaka H, et al: Restenosis after successful percutaneous transluminal coronary angioplasty: Serial angiographic follow-up of 229 patients. J Am Coll Cardiol 1988; 12:616–623.
24. Beatt K, Serruys PW, Luijten HE, et al: Restenosis after coronary angioplasty: The paradox of increased lumen diameter and restenosis. J Am Coll Cardiol 1992; 19:258–266.
25. Kent KM, Bentivoglio LG, Block PC, et al: Percutaneous transluminal coronary angioplasty: Report from the Registry of the National Heart, Lung and Blood Institute. Am J Cardiol 1982; 49:2011–2020.
26. Detre K, Holubkov R, Kelsey S, et al: Percutaneous transluminal coronary angioplasty in 1985–1986 and 1977–1981: The National Heart, Lung and Blood Institute Registry. N Engl J Med 1988; 318:265–270.
27. Hollman J, Gruentzig AR, Douglas JR, et al: Acute occlusion after percutaneous transluminal coronary angioplasty—a new approach. Circulation 1983; 68:725–732.
28. Zollikofer CL, Chain J, Salomonowitz E, et al: Percutaneous transluminal angioplasty of the aorta: Light and electron microscopic observations in normal and atherosclerotic rabbits. Radiology 1984; 151:355–363.
29. Ellis SG, Vandormael MG, Cowley MJ, et al: Coronary morphologic and clinical determinants of procedural outcome with angioplasty for multivessel disease: Implications for patient selection. Circulation 1990; 82:1193–1202.
30. Savage MP, Goldberg S, Hirshfeld JW, et al: Clinical and angiographic determinants of primary coronary angioplasty success. J Am Coll Cardiol 1991; 17:22–28.
31. Meier B, Gruentzig A, Hollman J, et al: Does length or eccentricity of coronary stenoses influence the outcome of transluminal dilatation? Circulation 1983; 67:497–499.
32. Ellis SG: Elective coronary angioplasty: Technique and complications. In Topol EJ (ed): Textbook of Interventional Cardiology. Philadelphia, WB Saunders, 1990, p 186–206.

directional atherectomy with coronary angioplasty in patients with coronary artery disease. N Engl J Med 1993; 329:221–227.

33. Bergelson BA, Jacobs AK, Cupples LA, et al: Prediction of risk for hemodynamic compromise during percutaneous coronary angioplasty. Am J Cardiol 1992; 70:1540–1545.

34. Califf RM, Phillips HR, Hindman MC, et al: Prognostic value of a coronary artery jeopardy score. J Am Coll Cardiol 1985; 5:1055–1063.

35. Park DD, Laramee LA, Teirstein P, et al: Major complications during PTCA: An analysis of 5413 cases [abstract]. J Am Coll Cardiol 1988; 11:237A.

36. Ellis SG, Roubin GS, King SB, et al: In-hospital cardiac mortality after acute closure after coronary angioplasty: Analysis of risk factors from 8207 procedures. J Am Coll Cardiol 1988; 11:211–216.

37. Marquis J, Schwartz L, Alridge H, et al: Acute coronary occlusion during percutaneous transluminal coronary angioplasty treated by redilatation of the occluded segment. J Am Coll Cardiol 1984; 4:1268–1271.

38. Sundram P, Harvey JR, Johnson RG, et al: Benefit of the perfusion catheter for emergency coronary artery grafting after failed percutaneous transluminal coronary angioplasty. Am J Cardiol 1989; 63:282–285.

39. Warner M, Chami Y, Johnson D, Crowley MJ: Directional coronary atherectomy for failed angioplasty due to occlusive coronary dissection. Cathet Cardiovasc Diagn 1991; 24:28–31.

40. Sigwart U, Urban P, Golf S, et al: Emergency stenting for acute occlusion after coronary balloon angioplasty. Circulation 1988; 78:1121–1127.

41. Roubin GS, Cannon AD, Agrawal SK, et al: Intracoronary stenting for acute and threatened closure complicating percutaneous transluminal coronary angioplasty. Circulation 1992; 85:916–927.

42. Hearn JA, King SB, Douglas JS, et al: Clinical and angiographic outcomes after coronary artery stenting for acute or threatened closure after percutaneous transluminal coronary angioplasty: Initial results with a balloon-expandable, stainless steel design. Circulation 1993; 88:2086–2096.

43. Serruys PW, Macaya C, de Jaegere P, et al: Interim analysis of the Bene stent trial [abstract]. Circulation 1993; 88(Part 2):I-594–I-590.

44. Cohen BM, Buchbinder M, Kozina J, et al: Rethrombosis during angioplasty in myocardial infarction and unstable syndromes: Efficacy of intracoronary urokinase and redilatation. Circulation 1988; 78(Suppl II):II-8–II-0.

45. Talley JD, Weintraub WS, Roubin GS, et al: Failed elective percutaneous transluminal coronary angioplasty requiring coronary artery bypass surgery: In-hospital and late clinical outcome at 5 years. Circulation 1990; 82:1203–1213.

46. Lazar HL, Faxon DP, Paone G, et al: Changing profiles of failed coronary angioplasty patients: Impact on surgical results. Ann Thorac Surg 1992; 53:269–273.

47. Muller DW, Shamir KJ, Ellis SG, Topol EJ: Peripheral vascular complications after conventional and complex percutaneous coronary intervention procedures. Am J Cardiol 1992; 69:63–68.

48. Saber RS, Edwards WD, Holmes DR, et al: Balloon angioplasty of aortocoronary saphenous vein bypass grafts: A histopathologic study of six grafts from five patients, with emphasis on restenosis and embolic complications. J Am Coll Cardiol 1988; 12:1501–1509.

49. Hartzler GO, Rutherford BD, McConahay DR: Retained percutaneous transluminal coronary angioplasty equipment components and their management. Am J Cardiol 1987; 60:1260–1264.

50. Watson LE: Snare-loop technique for removal of broken steerable PTCA wire. Cathet Cardiovasc Diagn 1987; 13:44–49.

51. Saffitz JE, Rose TE, Oaks JB, Roberts WC: Coronary arterial rupture during coronary angioplasty. Am J Cardiol 1983; 51:902–904.

52. Altman F, Yazdanfar S, Wertheimer J, et al: Cardiac tamponade following perforation of the left anterior descending coronary system during percutaneous transluminal coronary angioplasty: Successful treatment by pericardial drainage. Am Heart J 1986; 111:1196–1197.

53. Califf RM, Ohman EM, Frid DJ, et al: Restenosis: The clinical issues. In Topol EJ (ed): Textbook of Interventional Cardiology. Philadelphia, WB Saunders, 1990, pp 363–394.

54. Rensing BJ, Hermans WR, Strauss BH, Serruys PW: Regional differences in elastic recoil after percutaneous transluminal coronary angioplasty: A quantitative angiographic study. J Am Coll Cardiol 1991; 17:34B–38B.

55. Johnson DE, Hinohara T, Selmon MR, et al: Primary peripheral arterial stenoses and restenoses excised by transluminal atherectomy: A histopathologic study. J Am Coll Cardiol 1990; 15:419–425.

56. Liu MW, Roubin GS, King SB: Restenosis after coronary angioplasty: Potential biologic determinants and role of intimal hyperplasia. Circulation 1989; 79:1374–1387.

57. Thyberg J, Hedin U, Sjolund M, et al: Regulation of differentiated properties and proliferation of arterial smooth muscle cells. Arteriosclerosis 1990; 10:966–990.

58. Austin GE, Norman NB, Hollman J, et al: Intimal proliferation of smooth muscle cells as an explanation for recurrent coronary artery stenosis after percutaneous transluminal coronary angioplasty. J Am Coll Cardiol 1985; 6:369–375.

59. Rensing BJ, Hermans WRM, Deckers JW, et al: Lumen narrowing after percutaneous transluminal coronary balloon angioplasty follows a near-gaussian distribution: A quantitative angiographic study in 1,445 successfully dilated lesions. J Am Coll Cardiol 1992; 19:939–945.

60. Lambert M, Bonan R, Cote G, et al: Multiple coronary angioplasty: A model to discriminate systemic and procedural factors related to restenosis. J Am Coll Cardiol 1988; 12:310–314.

61. Margolis JR, Krieger R, Glemser E: Coronary angioplasty: Increased restenosis rate in insulin-dependent diabetics [abstract]. Circulation 1984; 70(Suppl II):II-175–II-170.

62. Desmarais RL, Ayers CR, Gimple LW, et al: Serum lipoprotein (a) levels as a risk factor for restenosis after coronary angioplasty [abstract]. Circulation 1993; 88 (Part 2):I-272–I-270.

63. de Groote P, Bauters C, Lablanche JM, et al: Coronary restenosis after double-vessel angioplasty in unstable angina [abstract]. Circulation 1991; 84(Suppl II):II-364–II-360.

64. Bertrand ME, Lablanche JM, Thieuleux FA, et al: Comparative results of percutaneous transluminal coronary angioplasty in patients with dynamic versus fixed coronary stenosis. J Am Coll Cardiol 1986; 8:504–508.

65. Lefkowitz CA, Ross BL, Schwartz L, et al: Superiority of tomographic thallium imaging for the detection of restenosis after percutaneous transluminal coronary angioplasty [abstract]. J Am Coll Cardiol 1988; 13:161A.

66. Bauters C, Lablanche JM, McFadden EP, et al: Clinical characteristics and angiographic follow-up of patients undergoing early or late repeat dilation for a first restenosis. J Am Coll Cardiol 1992; 20:845–848.

67. Bauters C, McFadden EP, Lablanche JM, et al: Restenosis rate after multiple percutaneous transluminal coronary angioplasty procedures at the same site: A quantitative angiographic study in consecutive patients undergoing a third angioplasty procedure for a second restenosis. Circulation 1993; 88:969–974.

Chapter 29

Coronary Plaque Ablation and Atherectomy
Methods and Results

MARK REISMAN
MAURICE BUCHBINDER
KIRK L. PETERSON

Percutaneous transluminal coronary angioplasty (PTCA) for treatment of flow-limiting coronary obstructions has evolved dramatically since its introduction in 1977. Improvements in balloon catheter and guide wire technology, coupled with an increased number of experienced interventional cardiologists, have led to higher success and lower complication rates. Despite these advances there remains a significant subset of lesions that, due to either morphology or location, are treated suboptimally with conventional balloon angioplasty. In addition, restenosis, the Achilles heel of percutaneous revascularization, continues to diminish the long-term effectiveness of these procedures. These limitations have provided the impetus for alternative transcatheter technologies that are aimed at plaque removal. High-speed rotational ablation, using the Rotablator system, and directional atherectomy, using the Simpson Athero-Cath (SCA) catheter, constitute the most extensively investigated and applied devices for plaque removal. This chapter aims to review the salient characteristics of these devices and their initial application in humans within the coronary arterial tree.

THE ROTABLATOR SYSTEM

The Rotablator system (Fig. 29–1) was invented by David Auth, PhD, and is manufactured by Heart Technology, Inc. (Redmond, WA). The components of the system include a nickel-plated, brass, elliptical burr (Fig. 29–2) that is coated with diamond microchips extending 20 to 30 μ from the leading surface. The burrs used in coronary applications are sized between 1.25 and 2.25 mm, in increments of 0.25 mm, with the exception of the 2.15-mm burr that was added before the development of large 9-French guiding catheters. The burr is welded to and driven by a long flexible, helical drive shaft. The burr and its continuation of the drive shaft have a 0.010-inch diameter core for the passage of the 0.009-inch guide wire.

The drive shaft is housed in a 4.3-French flexible Teflon sheath. The sheath protects the arterial tissue from potential injury caused by the spinning shaft and provides a conduit for normal saline to lubricate and cool the system. During rotation approximately 7 to 13 mL/min of saline are delivered to the distal end of the sheath.

The drive shaft is connected to the advancer unit that permits the independent advancement of the burr from the sheath by means of an advancer knob. The knob allows easy advancement and withdrawal of the burr from the lesion. The system is powered by compressed air or nitrogen. A turbine within the advancer spins the burr and the flexible drive shaft. It is designed with minimal rotational mass so that it can be started and stopped abruptly.

An operations console controls the gas turbine and therefore rotational speed of the burr (Fig. 29–3) with a foot pedal. Depressing the foot pedal initiates rotation of the burr and activates the brake in the advancer, preventing

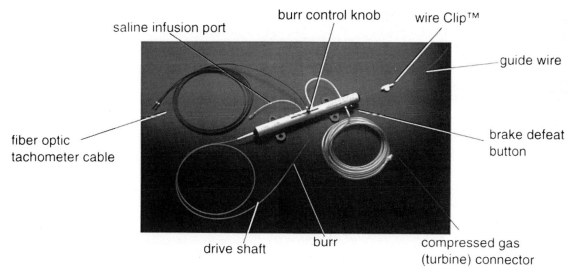

Figure 29–1. Components of the Rotablator system, disconnected from the operator's console.

the coaxial guide wire from spinning while the burr is rotating. The revolutions per minute (rpm) are measured with a fiberoptic light probe (tachometer) and are displayed on the console. The console also indicates the elapsed treatment time. During treatments, the device is generally activated between 160,000 and 180,000 rpm, depending on the burr size selected. In addition to the normal therapeutic speed of the turbine, a controlled, low-speed rotation of the burr (at 60,000 to 90,000 rpm) is possible using the Dynaglide mode. The Dynaglide mode is used during the intraprocedural exchange of Rotablator catheters.

The guide wire is a 0.009-inch diameter stainless steel monofilament that is soldered to a distal tip. The radiopaque platinum tip is 3.7 cm (type C) or 2.7 cm (type A), with the diameter of its distal end increasing to 0.017 inch. The central core continues into the platinum

tip of the stiff type A wire and it is therefore more like a conventional PTCA standard wire. The type C wire more closely resembles the conventional "floppy" guide wire systems. The burr is passed over the guide wire to a site just proximal to the lesion. The distal platinum tip of the guide wire must be advanced beyond the lesion site because the burr cannot pass over the larger-sized segment. A wireClip is attached to the proximal end of the guide wire to prevent it from spinning when the brake defeat is activated during withdrawal of the burr (during the exchange procedure). The wireClip has a dual purpose—it is also used as a torquing device.

The guiding catheter through which the guide wire and burr are advanced must possess an inner diameter that is 0.004 inch greater than the burr to provide clearance and facilitate advancement and withdrawal of the device. With currently available guiding catheters, the

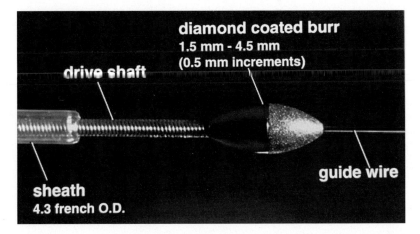

Figure 29–2. Distal end of Rotablator catheter, with the guide wire positioned through central diameter core.

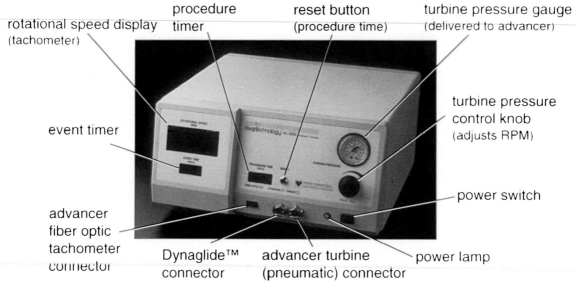

Figure 29–3. Operator's console for the Rotablator system.

1.25- to 2.0-mm burrs can be accommodated with an 8-French, 2.15- to 2.25-mm burrs with a 9-French, and 2.50-mm burrs with a 10-French guiding catheter.

Mechanism of Action

The two physical principles that enable the Rotablator system to effectively treat coronary artery lesions are differential cutting and orthogonal displacement of friction.

Differential Cutting

Differential cutting is defined as the ability to selectively cut one material while sparing and maintaining the integrity of another based on differences in substrate composition (Fig. 29–4). High-speed rotational ablation is a method of mechanical removal of plaque by cleaving small divots of material away from the substrate. The Rotablator system, using high-speed rotation with an abrasive element, removes or ablates inelastic components of the artery by pulverizing them into microparticulate matter while sparing elastic components from injury as they are deflected away from the device. Hard, calcific tissue is unable to deflect and is therefore cut as microfractures are generated at the intense point-pressure zone of the tissue. Lipid-rich tissue deposits, although soft, are inelastic and therefore are ablated. This principle is easily demonstrated by passing a knife gently across one's own skin and then fingernail. The fingernail will exhibit fine, pulverized debris fragments in front of the knife blade, whereas the skin sample will dive out of the way of the advancing edge and no cutting will occur. An-

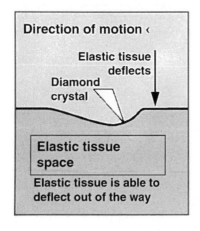

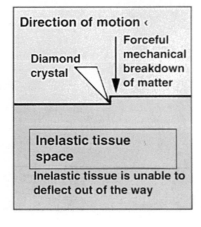

Figure 29–4. Principle of differential cutting.

other example is a razor that cuts whiskers but spares the elastic skin that deflects away from the advancing razor edge.

Orthogonal Displacement of Friction

The principle of orthogonal displacement of friction allows the easy passage of the burr through tortuous and diseased segments of the coronary tree. Friction normally occurs between sliding surfaces in contact and opposes the relative motion between them. The principle of orthogonal displacement of friction refers to the reduction of the effective friction in the direction of the artery by a relative motion in a plane perpendicular (or orthogonal) to that direction. The principle is exemplified by the removal of a cork from a bottle of wine. If the cork is twisted as it is pulled, the frictional force that opposes the cork's removal is spent resisting the twisting motion and the cork comes out much easier. The faster the cork is turned, the more easily it is withdrawn. In addition to providing movement through coronary arteries, this principle is useful in the exchange over the guide wire of one burr size for another. At a speed greater than 60,000 rpm, the longitudinal friction vector is virtually eliminated (reduced surface drag), and unimpeded advancement and withdrawal of the device are permitted.

Early Investigations

Initial investigations of the Rotablator system were performed (1) to define the effect of high-speed rotation of an abrasive element on the vascular integrity of normal and abnormal tissue; (2) to assess the impact of microparticulate debris on myocardium subtended by the vessel and determine the fate of these particles; (3) to assess the presence and relevance of microcavitations; and (4) to quantify the degree of luminal enlargement conferred by various burr sizes.

Effect on the Vessel Wall

One of the earliest studies of the effect of the Rotablator system on arteries was performed on 13 New Zealand white rabbits that were fed high-cholesterol diets for 2 weeks before undergoing iliac artery balloon denudation.[1] At 10 weeks, contrast angiography revealed greater than 60% arterial narrowing in the injured segments. These sites were then treated with the Rotablator system with the speed of rotation maintained at 150,000 rpm. After treatment, 11 of the 13 arteries showed angiographic increase in minimal luminal diameter, with an overall

significant improvement in percent diameter stenosis from 81.9% to 38.22% (mean, $P<.001$, paired t-test). Histologic sections demonstrated smooth-walled, patent lumina, with nearly total absence of endothelium, and various portions of the atheromatous intima missing. The internal elastic laminae were disrupted in some specimens, but medial injury was generally absent. When medial damage was present, it was evidenced by loss of the innermost (luminal) layer of smooth muscle cells. Intimal splits and medial dissections were not seen.

Ahn and associates[2] performed initial experiments on 68 cadaver arteries with atheromatous lesions involving the superficial femoral, popliteal, and tibial arteries. The specimens were studied angioscopically during treatment and with scanning electron and light microscopy after treatment. The histologic specimens revealed smooth, highly polished intraluminal surfaces denuded of intimal and endothelial cells. Verhoeff-van Gieson stains for elastin revealed occasional disruption of the internal elastic fibers but intact outer elastic fibers of the media and adventitial layers. No intimal dissections were observed.

Hansen and colleagues[3] validated the results just discussed with high-speed ablation of 11 normal canine coronary arteries. Postmortem examination revealed extensive intimal loss in treated segments, with superficial medial damage (never exceeding 40% of the total medial thickening) and a loss of 20% to 30% of the internal elastic membrane. No perforations were observed.

Finally, Fourrier and coworkers[4] used the Rotablator system on femoral arteries before the patient underwent femoral to popliteal artery bypass. The results were consistent with prior studies demonstrating removal of fibrous and calcified atherosclerotic plaque. The abraded surfaces were smooth and, importantly, free of thrombus. No arterial medial damage was noted after removal of the endothelium of adjacent walls. There was absence of dehiscence between plaque and media and only some surface irregularities were seen in areas where the Rotablator system was used at rotational speeds of less than 75,000 rpm.

The advent of intravascular ultrasonography and its recent refinement have provided an additional window into the lumen of arterial segments. Mintz and coworkers[5] analyzed images of 11 patients who were treated with the Rotablator system and subsequently evaluated with intravascular ultrasonography. Four patients demonstrated fissures, one had a dissection, and none had arterial expansion (defined as the area within the external elastic membrane at the angioplasty site greater than that of the proximal reference segment). Using three-dimensional reconstructions of cross-sectional images, smooth, tubular lumina were observed, especially in areas of the most dense calcium.

Potkin and associates[6] assessed the outcome of calcified versus noncalcified lesions treated with the Rotablator system and noted no evidence of dissections or arterial expansion in either group. In the calcified group, fewer than half of the patients had fissures, whereas the noncalcified group had no sign of fissures.

A study by Kovach and colleagues[7] examined 18 patients with calcified vessels and analyzed lumen and plaque cross-sectional areas using three-dimensional reconstruction of intravascular ultrasound images. Areas treated with high-speed rotational ablation had a significant increase in luminal diameter based on a decrease in cross-sectional plaque area. No evidence of vessel expansion was demonstrated, implying that ablation, not mechanical dilation or "dottering," is the mechanism by which larger lumina are obtained.

Finally, a recent investigation by Berkalp and coworkers[8] used intravascular ultrasonography to determine the effect of interventional devices on luminal shape and surface features. Results demonstrated the production of significantly different plaque surfaces and luminal shapes after treatment with PTCA, rotational ablation, and directional atherectomy. Vessel lumina were characterized as smooth and circular after rotational ablation, irregular in shape with flaps after directional atherectomy, and as having an increased incidence of deep dissections after PTCA.

One of the concerns in using high-speed rotational ablation is the impact of the procedure on sites proximal and distal to the treated segment. Quantitative coronary angiography (QCA) at 24-hour and 3- to 6-month follow-up revealed no changes in luminal dimensions at these sites after treatment, thus implying that accelerated atherosclerosis in adjacent "nondiseased" segments does not occur after burr rotation.[9]

Microparticulate Debris

The sharp, multifaceted diamond crystals rotating at high speed produce predictably sized particles as long as appropriate technique is applied. Microparticulate size is determined not only by the abrasive surface of the burr but also by the speed and pressure of the advancing cutting edge. Gentle, forward pressure applied

to the catheter minimizes the degree of penetration of the diamond "plows" and therefore will yield microparticles. This eliminates the need for an aspiration or collection apparatus. Figure 29–5 is a photomicrograph of the particles produced by the action of the Rotablator system, which are small enough to readily pass through the capillary system. Adjacent to the particles are normal human red blood cells measuring approximately 7 μ in diameter. A 5-μ calibration sphere is included in the figure for measurement reference. The larger particle masses that are seen are actually aggregates of smaller particles held together by surface tension and that easily break apart with gentle agitation.

The fate of the particles produced by the Rotablator system has been a major concern since initial investigations. In vitro studies using rabbit aorta segments of 3 to 5 cm in length were performed in which the vessels were treated with the Rotablator while undergoing continuous saline perfusion.[1] Macroscopic analysis revealed no large-sized particulate debris. Further examination by Coulter analysis with a fluorescence-activated cell sorter analyzer revealed that 1.5% to 2% of the particles were larger than 10 μ, whereas the average particle size was smaller than 5 μ. Prevosti and associates[10] demonstrated similar findings when using the Rotablator procedure on human atherosclerotic iliac arteries. Seventy-seven percent of the particles generated were smaller than 5 μ and 88% were smaller than 12 μ, with an average of 10^6 microparticles per milliliter.

To assess in vivo effects, particulate debris (human) was injected into the left circumflex artery of three dogs, and analysis of myocardial blood flow was performed using radiolabeled microspheres.[10] In two dogs there was no detectable change in myocardial blood flow after a 32-mL injection of noncalcified particulate debris. However, one dog was subjected to large boluses of 42 mL and 96 mL of heavily calcified debris, which reduced myocardial blood flow by 50% and 100% of control values, respectively. These quantities are approximately 10 to 30 times the volume produced from human coronary lesions. Particulate debris was further investigated by subjecting human cadaveric lower extremity vessels to high-speed rotational ablation and labeling the effluent with technetium 99m.[2] These radiolabeled particles were then injected into the common femoral artery of five dogs and scanned by nuclear scintigraphy. The study demonstrated that a few particles lodged harmlessly in the lower extremities, whereas most passed through the circulation and were cleared by the liver, lung, and spleen.

Microparticles

Particles smaller than red blood cells

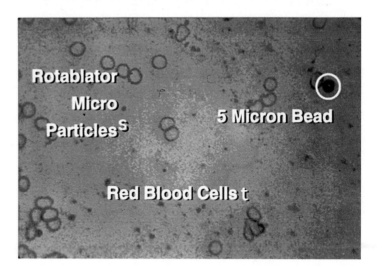

Figure 29–5. Photomicrograph of particles generated by the Rotablator. Note the comparison of their size with a 5-μ bead and red blood cells.

Friedman and coworkers[11] did a similar experiment by performing high-speed rotational ablation on human cadaveric coronary arteries. Debris was collected and injected into the left anterior descending artery of dogs. There were no significant changes in heart rate, left ventricular end-diastolic pressure, systolic blood pressure, coronary blood flow, or coronary flow reserve. Regional myocardial function was minimally reduced for 30 minutes after injection of the debris and complete recovery by 60 minutes was observed. Pathologic sections of the canine hearts had evidence of limited areas of necrotic myofibers of single cells and clusters of three or four cells. Further human clinical assessment of the effects of microparticles produced after rotational ablation was investigated using positron emission tomography.[12] Myocardial perfusion was evaluated in nine patients using ^{13}N ammonia. In all patients there was no evidence of procedure-related infarction by electrocardiography, creatinine phosphokinase (CPK) elevation, or clinical event. In two patients where myocardial perfusion was normal by positron emission tomography on polar maps, there was no significant change after therapy. In seven patients with impaired baseline myocardial perfusion, the perfusion improved after treatment. Concomitant left ventricular function was analyzed using echocardiography. Four patients had normal function that was unchanged after the procedure, and of five patients with hypokinesis, four demonstrated no change and one had improvement.

Finally, Pavlides and colleagues[13] studied 17 patients undergoing rotational ablation with electrocardiography, hemodynamic monitoring, and simultaneous transesophageal echocardiography. The results showed that the hemodynamic parameters and global left ventricular function remained unchanged during rotational ablation. Regional wall motion function in the distribution of the target coronary artery (assessed by wall motion score) was also shown to be unaffected during treatment.

In summary, these investigational studies suggest that the possible damage produced by the distal embolization of microparticles has not been realized. Extrapolation of these findings to the clinical setting would suggest that plaque ablation using the Rotablator system results in reliably small to moderate amounts of distal embolization of debris and should be accompanied by minimal effects on the myocardium subtended by the vessel.

Microcavitations

High-speed rotational ablation may cause the production of microcavitations, or bubbles. The mean pressure in blood is approximately 20 kPa and the atmospheric pressure is 100 kPa. To produce cavitations under these conditions, rotational speed of the Rotablator must exceed 14.7 m/sec. A 2-mm burr rotating at 160,000 rpm achieves a rotational speed of 16.7 m/sec, thus meeting the conditions necessary for microcavitation formation. In vitro experimentation to study bubble size after high-speed rotational ablation in fresh whole blood by Zotz and associates[14] measured a mean bubble size of 90 ± 33 μ. The bubble dimensions are large when compared with the 7-μ mean size of red blood cells. The collapse time of these cavitation bubbles was calculated to be very short, in the range of 10 seconds.

In the same investigation, Zotz and associates[14] also studied the in vivo production of microcavitations. Transthoracic and transesophageal echocardiograms were obtained before and after treatment from nine patients treated with the Rotablator system, with treatment intervals lasting 10 seconds, interrupted by 1 to 2 minutes of recovery. With the onset of high-speed rotational ablation, transient enhancement of echo contrast occurred in the area of myocardium supplied by the treated artery that disappeared immediately after burr rotation was stopped. It is unlikely that the myocardial contrast enhancement was the result of debris, because the opacification was transient and occurred before advancement of the device. No decrease in regional ejection fraction during or after rotational ablation occurred in any of the nine patients.

The impact of microcavitations on angiographic and clinical outcomes remains unclear. To date there is no evidence of deleterious effects. However, further studies evaluating their role may have relevant implications on the speed, burr sizing, and technique of using the Rotablator.

Efficiency of Ablation

The efficiency of debulking with the Rotablator system has been investigated using QCA. An early study using QCA on 109 patients in the Rotablator multicenter registry demonstrated that a predictable minimal luminal diameter can be achieved across the spectrum of burr sizes (ranging from 1.75 to 2.25 mm). Expressing this minimal luminal diameter as a burr ratio (defined as minimal luminal diameter/burr size), the immediate results are 0.72 ± 0.19 mm of the burr used (i.e., a 2-mm burr predicted a minimal luminal diameter of approximately 1.4 mm). When these lesion sites were then measured at 24-hour follow-up, the burr ratio increased to 0.84 ± 0.15 mm.

Safian and colleagues[15] performed a similar analysis of the efficiency of the Rotablator as well as the relationship of the burr size to the artery. Despite the fact that the burr was generally undersized for the artery (burr to artery ratio = 0.59), it was effective in achieving a

lumen close to the selected device size (0.9). This ratio was higher than that seen with other devices in the comparison (Fig. 29–6).

The increase in luminal diameter at 24 hours was confirmed by Reisman and associates[16] in an investigation on 186 patients. QCA was performed before, immediately after, and 24 hours after rotational ablation. There was no evidence of early partial reclosure at 24 hours (i.e., recoil) and, in fact, a gain in luminal dimensions was observed. This "late" gain is based on the relief of vasospasm, possibly also to increased flow through the vessel, and was noted irrespective of whether adjunctive balloon dilation was performed (Figs. 29–7 and 29–8).

Mintz and colleagues,[17] using intravascular ultrasonography, found that when the minimal lumen diameter was divided by the largest burr used, the ratio range was 0.93 to 1.45 (1.19 ± 0.19) for stand-alone procedures and 1.02 to 1.56 (1.30 ± 0.15, $P = $ NS) for Rotablator plus adjunct balloon angioplasty. Therefore, there appears, at least in this study, to be a trend toward a larger lumen than that expected from the size of the largest burr used. This was true regardless of the amount of calcium present and whether adjunctive balloon angioplasty was used. One possible explanation is that once the calcium is ablated, the vessel becomes "unbound," or released. An alternative explanation is that the orientation of the guide wire is responsible; that is, nonaxial ablation occurs, causing greater cross-sectional area ablation than the size of the device.

Clinical Results

One of the first reports on use of the Rotablator in the coronary circulation concerned an investigation conducted on 12 patients with focal discrete stenosis.[18] Ten of the 12 patients had a successful outcome with the minimal luminal diameter increased significantly from 0.72 ± 0.05 mm to 1.4 ± 0.3 mm ($P<.01$) after treatment. There were two failures secondary to inability to cross the lesion with the Rotablator guide wire. Of the 10 patients treated, five required adjunctive balloon angioplasty to improve the lumen to less than 30% residual stenosis. This was primarily the result of using small burrs (1.5 mm), the only size available in this preliminary trial. There were no major complications. One patient died several days after the procedure from a noncardiac-related event. Analysis of the treated left anterior descending artery lesion using scanning electron microscopy revealed a smooth segment with

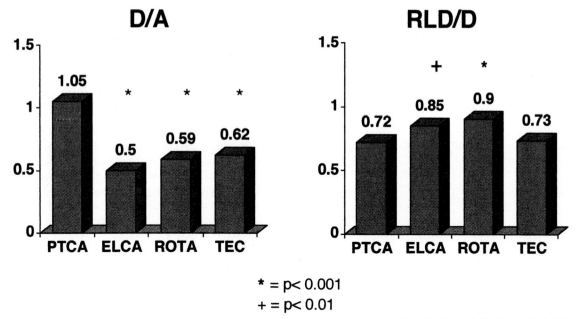

Figure 29–6. Comparison of ratio of size of device to size of artery (D/A) and residual lumen diameter/device ratio for percutaneous transluminal coronary (balloon) angioplasty (PTCA), excimer laser angioplasty (ELCA), rotablator (ROTA), and transluminal extraction atherectomy (TEC). (Data from Safian RD, Freed M, Lichtenberg A, et al: Are residual stenoses after excimer laser angioplasty and coronary atherectomy due to inefficient or small devices? Comparison with balloon angioplasty. J Am Coll Cardiol 1993; 22:1628–1634.)

thin furrows. There was no evidence of platelet deposition. Three of the patients who had right coronary artery lesions had transient (5- to 10-second) atrioventricular block, a problem now recognized to occur frequently when using the Rotablator in right coronary arteries or when lesions are located in left dominant circumflex arteries.

Based on encouraging early data, Teirstein and associates[19] evaluated the use of the Rotablator on lesions regarded as suboptimal for balloon angioplasty. Most patients in this study had lesions greater than 10 mm (71%), with a mean lesion length of 31 mm. Twenty-one percent were restenotic, and 10% were ostial lesions. The protocol considered adjunctive balloon angioplasty after rotational ablation a failure of therapy, a significantly different approach than is presently practiced.

Teirstein and associates[19] found that the Rotablator was capable of significant debulking in most lesions. The overall minimal luminal diameter increased from 0.77 to 1.51 mm, and mean stenosis was reduced from 80.6% to 36.7%. Of 10 procedural failures, four resulted from an inability to cross the lesion with the guide wire. One patient with a recent myocardial infarction had abrupt closure secondary to thrombotic occlusion. Four patients underwent

adjunctive PTCA—three for residual stenosis of greater than 50% and one for incessant vasospasm. In addition, a total of eight patients (19%) had CPK elevations greater than 200 U/L with greater than 2.2% CPK-MB. Of these eight patients, four had transient wall motion abnormalities that returned to baseline on follow-up left ventriculography. Angiographic follow-up (mean follow-up 6.2 ± 2.6 months) was obtained in 29 of the 32 patients treated (91%), with an overall restenosis rate of 59%.

Several limitations should be noted from this early experience. The first is the lack of adjunctive PTCA required in larger vessels not included in this protocol. In addition, procedural modifications have been implemented since the time of this study, including slow, gentle burr advancement based on minimizing drops in rpm and a gradual increase in burr sizes for complex lesions.

Multicenter Registry

The expansion of the Rotablator procedure as a multicenter investigation began in 1988 and included 18 centers. Initially, enrollment was reserved for those patients whose anatomy was suboptimal for standard balloon angioplasty. Also treated were patients who had previously

Table 29–1. **Demographics and Diagnoses of Patients in the Multicenter Rotablator Registry**

Variable	Number or Percentage
Demographics	
Number of procedures	2736
Number of lesions	3424
Males	71%
Females	29%
Average age	63.2 (range 30–87) yr
Diagnoses (Some Patients in More Than One Category)	
Multivessel disease	66%
Stable angina	43%
Unstable angina	43%

been treated with balloon angioplasty and, because of restenosis or failure to achieve an adequate result, were referred for Rotablator therapy. A broad spectrum of lesions was approached, a significant number of which were eccentric, calcified, and greater than 10 mm; a few were the less formidable type A and B_1 lesions.[20] As data accrued with favorable results and investigator experience with the device increased, intervention in more complex lesions was carried out, including total and subtotal chronic occlusions. Patients with acute myocardial infarction were excluded, as were patients with postinfarction angina because, mechanically, thrombus would be an inadequate substrate for the device. Also excluded were saphenous bypass grafts, lesions longer than 25 mm, and patients with ejection fractions less than 30%.

As of January 1993, the multicenter Rotablator registry included a total of 2499 patients involving 3424 lesions. Most subjects were males, with a mean age of 63 years (Table 29–1). The clinical antecedents consisted of a majority of patients with stable angina and multivessel disease with slightly less than half having had unstable angina. The lesions were predominantly located in the left anterior descending artery, followed by the right coronary and circumflex arteries (Fig. 29–9). Lesion morphology included 49% calcified, 69% eccentric, 28% bifurcated, and 66% de novo lesions, including those that had failed prior PTCA (Fig. 29–10). The lesions were focal in 76% of the cases, with 24% between 11 and 25 mm.

The procedural success rate was 85% with

the Rotablator system alone and increased to 95% with adjunctive balloon angioplasty. Figure 29–11 demonstrates the angiographic appearance of diffuse atherosclerotic disease in the left anterior descending coronary artery before and after rotational ablation. When assessing outcome based on complex lesion morphology, there were no significant differences compared with those lesions with more favorable characteristics (Fig. 29–12). Significant angiographic complications included a 0.7% perforation rate, 4% persistent occlusion, 13.7% dissections, and 1.1% closure after the procedure (Table 29–2). Major clinical complications included 1.1% myocardial infarction, 2.5% coronary artery bypass graft (CABG) surgery, and 1% death (Table 29–3). A further complication included CPK elevation in 5.8% of the patients. The restenosis rate was 50% in the 57% of the total population who underwent angiographic follow-up.

Recent Investigations

Several single-center and multicenter experiences have been published (Table 29–4). The data indicate the heterogeneity of results obtained with the Rotablator. This is partially due to the inconsistency in definitions of outcomes between centers, although operator experience, the approach toward burr sizing, and at what point during the evolution of technique the data were generated and collected may be responsible for the wide range.

A recent clinical trial conducted by Vandormael and colleagues[25] (Excimer Laser Angioplasty, Rotational Atherectomy, and Balloon Angioplasty for Complex Lesions [ERBAC] randomized study) compared immediate and 6-month outcomes of rotational atherectomy, excimer laser angioplasty (ELCA), and balloon angioplasty (PTCA) in patients with de novo type B or C lesions. Overall procedural success (<50% residual stenosis without death, Q wave myocardial infarction, or CABG) was attained in 91% of patients undergoing rotational ablation versus 80% with PTCA and 76% with ELCA. The rate of major complications at 2.3% was significantly lower in the rotational atherectomy group (vs. 6.2% and 4.8% in the ELCA and PTCA groups, respectively). Finally, the restenosis rate for rotational ablation of 55.6% was comparable with the 51.4% restenosis rate for

Figure 29–7. Quantitative coronary angiographic measurements of proximal reference, minimal luminal, and distal reference diameters before and immediately after rotational ablation, and at 24 hours after the procedure. Note the significant increase in the size of the artery at 24 hours.

Stand Alone High Speed Rotational Ablation
N = 94 patients

	Diagnostic				Immediately Post-Burr				24 Hours Follow-up			
	MEAN	±SD	Max	Min	MEAN	±SD	Max	Min	MEAN	±SD	Max	Min
Proximal Diameter	2.52	0.60	4.35	1.40	2.49	0.64	4.28	1.16	2.72	0.66	4.74	1.54
Minimum Diameter	0.74	0.27	1.62	0.24	1.42	0.32	2.93	0.55	1.72	0.35	2.79	0.97
Distal Diameter	2.31	0.52	3.77	1.28	2.24	0.51	3.57	1.23	2.50	0.53	4.06	1.53

* = p < 0.001 vs. Diagnostic and Post-Burr

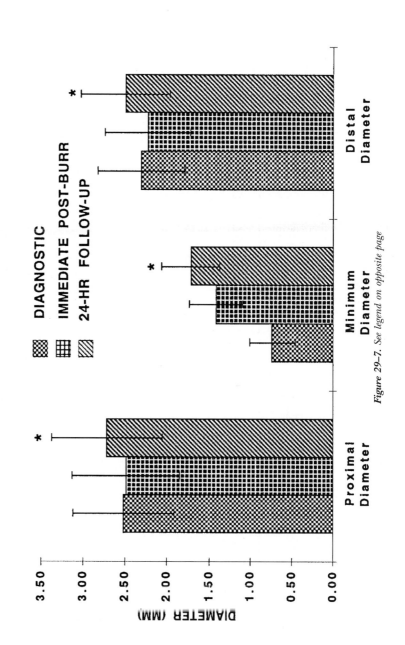

Figure 29-7. See legend on opposite page

Rotational Ablation with Adjunctive PTCA
N = 92 patients

	Diagnostic				Immediately Post-Burr/Balloon				24 Hours Follow-up			
	MEAN	±SD	Max	Min	MEAN	±SD	Max	Min	MEAN	±SD	Max	Min
Proximal Diameter	2.52	0.60	4.35	1.40	2.49	0.64	4.28	1.16	2.72	0.66	4.74	1.54
Minimum Diameter	0.74	0.27	1.62	0.24	1.42	0.32	2.93	0.55	1.72	0.35	2.79	0.97
Distal Diameter	2.31	0.52	3.77	1.28	2.24	0.51	3.57	1.23	2.50	0.53	4.06	1.53

* = p < 0.001 vs. Diagnostic and Post-Burr

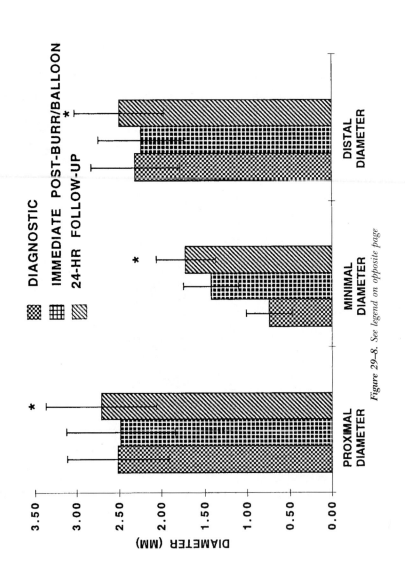

Figure 29–8. See legend on opposite page

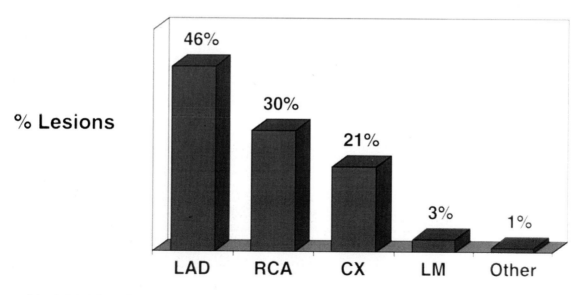

N=3424 Lesions

Figure 29–9. Anatomic location of lesions treated by rotational ablation in the Multicenter Registry of Heart Technology, Inc. LAD, left anterior descending; RCA, right coronary artery; CX, circumflex coronary artery or its branches; LM, left main coronary artery.

PTCA and lower than the 61.3% restenosis rate of ELCA.

Procedure

Preprocedural Management

The preparation before the performance of high-speed rotational ablation is similar to that for PTCA, but it differs in several important aspects: It is essential that the patient is well hydrated at the start of the procedure to ensure an appropriate arterial blood pressure. An adequate arterial pressure permits the use of generous amounts of intravenous nitroglycerin and is critical for diastolic coronary blood flow for clearance of microparticles. In most patients, a pulmonary artery catheter is not required. However, in high-risk patients such as those with compromised left ventricular function or frank congestive heart failure, and in patients where the treated artery subtends a large area of myocardium, continuous measurements of left ventricular end-diastolic pressure is warranted. Such monitoring may indicate compromised left ventricular function due to distal particulate matter prior to changes in arterial blood pres-

sure and indirectly correlate with the advent of subsequent slow or no flow if further ablation is performed with larger burrs.

Preprocedural Medication

In addition to sufficient hydration, premedication includes aspirin, 325 mg orally, and oral calcium channel blockers. Some operators administer verapamil or diltiazem directly into the coronary artery at the time of the procedure. Calcium channel blockers rather than β-blockers are recommended for several reasons. First, and foremost, calcium channel blockers may reduce the incidence of vasospasm, which occurs in approximately 15% of patients. β-Blockers have been controversial in patients undergoing rotational ablation. Although not systematically analyzed, many investigators believe that they are deleterious, possibly causing an increased propensity for vasospasm. Another consideration is that β-blockers have a negative inotropic effect and may decrease contractility, with a possible reduction in particulate clearance. Therefore, the current recommendation is to discontinue β-blockers and begin calcium channel blockers before the procedure.

Figure 29–8. Quantitative coronary angiographic measurements of proximal reference, minimal luminal, and distal reference diameters before and immediately after rotational ablation and adjunctive balloon dilation, and at 24 hours after the procedure. Note the significant increase in the size of the artery at 24 hours.

Lesion Characteristics

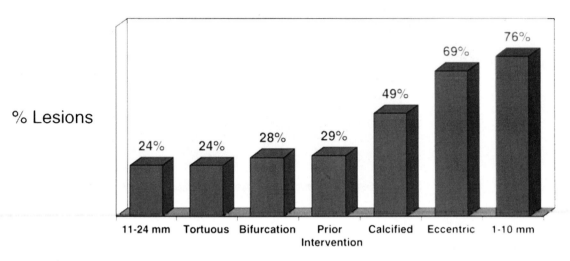

% Lesions

| 24% | 24% | 28% | 29% | 49% | 69% | 76% |

11-24 mm Tortuous Bifurcation Prior Intervention Calcified Eccentric 1-10 mm

N=3424 Lesions

Note: Some patients fell into more than one category

Figure 29–10. Characteristics of lesions treated by rotational ablation in the Multicenter Registry of Heart Technology, Inc.

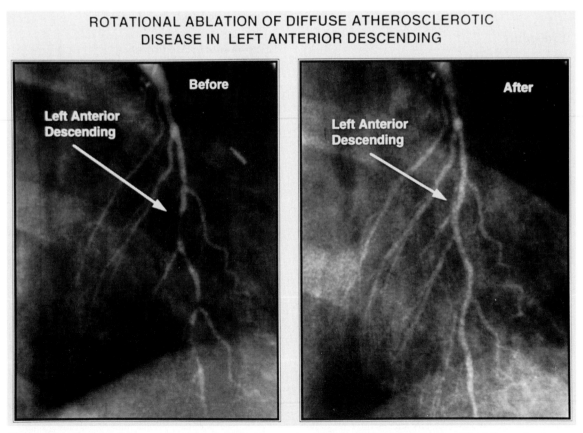

ROTATIONAL ABLATION OF DIFFUSE ATHEROSCLEROTIC DISEASE IN LEFT ANTERIOR DESCENDING

Figure 29–11. Example of the use of rotational ablation in a patient with complex, diffuse disease of the left anterior descending coronary artery.

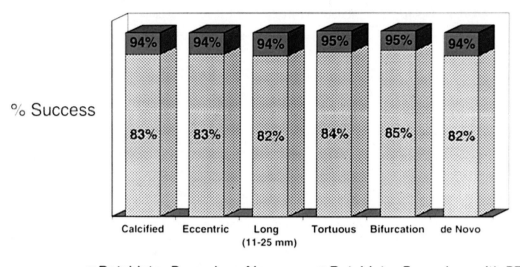

Figure 29–12. Percentage of cases with primary procedural success, according to preprocedure classification of lesion type.

Sedation is a concern during rotational atherectomy because patients often have chest pain immediately after the procedure. The particular pharmacologic regimen used varies among operators and catheterization laboratories. One regimen that has been successful is premedication with diazepam and diphenhydramine followed by intraprocedural sedation with morphine and fentanyl in 25-µg increments (up to a total of 125 µg).

Temporary Pacemaker

The high incidence of bradyarrhythmias and heart block during high-speed rotational ablation warrants the insertion of a temporary pacemaker catheter. Such problems occur most frequently during treatment of the right coronary,

dominant circumflex, and ostial left anterior descending arteries. In addition, it appears that patients treated with larger burrs (2.5 mm) are more prone to bradycardia. The slowing of heart rate usually occurs immediately after activation of the device, and, in most instances, returns to baseline rate shortly after the ablation is completed. The mechanism of this disturbance is unclear. Several theories have been advanced, including microcavitation or microparticulate embolization to conduction sensitive tissue, guide wire vibration, or a yet to be described reflex. The onset of atrioventricular block has also been seen during activation of the device in the guiding catheter.

Intraprocedural Medication

The intraprocedural medication regimen for the Rotablator system procedure consists of anticoagulation similar to that used with conven-

Table 29–2. **Complications Recognized by Angiography**

Complication	Rate (%)
Perforation	0.7
Abrupt closure in laboratory	
Transient (spasm)	1.1
Persistent (occlusion)	4.0
Abrupt closure after procedure	1.1
No flow	0.5
Flap/dissection	13.7
Thrombosis	1.6

N = 2736 procedures; some patients fit into more than one category.

Table 29–3. **Clinical Complications of Rotational Ablation**

Complication	Rate (%)
Death	1.0
Q wave myocardial infarction	1.1
CK-MB elevation	5.8
Coronary artery bypass graft surgery	2.5
Restenosis	50*

*57% rate of angiographic follow-up.

Table 29–4. Single-center Reports Versus Multicenter Registry on Use of Rotablator System

	Teirstein et al, 1991[19] (%) (n = 42)	Stertzer et al, 1993[21] (%) (n = 242)	Safian et al, 1993[22] (%) (n = 104)	MCR, 1994[23, 24] (%) (n = 2736)
Procedure success	76	94	75	95
Residual stenosis	37	—	30	31
Complications				
Q wave MI	0.0	2.5	4.8	1.1
NQ wave MI	19.0	11.0	2.9	5.8
CABG	2.0	0.8	1.9	2.5
Death	2.0	0.0	1.0	1.0
Restenosis	59	37.0	51.0	50.0

MI, myocardial infarction; NQ, non Q; CABG, coronary artery bypass graft surgery; MCR, multicenter registry.

tional angioplasty. There is generally a need for aggressive therapy with vasodilators and the need for analgesics.

Anticoagulation is generally achieved with 10,000 units of intravenous heparin followed by small boluses to maintain the activated clotting time longer than 350 seconds.

Although the frequency of severe vasospasm seems to be decreasing with recent modifications of technique, use of generous amounts of intravenous vasodilators during the procedure continues to be advocated. The most common technique is to give a small intracoronary bolus after each ablation run. The typical dose of nitroglycerin is 100 to 150 μg, although several smaller doses may accomplish the same effect with a less significant impact on systemic hemodynamics. The combination of maintained coronary blood flow with adequate diastolic pressure and vasodilation will yield the optimal result. In addition to nitroglycerin, verapamil and diltiazem are being tested for their ability to treat vasospasm. The effectiveness of these therapeutic measures relies on delivery to the treated segment and may be limited by decreased blood flow. Therefore, in instances of severe vasospasm, subselective distal injection through a balloon or transfer catheter may enhance the effect of the various vasodilators and may reduce the quantities required.

Although the use of vasopressors during Rotablator procedures is infrequent, they should be available and the catheterization laboratory personnel acquainted with their administration and dosages. Vasopressors such as dopamine should be easily accessible and administered in patients with hemodynamic compromise. In addition, some laboratories have phenylephrine, metaraminol, and epinephrine available.

The use of analgesics, on the other hand, is common during the procedure. Shortly after the ablation some patients have moderate to severe chest discomfort that requires attention.

The combination of diazepam with medications such as morphine and fentanyl has provided effective levels of patient comfort.

Rotablator Technique

The Rotablator technique has undergone several refinements since its earliest applications and continues to evolve as operators gain experience and results are reviewed.

The emphasis when selecting a guiding catheter for Rotablator procedures focuses primarily on coaxial alignment and secondarily on support. The guides for the left and right coronary arteries are chosen based on the inner luminal diameter necessary to accommodate the largest burr size predicted to be used. The curves are similar to those used in conventional angioplasty.

The coaxial position of the guiding catheter permits the tension applied to the guide wire to be transmitted along its length. This translates into smooth tracking of the device into the vessel. Failure of the burr to exit the guiding catheter despite significant tension on the guide wire is most commonly caused by improper alignment of the guide. For example, if the guiding catheter is intubated into the ostium but is not coaxial, it may be difficult to advance the device.

Once the appropriate burr has been selected, loaded onto the guide wire, and advanced just proximal to the Y connector, the device is tested outside the body. The speed should be set 10,000 to 20,000 rpm higher than that desired to treat the lesion. This higher speed accommodates for the friction that develops between the guide wire and drive shaft as a result of curves in the guiding catheter and tortuosity in the coronary arteries.

The burr is then advanced just proximal to the lesion into the "platforming segment" of the vessel. In this segment contrast should flow easily around the burr, indicating that the device is not in contact with the arterial wall. Prior to activation of the burr, all the forward tension or compression accumulated from advancing the device must be neutralized. This is accomplished by slightly pulling back the drive shaft. The release of tension can be verified by loosening the advancer knob and feeling no resistance when moving or "jiggling" the knob. If tension remains in the drive shaft, activation of the device will cause the burr to lurch forward, possibly resulting in a torsional dissection.

At this point, the burr is activated in the platforming segment and the "platform speed" (i.e., the speed proximal to the lesion) is adjusted based on burr size. Because larger burrs have a higher surface velocity than smaller burrs at the same rpm level, they are set at lower ablation speeds. The platform speed is 180,000 rpm for 1.25- to 2.0-mm burrs and 160,000 rpm for 2.15- to 2.5-mm burrs (Fig. 29–13).

The most recent and important modification to technique has focused on the gentle and careful advancement of the burr through the lesion based on rpm surveillance. The rotational speed should be maintained within 5000 rpm

of the platform speed. Aggressive forward pressure on the tissue, indicated by excessive drops in speed, could cause significant heat generation and deep tissue invagination by the diamond cutting surfaces. This could in turn result in damage to the vessel wall and formation of large particulate debris. In addition to monitoring the rotational speed, contrast agents should be injected intermittently to provide visual assessment during burr advancement. These injections identify the borders of the lesion, the cutting orientation of the device in tortuous segments, and the burr-to-artery relationship. If no egress of contrast agent is noted, the burr should be withdrawn proximally every 10 to 15 seconds to reestablish antegrade flow and particle clearance during the ablation. The contrast agent injections may also provide a secondary benefit by inducing a hyperemic environment.

Optimal ablation time is based on the integration of lesion morphology, distal runoff, and, most importantly, the clinical parameters of hemodynamics and patient discomfort. In general, 15 to 30 seconds per ablation run is recommended, with an interval between runs to allow for particle clearance, administration of vasodilators, and stabilization of hemodynamics. Sev-

High-Speed Rotary Sander

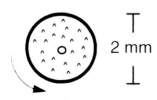

2 mm

Circumference ~ 6 mm

- at 180,000 rpm
  = 3000 rps

- 1,080,000 mm/min
  = 18 m/sec
  ~ 60 ft/sec
  ~ 45 mph

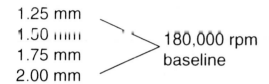

1.25 mm
1.50 mm
1.75 mm
2.00 mm
> 180,000 rpm
baseline

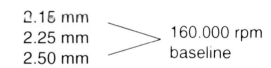

2.15 mm
2.25 mm
2.50 mm
> 160.000 rpm
baseline

Δ Decrement ≤ 5,000 RPM

Set baseline in normal segment 5-10 mm proximal to lesion being treated.

Figure 29–13. Guidelines for platform speed of rotational ablation, according to burr size. See text for details.

eral such runs may be performed until the lesion is completely treated. The final pass should be associated with minimal tactile resistance and no drop in rpm.

The final burr size is based on the operator's strategy for treatment. One strategy currently practiced treats arterial stenosis with small, undersized burrs, usually maintaining a burr-to-artery ratio of less than 0.6, followed by systematic balloon angioplasty. This method employs the concept of minimal debulking in which arterial compliance is increased and the lesion is thereby made more amenable to conventional balloon angioplasty. Often only a single burr is required. The second strategy incorporates the concept of maximal safe debulking, attempting to achieve a 0.70 to 0.85 burr-to-artery ratio and performing adjunctive balloon angioplasty only as necessary. This technique almost always requires the use of multiple burrs (frequently two) to successfully deploy large burr sizes. Adjunctive balloon angioplasty in this setting is often applied to relieve vasospasm and improve residual stenosis. With this strategy, application of oversized balloons at the lowest possible pressure is advocated in the hope that this will reduce the effects of barotrauma on the vessel wall.

Postprocedural Management

Postprocedural management includes the use of nitroglycerin (which is usually administered if hemodynamically tolerated after the first ablation) and fluids (normal saline) to maintain adequate hydration. The pacemaker is removed unless bradyarrhythmias persist after therapy, which occurs rarely.

It is not infrequent that, despite a coronary angiogram demonstrating an excellent result with thrombolysis in myocardial infarction (TIMI) grade 3 flow and patency of all arterial branches, the patient has persistent chest pain and electrocardiographic abnormalities, including ST elevation or depression. The general pattern is that the pain diminishes and is relieved within the first 20 minutes after the procedure, as normalization of the ST-T wave segments occurs. It is important to obtain a baseline for the intensity of pain to assess for later possible worsening of symptoms.

It is recommended that the patient be monitored in a telemetry setting overnight. In addition to nitroglycerin and fluids, medications consist of aspirin and calcium channel blockers. Intravascular sheaths are maintained overnight, but based on the angiographic result, this can be left to the discretion of the operator.

The issue of anticoagulation is controversial. In uncomplicated cases, heparin overnight is usually adequate. If there is evidence of dissection or thrombus, 48 to 72 hours of heparinization may be beneficial, and in patients with excessively long lesions or total occlusions, 72 hours should be considered.

Indications

One of the motivating factors that prompted investigation into the development of alternative devices included a desire to broaden the indications of percutaneous therapy. The Rotablator system addresses some of the limitations inherent to balloon dilation.

The broad range of lesion types treated as well as the high success and low complication rates reflects the versatility of the Rotablator system. Since the registry enrolled patients based on the discretion of the investigator (a nonrandomized approach), certain lesions have become the signature of the Rotablator system.

Recent data from New Approaches to Coronary Intervention (NACI) investigators show that, when assessing usage patterns of the various devices (including directional atherectomy, laser stents, and the transluminal extraction catheter), the Rotablator system was preferentially chosen for patient subsets consisting of eccentric, calcified lesions in vessels with small reference diameters.[26] The subsets discussed in the following sections have become the "signature" lesions of the Rotablator system.

Calcified Lesions

Lesions with fluoroscopically identified calcium comprise more than 50% of the Rotablator system multicenter registry. This percentage probably underestimates the number of these lesions because intravascular ultrasonography has demonstrated that a significant percentage of calcified lesions are not appreciated with conventional angiography.

Calcified lesions represent a subset in which the Rotablator system is optimally suited and other percutaneous methods have notable limitations. The ablation of calcified plaque creates a more compliant vessel and, therefore, mitigates the need for high-pressure balloon inflation if adjunctive balloon angioplasty is required. The high rate of success (>95%) and the low rates of complication (death 1.1%, CABG 2.0%, Q wave myocardial infarction 1.1%, and non–Q wave myocardial infarction 4.9%) reflect the suitability of rotational ablation as the treatment of choice for these lesions.

Sixty-seven patients from the multicenter registry had failed PTCA secondary to the inability to dilate their lesions despite inflation pressures exceeding 12 atm. After high-speed rotational ablation of these lesions the vessels became significantly more compliant, thus allowing adjunctive balloon angioplasty (at pressures less than 6 atm) to be performed in 80% of the cases. Successful results were achieved in 98% of the patients with less than 10 atm of pressure. An 82% angiographic follow-up demonstrated a restenosis rate of 36%.[32]

Calcified lesions can produce large amounts of microparticulate debris during ablation. Therefore, the lesion, the distal vessel, and myocardial function must be critically assessed before treatment. If the distal vascular bed is small and the lesion is heavily calcified, or moderately calcified with complex margins, the burr should be undersized with short (15-second) ablation runs. Stepping to a larger burr is based on angiographic appearance as well as coronary flow and hemodynamics. Severe chest discomfort may indicate inadequate particle clearance and should improve before stepping to a larger burr.

Ostial Lesions

Ostial lesions have always been difficult to treat with PTCA; this is reflected in a lower success rate and higher complication rate. Although the Rotablator system has been used in a limited number of these cases, there appear to be advantages with regard to positioning the device in true ostial lesions, the limited time the vessel is obstructed (as opposed to sometimes long inflations with PTCA), and removal of the typically fibrocalcific elements. The ostium is a site often considered for device synergy with directional atherectomy (Fig. 29–14).

Long Lesions

The procedural success in long lesions has undergone moderate improvement with the advent of lower profile balloons and the use of long balloons (> 20 mm), although with a restenosis rate exceeding 50%.[27] Orthogonal displacement of friction allows advancement of the Rotablator through the often tortuous and diffusely diseased segments. The treatment of diffuse lesions, especially when the distal bed has limited capacity, warrants special attention to avoid excessive plaque burden. This problem has been ameliorated with judicious selection of smaller burrs using a step approach and ablating the lesion in segments.

An investigation by Reisman and coworkers[28] examined long lesions treated with rotational ablation. Lesions were grouped according to lesion length (1 to 10 mm, 11 to 15 mm, and 15 to 25 mm). Procedural success ranged from 83% to 86% for stand-alone rotational ablation among the three groups and 92% to 97% for rotational ablation followed by PTCA. Complications among the three groups were low (Q wave myocardial infarction, 0% to 2.8%; CABG, 1.1% to 2.6%; and death, 0.6% to 2.1%). Overall rates of restenosis at angiographic follow-up ranged from 46% to 57%.

Chronic Total Occlusions

The percutaneous management of chronic total occlusions with balloon angioplasty has been reported in retrospective studies to have an overall success of approximately 60% with outcome predicated on operator experience, shorter occlusion duration, tapered morphology, and absence of bridging collaterals.[29] Whether these limitations can be extrapolated to the present Rotablator system is only speculative, although the small number of patients treated with high-speed rotational ablation indicates that the only constraint would be the ability to cross the lesion with a guide wire.

The advantage of the Rotablator system, in contrast with the requirements of conventional angioplasty and some other second-generation devices, is that it needs only to be proximal to the lesion rather than positioned in the segment. One concern when treating total occlusions with a collateral bed is the microparticle outflow with competing collateral flow. Although not systematically studied, there does not appear to be an increase in procedural or clinical complications.

Undilatable Lesions

The most complex spectrum of lesions is the subgroup that was not suitable for balloon angioplasty. In the National Heart, Lung, and Blood Institute Percutaneous Transluminal Coronary Angioplasty Registry, balloon angioplasty was unsuccessful, as defined by an inability to reduce the stenosis diameter greater than or equal to 20%, in 353 (12.2%) of 2892 lesions.[30] Sixty-five percent of these procedural failures were due to inability to position the balloon at the lesion, and 35% of the failures resulted from inability to adequately dilate the lesion. Kahn and associates[31] reported a higher overall success rate of 96%, although nearly 50% of the

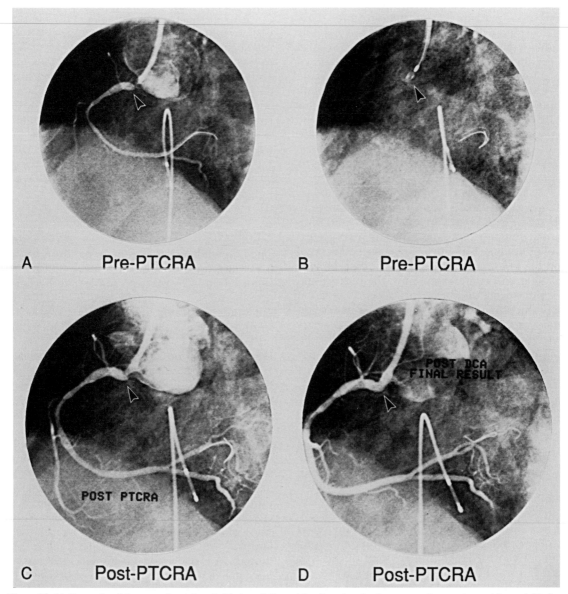

Figure 29–14. Example of the use of rotational ablation, followed by directional atherectomy in a patient with a calcified, tight stenosis at the ostium of the right coronary artery. PTCRA, percutaneous transluminal coronary rotational ablation; DCA, directional coronary atherectomy.

failures in this series were due to ineffective balloon dilation, despite appropriate positioning of the balloon at the lesion site. A more recent study, using the Rotablator, by Reisman and colleagues[32] reported an overall procedural success rate of 96% and a low incidence of complications (0% Q wave myocardial infarction, 1.5% CABG, and 0% deaths). The most prominent reasons for unsuccessful balloon angioplasty from a morphologic standpoint are lesions that are heavily calcified and cannot be dilated and eccentric lesions that have a contralateral wall that has normal vascu-

lar integrity, and therefore, yields more to dilation than the diseased wall. The latter is probably the mechanism for elastic recoil, a result of restitution of tone of the overexpanded normal segment. Also included are lesions that are unable to be crossed over with balloon catheters despite the most recent innovations in low-profile balloons. Approximately 10% of the lesions treated in the Rotablator multicenter registry have failed prior attempts with PTCA for one of these reasons. The high success and low complication rates sufficiently demonstrate a role for high-speed rotational ablation in these lesions.

Management of Complications

The application of high-speed rotational ablation may be associated with complications specific to this device and infrequently seen with balloon angioplasty. The operator and the entire catheterization staff should have a thorough understanding of these complications so that appropriate management can expedited. They include (1) vasospasm, (2) slow flow postablation, (3) dissection, (4) side branch occlusion, (5) hypotension, (6) bradycardia, and (7) thrombus.

Vasospasm

Coronary vasospasm is a frequent event following high-speed rotational ablation, and in most cases diffusely affects the vessel. The mechanism is unclear, and there does not seem to be a greater predilection for one vessel. Because the precise incidence is unknown and resolution almost uniform, it is difficult to determine the impact of changes in technique. Anecdotally, it appears that running the larger burrs at slower speeds and not permitting the drop in rpm to exceed 5000 has translated into fewer cases of severe, unremitting vasospasm.

The primary treatment is intracoronary nitroglycerin given in moderate doses (150 to 300 μg). Intracoronary calcium channel blockers are additional measures that have recently been used. These bolus injections over a 2- to 3-minute period are usually effective in breaking mild to moderate spasm. In the more recalcitrant cases of severe spasm, an alternative route of drug delivery is via a balloon catheter or any end-hole subselective device (i.e., transfer catheter) to administer the vasodilator directly to the site. The predominant calcium channel blockers in use include verapamil and diltiazem.

If the vasospasm is unresponsive to medical intervention either because of a refractory vessel or the hemodynamics not supportive for use of a vasodilator, the use of PTCA is effective in "mechanically" breaking the spasm. The method is to place a slightly oversized balloon and perform low-pressure inflations (<2 atm).

The continuation of high-speed ablation with larger burrs is acceptable (as opposed to after slow flow) after a significant bout of severe spasm relieved with vasodilators. If low-pressure balloon inflations were required to relieve the spasm, close inspection of the vessel is required to ensure no dissections have been created that would compromise further use of the Rotablator system.

Slow Flow

Slow flow and the more profound no reflow represent the most challenging adverse sequelae observed in approximately 5% of patients undergoing treatment with the Rotablator system. Slow flow is a diminution of flow by 1 or 2 TIMI grades from the baseline antegrade flow. *No flow* is defined as the cessation of flow into the distal coronary circulation of the treated vessel. The latter is appreciated angiographically by a contrast dye column with a back-and-forth movement, usually at or near the lesion site, but not infrequently proximal or distal to this segment. The possible mechanisms include an overwhelming amount of plaque burden, microparticulate aggregation, vasospasm, compromised myocardial contraction in the subtended vessel, and inadequate perfusion pressure. Slow flow and no reflow probably reflect a combination of these factors with one or more playing a predominant role. A retrospective analysis of a subgroup of patients from the multicenter registry correlated the treatment of long de novo lesions, long ablation times, and compromised myocardium in the subtended arterial zone to an increased incidence of slow flow.[33]

It is important to recognize slow and no reflow to separate them from abrupt closure because the latter angiographic complication has different treatments. An example is that cessation of flow due to abrupt closure from a severe dissection or flap would be treated with prolonged balloon inflations or deployment of an intravascular stent. The use of prolonged balloon inflations in the setting of slow flow (a nonstructural complication) would not improve the situation and instead would probably accelerate a worsening clinical picture. Vasospasm is sometimes difficult to differentiate from no reflow when severe. The difference is that coronary vasospasm typically responds to nitroglycerin. Also, if a balloon is deployed to mechanically break the spasms, the vessel (after treatment) will regain baseline flow characteristics.

Slow flow and no reflow are managed in a similar fashion, with the latter usually having a more deleterious hemodynamic impact and therefore more urgently requiring an intervention. The event is usually noted after retraction of the burr after a treatment. Once observed, no further ablation should be performed until the situation is resolved. The goal is to reduce the ischemic time interval. Initial steps include maintaining adequate perfusion pressure, either with aggressive hydration or vasopressors.

Intracoronary nitroglycerin should be vigorously administered as tolerated either through the guiding catheter or an end-hole subselective catheter. Other vasodilators such as verapamil have been used, but no one agent has demonstrated advantages over another. The use of high-pressure "blood" perfusion is also believed to be an asset in these situations. Blood perfusion is performed by withdrawing blood slowly from the side holes of the guiding catheter into the manifold syringe and forcefully reinfecting the blood through the guiding catheter. The rationale is that high-pressure injections accelerate particle clearance and increase perfusion to the myocardium ("poor man's" intra-aortic balloon pump). Adjunctive balloon angioplasty has also been shown to be beneficial in these situations. It is performed by choosing a balloon size that at low pressure will permit safe dilation in the distal coronary vessel. This can relieve any concomitant vasospasm and the balloon directed into the distal vessel may serve as a plunger to improve flow. If the patient does not respond adequately, there should be no hesitancy to place an intra-aortic balloon pump, because this frequently not only attends to the hemodynamics, but the augmented diastolic pressure benefits the coronary blood flow and clearance of microparticles.

In summary, the management of slow flow or no reflow requires the integration of several techniques. How aggressive the operator needs to be with either pharmacologic or mechanical intervention is typically mandated by the severity of the clinical parameters. Because slow flow and no reflow tend to worsen with time (a vicious cycle of low pressure causing further reduction in coronary flow), it is important to anticipate the possible deterioration and expedite the therapy as quickly as possible.

Once flow has been re-established the electrocardiogram often begins to normalize but generally does not return to the baseline pattern. The patient's chest pain begins to improve but usually requires time for complete resolution. Whether a CPK elevation occurs is usually dependent on the severity of the flow disturbance, that is, minimal slow flow to complete no reflow, and the amount of time that lapsed before its restoration.

Dissection

Angiographically visible dissections occur in approximately 15% of patients treated with the Rotablator system. There are several mechanisms that have been implicated in Rotablator-induced dissections. When using appropriate burr sizing in a step procedure, occasionally a dissection is seen that does not stain or compromise distal flow with the initial undersized device. Much debate has evolved over whether this represents an "underdone" result with the burr in which the surface of the plaque has been unroofed and the irregularity is the exposed inner aspects of the lesion, as seen in a splintered piece of wood. This may be consistent with results found by Mintz and coworkers[17] where 12 of 28 patients (43%) had fissures or dissections. When the dissections were noted with intravascular ultrasonography, they were typically superficial, located within an arc of calcified plaque, and had limited axial and circumferential extension. The management of this type of dissection ranges from the use of a larger burr to deployment of an oversized balloon at low pressures to "tack up" the tissue. The latter technique is more frequently used and presently recommended.

In instances when there is severe angulation at the exit of the lesion, a trend toward increased dissections has been noted. This may be secondary to the guide wire's stiffness and inability to conform to angles in the vessel. This would cause the orientation of the burr to be out of plane and result in tangential ablation, with cutting not based on differential mechanisms but on the resultant vector of the guide wire. Therefore, the wire may force the burr in a direction that, despite elasticity of the tissue, ablates the vessel because it cannot be deflected away from the burr. Another site where dissections appear to be more common is at a lesion at the ostium of a severely angulated circumflex artery. Again, it is the stiffness of the guide wire that forces the burr to preferentially rather than differentially ablate the lesion because the wire is eccentrically oriented. Therefore, in the case of an ostial circumflex on a severe bend or severe angles, it is advisable to undersize the burr to an approximately 0.5 to 0.6 burr-to-artery ratio and subsequently attempt to achieve the best result with adjunctive PTCA.

Side Branch Management

In most instances, side branch occlusion with the Rotablator system is secondary to the generation of microparticulate debris during ablation or vasospasm. This is in contrast with PTCA, in which it is often a result of the stretching of a common wall at a bifurcation point, with one vessel being dilated and the other impinging on the lumen. When operating the Rotablator system, secondary or protecting wires for bifurcated lesions cannot be used because of the cutting mechanism of the device. An example might be a lesion in the left anterior descending artery, where moderate to severe vasospasm may occur at the ostium of a diagonal. In the right coronary artery the problem usually involves small right ventricular branches that often have minimal electrocardiographic or hemodynamic consequences but cause the patient profound chest discomfort. Both situations generally respond to vasodilators, and in the case of the diagonal artery, if it does not improve over a reasonable period it is sometimes worthwhile to perform low-pressure balloon inflation at the site of the spasm. If it is possible to platform the burr distal to the takeoff of larger side branches, this is advisable because it will reduce the possibility of inducing vasospasm. In cases of abrupt closure of a side branch after high-speed ablation, the treatment should be initial attempts with vasodilators with a low threshold and progress to performing low-pressure PTCA after crossing the site with a second wire.

Summary

High-speed rotational ablation has come to have an important place in the armamentarium of interventional devices. It has expanded the indications for percutaneous therapy, primarily in lesions that because of calcific elements respond poorly to balloon dilation. As more experience is gained and the procedure further refined, this unique method of revascularization will be studied not only in the context of acute procedural results but with respect to whether it can impact restenosis rates.

THE SIMPSON ATHEROCATH DEVICE

The SCA, a directional coronary atherectomy (DCA) catheter, represents the first of the second-generation coronary interventional devices to be approved by the federal Food and Drug Administration (FDA). The impetus for its development, as with the Rotablator system, was to overcome the limitations of balloon angioplasty.[34] Specifically, its designers hoped to achieve a more predictable angiographic result by removing obstructive atheromatous plaque, to expand the application of percutaneous revascularization to more complex lesions, to reduce complications, and, finally, to possibly reduce the occurrence rate of restenosis.

History of Development

The idea of a DCA catheter purportedly was generated in the spring of 1980 after a failed

balloon angioplasty.[34] Subsequently, a Cope pleural needle biopsy device was used postmortem to shave off an obstructive plaque in a diseased left main coronary artery. Thereafter, a corporation was established to develop and manufacture a similar device for vascular use. After multiple engineering iterations and extensive tests in animals, an investigational device exemption (IDE) was granted by the FDA in 1986 to begin clinical testing in humans of the SCA (Devices for Vascular Intervention [DVI], Redwood City, CA). After initial successful application in humans at Sequoia Hospital in Northern California, the device received approval for broader testing in mid-1988. Eleven other institutions began to apply the device, and by November 1989 1032 lesions had been treated. The results from these initial applications led to full FDA approval in September 1990.[35] Since that time, the device has undergone major improvements, and as more data are analyzed, a better understanding of the benefits and limitations of its application have been realized.

Description of the Directional Coronary Atherectomy Device

The overall equipment for a DCA consists of a guiding catheter (9.5- to 11-French), the SCA, a motor drive unit, a rotating hemostatic valve, and an "indeflator." The SCA itself—a cutter within a housing—consists of several functional compartments; a distal nose cone for acceptance of the shaved atheromatous material, bioptome housing, cutter, supporting balloon, device shaft, and proximal assembly unit (Fig. 29–15). The distal end of the SCA has a radiopaque, gold-plated, rigid stainless steel housing mounted on a torque cable shaft that surrounds the central cutter and its cable. Over the length of the housing is a support balloon made of either Surlyn (SCA-1) or polyethylene terephthalate (SCA-EX) that serves to hold the device stable while the atheroma prolapses into the cutting chamber. The housing itself has a 9- to 10-mm window. The cutter spins at 2000 rpm and is advanced manually through the cutting chamber over a 0.014-inch guide wire. Three types of SCA devices are available (Table 29–5). Both SCA-1 and SCA-EX are distinguished by a housing length of 17 mm; the SCA-EX has a slightly smaller window size (9 as opposed to 10 mm, 120-degree arc), its balloon material is made of polyethylene terephthalate, and its nose cone consists of a polyurethane-covered spring coil. This latter component provides a smooth, tapered transition from the housing

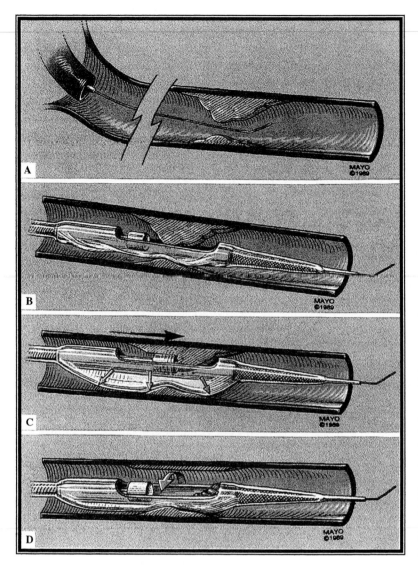

Figure 29–15. Diagrams of the use of the Simpson coronary athero-cath. *A,* Positioning of guide wire through the lumen of the lesion. *B,* Atherectomy catheter housing is advanced across the lesion. *C,* Low-pressure inflation of balloon to stabilize housing and cause protrusion of atheroma into path of cutting blade; the motorized cutting unit is slowly advanced. *D,* The unit is turned in a different direction to reposition the window, and the cutting operation is repeated. (From Kauffmann UP, Garratt KN, Vlietstra RE, Menke KK, Holmes DR Jr: Coronary atherectomy: First 50 patients at the Mayo Clinic. Mayo Clin Proc 1989; 64:747–752. By permission.)

unit to the distal tip and facilitates crossing a lesion. In addition, it functions as a storage compartment for excised tissue. The SCA-EX-SC device has a window length of 5 mm (short window) that facilitates passage through areas of tortuosity. The EX series of catheters is manufactured in three different housing sizes: 5 French (1.7 mm), 6 French (2.0 mm), and 7 French (2.3 mm).

Various improved versions of the DCA catheter are under development. These include positron emission tomographic large balloon devices for larger vessels, wider window devices to improve tissue excision, and sharper and stronger cutters to cut through calcified lesions. An ultrasound-guided atherectomy device, as well as a flexible housing with a new cutting method, is under development.

Mechanism of Action

The design of the DCA device is aimed, obviously, at removal of atherosclerotic plaque. Figure 29–15 demonstrates the integration of the cutting window and balloon to achieve this goal, along with directional control. Early on it was noted that application of the device was associated with a residual lumen that was relatively large and smooth.

The relation among the tissue removal, a possible dilation effect, and the final luminal dimension was investigated to evaluate the relative impact of the various mechanisms. Models using cylindrical models, based on angiograms and excised tissue weight, have been used to calculate the contribution of tissue removal versus balloon-device dilatory effect. Penny and co-

Table 29–5. Types of Simpson AtheroCath (SCA)

Type*	Housing Length (mm)	Window Size (mm)	Balloon Material	Nose Cone	Sizes (French)
SCA-1	17	10	Surlyn	Stiff, notched transition	5, 6, 7, 7G
SCA-EX	17	9	PET	Polyurethane, spring coil	5, 6, 7
SCA-EX SC	9	5	PET	Polyurethane, spring coil	5, 6, 7

*See text for abbreviations used in this column.
PET, polyethylene terephthalate.

workers[36] estimated that atherectomy excised one third of the obstructive tissue and that two thirds of the angiographic improvement was the result of stretching of the vessel wall. Scharaf and Williams[37] reported that there was transient increase in the size of the stenotic lumen merely by passage and withdrawal of the relatively large diameter (2- to 2.5-mm) rigid atherectomy device, a so-called Dotter effect. There may also be some luminal dilation brought about by inflation of the positioning balloon, a so-called Gruentzig effect. It has been estimated that atherectomy of a completely occluded 10-mm segment of a vessel 3 mm in diameter should yield approximately 70 mg of atheromatous tissue. In a study by Safian and colleagues,[38] however, the average tissue weight removed was only 18.5 mg and angiographic and clinical success were achieved after removal of as little as 6 mg of tissue. These results imply a synergy between the balloon and cutting mechanism of the atherectomy device that translates into larger luminal gains. This combination of stretching and plaque removal, and how the relative contribution of each fulfills the best outcome, requires further analysis.

Procedure

Deployment of the Device

The rigidity and high profile of the DCA requires specially designed guiding catheters. These large-lumen catheters provide the support necessary to advance the device across the lesion site. These guiding catheters, because of their larger size and firmness, demand care during intubation of the ostium to avoid excessive trauma to the artery. The guide wires are generally the types used for conventional balloon angioplasty, although several interventional cardiologists are performing the procedure with stiffer wires, available from several manufacturers. The guide wire is either manipulated down the artery as either a "bare wire" or preloaded into the DCA catheter. Once the wire is distal to the lesion, the DCA is advanced and often torqued as it traverses the vessel and is finally positioned at the lesion site. After excision of large numbers of plaque shavings that maximally fill the chamber, the guide wire may become fixed or "frozen" and will therefore be withdrawn with the device.

Plaque Excision

Several steps should be undertaken prior to tissue removal. These include the following:

• Confirm the device position with contrast agent injections using anatomic landmarks such as side branches
• Orient the cutting window toward the plaque
• Inflate the balloon with low pressure (0.5 to 1.0 atm)

The expanded balloon forces the plaque to protrude into the housing. The cutter is then retracted and the motor drive unit activated. The cutter is then slowly advanced over a 5- to 8-second interval. In the hands of an experienced operator, the slow advancement provides tactile feedback as to whether material is being excised; auditory feedback may indicate whether the device is being inhibited or meeting significant resistance from hard (calcified) plaque. The balloon is then deflated and the window reoriented by torquing the proximal end of the catheter; the balloon is then reinflated with low pressure before retraction of the cutter to the proximal end to avoid distal embolization by already excised tissue. The whole process is then repeated.

After serial cuts the operator may elect to use increased balloon pressures of 20 to 30 psi. This decision is often based on the relationship of the size of the artery to the device, the tactile feedback during the passing of the cutter, and the angiographic appearance. One somewhat crude but often helpful method to assist in whether higher pressures are required is to assess the amount of flow around the device as a guide. If the flow is attenuated by the device, this may indicate inadequate debulking that requires a more aggressive strategy. In most instances 8 to 12 cuts are made with one insertion of the device into the coronary artery; however, this is often controlled by the patient's degree of tolerance of myocardial ischemia. Eccentric plaque cuts should be made over an arc of approximately 180 degrees, and in concentric lesions the entire circumference of the vessel at the lesion site should be treated. The experienced operator should be able to position the device in ranges of about 45 degrees with reasonable reliability, allowing for smaller arcs of cuts with the implied benefit of acquiring more material. Once satisfied with the results, the DCA is retracted into the guiding catheter, taking care that the latter does not slip in, deeply intubating the ostium and possibly traumatizing the vessel.

Two further points require special attention: The first is the issue of predilation. Since the recent release of the more user-friendly SCA-EX device, a greater number of lesions can now be reached, although device size and stiffness are still limiting factors. The use of predilation with small balloon catheters is therefore occasionally needed to facilitate crossing the lesion with the device. In addition, predilation should be considered for calcified lesions, long lesions, and lesions located in distal segments. Another strategy showing significant promise is the combined use of high-speed rotational ablation with the Rotablator to remove inelastic substrate from the vessel and subsequent use of DCA to maximize luminal dimensions in larger vessels (see Fig. 29–14).

A further issue is the question of when the operator would be satisfied with the final result. This has been an evolving issue, but the debate appears to be leading to a more aggressive strategy, assuming safety, that provides a residual stenosis visually of less than 10%. A 10% residual stenosis visually at the end of a procedure usually translates to approximately 20% by QCA. Therefore, when a 20% to 30% stenosis remains, further atherectomy should be considered. If appropriate, a larger device can be applied. If the device is the largest, or because of anatomic reasons switching to a larger device is impossible, the application of balloon pressures in the range of 30 to 40 psi can be used.

Medications

The premedication regimen for DCA procedures is similar to that for PTCA. This includes aspirin, 325 mg before the procedure and continued daily after the procedure, and a calcium channel blocker. Heparinization is initiated with a bolus of 10,000 units and subsequent doses during the procedure are given to maintain an activated clotting time in excess of 350 seconds. The adjunctive use of intracoronary nitroglycerin, verapamil, or urokinase reflects the status of the treated vessel during the procedure. Specifically, the use of intracoronary urokinase for preexisting thrombus or diffusely diseased saphenous vein grafts may result in an improved outcome. The use of further adjuncts such as dextran has not been supported by clinical data.

Histopathology of Atherectomy Specimens

Analysis of excised tissue samples from native (de novo) lesions has revealed atherosclerotic plaque in 78% to 98%, media in about 39% to 69%, and adventitia in approximately 3% to 34%.[39-42] Fibrointimal proliferation can also be found in about 22% to 42% of primary lesions, whereas this pathologic finding is much more commonly present in restenotic lesions.[39-42] Table 29–6 lists these findings according to their citation in the literature.

A number of important conclusions have been drawn from the combined analyses of histopathologic specimens taken at the time of coronary atherectomy.[43] They include the following:

1. Intimal proliferation lesions after balloon angioplasty are histologically identical to those reported in autopsied patients
2. Restenotic lesion tissue is histologically identical to the intimal proliferation tissue after conventional balloon angioplasty
3. Restenotic lesion tissue after conventional balloon angioplasty does not consist solely of intimal proliferation
4. Deep-vessel wall components (media and adventitia) can be observed relatively frequently in patients undergoing directional atherectomy
5. De novo coronary stenotic lesions do not consist solely of atherosclerotic plaque but may contain intimal proliferative tissue

Atherectomy specimens have also been subjected to transmission electron microscopy that showed that smooth muscle cells were the predominant cells in both primary and restenotic lesions.[44] These cells have then been cultured and their degree of metabolic activation quantified. Inhibitors of the proliferative and migratory activity of these cultured smooth muscle cells, such as colchicine, have also been studied. Thus, cell cultures of atherectomy specimens will likely continue to have an important role to play in the investigation of the numerous approaches being taken to inhibit the restenosis process.

Table 29–6. Histologic Observations in Coronary Atherectomy Specimens

Tissue Features	De Novo Lesions (%)		
	Waller et al[39] *(n = 33)*	*Johnson et al*[40] *(n = 109)*	*Schnitt et al*[41, 42] *(n = 105)*
Atherosclerotic plaque ± thrombus	97	78	98
Intimal proliferation ± thrombus	0	22	42
Thrombus only	6		0
Calcified deposits	76	47	—
Vessel media	39	47	69
Vessel adventitia	3	20	34
	Restenosic Lesions (%)		
Atherosclerotic plaque ± thrombus	17	14	95
Intimal proliferation ± thrombus	17	86	91
Thrombus only	0	—	0
Calcified deposits	64	45	—
Vessel media	39	40	63
Vessel adventitia	0	17	20

Data from Waller BF, Johnson DE, Schitt SJ, et al: Histologic analysis of directional coronary atherectomy samples. Am J Cardiol 1993; 72:80E–87E.

Immediate and Near-term Results

Data accumulated from a multicenter investigational registry, as well as single-center studies, have demonstrated that the SCA device, when applied to a broad range of coronary artery lesion subsets, is safe and efficacious.

Ellis and associates[45] reviewed the use of DCA of 400 lesions in 378 patients and reported that the primary success rate was 87.8%, with ischemic complications occurring in 6.3% (emergency CABG surgery in 5.5%, myocardial infarction in 1.8%, and death in 1.0%). The complication rate was decidedly related to operator experience; other factors that presaged a complication included a lesion occurring at a relatively acute bend and a primary, rather than a restenotic, lesion.

The initial multicenter preapproval data base, compiled by DVI under their original IDE, compiled information on the use of the SCA device in 1069 lesions in 873 patients. These data revealed a relatively high (85%) primary success rate (defined as tissue removal, <50% residual stenosis, and no major complications). If the number of conventional balloon angioplasty after attempted DCA is included, the overall primary success rate rose to 92%. Complications after the introduction of the SCA catheter occurred in 4.1% of patients; dissection at the treated site was noted in 7.2% of patients.[46]

Popma and colleagues[47] reported the associated conditions with abrupt vessel closure after DCA in 1020 patients (1,140 lesions) at 14 participating clinical centers. *Abrupt occlusion* was defined as total occlusion or subtotal obstruc-

tion sufficient to cause evidence of myocardial ischemia. This problem eventuated in 43 procedures (4.2%) and most (79%) took place in the cardiac catheterization laboratory. Predictors of abrupt closure, by this definition, were (1) lesions in the right coronary artery ($P = .001$), (2) diffuse lesions ($P = .04$), and (3) de novo lesions ($P<.001$). Subsequent balloon angioplasty relieved the total obstruction in approximately one half of the cases of abrupt closure. Twenty-five of the 43 patients were referred for immediate CABG surgery.

Two randomized trials, both comparing DCA with transluminal coronary balloon angioplasty (TCBA), have now been concluded (Table 29–7).[48, 49] The Canadian Coronary Atherectomy Trial (CCAT) randomized 274 de novo lesions of the proximal one third of the left anterior descending coronary artery to either DCA or TCBA. Immediate angiographic success (<50 percent residual diameter stenosis, assessed quantitatively) was superior in the DCA group than in those who received TCBA (98% vs. 91%; $P = .01$). Complication rates did not differ between the two groups. However, there was a trend for a higher rate of emergency CABG surgery in the TCBA than in the DCA group (4.4% vs. 1.4%, respectively; $P = .17$).

In the Coronary Angioplasty Versus Excisional Atherectomy Trial (CAVEAT), 1012 patients, 500 treated with TCBA and 512 with DCA, were randomized. In contrast with CCAT, lesions for study and treatment were not constrained by their anatomic location; they only had to be treatable by either modality. Again, a higher procedural primary success rate (50% residual stenosis) was noted with DCA (88.6%)

Table 29–7. Immediate Procedural Results:
DCA Versus TCBA

Results	Coronary Angioplasty Versus Excisional Atherectomy[49] (CAVEAT) (%)	Canadian Coronary Atherectomy Trial[50] (CCAT) (%)
Primary success rate		
DCA	88.6	94
TCBA	80.3	88
Abrupt closure		
DCA	7	4.3
TCBA	3	5.1
Death		
DCA	0	0
TCBA	0.4	0
Emergency CABG		
DCA	3	1.4
TCBA	2	4.4
Myocardial infarction*		
DCA	19	4.3
TCBA	8	3.7
Freedom from adverse end-point		
DCA	89	91
TCBA	95	91

*Q wave or non–Q wave by electrocardiography or abnormal enzyme elevation.

DCA, directional coronary atherectomy; TCBA, transluminal coronary balloon angioplasty; CABG, coronary artery bypass graft.

than with TCBA (80.3%; $P = .001$). However, patients treated with TCBA, as opposed to DCA, were significantly less likely to experience a combined end-point of death, myocardial infarction, CABG surgery, or abrupt closure (6% vs. 11%; $P = .001$). Nevertheless, two patients in the TCBA group, as opposed to none in the DCA, died as a result of the procedure.

Restenosis and Long-term Results

The Sequoia Hospital group analyzed their long-term results in 332 lesions treated between 1986 and 1989.[50] Angiographic follow-up was accomplished in 280 (82.4%) of these lesions; using a definition of greater than 50% diameter obstruction, the overall restenosis was found to be 42% (30% for primary lesions, 28% in vessels with one previous angioplasty, and 47% in lesions with two or more previous angioplasties). Predictors of restenosis included hypertension; lesions 10 mm or less in diameter; noncalcified lesions; vessels 3 mm or less in diameter; and use of the smaller, 6-French cutting device. Similar long-term results were reported by the investigators at Beth Israel Hospital, Boston, in their series of patients treated between 1988 and 1991.[41] The angiographic follow-up rate at 6 months in 225 lesions was 77%; using again a

definition of greater than 50% residual diameter obstruction at follow-up, the restenosis rate was found to be 32%. If the post-DCA luminal diameter was greater than 3 mm, the restenosis was found to be 24%, providing the first observation that suggested that "bigger is better."

In the CAVEAT,[48] 862 and 959 eligible patients have undergone 6-month follow-up angiography. The angiographic restenosis rate (50% stenosis) trended toward a higher rate in the TCBA group (57%) than with the DCA group (50%; $P = .06$). The restenosis rate was significantly lower in proximal left anterior descending lesions with DCA (51%) than with TCBA (63%; $P = .04$). Immediately after treatment, the DCA group demonstrated a larger luminal diameter at the site of atherectomy or balloon dilation ($P<.001$); however, this significant difference was not sustained at the 6-month angiographic follow-up (Fig. 29–16). In a subgroup analysis, it was noted that a post-DCA stenosis of less than 20% was associated with a lower restenosis rate of 31%, again supporting the notion that a larger postprocedural lumen is desirable. Importantly, the larger luminal diameter immediately after the procedure in the DCA group did not translate into an improved clinical outcome at 6 months. To the contrary, primarily because of the higher rate of periprocedural myocardial infarction and death during 6 to 7 months of follow-up, the clinical probability of death and myocardial infarction was higher for DCA than for TCBA ($P = .007$).

The angiographic follow-up of patients in the CCAT[49] (97%; follow-up in 257 of the eligible 265 patients) demonstrated cumulative distribution curves of minimal luminal diameter that were very similar to those in CAVEAT. Again, the initially larger luminal diameter with DCA, as compared with TCBA, was not maintained on the 6-month follow-up examination. The restenosis rate (50% diameter stenosis) was found to be 46% for DCA and 43% for TCBA ($P = .71$).

Management of Complications

Several complications deserve special attention because the DCA device presents an alternative mechanism to obtain increased luminal dimensions.

The observed rate of occlusion in the DVI multicenter experience was 4.2%.[47] The factors associated with risk of abrupt closure were primary lesions, lesions in the right coronary artery, and lesions in diffusely diseased vessels. Procedural predictors were lesions that were attempted but not crossed with the device, in-

Angiographic Follow-up After Directional Coronary Atherectomy

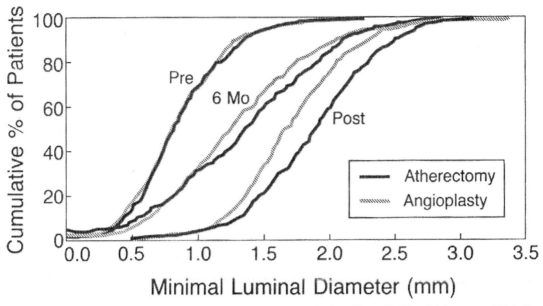

Figure 29–16. Quantitative angiographic data from the Coronary Angioplasty Versus Excisional Atherectomy Trial. Cumulative percentage of patients (vertical axis, directional atherectomy, and angioplasty cohorts) are plotted against the minimal luminal diameter before atherectomy, immediately after atherectomy, and at 6 months' follow-up. See text for discussion. (From Topol EJ, Leya F, Pinkertron CA, et al, for the CAVEAT Study Group: A comparison of directional atherectomy with coronary angioplaty in patients with coronary artery disease. N Engl J Med 1993; 329:221–227.)

ability to cut tissue, inadequate tissue removal, or dissection during the procedure. In addition, occlusion distal to the DCA site resulting from nose cone injury has been observed. The newer generation of devices should address this latter problem.

Perforation represents a complication with possible severe consequences. Despite the frequent incidence of deep wall resection, either of media (67%) or of adventitia (27%), the Sequoia Hospital experience had a rate of 1.3%. Cases should be selected judiciously, avoiding severely angulated lesions, dissections involving normal segments, and small vessels.

Finally, embolization is a concern secondary to dislodgement of debris or excised tissue that may escape from the cutting chamber. The incidence of distal embolization in native coronary arteries is less than 1%. The incidence in saphenous vein grafts occurred in 7.2% of 318 procedures.[51] The presence of diffuse disease is the one characteristic that increases the risk for this event.

Analysis of Outcome by Lesion Morphology

The impact of any new interventional device to succeed against conventional balloon angio-

plasty will be its ability to impact on acute outcome either by lowering the rate of complications in complex lesions or expanding the indications of percutaneous revascularization. The second method would be to lower restenosis rates significantly without jeopardizing the acute success rate. The success rate from the Sequoia Hospital experience of 447 lesions were analyzed to identify risk factors.[52] When categorizing lesions based on the American Heart Association–American College of Cardiology classification,[20] the primary success rate for types A and B was 93% and 87%, respectively ($P<.01$). The factors that limited success for the type B lesions were calcification, lesion length greater than 10 mm, and calcified restenotic lesions. Calcified lesions present difficulties for this device for several reasons: (1) an inability to reach the lesion because of increased vessel stiffness; (2) an inability to cross the lesion; and (3) an inadequate excision of tissue. Ellis and coworkers[45] analyzed the multicenter data and revealed that proximal tortuosity, bend stenosis, primary lesions, and calcification were predictors of higher risk of failure. The results of this study for success and complication rates were, respectively, type A (n = 176) 93% and 3.4%; type B (n = 148) 88% and 6%; and type B$_2$ (n = 72) 75% and 12.5%.

Eccentric lesions are a morphologic subset that should be particularly amenable to treatment with this device. Theoretically, extremely eccentric lesions should be excised selectively with this device with a directional approach. Despite the often complex nature of these lesions, the primary success rate has been 95%, with a CABG rate of 2.4%, and a postprocedural residual stenosis of 19%. The directional nature of the device may also be beneficial in treating ulcerations or dissected lesions.[45] Excision of these complex lesions can often salvage an otherwise deteriorating clinical course.

Directional atherectomy has also been applied to aorto-ostial lesions.[53] The success rate is 94% (100% in vein grafts and 89% of right coronary artery lesions) with a residual angiographic stenosis of 11%. However, the combination of difficult guide catheter placement and the high incidence of calcification at these locations can be problematic. The hybridization of DCA with Rotablator may be a more effective method of treating this difficult subset (see Fig. 29–14).

DCA has also been used as therapy for failed or suboptimal balloon angioplasty.[54] In 100 patients (103 lesions) combined from the Cleveland Clinic Foundation, the Medical College of Virginia, and the CAVEAT data base, DCA was successful (TIMI grade 3 flow, greater than 20% stenosis reduction without death, Q wave myocardial infarction, or CABG surgery) in 94 of 103 lesions (91.3%). The etiology of failed PTCA was primarily from dissection in 52 lesions (50.5%), "recoil" in 43 lesions (41.8%), and recurrent thrombosis in 8 lesions (7.8%). Complete vessel closure was noted in 23 lesions (22.3%). Although the use of DCA in vessels with significant dissections can be treated effectively with atherectomy, the risk of perforation may be higher if the dissection extends beyond the original plaque.

Summary

DCA represents a new device in our armamentarium to treat obstructive coronary arteries. The safety and efficacy achieved in the multicenter study and subsequent follow-up studies imply that it can be used as an alternative to balloon angioplasty. The question remains as to the additional benefit it portends at the expense of a more difficult device to use technically and its associated higher risks and costs.

The continued design advances of the device and greater clinical experience, coupled with improved imaging modalities, suggest that the role is still to be determined.

REFERENCES

1. Hansen DD, Auth DC, Vracko R, Ritchie JL: Rotational atherectomy in atherosclerotic rabbit iliac arteries. Am Heart J 1988; 115:160–165.
2. Ahn SS, Auth DC, Marcus DR, Moore WS: Removal of focal atheromatous lesions by angioscopically guided high-speed rotary atherectomy: Preliminary experimental observations. J Vasc Surg 1988; 7:292–300.
3. Hansen DH, Auth DC, Hall M, Ritchie JL: Rotational endarterectomy in normal canine coronary arteries: Preliminary report. J Am Coll Cardiol 1988; 11:1073–1077.
4. Fourrier JL, Stankowiak C, Lablanche JM, et al: Histopathology after rotational angioplasty of peripheral arteries in human beings [abstract]. J Am Coll Cardiol 1988; 11:109A.
5. Mintz GS, Potkin BN, Keren G, et al: Cross-sectional and three-dimensional intravascular ultrasound analysis of coronary artery geometry after rotational atherectomy [abstract]. Circulation 1991; 84:II-155.
6. Potkin BN, Mintz GS, Matar FA, et al: A mechanistic comparison of transcatheter therapies assessed by intravascular ultrasound [abstract]. Circulation 1991; 84: II-541.
7. Kovach JA, Mintz GS, Pichard AD, et al: Sequential intravascular ultrasound imaging characterizes mechanisms of lumen enlargement after rotational atherectomy [abstract]. Circulation 1992; 86:I-532.
8. Berkalp B, Nissen SE, De Franco AC, et al: Intravascular ultrasound demonstrates marked differences in surface and lumen shape following interventional devices [abstract]. Circulation 1994; 90:I-58.
9. Cowley M, Buchbinder M, Warth D, et al: Effect of coronary rotational atherectomy abrasion on vessel segments adjacent to treated lesions [abstract]. J Am Coll Cardiol 1992; 19:333A.
10. Prevosti LG, Cook JA, Unger EF, et al: Particulate debris from rotational atherectomy: Size distribution and physiologic effects [abstract]. Circulation 1988; 78:II-83.
11. Friedman HZ, Elliot MA, Gottlieb GJ, O'Neill WW: Mechanical rotary atherectomy: The effects of microparticle embolization on myocardial blood flow and function. J Int Cardiol 1989; 2:77–83.
12. Sherman CT, Brunken R, Chan A, Krivokapich J, Buchbinder M: Myocardial perfusion and segmental wall motion after coronary rotational atherectomy [abstract]. Circulation 1992; 86:I-652.
13. Pavlides GS, Hauser AM, Grines CL, et al: Clinical, hemodynamic, electrocardiographic, and mechanical events during nonocclusive coronary atherectomy and comparison with balloon angioplasty. Am J Cardiol 1992; 70:841–845.
14. Zotz RJ, Erbel R, Philipp A, et al: High-speed rotational angioplasty-induced echo contrast in vivo and in vitro optical analysis. Cathet Cardiovasc Diagn 1992; 26: 98–109.
15. Safian RD, Freed M, Lichtenberg A, et al: Are residual stenoses after excimer laser angioplasty and coronary atherectomy due to inefficient or small devices? Comparison with balloon angioplasty. J Am Coll Cardiol 1993; 22:1628–1634.
16. Reisman M, Buchbinder M, Bass T, et al: Improvement in coronary dimensions at early 24-hour follow-up after coronary rotational ablation: Implications for restenosis [abstract]. Circulation 1992; 86:I-332.
17. Mintz GS, Potkin BN, Keren G, et al: Intravascular ultrasound evaluation of the effect of rotational atherectomy in obstructive atherosclerotic coronary artery disease. Circulation 1992; 86:1383–1393.

18. Fourrier JL, Bertrand ME, Auth DC, et al: Percutaneous coronary rotational angioplasty in humans: Preliminary report. J Am Coll Cardiol 1989; 14:1278–1282.

19. Teirstein PS, Warth DC, Haq N, et al: High-speed rotational coronary atherectomy for patients with diffuse coronary artery disease. J Am Coll Cardiol 1991; 18:1694–1701.

20. Ryan TJ, Faxon DP, Gunnar RM, et al: Guidelines for percutaneous transluminal coronary angioplasty: A report of the American College of Cardiology/American Heart Association Task Force on Assessment of Diagnostic and Therapeutic Cardiovascular Procedures (Subcommittee on Percutaneous Transluminal Coronary Angioplasty). Circulation 1988; 78:486–502.

21. Stertzer SH, Rosenblum J, Shaw RE, et al: Coronary rotation ablation: Initial experience in 302 procedures. J Am Coll Cardiol 1993; 21:287–295.

22. Safian RD, Niazi KA, Strzelecki M, et al: Detailed angiographic analysis of high-speed mechanical rotational atherectomy in human coronary arteries. Circulation 1993; 88:961–968.

23. Ellis SG, Popma JJ, Buchbinder M, et al: Relation of clinical presentation, stenosis morphology, and operator technique to the procedural results of rotational atherectomy and rotational atherectomy-facilitated angioplasty. Circulation 1994; 89:882–892.

24. Warth DC, Leon MB, O'Neill W, et al: Rotational atherectomy multicenter registry: Acute results, complications, and 6-month angiographic follow-up in 709 patients. J Am Coll Cardiol 1994; 24:641–648.

25. Vandormael M, Reifart N, Pruesler W, et al: Immediate and 6-month follow-up outcomes following excimer laser angioplasty, rotational atherectomy, and balloon angioplasty for complex lesions: ERBAC randomized study. Symposium conducted at the German Rotablator Practitioner Meeting, Frankfurt, Germany, September 17, 1994.

26. Detre KM, Baim D, Buchbinder M, et al: Baseline characteristics and therapeutic goals in the New Approaches to Coronary Intervention (NACI) registry. Coron Artery Dis 1993;4:1013–1022.

27. Zidar JP, Jackman JD, Tenaglia AN, et al: Late outcome for PTCA of long coronary lesions using long angioplasty balloon catheters [abstract]. Circulation 1992; 86:I-512.

28. Reisman M, Cohen B, Warth D, et al: Outcome of long lesions treated with high-speed rotational ablation [abstract]. J Am Coll Cardiol 1993; 21:443A.

29. Maiello L, Colombo A, Gianrossi R, et al: Coronary angioplasty of chronic occlusions: Factors predictive of procedural success. Am Heart J 1992; 124:581–590.

30. Detre K, Holubkov R, Kelsey S, et al: Percutaneous transluminal coronary angioplasty in 1985–1986 and 1977–1981: The National Heart, Lung, and Blood Institute Registry. N Engl J Med 1988; 318:265–270.

31. Kahn JK, Hartzler GO: Frequency and causes of failure with contemporary balloon coronary angioplasty and implications for new technologies. Am J Cardiol 1990; 66:858–860.

32. Reisman M, Devlin P, Melikian J, et al: Undilatable noncompliant lesions treated with the Rotablator: Outcome and angiographic follow-up [abstract]. Circulation 1993; 88(Part 2): I-547.

33. Ellis SG, Franco I, Satler LF, Whitlow P: Slow reflow and coronary perforation after Rotablator therapy—incidence: Clinical, angiographic, and procedural predictors [abstract]. Circulation 1992; 86:I-652.

34. Simpson JB: How atherectomy began: A personal history. Am J Cardiol 1993; 72:3E–5E.

35. Baim DS, Hinohara T, Holmes D, et al: Results of directional coronary atherectomy during multicenter preapproval testing. Am J Cardiol 1993; 72:6E–11E.

36. Penny WF, Schmidt DA, Safian RD, et al: Insights into the mechanism of luminal improvement following directional coronary atherectomy. Am J Cardiol 1991; 67:435–437.

37. Scharaf BL, Williams DO: "Dotter" effect contributes to angiographic improvement following coronary atherectomy [abstract]. Circulation 1990; 82:III-310A

38. Safian RD, Gelbfish JS, Erny RE, et al: Coronary atherectomy: Clinical, angiographic, and histologic findings and some observations regarding potential mechanisms. Circulation 1990; 82:69–79.

39. Waller BF, Pinkerton CA, Kereiakes D, et al: Morphologic analysis of 506 coronary atherectomy specimens from 107 patients: Histologically similar findings of restenosis following primary balloon angioplasty versus primary atherectomy. J Am Coll Cardiol 1990; 15:197A.

40. Johnson DE, Hinohara T, Robertson GC, et al: Coronary vascular lesions resected by directional coronary atherectomy: The histopathology of 328 successfully excised primary and recurrent stenosis. Cited in ref. 43 as in press.

41. Fishman RF, Kuntz RE, Carrozza JP, et al: Long-term results of directional coronary atherectomy: Predictors of restenosis. J Am Coll Cardiol 1992; 20:1101–1110.

42. Schnitt SJ, Safian RD, Kuntz RE, et al: Histologic findings in specimens obtained by percutaneous directional coronary atherectomy. Hum Pathol 1992; 23:415–420.

43. Waller BF, Johnson DE, Schnitt SJ, et al: Histologic analysis of directional coronary atherectomy samples. Am J Cardiol 1993; 72:80E–87E.

44. Hofling B, Welsch U, Heimerl J, et al: Analysis of atherectomy specimens. Am J Cardiol 1993; 72:96E–107E.

45. Ellis SG, De Cesare NB, Pinkertron CA, et al: Relation of stenosis morphology and clinical presentation to the procedural results of directional coronary atherectomy. Circulation 1991; 84:644–653.

46. Baim DS, Hinohara T, Holmes D, et al: Results of directional coronary atherectomy during multicenter preapproval testing. Am J Cardiol 1993; 72:6E–11E.

47. Popma JJ, Topol EJ, Hinohara T, et al: Abrupt vessel closure after directional coronary atherectomy. J Am Coll Cardiol 1992; 19:1372–1379.

48. Topol EJ, Leya F, Pinkertron CA, et al, for the CAVEAT Study Group: A comparison of directional atherectomy with coronary angioplasty in patients with coronary artery disease. N Engl J Med 1993; 329:221–227.

49. Adelman AG, Cohen EA, Kimball BP, et al: A comparison of directional atherectomy with balloon angioplasty for lesions of the left anterior descending coronary artery. N Engl J Med 1993; 329:228–233.

50. Hinohara T, Robertson GC, Selmon MR, et al: Restenosis after directional coronary atherectomy. J Am Coll Cardiol 1992; 20:623–632.

51. Cowley MJ, Whitlow PL, Baim DS, et al: Directional coronary atherectomy of saphenous vein graft narrowings: Multicenter investigational experience. Am J Cardiol 1993; 72:30E–34E.

52. Hinohara T, Rowe MH, Robertson G, et al: Effect of lesion characteristics on outcome of directional coronary atherectomy. J Am Coll Cardiol 1991; 17:1112–1120.

53. Cowley MJ, DiSciascio G: Experience with directional coronary atherectomy since pre-market approval. Am J Cardiol 1993; 72:12E–20E.

54. McCluskey ER, Cowley M, Whitlow PL: Multicenter clinical experience with rescue atherectomy for failed angioplasty. Am J Cardiol 1993; 72:42E–46E.

Chapter 30

Coronary Stents
Types and Results

JONATHAN CLAGUE
ULRICH SIGWART

BACKGROUND

In recent years many improvements have been made in the technique of percutaneous transluminal coronary angioplasty (PTCA). The mechanism underlying this technique involves dilating a constricted artery, thereby producing cracks involving the arterial intima and media and often separating atherosclerotic plaques from the vessel wall. Therefore, by its nature, angioplasty is bound to lead to dissection of the arterial wall and subsequent vessel closure in a significant proportion of patients. Such acute occlusion has been said to occur in as many as 5% of patients.[1] This finding, plus the problem of restenosis, which in some series is as high as 35% within the first few months after the procedure, has led to the development of intravascular stents.[2, 3] The concept of stent implantation, therefore, arises from the need to treat abrupt vessel closure and prevent restenosis after angioplasty.

HISTORICAL PERSPECTIVE

Stents were first implanted in animals in 1968 by Charles Dotter.[4] He noted that if thrombosis could be avoided, the metal stents became covered with endothelial cells within a few days of implantation. Within 2 weeks stents were completely covered with endothelium. The endothelial covering was at maximum thickness after about 8 weeks and then regressed to a maximum thickness of approximately 300 nm. In the late 1970s Mass and associates[5] implanted a helical stainless steel stent in canine vena cava, common jugular, and iliac veins. A total of 52 implants were performed and in all instances implants remained free of thrombosis despite the low rate of blood flow in these structures. Attempts were made to implant similar devices into smaller arteries, but these were unsuccessful because the surface area of the device used was too large and tended to promote thrombosis. Accordingly, subsequent designs focused on the need to keep surface area to a minimum. In the early 1980s Gianturco and colleagues[6] designed a self-expanding, springlike stent that had the desirable characteristic of presenting only a small surface area to blood and was therefore less thrombogenic. In 1986 Palmaz and coworkers[7] published the first article describing a balloon-expandable device. The Palmaz stent is a stainless steel tube with longitudinal slots that expand to diamond-shaped holes. This stent is balloon expandable and has little elastic recoil. The device underwent thorough testing in dogs with promising results and was subsequently tested in humans in 1988.[8]

The first stent to be employed in humans was a self-expanding mesh stent (Wallstent). After extensive testing in animals the stent was deployed in human coronary and peripheral arteries by Sigwart and coworkers.[9] This stent is composed of elastic metal braids. In the relaxed state the stent is expanded. It is delivered to the stenosis in a nonexpanded form covered by a membrane. When the membrane is removed the stent expands to the size of the artery. The stent is deployed using a specially designed delivery device that permits release of the membrane in the appropriate position. This stent produces an excellent angiographic result but has temporarily fallen into disrepute because of an unacceptably high thrombosis rate reported in one series.[10]

The most popular stent in use is the Palmaz-Schatz stent, and more than 50,000 of these have now been deployed in human coronary arteries. This stent is balloon expandable, obviating the need for a special delivery device, and, long-term, the results appear to be relatively satisfactory.[11, 12]

CLASSIFICATION OF STENTS

Stents may be classified into two broad groups: permanent and temporary. All existing permanent stents have been made of metal alloys, either spring alloys for self-expanding stents or deformable alloys for balloon-expandable stents.

Permanent Stents

The Wallstent

The self-expanding mesh stent, Wallstent (Fig. 30–1), is the only self-expanding stent that has been used in human coronary arteries. A number of animal studies had previously demonstrated the efficacy of this stent. Accordingly, in 1986, implantation in human coronary arteries began.[9] Between 1986 and 1990, 265 patients received stents in five participating European centers. Angiographic follow-up was obtained in 218 patients (82%) and the angiograms were analyzed using a well-validated computerized system. Early occlusion was reported in 14% (native vessels 18% and bypass grafts 7%). The overall mortality rate during the study period was 9% for bypass grafts and 7% for native vessels. Restenosis rate was about 50% for bypass grafts and 25% for native vessels. In this study it became apparent that stents implanted in restenosed native vessels had a high in-hospital occlusion rate, particularly in patients with unstable angina. In fact, the risk of sudden occlusion in this scenario convinced the authors of the study that the left anterior descending artery should be stented only in bailout situations. This factor and the relatively high mortality rate when compared with PTCA give cause for concern; consequently, this stent became temporarily unavailable for clinical use.[10] This study has a number of serious shortcomings, including broad range of operator experience and a lack of strict anticoagulation regimen. It is likely that this stent has been criticized too early. In the right hands it remains most useful, particularly in large vessels and saphenous vein grafts where currently available balloon-expandable devices are either too small or too short.

The Gianturco-Roubin (Cook) Stent

The balloon expandable Gianturco-Roubin (Cook) stent was the first device to be used in bailout situations for acute vessel closure after PTCA. Its design features include flexibility and a lack of shortening during expansion, but it has the disadvantage of important strut thickness and having rather large spaces between its constituent wires.

In a study conducted at Emory University between September 1988 and December 1990, 100 stents were implanted in 93 patients.[13] All patients included in this study had abrupt, complete vessel closure after PTCA or evidence of imminent closure due to severe dissection. In this study patients were treated with aspirin, heparin, dipyridamole, calcium channel block-

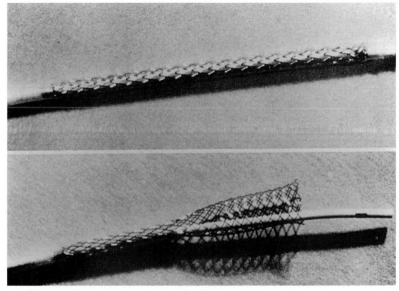

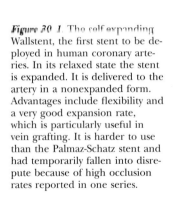

Figure 30–1. The self-expanding Wallstent, the first stent to be deployed in human coronary arteries. In its relaxed state the stent is expanded. It is delivered to the artery in a nonexpanded form. Advantages include flexibility and a very good expansion rate, which is particularly useful in vein grafting. It is harder to use than the Palmaz-Schatz stent and had temporarily fallen into disrepute because of high occlusion rates reported in one series.

ers, and dextran before the procedure, and intracoronary nitrates were infused before stent delivery. Dextran was continued after the stent placement, as was heparin (at least 1000 units/hr). After sheath removal, heparin was continued, and warfarin, aspirin, and dipyridamole were given for protracted periods after the procedure. One hundred and two patients with acute closure or threatened acute closure were included. A total of 104 PTCA procedures were performed and 109 stents were implanted. In nine patients stent delivery was impossible for various technical reasons. This left a total of 93 patients: 83 stents were in native coronaries and 10 in saphenous vein grafts. Ninety of the 93 stent placements were deemed angiographically successful at the time of the procedure. There were a total of five deaths, of which two were unrelated to the stent placements. Two died either as a result of stent placement or because of complications of anticoagulant therapy. The third died after coronary artery bypass grafting. Coronary artery bypass grafting before discharge was performed in 19%, and Q wave myocardial infarction occurred in 5.2%. A further 5.2% required repeat PTCA, and restenosis before discharge occurred in an additional 7.3%. This left 67 patients (74%) without complications. This trial was not designed to address the question of restenosis but to evaluate the efficacy of stents in acute-closure syndromes. However, angiographic follow-up was obtained in 50 patients at 6 months. Of these, 50% had restenosis. The restenosis rate was particularly high in saphenous vein grafts (100%). Circumflex arteries were also prone to restenosis (79%). Although the complication rates appear somewhat high in this study, it is important to note that the study focused on the patients with acute-closure syndromes, a condition associated with a high mortality rate.

The Wiktor Stent

The Wiktor stent (Fig. 30–2) was designed to overcome the major problem of radiopacity. The stent is composed of tantalum, a highly radiopaque metal with acceptable thrombogenicity. There are a few studies available using this stent. A recent multicenter study in patients with restenosis after PTCA demonstrated a restenosis rate of approximately 30% and an in-hospital acute-closure rate of 10%.[14]

The Advanced Catheter Systems MultiLink Stent System

The design concepts underlying the Advanced Catheter Systems (ACS) MultiLink metal stent were good structural support, low strut thickness, flexibility, and technically easy delivery.[15] Like the Palmaz-Schatz stent, this stent is also based on a stainless steel cylinder with gaps. The stent is flexible, with smaller gaps than the Palmaz-Schatz stent. The device is mounted on an elastic sleeve that covers the delivery balloon, thereby ensuring uniform expansion and balloon protection. The stent is covered by another sleeve designed to protect the stent during its delivery through the guiding catheter to the target area. Several diameters are available. The stent also comes in varying lengths, and unlike the Palmaz-Schatz stent it does not shorten during expansion. Extensive studies have been carried out in animals, but the human experience is so far limited to rigorous trials (WEST [West European Stent Trial]).

The Palmaz-Schatz Stent

The Palmaz-Schatz Stent (Fig. 30–3) is based on a stainless steel cylinder 15 mm in length and 1.6 mm in diameter. Multiple rows of rectangles are excised from the tube so that when the stent expands these become diamond shaped, permitting expansion to a maximum diameter of 5 or 6 mm. The stent is mounted on a standard angioplasty balloon that is then passed through an 8-French guiding catheter, over a 0.014-inch PTCA guide wire, and into the target vessel. The stent is delivered to the predilated lesion and deployed with a single balloon inflation. As is the case with the self-expanding stent, the Palmaz-Schatz stent also tends to shorten

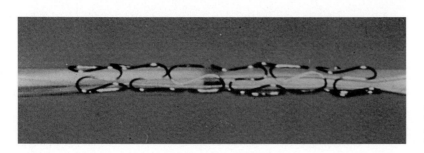

Figure 30–2. The Wiktor stent, composed of tantalum and designed to overcome the problem of lack of radiopacity.

with expansion. This reduces its value in very large vessels (4 to 6 mm) because at this diameter the stent is shortened to only 11 mm. Up to recently, the stent has been available in only one length, which makes it difficult to deal with longer lesions, particularly as a number of investigations have now highlighted the increased risk of restenosis with the use of multiple stents.[16, 17] A way of overcoming this difficulty is to mount two stents on one long balloon. Initial results with this technique are promising.[18]

The Palmaz-Schatz stent (PS 153) consists of two 7-mm-long rigid segments joined by a 1-mm-long flexible strut. This design permits more efficient delivery to tortuous target vessels than the rigid design. However, the gap between the two articulated segments appears to favor the occurrence of restenosis.[19, 20] Ways of overcoming this problem include making stents of differing lengths available or eliminating the gap while maintaining articulation between two segments. The new designs (PS 104, PS 153A, and PS 204C) are now available in Europe. Another problem with this stent is that difficulties are encountered in traversing small-caliber and diseased coronary arteries with the balloon stent assembly. This has resulted in failure of stent delivery in as many as 5% of patients and stent embolization.[21] These problems can be obviated by the use of a protective sheath that can be withdrawn when the stent is in place.[22] An alternative method is to pressurize the angioplasty balloon to 0.2 to 0.3 atm. This increases the diameter of the balloon distal and proximal to the stent, preventing the loss of the stent. If this method is employed, stent delivery can be achieved in most patients without the use of the protective sheath.

Temporary Stents

Catheter-mounted Temporary Stents

PERFUSION BALLOONS. Theoretically, perfusion balloons are acting as catheter-mounted temporary stents. Although perfusion balloons are helpful in the treatment of acute dissection after angioplasty, several problems associated with their use have engendered the design of alternative devices. A major problem with perfusion balloons is the potential occlusion of large side branches in close proximity to the stenosis. If the balloon remains inflated longer than 1 hour, side branches may be lost, leading to a variable amount of myocardial infarction. In addition, perfusion balloons do not permit enough blood to pass to the distal artery to guarantee maintenance of myocardial viability. Typically, only 60 mL of blood per minute reaches the distal artery.[23] These problems have led to the design of alternative devices.

FLOW SUPPORT CATHETER. This stent is designed in the form of a wire basket that expands by shortening of its long axis, which is achieved as a screw mechanism at the proximal end of the catheter. This device permits excellent perfusion of distal segments in side branches, but long-term results are less encouraging. In a multicenter trial published in 1992,[24] 37 patients underwent insertion of this device after reduction of coronary flow during angioplasty. Only 25% of the results were considered satisfactory

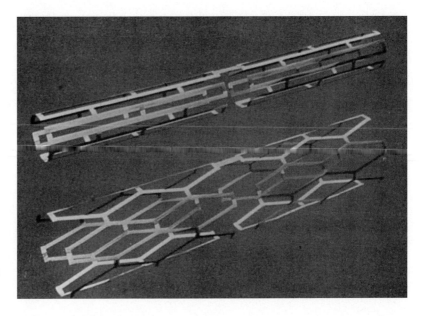

Figure 30–3. The Palmaz-Schatz stent, the most popular type in use, combines ease of deployment with acceptable complication rates. The device is shown in its expanded and nonexpanded forms.

at the end of the procedure (30 to 60 minutes). More than 60% needed additional treatment.

Retrievable Temporary Stents

The retrievable temporary (heat-activated) type of stent is constructed of titanium and nickel. It is delivered by balloon expansion. Injection of either warm saline or contrast medium into the relevant coronary artery forces the stent to collapse onto a catheter, thus permitting its retrieval.[25] The results of clinical trials are awaited.

Biodegradable Mesh Stents

Several biodegradable mesh stent devices are currently being tested.[26-28] These are constructed with polymers that are designed to survive for varying lengths of time. An attractive theoretical advantage of such a device is that drugs designed to prevent restenosis can be incorporated into the polymers and released slowly. So far, only results from animal studies are available, but these appear to be promising. A major problem with such devices is that they tend to be bulkier than metal stents and therefore more thrombogenic. They also appear to induce a greater inflammatory response in the arterial wall.

TECHNIQUE OF STENT DEPLOYMENT

The Palmaz-Schatz stent is the most popular stent in current clinical use and therefore the technique of deploying this stent is described in detail. Eight-French guiding catheters with an internal diameter larger than 0.079 inch are used most frequently. Several views of the target vessel should be obtained. If possible, markers such as arterial branches or surgical clips should be used to help localize the target lesion. The lesion should be crossed with a 0.014-inch guide wire. Generally, vessels with a diameter smaller than 3 mm are not suitable for stenting. The lesion is normally predilated with a slightly undersized balloon. The reason for underdilating is to prevent excessive disruption of the lesion before stent deployment. The balloon should then be removed, leaving the guide wire in place (using either a trapper device or an exchange-length guide wire). The stent is then placed on the balloon and crimped. This can either be done with a crimping device supplied by the manufacturer or, usually more satisfactorily, by hand. The balloon is inflated to 0.2 to 0.3 atm and then placed in the appropriate coronary artery and across the target lesion.

Great care should be taken to accurately place the stent. The stent is deployed with a single balloon inflation to a pressure necessary to ensure full, uniform balloon expansion (this usually takes 15 seconds). The balloon is deflated and withdrawn, leaving the guide wire across the lesion. A repeat angiogram should then be performed and, normally, the stented segment may be dilated with larger sized, preferably shorter, balloons at high pressure.

Before the procedure the patient should be prescribed aspirin. Throughout the procedure the patient should be given intravenous heparin to keep the activated clotting time greater than 300 seconds. If there is any indication of thrombus, either before or after stent deployment, intracoronary thrombolytic agents (usually urokinase) should be administered. After stent delivery intravenous dextran is often administered (50 mL/hr for 24 hours), although this is no longer considered mandatory. Once the patient returns to the unit the sheath should be removed when the activated clotting time is less than 180 seconds. After sheath removal hemostasis should be achieved with manual compression or with a groin clamp. In our institution the Femostop device has been employed with great success. It is our practice to leave the Femostop inflated at low pressure (30 to 40 mm Hg) for 4 to 6 hours. Until 1984 the following management was used in most institutions: Once hemostasis had been satisfactorily achieved (usually 2 hours after sheath removal), intravenous heparin was administered sufficient to keep the partial thromboplastin time between 80 and 100 seconds. Heparin infusion was continued for 5 days. On the same day the patient was commenced on warfarin. The patient was given sufficient warfarin to keep the prothrombin time greater than 16 seconds. The prothrombin time was maintained between 16 and 18 seconds for 3 months after stenting, at which point warfarin was discontinued. Dipyridamole, 75 mg three times daily, was also continued for 3 months and low-dose aspirin was continued indefinitely. Patients were also normally prescribed a calcium channel blocking agent for 3 months.

Most clinicians agree now that stent thrombosis is a function of the primary result. Therefore, no anticoagulation is deemed necessary after optimal stent placement. Ticlopidine has become popular in some countries.

Even with meticulous care of the access site, complications (including bleeding, pseudoaneurysms and hematomas) occur in approximately 8% to 10% of patients,[29] although our preliminary experience is that the complication rate is much lower if the Femostop device is used. In most studies there is a 2% to 6% risk of subacute closure (occurring after 24 hours after stent deployment). This complication is potentially life threatening, and there should be a low threshold to repeat coronary angiography, especially during the first 2 weeks after the procedure (although this should be balanced against the potential local complications associated with repeat angiography in fully anticoagulated patients). Treatment strategies include intracoronary thrombolysis, repeat PTCA, or bypass surgery. Intravenous thrombolytic therapy may be effective provided the femoral artery puncture site is secured with a Femostop. Most centers recommend repeat coronary arteriography 6 months after stenting, a stress test 1 month after the procedure, and a thallium stress test 3 months after the procedure.

INDICATIONS FOR STENTING

Unsatisfactory PTCA Result or Abrupt Closure

Stenting is the treatment of choice for abrupt closure after angioplasty in vessels of 3 mm or more in diameter.[30-34] When possible, the dissection should be covered completely; however, if the dissection is extensive, the entry site should be sealed. The temptation to deploy multiple stents should be resisted. Stent deployment for abrupt closure as a result of dissection after PTCA carries a higher restenosis rate than does primary stenting. In most studies this appears to be approximately 30%.[17, 35-38] It is likely that this high restenosis rate is the result of repeated trauma to the arterial wall by multiple balloon inflations. For this reason it is prudent to deploy the stent soon after the problem has been diagnosed. Subacute-closure rates are also higher in this group, and in some series the rate approaches 30%.[37, 38] The results of studies on stenting for acute closure are therefore disappointing. Several factors are likely to be responsible, including unnecessary delay in stent deployment, use of short stents, and implantation in arteries of less than 3 mm in diameter.

Restenosis After PTCA

In 1991 Schatz and colleagues[21] reviewed the first 213 patients with successfully implanted Palmaz-Schatz stents in native coronary arteries. The restenosis rate at 4 to 6 months was 20% in patients with single stents and 50% in patients with multiple stents. Clinical restenosis (requiring repeat PTCA or bypass surgery) oc-

curred in approximately half of the patients with angiographic restenosis.[19]

In another study,[39] 79 patients underwent successful implantations of a single Palmaz-Schatz stent. In approximately 30% of this group the main indication for stenting was restenosis after PTCA. At follow-up angiographic restenosis was observed in 15.2% of patients. The restenosis rate was highest in left anterior descending artery stents and lowest in right coronary artery stents.[39] Fewer data are available for the other types of stents, but restenosis rates of approximately 13% for the self-expanding Wallstent were documented.[9] The Wiktor and the Strecker stents were much less successful in this context.[14, 40, 41] In a recent study involving the Palmaz-Schatz stent a restenosis rate of 5.6% was quoted if the initial result after stenting was ideal.[42]

Two major randomized trials of primary stenting with the Palmaz-Schatz stent have been reported: the Benestent study in Europe[11] and the Stent Restenosis Study (STRESS trial) in the United States.[12] These trials are designed to assess hospital outcomes and the restenosis rate after primary stenting as compared with PTCA alone. All patients in these studies were investigated by quantitative angiography after 6 months. Based on these studies, it is clear that the results after primary stenting are significantly better than after PTCA alone. Patients with stents appear to have fewer repeat interventions and fewer in-hospital complications. However, stent patients stayed in the hospital longer and local complications were more frequent. In the Benestent trial,[11] the mean ($\pm$SD) minimal luminal diameters immediately after the procedure were 2.48 $\pm$ 0.39 mm in the stent group and 2.05 $\pm$ 0.33 mm in the angioplasty group; at follow-up angiography, the diameters were 1.82 $\pm$ 0.64 mm in the stent group and 1.73 $\pm$ 0.55 mm in the angioplasty group ($P = 0.09$). These values correspond to restenosis rates (diameter of stenosis, 50%) of 22% and 32%, respectively ($P = 0.02$). In the STRESS investigation,[12] patients who underwent stent placement had a higher rate of procedure success than those who underwent PTCA alone (96.1% vs. 89.6% respectively; $P = 0.011$), and a greater immediate increase in the luminal diameter (1.72 $\pm$ 0.46 vs. 1.23 $\pm$ 0.48 mm; $P<0.0001$). At 6 months' angiographic follow-up, the patients with stented lesions continued to have a larger luminal diameter (1.74 $\pm$ 0.60 vs. 1.56 $\pm$ 0.65 mm; $P = 0.007$) and a lower rate of restenosis (31.6% vs. 42.1%; $P = 0.046$) than those patients undergoing PTCA alone.

Saphenous Vein Graft Stenosis

Venous bypass grafts appear to be subject to complex pathologic changes. The grafts undergo fibrous proliferation, which can lead to the development of extremely rigid structures that are extremely hard to dilate.[43] Another significant problem is stenosis at the anastomotic site. Balloon angioplasty on venous conduits is associated with a high restenosis rate, particularly in the proximal and mid-portion (approximately 60%).[44] There is now considerable experience with the Palmaz-Schatz stent in this context. Leon and associates[45] reviewed the outcomes in 90 patients. The mean age of the venous grafts stented was 85 years; 59% of the patients had undergone previous PTCA of the lesion stented. Early angiographic follow-up (3 months after the procedure) demonstrated angiographic restenosis in only 17% of patients. In another multicenter trial the restenosis rate after primary stent insertion was as low as 14%.[46] Although this is higher than in native coronary arteries, it is a considerable improvement over PTCA alone. Stenting of ostial lesions appears to be particularly promising. Stenting in this context appears to have low complication and high success rates, although no definitive studies have been published. An example of the effects of stenting in saphenous vein grafts is shown in Figure 30–4.

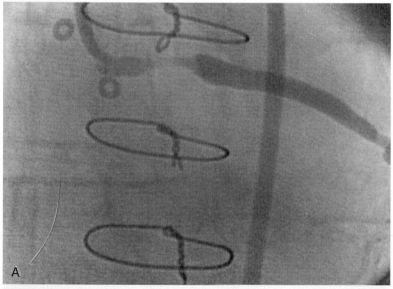

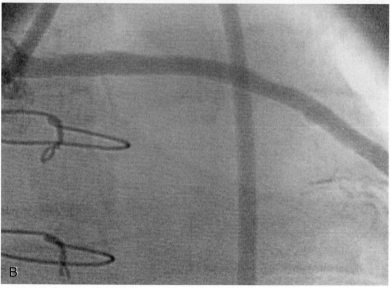

Figure 30–4. Stenting of vein grafts. Managing stenosis within saphenous vein grafts is a particularly challenging problem. Percutaneous transluminal coronary angioplasty is not too successful, but stent deployment is promising to be a useful technique. *A,* Before stent deployment. *B,* After stent placement. The figure shows an example of the excellent angiographic results that can be achieved with stents (in this instance, the self-expanding Wallstent). Whether these results can be translated into long-term clinical benefits to the patient remains to be proven.

CONCLUSION

Numerous angioplasty techniques are available, including atherectomy, lasers, and stenting. Of all these, stenting holds the most promise. Since the first deployment of a self-expanding stent in a human coronary artery in 1986, research has progressed and now stenting can be considered as a primary procedure in certain conditions. Of all the stents that have been tested over the last 9 years, the largest experience is with the Palmaz-Schatz stent. New stent designs under investigation are likely to improve outcomes still further. The next generation of stents is likely to incorporate chemical or cellular bonding of biologically active substances to facilitate continuous delivery of drugs to the defective vessel. Such drugs may include an anticoagulant or antiproliferative agent designed to overcome the problem of early stent thrombosis and later restenosis. Stents are likely to find an even greater role in the management of saphenous vein graft stenosis where the results of angioplasty are so disappointing.

REFERENCES

1. Ellis SG, Roubin GS, King SB, et al: In-hospital cardiac mortality after acute closure after coronary angioplasty: Analysis of risk factors from 8207 procedures. J Am Coll Cardiol 1988; 11:211–216.
2. Kaltenbach M, Kober G, Scherer D, Vallbracht C: Recurrence rate after successful coronary angioplasty. Eur Heart J 1985; 6:276–281.
3. Leimgruber PP, Roubin GS, Hollman J, et al: Restenosis after successful coronary angioplasty in patients with single-vessel disease. Circulation 1986; 73:710–717.
4. Dotter CT: Transluminally placed coil spring arterial tube grafts: Long-term patency in canine popliteal artery. Invest Radiol 1969; 4:329–332.
5. Mass D, Zollikofer CL, Largiader F, Senning A: Radiological follow-up of transluminally inserted vascular endoprostheses: An experimental study using expanding spirals. Radiology 1984; 152:639–663.
6. Gianturco C, Wright KC, Wallace S, et al: Percutaneous endovascular stents: An experimental evaluation. Radiology 1982; 156:169–172.
7. Palmaz JC, Windeler SAM, Garcia FM, et al: Atherosclerotic rabbit aortas: Expandable intraluminal grafting. Radiology 1986; 160:793–796.
8. Palmaz JC, Sibbitt RR, Reuter SR, et al: Expandable intraluminal graft: A preliminary study. Radiology 1985; 156:73–77.
9. Sigwart U, Puel J, Mirkovitch V, et al: Intravascular stents to prevent occlusion and restenosis after transluminal angioplasty. N Engl J Med 1987; 316:701–706.
10. Serruys PW, Strauss BH, Beatt KJ, et al: Angiographic follow-up after placement of a self-expanding coronary artery stent. N Engl J Med 1991; 324:13–17.
11. Serruys PW, de Jaegere P, Kiemeneij C: A comparison of balloon-expandable stent implantation with balloon angioplasty in patients with coronary artery disease. N Engl J Med 1994; 331:489–495.
12. Fischman DL, Leon MB, Baim DS: A randomized comparison of coronary stent placement and balloon angioplasty in the treatment of coronary artery disease. N Engl J Med 1994; 331:496–501.
13. Haren JA, King SB III, Douglas JS Jr, et al: Intracoronary stenting during percutaneous transluminal coronary angioplasty. Circulation 1990; 81(Suppl 4):92–100.
14. de Jaegere PP, Serruys PW, Bertrand M, et al: Wiktor stent implantation in patients with restenosis following balloon angioplasty of a native coronary artery. Am J Cardiol 1992; 69:598–602.
15. Sigwart U, Khosravi F, Virmani R, et al: Ein neuer: Balloon-expandierbarer, flexibler stent. Z Kardiol 1993; 71:219.
16. Fajadet J, Marco J, Cassagneau B, et al: Multiple intracoronary balloon expandable stent: Early experience. Eur Heart J 1990; 11:370.
17. Fajadet J, Marco J, Cassagneau B, et al: Coronary stenting with the Palmaz-Schatz stent: The Clinique Pasteur Interventional Cardiology Unit experience. In Sigwart U, Frank GI (eds): Coronary Stent. New York, Springer-Verlag, 1992, pp 57–77.
18. Nordrehaug JE, Priestley K, Rickards AF, et al: Simultaneous implantation of two Palmaz-Schatz stents mounted on a long angioplasty balloon. J Intervent Cardiol 1994; 7:161–164.
19. Zeiher A, Holnloser S, Fassbender S, et al: Intracoronary ultrasound morphology following interventional therapy in coronary heart disease. Eur Heart J 1992; 13:308.
20. George G, Erbel R, Ge T, et al: Intravascular ultrasound after stent implantation: Can stent recoil or compression occur? Eur Heart J 1992; 13:308.
21. Schatz RA, Baim DS, Leon M, et al: Clinical experience with the Palmaz-Schatz coronary stent: Initial results of a multicenter study. Circulation 1991; 83:148–161.
22. Baim DS, Bailey S, Curry C, et al: Improved success and safety of Palmaz-Schatz coronary stenting with a new delivery system [abstract]. Circulation 1990; 82(Suppl 3):657.
23. Stack RS, Quigley PJ, Collins G, Phillips HR: Perfusion balloon catheter. Am J Cardiol 1988; 61:77G–80G.
24. Whitlow P, Gaspard P, Kent K, et al: Improvement of coronary dissection with a removal flow support catheter. J Am Cardiol 1992; 19:217.
25. Mehan JK, Neal LE, Robert L, Hess JP, et al: Implantation and recovery of balloon-delivered removable stents. J Am Coll Cardiol 1992; 19:218a.
26. Schwartz RS, Murphy JG, Edwards WD, Holmes DR: Bioabsorbable, drug-eluting, intracoronary stents: Design and future applications. In Sigwart U, Frank GI (eds): Coronary Stents. New York, Springer-Verlag, 1992, pp 135–154.
27. Gammon RS, Chapman GD, Bauman RP, Stack RS: Bioabsorbable endovascular stent prostheses. In Sigwart U, Frank GI (eds): Coronary Stents. New York, Springer-Verlag, 1992, pp 155–167.
28. van der Giessen WJ, Slager CJ, van Beusekom HM, et al: Development of a polymer endovascular prosthesis and its implantation in porcine arteries. J Intervent Cardiol 1992; 5:175–185.
29. Levine MJ, Leonard BM, Burke JA, et al: Clinical and angiographic results of balloon-expandable intracoronary stents in right coronary artery stenoses. J Am Coll Cardiol 1990; 16:332–339.
30. Sigwart U, Urban P, Golf S, et al: Emergency stenting for acute occlusion after coronary balloon angioplasty. Circulation 1988; 72:1121–1127.
31. Strauss BH, Serruys PW, Bertrand ME, et al: Quantitative angiographic follow-up of the coronary Wallstent in native vessels and bypass grafts: The evolving European

experience from March 1986 to March 1990. Am J Cardiol 1992; 69:475–481.

32. Roubin GS, Cannon AD, Agraval SK, et al: Intracoronary stenting for acute and threatened closure complicating percutaneous transluminal coronary angioplasty. Circulation 1992; 85:916–927.

33. Goy JJ, Sigwart U, Vogt P, et al: Long-term clinical and angiographic follow-up of patients treated with the self-expanding coronary stent for acute occlusion during balloon angioplasty of the right coronary artery. J Am Coll Cardiol 1992; 19;1593–1596.

34. Satler LF, Leon MB, Kent KM, Pichard AD: Strategies for acute occlusion after coronary angioplasty [editorial]. J Am Coll Cardiol 1992; 19:936–938.

35. Roubin GS, Pinkerton CA: Gianturco-Roubin stent: Development and investigation. *In* Sigwart U, Frank GI (eds): Coronary Stents. New York, Springer-Verlag, 1992, pp 79–99.

36. Haude M, Erbel R, Straub U, et al: Results of intracoronary stents for management of coronary dissection after balloon angioplasty. J Am Coll Cardiol 1991; 67:691–696.

37. Urban P, Sigwart U: The self-expanding mesh stent. *In* Sigwart U, Frank GI (eds): Coronary Stents. New York, Springer-Verlag, 1992, pp 21–44.

38. Schatz RA, Goldberg S, Leon M: Coronary stenting following suboptimal coronary angioplasty results [abstract]. Circulation 1990; 82(Suppl 3):III-540.

39. Fajadet JC, Marco J, Cassagneau BG, et al: Restenosis following successful single Palmaz-Schatz stent implantation [abstract]. Circulation 1990; 82(Suppl 3):314.

40. Beytien C, Terres W, Kupper W, Hamm C: In vitro model to test the thrombogenicity of coronary stents. Eur Heart J 1992; 13:266.

41. Geschwind H, Nakamura F, Kvasnicka J, et al: Coronary Strecker stent: Does it look promising? Angiology 1992; 43:272–273.

42. Ellis S, Savage M, Fischman D, et al: Restenosis after placement of Palmaz-Schatz stent in native coronary arteries: Initial results of a multicenter experience. Circulation 1992; 86:1836–1844.

43. Kalan JM, Roberts CW: Morphologic findings in saphenous veins used as coronary arterial bypass conduits for longer than 1 year: Necropsy analysis of 53 patients 123 saphenous veins and 1865 5-mm segments of veins. *In* Yacoub M, Pepper JR (eds): Annals of Cardiac Surgery. Philadelphia, Current Science, 1992, p 152.

44. Kussmaul WG: Percutaneous angioplasty of coronary bypass grafts: An emerging consensus. Cathet Cardiovasc Diag 1988; 15:1–4

45. Leon MB, Pichard AD, Baim DS, et al: Early results of stent implantation in aortocoronary saphenous vein grafts. Circulation 1990; 82(Suppl 3):679.

46. Leon MB, Ellis SG, Pichard AD, et al: Stents may be the preferred treatment for focal aortocoronary vein graft disease. Circulation 1991; 84(Suppl 4):II-249.

Chapter 31

Supported Circulation in the Cardiac Catheterization Laboratory

BRIAN E. JASKI
KELLY R. BRANCH

Every body continues in its state of rest, or of uniform motion . . . unless it is compelled to change that state by forces acting upon it.

SIR ISAAC NEWTON, 1687

OVERVIEW

The heart functions as a circulatory pump by conversion of biochemical energy to pressure-volume work through oxidative phosphorylation and utilization of adenosine triphosphate by actin and myosin. Inadequate delivery of oxygen to the heart and other vital organs can initiate a downhill spiral of organ dysfunction, tissue necrosis, and death. When primary cardiac dysfunction results in hemodynamic compromise, myocardial reserve can be recruited through endogenous or exogenous inotropic stimulation but at the potential cost of myocardial ischemia. Mechanical support devices supplement myocardial biochemical reserve with hydraulic energy derived from external electrical sources (Fig. 31–1). This chapter emphasizes the relative benefits and risks of these mechanical support devices that are rapidly evolving to maintain the circulation, reduce left ventricular ischemia, or both during diagnostic and therapeutic interventions in the cardiac catheterization laboratory.

Mechanical cardiovascular support in the form of cardiopulmonary bypass was initially developed for the cardiac surgery operating room more than 4 decades ago. Currently, mechanical circulatory support devices can be placed in the cardiac catheterization laboratory with percutaneous techniques facilitated by ra-diographic guidance (Table 31–1). After the clinical success in resuscitation of patients with acute hemodynamic compromise, use of mechanical support devices was extended to standby or prophylactic applications during high-risk catheterization procedures (Fig. 31–2). In the future, cardiac catheterization evaluation of patients with chronically implanted ventricular assist devices (VADs) or total artificial hearts may also be important.

History

Initially conceived for patients with acute pulmonary embolism, cardiopulmonary bypass was first successfully applied by Gibbon in 1953.[1] Blood was oxygenated outside the body and flow was maintained with roller-type pumps (termed *extracorporeal circulation*) during an operation to correct a congenital atrial septal defect. Kirklin and associates[2] continued this research to create a design for the operating room similar to current portable models. At present, rapid percutaneous institution of cardiopulmonary support (CPS) can be initiated in almost any part of the acute care hospital.

The need for rapidly instituted and less-invasive support devices for acute heart failure in the 1960s spawned development of the intra-aortic balloon pump (IABP). The first counter-pulsatile device by Clauss and colleagues[3] decreased systolic aortic pressure and left ventricular afterload through the rapid removal of aortic blood to an external console. Blood was pumped back to the aorta during diastole to increase total cardiac output. Although conceptually sound, blood handling limited sustained support. Based on this concept, the first IABP was developed and tested in dogs in 1962 by Dr. Willem Kolff at the Cleveland Clinic.[4]

A

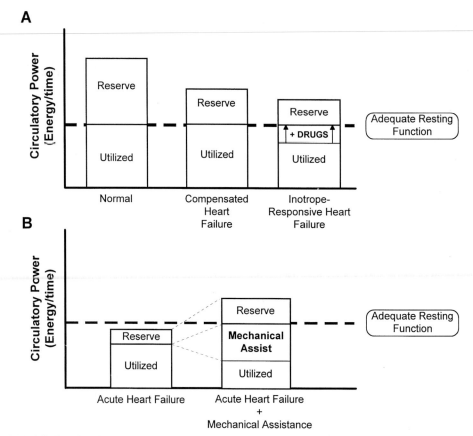

B

Figure 31–1. Model of cardiac function in patients without cardiac dysfunction compared with compensated and decompensated heart failure. Circulatory power can be considered a measure of both utilized and potential reserve left ventricular function delivered to the systemic circulation under ideal loading conditions. *A,* Compensated heart failure, compared with normal cardiac function, reveals a decreased circulatory reserve. Inotropic stimulation of the heart may recruit additional myocardial reserve for maintaining adequate function but at the potential risk of increased myocardial ischemia or ventricular arrhythmias. *B,* Acute heart failure decreases left ventricular reserve below an adequate resting level. Mechanical assistance increases total circulatory function to allow (1) maintenance of adequate circulatory function; (2) a decrease in utilized cardiac function; and (3) an increase in cardiac reserve.

Kantrowitz and colleagues,[5] using a single-lumen balloon and a femoral cutdown for insertion, successfully resuscitated two patients in cardiogenic shock after acute myocardial infarction in 1968. Subsequent clinical pathologic studies by Page and colleagues[6] in patients undergoing autopsy after fatal myocardial infarction correlated death due to cardiogenic shock with the amount of loss of viable myocardium. These findings encouraged the application of mechanical support in acute myocardial infarction to salvage myocardium and improve prognosis. Design changes led to the multiple-lumen polyurethane balloon and percutaneous insertion technique accompanied by improved patient hemodynamic monitoring and pediatric use. Recently, two investigational devices that target more specific levels of support for either acute myocardial ischemia (synchronized coronary sinus retroperfusion [SRP]) or profound left ventricular failure (Hemopump) have been evaluated (see Table 31–1).

Patients with sustained, profound cardiac damage require devices capable of high flows and long-term circulatory support. The first total artificial heart used clinically was developed at Baylor School of Medicine and was used by Dr. Denton Cooley as a bridge to transplantation in 1970.[7] The Jarvik-7 heart was developed as a permanent heart replacement device by Dr. William DeVries and coworkers and was used for 61 days in 1982.[8] However, thromboembolic complications, infections, and poor data reporting to the Food and Drug Administration (FDA) limited the use of the device even as a short-term bridge to transplantation and ultimately led to its removal from clinical trials. Research development continues on prototypes of totally implanted total artificial hearts.

VADs were first applied in 1971 as a tempo-

Table 31–1. **Percutaneous Mechanical Devices for Use in the Cardiac Catheterization Laboratory**

Device	Access	Size	Features	Duration
Intra-aortic balloon pump	Femoral artery	*Sheath:* 11.5–12.5 French *Catheter:* 9.5–10 French	↓ Myocardial oxygen demand ↑ Coronary and peripheral perfusion Relative ease of placement and low incidence of vascular complications Limited in presence of tachyarrhythmias	1 month +
Cardiopulmonary support	*Arterial:* Femoral artery *Venous:* Femoral vein Internal jugular vein	*Arterial:* 15–21 French *Venous:* 18–21 French	Capable of total circulatory support without stable ECG or residual LV function ↓ Myocardial oxygen demand Large catheter size ↑ vascular complications Abrupt closure: needs autoperfusion catheter/ stent to protect myocardium	3 days +
Synchronized coronary sinus retroperfusion	Internal jugular vein and femoral artery	*Arterial:* 8 French *Venous:* 8.5 French	Able to perfuse myocardium despite total coronary artery occlusion or PTCA inflation May improve drug delivery to myocardium Perfusion specific for LAD distribution Not commercially available	During procedure only
Hemopump	Femoral artery	*Sheath:* 14 French	Total LV support independent of cardiac rhythm or LV function No data with percutaneous (14-French) device Investigational	1 week +

LV, left ventricular; ECG, electrocardiogram; PTCA, percutaneous transluminal coronary angioplasty; LAD, left anterior descending.

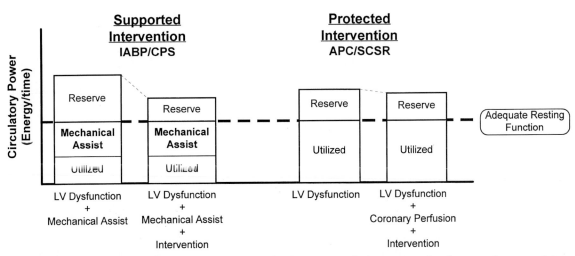

Figure 31–2. Effects of percutaneous revascularization on circulatory power during supported and protected coronary interventions. *Supported Intervention:* Mechanical assistance maintains adequate function during interventions that may compromise the myocardial contribution to total systemic circulatory reserve. *Protected Intervention:* The device does not directly support the systemic circulation but may protect the myocardium from ischemic insult and associated reductions in cardiac function due to acute ischemia. IABP, intra-aortic balloon pump; CPS, cardiopulmonary support; APC, autoperfusion catheter; SCSR, synchronized coronary sinus retroperfusion.

rary extracorporeal assist to native cardiac output in patients with acute cardiogenic shock with little or no residual cardiac function after cardiac surgery.[9] Newer implanted designs have lower thromboembolic risks and allow extended VAD support. Patients can participate in exercise rehabilitation after left VAD (LVAD) implantation during cardiac recovery or as a bridge to transplantation.[10, 11] These designs have supported patients for 500 days or longer and may be available for permanent implantation in the future.[12]

CONSIDERATION OF MECHANICAL SUPPORT

The need for mechanical circulatory assistance is based on a clinical and hemodynamic profile of cardiac failure that depends on the cause of cardiac failure as well as the pace of hemodynamic deterioration. In the cardiac catheterization laboratory, mechanical support may be indicated for anticipated risk associated with a diagnostic or therapeutic intervention as well as manifest cardiac decompensation (see Figs. 31–1 and 31–2).

Within 6 seconds after the onset of a coronary artery balloon occlusion, regional myocardial contraction may become biphasic with premature systolic relaxation associated with decreases in measures of global left ventricular contractility, including peak positive maximum rate of tension development and maximum consumption.[13] By 40 seconds, regional myocardial motion may exhibit pansystolic dyskinesis associated with decreased peak systolic and increased end-diastolic left ventricular pressures.[13, 14] When a coronary intervention results in a significant portion of the myocardium being dysfunctional either from ischemia or previous infarction, marked chest discomfort, profound hypotension, or life-threatening arrhythmias

may result even though the ischemic insult is "reversible." Newer niche devices such as directional atherectomy and coronary stenting can be associated with increased myocardial ischemia as a result of increased catheter size and device-specific potential for vessel luminal occlusion.[15, 16]

When acute hemodynamic instability is present, use of the IABP, CPS, or other assist device should be considered an adjunct to volume repletion, vasodilatory, and inotropic therapy. Because of the potential for increasing myocardial oxygen consumption ($M\dot{V}O_2$) with inotropic stimulation, mechanical assistance may allow increased salvage of myocardium. Algorithms for pharmacologic and mechanical support for patient resuscitation are shown in Figures 31–3 and 31–4. Contemporary indications and contraindications for IABP and CPS are detailed in Table 31–2.

INTRA-AORTIC BALLOON PUMP

Theory

Coincident with cardiac diastole, IABP inflation displaces blood volume within the aorta to increase total systemic and myocardial blood flow. Systolic compression of coronary resistance vessels leads to a normal ratio of resting diastolic to systolic coronary blood flow of approximately 6:1.[17] Augmentation of diastolic coronary perfusion pressure specifically improves depressed myocardial oxygen delivery during the phase of the cardiac cycle when coronary vascular impedance is low. Deflation of the balloon during systole diminishes total aortic volume, thereby decreasing left ventricular afterload and $M\dot{V}O_2$. Improvement in the myocardial demand to delivery ratio may enhance left ventricular viability and performance (Fig. 31–5).

EFFECTS OF IABP ON HEMODYNAMICS. IABP support has been shown to reduce myocardial oxy-

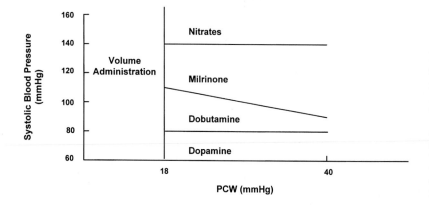

Figure 31–3. Example of approach to pharmacologic intervention for patients with acute hemodynamic compromise. Intravascular depletion should be considered initially in all patients. Greater potential myocardial ischemia and ventricular arrythmias may be anticipated when greater inotropic stimulation is necessary to maintain adequate circulatory flow and arterial pressure.

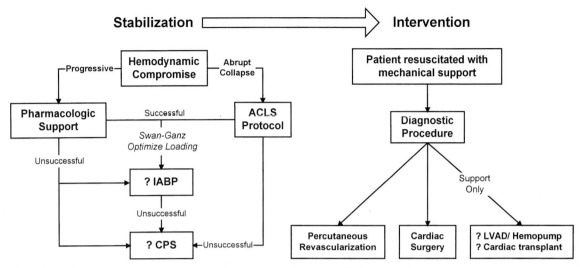

Figure 31–4. Example of emergent mechanical assistance algorithm. *Stabilization:* Etiology and rate of acute hemodynamic compromise determines whether initial treatment is with conventional intravenous therapy or with ACLS protocol. Patients refractory to initial pharmacologic therapies should be considered for CPS. *Intervention:* After resuscitation and stabilization, diagnostic and therapeutic procedures can then be performed. ACLS, advanced cardiac life support; CPS, cardiopulmonary support; IABP, intra-aortic balloon pump; LVAD, left ventricular assist device.

gen demand in ischemic myocardium.[4, 18–20] Studies of IABP patients have confirmed decreases in systolic blood pressure and increases in diastolic pressure during balloon pumping.[19–22] Increased total cardiac output and decreased myocardial lactate production are consistent with an improved cardiac oxygen balance and a return of the myocardium to aerobic metabolism.[21]

EFFECTS OF IABP ON CORONARY BLOOD FLOW. Reports of changes in coronary blood flow during IABP support are variable but are probably dependent on the subgroup of patients studied. In patients with cardiogenic shock, diastolic augmentation may increase total blood flow to the myocardium and improve oxygen delivery to the left ventricle.[23]

Coronary flow in patients with unstable an-

Table 31–2. Indications and Contraindications for IABP and CPS

Device	Indications	Contraindications
IABP	Cardiogenic shock despite inotropic therapy	Aortic aneurysms or dissection
	Elective interventional use	Aortic valve insufficiency
	High-Risk PTCA with LVEF <30%	Obstructive peripheral vascular disease
	High-risk PTCA of "protected" left main coronary or only	Inability to insert cannulas
	patent vessel	Wire may assist placement into aorta
	Urgent PTCA in acute myocardial infarction with LVEF <30%	Unstable cardiac rhythm
	Acute myocardial infarction complicated by mitral regurgitation	Little or no native cardiac output
	or ventricular septal defect	
	Acute myocarditis associated with shock	
CPS	Cardiogenic shock despite IABP and inotropes	No correctable pathology
	Cardiac arrest	Unwitnessed arrest, prolonged CPR
	Elective interventional use	Severe aortic insufficiency
	CPS on standby ± primed	Obstructive peripheral vascular disease
	PTCA with LVEF <30% and/or target vessels supplying 50%	Inability to insert cannulas
	of remaining viable myocardium	Contraindications to percutaneous insertion
	PTCA of only patent vessel	Bleeding diathesis
	Valvuloplasty with LVEF <25%	Severe obesity
	Prophylactic CPS	
	PTCA with LVEF <20%	
	Hemodynamic instability during coronary intervention	
	despite IABP	

IABP, intra-aortic balloon pump; CPS, cardiopulmonary support; PTCA, percutaneous transluminal coronary angioplasty; LVEF, left ventricular ejection fraction; CPR, cardiopulmonary resuscitation.

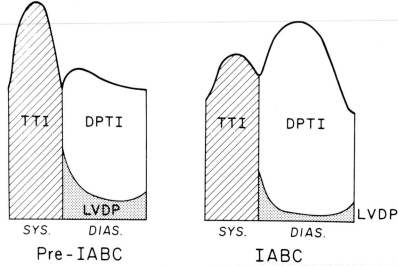

Figure 31–5. During cardiogenic shock, IABC decreases TTI, a measure of myocardial oxygen consumption, and augments DPTI. The endocardial viability ratio (DPTI/TTI) and the coronary perfusion gradient (DPTI/LVDP) are increased with IABC consistent with diminished myocardial oxygen demand and improved oxygen supply. TTI, tension-time index; DPTI, diastolic pressure-time index; IABC, intra-aortic balloon counterpulsation; LVDP, left ventricular diastolic pressure; SYS, systolic; DIAS, diastolic. (From Amsterdam EA, Awan NA, Lee G, et al: Intra-aortic balloon counterpulsation: Rationale, application, and results. *In* Rackley CE [ed]: Critical Care Cardiology. Philadelphia, FA Davis, 1981.)

gina without cardiogenic shock measured by coronary sinus thermodilution techniques increased in one study[24] but decreased slightly in another,[20] despite increased diastolic pressures with balloon counterpulsation. In similar patients with severe coronary disease, total coronary flow measured by radionuclide washout[22] decreased, whereas Doppler guide wire velocity[25] and coronary pressure measurements distal to the lesion site[26] did not change significantly with initiation of intra-aortic balloon counterpulsation. Kern and associates[25] found that coronary blood velocity past critical stenoses (mean 95% stenosis) increased significantly with IABP support only after percutaneous transluminal coronary angioplasty (PTCA) dilation of the artery.

EFFECTS OF IABP WITH COMPLETE CORONARY OCCLUSION. Laas and colleagues,[27] in an experimental pig model of acute myocardial infarction, instituted IABP pumping after 1 hour of left anterior descending coronary artery ligation. Although mean arterial pressure (MAP) and cardiac output both increased with balloon pumping, nitroblue tetrazolium staining of the infarct area did not differ significantly from controls, suggesting no change in oxygen availability to regions supplied by an occluded artery. Thus, patients with total occlusion of an infarct-related artery without established collateral circulation may not achieve myocardial salvage from IABP without revascularization.

SUMMARY OF IABP SUPPORT AND CORONARY BLOOD FLOW. Generally, increased diastolic coro-

nary perfusion pressure during IABP support may be expected to increase blood flow to the myocardium unless either (1) coronary vascular autoregulation increases coronary vascular resistance secondary to decreased myocardial oxygen demand or (2) total vessel occlusion is present with little collateralization. In patients without cardiogenic shock, the beneficial effects of IABP on the myocardium seem to be primarily related to left ventricular unloading rather than augmentation of coronary flow.

Technique (Table 31–3)

INSERTION. In the cardiac catheterization laboratory, IABP support is initiated by percutaneous catheter insertion using fluoroscopic guidance. From the femoral artery, a J-type 0.032-inch guide wire is inserted into the abdominal aorta. An 8-French sheath or dilator is

Table 31–3. **Technique for Insertion of Intra-aortic Balloon Pump**

1. Percutaneous access into femoral artery
2. Insert J-type 0.032-inch guide wire into abdominal aorta
3. Place 8-French dilator and exchange for 11.5–12.5-French introducer sheath over wire
4. Insert balloon and, using fluoroscopic guidance, advance balloon and wire to aorta, just distal to left subclavian artery (third intercostal space)
5. Administer heparin
6. Start balloon counterpulsation

initially placed and then exchanged for a 12-French balloon introducer sheath. If placement of the wire is difficult, the balloon catheter is advanced over the guide wire into the abdominal aorta. Otherwise, the wire is removed and the wire and balloon are advanced up the aorta to a level just distal to the left subclavian artery (third intercostal space) where the position is checked by fluoroscopy. Generally, balloon pumping is initiated with either intravenous heparin or dextran administered.

OPERATION AND MONITORING. During diastole, the console pumps helium or carbon dioxide into the balloon through intraluminal holes in the catheter. The balloon gas is then actively drawn out into the console just before systole. The rate of gas evacuation differs by manufacturer and catheter size but determines the maximal output for an IABP at higher heart rates.

Adjustment of the IABP to inflate throughout cardiac diastole (counterpulsation) is important to obtain maximal hemodynamic benefit.[28] The console initiates inflation after a manually or electronically determined interval after the occurrence of the electrocardiographic R wave or arterial pressure peak. Depending on the type of console, deflation can occur either at the onset of the next R wave (real timing) or after an operator-set or electronically calculated interval after the onset of balloon inflation (conventional timing). Because the interval between electrical (QRS complex) and mechanical events (e.g., aortic valve opening) varies little with changes in heart rate or rhythm, newer designs use real timing to permit correct deflation and inflation independent of heart rate or operator manipulation. Real timing may also operate effectively with irregular cardiac rhythms having an identifiable R wave (e.g., atrial fibrillation and premature ventricular contractions).[29] Real timing, however, can be mechanically limited by the ability of the console to evacuate the balloon gas before aortic ejection to prevent balloon obstruction to aortic outflow. A comprehensive review of IABP timing is provided by Quaal.[28]

REMOVAL. After a successful procedure with elective balloon support, the balloon and sheath are typically pulled 4 hours after anticoagulation has been discontinued. After high-risk PTCA, the balloon pump can be pulled with the use of a mechanical compression device such as the Femostop to sustain femoral pressure without discontinuation of heparin. In patients with persistent cardiogenic shock after the procedure, weaning should be attempted only when the clinical appearance of the patient is satisfactory and evidence of the low-output syndrome no longer persists using clinical criteria.[30] Patients who deteriorate hemodynamically with attempts to wean off the pump suggest balloon dependency and may require further procedures, including additional revascularization, or VAD placement.

Indications (see Table 31–2)

CARDIOGENIC SHOCK. Multiple authors have suggested quantitative guidelines to define an impaired circulatory state requiring an IABP.[31–34] Among these are a "shock box" by Bolooki where indications are categorized by comparing stroke work index* and PCWP[35] or use of a hemodynamic diagram with systolic blood pressure and PCWP in the setting of a low-output state similar to Figure 31–3. Both are analogous suggesting generally that patients on inotropes with clinical low-output syndrome despite adequate or elevated left heart filling pressures and a low arterial pressure may benefit from IABP support.

An early multicenter study[21] in 1973 of 87 patients with cardiogenic shock secondary to acute myocardial infarction supported with IABP reported an acute survival of 40% during balloon assistance; 17% survived to be discharged. The poor survival was probably the result of patient selection and late institution of support, as well as inexperience with this early design. A more recent, larger experience with the IABP found that 83% of patients survived hospitalization when applied with an intervention during a multicenter trial of 84 patients with cardiogenic shock.[36] Early institution of IABP support, greater experience with the device, and aggressive interventions rather than medical therapy alone during hemodynamic collapse probably contributed to higher survival. Other studies have revealed similar survival rates ranging from 60% to 100%.[37–41]

ELECTIVE USE OF IABP IN THE SETTING OF HIGH-RISK ANGIOPLASTY. Although widely used, the indications for IABP prophylactic support as an adjunct for patients undergoing PTCA are not definite. Szatmary and coworkers[42] first successfully supported 16 "high-risk" PTCA patients with unstable angina complicated by hypotension (systolic pressure <100 mm Hg) or poor left ventricular function (left ventricular

---

*(MAP – PCWP) · (stroke volume ÷ BSA), where MAP is mean arterial pressure, PCWP is pulmonary capillary wedge pressure, and BSA is body surface area.

ejection fraction [LVEF] <40%), or both. PTCA success was 96%. Other studies have reported 90%[43] and 100%[44] PTCA success rates in patients with poor ventricular function (LVEF <40%) or with multivessel disease, including those where multiple vessel dilations were necessary.

In a recent study by Kahn and associates,[40] prophylactic IABP support was instituted for high-risk angioplasty in 28 patients with a mean ejection fraction of 24%. Multivessel angioplasty was performed in 21 patients and a 96% PTCA dilation success rate was obtained with no deaths or infarctions within 72 hours. Although the retrospective study lacked a set protocol for patient selection, the authors suggest that patients with an LVEF of less than 30% or undergoing PTCA of either the only patent vessel or the left main coronary artery may benefit from IABP. The authors proposed that a randomized study of PTCA with prophylactic IABP or CPS may be useful in better defining the role of different methods of supported angioplasty. Thus, acute ischemia, multivessel disease, and left ventricular function may indicate a need for IABP insertion, although the degree of left ventricular dysfunction that suggests IABP insertion over CPS is not defined. Our practice is to consider prophylactic IABP placement before coronary intervention when there is a recent clinical history of heart failure associated with multivessel disease, or an LVEF of less than 30%.

IABP USE WITH ACUTE MYOCARDIAL INFARCTION. During acute myocardial infarction PTCA, patient stability may also be facilitated by IABP placement when the ejection fraction is less than 30%.[40] In acute myocardial infarction patients undergoing immediate or rescue PTCA after either tissue plasminogen activator[39] or intracoronary urokinase[39, 41] thrombolytic therapy, emergent placement of the balloon pump was associated with a lower incidence of subsequent subacute closure of the vessel (2.4% and 5%, respectively) compared with patients without IABP support (17.7% and 13%, respectively). A trend toward improvement in global left ventricular function in patients treated with IABP was seen in one study.[41] At this time, a prospective, randomized trial is in progress (Primary Angioplasty in Myocardial Infarction Study, Part II) to better define the role of IABP-supported PTCA patients with acute myocardial infarction.

IABP USE DURING HEMODYNAMIC COMPROMISE SECONDARY TO MITRAL REGURGITATION OR VENTRICULAR SEPTAL DEFECT. For patients with acute myocardial infarction complicated by mitral regurgi-

tation or ventricular septal defect, IABP provides at least transient hemodynamic improvement and has been used as a bridge to surgical intervention. During cardiac systole, IABP deflation decreases aortic volume and pressure to decrease aortic impedance. This increases left ventricular ejection into the aorta rather than retrograde to the left atrium with mitral regurgitation or shunting to the right ventricle with septal defects. The optimal timing of surgical repair of an infarct-related ventricular septal defect after placement of an IABP has remained controversial, although the results of a series with surgical intervention immediately after IABP placement and cardiac catheterization evaluation have yielded encouraging survival outcomes.[45]

ACUTE MYOCARDITIS. Catheterization is often necessary in suspected acute myocarditis to exclude contributing coronary artery disease as well as to document the histologic presence of myocarditis with endomyocardial biopsy. Ventricular failure associated with acute myocarditis may be refractory to pharmacologic therapy but responsive and reversible after stabilization with IABP placement.[46] Indeed, with an acute onset of idiopathic heart failure, even in the absence of biopsy evidence of active myocarditis, sustained ventricular mechanical support may be associated with ventricular recovery and obviate the need for urgent cardiac transplant.[47]

LIMITATIONS OF IABP COUNTERPULSATION. Because of the relatively low contribution of the device to cardiac output,[21] successful intra-aortic balloon support requires residual cardiac function to maintain tissue oxygen delivery. Patients with profound low output and little recruitable cardiac reserve may not increase total cardiac output to levels consistent with adequate tissue perfusion.

Because the console identifies electrocardiographic or arterial pressure peaks as signals to deflate the balloon, irregular rhythms such as rapid atrial fibrillation and recurrent high-grade ventricular ectopy may inhibit optimal synchronization and limit adequate balloon pump function. Patients after a cardiac arrest have responded poorly to IABP assistance,[36, 48] requiring resuscitation with cardiopulmonary bypass in one report of IABP-supported patients.[48]

Contraindications and Complications

Contraindications for IABP insertion are listed in Table 31-2. Significant aortic aneurysms and dissections are contraindications because of an increased risk of aortic rupture. Marked aortic valve insufficiency is also a contraindication because increased diastolic pressure during balloon inflation may increase reflux into the left ventricle.

Recent (<48 hours) treatment with intravenous thrombolytics should be considered a relative contraindication, as for any percutaneous procedure. In a study with patients given intravenous thrombolytic therapy for acute myocardial infarction,[39] a substantial increase in bleeding complications was associated with IABP insertion (59% with IABP vs. 17% without IABP support). Thrombolytic therapy should not prevent insertion, however, if appropriate hemodynamic conditions are present.

Institution of the device in patients with peripheral vascular disease is a relative contraindication because catheter insertion may be impossible. Calcified arterial lesions may damage the integrity of the balloon, causing it to fail during support, or the large sheath size may inhibit distal blood flow to the leg. Complications with contemporary intra-aortic balloon insertion have been reduced compared with early designs,[21, 49, 50] although the incidence of peripheral vascular morbidity and leg ischemia with percutaneous insertion still ranges from 11% to 21%.[37-40] Thus, leg ischemia remains the primary complication of IABP support. In reports with percutaneous IABP insertion, strong predictors of leg ischemia include peripheral vascular disease[38, 39, 40, 51]; smoking[37]; diabetes[38]; and female gender,[51] presumably as a result of smaller leg vessel diameters. In patients at high risk for ischemia, performance of iliofemoral contrast angiography before IABP insertion may assist in the decision to initiate IABP counterpulsation and may be used to guide insertion site selection and aortic wire placement.

CARDIOPULMONARY SUPPORT

Theory

A portable extracorporeal life support system (ECLS) (Fig. 31–6) comprised of a pump, heat exchanger, and an oxygenator is analogous in design to the heart-lung machine used during open heart surgery. Deoxygenated blood flows from the venous circulation through a polyvinylchloride (PVC) cannula and tubing to an external centrifugal pump mounted on the CPS cart. Blood enters the apex of the pump where smooth-surfaced, internal rotating cones trans-

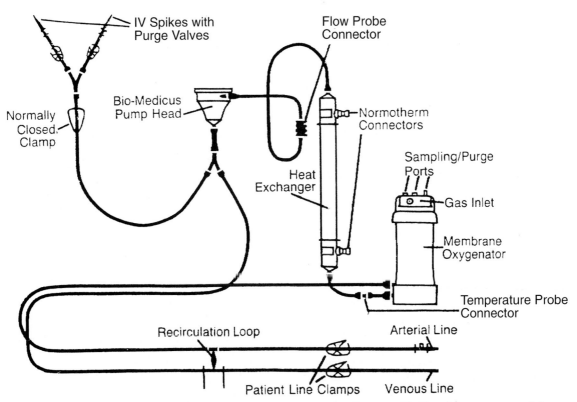

Figure 31–6. Schematic diagram of cardiopulmonary support circuit. (From Tommaso CL: Use of the percutaneously inserted cardiopulmonary bypass in the cardiac catheterization laboratory. Cathet Cardiovasc Diagn 1990; 20:32–38.)

fer centrifugal energy to the blood to force it outward at increased speeds. The accelerated blood is allowed to "escape" at the widest part of the pump while blood is drawn in at the apex of the spinning cones to replace the expelled volume.

The accelerated blood passes through a heat exchanger where the blood is warmed to physiologic temperatures by circulating water and an electromagnetic flow probe estimates total CPS output. The blood then passes into a membrane oxygenator for gas exchange. Oxygen circulating through hollow fibers diffuses across a large membrane surface area and is exchanged for carbon dioxide in the passing blood. Blood exiting the membrane oxygenator circulates to the arterial cannula and returns to the patient's arterial circulation.

EFFECTS OF CPS ON REGIONAL MYOCARDIAL FUNCTION. In a study of 20 CPS-supported patients by Pavlides and colleagues,[52] echocardiographic wall motion in myocardial regions supplied by stenotic vessels worsened after initiation of cardiopulmonary bypass despite reductions in determinants of global MVO_2 and increased mean diastolic coronary perfusion pressure. Possible explanations for this paradoxical finding include an observed reduction in oxygen-carrying capacity of blood (hematocrit decreased from 41.4% to 27.9% secondary to hemodilution) or to the release of vasoactive substances by cardiopulmonary bypass that could lead to coronary steal. Furthermore, during transient balloon coronary occlusion, CPS has not been found to blunt the rate of ischemic wall motion changes.[53] Thus, when CPS is required for bailout of ischemic hemodynamic collapse, restoration of compromised regional blood flow through use of an autoperfusion catheter or stent should still be attempted to limit irreversible myonecrosis if surgical myocardial revascularization may be delayed (e.g., redo sternotomy). Additional options to contribute to myocardial salvage on CPS include cooling of the patient, retrograde coronary sinus perfusion of arterial blood, or pharmacologic β-blockade.

Rapidly applied venoarterial bypass using CPS lowers the systemic venous pressure while increasing systemic arterial pressure. In patients with preserved transpulmonary flow, aortic insufficiency, or significant bronchial flow, the compromised left ventricle may become distended as a result of increased left ventricular volume and higher afterload. IABP counterpulsation may provide pulsatile flow to diminish left ventricular afterload and ameliorate this potential problem.[54]

Technique (Table 31–4)

INSERTION. Before elective or emergent CPS institution, a team trained in the use of CPS must be assembled and include a cardiologist for insertion of the cannulas and Swan-Ganz monitoring, a perfusionist or a clinician trained in CPS operation, and possibly an anesthesiologist for potential intubation. Peripheral pulses should be checked in both legs according to standard catheterization preparation.

Commercially available systems include the portable Bard CPS system (C. R. Bard, Inc., Billerica, MA) and the Medtronic system (Medtronic, Inc., Prairie, MN) . In our center, Carmeda heparin-bonded PVC cannulas (15- to 21-French arterial, 21-French venous; Medtronic, Inc.) are primarily used. For patients who require jugular venous cannula insertion, the 15-French arterial cannula may be used. Traditionally, PVC cannulas and tubing without bonded anticoagulants have been used successfully (18- to 20-French; Bard, Inc.) and are still standard for most portable CPS systems.

In the cardiac catheterization laboratory, vascular access should be through the femoral artery and vein. Insertion of a short cannula through the right internal jugular vein may be

Table 31–4. **Technique for Insertion of Cardiopulmonary Support**

1. Swan-Ganz catheter insertion should precede or follow CPS insertion for right heart hemodynamic monitoring
2. Place CPS cannulas, tubing, and oxygenator on patient to allow easy access
3. Percutaneous access into femoral artery and femoral or internal jugular vein
4. Perform contrast angiography (8 mL/sec for 20 mL total) at bifurcation of aorta for visualization of best arterial cannula site for elective use
5. Dilate femoral artery with either successive sheath insertion (8-French → 14-French → 17–20-French cannula) or direct exchange for arterial cannula. Have assistant apply gentle back-and-forth motion of guide wire to detect kinking of wire during cannula placement
6. Insert 0.038-inch stiff J-type wire into vein and advance to right atrium under fluoroscopic guidance
7. Advance venous 14-French dilator
8. Insert venous cannula and advance to mid-right atrium using fluoroscopic guidance
9. Give heparin
10. Eliminate all air in arterial cannula by circulating saline through arteriovenous crossbridge with arterial tubing clamp open (Fig. 31–6). Aspirate remaining air through distal arterial tubing stopcock.
11. Connect cannulas to system and initiate pumping as per perfusion protocol
12. Sew cannulas into place with no. 0 or 00 silk

CPS, cardiopulmonary support.

used for patients with deep venous thrombosis or a history of inferior vena cava filter placement. Insertion of a Swan-Ganz catheter should precede or follow CPS placement for monitoring of right-sided cardiac hemodynamics. Because systemic blood flow is nonpulsatile, arterial pressures must be monitored with a transducer, preferably at a site separate from the opposite femoral artery when available (e.g., a coronary guide catheter). If necessary during emergent use, arterial pressure can be estimated with an arterial cuff occluding a brachial or radial artery Doppler signal before insertion of a separate arterial line.

Six- to 8-French sheaths are placed in both femoral arteries and the right femoral vein before cannula insertion. Bilateral iliofemoral angiography contrast performed from the distal abdominal aorta at 8 mL/sec for a total of 20 mL allows selection of the best vascular access site for elective placement of the arterial cannula.

Arterial and venous vessels can be successively dilated for cannula insertion (8- to 14-French to 17- to 21-French), or cannula dilators can be directly inserted over a 0.038-inch stiff J-tip wire. An assistant applying a gentle back-and-forth motion of the guide wire during cannula advancement will detect kinking of the wire if resistance is encountered and prevent vessel perforation. A 0.038-inch stiff J-tip wire is then passed through the femoral venous sheath and guided to the right atrium for placement of the venous cannula. The venous cannula is advanced to the mid-right atrium under fluoroscopic guidance. Heparin (20,000 units) is then given. After placement, the cannulas should be sewn into place with no. 0 or 00 silk. Careful elimination of all air in the arterial cannula and tubing can be achieved by circulating saline through the arteriovenous crossbridge with the arterial tubing clamp open and aspiration of any remaining air through a stopcock on the distal arterial tubing with a 60-mL syringe. Air in the venous cannula or tubing is eliminated as blood passes through the oxygenator.

When a patient deteriorates despite IABP support, the operator may need to "upgrade" the patient's support to CPS. It is important to have a 0.032-inch wire available for this exchange to match maximum IABP lumen size. Use of a 12- to 14-French intermediate dilator allows exchange to a 0.038-inch stiffer guide wire prior to CPS cannula placement.

OPERATION AND MONITORING. Hemodynamics are monitored by Swan-Ganz and arterial pressure measurement. For elective use, CPS is started at 2 to 3 L/min for 4 minutes, or until hemodynamics are adequate (PCWP <20 mm Hg). PCWP may paradoxically increase with higher CPS flow as a result of increased afterload on the compromised left ventricle. Left ventricular size and mechanical defects may be assessed with echocardiography. Measurement of arterial and mixed venous blood gases is often useful to assess tissue oxygenation. Thermodilution cardiac output measurements, however, are not useful during CPS operation.

After adequate recovery or completion of the procedure, the patient is weaned off the pump (if possible). The Cell Saver is used by the perfusionist or CPS operator, and blood is returned to the patient as CPS is discontinued.

REMOVAL. The cannulas are usually clamped for 6 to 12 hours before removal. When the partial thromboplastin time is less than 70 seconds or the activated clotting time is less than 160 seconds, sheaths are removed with a Femostop device such that femoral pulses are still obtainable by Doppler. One to 2 hours of pressure are generally necessary, although as long as 12 hours is possible without the need for vascular repair. Following emergent placement, it is often appropriate to remove cannulas with direct vascular repair to avoid potential risk of deep venous thrombosis or pseudoaneurysm. Swan-Ganz and arterial lines can be removed the day after cannula removal.

Indications (see Table 31–2)

EMERGENT USE OF CPS. Emergent institution of CPS should be considered in rapid circulatory collapse refractory to advanced cardiac life support (ACLS). Symptoms of refractory clinical cardiogenic shock despite inotropes and IABP support also imply the potential need for CPS if reversible pathology is present or the patient is a candidate for cardiac transplantation.

Litzie and colleagues[55] reported on the initial emergent use of the portable CPS machine outside the operating room in 1987. Shawl and coworkers[56] reported salvage of 4 of 7 patients with cardiac arrest in the cardiac catheterization laboratory who survived longer than 6 months after coronary bypass or PTCA. In a larger study, Reichman and coworkers[57] reported that 18 of 36 patients (50%) placed emergently on portable CPS were able to be weaned after cardiovascular collapse in the cardiac catheterization laboratory. Six patients survived longer than 60 days after CPS initiation. Similarly, Overlie and associates[58] weaned 15 of 35 patients in cardiac arrest, with 8 patients surviving long term.

ELECTIVE USE OF CPS. Prophylactic use of the device may be considered during high-risk PTCA or valvuloplasty.[59] Formation of a national registry allowed the investigation of CPS-supported angioplasty in a large number of patients. Vogel and colleagues[60] showed a 95% angioplasty success in 105 patients prophylactically supported with CPS. The in-hospital mortality rate was 7.6%, with most of the deaths occurring in patients older than 75 years or with left main coronary artery disease. In a recent update, 389 patients undergoing supported angioplasty were compared with 180 patients with CPS on standby.[61] Only 5 patients (2.8%) in the standby group had prophylactic placement of an IABP. Overall, there was no significant difference in mortality rates between the two groups. However, in patients with an LVEF of less than 20%, prophylactic CPS was associated with a significantly decreased mortality (4.8% vs. 18.8%), although morbidity still remained high (41%) compared with standby CPS (9.4%). The study suggests that patients with an LVEF of less than 20% may benefit from prophylactic CPS despite the risk of increased morbidity.

Currently, CPS may be considered prophylactically for patients during (1) PTCA with an LVEF of less than 20%; (2) PTCA of only patent coronary vessel; (3) hemodynamic instability during previous coronary intervention; or (4) valvuloplasty with an LVEF of less than 25%. Use of IABP with the availability of standby upgrade to CPS seems appropriate with an LVEF of 20% or higher. For standby use, the system may or may not be primed before the procedure, depending on the anticipated risk of the procedure. Self-primed (permanently primed) models are being investigated.

Contraindications and Complications

Contraindications for CPS support are listed in Table 31–2. In patients without correctable pathology, CPS initiation can resuscitate the patient neurologically but necessitate subsequent termination of support and death. Thus, careful consideration of whether a patient may be a potential candidate for cardiac transplantation may be appropriate before placement of CPS. Severe aortic insufficiency is also a relative contraindication to CPS use because reflux into the left ventricle during CPS support could aggravate pulmonary edema and increase $M\dot{V}o_2$.

Even more than with IABP placement, peripheral vascular disease may prevent percutaneous insertion of the large cannulas required. Complications including vascular hemorrhage, leg ischemia, or aortic dissection can result. In the multicenter report by Vogel and coworkers,[60] morbidity due to arteriovenous cannulation was noted in 41 of the 105 patients predominantly as a result of vascular complications or the need for blood transfusions. Similarly, Teirstein and associates[61] reported that 42% of patients supported prophylactically with CPS had femoral site complications or required blood transfusions compared with only 11.7% of patients with standby CPS. Acute limb ischemia in a patient dependent on CPS may be treated with surgical iliofemoral bypass of the arterial cannula in the affected leg. Newer designs with smaller cannula sizes and heparin-bonded tubing (Carmeda, Medtronic, Inc., Anaheim, CA) may decrease the relatively high number of complications in the future.

Risk of central nervous system or other embolic events has been uncommon after initiation of retrograde femoral artery perfusion.[60] If percutaneous insertion is not possible, as in a severely obese patient, or unsafe because of a known bleeding diathesis, a femoral cutdown by a vascular surgeon or qualified clinician may still allow safe insertion of the cannulas.

Duration of CPS may limit its use during a potentially reversible myocardial injury or as a bridge to cardiac transplantation. Hemodynamic recovery is usually within 48 hours, after which the risk of hemolysis and embolic events may increase.[62] If patients are not appropriate candidates for interventions including LVAD placement, the decision for the initiation of CPS support should be carefully considered.

CORONARY SINUS RETROPERFUSION

Theory

Synchronized coronary SRP is a technique to deliver oxygenated blood retrograde from the coronary sinus to ischemic myocardium that has obtained preliminary approval by the FDA for left anterior descending artery interventions. Analogous to the timing of the IABP, oxygenated blood flow into the coronary circulation is augmented during cardiac diastole, when coronary vascular conductance and capacitance are highest, while allowing normal venous drainage to occur during systole. Goals of retroperfusion include improvement in myocardial recovery associated with an ischemic insult and more rapid and direct delivery of drugs to the myocardium.[63]

The retroperfusion system (Retroperfusion Systems, Inc., Irvine, CA) consists of a specially designed 8.5-French triple-lumen coronary sinus catheter with a balloon tip, an external console and pump, and an 8-French femoral arterial catheter with end and side holes for oxygenated blood aspiration. Arterial blood is withdrawn from the femoral artery through the arterial catheter to a disposable pump chamber (cassette) housed in the external console. Electrocardiographic information is processed by the pump console and, using an algorithm relating diastolic duration and changes in heart rate, synchronizes the start of diastole and infusion of blood. Coinciding with the beginning of diastole, compressed gas (carbon dioxide) inflates the balloon tip of the retroperfusion catheter, preventing coronary venous drainage and reflux of delivered arterial blood to maximize retrograde delivery (Fig. 31–7). Blood infusion may be extended over more than one cardiac cycle when a single pump stroke is insufficient to fill the venous volume or increase coronary sinus pressure (e.g., during tachycardia). Deflation of the balloon and cessation of arterial blood pumping during systole permit normal cardiac venous drainage. Depending on the total volume of the pumping cassette, SRP is capable of a maximum of 96 to 250 mL/min of retrograde flow.

Technique

Preparation for SRP institution includes standard sterile preparation for percutaneous access of both femoral artery systems as well as the site for SRP catheter insertion, usually the right internal jugular vein, although subclavian and brachial veins have also been used. Using fluoroscopic guidance, the 8.5-French retroperfusion catheter is inserted from the jugular vein and advanced into the coronary sinus. A 0.035-inch J-tip guide wire may assist placement, if needed. The catheter is advanced to a nonoccluding position in the great cardiac vein to allow normal venous drainage during balloon deflation. Hand injection of radiopaque contrast agent allows visualization of placement and the degree of venous reflux. The catheter is attached to the disposable pump cassette to allow infusion of arterial blood and carbon dioxide for balloon inflation. A side-hole tip in the catheter allows monitoring of coronary venous pressure during pumping.

The 8-French arterial catheter is placed in the femoral artery not used for PTCA access and is attached to the inflow side of the pumping cassette. A motor-driven piston pumps oxy-

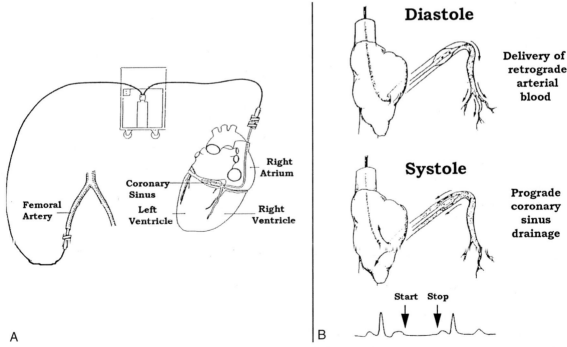

A

B

Figure 31–7. A, Diagram of synchronized coronary venous retroperfusion circuit. B, *upper:* Computer processing of the electrocardiographic signal controls diastolic arterial blood infusion and balloon tip inflation timing for maximal retrograde coronary sinus flow; *lower:* Onset of systole ends blood infusion and deflation of catheter balloon to allow normal systolic coronary sinus drainage. (*A* and *B* courtesy of Retroperfusion, Inc., Irvine, CA.)

genated arterial blood to the retroperfusion catheter at the operator-set flow rate. Unidirectional flow is controlled by integrated valves on the pump cassette. Adequate function of the system may be monitored by electrocardiogram, central or coronary venous pressure, and balloon pressure displays on the external pumping console.

Indications

SRP FOR ACUTE MYOCARDIAL ISCHEMIA. In an animal model, infarct size measured by nitroblue tetrazolium was reduced 84% with retroperfusion in baboons begun 15 minutes after total left anterior descending artery occlusion.[64] Similarly, infarct size was reduced 70%[65] and 67%[66] in dogs with total left anterior descending artery occlusion, and in one study, metabolism was maintained in the risk-zone myocardium as measured by positron emission tomography.[65] Gore and colleagues[67] reported the first clinical use of synchronized retroperfusion in five patients with unstable angina refractory to medical therapy. Institution of venous retroperfusion significantly reduced the number of anginal episodes and the need for nitroglycerin while stabilizing patients for diagnostic or therapeutic intervention.

In a recent study, Barnett and coworkers[68] used SRP in 15 intensive care unit patients with unstable angina refractory to pharmacologic therapy (n = 12) or with myocardial infarction with contraindications to thrombolytic therapy (n = 3; 2 posterior, 1 inferolateral). With SRP, full relief of ischemic pain and decreases in electrocardiographic ST segment deviations were noted in most patients. Echocardiographic systolic wall motion significantly improved in ischemic areas. In two patients who were refractory to IABP counterpulsation, SRP led to improved systemic hemodynamics when used as an adjunct to IABP support. All patients were successfully supported to PTCA (n = 7) or coronary artery bypass grafting (n = 5) interventions or maintained on medical therapy (n = 3). This suggests that SRP may reduce myocardial ischemia and improve ventricular function during acute ischemic syndromes.

ELECTIVE SRP DURING PTCA. Use of the system may be beneficial for patients during total left anterior descending coronary artery occlusion or left main artery disease,[69] especially during prolonged PTCA balloon inflations.[70] Compared with autoperfusion catheters, retroperfusion may improve outcome by maintaining flow to side branches occluded by the balloon, especially in patients with little collateral circulation.

In larger, more recent studies, anginal pain[71, 72] and ST segment changes decreased[71–73] during PTCA balloon inflation with retroperfusion support as compared with nonsupported inflations. Global left ventricular function determined by echocardiography was also preserved during retroperfusion-supported inflations.[70, 71, 73]

Remarkably, no deaths have been reported during 350 consecutive SRP procedures (E. Corday, personal communication). Nevertheless, concerns regarding possible coronary venous perforation, myocardial edema, and peripheral arterial complications may limit its widespread use in the immediate future.

LIMITATIONS OF SRP. Venous drainage of the left anterior descending coronary artery occurs almost exclusively through the great cardiac vein and coronary sinus.[17] However, venous drainage from the right and, to a lesser extent, the circumflex arteries enters chambers of the heart through thebesian vessels rather than the coronary sinus. It is unlikely that venous retroperfusion through the coronary sinus will have a comparable salutary effect with circumflex or right coronary artery ischemia except in patients with established left-to-right collateral flow. Newer designs with larger balloon sizes to allow more proximal placement of the SRP catheter may allow broader applications.

Contraindications and Complications

Obstructive peripheral vascular disease preventing insertion of the arterial aspiration catheter and interventional (e.g., PTCA) catheter is a contraindication to retroperfusion insertion. Technical ability to cannulate the coronary sinus is also necessary for this support to be initiated.

HEMOPUMP

Theory

The goals of the Hemopump LVAD are to maintain tissue perfusion while reducing $M\dot{V}O_2$ to allow recovery of viable myocardium. Although investigational, the Hemopump may serve as an intermediate level of support for patients who require more support than the IABP alone but not complete cardiopulmonary bypass. The percutaneous device is not presently available in the United States but is undergoing clinical testing in Europe. Previous experience in this country with a 21-French device required surgical cutdown for insertion.

The current design of the pump for percutaneous catheterization use is a 14-French catheter-mounted, nonpulsatile device inserted into the femoral artery and advanced retrograde into the left ventricle across the aortic valve. Blood is removed from the left ventricle and expelled into the aorta by a single Archimedes-type vane screw (impeller) rotating at a rate of 15,000 to 27,000 rpm housed in a silicone tube. The impeller is rotated via a continuously irrigated drive shaft connected to an external motor to allow a maximum of 2.5 L/min (14-French) or 3.5 L/min (21-French) of flow. Maximum flow rate is partly dependent on arterial pressure. In the past, the Hemopump was approved for use as long as 1 week.

EFFECTS OF HEMOPUMP SUPPORT ON HEMODYNAMICS. A report compiled by Wampler and Riehle[74] of 87 patients with cardiogenic shock showed an increase in cardiac index from a mean of 1.7 to 2.3 L/min/m² after 24 hours of pump operation. Patients who survived to weaning had a mean cardiac index of 2.8 L/min/m². MAP rose from 57 to 62 mm Hg. Mean PCWP decreased from 25 to 15 mm Hg after 24 hours of Hemopump assistance.

EFFECTS OF HEMOPUMP SUPPORT ON CORONARY BLOOD FLOW. In a study by Shiiya and colleagues[75] of dogs with a ligated left anterior descending artery, left circumflex coronary artery blood Doppler velocity did not increase with Hemopump support even though the ratio of myocardial oxygen supply to demand increased with mechanical support. In a similar canine model, Smalling and associates[76] found that coronary flow in nonischemic regions, as measured by microsphere injection, remained unchanged with Hemopump initiation but increased in the ischemic region supplied by the ligated left anterior descending artery. Further, infarct size was significantly lower with Hemopump support (mean = 21.7% region infarcted) than control (62.6%) or IABP counterpulsation (27%).

Technique

Percutaneous Hemopump insertion is currently under investigation but is assumed to be similar to standard percutaneous techniques. Retrograde crossing of the aortic valve with the 21-French device can be achieved with either direct prolapse of the distal inflow cannula or facilitated with a J guide wire or pigtail passed through aspiration holes close to the end of the cannula. A radiographic image of proper placement Hemopump is shown in Figure 31–8.

Indications

CARDIOGENIC SHOCK COMPLICATING ACUTE MYOCARDIAL INFARCTION. Generally, the Hemopump could be used in situations in which sufficient output may not be obtained with IABP support or IABP counterpulsation has failed but initiation of CPS or placement of an LVAD is not

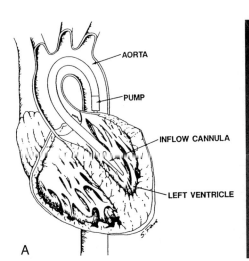
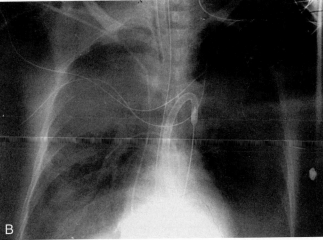

Figure 31–8. A, Diagram of proper placement of Hemopump in the left ventricle. B, Fluoroscopic image of proper Hemopump device placement into the left ventricle. Blood is expelled at the level of the radiopaque band in the proximal aorta.

warranted. The 1-week support duration limit makes the device attractive for patients with low-output syndrome but acute recoverable ventricular function. Patients who fail to wean from cardiopulmonary bypass in the operating room may benefit from the larger 21-French device.[77-79] The previous investigational protocol limited patient selection to critically ill patients meeting the following criteria of cardiogenic shock: (1) a cardiac index of less than 2 L/min/m²; (2) PCWP greater than 18 mm Hg; and (3) systolic blood pressure lower than 90 mm Hg or a left ventricular work index less than 1500 gm·m⁻²·min⁻¹ despite inotrope and IABP support.[78]

All reported studies have used the 21-French device. Five of seven patients with cardiogenic shock survived with the first clinical use of the device in 1988.[79] In a recent follow-up multicenter trial of patients with cardiogenic shock, 31.7% survived 30 days or longer.[78]

Baldwin and colleagues[80] reported a long-term follow-up of 10 patients, 8 with cardiogenic shock and 2 with acute allograft rejection. The mean duration of support was 71 hours. There were 8 survivors with a mean of 21 months after Hemopump support. Four patients were New York Heart Association class I and 4 were class II. Adverse long-term effects of Hemopump insertion were not noted in any patient.

ACUTE CARDIAC ALLOGRAFT FAILURE. In a study by Wiebalck and coworkers,[81] two patients were successfully supported to retransplantation with no long-term sequelae resulting from Hemopump support. In the event of cardiac transplant graft failure, patients have been supported by the Hemopump until recovery of cardiac native function.[80]

ELECTIVE HEMOPUMP SUPPORT. Only one study of supported angioplasty in patients unsuitable for surgery has been reported with the 21-French Hemopump.[82] Of patients supported with the device during high-risk PTCA, all angioplasties were successful and no acute deaths were reported. However, the percutaneous device has not been used for this purpose.

Contraindications and Complications

Contraindications to Hemopump insertion include evidence of significant aortic valve disease or aortic aneurysm or dissection. Preexisting blood dyscrasia may be potentially associated with increased hemolysis with pump function. Previous implantation of a mechanical prosthetic aortic valve is also a contraindication because of the inability to pass the catheter into the left ventricle. Because of possible thromboembolic complications, the presence of a mural left ventricular thrombus may contraindicate Hemopump insertion. As with other devices, peripheral vascular disease may prevent insertion of the device and should also be considered a relative contraindication to Hemopump initiation.

The surgically implanted version was not convenient for cardiac catheterization during emergent diagnostic or therapeutic interventions. The requirement of a femoral cutdown and anastomosis of a Dacron graft to the femoral artery precluded rapid insertion. Additional disadvantages included the large catheter size (21-French) and the relatively high failure insertion rate of the device (24.1%).[74] Total complications with the 21-French Hemopump have primarily been related to thrombocytopenia (11.5%), thromboembolism (10.3%), hemolysis (9.2%), and vascular morbidity (6.9%).[74] Positioning of the pump in the left ventricle can be associated with dysrhythmias and could potentially cause aortic regurgitation secondary to aortic valve prolapse.

The percutaneous Hemopump is just beginning clinical investigation. It is likely that the risk of percutaneous insertion will be at least as high as that associated with insertion of IABP pumps. Compared with the maximal 3.5-L/min flow of the surgically inserted Hemopump, the percutaneous pump is capable of peak flows of only 2.5 L/min. This decrease in potential output may limit its usefulness in situations of hemodynamic collapse, although it is in the range of flows typically used for elective CPS support.

ADDITIONAL MECHANICAL SUPPORT

Patients suitable for cardiac transplantation with hemodynamic collapse unable to wean from mechanical support may be bridged to transplantation with more invasive devices such as the total artificial heart and VAD.[83] The total artificial heart, however, is presently limited in clinical trials and future availability remains uncertain.

Many types of VADs for recovery from acute postcardiotomy cardiogenic shock or as a bridge to transplantation have been used clinically for several decades.[84, 85] The VAD unloads and assumes the pumping function of a ventricle to maintain adequate systemic blood flow with little or no ventricular contribution. The VAD may support the right (RVAD) or the left (LVAD) ventricle, or both, and can deliver total output of as high as 10 L/min. VAD insertion, however, requires a sternotomy, advanced personnel training and monitoring equipment, and availability of the device (because few are available for general use). Recent long-term support with implantable LVADs suggests that chronic support as an alternative to heart transplantation may soon be possible with these devices.[10, 11]

In patients implanted with the LVAD, exercise rehabilitation may improve their overall physical state to enhance their transplant operative survival and long-term prognosis. Diagnostic evaluation may be appropriate in the catheterization laboratory setting (Fig. 31–9) to assess pump function or to characterize rehabilitation of the native heart and LVAD complex with exercise testing.[86] In the future, if exercise performance is comparable with the activities of daily living, LVAD patients may be deemed physically suitable for chronic outpatient support either before transplantation or as an alternative to cardiac transplantation.

FUTURE CONSIDERATIONS

With the expanding role of the cardiac catheterization laboratory in the diagnosis and treatment of high-risk cardiac patients, devices capable of sustaining myocardial function and systemic hemodynamics will continue to be needed for use in the catheterization laboratory. Future designs should include (1) lower profile catheters to allow insertion of the device in patients with moderate to severe peripheral vascular disease and to reduce the incidence of vascular injury; (2) more powerful devices that provide greater circulatory reserve for high-risk patients; and (3) techniques to permit greater ease of use, including insertion and operation of the device to facilitate rapid institution of support in cases of emergent hemodynamic decompensation.

In an individual patient, better methods are

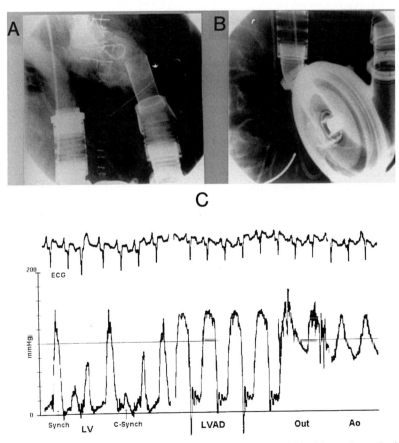

Figure 31–9. A, Left ventricular angiogram of left ventricular assisted device (LVAD) with a catheter in the left ventricle. *B,* Fluoroscopy of catheter inside LVAD for pressure measurements. *C,* Sequential left ventricular (LV), LVAD, outflow conduit (Out), and aortic (Ao) pressure tracings at rest.

needed to characterize the myocardial and hemodynamic stress associated with a planned intervention in comparison with the resting cardiac function and circulatory reserve present. With these methods, an appropriate mechanical device could be selected that balances benefit versus potential risk of any level of support.

REFERENCES

1. Gibbon JH Jr: Application of a mechanical heart and lung apparatus to cardiac surgery. Minn Med 1954; 37:171–180.
2. Kirklin JW, DuShane JW, Patrick RT, et al: Intra-cardiac surgery with the aid of a mechanical pump oxygenator (Gibbon type): Report of eight cases. Proc Staff Meet Mayo Clin 1955; 30:201–206.
3. Clauss RH, Birtwell WC, Albertal G, et al: Assisted circulation. Part I. The arterial counterpulsator. J Thorac Cardiovasc Surg 1961; 41:447–458.
4. Moulopoulos SD, Topaz S, Kolff WJ: Diastolic balloon pumping (with carbon dioxide) in the aorta: A mechanical assistance to the failing circulation. Am Heart J 1962; 63:669–675.
5. Kantrowitz A, Tjonneland S, Freed PS, et al: Initial clinical experience with intra-aortic balloon pumping in cardiogenic shock. JAMA 1968; 203:113–118.
6. Page DL, Caulfield JB, Kastor JA, et al: Myocardial changes associated with cardiogenic shock. N Engl J Med 1975; 285:133–137.
7. Cooley DA: The first implantation of an artificial heart: Reflections and observations. Transplant Proc 1973; 5:1135–1137.
8. DeVries WC, Anderson JL, Joyce LD, et al: Clinical use of the total artificial heart. N Engl J Med 1984; 310:273–278.
9. DeBakey ME: Left ventricular bypass pump for cardiac assistance: Clinical experience. Am J Cardiol 1971; 27:3–11.
10. Frazier OH, Rose EA, Macmanus Q, et al: Multicenter clinical evaluation of the HeartMate 1000 IP left ventricular assist device. Ann Thorac Surg 1992; 53:1080–1090.
11. Daniel MA, Lee J, LaForge DH, et al: Clinical evaluation of the Novacor totally implantable ventricular assist system. ASAIO Trans 1991; 37:M423–M425.
12. Frazier OH, La Francesca S, Radovancevic B, et al: Battery-powered LVAD for patients awaiting heart transplantation [abstract]. J Heart Lung Transplant 1993; 12(Part 2):S99.
13. Jaski BE, Serruys PW, Katent HT, Meij S: Epicardial wall motion and left ventricular function during coronary graft angioplasty in humans. J Am Coll Cardiol 1985; 6:695–700.
14. Serruys PW, Wijns W, van der Brandt M, et al: Left ventricular performance, regional blood flow, wall motion, and lactate metabolism during transluminal angioplasty. Circulation 1984; 70:25–36.
15. Topol EJ, Leya F, Pinkerton CA, et al: A comparison of directional atherectomy with coronary angioplasty in patients with coronary artery disease—The CAVEAT Study Group. N Engl J Med 1993; 329:221–227.
16. Serruys PW, Keane D: The bailout stent: Is a friend in need always a friend indeed? Circulation 1993; 88:2455–2457.
17. Marcus ML: The Coronary Circulation in Health and Disease. New York, McGraw-Hill, 1983.
18. Gewirtz H, Ohley W, Williams DO, et al: Effect of intra-

19. aortic balloon counterpulsation on regional myocardial blood flow and oxygen consumption in the presence of coronary artery stenosis: Observations in an awake animal model. Am J Cardiol 1982; 50:829–837.
19. Leinbach RC, Buckley MJ, Austen WG, et al: Effects of intra-aortic balloon pumping on coronary flow and metabolism in man. Circulation 1971; 43(Suppl 1):1-77–1-88.
20. Williams DO, Korr KS, Gewirtz H, Most AS: The effect of intra-aortic balloon counterpulsation on regional myocardial blood flow in patients with unstable angina. Circulation 1983; 66:593–597.
21. Scheidt S, Wilner G, Mueller H, et al: Intra-aortic balloon counterpulsation in cardiogenic shock. N Engl J Med 1973; 288:979–984.
22. Port SC, Patel S, Schmidt DH: Effects of intra-aortic balloon counterpulsation on myocardial blood flow in patients with severe coronary artery disease. J Am Coll Cardiol 1984; 3:1367–1374.
23. Mueller H, Ayres SM, Conklin EF, et al: The effect of intra-aortic counterpulsation on cardiac performance and metabolism in shock associated with acute myocardial infarction. J Clin Invest 1971; 50:1885–1900.
24. Fuchs RM, Brin KP, Brinker JA, et al: Augmentation of regional coronary blood flow by intra-aortic balloon counterpulsation in patients with unstable angina. Circulation 1983; 68:117–123.
25. Kern MJ, Aguirre F, Bach R, et al: Augmentation of coronary blood flow by intra-aortic balloon pumping in patients after coronary angioplasty. Circulation 1993; 87:500–511.
26. MacDonald RG, Hill JA, Feldman RL: Failure of intra-aortic balloon counterpulsation to augment distal coronary perfusion pressure during percutaneous transluminal coronary angioplasty. Am J Cardiol 1987; 59:359–361.
27. Laas J, Campbell CD, Takanashi Y, et al: Failure of intra-aortic balloon pumping to reduce experimental myocardial infarct size in swine. J Thorac Cardiovasc Surg 1980; 80:85–93.
28. Quaal S: Conventional timing using the arterial pressure waveform. In Quaal S (ed): Comprehensive Intra-aortic Balloon Counterpulsation. St. Louis, CV Mosby, 1993, pp 246–259.
29. Cadwell CA, Tyson G: Real timing. In Quaal S (ed): Comprehensive Intra-aortic Balloon Counterpulsation. St. Louis, CV Mosby, 1993, pp 281–294.
30. Kantrowitz A, Cardona RR, Freed PS: Weaning from the intra-aortic balloon pump. In Quaal S (ed): Comprehensive Intra-aortic Balloon Counterpulsation. St. Louis, CV Mosby, 1993, pp 398–407.
31. Clements SD, Story WE, Hurst JW, et al: Ruptured papillary muscle: Clinical presentation, diagnosis and treatment. Clin Cardiol 1985; 88:93–103.
32. Quaal SJ: Indications. In Quaal S (ed): Comprehensive Intra-aortic Balloon Counterpulsation. St. Louis, CV Mosby, 1993, pp 118–143.
33. Bolooki H: Emergency cardiac procedures in patients in cardiogenic shock due to complications of coronary artery disease. Circulation 1989; 79:1137–1148.
34. Murphy DA, Craver JM, Jones EL, et al: Surgical management of acute myocardial ischemia after percutaneous transluminal coronary angioplasty. J Thorac Cardiovasc Surg 1984; 87:332–339.
35. Bolooki H: Clinical Application of the Intra-aortic Balloon Pump. Mount Kisko, NY, Futura, 1984.
36. Alcan KE, Stertzer SH, Wallsh E, et al: Current status of intra-aortic balloon counterpulsation in critical care cardiology. Critical Care Med 1984; 12:489–495.
37. Mackenzie DJ, Wagner WH, Kulber DA, et al: Vascular

complications of the intra-aortic balloon pump. Am J Surg 1992; 164:517–521.

38. Eltchaninoff H, Dimas AP, Whitlow PL: Complications associated with percutaneous placement of intra-aortic balloon counterpulsation. Am J Cardiol 1993; 71:328–332.

39. Ohman EM, Califf RM, George BS, et al: The use of the intra-aortic balloon pumping as an adjunct to reperfusion therapy in acute myocardial infarction—The Thrombolysis and Angioplasty in Myocardial Infarction (TAMI) Study Group. Am Heart J 1991; 121:895–901.

40. Kahn JK, Rutherford BD, McConahay DR, et al: Supported "high-risk" coronary angioplasty using intra-aortic balloon pump counterpulsation. J Am Coll Cardiol 1990; 15:1151–1155.

41. Ishihara M, Sato H, Tateishi H, et al: Intra-aortic balloon pumping as the postangioplasty strategy in acute myocardial infarction. Am Heart J 1991; 122:385–389.

42. Szatmary LJ, Marco J, Fajadet J, Caster L: The combined use of diastolic counterpulsation and coronary dilation in unstable angina due to multivessel disease under unstable hemodynamic conditions. Int J Cardiol 1988; 19:59–66.

43. Voudris V, Marco J, Morice MC, et al: "High-risk" percutaneous transluminal coronary angioplasty with preventative intra-aortic balloon pump counterpulsation. Cathet Cardiovasc Diagn 1990; 19:160–164.

44. Kreidieh L, Davies DW, Lim R, et al: High-risk coronary angioplasty with elective intra-aortic balloon pump support. Int J Cardiol 1992; 35:147–152.

45. Scanlon PJ, Montoya A, Johnson SA, et al: Urgent surgery for ventricular septal rupture complicating acute myocardial infarction. Circulation 1985; 72(Suppl 2):II-185–II-190.

46. Chaudary S, Jaski BE: Fulminant mumps myocarditis. Ann Intern Med 1989; 110:569–570.

47. Dembitsky WP, Moore CH, Holman WL, et al: Successful mechanical circulatory support for noncoronary shock. J Heart Lung Transplant 1992; 11:129–135.

48. Phillips SJ: Percutaneous cardiopulmonary bypass and innovations on clinical counterpulsation. Crit Care Clin 1986; 2:297–318.

49. McEnany MT, Kay HR, Buckley MJ: Clinical experience with intra-aortic balloon pump support in 728 patients. Circulation 1978; 58(Suppl 1):I125–I132.

50. Martin RS III, Moncure AC, Buckley MJ, et al: Complications of percutaneous intra-aortic balloon insertion. J Thorac Cardiovasc Surg 1983; 85:186–190.

51. Gottlieb SO, Brinker JA, Borkon AM, et al: Identification of patients at high risk for complications of intra-aortic balloon counterpulsation: A multivariate risk factor analysis. Am J Cardiol 1984; 53:1135–1139.

52. Pavlides GS, Hauser AM, Stack RK, et al: Effect of peripheral cardiopulmonary bypass on left ventricular size, afterload, and myocardial function during elective supported coronary angioplasty. J Am Coll Cardiol 1991; 18:499–505.

53. Geannopoulos CJ, Leya FS, Johnson SA, et al: Effect of cardiopulmonary support on regional and global left ventricular function during transient coronary occlusion. Am Heart J 1991; 122:34–43.

54. Phillips SJ, Zeff, RH, Kongtahworn C, et al: Benefits of combined cardiopulmonary balloon pumping and percutaneous cardiopulmonary bypass. Ann Thorac Surg 1992; 54:908–910.

55. Litzie AK, Roberts CP: Emergency femorofemoral cardiopulmonary bypass. Proc Am Acad CV Perfusion 1987; 8:60–5.

56. Shawl FA, Domanski MJ, Wish MH, et al: Emergency cardiopulmonary bypass support in patients with cardiac arrest in the catheterization laboratory. Cathet Cardiovasc Diagn 1990; 19:8–12.

57. Reichman RT, Joyo CI, Dembitsky WP, et al: Improved patient survival after cardiac arrest using a cardiopulmonary support system. Ann Thorac Surg 1990; 49:101–104.

58. Overlie PA: Emergency use of portable cardiopulmonary bypass. Cathet Cardiovasc Diagn 1990; 20:27–31.

59. Vogel RA, Tommaso CL, Gundry SR: Initial experience with coronary angioplasty and aortic valvuloplasty using elective semipercutaneous cardiopulmonary support. Am J Cardiol 1988; 62:811–813.

60. Vogel RA, Shawl F, Tommaso C, et al: Initial report of the National Registry of Elective Cardiopulmonary Bypass Supported Coronary Angioplasty. J Am Coll Cardiol 1990; 15:23–29.

61. Teirstein PS, Vogel RA, Dorros G, et al: Prophylactic versus standby cardiopulmonary support for high-risk percutaneous transluminal coronary angioplasty. J Am Coll Cardiol 1993; 21:590–596.

62. Dembitsy WP, Moreno-Cabral RJ, Adamson RM, Daily PO: Emergency resuscitation using portable extracorporeal membrane oxygenation. Ann Thorac Surg 1993; 55:304–309.

63. Corday E, Haendchen RV: Seminar on coronary venous delivery systems for support and salvage of jeopardized ischemic myocardium. Part I. J Am Coll Cardiol 1991; 18:1253–1256.

64. Smith GT, Geary GG, Blanchard W, McNamara JJ: Reduction in infarct size by synchronized selective coronary venous retroperfusion of arterialized blood. Am J Cardiol 1981; 48:1064–1070.

65. O'Byrne GT, Nienaber CA, Miyazaki A, et al: Positron emission tomography demonstrates that coronary sinus retroperfusion can restore regional myocardial perfusion and preserve metabolism. J Am Coll Cardiol 1991; 18:257–270.

66. Drury JK, Yamazaki S, Fishbein MC, et al: Synchronized diastolic coronary venous retroperfusion: Results of a preclinical safety and efficacy study. J Am Coll Cardiol 1985; 6:328–335.

67. Gore JM, Weiner BH, Benotti JR, et al: Preliminary experience with synchronized coronary sinus retroperfusion in humans. Circulation 1986; 74:381–388.

68. Barnett JC, Freedman RJ, Touchon RC, Mesner MR: Coronary venous retroperfusion of arterial blood for the treatment of acute myocardial ischemia. Cathet Cardiovasc Diagn 1993; 28:206–213.

69. Nanto S, Nishida K, Hirayama A, et al: Supported angioplasty with synchronized retroperfusion in high-risk patients with left main trunk or near-left main trunk obstruction. Am Heart J 1993; 125:301–309.

70. Constantini C, Sampaolesi A, Serra CM, et al: Coronary venous retroperfusion support during high-risk angioplasty in patients with unstable angina: Preliminary experience. J Am Coll Cardiol 1991; 18:283–292.

71. Berland J, Farcot JC, Barrier A, et al: Coronary venous synchronized retroperfusion during percutaneous transluminal angioplasty of left anterior descending coronary artery. Circulation 1990; 81(Suppl 4):IV-35–IV-42.

72. Kar S, Drury JK, Hajduczki L, et al: Synchronized coronary sinus retroperfusion for support and salvage of ischemic myocardium during elective and failed angioplasty. J Am Coll Cardiol 1991; 18:271–282.

73. Incovati RL, Tauberg SG, Pecora MJ, et al: Clinical applications of coronary sinus retroperfusion during high-risk percutaneous transluminal coronary angioplasty. J Am Coll Card 1993; 22:127–134.

74. Wampler RK, Riehle RA: Clinical experience with the Hemopump left ventricular assist device. In Shawl F

(ed): Supported Complex and High-Risk Coronary Angioplasty. Boston, Kluwer, 1991, pp 1–10.

75. Shiiya N, Zelinsky R, Deleuze PH, Loisance DY: Changes in hemodynamics and coronary blood flow during left ventricular assistance with the Hemopump. Ann Thorac Surg 1992; 53:1074–1079.

76. Smalling RW, Cassidy DB, Barrett R, et al: Improved regional myocardial blood flow, left ventricular unloading, and infarct salvage using an axial-flow, transvalvular left ventricular assist device: A comparison with intra-aortic balloon counterpulsation and reperfusion alone in a canine infarction model. Circulation 1992; 85:1152–1159.

77. Burnett CM, Vega JD, Radovancevic B, et al: Improved survival after Hemopump insertion in patients experiencing postcardiotomy cardiogenic shock during cardiopulmonary bypass. ASAIO Trans 1990; 36:M626–M629.

78. Wampler RK, Frazier OH, Lansing AM, et al: Treatment of cardiogenic shock with the Hemopump left ventricular assist device. Ann Thorac Surg 1991; 52:506–513.

79. Frazier OH, Wampler RK, Duncan JM, et al: First human use of the Hemopump, a catheter-mounted ventricular assist device. Ann Thorac Surg 1990; 49:299–304.

80. Baldwin RT, Radovancevic B, Duncan JM, et al: Quality of life in long-term survivors of the Hemopump left ventricular assist device. ASAIO Trans 1991; 37:M422–423.

81. Wiebalck AC, Wouters PF, Waldenberger FR, et al: Left ventricular assist with an axial flow pump (Hemopump): Clinical application. Ann Thorac Surg 1993; 55:1141–1146.

82. Loisance D, Deleuze P, Dubois-Rande JL, et al: Hemopump ventricular support for patients undergoing high-risk coronary angioplasty. ASAIO Trans 1990; 36:M623–626.

83. Pae WE, Pierce WS, Myers JL, et al: Staged cardiac transplantation: Total artificial heart or ventricular assist pump? Circulation 1988; 78(Suppl 3):III-66–III-72.

84. Hill DJ: Bridging to cardiac transplantation. Ann Thorac Surg 1989; 47:167–171.

85. Adamson RM, Dembitsky WP, Reichman RT, et al: Mechanical support: Assist or nemesis. J Thorac Cardiovasc Surg 1989; 98:915–921.

86. Jaski BE, Branch KR, Adamson R, et al: Exercise hemodynamics during long-term implantation of a left ventricular assist device in patients awaiting heart transplant. J Am Coll Cardiol 1993; 80:1574–1580.

Chapter 32

Catheter Balloon Valvuloplasty

KIRK L. PETERSON

Following the development of coronary balloon angioplasty in 1977, percutaneous catheter balloon valvuloplasty emerged in the 1980s and 1990s as a therapeutic procedure for relief of valvular obstruction. The technique was first reported in 1982 as useful for relief of pulmonary valve stenosis.[1, 2] It has now been applied successfully to all four cardiac valves,[3–8] membranous subaortic stenosis,[9] bioprosthetic valves,[10–13] and coarctation of the aorta.[14]

Over the last decade the techniques and equipment for the performance of balloon valvuloplasty have evolved, and they remain dynamic. In this chapter, the past and current techniques for catheter balloon valvuloplasty, as applied in the United States, are presented. Approaches to the performance of valve dilation that are of historical interest alone are not considered except in parenthetic fashion. Because of the relevance to patient selection and indications for the procedure, information on the immediate, near-term, and, when available, long-term results of catheter balloon valvuloplasty also are reviewed.

MITRAL STENOSIS

Mechanism of Action and Indications

The potential of balloon catheters, by application of circumferential tension, to relieve mitral stenosis is inherent in the pathologic process underlying valve obstruction and the previous success of closed surgical commissurotomy.[15–21]

As discussed in Chapter 18, mitral stenosis is most commonly related to late pathologic sequelae of rheumatic valvulitis, although the degenerative calcification of aging, congenital mitral stenosis, and a few other rare causes (Whipple's disease and carcinoid syndrome) may infrequently be operative. Commissurotomy is feasible in those pathologic states when the primary cause of the valve orifice narrowing is commissural fusion. Much less success can be anticipated if mitral valve obstruction is related to thickening and fibrosis of the valve leaflets; thickening, fusion, and retraction of the chordae; and calcification of the leaflets and valve annulus.

Justification for performance of a catheter balloon valvuloplasty resides in the relative risk of the procedure versus its potential for improvement of symptomatic status and improvement in natural history. Other factors that would justify the procedure include the presence of significant pulmonary hypertension at rest, clearly related to mitral valve obstruction, or recurrent systemic thromboemboli during anticoagulant therapy. A less certain indication would be the potential for avoidance or delay in the development of atrial fibrillation.

Prevalvuloplasty Evaluation

Before catheter balloon mitral valvuloplasty is performed, the two most important diagnostic modalities that should be reviewed are (1) two-dimensional echocardiography with Doppler velocity recordings and pseudocolor imaging and (2) right- and left-sided heart catheterization and left ventriculography.

DOPPLER AND TWO-DIMENSIONAL ECHOCARDIOGRAPHY. Two-dimensional echocardiographic images should initially be obtained by transcutaneous imaging; however, if they are of insufficient quality, then a transesophageal examination is valuable to see more clearly the anatomy of the mitral valve and its supporting structures and to detect the presence or absence of clots in the left atrial cavity or appendage. The ultrasonographic images of the mitral valve orifice can be directly planimetered to assess the cross-sectional area. Left ventricular and left atrial chamber sizes, pulmonary artery diameter, and right ventricular and right atrial sizes are useful references for the severity of the hemodynamic burden imposed by mitral stenosis. Doppler velocity recordings, with measurement of the mitral valve diastolic pressure gradient from the modified Bernoulli relation and mitral valve area from the pressure half-time method, are particularly useful for estimating the severity of valve obstruction. Color Doppler recordings are of importance for assessing the coexistence of mitral regurgitation.

In like fashion to observations that echocardiographic characteristics predict suitability for operative mitral commissurotomy,[22] Reid and associates reported the same for catheter balloon mitral valvuloplasty.[23] The group at the Massachusetts General Hospital has popularized a predictive scoring system that assesses the severity of four morphologic features (Table 32–1), including leaflet mobility, valvular calcification, subvalvular thickening, and leaflet thickening.[24–26] This same group has also reported that immediate and long-term results of mitral valvuloplasty are not as successful in patients with fluoroscopically visible mitral valve calcification as in those without calcification.[27]

CATHETERIZATION AND ANGIOGRAPHIC DATA. The physiologic data obtained at cardiac catheterization document the severity of the mitral valve obstruction, and the left ventriculogram is often useful for assessing valve leaflet mobility, degree of calcification, and the degree of subvalvular disease (see Chapter 18).

Procedural Technique

Several techniques and types of balloon catheters have been developed for realization of valve orifice dilation. In 1984, Inoue and associates described an asymmetric, volume-adjustable, compliant balloon that was inserted through the mitral orifice using the transseptal approach.[4] Then in 1985 Lock and colleagues described the successful use of a symmetric, sausage-shaped balloon that was again inserted transseptally.[5] The first description of the application of two balloons in tandem was by Al Zaibag and coworkers in 1986.[28] Subsequently, Babic and associates reported on a retrograde arterial method for inserting either a single- or double-balloon catheter assembly across the mitral valve by way of the left ventricle.[29, 30] A further design, used primarily in Europe, has been the bifoil or trefoil balloon catheter, where more than one balloon is mounted on a single catheter shaft.

Although more difficult a procedure to perform, the double-balloon technique has the following general advantages: (1) two smaller balloons, rather than one larger one, are easier to insert into an extremity vessel; (2) use of two balloons extends the range of patients that are treatable with balloon dilation; and (3) double-balloon catheters do not completely occlude the valve orifice during inflation.

In the United States the two most commonly used approaches have been the insertion transseptally of two balloon catheters antegrade across the mitral valve and the use of the Inoue balloon catheter, also inserted transseptally. Both techniques mandate skill and experience in performing transseptal catheterization of the left atrium (see Chapter 2).

DOUBLE BALLOON. To get two balloon catheters across a single atrial septal puncture site (Fig. 32–1), it is helpful to predilate multiple times the puncture site with an 8-mm balloon before attempting to pass the larger valvular

Table 32–1. **Echocardiographic Criteria for Mitral Balloon Valvuloplasty**

Score*	Valve Leaflet Mobility	Valvular Calcification	Subvalvular Thickening	Valve Leaflet Thickening
0	Normal, highly mobile	None	None	None
1	Only leaflet tips restricted	Leaflet margins	Minimal	Minimal
2	Mid-leaflets and base have normal mobility	Scattered	One third of chordal length	Considerable, at margins only
3	Valve moves only from base; tips and mid-section are stiff	Ca^{2+} noted into mid-leaflets	Two thirds of chordal length	Thickening (5–8 mm) noted of full leaflet
4	Minimal forward motion during diastole	Ca^{2+} throughout full length of chordae	Thickening and shortening of all chordae	Massive increase (8–10 mm) noted of full leaflet

*Total score = 0–16.

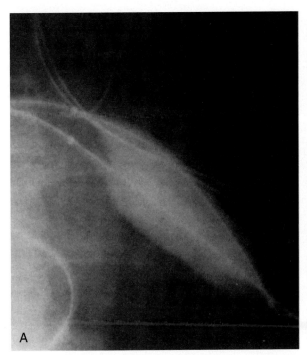
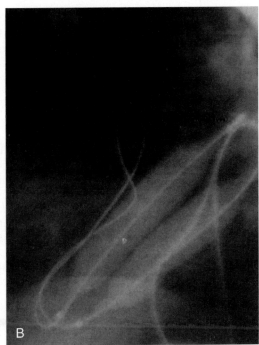

Figure 32–1. Two balloon catheters inflated simultaneously while positioned across the mitral valve, shown in the antero-posterior *(A)* and left lateral *(B)* projections. (From Mullins CE, Nihill MR, Vick GW, et al: Double-balloon technique for dilation of valvular or vessel stenosis in congenital and acquired heart disease. J Am Coll Cardiol 1987; 10:110. Reprinted with permission from the American College of Cardiology.)

balloon catheters themselves (in sequential fashion) across the septum and through the mitral valve orifice.

In our laboratories we use the Mullins sheath, positioned just into the inflow of the left ventricle, as a conduit for positioning one or two guide wires into the left ventricle. These J-guide wires are gradually curved near their insertion end and are positioned at the apex of the left ventricle with their tips curved back toward the mitral valve orifice. Considerable ventricular ectopy is normally encountered during the process of positioning these guide wires. Alternatively, a double-lumen balloon flotation catheter can be first floated through the left ventricle into the ascending and descending thoracic aorta; this catheter is then used as a conduit to position guide wires into the descending aorta. During the subsequent phases of the procedure, however, great care must be exercised to avoid cinching up these guide wires against the mitral valve and rupturing the anterior leaflet.

Slow insertion of the balloon catheter(s) across the valve is accomplished by using a coaxial, reverse friction movement where one person puts gentle traction on the wire while a second advances the balloon catheter. Care is taken to be certain that the guide wire does not loop up into the left atrium or that the loop at

the apex of the left ventricle becomes uncoiled. We prefer to position the balloon(s) across the mitral valve in the right anterior oblique position where we can readily visualize the atrioventricular groove and the anatomic position of the mitral valve. Occasionally, with the double-balloon technique, both catheters cannot be advanced across a tight orifice until a dilation with a single balloon has first been accomplished.

Several precautions are important during the course of inflating and deflating the balloons. First, in some instances during the course of inflation the balloon tends to project forcefully toward the apex and can perforate the left ventricle at that location despite the presence of the curved guide wire. Second, care must be exercised that the proximal end of the balloon is free of the interatrial septum at the time of inflation, otherwise, a considerably larger atrial septal defect may be created. Finally, before attempts are made to withdraw the balloon(s) out of the left atrium, they should be fully deflated. We find it useful that two other assistants, other than the operators themselves, act to inflate and deflate the balloons on command.

SINGLE BALLOON (INOUE). The Inoue balloon catheter differs significantly from the conventional balloon catheters described earlier. It is made of two layers of latex with a nylon mesh interposed. The latex lends elasticity and high compliance to the balloon, whereas the nylon mesh serves to limit the maximum inflated diameter of the balloon and control its inflation characteristics. The balloon expands with inflation in three stages (Fig. 32–2): (1) initially, the distal end of the balloon inflates; (2) the proximal half of the balloon inflates, creating a dumbbell shape, with the waist positioned right at the plane of the mitral valve; and (3) once positioned at the mitral valve plane with the distal end into the left ventricle and the proximal end in the left atrium, the middle portion inflates and creates circumferential tension along the fused commissures. Because the Inoue balloon can be inflated over a broad range of diameters, multiple inflations are often made with progressively larger balloon diameters to effect an optimal result.

PREPARATION OF THE INOUE BALLOON.[31] This balloon catheter is packaged with the compo-nents necessary for valve dilation, including (1) a 0.025-inch spring exchange guide wire; (2) a relatively rigid 14-French dilator; (3) a metal tube for stretching the calipers used to measure the balloon diameter; (4) an inflation syringe, calibrated in milliliters; and (5) a stylet used to negotiate the balloon through the mitral valve orifice. Dilute contrast (2:1) is injected into the vent lumen to remove air from the inflation-deflation channel into the balloon. The calibrated inflation syringe is then filled up to the equivalent of the smallest balloon diameter (24 mm). The syringe is then connected to the inflation port, and the balloon is inflated over 10 to 20 seconds so that the nylon mesh is stretched slowly and without a chance for rupture; the balloon is then deflated passively. Then, the balloon is inflated rapidly, and the diameter is measured to verify that the precalibrated inflation syringe produces the minimum inflated diameter. Adjustments are made in the inflation volume, as necessary, to achieve the desired balloon diameter as measured by the

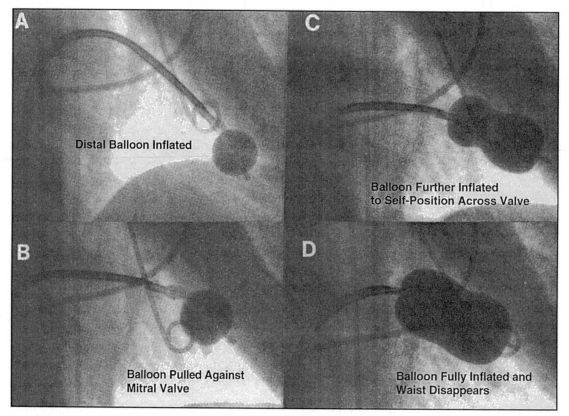

Figure 32–2. Progressive stages of the inflation of an Inoue mitral balloon valvuloplasty catheter. A pigtail catheter has also been passed retrograde across the aortic valve into the left ventricle. *A,* The balloon, only the distal portion partially inflated, is passed across the mitral valve. *B,* The distal portion is inflated further and then pulled back until it engages the mitral valve. *C,* The balloon is partially inflated further, allowing it to self-position across the mitral valve orifice. *D,* The balloon is fully inflated, and with disappearance of the narrow "waist" the commissures are opened. (From Feldman T, Carroll JD: The Inoue balloon for percutaneous mitral commissurotomy. Cardio Intervent 1992; 2:13–19.)

calipers. The syringe is subsequently filled to an amount equivalent to the maximal nominal inflated size, and again the balloon is inflated and tested to ensure that the maximum size dimension is achieved.

Next, the stretching metal tube (Fig. 32–3) is inserted into the central lumen and pushed down the balloon catheter until it locks into the metal hub at the balloon's proximal end. The hub and tube are advanced into the balloon catheter until the plastic Luer lock is engaged. After this procedure, the balloon is left in its stretched form.

BALLOON CATHETER (INOUE) PASSAGE (see Fig. 32–3). An initial step is to pass through the Mullins sheath (USCI, Billerica, MA) a 0.025-inch guide wire that is then curled near the roof of the left atrium. The Mullins sheath is removed, and the 14-French plastic dilator is advanced over the guide wire until it passes through the interatrial septum. This dilating maneuver is often profitably repeated three or four times. The balloon catheter subsequently is exchanged over the guide wire for the dilator and advanced through the skin, the interatrial septum, and into the left atrium. The balloon must be allowed to resume its unstretched configuration to avoid puncturing the roof of the left atrium with the stiff slenderizing tube. This is accomplished by disengaging the stretching metal tube from the catheter metal hub (see Fig. 32–3, panels 3 through 5) at the time that the tip of the balloon catheter has passed across the interatrial septum. Also, the plastic Luer lock is now disconnected, a maneuver that allows the balloon to shorten and assume its larger deflated profile. At this juncture the balloon should track the coil of the spring guide wire (see Fig. 32–3, panel 6) and curl down toward the orifice of the mitral valve. The stretching metal tube and spring guide wire are removed, cleaned, and saved until the end of the procedure.

Once the transmitral gradient is again registered, the balloon catheter is then stiffened by introducing the steering stylet, the balloon partially inflated with 3 to 8 mL of dilute contrast medium, and then the assembly is rotated counterclockwise in the right anterior oblique projection (see Fig. 32–2). The balloon should then seek out the mitral orifice and pass into the left ventricle; as it does so, the stylet is withdrawn about 10 cm. Thereafter, the distal half is inflated somewhat more and pulled back until it engages the mitral valve (see Fig. 32–2B). The proximal half of the balloon is then inflated partially, and when the position of the balloon appears correct, the inflation is com-

pleted (see Fig. 32–2C and D). Hypotension may occur as the balloon apparatus obstructs further a stenotic orifice, but provided the procedure of inflation and deflation is performed expeditiously, the hemodynamic embarrassment lasts no longer than 10 to 20 seconds.

As the balloon deflates, it usually retracts back into the left atrium; if not then gentle clockwise rotation brings this about. Gradient assessment is again performed, along with cardiac output determinations, to calculate the change in valve orifice area. A Doppler and two-dimensional echocardiographic assessment can also be done at this point to assess any worsening of mitral regurgitation. If the result is considered unsatisfactory, further inflations are undertaken using a 1-mm augmentation of balloon diameter size at full inflation.

BALLOON CATHETER WITHDRAWAL. Before making a final pull-back of the balloon catheter across the interatrial septum, it is important to take a terminal thermodilution cardiac output reading; if done after the pull-back, and while there is significant left-to-right shunting across the iatrogenic atrial septal defect, then the thermodilution measurement may overestimate true transmitral diastolic flow and exaggerate the orifice size.[32]

CAVEATS ABOUT BOTH DOUBLE-BALLOON AND SINGLE-BALLOON TECHNIQUES. With either double-balloon or single-balloon approaches, the ease with which a catheter balloon mitral valvotomy can be performed is dependent on the ready movement of the catheter(s) through the venotomy at the right groin, the site of puncture of the interatrial septum, the adequacy of the hole in the interatrial septum, the size of the left atrium, and the stability of the guide wire(s) in the left atrium and left ventricle. Successful completion of the procedure requires a high degree of operator concentration and alertness, comfortable and coordinated interaction between the primary and secondary operators, and meticulous attention to proper technique.

If the balloon catheter binds as it passes through the percutaneous puncture and venotomy in the right groin, it is advisable to redilate the area with a straight clamp and/or larger dilator. If the angle of entry into the vein is relatively steep, then use of a 14-French sheath will facilitate passage of the balloon catheter assembly.

Some patients with mitral stenosis have a markedly enlarged left atrium that displaces the interatrial septum into a plane that is near parallel with that of the transseptal needle apparatus. In this circumstance, as the needle is ad-

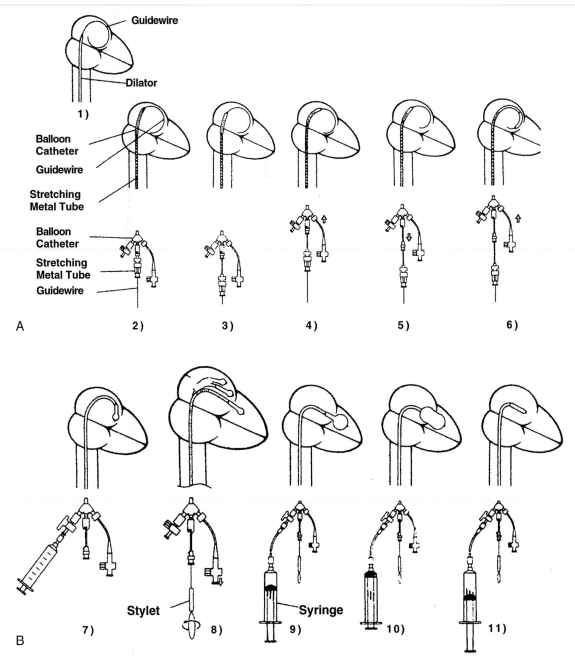

Figure 32–3. A and B, Illustration of the Inoue balloon mitral valvotomy procedure. 1. After a spring guide wire is introduced into the left atrium via the Mullins sheath, the interatrial septum is dilated using a rigid 14-French plastic dilator. 2. The elongated balloon catheter is advanced over the wire through the interatrial septum. 3. The stretching metal tube is partially withdrawn, allowing the balloon to shorten and curl within the left atrium. 4. The balloon is advanced through the interatrial septum. 5. The stretching metal tube and balloon straightening device are further withdrawn. 6. The balloon is advanced beyond the mitral orifice. 7. The balloon's distal portion is partially inflated with a contrast medium–saline mixture. 8. With a counterclockwise rotation of the stylet, slight advancement of the catheter shaft, and withdrawal of the stylet, the balloon is directed through the mitral orifice into the left ventricle. 9. The partially inflated balloon is withdrawn against the mitral orifice, fully and rapidly inflated (10.), and allowed to deflate. 11. After deflation, usually the balloon passively returns to the left atrium from the left ventricle. (Courtesy of Toray Industries, Tokyo, Japan.)

vanced forward, it tends to dissect the interatrial septum (Fig. 32–4A and B). Kyphoscoliosis or an atrial septal aneurysm can also significantly complicate finding the foramen ovale for the transseptal needle puncture. Simultaneous echocardiography has been found useful in guiding the locale for the puncture site.[33–39] Despite advantages of simplicity and noninvasiveness, transthoracic echocardiography interferes with simultaneous fluoroscopic imaging, exposes the echocardiographer to irradiation, and inhibits preservation of a sterile field. Transesophageal echocardiography gives high-quality images of the interatrial septum; nevertheless, this approach has the inherent risks of esophageal injury and lung aspiration, and the invasive nature of the procedure can be uncomfortable and stressful for the patient. Intracardiac echocardiography, using an 8-French catheter with a field depth radius of 4 to 8 cm appears to be particularly promising for facilitating the safe and comfortable performance of transseptal left atrial catheterization in patients with complex problems (Fig. 32–5A–D).[38, 39]

If passage of double-balloon catheters through the interatrial septum is problematic, then redilation of the hole, four to five times, with an 8- to 10-mm balloon is useful, or in the case of the single balloon technique, reapplication of the Inoue 14-French dilator often facilitates subsequent passage.

Whenever the puncture in the interatrial septum is relatively high and anterior, the balloon catheter assembly may be difficult to manipulate toward the orifice of the mitral valve. A useful approach, as shown in Figure 32–6, is to torque the catheter clockwise and loop the assembly off the roof of the left atrium. The leading end of the catheter will often then be directed in toward the mitral valve orifice. Once the balloon has crossed the mitral valve, the loop can then either be pulled down or, alternatively, left in place during the valve dilations.

Results of Mitral Catheter Balloon Valvuloplasty

Approximately a decade of experience with mitral catheter balloon valvuloplasty has revealed it to be an excellent procedure in well-selected patients for short-term and long-term relief of the hemodynamic consequences of mitral valve obstruction (Fig. 32–7). Less optimal results, however, have been noted in those patients with more severe valvular and subvalvular deformity, as evaluated by echocardiographic criteria (see earlier). These latter patients have a less optimal immediate result[23, 25, 26, 40–43] a higher incidence of restenosis, and a higher cardiovascular event rate during follow-up.

IMMEDIATE AND SHORT-TERM. The National Heart, Lung, and Blood Institute (NHLBI) organized a multicenter registry of 24 cooperating

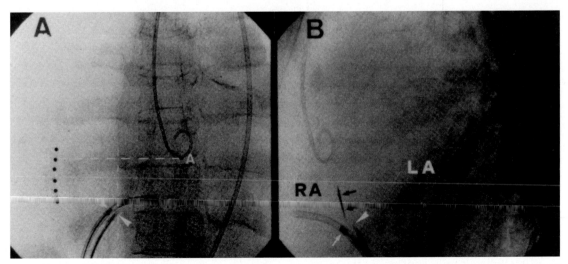

Figure 32–4. Patient with large left atrium undergoing transseptal catheterization. *A,* In frontal plane, a pigtail catheter (A) is positioned in the root of the ascending aorta; a dotted line marks the rightward boundary of the right atrium. The transseptal needle is positioned at the puncture site *(white arrowhead)* on the vertical "midline," a point equidistant from the aortic valve and the right atrial edge. *B,* Lateral fluoroscopic view, showing right atrium (RA) compressed by a large left atrium (LA) and catheter ultrasound catheter transducer within a Mullins sheath. A small dissection is present from the initial puncture, as evidenced by contrast stain *(black arrows)* within the interatrial septum. (From Hung JS, Fu M, Yeh KH, et al: Usefulness of intracardiac echocardiography in complex transseptal catheterization during percutaneous transvenous mitral commissurotomy. Mayo Clin Proc 1996; 71:134–140.)

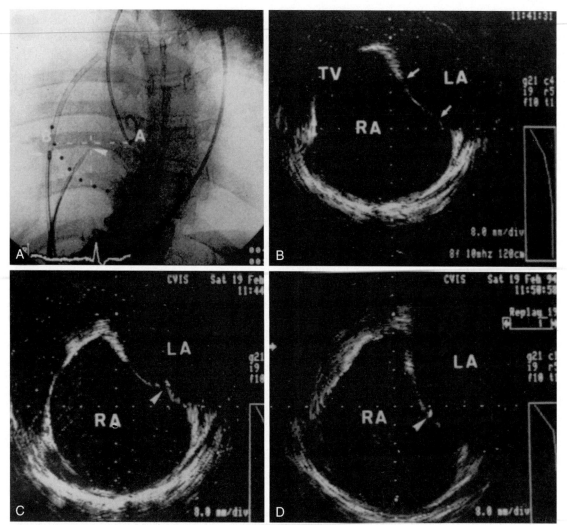

Figure 32–5. Use of intracardiac catheter ultrasound imaging of the interatrial septum to facilitate transseptal puncture during mitral balloon valvuloplasty procedure in a patient with kyphoscoliosis. *A,* Frontal fluoroscopic view, showing selection of puncture site *(white arrowhead)* on vertical "midline." The catheter ultrasound transducer is seen within the Mullins sheath. *B,* Intracardiac ultrasound image, demonstrating tricuspid valve (TV) and interatrial septum *(arrows),* bulging slightly toward the right atrium (RA). *C,* Indentation is created at thin-walled fossa ovalis when catheter and needle tip *(arrowhead)* are pressed firmly against the septum. *D,* After insertion of catheter into left atrium (LA), septal indentation is no longer present. The catheter and needle tip are shown as an echogenic point *(arrowhead)* in *C* and *D.* (From Hung JS, Fu M, Yeh KH, et al: Usefulness of intracardiac echocardiography in complex transseptal catheterization during percutaneous transvenous mitral commissurotomy. Mayo Clin Proc 1996; 71:134–140.)

centers in the late 1980s, and the hemodynamic and Doppler and two-dimensional echocardiographic results from this cumulative experience in 738 patients are provided in Table 32–2.[44, 45] Double-balloon dilation, as opposed to only a single-balloon (non-Inoue) dilation, gave a superior immediate result, confirming the experience reported from single centers.[26, 46, 47] The incidence of significant interatrial shunts was more frequent in the double-balloon, as opposed to, single-balloon patients ($P = 0.04$). In this combined series the average mitral valve area after final dilation using two balloons was

2.0 ± 0.8 cm^2 by the Gorlin equation (Fig. 32–8) and 1.8 ± 0.5 cm^2 by the Doppler pressure half-time method. The increase in mitral valve area was only weakly related to echo score when the latter was treated as a continuous variable. If treated as a categorical dichotomous variable, those patients with the lower echo scores[4–8] had somewhat greater mean increases in mitral valve area (1.0 ± 0.7 cm^2) as compared with those patients with the higher scores of 9 to 16 (0.85 ± 0.6 cm^2; $P = 0.004$). Other continuous variables that predicted a more successful result included younger age, lower pul-

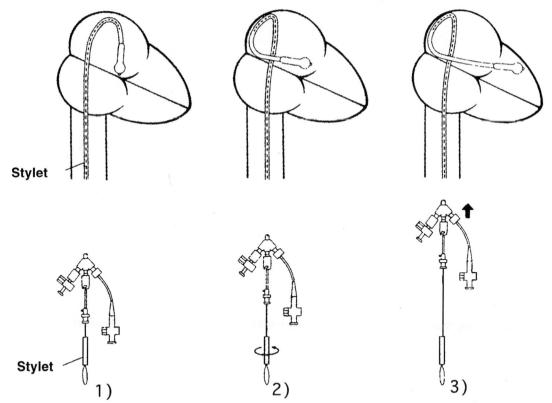

Stylet

Stylet

1)   **2)**   **3)**

Figure 32–6. Alternative approach to advancement of mitral balloon valvuloplasty catheter across the mitral valve. **1.** The balloon is introduced into the left atrium in the usual manner and guided past the mitral orifice. **2.** With a clockwise rotation of the stylet and catheter shaft, a loop is created that directs the balloon off the posterior left atrial wall. **3.** Withdrawal of the stylet and advancement of the catheter shaft directs the balloon catheter across the mitral valve into the left ventricle. (Courtesy of Toray Industries, Tokyo, Japan.)

monary artery pressure, and treatment with larger balloons. Categorical variables that were associated with a final valve orifice size of more than 1.5 cm^2 included were a lower New York Heart Association (NYHA) classification and normal sinus rhythm predilation, double-balloon technique, and absence of mitral valve calcification. At the 30-day follow-up, 4% of the patients with completed procedures were referred for mitral valve surgery, 3% had died, and 83% reported that their condition had improved.

LONGER-TERM. The 6-month follow-up of NHLBI registry patients in relation to echo morphology score has also been reported.[48] A multiple regression analysis revealed that the mitral valve area after balloon valvuloplasty could be predicted by the preprocedure mitral valve area ($P<0.001$), left atrial size ($P = 0.01$), balloon diameter ($P = 0.02$), cardiac output ($P = 0.004$), and leaflet mobility ($P = 0.01$). The total morphology score, leaflet thickness, calcification, and subvalvular disease were not important univariate or multivariate predictors

of the ultimate result of mitral balloon valvuloplasty.

The group from the Massachusetts General Hospital (MGH) reported their single-center experience in 1989.[26] In this analysis there was a significant difference in the ultimate mitral valve area attained between those patients below and above an echocardiographic "score" of 8 ($P<0.01$). Also, in a longer-term follow-up in a group of 37 patients, there appeared to be a restenosis rate of only 4% (1/27) in those with an echocardiographic score of 8 or less whereas the rate was 70% (7/10) in those patients with a score higher than 8. Palacios later described results in 320 patients after single-balloon and double-balloon valvotomy and reported an event-free survival of 77%, with 19% requiring mitral valve replacement at 2 years.[49] The 3-year event-free survival was 70%. By comparison, those patients with an MGH echocardiographic score higher than 8 had less favorable results with a 3-year event-free survival of 46%.

BALLOON VALVULOPLASTY AFTER PREVIOUS SURGICAL COMMISSUROTOMY. An important group of

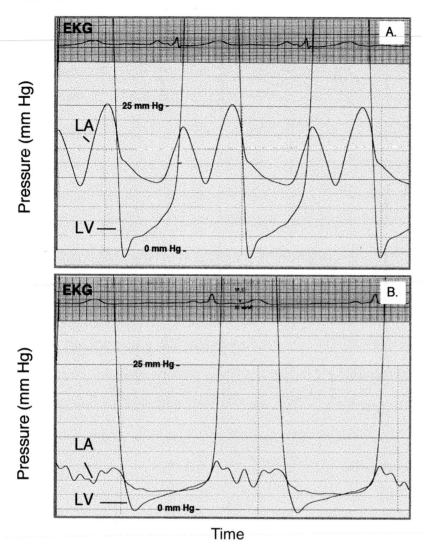

Figure 32-7. Left ventricular (LV) and left atrial (LA) pressure pulses recorded before *(A)* and after *(B)* successful mitral balloon valvuloplasty. Note the significant reduction of the diastolic pressure gradient. (Courtesy of Rainaldo Beyer, MD, University of California, San Diego.)

patients with mitral stenosis is the subset that has previously undergone a surgical commissurotomy. Hemodynamically significant restenosis often occurs within 5 to 15 years and compels a repeat intervention.[19, 50–52] The investigators of the NHLBI compiled a registry of 133 patients who underwent balloon mitral commissurotomy after a previous surgical commissurotomy and found little difference in the hemodynamic result, complication, or functional status as compared with those patients without a previous surgical commissurotomy.[52] The 6-month mortality rate was low (0% to 1% for both groups; P = NS), and 80% of cases were found to be in NYHA functional class I or II at that time. In the previous surgical commissurotomy group, the mitral valve area averaged 1.0 ± 0.3 cm² before and 1.8 ± 0.8 cm² after the balloon dilation; the comparable values in the patients with no prior commissurotomy were 1.0 ± 0.4

cm² and 2.0 ± 0.8 cm², respectively (see Fig. 32–8). Balloon mitral valvuloplasty after previous surgical commissurotomy produced a significant reduction in transvalvular gradient from 13 ± 5 to 6 ± 3 mm Hg ($P<0.0001$). The multivariate predictors of improvement in 6-month clinical status were the experience of the center (P = 0.006), a lower echocardiographic score (P = 0.001), and a lower left ventricular end-diastolic pressure (P = 0.008).

INOUE BALLOON VALVULOPLASTY. The results of Inoue balloon valvotomy have been reported from both North America and other countries.[53–60] Initially the safety and efficacy of this approach were well documented in reports from Japan and China.[53, 54] Thereafter, the multicenter results in 200 procedures performed in North America were reported,[55] and the multicenter results in 4832 patients treated

Table 32–2. National Heart, Blood, and Lung Institute Balloon Valvuloplasty Registry Results

Hemodynamic Results of Completed Balloon Mitral Commissurotomy

	MV Gradient (mm Hg)	MV Area (cm²)	Mean LA Pressure (mm Hg)	Cardiac Output (L/min)	Mean PA Pressure (mm Hg)	Increased MR (%)	L-R Shunt (Qp/Qs ratio >1.5) (%)
Single balloon							
n =	121	99	86	98	75	52	49
Before	14 ± 6	0.9 ± 0.4	26 ± 7	3.9 ± 1.2	40 ± 14		
After	7 ± 3*	1.7 ± 0.7*	19 ± 6*	4.5 ± 1.2*	34 ± 12*	4	2
Double balloon							
n =	559	557	538	553	511	493	440
Before	14 ± 6	1.0 ± 0.3	25 ± 7	4.1 ± 1.2	35 ± 13		
After	6 ± 3*	2.0 ± 0.8*	16 ± 7*	4.5 ± 1.4*	29 ± 11*	12	12

Echocardiographic/Doppler Hemodynamic Results

	MV Gradient (mm Hg)	MV Area (2-D planimeter) (cm²)	MV area ($t_{1/2}$) (cm²)	LA Size (L/min)
Single balloon				
n =	89	38	92	88
Before	9 ± 4	1.1 ± 0.5	1.1 ± 0.3	54 ± 12
After	6 ± 3*	1.6 ± 0.4*	1.6 ± 0.5*	52 ± 10†
Double balloon				
n =	58	307	421	476
Before	10 ± 4	1.1 ± 0.3	1.1 ± 0.3	52 ± 9
After	5 ± 2*	1.7 ± 0.5*	1.8 ± 0.5*	49 ± 8*

*$P < 0.0001$ vs. before.
†$P < 0.05$ vs. before.
MV, mitral valve; LA, left atrial; PA, pulmonary artery; MR, mitral regurgitation; L-R, left-to-right; 2-D, two-dimensional.

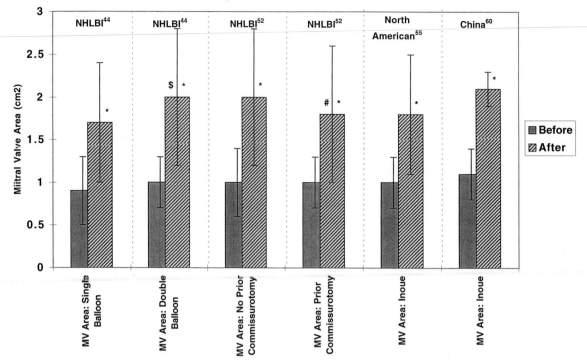

Figure 32–8. Compilation of changes in mitral valve orifice area immediately following mitral balloon valvuloplasty, as reported in selected registries of patients. Note that final result is quite comparable irrespective of technique and prior surgical commissurotomy.

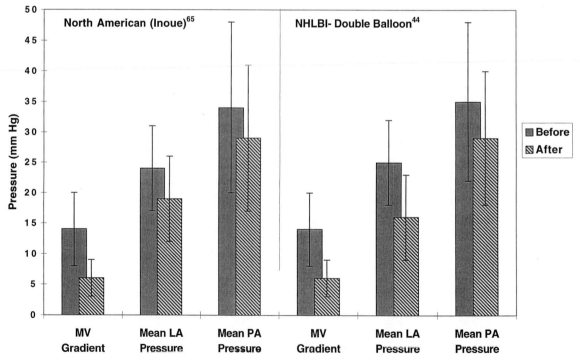

Figure 32–9. Compilation of changes in relevant pressure measurements immediately following mitral balloon valvuloplasty, as reported in selected registries of patients. Use of the Inoue mitral balloon catheter results are shown in the left panel, and the results of the conventional double-balloon technique are shown in the right panel.

in China have been compiled and reported.[60] The hemodynamic data and early restenosis rates were similar to those reported by investigators compiling the results of single-balloon and double-balloon techniques, using the Mansfield balloon catheters.[44, 45, 61, 62]

As shown in Figure 32–9, in the North American Registry the mean transmitral gradient fell from 14 ± 6 to 6 ± 3 mm Hg ($P<0.001$), and the mean mitral valve area increased from 1.0 ± 0.3 to 1.8 ± 0.7 cm^2 ($P<0.01$).[55] These results are closely comparable with those reported by the NHLBI Registry investigators. As in other reports, the total echocardiographic valvular score had only a weak correlation with immediate outcome and was not significant in multivariate analysis (Fig. 32–10). Important determinants of successful procedures were the presence of a relatively high prevalvotomy gradient and a small preprocedure valve area.

The same North American multicenter Inoue registry investigators have reported results in 72 patients (of a total of 550 in the registry) with severe valvular and subvalvular deformity (MGH echo score ≥10).[63] The mitral valve area increased from 0.9 ± 0.3 to 1.5 ± 0.5 cm^2, and an immediate satisfactory result was obtained in 46 subjects (64%). Over a mean follow-up of 22.9 ± 11 months, the cardiovascular event rate (mitral valve replacement, repeat valvotomy, and death) was relatively high (actuarial 3-year event-free survival of 42%) compared with other patients in the registry.

Complications of Mitral Balloon Valvuloplasty

The major complications of mitral balloon valvuloplasty are listed in Table 32–3. Creation of an atrial septal defect has been the most common complication, varying between 0.1% and 18%, depending on the criteria used for a significant shunt. Use of a smaller balloon (5 ver-

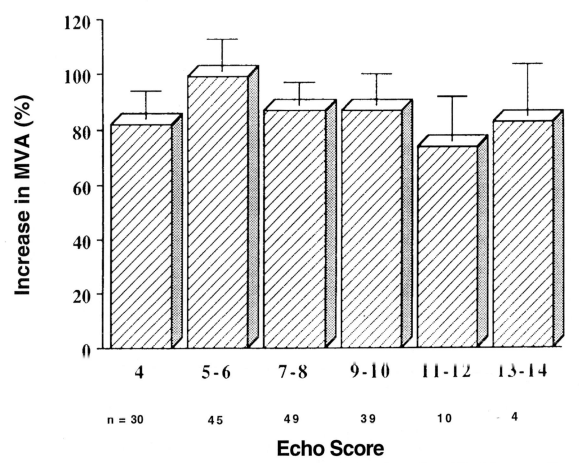

Figure 32–10. Relation between mitral valve "echo score," compiled by the Massachusetts General Hospital system, and increase in mitral valve area (percentage) following Inoue mitral balloon valvuloplasty. Note the relatively weak correlation. (From Herrmann HC, Ramaswamy K, Isner JM, et al: Factors influencing immediate results, complications, and short-term follow-up status after Inoue balloon mitral valvotomy: A North American multicenter study. Am Heart J 1992; 124:160–166.)

Table 32–3. **Incidence of Complications of Mitral Valve Balloon Commissurotomy: Registry Results**

Type	Standard Balloon(s) (%)	Registry and Reference	Inoue Balloon (%)	Registry and Reference
Death (1–30-day follow-up)	2.7	M-Heart[61]	0.5–1.4	North American[55, 64]
	3.3 (30-day)	NHLBI[44]		
	1.1 (1-day)	NHLBI[45]	0.12	China[60]
Cardiac perforation	9.3	M-Heart[61]	1.5	North American[55]
	3.7	NHLBI[52]		
Tamponade	6.7	M-Heart[61]	1.0	North American[55]
	3.7	NHLBI[52]	0.8	China
Systemic embolism	2.1	M-Heart[61]	2.0	North American[55]
	2.7	NHLBI[52]	0.5	China[60]
Interatrial shunt	18	M-Heart[61]	2.8*	North American[55]
	12	NHLBI[44]		
	9.6	NHLBI[52]	0.1‡	China[60]
Severe worsening of mitral leakage	8	M-Heart[61]	2.4†	North American[55]
	3.3	NHLBI[52]	1.4	China[60]
Cardiac arrhythmias				
Requiring treatment	9.6	NHLBI[52]	2.4	North American[55]
Conduction disturbance	5.3	M-Heart[61]		
Blood transfusion	6.7	M-Heart[61]		
	8.6	NHLBI[52]		
Prolonged hypotension	4	M-Heart[61]		
	6.8	NHLBI[52]		
Vascular injury or hematoma	0.5	NHLBI[52]	1.8	North American[65]
Emergency or subsequent surgery	6.7	M-Heart[61]	0.3	China[60]
	4	NHLBI[44]		

M-Heart Registry: n = 74 patients (75 procedures) enrolled between May 1986 and January 1989.
NHLBI Registry: n = 738 patients enrolled between November 1, 1987, and October 31, 1989.
North American Registry: n = 200 patients enrolled between June 1989 to May 1991. *Q_p:Q_s ratio ≥ 2.0; †Regurgitation increase ≥ 3 grades. Reference 64 includes results on 290 patients.
China Registry: n = 4832 patients enrolled between November 1985 and January 1994. ‡"Lutembacher" syndrome.

sus 8 mm) to dilate the interatrial septum has significantly reduced this complication in one group's experience.[61]

The incidence of death directly related to the procedure has been reported as 0% to 2.7% and compares favorably with surgical series of either closed or open commissurotomy. Mortality rates have improved as experience with the procedure has accumulated and patient selection refined. Death rates at 30 days after the procedure have been reported as 3.3% in the NHLBI registry.[44]

Perforation of the heart during atrial transseptal puncture, or subsequent passage and inflation or the balloon catheters, represents another significant risk and highlights the importance of experience in performing acute periocardiocentesis and surgical standby for chest exploration. Left ventricular perforation is decidedly more common with the double-balloon technique than with use of the Inoue single-balloon approach.[65] Other serious complications include embolization of either thrombotic or calcific material and the induction of ventricular arrhythmias requiring cardioversion. Induction of worsened mitral regurgitation, usually caused by rupture of a chordal structure, is a further serious complication.

COMPARISON OF MITRAL BALLOON VALVULOPLASTY WITH SURGICAL COMMISSUROTOMY. Turi and colleagues performed a prospective, randomized trial that compared percutaneous balloon commissurotomy with surgical closed commissurotomy in 40 patients (20 in each group) with severe rheumatic mitral stenosis.[66] Both at a 1-week and at an 8-month follow-up evaluation no significant difference was found between the two groups as assessed by mitral valve area. Subsequently, these same authors reported on a second randomized, prospective trial that compared percutaneous balloon valvuloplasty with open surgical commissurotomy.[67] In this study 60 patients were enrolled, 30 patients in each group. Both groups demonstrated an initial improvement of the mitral valve area to 2.0 to 2.1 cm². Although improvement was maintained in both groups at 3 years' follow-up, the mitral valve areas were greater in the patients in the balloon valvuloplasty group (2.4 ± 0.6 cm² versus 1.8 ± 0.4 cm² in the surgery group; $P<0.001$). Restenosis rates were comparable in the two groups at 3 years' follow-up.

SUMMARY. Reports emanating from both multicenter registries and large single-center experiences suggest that both double-balloon and single (Inoue)-balloon catheter techniques are capable of significantly improving mitral stenosis to a postprocedure valve area of approximately 1.7 to 2.1 cm². A randomized trial that compares these two technical approaches has not been accomplished. Accumulated clinical experience suggests that both the conventional and Inoue approaches have advantages and disadvantages. The Inoue device, with its segmental hourglass inflation profile, is attractive because of the ease of positioning across the valve, the reduced risk of ventricular perforation, tip steerability to assist in crossing the valve, design that allows progressively larger balloon inflations, rapid inflation-deflation times, and the ability to measure left atrial pressure through the central lumen after each inflation. The double-balloon approach probably provides a slightly yet significantly greater valve orifice area as an end result, but the procedure is technically more demanding and time consuming and exhibits a higher complication rate. In randomized studies, balloon dilation provides results comparable with either closed or open surgical commissurotomy while avoiding a thoracotomy and at significantly reduced cost. Although not without risk, balloon mitral valvuloplasty should be considered for all patients with favorable mitral valve pathoanatomy.

AORTIC STENOSIS

Mechanism of Action and Indications

In like fashion to mitral valvuloplasty, the usefulness of balloon catheters for relief of aortic valvular stenosis is inherent in the pathologic processes underlying the obstruction. Other elements in addition to commissural fusion are operative in the pathogenesis of valvular aortic stenosis, including congenital malformation (particularly the bicuspid valve[68, 69]), calcification,[70] and stiffening and thickening of the valve leaflets. Thus, the immediate success of the dilation depends on the architecture and pliability of the valve as it is influenced by age, the size of the arc of attachment of the valve leaflets, and the degree of calcification.

Some authors have questioned whether aortic balloon dilation has a salutary effect on valve orifice area. Robicsek and Harbold performed balloon valvotomy on 16 patients whose aortic valves were exposed at the operating table.[71] Careful planimetric measurement of the valve orifice area, before and after dilation, failed to reveal significant augmentation of valve orifice area in any of the patients. In contrast, balloon

valvuloplasty performed postmortem on fresh specimens of adult aortic stenosis indicated that orifice augmentation occurred by three mechanisms, including stretch of valve tissue, rupture of commissural fusion, and fracture of calcific deposits.[72] The last two mechanisms, in particular, were noted to cause an increased opening of the valve leaflets. If stretching of valve tissue alone occurs, there may be only temporary hemodynamic improvement, measured in hours, owing to elastic recoil.[73] Calcific emboli appear not to occur with significant frequency because they remain embedded in the valve leaflets.

Because of the significant success of prosthetic aortic valve replacement and the relatively low operative mortality rate in most adult patients with aortic stenosis,[74–79] as well as the relatively high rate of hemodynamic evidence of restenosis after dilation,[80–82] balloon valvuloplasty is firmly indicated in adult patients in only a few subjects, including the following:

1. Those with a limited life span due to noncardiac illness (e.g., metastatic malignant disease)

2. Those for whom cardiac surgery is undesirable for reasons of mental incapacity, inability to attend to one's own needs, or advanced age (this indication should be individualized)

3. Those with an increased operative risk for aortic valve replacement due to a major noncardiac illness (e.g., advanced chronic obstructive lung disease)

4. Those with an urgent indication for noncardiac surgery that would be complicated by the coexistence of severe valvular aortic stenosis

5. Those with advanced heart failure, or cardiogenic shock, in whom a "bridge" dilation of the aortic valve allows improvement in overall clinical condition before a prosthetic valve replacement is performed

6. Those in whom there are signs of significant left ventricular dysfunction but in whom the severity and role of aortic valvular stenosis are ambiguous

In pediatric patients balloon aortic valvuloplasty can palliate significant valve obstruction with much longer-lasting success and may delay the time for valve replacement until adulthood and full growth is reached.[83]

Prevalvuloplasty Evaluation

Before performance of catheter balloon aortic valvuloplasty, the clinical status of the patient, relevant physical findings, two-dimensional echocardiography with Doppler recording and imaging, as well as cardiac catheterization data and angiography, should be carefully reviewed.

DOPPLER AND TWO-DIMENSIONAL ECHOCARDIOGRAPHY. Two-dimensional echocardiography and Doppler velocity data now play a major role in the assessment of the severity of aortic valvular stenosis. The techniques are also important in ruling out coexistent obstruction at the subvalvular level (fixed or dynamic related to hypertrophic obstructive cardiomyopathy). They also are helpful in establishing the temporal changes in left ventricular function, the efficacy of the dilation on the severity of obstruction, and the coexistence of aortic regurgitation both before and after the balloon dilation. Using the modified Bernoulli equation, the aortic valve pressure gradient (mean and peak instantaneous) can be accurately estimated from continuous wave recordings of ascending aortic velocities[84]; the orifice area also can be closely estimated from the continuity equation (see Chapter 18).[85] These data are then correlated with the direct pressure measurements and the Gorlin valve orifice area calculation made at the time of a diagnostic cardiac catheterization. Because under ideal experimental conditions,[86] the correlation of the continuity equation and the Gorlin calculation is 0.74, with a standard error of the estimate of 0.12 cm², we recommend that patients not be referred for a valvuloplasty procedure based on two-dimensional echocardiographic and Doppler data alone. Others have expressed a similar opinion, based on review of correlated data obtained in humans.[87] Moreover, because most candidates for aortic balloon valvuloplasty are adults with possible coronary heart disease, they need coronary angiography performed before a therapeutic intervention. In these patients, we measure routinely at the time of the left-sided heart catheterization an aortic transvalvular pressure gradient and cardiac output and then calculate the Gorlin equation orifice size. Nevertheless, there is considerable controversy and difference of opinion about this recommendation and practice.[88-90]

CATHETERIZATION AND ANGIOGRAPHIC DATA. The approaches to obtaining reliable hemodynamic assessment of the severity of valvular aortic stenosis are discussed in Chapter 18. To reiterate, we prefer to obtain a simultaneous pressure measurement in the left ventricle and ascending aorta in close proximity to the time that cardiac output determinations are performed.

Procedural Technique

Several approaches have been used to place one or more balloon catheters across a stenotic aortic valve, including the retrograde percutaneous approach, a retrograde direct-arterial entry approach, and an antegrade approach via a transseptal catheterization of the left heart.

RETROGRADE PERCUTANEOUS APPROACH. A percutaneous retrograde entry into the left ventricle, through the right or left femoral artery, is performed by standard techniques (see Chapter 2), using a 14-French sheath (Cook, UMI, or Schneider Medintag) in the artery. An extra stiff 0.038-inch guide wire (Cook or Schneider Medintag) is then looped at the apex of the left ventricle so that its J-shaped tip curls back toward the inflow of the left ventricle and so as to minimize ventricular ectopy. Preshaping of the wire before its insertion helps achieve this configuration. While the guide wire is held firmly in place, the retrograde catheter is then withdrawn and exchanged for a single dilating catheter that is 15 to 23 mm wide when fully inflated. Choice of balloon size can be profitably dictated by analysis of the aortic annulus size by echocardiography. It is preferable that the operator begin with a smaller-size rather than larger-size balloon. Multiple inflations are performed with each size balloon until it appears that the balloon is fully inflated and there is no longer a waist during inflation at the level of the aortic annulus (Fig. 32–11). Undersized balloons are frequently propelled into the aorta during ventricular ejection. Alternatively, with balloons not held in place, the catheter may move abruptly toward the left ventricular apex as it is inflated. The operator must be vigilant to watch for these potential movements. The balloon is quickly deflated if there is severe hypotension, severe arrhythmias, a presyncopal or seizure state, or abrupt ST-segment shifts. Atropine, 0.6 mg, given intravenously, is useful as prophylaxis against bradycardia during the balloon inflation.

ANTEGRADE TRANSSEPTAL APPROACH. In some patients with severe peripheral vascular disease, abdominal aortic disease, or severe iliac tortuosity, the retrograde approach may be technically difficult. An alternative approach to the left ventricle is using the transseptal atrial puncture (Brockenbrough modified needle) and a Mullins sheath. Once the sheath is placed safely into the left atrium and the patient heparinized, a CO_2-filled balloon flotation catheter (Arrow International, Reading, PA) is floated across the mitral valve and through the left ventricle into the aorta. If there is difficulty in passing the catheter through the stenotic aortic orifice, partial deflation of the balloon is helpful, or a flexible 0.025-inch guide wire may be helpful in

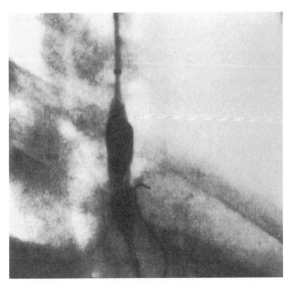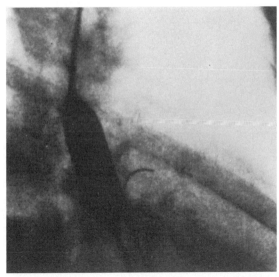

Figure 32–11. Correct positioning of a 15-mm balloon catheter across the aortic valve in a patient with aortic stenosis. *Left panel,* Demonstration of early inflation; the indentation from the calcified stenotic valve is clearly seen. *Right panel,* Demonstration of disappearance of the indentation at full inflation. (From Cribier A, Savin T, Berland J, et al: Percutaneous transluminal balloon valvuloplasty of adult aortic stenosis: Report of 92 cases. J Am Coll Cardiol 1987; 9:381–386. Reprinted with permission from the American College of Cardiology.)

traversing the aortic valve. Once the balloon catheter is well into the ascending aorta, a 0.038-inch exchange wire is advanced through the balloon catheter into the descending thoracic aorta. The Mullins sheath and balloon catheter are then removed, with the exchange wire held firmly in place. One must also be careful that the exchange wire remains looped in the left ventricle and does not cinch up against the anterior leaflet of the mitral valve. The interatrial septum is next dilated with a 5-mm balloon catheter and then exchanged for the balloon valvuloplasty catheter (15 to 23 mm). As with the retrograde approach, multiple inflations are performed until the balloon appears fully inflated and transient hypotension occurs. Repeat hemodynamic measurements are then made using standard catheters inserted over the guide wire.

OTHER ALTERNATIVE APPROACHES. Some patients in whom the percutaneous femoral approach is not feasible can be approached using a direct cutdown over the brachial artery, provided its lumen is sufficiently large. Again, a 14-French sheath is inserted into the brachial arteriotomy that is then repaired at the end of the procedure. Some operators also prefer to have surgical assistance in making a direct cutdown on the femoral artery that is then repaired under direct vision after the completion of procedure. These latter approaches have the advantage that bleeding can more readily be controlled.

In a few patients there appears to be no measurable impact of the balloon dilation using a single-balloon catheter. In this situation, some operators have used a double-balloon technique,[91–93] where either two balloon catheters are inserted sequentially through the same sheath using two guide wires, or inserted through two separate vascular accesses, such as both femoral arteries, one femoral artery and a brachial artery cutdown.

The leading French investigators in balloon aortic valvuloplasty have reported on the use of a specially designed balloon catheter with three lumina and a distal pigtail tip (Boston Scientific, Inc.), Figure 32–12.[94] One lumen upstream to the balloon is used to record ascending aortic pressure; a distal lumen is used to record left ventricular pressure and inject contrast material. The balloon itself is double sized and is inflated through the third lumen. The proximal balloon segment is 3.5 cm long and 20 mm wide when inflated, and the distal segment is 2 cm long and 15 mm wide when inflated. Other catheters with modifications of these segment sizes have also been made. This catheter allows sequential dilation of the valve, first with the smaller distal segment of the balloon followed by a dilation with the larger proximal segment. The transvalvular gradient is readily measured by removing the guide wire and leaving the pigtail tip into the left ventricle. Use of this balloon has significantly reduced procedure time and purportedly improves the hemodynamic results.[94]

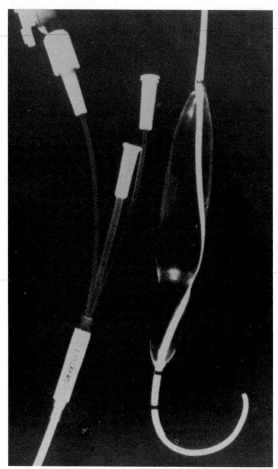

Figure 32–12. A triple-lumen, double-size (15- and 20-mm) Mansfield balloon catheter for aortic valvuloplasty. (From Cribier A, Gerber LI, Letac B: Aortic valvuloplasty. *In* Topol EJ [ed]: Textbook of Interventional Cardiology, Update 3. Philadelphia, WB Saunders, 1991, pp 43–58.)

Results of Aortic Balloon Valvuloplasty

IMMEDIATE RESULTS. A number of series have been reported on the initial hemodynamic results and early follow-up (an aggregate of >1000 patients).[94–101] The largest series reported from the United States has been the accumulated experience between November 1, 1987, and November 1, 1989, from 24 clinical sites that were tabulated in the NHLBI Balloon Valvuloplasty Registry.[101] This patient population was symptomatic and elderly; 76% were in NYHA functional class III or IV, 34% exhibited syncope or presyncope, and 23% exhibited Canadian Heart Association class III or IV angina pectoris, while 83% were older than 70 years of age. Eighty per cent of the cohort seen by a cardiothoracic surgeon were believed to be poor candidates for aortic valve replacement. Immediately after balloon dilation, the aortic valve area increased

from 0.5 ± 0.2 cm^2 to 0.8 ± 0.3 cm^2 ($P<0.0001$), accompanied by a fall in the mean and peak aortic valve gradients from 55 ± 21 and 65 ± 28 to 29 ± 13 and 31 ± 18 mm Hg, respectively (both $P<0.0001$; Fig. 32–13). Thus, the mean valvular gradient is reduced approximately in half, and the aortic valve area increased by about 65%. However, the final absolute aortic valve area remained in the range of 0.7 to 0.9 cm^2.

The Mansfield Scientific Aortic Valvuloplasty Registry, enrolling patients between December 1, 1986, and October 30, 1987, revealed similar data with the aortic valve area increasing from 0.50 ± 0.18 to 0.82 ± 0.30 cm^2, and the mean aortic valve gradient diminishing from 60 ± 23 to 30 ± 13 mm Hg (see Fig. 32–13).[100]

The Rouen, France, series included 363 patients that were treated over a period of approximately 3 years.[93] These investigators achieved somewhat better results overall. In 182 patients treated with the original balloon catheters (and generally smaller sizes), the aortic valve orifice area increased from 0.53 to 0.92 cm^2. Those 181 patients treated with an updated technique (specific three-lumen balloon catheter, extra-stiff guide wires, and 14-French sheath) were observed to have an increase in aortic valve orifice area from 0.57 to 1.01 cm^2 (see Fig. 32–13).

Even though these immediate results showed only modest improvement in aortic valve orifice area, most patients demonstrated marked improvement in symptoms by the time of hospital discharge.

FACTORS THAT PREDICT IMMEDIATE RESULTS. The most potent predictor of the immediate result following catheter balloon aortic valvuloplasty has been the predilation orifice area. This observation is consistent with the fact that the technique usually gives a fixed augmentation of orifice area of approximately 0.2 to 0.4 cm^2. Other factors that may impact on the immediate result include bicuspid versus tricuspid valves (the latter appear to get a better result),[102, 103] a rheumatic etiology (areas are larger after dilation),[104] and age (children and young adults attain a larger orifice area that is sustained for a longer period).[105, 106]

INTERMEDIATE RESULTS. Most available studies would suggest that the immediate improvement in aortic valve area with balloon aortic valvuloplasty lasts for a relatively short period (6 to 9 months). The Mansfield Scientific Aortic Valvuloplasty Registry Investigators reported on a select group of 95 patients in whom follow-up cardiac catheterization was obtained.[81] The aortic valve orifice area increased initially from 0.56

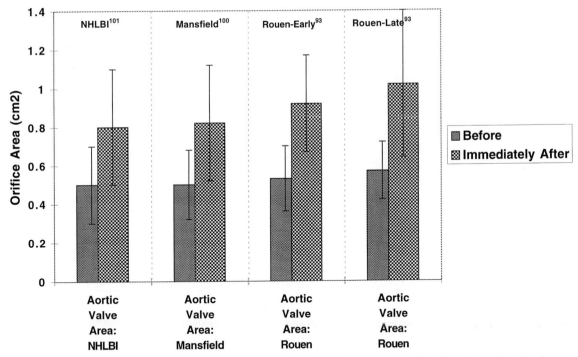

Figure 32–13. Compilation of immediate effect of balloon aortic valvuloplasty, as reported in selected registries of patients. Note that all series reveal only a modest increase in valve orifice area.

± 0.16 to 0.87 ± 0.27 cm² but then regressed to 0.63 ± 0.25 cm² at follow-up catheterization (Fig. 32–14). The average pressure gradients moved concordantly.

In a small group of 71 patients, 41 of whom agreed to late recatheterization at 6 months, Harrison and colleagues found that 76% of the 41 patients exhibited valvular restenosis.[82] Before valvuloplasty the valve area was 0.51 ± 0.14 cm², immediately after 0.81 ± 0.19 cm², and then at 6 months was found to be 0.58 ± 0.16 cm². Analysis of left ventricular function in these same 41 patients suggested that end-diastolic volume was reduced as compared with prevalvuloplasty but was significantly improved in 9 of 15 patients with a baseline ejection fraction of less than 50%.

LONGER-TERM RESULTS. The longer-term outcome of patients undergoing balloon aortic valvuloplasty has only recently been more fully described.[107] Previous studies were limited by analysis of only short-term and mid-term outcomes and failure to follow serially the same cohort of patients.[108] In the 165 patients followed at the Duke University Medical Center for 1 to 6 years after balloon aortic valvuloplasty, 152 (93%) died or underwent aortic valve replacement, and 99 (60%) died of cardiac-related causes. The probability of an event-free survival (freedom from death, aortic valve re-

placement, or repeat balloon aortic valvuloplasty) 1, 2, and 3 years after valvuloplasty was 40%, 19%, and 6%, respectively (Fig. 32–15). In contrast, in a subset of 42 patients who underwent aortic valve replacement after balloon aortic valvuloplasty, the probability of survival was 84%. It was concluded from these observations that the natural history of valvular aortic stenosis, treated with balloon aortic valvuloplasty, is little changed, if any, from that of untreated aortic stenosis. In fact, the outcomes in these 165 treated patients, excluding those who subsequently underwent aortic valve replacement, were quite comparable with those reported by O'Keefe and coworkers in a group of candidates for balloon valvuloplasty who did not undergo the procedure.[109] In this latter cohort, they found that the 1-year, 2-year, and 3-year actuarial survival rate of 50 untreated elderly patients (mean age 77 years) was 57%, 37%, and 25%, respectively; the corresponding survival rates in the balloon-treated patients from Duke were 52%, 31%, and 18%.

Complications of Balloon Aortic Valvuloplasty

The major complications, as reported by the major series of balloon aortic valvuloplasty, are listed in Table 32–4.

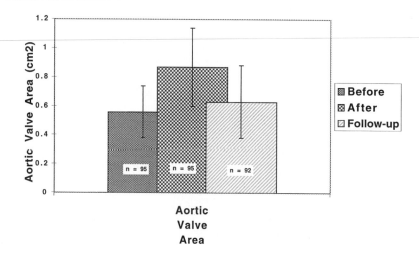

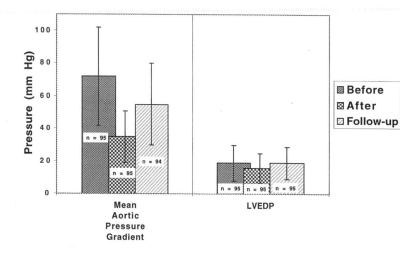

Figure 32–14. Hemodynamic changes at 6-month follow-up cardiac catheterization in selected series of patients from Mansfield Scientific Aortic Valvuloplasty Registry.[81]

Table 32–4. Incidence of Complications of Aortic Valve Balloon Commissurotomy: Registry Results

Type	Standard Balloon(s) (%)	Registry and Reference
Death (1–30-day follow-up)	4.9	Mansfield Scientific[100]
	3.3 (30-day)	French[94]
	2.5 (1-day)	NHLBI[101]
Cardiac perforation	1.8	Mansfield Scientific[100]
Tamponade	1.8	Mansfield Scientific[100]
	1.0	NHLBI[101]
Systemic embolism	2.2	Mansfield Scientific[100]
	2.0	NHLBI[101]
Severe worsening of aortic leakage	2.1	Mansfield Scientific[100]
	1.0	NHLBI[101]
Cardiac arrhythmias requiring treatment	0.8	Mansfield Scientific[100]
	10	NHLBI[101]
Blood transfusion	23	NHLBI[101]
Prolonged hypotension	8.0	NHLBI[101]
Vascular injury or hematoma	11	Mansfield Scientific[100]
	11.8	NHLBI[101]
Emergency surgery	0.8	NHLBI[101]

Mansfield Scientific Aortic Vavuloplasty Registry: n = 492 patients enrolled between December 1, 1986, and October 30, 1987.
NHLBI Registry: n = 674 patients enrolled between November 1, 1987, and November 1, 1989.

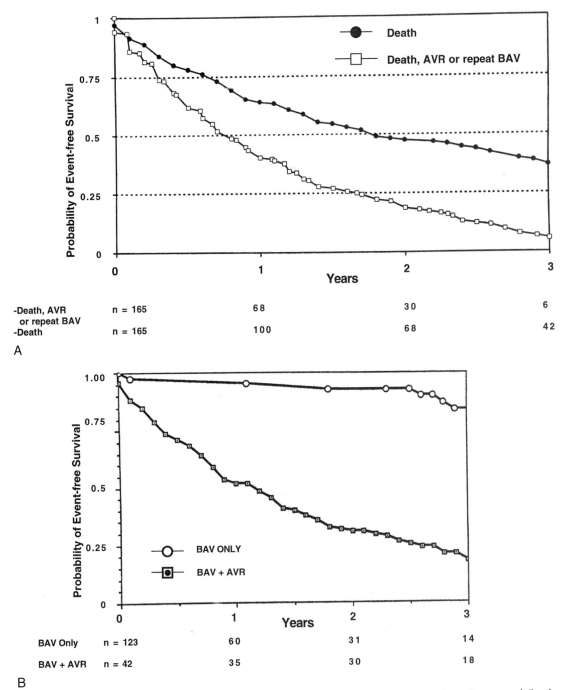

Figure 32–15. *A,* Actuarial and event-free survival in patients undergoing balloon aortic valvuloplasty. Events are defined as death, aortic valve replacement (AVR), or a second balloon aortic valvuloplasty (repeat BAV). *B,* Actuarial survival from the date of balloon aortic valvuloplasty in patients who subsequently underwent aortic valve replacement (BAV + AVR) and those treated by balloon aortic valvuloplasty alone (BAV only). (*A* and *B* modified from Lieberman EB, Bashore TM, Hermiller JB: Balloon aortic valvuloplasty in adults: Failure of procedure to improve long-term survival. J Am Coll Cardiol 1995; 26:1522–1528. Reprinted with permission from the American College of Cardiology.)

Death occurring during the hospitalization has been relatively low at 2.8% to 8.9%, considering the age of the patients treated and their deteriorating clinical status at the time of the dilation.[87] Death rates during the first 24 hours directly related to the procedure have varied between 2.5% and 4.9% in the registries that have been compiled (see Table 32–4). Death rates have also been shown to reduce significantly with operator experience; Cribier and associates demonstrated a reduction in mortality from 5% to 3% with increasing operator experience and use of newer equipment.[94] The causes of death cover a broad spectrum and include persistent hypotension, congestive heart failure with pulmonary edema, new and acute aortic regurgitation, left ventricular perforation with tamponade, bradyarrhythmias and tachyarrhythmias, tearing of the mitral valve apparatus, cerebrovascular accident, renal failure, and sepsis.[87]

Investigators of the NHLBI Registry[101] compiled other types of morbidity following balloon aortic valvuloplasty, including the need for transfusion (23%), the need for vascular surgical intervention (7%), cerebrovascular accident (3%), cardiogenic shock (3%), myocardial infarction (2%), systemic embolus (2%), emergent cardiac surgery (1%), and acute tubular necrosis (1%). Although 35 of 674 patients had vascular surgery, in some institutions this was an elective procedure and probably overrepresents the actual incidence of vascular injury.

SUMMARY. Although a useful palliative technique in highly selected patients with severe aortic stenosis, balloon aortic valvuloplasty provides only a modest initial improvement in valve orifice size and is associated with a high restenosis rate over the first 6 months of follow-up. Moreover, the long-term event-free and actuarial survival of patients who have undergone aortic valvuloplasty is quite unfavorable and resembles strongly the documented natural history of untreated aortic stenosis. If possible, patients with severe aortic stenosis should be referred for prosthetic valve replacement. In those patients for whom this course is not advisable, balloon aortic valvuloplasty can be used to palliate briefly the consequences of the valve obstruction.

TRICUSPID STENOSIS

Indications, Technique, and Preliminary Results

As indicated in Chapter 18, tricuspid stenosis by itself is a relatively uncommon lesion. In those countries where rheumatic valvular disease is still quite prevalent, tricuspid stenosis may be seen in association with rheumatic disease of the mitral and aortic valves. Catheter balloon commissurotomy has been performed successfully in such patients and serves as a potential alternative to surgical commissurotomy. Because the reported experience with this technique is quite limited, it is not possible to clearly delineate the indications and results of the procedure. In the few cases reported,[110–112] a double-balloon technique has been used, and there has been significant relief of the diastolic pressure gradient. However, in one of the reported cases there was a significant worsening of tricuspid regurgitation after double-balloon dilation with two 20-mm diameter balloon catheters.[113]

PULMONIC STENOSIS

Indications and Preprocedure Evaluation

Following its first description in 1982,[1] experience with balloon catheter dilation of pulmonary valve stenosis has confirmed its effectiveness and made it the treatment of choice in those patients believed to be candidates for relief of the obstruction. Pulmonic stenosis is almost always congenital in origin. Balloon dilation is indicated in those patients with symptoms of right-sided heart dysfunction. Asymptomatic patients with a transvalvular gradient of more than 80 mm Hg or a right ventricular systolic pressure of more than 130 mm Hg are also considered to be candidates for relief of their stenosis. Finally, patients with a moderate systolic pressure gradient (50 to 80 mm Hg) who have signs of hemodynamic dysfunction of the right heart may also be considered for balloon dilation.

As with mitral commissurotomy, balloon dilation of the pulmonary valve is most successful in those patients with commissural fusion and minimal dysplasia of the other elements of the valve. This condition can be visualized either by right ventricular angiography ("doming" of the pulmonic valve; see Chapter 25) or by use of two-dimensional echocardiography.

Procedural Technique

To accomplish pulmonary valve dilation, the valve is first crossed with a guide wire and endhole catheter. The latter is then exchanged for a balloon catheter that is advanced over the guide wire and positioned across the pulmonary valve. Under fluoroscopic control, the balloon is inflated with diluted iodinated contrast agent; the waist produced in the partially inflated balloon serves to indicate satisfactory balloon positioning. Then during full balloon inflation, the waist should be observed to disappear as the commissures split. In some patients, particularly large adolescents or adults, it may be necessary to use the double-balloon technique to get a satisfactory result. In this instance, two guide wires are positioned across the valve, and the two balloon catheters are then advanced sequentially through the orifice before they are inflated. The ultimate balloon diameters are chosen in reference to the pulmonary valve diameter. This latter dimension can be obtained either through use of two-dimensional echocardiography or by a well-calibrated right ventricular contrast angiogram. Usually, satisfactory relief of obstruction is obtained by using balloons that during inflation are equivalent to a balloon to pulmonary valve annulus ratio of 1.1 to 1.5.[114-116]

Following the final balloon inflation, the balloon catheter is removed and exchanged for an end-hole catheter through which a pressure gradient can again be measured.

Results of Pulmonary Balloon Valvuloplasty

IMMEDIATE AND LONG-TERM RESULTS. A number of series have now been reported in both children and adults that confirm the efficacy of balloon pulmonary valvulotomy (Fig. 32–16).[117-124] Moreover, longer-term follow up has revealed a restenosis rate of 0% to 10%, a range considerably more favorable than for balloon valvuloplasty for either mitral or aortic stenosis.[117-123]

Complications of Pulmonary Balloon Valvuloplasty

Balloon pulmonary valvuloplasty is usually performed with few complications. Because of the proximity of the atrioventricular node to the tricuspid valve, use of longer balloons (>4 to 5 cm long) can be associated with transient second-degree or third-degree atrioventricular block. In fact, use of longer balloons is discouraged because of the potential for traumatizing the tricuspid valve or its subvalvular apparatus during the course of dilating the pulmonic valve. Significant tricuspid regurgitation caused

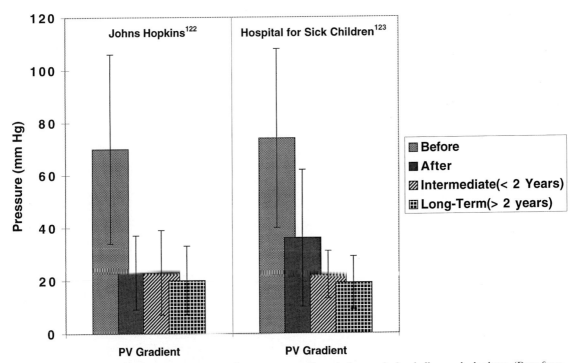

Figure 32–16. Changes over time in pulmonary valve pressure gradient, before and after balloon valvuloplasty. (Data from Reference 122 [McCrindle BW, Kan JS: Long-term results after balloon pulmonary valvuloplasty. Circulation 1991; 83:1915–1922]; and Reference 123 [Masura J, Burch M, Deanfield JE, Sullivan ID: Five-year follow-up after balloon pulmonary valvuloplasty. J Am Coll Cardiol 1993; 21:132–136].)

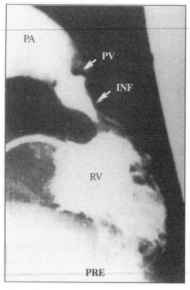 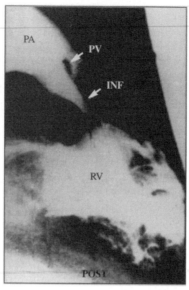 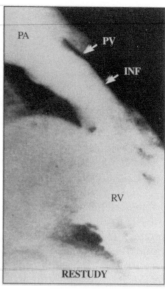

Figure 32–17. Right lateral angiographic views of right ventricular contrast medium injections in patient with pulmonary valvular stenosis. Films recorded before balloon dilation *(left)*, immediately after *(middle)*, and at restudy 6 months later *(right)*. Note resolution of the narrowing at the infundibular level after relief of the pulmonic valve obstruction. PV, pulmonary valve; INF, infundibulum; PA, pulmonary artery; RV, right ventricle. (From Sullivan ID, Burch M: Balloon dilation for pulmonary valve stenosis. Prim Cardiol 1995; 21:23–27.)

by this complication has been reported.[119] Pulmonic regurgitation by Doppler imaging is commonly seen after pulmonary valvuloplasty, but, if present, is usually not clinically significant.

COEXISTENT SUBVALVULAR OR INFUNDIBULAR NARROWING. In 20% to 25% of patients with valvular pulmonic stenosis there is also a measurable outflow tract gradient.[125] Immediately after balloon pulmonary valvuloplasty, 62% of these gradients persisted and 38% had resolved. Most of those that persisted immediately after dilation resolved by 10 months' follow-up, and the remainder were significantly reduced. Others have noted resolution of postdilation outflow tract gradients at the time of late follow-up (Fig. 32–17).[118, 126] Until the hypertrophy regresses in the outflow tract following successful balloon pulmonary valvuloplasty, it is often advisable to place the patient on a β+-adrenergic blocking agent.

SUMMARY. Balloon dilation has proven to be a highly effective technique for relief of pulmonary valve obstruction. The initial complication rate is low, and the results appear to be sustained at 5 years' follow-up. Pulmonary valve insufficiency is a frequent by-product of the dilation but generally is of no hemodynamic or clinical consequence. Subvalvular obstruction due to outflow tract hypertrophy is often present both before and after valve dilation; it appears to regress and ultimately disappear in most patients.

REFERENCES

1. Kan JS, White RI, Mitchell SE, et al: Percutaneous balloon valvuloplasty: A new method for treating congenital pulmonary valve stenosis. N Engl J Med 1982; 307:540–542.
2. Pepine CJ, Gessner IH, Feldman RL: Percutaneous balloon valvuloplasty for pulmonary valve stenosis in the adult. Am J Cardiol 1982; 50:1442–1445.
3. Lababidi Z, Wu JR, Walls JT: Percutaneous balloon aortic valvuloplasty: Results in 23 patients. Am J Cardiol 1984; 53:194.
4. Inoue K, Ouraki TN, Nakamura T, et al: Clinical application of transvenous mitral commissurotomy by a new balloon catheter. J Thorac Cardiovasc Surg 1984; 87:394.
5. Lock JE, Khalilullah M, Shrivastava S, et al: Percutaneous catheter commissurotomy in rheumatic mitral stenosis. N Engl J Med 1985; 313:1515.
6. Cribier A, Saoudi N, Berland J, et al: Percutaneous transluminal valvuloplasty of acquired aortic stenosis in elderly patients: An alternative to valve replacement? Lancet 1986; 1:63–67.
7. Al Zaibag MA, Ribeiro PA, Al Kasab S: Percutaneous balloon valvotomy in tricuspid stenosis. Br Heart J 1987; 57:51.
8. Ribeiro PA, Al Zaibag MA, Al Kasab SA, et al: Percutaneous double balloon valvotomy in tricuspid stenosis. Am J Cardiol 1988; 61:660.
9. de Lezo JS, Pan M, Sancho M, et al: Percutaneous transluminal balloon dilatation of discrete subaortic stenosis. Am J Cardiol 1986; 58:619.
10. Waldman JD, Schoen FJ, Kirkpatrick SE, et al: Balloon dilatation of porcine bioprosthetic valve in the pulmonary position. Circulation 1987; 76:109.
11. McKay CR, Waller BF, Hong R, et al: Problems encountered with catheter balloon valvuloplasty of bioprosthetic aortic valves. Am Heart J 1988; 115:463.
12. Calvo OL, Sobrino N, Gamallo C, et al: Balloon percu-

taneous valvuloplasty for stenotic bioprosthetic valves in mitral position. Am J Cardiol 1987; 60:736.

13. Feit F, Stecy PJ, Nachamie MS: Percutaneous balloon valvuloplasty for stenosis of a porcine bioprosthesis in the tricuspid valve position. Am J Cardiol 1986; 58:363.

14. Lock JE, Bass JL, Amplatz K, et al: Balloon dilatation angioplasty of aortic coarctations in infants and children. Circulation 1983; 68:109.

15. Hoeksema TD, Wallace RB, Kirklin JW. Closed mitral commissurotomy: Recent results in 291 cases. Am J Cardiol 1966; 17:825–828.

16. Mullin EM, Glancy DL, Higgs LM, et al: Current results of operation for mitral stenosis: Clinical and hemodynamic assessments in 124 consecutive patients treated by closed commissurotomy, open commissurotomy, or valve replacement. Circulation 1972; 46:298–308.

17. Ellis LB, Singh JB, Morales DD, et al: Fifteen to twenty-year study of one thousand patients undergoing closed mitral valvuloplasty. Circulation 1973; 48:357–364.

18. Nathaniels EK, Moncure AC, Scannell JG. A fifteen-year follow-up study of closed mitral valvuloplasty. Ann Thorac Surg 1970; 10:27–36.

19. John S, Bashi VV, Jairaj PS, et al: Closed mitral valvotomy: Early results and long-term follow-up of 3,724 consecutive patients. Circulation 1983; 68:891–896.

20. Morrow AG, DuPlessis LA, Wilcox BR: Hemodynamic studies after mitral commissurotomy. Surgery 1963; 54:463–470.

21. Feigenbaum H, Linback RE, Nasser WK: Hemodynamic studies before and after instrumental mitral commissurotomy: A reappraisal of the pathophysiology of mitral stenosis and the efficacy of mitral valvotomy. Circulation 1968; 38:261–276.

22. Nanda N, Gramiak R, Shah PM, et al: Mitral commissurotomy versus replacement: Preoperative evaluation of echocardiography. Circulation 1975; 51:263–267.

23. Reid CL, McKay CR, Chandraratna PAN, et al: Mechanisms of increase in mitral valve area and influence of anatomic features in double-balloon, catheter balloon valvuloplasty in adults with rheumatic mitral stenosis: A Doppler and two-dimensional echocardiographic study. Circulation 1987; 76:628–636.

24. Abascal VM, Wilkins GT, Choong CY, et al: Mitral regurgitation after percutaneous balloon mitral valvuloplasty in adults: Evaluation by pulsed Doppler echocardiography. J Am Coll Cardiol 1988; 11:257–263.

25. Wilkins GT, Weyman AE, Abascal VM, et al: Percutaneous balloon dilatation of the mitral valve: An analysis of echocardiographic variables related to outcome and the mechanism of dilatation. Br Heart J 1988; 60:299–308.

26. Palacios IG, Block PC, Wilkins GT, Weyman AE: Follow-up of patients undergoing percutaneous mitral balloon valvotomy. Circulation 1989; 79:573–579.

27. Tuzcu EM, Block PC, Griffin B, et al: Percutaneous mitral balloon valvotomy in patients with calcific mitral stenosis: Immediate and long-term outcome. J Am Coll Cardiol 1994; 23:1604–1609.

28. Al Zaibag MA, Ribeiro PA, Kasab SA, et al: Percutaneous double-balloon mitral valvotomy for rheumatic mitral valve stenosis. Lancet 1986; 1:757i–761.

29. Babic UU, Pejcic P, Djurisic Z, et al: Percutaneous transarterial balloon valvuloplasty for mitral valve stenosis. Am J Cardiol 1986; 57:1101–1104.

30. Babic UU, Dorros G, Pejcic P, et al: Percutaneous mitral valvuloplasty: Retrograde, transarterial double-balloon technique utilizing the transseptal approach. Cathet Cardiovasc Diagn 1988; 14:229–237.

31. Feldman T, Carroll JD: The Inoue balloon for percutaneous mitral commissurotomy. Cardio Intervent 1992; 2:13–19.

32. Petrossian GA, Tuzcu EM, Ziskind AA, et al: Atrial septal occlusion improves the accuracy of mitral valve area determination following percutaneous mitral balloon valvotomy. Cathet Cardiovasc Diagn 1991; 22:21–24.

33. Kronzon I, Glassman E, Cohen M, Winer H. Use of two-dimensional echocardiography during transseptal cardiac catheterization. J Am Coll Cardiol 1984; 4:425–428.

34. Ballal RS, Mahan EF III, Nanda NC, Dean LS: Utility of transesophageal echocardiography in interatrial septal puncture during percutaneous mitral balloon commissurotomy. Am J Cardiol 1990; 66:230–232.

35. Kronzon I, Tunick PA, Schwinger ME, Slater J, Glassman E: Transesophageal echocardiography during percutaneous mitral valvuloplasty. J Am Soc Echocardiogr 1989; 2:380–385.

36. Goldstein SA, Campbell A, Mintz GS, et al: Feasibility of on-line transesophageal echocardiography during balloon mitral valvulotomy: Experience with 93 patients. J Heart Valve Dis 1994; 3:136–148.

37. Kyo S, Omoto R, Mototyama T, et al: Transesophageal echocardiography during catheter interventions. In Maurer G (ed): Transesophageal Echocardiography. New York, McGraw-Hill, 1994, pp 215–233.

38. Hung JS, Fu M, Yeh KH, et al: Usefulness of intracardiac echocardiography in transseptal puncture during percutaneous transvenous mitral commissurotomy. Am J Cardiol 1993; 72:853–854.

39. Hung JS, Fu M, Yeh KH, et al: Usefulness of intracardiac echocardiography in complex transseptal catheterization during percutaneous transvenous mitral commissurotomy. Mayo Clin Proc 1996; 71:134–140.

40. Reid CL, Chandraratna AN, Kawanishi DT, et al: Influence of mitral valve morphology on double-balloon catheter balloon valvuloplasty in patients with mitral stenosis. Circulation 1989; 80:515–524.

41. Hermann HC, Wilkins GT, Abascal VM, et al: Percutaneous balloon mitral valvotomy for patients with mitral stenosis. J Thorac Cardiovasc Surg 1988; 96:33–38.

42. Vahanian A, Michel PL Cormier B, et al: Results of percutaneous mitral commissurotomy in 200 patients. Am J Cardiol 1989; 63:847–852.

43. Abascal VM, Wilkins GT, O'Shea JP, et al: Prediction of successful outcome in 130 patients undergoing percutaneous balloon mitral valvotomy. Circulation 1990; 82:448–456.

44. NHLBI Balloon Valvuloplasty Registry Participants: Multicenter experience with balloon mitral commissurotomy. Circulation 1992; 85:448–461.

45. NHLBI Balloon Valvuloplasty Registry Participants: Complications and mortality of percutaneous balloon mitral commissurotomy: A report from the National Heart, Lung, and Blood Institute Balloon Valvuloplasty Registry. Circulation, 1992; 85:2014–2024.

46. McKay CR, Kawanishi DT, Rahimtoola Sh: Catheter balloon valvuloplasty of the mitral valve using a double-balloon technique: Early hemodynamic results. JAMA 1987; 257:1753–1761.

47. Chen C, Wang Y, Quing D, et al: Percutaneous balloon dilatation by a new sequential single- and double-balloon technique. Am Heart J 1988; 116:1161–1167.

48. Reid CL, Otto CM, Davis KB, et al: Influence of mitral valve morphology on mitral balloon commissurotomy: Immediate and six-month results from the NHLBI Balloon Valvuloplasty Registry. Am Heart J 1992; 124:657–664.

49. Palacios IG: Balloon mitral valvuloplasty: What are the long-term outcomes? Choices Cardiol 1993; 22:783–789.

50. Harken DE, Black H, Taylor WJ, et al: Reoperation for mitral stenosis: A discussion of postoperative deteriora-

tion and methods of improving initial and secondary operations. Circulation 1961; 23:7–12.

51. Gross RI, Cunningham JN, Snively, et al: Long-term results of open radical mitral commissurotomy: Ten-year follow-up study of 202 patients. Am J Cardiol 1981; 47:821–825.

52. Davidson CJ, Bashore TM, Mickel M, et al: Balloon mitral commissurotomy after previous surgical commissurotomy. Circulation 1992; 86:91–99.

53. Nobuyoshi M, Hamasaki N, Kimura T, et al: Indications, complications, and short-term clinical outcome of percutaneous transvenous mitral commissurotomy. Circulation 1989; 80:782–792.

54. Hung JS, Chern MS, Wujj, et al: Short- and long-term results of catheter balloon percutaneous transvenous mitral commissurotomy. Am J Cardiol 1991; 67:854–862.

55. Herrmann HC, Ramaswamy K, Isner JM, et al: Factors influencing immediate results, complications, and short-term follow-up status after Inoue balloon mitral valvotomy: A North American multicenter study. Am Heart J 1992; 124:160–166.

56. Feldman T, Carroll JD, Isner JM, et al: Effect of valve deformity on results and mitral regurgitation after Inoue balloon commissurotomy. Circulation 1992; 85:180–187.

57. Chen CR, Cheng TO, Chen JY, et al: Long-term results of percutaneous mitral valvuloplasty with the Inoue balloon catheter. Am J Cardiol 1992; 70:1445–1448.

58. Sharma S, Loya Y, Desai DM, Pinto Rj: Percutaneous mitral valvotomy using Inoue and double-balloon technique: Comparison of clinical and hemodynamic short-term results in 350 cases. Cathet Cardiovasc Diagn 1993; 29:18–23.

59. Park SJ, Kin JJ, Park SW, et al: Immediate and one-year results of percutaneous mitral balloon valvuloplasty using Inoue and double-balloon techniques. Am J Cardiol 1993; 71:938–943.

60. Chen C-R, Cheng TO, for the Multicenter Study Group: Percutaneous balloon mitral valvuloplasty by the Inoue technique: A multicenter study of 4832 patients in China. Am Heart J 1995; 129:1197–1203.

61. Herrmann HC, Kleaveland JP, Hill JA, et al: The M-Heart percutaneous balloon mitral valvuloplasty registry: Initial results and early follow-up. J Am Coll Cardiol 1990; 15:1221–1226.

62. Tuzcu EM, Block PC, Palacios IF: Comparison of early versus late experience with percutaneous mitral balloon valvuloplasty. J Am Coll Cardiol 1991; 17:1121–1124.

63. Post JR, Feldman T, Isner J, Herrmann HC: Inoue balloon mitral valvotomy in patients with severe valvular and subvalvular deformity. J Am Coll Cardiol 1995; 25:1129–1136.

64. Feldman T: Hemodynamic results, clinical outcome, and complications of Inoue balloon mitral valvotomy. Cathet Cardiovasc Diagn, 1994; 2(Suppl):2–7.

65. Feldman T, Carroll JD: The Inoue balloon for percutaneous mitral commissurotomy. Cardio Intervent 1992; 2:13–19.

66. Turi ZG, Reyes VP, Raju BS, et al: Percutaneous balloon versus surgical closed commissurotomy for mitral stenosis: A prospective, randomized trial. Circulation 1991; 83:1179–1185.

67. Reyes VP, Raju BS, Wynne J, et al: Percutaneous balloon valvuloplasty compared with open surgical commissurotomy for mitral stenosis. N Engl J Med 1994; 331:961–967.

68. Subramanian R, Olson LJ, Edwards WD: Surgical pathology of pure aortic stenosis: A study of 374 cases. Mayo Clin Proc 1984; 59:683–690.

69. Peterson MD, Roach RM, Edwards JE: Types of aortic stenosis in surgically removed valves. Arch Pathol Lab Med 1985; 109:829–832.

70. Selzer A: Changing aspects of the natural history of valvular aortic stenosis. N Engl J Med 1987; 317:91–98.

71. Robicsek F, Harbold NB: Limited value of balloon dilatation in calcified aortic stenosis in adults: Direct observations during open heart surgery. Am J Cardiol 1987; 60:857–864.

72. Letac B, Gerber LI, Koning R: Insights on the mechanism of balloon valvuloplasty in aortic stenosis. Am J Cardiol 1988; 62:1241–1247.

73. Davidson CJ, Harpole DA, Kisslo K, et al: Analysis of the early rise in aortic transvalvular gradient after aortic valvuloplasty. Am Heart J 1989; 117:411–417.

74. Stephenson LW, Edie RN, Harken AH, et al: Combined aortic and mitral valve replacement: Changes in practice and prognosis. Circulation 1984; 69:640–644.

75. Magovern JA, Pennock JL, Campbell DB, et al: Aortic valve replacement and combined aortic valve replacement and coronary artery bypass grafting: Predicting high-risk groups. J Am Coll Cardiol 1987; 9:38–43.

76. Mullany CJ, Elveback LR, Frye RL, et al: Coronary artery disease and its management: Influence on survival in patients undergoing aortic valve replacement. J Am Coll Cardiol 1987; 10:66–72.

77. Galloway, AC, Colvin SB, Grossi EA, et al: Ten-year experience with aortic valve replacement in 482 patients 70 years of age or older: Operative risk and long-term results. Ann Thorac Surg 1990; 49:84–93.

78. Culliford AT, Galloway AC, Colvin SB, et al: Aortic valve replacement for aortic stenosis in persons 80 years of age and over. Am J Cardiol 1991; 67:1256–1260.

79. Teoh KH, Weisel RD, Ivanou J, Slattery SA: Survival and valve failure after aortic valve replacement. Ann Thorac Surg 1991; 52:270–275.

80. Harrison JK, Davidson CJ, Leithe ME, et al: Serial left ventricular performance evaluated by cardiac catheterization before, immediately after, and at 6 months after balloon aortic valvuloplasty. J Am Coll Cardiol 1990; 16:1351–1358.

81. Bashore TM, Davidson CJ, Mansfield Scientific Aortic Valvuloplasty Registry Investigators: Follow-up recatheterization after balloon aortic valvuloplasty. J Am Coll Cardiol 1991; 17:1188–1195.

82. Harpole DH, Davidson CJ, Skelton TN, et al: Early and later changes in left ventricular systolic performance after percutaneous aortic balloon valvuloplasty. Am J Cardiol 1990; 66:327–332.

83. Wisenburg M, Cromme-Dijkhuis AH, Frohn-Mulder IME, Hess J: Short- and mid-term results of balloon valvuloplasty for valvular aortic stenosis in children. Am J Cardiol 1992; 69:945–950.

84. Hatle L, Angelsen BA, Tromsdal A: Noninvasive assessment of aortic stenosis by Doppler ultrasound. Br Heart J 1980; 43:284–292.

85. Skjaerpe T, Hegrenaes L, Hatle L: Noninvasive estimation of valve area in patients with aortic stenosis by Doppler ultrasound and two-dimensional echocardiography. Circulation 1985; 72:810–818.

86. Burwash IG, Thomas DD, Sadahiro M, et al: Dependence of Gorlin formula and continuity equation valve areas on transvalvular volume flow rate in valvular aortic stenosis. Circulation 1994; 89:827–835.

87. Kulick DL, Kawanishi DT, Reid CL, Rahimtoola SH: Catheter balloon valvuloplasty in adults: Aortic stenosis. Curr Probl Cardiol 1990, 15:362.

88. Miller FA Jr: Aortic stenosis: Most cases no longer require invasive hemodynamic study [editorial]. J Am Coll Cardiol 1989; 13:551–553.

89. Nishimura RA, Tajik AJ: Quantitative hemodynamics by Doppler echocardiography: A noninvasive alternative to cardiac catheterization. Prog Cardiovasc Dis 1994; 36:309–342.

90. Roger VL, Tajik AJ, Reeder GS, et al: Effect of Doppler echocardiography on utilization of hemodynamic cardiac catheterization in preoperative evaluation of aortic stenosis. Mayo Clin Proc 1996; 71:141–149.

91. Dorros G, Lewin RF, King JF, et al: Percutaneous transluminal valvuloplasty in calcific aortic stenosis: The double-balloon technique. Cathet Cardiovasc Diagn 1987; 13:151–156.

92. Isner JM, Deeb NS, Desnoyers MR, et al: Dual-balloon technique for valvuloplasty of aortic stenosis in adults. Am J Cardiol 1988; 61:583–589.

93. Fields CD, Lucas A, Desnoyers M, et al: Dual-balloon aortic valvuloplasty, despite augmenting acute hemodynamic improvement, fails to prevent post-valvuloplasty restenosis [abstract]. J Am Coll Cardiol 1989; 13:148A.

94. Cribier A, Gerber LI, Letac B: Aortic valvuloplasty. *In* Topol EJ (ed): Textbook of Interventional Cardiology, Update 3. Philadelphia, WB Saunders, 1991, pp 43–58.

95. Letac B, Cribier A, Koning R, et al: Results of percutaneous transluminal valvuloplasty in 218 adults with valvular aortic stenosis. Am J Cardiol 1988; 62:598–605.

96. Letac B, Cribier A, Koning R: Treatment of acquired aortic stenosis in adults by percutaneous valvuloplasty with balloon catheterization: Experience of 245 cases. Arch Mal Coeur 1989; 82:17–25.

97. Safian RD, Berman AD, Diver DJ, et al: Balloon aortic valvuloplasty in 170 consecutive patients. N Engl J Med 1989; 319:125–130.

98. Holmes DR, Nishimura RA, Reeder GS: In-hospital mortality after balloon aortic valvuloplasty: Frequency and associated factors. J Am Coll Cardiol 1991; 17:189–192.

99. O'Neill WW: Seminar on balloon aortic valvuloplasty. J Am Coll Cardiol 1991; 17:187–188.

100. McKay RG: The Mansfield Scientific Aortic Valvuloplaty Registry: Overview of acute hemodynamic results and procedural complications. J Am Coll Cardiol 1991; 17:485–491.

101. NHLBI Balloon Valvuloplasty Registry Participants: Percutaneous balloon aortic valvuloplasty: Acute and 30-day follow-up results in 674 patients from the NHLBI Balloon Valvuloplasty Registry. Circulation 1991; 84:2383–2397.

102. Salem DN, Isner FJM: Percutaneous aortic valvuloplasty. Chest 1987; 92:326–329.

103. Isner JM: Aortic valvuloplasty: Are balloon dilated valves all they are "cracked" up to be? Mayo Clin Proc 1988; 63:830–834.

104. Ruiz CE, Allen JW, Lau FYK: Different immediate and long-term outcome after percutaneous balloon valvuloplasty for severe aortic stenosis, contingent upon the type of valve [abstract]. J Am Coll Cardiol 1989; 13:54A.

105. Walls JT, Lababidi Z, Curtis JJ, et al: Assessment of percutaneous balloon pulmonary and aortic valvuloplasty. J Thorac Cardiovasc Surg 1984; 88:352–356.

106. Meliones JN, Beekman RH, Rocchini AP, et al: Balloon valvuloplasty for recurrent aortic stenosis after surgical valvotomy in childhood: Immediate and follow-up studies. J Am Coll Cardiol 1989; 13:1106–1110.

107. Lieberman EB, Bashore TM, Hermiller JB: Balloon aortic valvuloplasty in adults: Failure of procedure to improve long-term survival. J Am Coll Cardiol 1995; 26:1522–1528.

108. Kuntz RE, Tosteson ANA, Berman AD, et al: Preditors of event-free survival after balloon aortic valvuloplasty. N Engl J Med 1991; 325:17–23.

109. O'Keefe JH, Vlietstra RE, Bailey KR, Holmes DR: Natural history of candidates for balloon aortic valvuloplasty. Mayo Clin Proc 1987; 62:986–991.

110. Mullins CE, Nihil MR, Vick GW, et al: Double-balloon technique for dilation of valvular or vessel stenosis in congenital and acquired heart disease. J Am Coll Cardiiol 1987; 10:107–114.

111. Khalilullah M, Tyagi S, Yadav BS, et al: Double-balloon valvuloplasty of tricuspid stenosis. Am Heart J 1987; 114:1232–1233.

112. Zaibag MA, Ribeiro P, Kasab SA: Percutaneous balloon valvotomy in tricuspid stenosis. Br Heart J 1987; 57:51–53.

113. Bourdillon PDV, Hookman LD, Morris SN, et al: Percutaneous balloon valvuloplasty for tricuspid stenosis: Hemodynamic and pathologic findings. Am Heart J 1989; 117:492–495.

114. Lo RNS, Leung MP, Yung TC, Chan Ch: Variability of the diameter of the pulmonary outflow tract and its relation to balloon valvuloplasty for congenital pulmonary valvular stenosis. Cardiol Young 1993; 3:111–117.

115. Radtke W, Keane JF, Fellows KE, et al: Percutaneous balloon valvuloplasty of congenital pulmonary stenosis using oversized balloons. J Am Coll Cardiol 1986; 8:909–915.

116. Rao PS: How big a balloon and how many balloons for pulmonary valvuloplasty? Am Heart J 1988; 116:577–580.

117. Kvesilis DA, Rocchini AP, Snider AR, et al: Results of balloon valvuloplasty in the treatment of congenital valvular pulmonary stenosis in children. Am J Cardiol 1985; 56:527–532.

118. Mullins CE, Ludomirsky A, O'Laughlin MP, et al: Balloon valvuloplasty for pulmonic valve stenosis—two-year follow-up: Hemodynamic and Doppler evaluation. Cathet Cardiovasc Diagn 1988; 14:76–81.

119. Fawzy ME, Mercer EN, Dunn B: Late results of pulmonary balloon valvuloplasty in adults using double-balloon techniques. J Intervent Cardiol 1988; 1:35–42.

120. Al Kasab S, Ribeiro PA, Al Zaibag M, et al: Percutaneous double-balloon pulmonary valvotomy in adults: One to two-year follow-up. Am J Cardiol 1988; 62:822–824.

121. Rao PS, Fawzy ME, Solymar L, et al: Long-term results of balloon pulmonary valvuloplasty of valvular pulmonic stenosis. Am Heart J 1988; 115:1291–1296.

122. McCrindle BW, Kan JS: Long-term results after balloon pulmonary valvuloplasty. Circulation 1991; 83:1915–1922.

123. Masura J, Burch M, Deanfield JE, Sullivan ID: Five-year follow-up after balloon pulmonary valvuloplasty. J Am Coll Cardiol 1993; 21:132–136.

124. Marantz PM, Huhta JC, Mullins CE, et al: Results of balloon valvuloplasty in typical and dysplastic pulmonary valve stenosis: Doppler echocardiographic follow-up. J Am Coll Cardiol 1988; 12:476–479.

125. Thapar MK, Rao PS: Significance of infundibular obstruction following balloon valvuloplasty for valvular pulmonic stenosis. Am Heart J 1989; 118:99–103.

126. Fawzy ME, Mercer EN, Dunn B, et al: Regression of infundibular pulmonary stenosis after successful balloon pulmonary valvuloplasty in adults [abstract]. J Am Coll Cardiol 1989; 13:56A.

Chapter 33

Cardiac Pacing
Modes, Indications, and Implantation Techniques

JÜRG SCHLAEPFER
LUKAS KAPPENBERGER

Beginning with the first permanent pacemaker implantation 35 years ago,[1] clinical cardiac pacing and pacemaker technology have evolved rapidly. The initial pacemaker in the late 1950s was an asynchronous, ventricular stimulator that provided fixed ventricular rhythm to prevent syncope or sudden death.[2, 3] Since then, marked progress in pacemaker technology has led to the development of multifunction devices that are highly reliable. At the same time, indications for pacemaker therapy have expanded, giving cardiac patients an improved survival and quality of life. This chapter focuses on the important practical aspects in clinical cardiac pacing without dealing with antitachycardia pacemakers or intracardiac defibrillators.

PACEMAKER CODE

The nomenclature for pacemaker modes accepted for international use is provided by the North American Society of Pacing and Electrophysiology (NASPE) and the British Pacing and Electrophysiology group (BPEG) and is known as the *NBG* (NASPE/BPEG generic) *code.*[4] It is a five-letter code, but the first three letters describing exclusively the antibradyarrhythmia function are the most frequently used (Table 33–1). The first letter indicates the cardiac chamber(s) paced; the second letter defines the chamber(s) sensed (*A* is used for atrium, *V* is for ventricle, and *D* is for dual chambers); and the third letter refers to the pacemaker response to a sensed event (*T* is for triggered, *I* is for inhibited, and *D* is for dual mode of response). The fourth letter refers to both the degree of programmability and the rate modulation *(R)*, and the fifth letter is reserved for antitachyarrhythmia functions.

CHOICE OF PACEMAKER MODE

The choice of pacemaker mode should allow the pacemaker to restore (as much as possible) the physiologic and hemodynamic characteristics of sinus rhythm.[5–8] Before pacemaker im-

Table 33–1. **The NASPE/BPEG Generic Pacemaker Code**

Position	Category	Code
I and II	Chamber(s) Paced	O = None A = Atrium V = Ventricle D = Dual (A+V)
	Sensed	O = None A = Atrium V = Ventricle D = Dual (A+V)
III	Response to sensing	O = None T = Triggered I = Inhibited D = Dual (T+I)
IV	Programmability and rate modulation	O = None P = Simple programmable M = Multiprogrammable C = Communicating R = Rate modulation
V	Antitachyarrhythmia function(s)	O = None P = Pacing S = Shock D = Dual (P+S)

plantation, clinical data and the various pacemaker features available must be known to select the best device for a given patient.

The patient's status (including usual level of physical activity, emotional status, cardiac function and left ventricular ejection fraction, the presence of other concomitant diseases, the specific cardiac rhythm or conduction disturbances, the use of any drug, or the presence of any metabolic disturbance slowing sinus node activity or atrioventricular nodal conduction) should be checked and known before implantation.[5, 9] Holter monitoring, an exercise stress test, or an electrophysiologic study may be required to determine the dominant rhythm and whether or not sinus node chronotropic incompetence or intermittent atrioventricular block is present.

Several available features of the pacemaker include rate modulation, atrioventricular synchrony, and hysteresis.[8]

Rate Modulation

During exercise, an appropriate increase in cardiac output is achieved mainly by an increment in heart rate and, to a lesser extent, in stroke volume.[10, 11] The sinus node is the best sensor of metabolic requirements when its function is preserved.[11] In patients unable to adapt their heart rate to metabolic demand, rate-responsive pacing significantly increases cardiac output during exercise, improving exercise tolerance and quality of life.

Rate-adaptive pacemakers use various types of biosensors responding to physical (muscular activity, acceleration, temperature), chemical (pH, venous oxygen saturation) or electrical signals (respiratory rate, right ventricular stoke volume, QT interval) to accommodate the heart rate to metabolic requirements.[5, 12] The ideal sensor should mimic the normal cardiac response and thus should be (1) sensitive (responsive to all physiologic stimuli, such as exercise and emotion); (2) specific (nonresponsive to environmental noise, passive motion, respiration, and cough); (3) proportional (adapted to the level of the physiologic demand); and (4) quickly responsive (without lag to increasing or decreasing demand).[13] Such an ideal sensor, properly responding to metabolic needs in all circumstances, remains to be developed. A combination of various sensors (multisensor systems) will hopefully offer a better adaptation of heart rate to physiologic demand in the future.[11, 14-16]

In clinical practice, rate-responsive pacing is particularly useful in patients with sinus node chronotropic incompetence or in patients with atrial fibrillation and slow ventricular response. On the other hand, patients with preserved sinus node chronotropy and atrioventricular block may use their spontaneous sinus activity and benefit the most from placement of an atrial sensing pacemaker with triggered ventricular pacing.

Atrioventricular Synchrony

Atrial systole contributes to about 20% to 30% of resting cardiac output in the normal heart.[11, 17-19] Although still controversial, the hemodynamic benefits of atrioventricular synchrony seem to persist during exercise.[2, 3, 10-12, 17] However, the atrial contribution to cardiac output may diminish at higher rates and is dependent on several factors such as the presence of underlying heart disease, ventricular compliance and filling pressures, and autonomic tone.[11] Atrioventricular synchrony is particularly useful in patients with diastolic left ventricular dysfunction[19] such as those with aortic stenosis and hypertensive heart disease, in which loss of atrioventricular synchrony may result in reduction of cardiac output and clinical signs of heart failure.

The optimal atrioventricular interval differs depending on whether a P wave is sensed or paced. Several studies have shown that optimizing the atrioventricular delay interval for both sensed and paced P waves results in a significant increase in resting cardiac output compared with a fixed atrioventricular delay.[20]

Some dual-chamber pacemakers allow selection of a rate-adaptive atrioventricular delay during exercise.[11] Although the hemodynamic benefit may be difficult to prove, this may prevent pacemaker-mediated tachycardia by allowing a longer post-ventricular atrial refractory period without limiting the maximal tracking rate.[10]

Preservation of a normal ventricular contraction pattern, as in AAI pacing mode, may allow better hemodynamic tolerance than both VVI or DDD pacing mode, in which ventricular activation is initiated in the right ventricular apex.[21] This may result in delayed ventricular contraction and septal motion abnormalities that could further compromise cardiac output in failing left ventricles.

Hysteresis

Hysteresis (Fig. 33–1) is defined by a pacing rate that is faster than the sensing rate (or escape interval).[8, 19] This feature enables maintenance

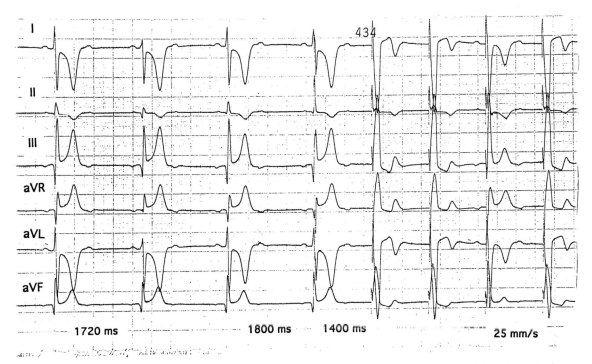

Figure 33–1. Hysteresis phenomenon. Peripheral leads of a surface electrocardiogram showing complete atrioventricular block with a ventricular escape rhythm (basic cycle length is 1720 msec = 35 beats/min). Following a longer spontaneous RR interval of 1800 msec, ventricular pacing is initiated at a basic cycle length of 1200 msec (50 beats/min). Note the giant T wave inversion in leads I and aVL caused by ventricular pacing (Chatterjee phenomenon).

of spontaneous sinus rhythm at a rate lower than the pacing rate if the patient remains asymptomatic. Its use should be restricted to patients with episodic symptomatic bradycardia or with frequent extrasystoles with compensatory pauses triggering pacemaker escape rhythm.

CLINICAL INDICATIONS FOR PACING

In 1989, sinus node disease accounted for 48% of primary pacemaker implantations in the United States, atrioventricular node and His-Purkinje conduction disorders for 45%, drug-induced bradycardia for 4%, and supraventricular and ventricular tachycardia for 2%.[22]

An American College of Cardiology–American Heart Association report provides guidelines for pacemaker implantation based on "current evidence in relation to both knowledge of the natural history of disorders of cardiac rhythm and characteristics of available devices."[5] Indications for permanent pacing have been grouped in three classes, summarized as follows:

Class I: Conditions in which there is general agreement that permanent pacemakers should be implanted

Class II: Conditions in which permanent pacemakers are frequently used, but there is divergence of opinion about whether they are needed

Class III: Conditions in which there is general agreement that pacemakers are unnecessary

MAIN CLASS I INDICATIONS. The main class I indications include the following:

Complete heart block (permanent or not) associated with any one of the following complications: symptomatic bradycardia; congestive heart failure; documented periods of asystole longer than 2 to 3 seconds or any escape rhythm less than 40 beats/min in symptom-free patients; after atrioventricular junction ablation

Second-degree atrioventricular block (permanent or not) with symptomatic bradycardia

Atrial tachyarrhythmia with complete or advanced heart block and bradycardia associated with symptoms or congestive heart failure (bradycardia must not be related to drugs known to impair atrioventricular conduction)

Bifascicular block with intermittent complete heart block associated with symptomatic bradycardia

Sinus node dysfunction with documented symptomatic bradycardia

MAIN CLASS II INDICATIONS. The main class II indications include the following:

Asymptomatic permanent or intermittent complete heart block with ventricular rates of 40 beats/min or higher

Asymptomatic type II second-degree atrioventricular block

Asymptomatic intrahisian or infrahisian type I, second-degree atrioventricular block

Bifascicular or trifascicular block with syncope not proved to be due to complete heart block but without other known causes of syncope

Marked prolongation of the HV interval (>100 msec)

Pacing-induced infrahisian block

Sinus node dysfunction with heart rate less than 40 beats/min without documentation of a clear association between significant symptoms consistent with bradycardia and the actual presence of bradycardia

MAIN CLASS III INDICATIONS. The main class III indications include the following:

First-degree atrioventricular block

Asymptomatic type I second-degree atrioventricular block at the suprahisian level

Fascicular block without atrioventricular block or symptoms

Fascicular block with first-degree atrioventricular block without symptoms

Sinus node dysfunction in asymptomatic patients

Sinus node dysfunction in patients in whom symptoms suggestive of bradycardia are clearly documented not to be associated with a slow heart rate

This report[5] also emphasizes the importance of a complete analysis of the medical, emotional, and mental state of each patient, as well as an understanding of the underlying cardiac rhythm or conduction disturbances, before each pacemaker implantation.

Correct interpretation of the electrocardiogram and recognition of transient conduction or rhythm disturbances (e.g., secondary to medications or to acute myocardial infarction) avoid unnecessary pacemaker implantation.[6, 7]

Sinus Node Disease

In patients with sick sinus disease, permanent pacing may not improve survival, but symptoms related to bradycardia are relieved.[5, 23] Several retrospective studies have shown a deleterious effect of single-chamber ventricular pacing in patients with sick sinus syndrome. In these studies, atrial and sequential atrioventricular pacing both may reduce the incidence of chronic atrial fibrillation, the risk of stroke, the incidence of congestive heart failure, and the overall mortality as compared with VVI pacing.[3, 24–30] These differences in clinical outcome are mainly attributed to the loss of atrial kick and to a high rate of retrograde ventriculoatrial conduction (as high as 70%) in patients with VVI pacing, leading to atrial distension and electrical instability and to the clinical complications described in the previous section. However, in a recent retrospective study including 507 patients with sick sinus syndrome, Sgarbossa and associates[31] showed that occurrence of chronic atrial fibrillation and stroke was strongly determined by clinical variables and only secondarily by ventricular single-chamber pacing. In their study, ventricular pacing mode was predictive of recurrent atrial fibrillation only in patients with, but not in those without, preimplant paroxysmal atrial fibrillation.

To the best of our knowledge, only one prospective study has shown a better outcome with AAI pacing as compared with VVI pacing in patients with sick sinus syndrome.[32] This finding remains to be confirmed by a multicenter prospective, randomized trial.[31, 33, 34]

In patients with sick sinus syndrome, occurrence of life-threatening atrioventricular conduction defects is rare under AAI pacing (with an annual incidence of about 0.2% to 3%).[24, 26, 29, 30] Others report, however, atrioventricular conduction disturbances in as much as 14% of sick sinus disease.[35] With careful patient selection, AAI or AAIR pacing (in the presence of sinus node chronotropic incompetence) should be used. If atrioventricular conduction disturbances are suspected or proven, a DDD pacemaker must be implanted.

Atrioventricular Conduction Disturbances

Permanent pacing improves survival in patients with advanced heart block.[4, 5, 36] However, survival is related to the age of the patient at implantation and to the severity of the underlying heart disease.[36, 37] Furthermore, two studies suggest that fixed-rate single-chamber ventricular pacing may adversely influence prognosis for patients with atrioventricular block and congestive heart failure compared with atrial synchronous pacing[37, 38] and that atrioventricular synchrony should be preserved in such patients.

Before pacemaker implantation, sinus node function should be tested to determine if a rate-adaptive device is necessary.

Atrial Arrhythmias

As suggested by Sutton,[29] unless the atria are in chronic fibrillation, they should be paced, because atrial pacing may stabilize the spontaneous atrial activity and reduce the incidence of bradycardia-dependent atrial fibrillations. In chronic atrial fibrillation with slow ventricular response, the best choice may be a VVIR pacemaker.

Overall, according to the most recent implantation guidelines for antibradycardia pacemakers,[8, 39, 40] permanent atrial fibrillation appears to be the sole contraindication to dual-chamber pacing. Whereas 70% of all new pacemakers implanted worldwide are still single-chamber devices,[22, 40] strict application of these guidelines would reduce their use to about 15% of the total number of pacemakers implanted,[40] resulting in a significant increase in pacing costs.[39] On the other hand, inappropriate pacing mode selection may also be costly in the long term because of worse clinical outcome. Prospective studies should evaluate pacemaker indications in terms of long-term clinical benefits and costs.

CLINICAL CARDIAC PACING IN SPECIAL INDICATIONS

In the carotid sinus syndrome, symptoms may be due to excessive bradycardia in the cardioinhibitory form (60%), to severe hypotension in the cardiodepressive form (10%), or to both mechanisms in the mixed form (30%).[41]

Pacing is indicated after recurrent syncopal episodes or after a single episode resulting in conditions such as fractures, burns, and head trauma.[5, 41] However, optimal pacing may not totally eliminate symptoms in the presence of an associated vasodepressor component. Atrial pacing alone should be avoided because of frequent associated reflex-induced atrioventricular block. Single-chamber ventricular pacing should be considered only in the absence of retrograde ventriculoatrial conduction or hypotension due to the pacemaker syndrome. Dual-chamber pacing is the most effective therapy in most patients with symptomatic bradycardia.[41]

Vasovagal Syncope

Vasovagal syncope is a recurrent episode of hypotension and bradycardia often occurring in young patients that usually has a benign clinical course. Thus, patients and physicians may be reluctant to consider the use of a pacemaker as the first therapeutic choice.[42] As in the carotid sinus syndrome previously discussed, and according to the American College of Cardiology–American Heart Association Task Force guidelines, pacing is indicated only in severely affected patients with recurrent vasovagal syncope due to marked bradycardia and not in those with predominant vasodilation (class II indication).[5, 42] However, the place of cardiac pacing in vasovagal syncope remains to be defined.[42, 43] Fitzpatrick and associates[44] showed a significant clinical improvement after dual-chamber pacing in 85% of patients with vasovagal syncope and marked sinus bradycardia. On the other hand, Sra and colleagues[45] demonstrated that most such patients could be successfully treated medically and that dual-chamber pacing was not as effective. Significant differences in the subjects' age between the two studies may explain these opposite conclusions. To better evaluate indications for cardiac pacing in patients with vasovagal syncope, the Vasovagal Syncope International Study (VASIS) is presently underway.

Dilated Cardiomyopathy

Beneficial effects of dual-chamber pacing, with short atrioventricular delay, were recently demonstrated in patients with dilated cardiomyopathy.[46–48] In a small group of patients with end-stage, drug-resistant dilated cardiomyopathy, Hochleitner and associates[46, 47] showed that dual-chamber pacing with short atrioventricular delay (100 msec) induced a significant increase in left ventricular ejection fraction associated with a reduction in heart size, mainly attributed to decreased left atrial and right ventricular dimensions. At the same time, both systolic and diastolic blood pressures increased, whereas no changes were observed in fractional fiber shortening. Clinically, New York Heart Association functional class improved. After pacemaker implantation, no patient needed rehospitalization or died from worsening heart failure. Death was mainly sudden, leading the authors to suggest that dual-chamber pacing prevented death mostly from worsening pump failure.[47] These positive results were attributed to several factors: a decrease in preload and afterload, a regression in mitral regurgitation, and a better coordination of atrial and ventricular contraction, possibly sparing the damaged cardiac muscle. Clinical improvement was maintained at long-term follow-up (as long as 5 years).

In another study, Brecker and colleagues[48] also showed a beneficial effect of dual-chamber pacing with a very short atrioventricular delay in a small number of patients with dilated cardiomyopathy and functional mitral or tricuspid regurgitation. Most improvement was noted at the shortest atrioventricular interval: duration of mitral and tricuspid regurgitation significantly decreased while their presystolic component disappeared, leading to an increase in ventricular filling time, forward cardiac output, and exercise duration.

These preliminary results, obtained in a limited number of subjects, suggest that pacing may be considered as a therapeutic option in patients with dilated cardiomyopathy.[43] However, these studies need to be confirmed and extended to better define which pacing mode should be used and to better understand the pathophysiologic mechanisms responsible for hemodynamic and clinical improvement in such patients.[49]

Obstructive Cardiomyopathy

Several studies have shown that dual-chamber pacing may relieve symptoms in patients with drug-resistant obstructive hypertrophic cardiomyopathy.[50-52] Dual-chamber pacing significantly reduces the left ventricular outflow tract gradient and results in improvement in functional status and in reduction of both angina and dyspnea.[50-53] Maintenance of atrioventricular synchrony allows optimal left ventricular filling. The observed decrease in outflow tract gradient is probably secondary to an alteration in the ventricular contraction pattern because apical emptying precedes septal contraction during apical stimulation.[51] A total capture of the left ventricle from the right ventricular apex is mandatory to obtain the expected hemodynamic improvement and is achieved by programming a shorter atrioventricular delay than the spontaneous atrioventricular delay at all times and activities. Additional drug treatment with a slowing effect on atrioventricular node conduction may help maintain complete left ventricular capture from the right ventricular apex. These studies suggest that dual-chamber pacing could be an alternative to surgery in hypertrophic cardiomyopathy, but this conclusion is limited by the small number of patients included. Prospective studies will evaluate more extensively the long-term efficacy of this therapeutic approach and its place in the management of these patients.[54]

IMPLANTATION TECHNIQUES

Transvenously implanted electrodes and infraclavicular pacemaker pockets account for more than 95% of all permanent implantations; thoracotomy with epicardial electrodes implantation and abdominal pockets is usually limited to patients undergoing thoracotomy for other reasons, mainly open heart surgery, and to children.[55, 56] A sterile environment is mandatory for implantation, usually performed either in a catheterization laboratory or in an operating room. Life support equipment has to be immediately available during the procedure.[57]

Transvenous approaches are most commonly cephalic or subclavian and more rarely jugular. After preparation and draping with a sterile field and infiltration with a local anesthetic agent, a 5- to 10-cm incision beginning 1 cm lateral to the deltopectoral groove is performed two fingerbreadths below and parallel to the clavicle. Dissection is made down to the prepectoral fascia, and a pocket is prepared medially for the pulse generator. Depending on the operator's experience, the institution's guidelines, and the patient's status, a cephalic or a subclavian approach may be used for lead(s) placement. The cephalic approach includes dissection of the connective and fat tissue of the deltopectoral groove, allowing isolation of the vein, which is distally ligated; a venotomy is then performed for lead(s) insertion. For the subclavian approach, a modified Seldinger approach is used, the subclavian vein being entered usually through the infraclavicular incision with a needle at the junction of the inner and middle thirds of the clavicle. The subclavian approach has a higher complication rate, including pneumothorax, traumatic arterial puncture with possible hemothorax, and air embolism.[58] For ventricular lead placement, the right ventricular apex is usually selected. Radioscopic oblique view or QRS morphology during ventricular pacing may be useful to ensure proper lead position. The atrial lead may be positioned in the appendage or elsewhere on the atrial wall depending on the type of lead selected (J shaped; with active or passive fixation), the patient's status, or the operator's experience. For dual-chamber pacemakers, both leads may be inserted in the same vein or in two different veins. However, in selected patients, single-lead VDD pacing modalities may be used to simplify the implantation procedure; this system allows ventricular pacing in response to a sensed atrial event using a "floating" electrode located in the intra-atrial part of the single implanted lead.[59, 60]

After lead(s) placement, pacing and sensing thresholds are measured. At 0.5-msec pulse duration, acute pacing threshold should be 1 V or less in the ventricle and 1.5 V or less in the atrium; the amplitude of the local electrogram to ensure reliable sensing should be higher than 6 mV in the ventricle and higher than 1.5 mV in the atrium. Pacing and sensing thresholds may be influenced by several factors, including myocardial infarction, antiarrhythmic drug therapy, and electrolyte disturbances. Lead impedance is also assessed, usually ranging from 300 to 800 Ω, depending on design and material. After appropriate positioning with satisfactory electrical measurements, the leads are tightly sutured to the vessel or fascia of the muscle and then properly connected to the pulse generator that is to be placed in the already prepared pocket. Finally, we recommend closure of the pocket, subcutaneous tissue, and skin in two or three layers. On the following day, the entire system is checked using a 12-lead electrocardiogram, an anteroposterior (Fig. 33–2) and a lateral chest radiograph (Fig. 33–3), and a complete interrogation of the device to ensure proper function of the pacing system and its adaptation to the individual needs. Patients are usually discharged 1 or 2 days after implantation.

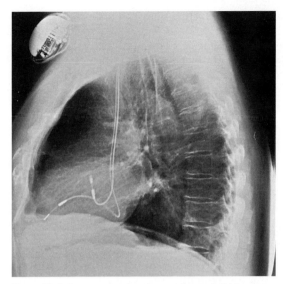

Figure 33–2. Anteroposterior chest radiograph 24 hours after permanent transvenous dual-chamber pacemaker implantation. The tip of the ventricular lead is at the right ventricular apex, and the tip of the atrial lead at the anterolateral wall of the right atrium. Both leads were introduced through the subclavian vein.

COMPLICATIONS OF PERMANENT TRANSVENOUS PACING

General Complications

The overall complication rate of permanent transvenous pacing approximates 5%.[6, 61] Complications are the result of venous access (pneumothorax and hemothorax), lead placement (arrhythmias, perforation of the heart, and displacement), thrombosis and embolism, and generator failure (misconnection, migration, erosion, and infection).[6, 55]

Clinically inapparent venous thrombosis of the upper arm and shoulder is present in 25% to 40% of patients with transvenous pacemakers.[6, 62] The most common site of venous obstruction is the subclavian vein proximal to the cephalic vein.[63] Symptomatic thrombosis of the upper extremities and central veins affects only 1% to 5% of patients.[6, 63] Pacemaker-induced superior vena cava syndrome is rare, with a 1% to 3% incidence.[63] Pulmonary embolism in a patient with a pacemaker is uncommon and should raise a suspicion of thrombosis on the pacing lead as the source.[6]

Infection rates of the pacemaker pocket or the endocardial lead, or both, are estimated to be between 1% and 7%.[6] Clinically, the infection may present as local infection, septicemia, or endocarditis. The pacemaker pocket is the most frequent site of entry, with subsequent involvement of the pacing wire. In the presence of infection, removal of the complete pacing apparatus is mandatory. The mortality rate when infected material is left in place may be as high as 66%.[63]

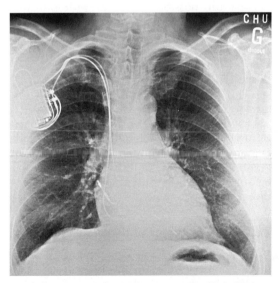

Figure 33–3. Lateral view of the same patient as in Figure 33–1, confirming good positioning of both leads.

Several factors may influence the complication rate: the operator's experience, the method of lead placement (subclavian versus cephalic approach), and the use of dual-chamber pacing. Overall, the complication rate increases if fewer than 12 implantations are performed during 1 year by one physician.[61]

Pacemaker Syndrome in a VVI Pacemaker

Single-chamber ventricular pacing may lead to the pacemaker syndrome, considered as an iatrogenic complication by some authors.[64] Its incidence varies between 7% to 20% in patients paced in the VVI mode.[2, 5, 65] It is mainly caused by the loss of atrioventricular synchrony and the persistence of ventriculoatrial conduction from the paced ventricle, which is found in about 20% of patients with complete anterograde atrioventricular block and in 60% to 70% of patients with sinus node disease.[30] Subsequent atrial distension may initiate inappropriate vascular dilation,[66] possibly mediated, among other factors, by the atrial natriuretic factor.[65] Hypotension may also be due to the loss of atrial kick, causing a decrease in stroke volume at the onset of single-chamber ventricular pacing.[3] Associated symptoms include syncope, presyncope, dyspnea in the severe form, fatigue, palpitations, or neck pulsations in milder cases. All these symptoms usually disappear during restoration of atrioventricular synchrony with atrial or dual-chamber pacing.

Dual-Chamber Pacemaker Problems

Complications related to dual-chamber pacing include the possible problems with the atrial lead, loss of atrial pacing or sensing, and recurrent or persistent atrial tachyarrhythmias. This may necessitate, in as many as 18% of cases over a mean period of 3 years, reprogramming out of the DDD mode.[64]

Pacemaker-mediated tachycardia or endless-loop tachycardia occurs when pacemakers track retrograde atrial activity due to a paced ventricular event or a spontaneous ventricular extrasystole. It usually occurs at the programmed upper rate of the pacemaker and may be solved with appropriate reprogramming of the device.[3, 64]

Technical Problems and Follow-up

As demonstrated in this chapter, the evolution of pacemaker treatment has been tremendous over the last decades. The battery life span has increased from a few months to an average of more than 6 years, lasting as long as 12 years with appropriate programming, and circuitry failure is an extremely rare event.

In conclusion, pacemaker therapy has become a simple, yet highly sophisticated tool in the hands of the cardiologist or cardiac surgeon. It has been used for the improvement of severe symptoms and quality of life of millions of patients; however, the indications should be carefully evaluated to prevent overuse.

REFERENCES

1. Elmquist R, Senning A: An implantable pacemaker for the heart. *In* Smyth CN (ed): Medical Electronics. Proceedings of the Second International Conference on Medical Electrical Engeneering. London, Illife & Sons, 1959, p 253.
2. Furman S: The present status of cardiac pacing. Herz 1991; 16:171–181.
3. Shakespeare CF, Camm AJ: Benefits of the advances in cardiac pacemaker technology. Clin Cardiol 1992; 15:601–606.
4. Bernstein A, Camm J, Fletcher R, et al: The NASPE/BPEG generic pacemaker code for antibradyarrhythmia and adaptive-rate pacing and antitachyarrhythmia devices. PACE Pacing Clin Electrophysiol 1987; 10:794–799.
5. Dreifus LS, Fish C, Griffin JC, et al: Guidelines for implantation of cardiac pacemakers and antiarrhythmia devices: A report of the American College of Cardiology/American Heart Association Task Force on Assessment of Diagnostic and Therapeutic Cardiovascular Procedures (Committee on Pacemaker Implantation). J Am Coll Cardiol 1991; 18:1–13.
6. Phibbs B, Marriott HJL: Complications of permanent transvenous pacing. N Engl J Med 1985; 312:1428–1432.
7. Greenspan AM, Kay HR, Berger BC, et al: Incidence of unwarranted implantation of permanent cardiac pacemakers in a large medical population. N Engl J Med 1988; 318:158–163.
8. Clarke M, Sutton R, Ward D, et al: Recommendations for pacemaker prescription for symptomatic bradycardia. Br Heart J 1991; 66:185–191.
9. Bernstein AD, Parsonnet V: Strategies for mode selection in antibradyarrhythmia pacing. Cardiol Clin 1992; 10:719–734.
10. Nordlander R, Hedman A: Hemodynamics and exercise capacity during pacemaker stimulation. Herz 1991; 16:149–157.
11. Maloney JD, Helguera ME, Woscoboinik JR: Physiology of rate responsive pacing. Cardiol Clin 1992; 10:619–633.
12. Furman S: Rate-modulated pacing. Circulation 1990; 82:1081–1094.
13. Chirife R: Physiological principles of a new method for rate-responsive pacing using the pre-ejection interval. PACE Pacing Clin Electrophysiol 1988; 11:1545–1554.
14. Alt E: Implantable devices—pending issues and future trends. PACE Pacing Clin Electrophysiol 1990; 13:1079–1081.
15. Katritsis D, Camm AJ: Adaptive-rate pacemakers: Comparison of sensors and clinical experience. Cardiol Clin 1992; 10:671–690.
16. Kappenberger L: Technical improvements in sensors for rate-adaptive pacemakers. Am Heart J 1994; 127:1022–1026.

17. Kappenberger L, Gloor HO, Babotai I, et al: Hemodynamic effects of atrial synchronization in acute and long-term ventricular pacing. PACE Pacing Clin Electrophysiol 1982; 5:639–645.

18. Baig MW, Perrin EJ: The hemodynamics of cardiac pacing: Clinical and physiological aspects. Prog Cardiovasc Dis 1991; 33:283–298.

19. Barold SS, Zipes DP: Cardiac pacemakers and antiarrhythmic devices. *In* Braunwald E (ed): Heart Disease, 4th ed. Philadelphia, WB Saunders, 1992, pp 726–755.

20. Janosick DL, Pearson AC, Buckingham TA, et al: The hemodynamic benefit of differential atrioventricular delay intervals for sensed and paced atrial events during physiologic pacing. J Am Coll Cardiol 1989; 14:499–507.

21. Rosenqvist M, Isaaz K, Botvinik EH, et al: Relative importance of activation sequence compared to atrioventricular synchrony in left ventricular function. Am J Cardiol 1991; 67:148–156.

22. Bernstein AD, Parsonnet V: Survey of cardiac pacing in the United States in 1989. Am J Cardiol 1992; 69:331–338.

23. Shaw DB, Holman RR, Gowers JI: Survival in sinoatrial disorders (sick sinus syndrome). Br Med J 1980; 280:139–141.

24. Stangl K, Seitz K, Wirtzfeld A, et al: Differences between atrial single-chamber pacing (AAI) and ventricular single-chamber pacing (W I) with respect to prognosis and antiarrhythmic effect in patients with sick sinus syndrome. PACE Pacing Clin Electrophysiol 1990; 13:2080–2085.

25. Rosenqvist M, Brandt J, Schuller H: Long-term pacing in sinus node disease: Effects of stimulation mode on cardiovascular morbidity and mortality. Am Heart J 1988; 116:16–22.

26. Sasaki Y, Shimotori M, Akahane K, et al: Long-term follow-up of patients with sick sinus syndrome: A comparison of clinical aspects among unpaced, ventricular inhibited paced, and physiologically paced groups. PACE Pacing Clin Electrophysiol 1988; 11:1575–1583.

27. Feuer JM, Shandling AH, Messenger JC, et al: Influence of cardiac pacing mode on the long-term development of fibrillation. Am J Cardiol 1989; 64:1376–1379.

28. Hesselson AB, Parsonnet V, Bernstein AD, Bonavita G: Deleterious effects of long-term single-chamber ventricular pacing in patients with sick sinus syndrome: The hidden benefits of dual-chamber pacing. J Am Coll Cardiol 1992; 19:1542–1549.

29. Sutton R: Pacing in atrial arrhythmias. PACE Pacing Clin Electrophysiol 1990; 13:1823–1827.

30. Grimm W, Langenfeld H, Maisch B, Kochsiek K: Symptoms, cardiovascular risk profile, and spontaneous ECG in paced patients: A five-year follow-up study. PACE Pacing Clin Electrophysiol 1990; 13:2086–2090.

31. Sgarbossa EB, Pinski SL, Maloney JD, et al: Chronic atrial fibrillation and stroke in paced patients with sick sinus syndrome: Relevance of clinical characteristics and pacing modalities. Circulation 1993; 88:1045–1053.

32. Andersen HR, Thuesen L, Bagger JP, et al: Atrial versus ventricular pacing in sick sinus syndrome: A prospective, randomized trial in 225 consecutive patients [abstract]. Eur Heart J 1993; 14(Suppl):252.

33. Lamas GA, Estes NM III, Schneller S, Flaker GC: Does dual-chamber or atrial pacing prevent atrial fibrillation? The need for a randomized, controlled trial. PACE Pacing Clin Electrophysiol 1992; 15:1109–1113.

34. Sgarbossa EB, Pinski SL, Maloney JD: The role of pacing modality in determining long-term survival in the sick sinus syndrome. Ann Intern Med 1993; 119:359–365.

35. Fromer M, Kappenberger L, Steinbrunn W: Zur binoda-

len Erkrankung: Kranker Sinusknoten und AV Block. Z Kardiol 1983; 72:410–413.

36. Rosenqvist M, Nordlander R: Survival in patients with permanent pacemakers. Cardiol Clin 1992; 10:691–703.

37. Linde-Edelstam C, Gullberg B, Norlander R, et al: Longevity in patients with high-degree atrioventricular block paced in the atrial synchronous or the fixed-rate ventricular-inhibited mode. PACE Pacing Clin Electrophysiol 1992; 15:304–313.

38. Alpert MA, Curtis JJ, Sanfelippo JF, et al: Comparative survival after permanent ventricular and dual-chamber pacing for patients with chronic high-degree atrioventricular block with and without preexistent congestive heart failure. J Am Coll Cardiol 1986; 7:925–932.

39. Petch MC: Who needs a dual-chamber pacing?. Br Med J 1993; 307:215–216.

40. Barold SS: Rate-adaptive cardiac pacing: Cost versus technology versus patient benefit. Am Heart J 1993; 126:1828–1834.

41. Katritsis D, Ward DE, Camm AJ: Can we treat carotid sinus syndrome? PACE Pacing Clin Electrophysiol 1991; 14:1367–1374.

42. Benditt DG: Cardiac pacing in carotid sinus syndrome and vasovagal syncope. Cardiology 1993; 10:11–14.

43. Barold SS: Cardiac pacing in special and complex situations. Cardiol Clin 1992; 10:573–591.

44. Fitzpatrick A, Theodorakis G, Ahmed R, Sutton WR: Dual-chamber pacing aborts vasovagal syncope induced by head-up 60-degree tilt. PACE Pacing Clin Electrophysiol 1991; 14:13–19.

45. Sra JS, Jazayeri MR, Avitall B, et al: Comparison of cardiac pacing with drug therapy in the treatment of neurocardiogenic (vasovagal) syncope with bradycardia or asystole. N Engl J Med 1993; 328:1085–1090.

46. Hochleitner M, Hortnagl H, Ng C-K, et al: Usefulness of physiologic dual-chamber pacing in drug-resistant idiopathic dilated cardiomyopathy. Am J Cardiol 1990; 66:198–202.

47. Hochleitner M, Hortnagl H, Hortnagl H, et al: Long-term efficacy of physiologic dual-chamber pacing in the treatment of end-stage idiopathic dilated cardiomyopathy. Am J Cardiol 1992; 70:1320–1325.

48. Brecker SJD, Xiao HB, Sparrow J, Gibson DG: Effects of dual-chamber pacing with short atrioventricular delay in dilated cardiomyopathy. Lancet 1992; 340:1308–1312.

49. Iskandrian AS: Pacemaker therapy in congestive heart failure. Am J Cardiol 1990; 66:223–224.

50. McDonald K, McWilliams E, O'Keefe B, Maurer B: Functional assessment of patients treated with permanent dual-chamber pacing as a primary treatment for hypertrophic cardiomyopathy. Eur Heart J 1988; 9:893–898.

51. Jeanrenaud X, Goy JJ, Kappenberger L: Effects of dual-chamber pacing in hypertrophic cardiomyopathy. Lancet 1992; 339:1318–1323.

52. Fananapazir L, Cannon RO III, Tripodi D, Panza JA: Impact of dual-chamber permanent pacing in patients with obstructive hypertrophic cardiomyopathy with symptoms refractory to verapamil and β-adrenergic blocker therapy. Circulation 1992; 85:2149–2161.

53. McDonald KM, Maurer B: Permanent pacing as a treatment for hypertrophic cardiomyopathy. Am J Cardiol 1991; 68:108–110.

54. Nishimura RA, Danielson GK: Dual-chamber pacing for hypertrophic obstructive cardiomyopathy: Has its time come? Br Heart J 1993; 70:301–303.

55. Midei M, Brinker J: Pacemaker implantation. *In* Ellenbogen KA (ed): Cardiac Pacing. Boston, Blackwell Scientific, 1992, pp 211–262.

56. Holmes DR: Permanent pacemaker implantation. *In*

Furman S, Hayes DL, Holmes DR (eds): A Practice of Cardiac Pacing. Mount Kisco, NY, Futura Publishing, 1986, pp 97–127.

57. Parsonnet V, Furman S, Smyth NPD, Bilitch M: Optimal resources for implantable cardiac pacemakers. Circulation 1983; 68:226A–244A.

58. Mueller X, Sadeghi H, Kappenberger L: Complications after single- versus dual-chamber pacemaker implantation. PACE Pacing Clin Electrophysiol 1990; 13:711–714.

59. Curzio G: A multicenter evaluation of a single-pass lead VDD pacing system. Multicenter Study Group. PACE Pacing Clin Electrophysiol 1991; 14:434–442.

60. Varriale P, Chryssos BE: Atrial sensing performance of the single-lead VDD pacemaker during exercise. J Am Coll Cardiol 1993; 22:1854–1857.

61. Parsonnet V, Bernstein AD, Lindsay B: Pacemaker implantation complication rates: An analysis of some contributing factors. J Am Coll Cardiol 1989; 13:917–921.

62. Spitell PC, Hayes DL: Venous complications after insertion of a transvenous pacemaker. Mayo Clin Proc 1992; 67:258–265.

63. Byrd CL, Schwartz SJ, Hedin N: Lead extraction: Indications and techniques. Cardiol Clin 1992; 10:735–748.

64. Gross JN, Moser S, Benedek Z, et al: DDD pacing mode survival in patients with a dual-chamber pacemaker. J Am Coll Cardiol 1992; 19:1536–1541.

65. Travill C, Sutton R: Pacemaker syndrome: An iatrogenic condition. Br Heart J 1992; 68:163–166.

66. Ellenbogen KA, Thames MD, Mohanty PK, et al: New insights into pacemaker syndrome gained from hemodynamic, humoral, and vascular responses during ventriculoatrial pacing. Am J Cardiol 1990; 65:53–59.

Chapter 34

Implantable Cardioverter-Defibrillators

MARTIN FROMER
LUKAS KAPPENBERGER

Implantable cardioverter-defibrillators (ICDs) are electronic devices designed to terminate ventricular tachycardia or ventricular fibrillation by an electronic intervention, i.e., pacing or cardioversion for ventricular tachycardia and defibrillation for ventricular fibrillation.

RATIONALE OF ICD THERAPY

Holter monitor recordings of patients dying from sudden cardiac death have shown that in patients with coronary artery disease ventricular tachycardia preceded ventricular fibrillation in most patients (62%): in 8.2%, primary ventricular fibrillation occurred; in 12.7%, polymorphic ventricular tachycardia (like torsade de pointes) was noted; and in 16.5%, bradycardia and asystole led to sudden cardiac death.[1] In patients with cardiomyopathy the major arrhythmias leading to sudden cardiac death appear to be asystole and bradycardia.[2, 3] Thus, if sudden cardiac death is to be prevented by an electronic device, the intervention perforce must terminate ventricular tachycardia, ventricular fibrillation, bradycardia, and asystole. Most patients who are victims of sudden cardiac death have coronary artery disease, followed second by patients with dilated or hypertrophic cardiomyopathy.[4] It has been estimated that in the United States 300,000 to 450,000 sudden cardiac deaths occur each year.[5, 6] From community intervention programs it is known that early intervention with external defibrillation improves the survival rate.[7] Automatic ICD therapy has the advantage of ensuring early intervention.

Patients considered to be at high risk show the following features: (1) multiple myocardial infarctions, (2) reduced left ventricular pump function,[8] (3) decreased exercise tolerance,[9] (4) therapy with antiarrhythmic drugs,[10] (5) syncope or presyncope,[11] (6) inducible ventricular tachycardia,[12] (7) ventricular premature contractions on Holter recordings,[8] and recording of late potentials by signal-averaged electrocardiograms.[13, 14] Careful clinical evaluation of patients in these high-risk subsets helps identify candidates for ICD therapy.

HISTORICAL REVIEW OF ICD THERAPY

The experience with external defibrillation gained in the 1960s encouraged development of implantable devices. Schuder and associates[15] and Mirowski and colleagues[16–18] were pioneers in research and design. Mirowski as well as others realized that time is a critical factor in the successful termination of ventricular fibrillation. Investigations were initially directed toward a system with transvenous electrodes (a bielectrode system). For the detection of ventricular fibrillation or ventricular tachycardia, Mirowski and Mower[16] initially tested a pressure transducer placed on a right ventricular electrode. The defibrillation shock was delivered between the right ventricular and the subcutaneous, epicostal electrodes. Subsequently, a transvenous system with two electrodes positioned within the right heart was successfully tested.[17] Schuder and associates[15] proposed an electrode system in the right ventricular apex and superior vena cava, using truncated exponential waveforms that required less energy for successful defibrillation than rectangular pulses. Stable right ventricular electrode positions were difficult to achieve. Therefore, in subsequent studies a right ventricular cup electrode was used as the cathode in canine implants. Because of uncertain defibrillation efficacy with the available capacitor, pulse, and electrode technology, epicardial patch electrodes were subsequently developed and in 1979 to 1980 were successfully implanted in humans.[18] The first and second generation of implantable defibrillators delivered defibrillation and cardioversion by means of epicardial electrode systems or a combination of epicardial and intracardiac electrodes.[19-22] Third-generation devices typically can provide pacing, cardioversion, and defibrillation[23] and use a variety of electrodes, including epicardial patches, intracardiac electrodes, or a hybrid system.

Pacing is used for two purposes: (1) to prevent bradycardia and (2) to overdrive an underlying tachycardia. Antibradycardia pacing is an important function inasmuch as bradycardia in these patients may be the result of antiarrhythmic drug therapy, an underlying conduction disorder, or sinus node dysfunction, or it may occur after a defibrillatory shock. Antitachycardia overdrive pacing is an important adjunctive function in third-generation ICDs because it has the advantage of being painless. However, there is an inherent risk of destabilizing ventricular tachycardia and inducing ventricular flutter or fibrillation (Fig. 34–1).[24, 25] Destabilization of ventricular tachycardia into ventricular fibrillation may occur even with low-energy cardioversion pulses[25, 26] (Fig. 34–2). Although antitachycardia pacing has been used for many years to terminate ventricular tachycardia in well-selected patients, sudden cardiac death in patients with only antitachycardia pacing devices has been reported.[27-30] Therefore, antitachycardia pacing is now incorporated into devices that

offer automatic back-up cardioversion and defibrillation, so-called tiered therapy.[31-32]

THE CONCEPT OF HIERARCHICAL, TIERED THERAPY

A universal device prevents bradycardia by pacing and terminates ventricular tachycardia or ventricular fibrillation by pacing, cardioversion, and defibrillation, respectively. Figure 34–3 displays the various functions incorporated into this relatively complicated device.

Appropriate algorithms link antitachycardia pacing, cardioversion, and defibrillation capabilities and allow their programming in a hierarchical sequence.[23] This multiprogrammability of device response offers an individual approach for electrical therapy, fine tuned to the pattern of the arrhythmia and the observed responses.[32] Given a hemodynamically stable ventricular tachycardia, therapy would start with antitachycardia pacing and in case of nonresponse or acceleration, the next programmed step may consist of a low-energy cardioversion pulse. If the pulse is not effective, a subsequent, high-energy cardioversion pulse may be delivered (Fig. 34–4). In case of degeneration to ventricular fibrillation, several defibrillation discharges are delivered.[32] This staged therapy requires that various rate-detection windows are provided. Therefore, tiered-therapy devices use various independently preprogrammable detection

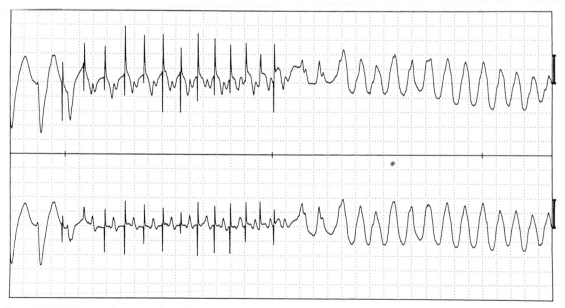

Figure 34–1. Holter monitor recording of a spontaneous ventricular tachycardia episode accelerated to ventricular flutter by rapid antitachycardia overdrive pacing. Not shown is the automatic termination of this flutter episode by internal defibrillation. Paper speed, 25 mm/sec.

PCD 7216 A

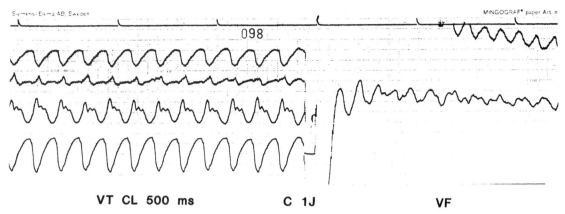

Figure 34–2. Shown is an acceleration of ventricular tachycardia (VT) to ventricular fibrillation by low-energy cardioversion. VT CL, ventricular tachycardia cycle length; C, cardioversion; VF, ventricular fibrillation; J, joule. Paper speed, 25 mm/sec.

zones. To each zone and tachycardia detection interval a therapeutic intervention can be assigned. In fact, a tiered-therapy device has (1) a programmable zone for bradycardia pacing; (2) a zone where the rate is considered to be normal and no interventions occurs; (3) a zone where the rate is considered to represent ventricular tachycardia; and (4) a cutoff rate from where any rhythm is treated as ventricular fibrillation. A tachycardia zone can be subdivided further into a slow or fast rate tachycardia zone and pacing therapies can be reserved for the slow rate tachycardia zone, whereas electrical shock therapy is chosen for the fast rate tachy-

cardia zone. Therapies are based mainly on rate criteria, but QRS duration criteria may also be incorporated. Hemodynamic sensors are not yet available. A tachycardia is considered terminated after a predetermined number of intervals are detected within the normal or slow rate zone.

An unsolved problem is the triggering of a device response by supraventricular arrhythmias, mainly atrial fibrillation-flutter with rapid ventricular response rate or sinus tachycardia during exertional stress. To avoid inappropriate interventions, additional algorithms are available. These algorithms consider sudden onset

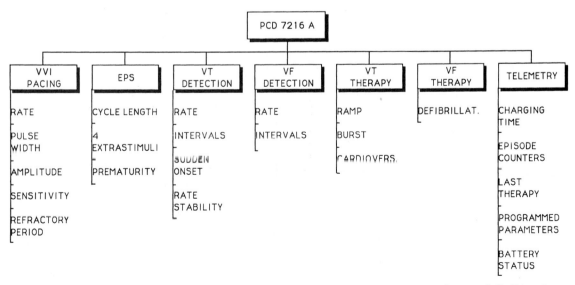

Figure 34–3. An example of the various programmable sections of a third-generation pacer, cardioverter-defibrillator, in this model the Medtronic PCD 7216 A. EPS, electrophysiologic study; VT, ventricular tachycardia; VF, ventricular fibrillation; VVI, ventricular on demand pacing.

PCD 7216 A

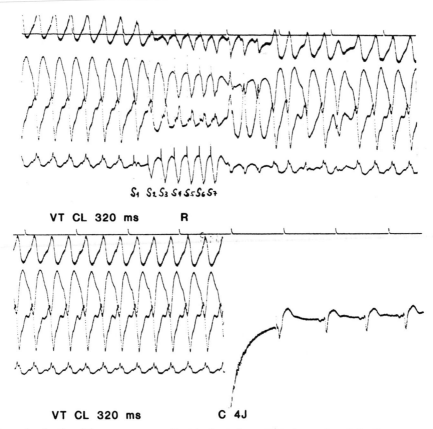

Figure 34–4. Example of a tiered-therapy sequence. Ventricular tachycardia is detected, and the first sequence consists of overdrive pacing; seven stimuli are delivered that result in an acceleration of ventricular tachycardia. However, the initial monomorphic ventricular tachycardia re-emerges and is automatically redetected by the device. On redetection, a cardioversion pulse of 4 J is delivered and results in restoration of sinus rhythm. The first beat after the cardioversion pulse is a paced complex. See Figure 34–2 for abbreviations. R, ramp pacing.

or rate stability, or both. Ventricular tachycardia is considered to be stable in cycle length and its onset to be sudden. Nevertheless, it has been shown that ventricular tachycardia may demonstrate considerable variation of its cycle length,[33] as well as a gradual onset in some instances. Although these algorithms may improve the specificity of device response, the trade-off is often a decrease in sensitivity. Inappropriate device response exposes the patient to some serious and yet unresolved problems: (1) unnecessary discomfort and pain due to spurious cardioversion or defibrillation discharges, and (2) the risk of provoking true ventricular tachyarrhythmias by antitachycardia pacing or low-energy cardioversion. In a few instances, such an intervention has caused documented deleterious ventricular tachyarrhythmias. Analogous to drug therapy, one may call these events a proarrhythmic effect of device therapy. In addition, atrial fibrillation can be provoked by de-

vice intervention, occurring mainly after cardioversion or defibrillation discharges (Fig. 34–5). This may again provoke device responses. Improved memory function of the latest devices has facilitated the detection and understanding of these undesirable situations, and device programming usually solves the problem. Device responses to supraventricular arrhythmias are the expression of the lack of specificity of arrhythmia detection algorithms. In some instances drug therapy is required to prevent either sinus tachycardia or rapid ventricular response during atrial fibrillation. Atrioventricular node ablation might be useful in some patients.

When automatic ICD therapy was first used, symptoms such as presyncope, syncope, and palpitations before shock delivery determined the appropriateness of device intervention. Shocks delivered in the absence of such symptoms were considered to be inappropriate. The estimation

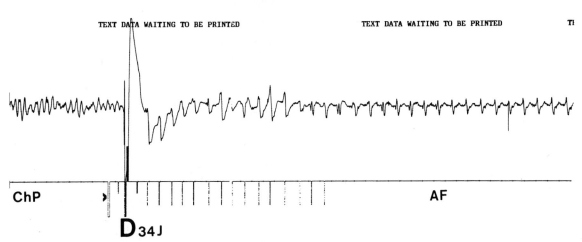

Figure 34–5. The initiation of atrial fibrillation (AF) after automatic internal defibrillation. A defibrillation pulse of 34 J is delivered that initially converts ventricular fibrillation to polymorphic ventricular tachycardia, which is followed by an episode of rapid AF. During this time the capacitors are charged after ventricular fibrillation has been detected. ChP, charging period, D, defibrillation; J, joule.

of appropriateness based on symptoms is less conclusive in patients with third-generation devices. If ventricular tachycardia is treated initially by antitachycardia pacing, which is painless, the intervention remains unnoticed by the patient. Third-generation ICDs offer information on detected arrhythmia and triggered device function.[33] In some devices the stored information includes a predetermined number of digitized RR intervals immediately before and after device intervention[33, 34] (see Fig. 34–7), and in the latest devices, ventricular electrograms can be retrieved. This information, together with deductive reasoning, allows a quite accurate interpretation of the appropriateness of device intervention, provides documentation of the incidence of asymptomatic interventions, and guides further programming of the device for the individual patient.

INDICATIONS FOR ICD THERAPY

In 1980, during the first clinical investigation of ICDs, only patients who had experienced two cardiac arrests while on therapy with antiarrhythmic drugs were candidates for ICD implantation. Since then the indications have greatly expanded, and, in general, an ICD is recommended in the patient with sustained ventricular tachycardia or ventricular fibrillation if the following conditions are met[35]:

1. Electrophysiologic or other testing cannot be used to predict efficacy of treatment

or

2. There are recurrent episodes of ventricular tachycardia or ventricular fibrillation while on therapy

or

3. There is persistent inducibility of sustained ventricular tachycardia or ventricular fibrillation at the time of electrophysiologic study or during Holter monitoring or after catheter ablation or surgical intervention

ICD therapy is a valuable important option in patients with syncope or presyncope in whom electrophysiologic testing or Holter monitoring could not demonstrate an arrhythmic event but in whom a sustained ventricular tachyarrhythmia was documented. ICD therapy has also to be considered in patients with a history of syncope, presyncope, and an otherwise proven arrhythmogenic substrate such as right ventricular dysplasia, cardiomyopathy, and myocardial infarction.

IMPLANTATION OF AUTOMATIC DEFIBRILLATORS

Before implantation of automatic defibrillators, diagnostic investigations of a potential candidate customarily include the following:

• Routine clinical and laboratory examinations
• Exclusion of potentially reversible arrhythmogenic factors
• Holter electrocardiogram, treadmill stress testing, and echocardiography

- Coronary angiography and left ventriculography
- Invasive electrophysiologic study

The purpose of these investigations is to analyze whether potentially reversible factors are present that might influence the arrhythmia profile and whether the patient could potentially benefit from a surgical intervention or a catheter ablation procedure.

ICDs are implanted during general anesthesia. To implant epicardial patch electrodes, a midline sternotomy is the usual approach. Modifications of this approach, however, include a subxiphoid incision, a modified sternotomy, or a left lateral thoracotomy.[20] The transvenous approach is similar to the insertion of standard pacemaker leads with a cutdown over the subclavian or cephalic veins, or both. The cathode is positioned at the right ventricular apex and the anode at the superior vena caval–right atrial junction.[36, 37] In transvenous systems the tip of the cathode also includes a bipolar sensing-pacing electrode as well. In systems with epicardial patches, sensing and pacing are done either by epicardial screw-in electrodes or by the insertion of a transvenous electrode placed at the right ventricular apex. In an unidirectional shock configuration, the shock is delivered between the cathode and the anode. If such a configuration does not provide reliable, efficacious defibrillation, an additional electrode has to be implanted. This electrode, which can be large (Fig. 34–6), is positioned subcutaneously on the left side of the chest. Epicardial patch electrodes are less commonly used. The additional anode provides the option of bidirectional shock, which may achieve defibrillation with less energy than a unidirectional shock. The ICD unit itself is usually implanted in the abdominal wall and the leads are connected to the "can" via tunneling. The device may also be implanted in the pectoral area, as shown in recent studies.[38] In the future, general anesthesia may be required only for testing defibrillation thresholds.

Intraoperative testing of the functions of third-generation devices consists of the evaluation of pacing and sensing, as in usual pacemaker therapy. Adequate R wave amplitude (>5 mV), and slew-rate (>0.75 V/sec) are important to ensure proper sensing during ventricular fibrillation. Sensing of induced ventricular fibrillation and efficacy of defibrillation are tested according to a protocol.[23] For the induction of ventricular fibrillation several methods are used: stimulation of the heart with high-frequency alternating current, rapid burst pacing, or dis-

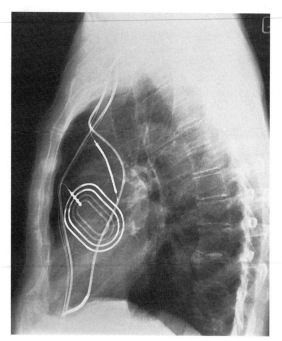

Figure 34–6. Radiograph of a patient with a hybrid nonthoracotomy lead system, consisting of a vena cava superior lead, a right ventricular apex lead, and an epicostal subcutaneous patch. This triple-electrode system allows a bidirectional pulse pathway to lower the defibrillation energy requirements.

charge of a low-energy T wave shock. In some patients induction of sustained ventricular fibrillation is difficult to achieve. This may lead to prolonged trials to induce ventricular fibrillation, ultimately increasing the risk of the procedure. The defibrillation threshold should reflect the lowest energy that allowed repeated successful defibrillation. A safety margin between the defibrillation threshold and the maximum output of the device of 10 J should be respected. It is recommended that the antifibrillation function of the device be activated when the patient leaves the operating room.

POSTOPERATIVE CARE

Postoperatively, the patient should be monitored for 2 to 3 days, because ventricular and supraventricular arrhythmias commonly occur. Chest radiographs should be used to document electrode and device position. Antiplatelet and anticoagulant therapy should be withheld until wound healing is ensured. Before discharge, a stress test should be conducted to ensure that muscle noise or sinus tachycardia does not trigger device function. Antibiotic prophylaxis is continued in our institution until the patient is discharged. Wound seroma and hematoma are not infrequent and need careful follow-up.

Before discharge, a complete interrogation and follow-up check of the ICD should be done, and its efficacy in detection and termination of ventricular fibrillation should be demonstrated again. This testing requires sedation of the patient but usually not general anesthesia. A chest radiograph is important to document electrode and device position. It is also important to instruct the patient about what to do and whom to inform in case of device discharges. Car driving by the patient should be forbidden.

Perioperative mortality is greatly influenced by patient-related as well as surgical-related factors. Patient-related factors include clinical stability, cardiac decompensation, as well as other organ functions known to influence mortality and morbidity in procedures requiring general anesthesia. Surgical-related factors include the approach used for placement of the electrodes and procedure-related complications, such as infection, bleeding, perforation of cardiac tissue, and displacement of electrodes. Placement of epicardial patches has a higher mortality than placement of transvenous leads (8% vs. 1% in some series, respectively).

Postoperative complications are related to the surgical procedure or to the underlying cardiac and rhythm disorders of the patient. Surgical problems include dislocation and retraction of leads, crinkling of patches, and infection in and around any part of the ICD system.[19, 21, 22]

Among the most serious postoperative problems are infection, arrhythmia storms, and cardiac dysfunction. Infections are usually treated by guided antibiotic therapy as well as removing the whole implanted material; the management of such a situation is difficult. Prevention of infection requires a clean surgical technique with prevention of hematoma and seroma and prophylaxis with antibiotics. Arrhythmia storms may occur either as ventricular tachyarrhythmias or as supraventricular tachyarrhythmias. They may require deactivation of the device, heavy sedation of the patient, and antiarrhythmic therapy. Myocardial decompensation with congestive heart failure requires symptomatic therapy and is an important proarrhythmic cofactor.

VT data

```
LAST EPISODE DETECTION SEQUENCE:
 -19. R-R INTERVAL- 260 MS
 -18. R-R INTERVAL- 250 MS
 -17. R-R INTERVAL- 230 MS
 -16. R-R INTERVAL- 260 MS          +1. R-R INTERVAL- 890 MS
 -15. R-R INTERVAL- 230 MS          +2. R-R INTERVAL- 890 MS
 -14. R-R INTERVAL- 260 MS          +3. R-R INTERVAL- 920 MS
 -13. R-R INTERVAL- 230 MS          +4. R-R INTERVAL- 870 MS
 -12. R-R INTERVAL- 250 MS          +5. R-R INTERVAL- 860 MS
 -11. R-R INTERVAL- 240 MS          +6. R-R INTERVAL- 860 MS
 -10. R-R INTERVAL- 260 MS          +7. R-R INTERVAL- 860 MS
  -9. R-R INTERVAL- 230 MS          +8. R-R INTERVAL- 780 MS
  -8. R-R INTERVAL- 260 MS          +9. R-R INTERVAL- 750 MS
  -7. R-R INTERVAL- 230 MS         +10. R-R INTERVAL- 760 MS
  -6. R-R INTERVAL- 250 MS         +10. THERAPY WAS SUCCESSFUL
  5. R-R INTERVAL- 240 MS
  -4. R-R INTERVAL- 260 MS
  -3. R-R INTERVAL- 230 MS
  -2. R-R INTERVAL- 260 MS         Patient # 6
  -1. R-R INTERVAL- 230 MS
  -0. R-R INTERVAL- 250 MS
  -0. VT DETECTED
```

Figure 34-7. Example of a memory printout. The device records the 19 RR intervals preceding the detection of ventricular tachycardia (VT) and the 10 intervals after therapy. It indicates that therapy was successful. In this specific instance ventricular flutter with a cycle length around 250 msec is detected, and after therapy discharge RR intervals between 760 and 890 msec are sensed. It is concluded that sinus rhythm has been re-established after therapy.

FOLLOW-UP OF PATIENTS AND DEVICES

Clinical follow-up is usually carried out at regular intervals to check patient status and device function. It includes interrogation of the device for battery status and lead status data, pacing and sensing functions, and printout of therapy-related data (Fig. 34–7); charging of the capacitors; or electrophysiologic studies using the programmed stimulation features of the implanted device and other means. A clinical follow-up includes arrhythmia history, data on cardiac therapy, and counseling of the patient. Changes in antiarrhythmic therapy may influence device action.

FUTURE DIRECTIONS

Implantation of devices will soon be easier through reduction in device volume and the use of a single electrode. However, evolution of these devices to universal antiarrhythmia units will include dual-chamber pacing and atrial defibrillation and therefore may become quite complex. The purpose of the device therapy is to provide specific and well-targeted antiarrhythmic therapy and to avoid inappropriate discharge or proarrhythmic device effects.

REFERENCES

1. Bayes de Luna A, Coumel P, Leclercq J: Ambulatory sudden cardiac death: Mechanisms of production of fatal arrhythmia on the basis of data from 157 cases. Am Heart J 1989; 117:151–159.
2. Kjekshus J: Arrhythmias and mortality in congestive heart failure. Am J Cardiol 1990; 65:421–481.
3. Luu M, Stevenson WG, Stevenson LW, et al: Diverse mechanisms of unexpected cardiac arrest in advanced heart failure. Circulation 1989; 80:1675–1680.
4. Roberts WC: Sudden cardiac death: Definitions and causes. Am J Cardiol 1986; 57:1410–1413.
5. Lown B: Sudden cardiac death—1978. Circulation 1979; 60:1593–1599.
6. Lown B: Sudden cardiac death: The major challenge confronting contemporary cardiology. Am J Cardiol 1979; 43:313–328.
7. Dalzell GWN, Cunningham SR, Wislon CM, et al: Ventricular defibrillation: The Belfast experience. Br Heart J 1987; 58:441–446.
8. Gomes JA, Winters SL, Stewart D, et al: A new noninvasive index to predict sustained ventricular tachycardia and sudden death in the first year after myocardial infarction; based on signal-averaged electrocardiogram, radionuclide ejection fraction, and Holter monitoring. J Am Coll Cardiol 1987; 10:349–357.
9. Gillespie JA, Moss AJ: Postinfarction risk profiling: Past, present and future considerations. J Am Coll Cardiol 1986; 8:50–51.
10. Ruskin JN, DiMarco JP, Garan H: Out-of-hospital cardiac arrest: Electrophysiolgic observations and selection of long-term antiarrhythmic therapy. N Engl J Med 1980; 303:607–613.
11. Brugada P, Talajic M, Mulleneers R, Wellens HJJ: The value of the clinical history to assess prognosis of patients with ventricular tachycardia or ventricular fibrillation after myocardial infarction. Eur Heart J 1989; 10:747–752.
12. Wilber DJ, Garan H, Finkelstein D, et al: Out-of-hospital cardiac arrest: Use of electrophysiologic testing in prediction of long-term outcome. N Engl J Med 1988; 318:19–24.
13. Breithardt G, Borggreffe M: Recent advances in the identification of patients at risk of ventricular tachyarrhythmias: Role of ventricular late potentials. Circulation 1987; 75:1091–1096.
14. Kuchar DL, Thorburn CW, Sammuel NL: Late potentials detected after myocardial infarction: Natural history and prognostic significance. Circulation 1986; 74:1280–1289.
15. Schuder JC, Stoeckle H, West JA, Keskar PY: Relationship between electrode geometry and effectiveness of ventricular defibrillation in the dog with catheter having one electrode in right ventricle and other electrode in superior vena cava, or external jugular vein, or both. Cardiovasc Res 1973; 7:629–637.
16. Mirowski M, Mower MM: Hemodynamic sensors for implantable defibrillators. J Am Coll Cardiol 1990; 15:656–657.
17. Mirowski M, Mower MM, Gott VL, Brawley RK: Feasibility and effectiveness of low-energy catheter defibrillation in man. Circulation 1973; 47:79–85.
18. Mirowski M, Reid PR, Mower MM, et al: Termination of malignant ventricular tachycardia with an implantable automatic defibrillator in human beings. N Engl J Med 1980; 303:322–324.
19. Winkle RA, Stinson EB, Echt DS, et al: Practical aspects of automatic cardioverter/defibrillator implantation. Am Heart J 1984; 108:1335–1346.
20. Lawrie GM, Griffin JC, Wyndham CRC: Epicardial implantation of the automatic implantable defibrillator by left subcostal thoracotomy. PACE Pacing Clin Electrophysiol 1984; 7:1370–1374.
21. Echt DS, Armstrong K, Schmidt P, et al: Clinical experience, complications, and survival in 70 patients with the automatic implantable cardioverter/defibrillator. Circulation 1985; 71:289–296.
22. Marchlinski FE, Flores BT, Buxton AE, et al: The automatic implantable cardioverter-defibrillator: Efficacy, complications, and device failures. Ann Intern Med 1986; 104:481–488.
23. Fromer M, Schlapfer J, Fischer A, Kappenberger L: Experience with a new implantable pacer-, cardioverter-, defibrillator for the therapy of recurrent sustained ventricular tachyarrhythmias: A step toward a universal tachyarrhythmia control device. PACE Pacing Clin Electrophysiol 1991; 14:1288–1298.
24. Newman DM, Lee MA, Herre JM, et al: Permanent antitachycardia pacemaker therapy for ventricular tachycardia. PACE Pacing Clin Electrophysiol 1989; 12:1387–1395.
25. Saksena S, Chandran P, Shah Y, et al: Comparative efficacy of transvenous cardioversion and pacing in patients with sustained ventricular tachycardia: A prospective, randomized, crossover study. Circulation 1985; 72:153–160.
26. Ciccone JM, Saksena S, Shah Y, Pantopoulos D: A prospective, randomized study of the clinical efficacy and safety of transvenous cardioversion for termination of ventricular tachycardia. Circulation 1985; 71:571–578.
27. Fisher JD, Mehra R, Furman S: Termination of ventricu-

lar tachycardia with bursts of rapid ventricular pacing. Am J Cardiol 1978; 41:94–102.

28. Zipes DP, Prystowsky EN, Miles WM, Heger JJ: Initial experience with Symbios model 7008 pacemaker. PACE Pacing Clin Electrophysiol 1984; 7:1301–1306.

29. Ruskin JN, Garan H, Harthorne JW: Permanent radio-frequency ventricular pacing for management of drug-resistant ventricular tachycardia. Am J Cardiol 1980; 46:317–321.

30. Kappenberger L, Sowton E: Programmed stimulation for long-term treatment and noninvasive investigation of recurrent tachycardia. Lancet 1981; 1:909–914.

31. Haluska EA, Whistler SJ, Calfee RJ: A hierarchical approach to the treatment of ventricular tachycardias. PACE Pacing Clin Electrophysiol 1986; 9:1320–1324.

32. Fromer M, Brachmann J, Block M, et al: Efficacy of automatic multimodal device therapy for ventricular tachyarrhythmias as delivered by a new implantable pacing cardioverter-defibrillator: Results of a European multicenter study incorporating 102 implants. Circulation 1992; 86:363–374.

33. Fromer M, Kus T, Nadeau R, Shenasa M: Oscillation of ventricular tachycardia cycle length [abstract]. PACE Pacing Clin Electrophysiol 1987; 10:593.

34. Saksena S, Mehta D, Krol RB, et al: Experience with a third-generation implantable cardioverter-defibrillator. Am J Cardiol 1991; 67:1375–1384.

35. Lehmann MH, Saksena S.: Implantable cardioverter-defibrillator in cardiovascular practice: Report of the Policy Conference of the North American Society of Pacing and Electrophysiology. PACE Pacing Clin Electrophysiol 1991; 14:969–979.

36. Saksena S, Parsonnet V: Implantation of a cardioverter-defibrillator without thoracotomy using a triple electrode system. JAMA 1988; 259:69–72.

37. Brooks R, Garan H, Torchiana D, et al: Determinants of successful nonthoracotomy cardioverter-defibrillator implantation: Experience in 101 patients using two different lead systems. J Am Coll Cardiol 1993; 22:1835–1842.

38. Bardy GH, Hofer B, Johnson G, et al: Implantable transvenous cardioverter-defibrillators. Circulation 1993; 87:1152–1168.

Chapter 35

Catheter Retrieval of Foreign Objects

BRUNO COTTER
PASCAL NICOD

Since Meyers[1] first introduced intravascular catheters in 1945, their use for diagnostic and therapeutic purposes has become a common source of foreign body embolization into the heart and the great vessels.[2] In 1954, Turner and Sommers[3] described the first case of embolization of an intravenous catheter in a patient. Subsequently, in 1971, Burri and associates[4] reviewed 112 published cases and reported a 1% incidence of catheter embolization. In 1978, Burri and Ahnefeld[5] found a 0.1% incidence of embolization after insertion of central venous catheters. This incidence may be underestimated, because not all cases are reported in the literature. Breakage of a polyethylene central venous conduit on a needle introducer accounts for about 80% of all foreign object embolization.[6] Other objects include Swan-Ganz catheters, hyperalimentation catheters, cardiac stimulators, pacemaker electrodes, angioplasty components, vascular stents, caval filters, broken needles in drug addicts, and foreign projectiles.[7]

SITE OF EMBOLIZATION

Most intravascular foreign bodies embolize to the superior vena cava, the right atrium, the right ventricle, or the pulmonary arteries.[8-17] There is, however, an increasing number of reports in the literature of embolized foreign bodies in the aorta and its branches, the left ventricle, or the coronary arteries resulting from the development of interventional cardiology and radiology.[18-37]

The site of embolization differs depending on the nature of the foreign body, the site of introduction in the vascular system, and the position of the patient at the time of the incident. The distal end of a long catheter tends to lodge against the right ventricular wall while its proximal end remains in the superior vena cava or the right atrium.[3, 7, 38] Shorter fragments tend to migrate more distally to the pulmonary arteries, where they are more difficult to retrieve.[14, 39, 40] Seldom does a catheter fragment breaking off in an upper extremity or thoracic vein end up in the inferior vena cava or the hepatic veins.[38] Migration of venous catheters from the lower extremities is uncommon and occurs preferentially into the right heart or the inferior vena cava and rarely into the superior vena cava or the hepatic veins.[11, 38]

RISKS AND COMPLICATIONS

As case reports have accumulated, it has become apparent that failure to remove foreign bodies can result in serious complications (40% to 70% of cases) and/or death (24% to 38%), according to various studies.[9, 21] The risk appears to be highest when the foreign body is located in the right heart (80% of serious complications), moderate when located in the pulmonary arteries (66%), and mild when localized in the distal portions of the pulmonary tree (2%).[9, 41] There are two major groups of complications: (1) those due to mechanical irritation, such as cardiac arrhythmias and arrest, inflammation of the cardiac vascular walls, and perforation of heart valves or myocardium[9]; and (2) those resulting from thrombus formation around the catheter, subsequent embolization, and associated infections. Significant morbidity and mortality can be associated with pulmonary embolization, bacterial and fungal endocarditis, mycotic aneurysms, multiple abscesses, septic thrombophlebitis, and septicemia. Whereas arrhythmias usually occur within a few hours of embolization, thrombosis and infections can be either early or late complications.[2, 9, 21]

Because the presence of intracardiac foreign bodies has a poor prognosis, the foreign bodies must be removed as soon as possible. Considering the risk of major surgical interventions (a mortality of 4% has been reported),[42] percutaneous retrieval techniques offer a simple, inexpensive, and fast approach to remove foreign bodies and should be tried first.

In 1964, Thomas and associates[15] published the first report of nonsurgical retrieval of a foreign body from the right atrium and the inferior vena cava. In 1969, Curry[43] described the snare loop method for percutaneous retrieval of intravascular foreign bodies. Two years later, a review of the literature by Dotter and colleagues[44] reported 29 cases of nonsurgical retrieval of embolized intravascular foreign bodies. In their review of the literature, in 1991, Dondelinger and colleagues[7] reported a success rate for percutaneous retrieval of foreign bodies varying between 71% and 100%. Since then, with the increasing use of catheters for diagnostic and interventional procedures, several novel methods have been described and used routinely.

METHODS FOR RETRIEVAL OF EMBOLIZED FOREIGN BODIES

Several methods have been developed for the removal of the wide variety of foreign bodies that may embolize into the cardiovascular system. All methods use either a snare or a basket when a free catheter end is available for grasping or a hook or forceps when the catheter adheres to the cardiac or vascular walls.[2] The large number of case reports and technical descriptions on a variety of instruments or devices

suggests that no particular technique has proved to be superior in all cases.

The Snare Loop

The snare loop technique is the method of choice in most patients in both the venous and arterial systems because of its simplicity, flexibility, and availability (Fig. 35–1).[20, 26, 28, 29, 31, 33, 37, 40, 42, 45–50] Snare loop sets are available commercially (Cook, Inc., Bloomington, IN) or may be made with standard materials in the catheterization laboratory. The sets are of two types:

1. The adult set, which consists of a 100-cm-long 8-French catheter used as the delivery system and a 300-cm-long guide wire (0.021 mm in outer diameter) folded to form a 150-cm-long snare.

2. The pediatric set, which consists of a smaller (6.3-French) 45-cm-long catheter and a 125-cm-long guide wire (0.018 mm in outer diameter) folded to make a 62.5-cm-long snare.

The folded snare is introduced in the guiding catheter. The catheter is then advanced, with the snare folded inside to avoid injury to the vessels or the cardiac walls. The desired snare loop is formed by advancing or withdrawing one end of the guide wire. The snare loop technique is effective if the embolized foreign body has a free end for snaring. Otherwise, this device usually does not work.

The patient is positioned under fluoroscopy for optimal visualization of the foreign body. Evaluation includes locating both ends of the foreign body and determining its length and size. The snare loop is held in such a way that it is shown under fluoroscopy as a straight line

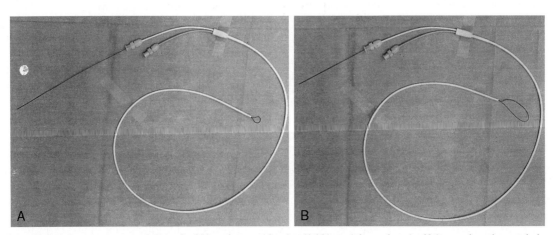

Figure 35–1. A, Loop snare, consisting of a 300-cm-long guide wire (0.021 mm) looped on itself, inserted, and extended a short distance outside the end of an 8-French catheter. B, Adjustment of the size of the loop snare outside the distal end of the delivery catheter by advancing the wire from the proximal hub of the catheter. Once the loop has surrounded a foreign object, the loop is tightened, and the object is secured by advancing the catheter forward over the wire.

or a closed loop, confirming its perpendicular plane in relation to the catheter fragment. The next step is to ensure that the snare has encircled the foreign body. The guiding catheter is advanced on the snare, causing the catheter fragment to bend when the snare is engaged. Withdrawing the snare loop instead of advancing the guiding catheter over the snare is not recommended because the loop may disengage from the catheter fragment during the maneuver.

Next, the guide wire is held in a fixed position while the tip of the introducing catheter is further advanced to trap the broken fragment. Smith and Durkos's technique can be used if the stiff folded end of the snare cannot make a smooth loop outside the delivery system.[51] With this technique, the tip of the catheter is placed beyond the foreign body and the folded guide wire is introduced into the catheter. When the wire loop is beyond the distal end of the foreign body, the catheter is withdrawn over the wire loop.

In small vessels, a tight snare loop is used; in larger vessels or in a cardiac chamber, a wider or even a redundant loop is used. Dotter and coworkers[44] suggested that the use of a redundant snare loop facilitated retrieval of foreign bodies in the right atrium. This technique seems to be helpful particularly when the position of the foreign body cannot be precisely determined.

Other Methods

If the snare loop cannot be placed around the foreign body, several other methods may be used. These include the use of a curve-tipped retrieval catheter, with a redundant wire loop.[44] Hubert and coworkers[52] described a modified snare technique, originally used for transcolonic removal of colonic polyps, to retrieve intravascular foreign bodies. The key difference from other snare techniques is the use of a wire snare with a crimp in its mid-portion that enables the formation of a loop in a plane perpendicular to the axial direction of the guiding catheter. With this technique, they have removed a variety of objects from the right heart and pulmonary arteries in four patients.

EXAMPLES OF PERCUTANEOUS RETRIEVAL OF FOREIGN BODIES USING THE SNARE LOOP

Retrieval from the Coronary Arteries

Serota and associates[33] described a 73-year-old man with previous coronary bypass surgery who was admitted for percutaneous angioplasty of a 90% stenosis at the level of the distal graft anastomosis to the right coronary artery. The right coronary artery bypass graft was engaged using an 8-French multipurpose guiding catheter. After dilation at high pressure using an over-the-wire system with a 3.5-mm balloon, a significant residual stenosis persisted. In an attempt to improve the results, the over-the-wire balloon was removed and two 2.5-mm USCI (Billerica, MA) New Probe balloon catheters were inserted side by side across the lesion through the same guiding catheter. After successful dilation, the distal 2-cm radiopaque tip of one balloon broke and remained across the dilation site. A 4-French USCI probing catheter was advanced proximal to the retained balloon fragment over a 0.014-inch high-torque floppy guide wire (USCI). The high-torque floppy wire was then withdrawn.

Using the same wire, a snare was fashioned by looping the distal 5 cm back on itself. The tip of the distal loop was given a 30-degree angle to facilitate maneuvering. The snare was then introduced into the probing catheter and advanced 1 cm outside the tip of the catheter. A gentle back-and-forth rotating motion of the snare at the level of the dislodged balloon fragment was used until it was entrapped. Slow withdrawal of the snare wire back into the probing catheter provided a firm grip. To prevent accidental release of the loop, the proximal end of the wire was secured to the hub of the probing catheter using a clamp before the system was withdrawn from the guiding catheter. Postprocedure angiography demonstrated adequate perfusion to the right coronary artery graft and its branches with no evidence of intimal dissection or occlusion. The patient's later course was uneventful.

The same technique was successfully used in two additional patients. In one patient, a broken USCI probe 3-mm balloon and its attached tip were snared at the level of the mid-left anterior descending artery segment diagonal bifurcation. The loop was accidentally released and the broken fragment had to be removed by another snare at the level of the ostium of the main coronary artery. In the other patient, a broken USCI New Probe 3-mm balloon catheter wire tip was successfully retrieved from the distal right coronary artery posterolateral branch bifurcation.[33]

Hartzler and colleagues[24] have reported removal of two retained intracoronary angioplasty wires by gradual withdrawal of an adjacent inflated balloon.

Retrieval from the Left Ventricle

Keltai and Meier[26] reported the retrieval of a broken guide wire from the left ventricle in a 81-year-old woman who underwent aortic balloon valvuloplasty. The pigtail catheter positioned in the left ventricle was exchanged for a valvuloplasty catheter (trefoil 3 × 9 mm) using a stiff 0.020-inch, 280-cm-long exchange wire with a flexible distal end. The rapid back-and-forth motion of the balloon during inflation resulted in kinking and breakage of the distal 15 cm of the guide wire. In view of the thrombogenicity of a left ventricular foreign body and the risk of embolization, immediate removal was considered mandatory. First, a Dormia ureteral stone-catching basket was introduced into the left ventricle through a guiding catheter, but it failed to catch the wire, which appeared to be anchored at both ends within the papillary muscles. Then a wire snare was introduced through an 8-French Judkins right coronary guiding catheter. Several attempts to catch a free end of the guide wire were unsuccessful. Finally, after freeing one end of the wire fragment with the tip of the guiding catheter, the snare entrapped the broken catheter, which could be pulled into the guiding catheter and removed through the femoral introducer sheath. The clinical course was uneventful, and the patient left the hospital 3 days after the procedure.

Retrieval from the Pulmonary Arteries

Bogart and colleagues[45] described a 59-year-old man who underwent aortocoronary bypass surgery. Postoperatively, a small catheter fragment embolized from the left subclavian vein to the left pulmonary artery. The patient was taken to the cardiac catheterization laboratory and a 9-French angioplasty sheath was introduced into the right femoral vein by the Seldinger technique. A snare was devised using an 8-French multipurpose catheter and a 0.038-inch movable core J-wire. The latter was introduced into the catheter and the core of the wire was then sutured to the side hole of the multipurpose catheter, taking care not to entrap the wire in the catheter. This created a variable snare loop that could be controlled by moving the wire in and out of the catheter. The catheter was then advanced under fluoroscopic guidance into the left pulmonary artery. The device was maneuvered easily and the end of the catheter fragment was secured using the snare, allowing the fragment to be removed through the right femoral vein.

The Basket Snare

The basket snare is composed of multiple parallel metallic wires and is introduced through an outer Teflon catheter (Fig. 35–2). Two types are available:

1. The Dotter retrieval set, which consists of a 100-cm-long, 8-French Teflon catheter and a basket formed by helicoid stainless steel wires with long handles.
2. The Dormia ureteric set, which is used to retrieve ureteral stones. Because of its small outside diameter (1.6 mm), this set is useful in pediatric patients.

The catheter containing the basket is opened and closed by sliding it in and out of the distal end of the guiding catheter. When the foreign body is trapped, the basket and the catheter are removed together. This maneuver gives directional control to advance the basket over the end of the foreign body.[10] The basket is particularly useful for retrieving nonopaque broken catheters (Fig. 35–3) or nonlinear foreign bodies. It is also useful when the plane of the catheter fragment cannot be determined. In such instances, the multiple planes of sweep by the basket increase the chances of success. Better results can be obtained if the width of the basket approximates the diameter of the vessel at the level of the entrapped foreign body. This may also prevent further downstream migration. One problem with this technique is the risk of vascular injury with the rigid basket tip. Also, the diameter of the open basket is small, limiting its use in large structures such as the cardiac chambers.

The Hook System

The hook system uses a hook-tipped catheter with a 180-degree curve in the distal end. It is especially helpful when the foreign body does not have a free end for snaring. The hook-tipped catheter alone or in combination with a guide wire deflector has been used successfully in many instances.[12, 53, 54] Because the hook-tipped catheter may open in iliac veins or narrowed vessels, the foreign body may be transferred from the hook-tipped catheter introduced in the contralateral femoral vessel. When the broken catheter fragment adheres firmly to the heart or blood vessels, the hook catheter may have insufficient resilience to pull the foreign body. In such instances, the combination of a hook-tipped catheter and a guide wire deflector may have to be used. Another alternative is to snare the tip of the hooked catheter by

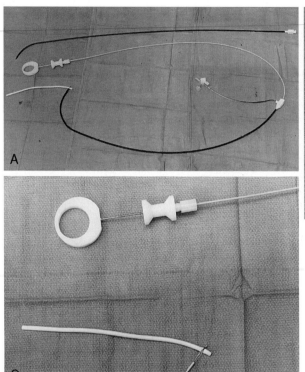

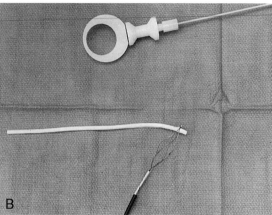

Figure 35-2. *A,* A basket retrieval system consisting of an outer guiding catheter through which is inserted the collapsible basket made of helicoid stainless steel wires. *B,* An enlarged view of the basket while expanded and passed over the end of an intravascular introducer that had previously embolized to the right ventricular outflow tract, extending into the main pulmonary artery (see Fig. 35-3). *C,* Enlarged view of the basket collapsed around the end of the intravascular introducer. The same maneuver was used to snare the foreign object and pull it to the outside of the body through a vascular introducer in the right femoral vein.

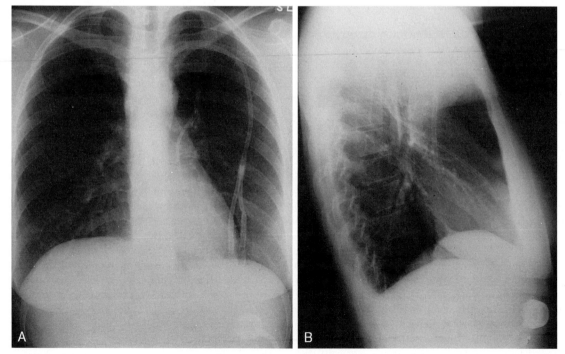

Figure 35-3. *A,* Standard posteroanterior chest roentgenogram showing a piece of a vascular intracatheter that had embolized into the right ventricular outflow tract, extending into the main pulmonary artery. *B,* A lateral chest roentgenogram of the same patient demonstrating the intracatheter fragment situated in the right ventricle and main pulmonary artery.

a loop.[38] One problem with the hook-tipped catheter is the risk of perforation of the vessel or cardiac wall, particularly when it is reinforced by a guide wire deflector system.

Repositioning the foreign devices has also been successfully done using pigtail catheters.[39] A snare loop can then be used to remove the catheter brought in a more favorable position.

The Pass-over Technique

Sometimes foreign bodies are wedged in small vessels such as branches of the pulmonary tree. In such instances, either the foreign body can be brought to a more accessible position by a balloon catheter or the pass-over technique can be used. A guide wire is passed through the broken catheter fragment using a large-bore guiding angiographic catheter. Subsequently, the catheter is gently advanced over the broken fragment. The captured foreign body, the guide wire, and the angiographic catheter are then removed altogether.[2]

Endoscopic Forceps

The endoscopic forceps method used in the cardiovascular system is identical to the one used in the bronchi, the esophagus, and the urinary tract. Various devices can be used: (1) a standard biopsy forceps; (2) a biopsy forceps with an ellipsoid mouth; (3) a grasping forceps with a rat-tooth mouth; (4) a grasping forceps with an alligator mouth; and (5) a grasping forceps with a W shape. These instruments have an excellent grasping ability and are helpful when the foreign bodies do not have a free end, excluding the use of snare loops or baskets. The fragment is caught by the jaws and pulled out through the catheter. Vascular bends and curves limit the use of rigid or semirigid forceps.[2, 14, 30, 38, 55]

REFERENCES

1. Meyers L: Intravenous catheterization. Am J Nurs 1945; 45:930–933.
2. Gerlock AJ, Mirfakhraee M: Retrieval of intravascular foreign bodies. J Thorac Imaging 1987; 2:52–60.
3. Turner DD, Sommers SC: Accidental passage of a poly-ethylene catheter from cubital vein to right atrium. N Engl J Med 1954; 251:744–745.
4. Burri C, Henkeneyer H, Passler HH: Katheterembolien. Schweiz Med Wochenschr 1971; 101:1537–1539.
5. Burri C, Ahnefeld FW: Complications of caval catheterization. In: The Caval Catheter. Berlin, Springer Verlag, 1978, pp 53–60.
6. Bloomfield DA: The nonsurgical retrieval of intracardiac foreign bodies: An international survey. Cathet Cardiovasc Diagn 1978; 4:1–14.
7. Dondelinger RF, Lepoutre B, Kurdziel JC: Percutaneous vascular foreign body retrieval: Experience of an 11-year period. Eur J Radiol 1991; 12:4–10.
8. Cho S-R, Tisnado J, Beachley MC, et al: Percutaneous unknotting of intravascular catheters and retrieval of catheter fragments. AJR Am J Roentgenol 1983; 141:397–402.
9. Clavier E, Laissy JP, Annoot-Ostyn B, et al: Percutaneous recovery of catheters migrated in the vascular system. J Radiol 1991; 72:171–175.
10. Harnick E, Rohmer J: Atraumatic retrieval of catheter fragment from the central circulation of children. Eur J Cardiol 1974; 1:421–422.
11. Kim SH, Song IS, Kim JH, et al: Retrieval of a guidewire introducer by catheter-capture from the proximal inferior vena cava [technical note]. Cardiovasc Intervent Radiol 1991; 14:252–253.
12. McSweeney WJ, Schwatz DC: Retrieval of a catheter foreign body from the right heart using a guidewire deflector system. Radiology 1971; 100:61–62.
13. Radojkovic S, Kamenica S, Jasovic M, Draganic M: Catheter-aided extraction of a steel coil accidentally lodged in the right ventricle. Cardiovasc Intervent Radiol 1980; 3:153–155.
14. Tanaka M, Iyomasa Y: Nonsurgical technique for removal of catheter fragments from the pulmonary artery. Cathet Cardiovasc Diagn 1983; 9:109–112.
15. Thomas JS, Sinclair-Smith B, Bloomfield D: Nonsurgical retrieval of a broken segment of steel spring guide from right atrium and inferior vena cava. Circulation 1964; 30:106–108.
16. Tsai FY, Myers TV, Ashraf A, Shah DC: Aberrant placement of a Kimray-Greenfield filter in the right atrium: Percutaneous retrieval. Radiology 1988; 167:423–424.
17. Yakes WF: Percutaneous retrieval of Kimray-Greenfield filter from right atrium and placement in inferior vena cava. Radiology 1988; 169:849–851.
18. Chuang VP: Nonoperative retrieval of Gianturco coils from abdominal aorta. AJR Am J Roentgenol 1979; 132:996–997.
19. Colombo A, Skinner JM: Balloon entrapment in a coronary artery: Potential serious complications of balloon rupture. Cathet Cardiovasc Diagn 1990; 19:23–25.
20. Davies RP, Voyovodic F: Percutaneous retrieval of a partially expanded iliac artery stent [case report]. Cardiovasc Intervent Radiol 1992; 15:120–122.
21. Feldman RL, Trice WA, Hennemann WW III, Furst A: Retrieval of a fractured USCI probe tip from a diseased coronary artery using another fixed-wire balloon catheter, the Cordis Orion. Cathet Cardiovasc Diagn 1990; 19:257–263.
22. Fjalling M, List AR: Transvascular retrieval of an accidentally ejected tip occluder and wire. Cardiovasc Intervent Radiol 1982; 5:34–36.
23. Ghosh PK, Alber G, Schistek R, Unger F: Rupture of guidewire during percutaneous transluminal coronary angioplasty: Mechanics and management. J Thorac Cardiovasc Surg 1989, 57:407–409.
24. Hartzler GO, Rutherford BD, McConahay DR: Retained percutaneous transluminal coronary angioplasty equipment components and their management. Am J Cardiol 1987; 60:1260–1264.
25. Juilliere Y, Danchin N, Amrein D, et al: Proximal rup ture and intracoronary entrapment of a rotating device during low-speed rotational coronary angioplasty. Cathet Cardiovasc Diagn 1991; 23:34–36.
26. Keltai M, Meier B: Percutaneous retrieval of foreign body from the left ventricular cavity. Cathet Cardiovasc Diagn 1987; 13:405–406.
27. Krone RJ: Successful percutaneous removal of retained

broken coronary angioplasty guidewire. Cathet Cardiovasc Diagn 1986; 12:409–410.

28. Marcuzzi DW, Chisholm RJ: Percutaneous retrieval of
an embolized arterial sheath. AJR Am J Roentgenol
1991; 157:873–874.

29. Mclvor ME, Kaufman SL, Satre R, et al: Search and
retrieval of a radiolucent foreign object. Cathet Cardiovasc Diagn 1989; 16:19–23.

30. Mintz GS, Bemis E, Unwala M, et al: An alternative
method for transcatheter retrieval of intracoronary angioplasty equipment fragments. Cathet Cardiovasc Diagn 1990; 20:247–250.

31. Rao VRK, Rout D, Sapru RP: Retrieval of a broken
catheter from the aorta without operation. Neuroradiol-
ogy 1982; 22:263–265.

32. Reddy CVR, Khan R, Feit A, et al: Catheter separation
during coronary angiography. Cathet Cardiovasc Diagn
1983; 9:417–419.

33. Serota H, Deligonul U, Lew B, et al: Improved method
for transcatheter retrieval of intracoronary detached
angioplasty guidewire segments. Cathet Cardiovasc Diagn 1989; 17:248–251.

34. Sharma RP, Shetty PC, Burke TH, Burke MW: Separation of a ruptured angioplasty balloon with successful
percutaneous retrieval [case report]. Angiology 1990;
41:753–756.

35. Steele PM, Holmes DR Jr, Mankin HT, Schaff HV:
Intravascular retrieval of broken guide wire from the
ascending aorta after percutaneous transluminal coronary angioplasty. Cathet Cardiovasc Diagn 1985;
11:623–628.

36. Travelli R, Cogbill TH: Retrieval of a 4-French diagnostic catheter fragment from the common carotid artery
by using a stone basket. AJR Am J Roentgenol 1991;
156:1105–1106.

37. Watson LE: Snare loop technique for removal of broken
steerable PTCA wire. Cathet Cardiovasc Diagn 1987;
13:405–406.

38. Uflacker R, Lima S, Melichar AC: Intravascular foreign
bodies: Percutaneous retrieval. Radiology 1986;
160:731–735.

39. Auge JM, Oriol A, Serra C, Crexells C: The use of
pigtail catheters for retrieval of foreign bodies from the
cardiovascular system. Cathet Cardiovasc Diagn 1984;
10:625–628.

40. Furui S, Yamauchi T, Makita K, et al: Intravascular
foreign bodies: Loop-snare retrieval system with a three-
lumen catheter. Radiology 1992; 182:283–284.

41. Fischer RG, Ferreyro R: Evaluation of current techniques for nonsurgical removal of intravascular iatrogenic foreign bodies. AJR Am J Roentgenology 1978;
130:541–548.

42. Chung KJ, Chernoff HL, Leape LL, Kreidberg MB:
Transfemoral snaring of broken catheters from the
right heart in small infants. Cathet Cardiovasc Diagn
1980; 6:331–335.

43. Curry JL: Recovery of detached intravascular catheter
or guidewire fragments: A proposed method. AJR Am J
Roentgenol 1969; 105:894–896.

44. Dotter CT, Rosch J, Bilbao MK: Transluminal extraction
of catheter and guide fragments from the heart and
great vessels: Twenty-nine collected cases. AJR Am J
Roentgenol 1971; 111:467–472.

45. Bogart DB, Earnest JB, Miller JT: Foreign body retrieval
using simple snare device. Cathet Cardiovasc Diagn
1990; 19:248–250.

46. Hartnell GG: Homemade snare for removal of foreign
bodies [letter to the editor]. Radiology 1991; 181:903–
904.

47. Huston J, Nicholas GG, Weinstein AJ: Transvenous
"rescue" of a Kimray-Greenfield filter from the right
atrium. J Cardiovasc Surg 1990; 31:313–314.

48. Lybecker H, Andersen C, Hansen MK: Transvenous
retrieval of intracardiac catheter fragments. Acta Anae-
sthesiol Scand 1989; 33:565–567.

49. Metha AB, Goldman JM, Hemingway AP, Allison DJ:
Percutaneous retrieval of catheter fragments from the
heart and great vessels: Five cases. Br Med J 1983;
286:937.

50. Yedlicka JW Jr, Carlson JE, Hunter DW, et al: Nitinol
gooseneck snare for removal of foreign bodies: Experimental study and clinical evaluation. Radiology 1991;
178:691–693.

51. Smith DC, Durkos JL: An improved ruptured-balloon
retrieval set. Radiology 1982; 144:430–431.

52. Hubert JW, Krone RJ, Shatz BA, Susman N: An improved snare system for the nonsurgical retrieval of
intravascular foreign bodies. Cathet Cardiovasc Diagn
1980; 6:405–411.

53. Gerlock AJ: Guidewire deflector system removal of catheter foreign body retained in the right heart for six
months. J Trauma 1975; 9:830–832.

54. Rossi P: "Hook catheters" technique for transfemoral
removal of foreign body from the right side of the
heart. AJR Am J Roentgenol 1979; 109:101–106.

55. Shaw TRD: Removal of embolized catheters using flexible endoscopy forceps. Br Heart J 1982; 48:497–500.

INDEX

Note: Page numbers in *italics* refer to illustrations; page numbers followed by t refer to tables.